Oxford Textbook of

Rheumatoid Arthritis

OXFORD TEXTBOOKS IN RHEUMATOLOGY

Oxford Textbook of Rheumatoid Arthritis
Edited by David L. Scott, James Galloway, Andrew Cope, Arthur Pratt, and Vibeke Strand

Oxford Textbook of Psoriatic Arthritis
Edited by Oliver FitzGerald and Dafna Gladman

Oxford Textbook of Osteoarthritis and Crystal Arthropathy, 3rd edition
Edited by Michael Doherty, David J. Hunter, Hans Bijlsma, Nigel Arden, and Nicola Dalbeth

Oxford Textbook of Axial Spondyloarthritis
Edited by Robert Inman and Joachim Sieper

Oxford Textbook of Clinical and Biochemical Disorders of the Skeleton, 2nd edition
Edited by Roger Smith and Paul Wordsworth

Oxford Textbook of Vasculitis, 3rd edition
Edited by Gene V. Ball, Barri J. Fessler, and S. Louis Bridges, Jnr.

Oxford Textbook of
Rheumatoid Arthritis

EDITED BY

David L. Scott

Professor of Clinical Rheumatology, King's College London, London, UK

James Galloway

*Senior Lecturer in Rheumatology, King's College London and
Honorary Consultant Rheumatologist, King's College London, London, UK*

Andrew Cope

*Versus Arthritis Professor of Rheumatology, King's College London and
Honorary Consultant Rheumatologist, Guy's and St Thomas' Hospital, London, UK*

Arthur G. Pratt

*Clinical Senior Lecturer in Rheumatology, Newcastle University and
Honorary Consultant Rheumatologist, Freeman Hospital, Newcastle, UK*

Vibeke Strand

*Biopharmaceutical Consultant and Adjunct Clinical Professor, Division of
Immunology and Rheumatology, Stanford University, Palo Alto, USA*

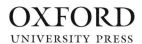

OXFORD
UNIVERSITY PRESS

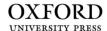

Great Clarendon Street, Oxford, OX2 6DP,
United Kingdom

Oxford University Press is a department of the University of Oxford.
It furthers the University's objective of excellence in research, scholarship,
and education by publishing worldwide. Oxford is a registered trade mark of
Oxford University Press in the UK and in certain other countries

First Edition published in 2020

Impression: 1

Published in the United States of America by Oxford University Press
198 Madison Avenue, New York, NY 10016, United States of America

British Library Cataloguing in Publication Data

Data available

Library of Congress Control Number: 2018933144

ISBN 978–0–19–883143–3

Printed in Great Britain by
Bell & Bain Ltd., Glasgow

Foreword

This textbook brings together current opinion about rheumatoid arthritis in 46 diverse chapters. It has involved five editors and over 90 authors have contributed to the various chapters. The size and relative complexity of the text highlights the enormous advances which have taken place in our understanding of rheumatoid arthritis in recent years. The volume of research in the field has expanded dramatically during the last decade. In the last 10 years over 40,000 papers have been published either completely or partially about rheumatoid arthritis. These papers have included over 4000 original contributions reporting about clinical trials in the field.

One key driving factor to this vast research output has been the development of biologic treatments for rheumatoid arthritis. These drugs have pushed forward both research and clinical practice. But just as the biologics revolution has started to fade in its intensity, with these therapies becoming well established treatments, and also becoming available as biosimilars, a whole new therapeutic area has opened. This has centred on the development and introduction of Janus Kinase inhibitors, which are novel and very different types of targeted treatments. These and other recent therapeutic developments have been characterised by providing treatments which are effective and relatively safe, but which are also expensive. Over time they have changed the face of rheumatoid arthritis. Nevertheless at the level of the individual patient rheumatoid arthritis continues to be a major personal challenge. There remains a pressing need for more research and development.

The book captures many of these recent changes in its eight broad sections. These sections start with history, epidemiology and diagnosis. They end with management and outcomes. Between these are sections on pathogenesis, clinical presentation, disease assessment, impact on life, non-drug treatments and drug treatments. Each section contains a range of chapters, written by leading international experts in their fields. The range of topics included means that the book has needed an editorial team of diverse interests and expertise, ranging from laboratory studies through clinical trials to outcome studies and disease registers.

Over time diseases change. This pattern of transformation is seen for rheumatoid arthritis as much as many other disorders. Whether or not the disease we see today is the same as the arthritis seen in years gone by is debatable. The modern diagnostic criteria, outlined by Daniel Aletaha and Helga Radner in Chapter 2 are somewhat different from the historic criteria. But many other things also change. There are more rheumatologists so todays' specialists will inevitably see a different spectrum of patients to those seen historically. And effective treatments are usually given soon after disease onset, changing the clinical course of the disease. In any event we need to focus on current patients and let the past go. The chapters on epidemiology and risk factors place the disease in context and highlight its continuing importance to society as a whole. Although prevention is currently unachievable, the identification of potentially modifiable risks such as smoking has been crucial for understanding the drivers of the disease.

The six chapters on pathogenesis span a range of complex and overlapping themes. It includes sections on fibroblasts, lymphocytes, cytokines, autoantibodies and bone and cartilage destruction. Not only is the pathogenesis of rheumatoid arthritis complex, but our views on its nature are for ever metamorphosing. Whether rheumatoid is principally a disorder of the synovium itself or an immunologically driven disease remains unresolved. It is equally uncertain if it is a single disease with a broad spectrum or a group of related disorders, with varying degrees of antibody formation. But irrespective of these considerations, increasing knowledge of the pathogenesis of rheumatoid disease has facilitated the development of many new drug treatments over the years, which all target different parts of the pathogenic cascade.

The section on clinical presentation combines classical descriptions of the disease, its extra-articular features and its comorbidities with a chapter describing pre-rheumatoid, which is a relatively new concept. Whether or not treatments will be used in the future to prevent the onset of rheumatoid arthritis in patients with pre-rheumatoid features is at the centre of ongoing research in the field. Understanding the features of pre-rheumatoid, and the strengths and weaknesses of knowledge in this field is vital when deciding about potential interventions with drug treatments.

Disease assessment naturally follows the section on clinical features. It spans conventional clinical assessments, a range of imaging approaches and synovial biopsies. Conventional clinical assessments and radiology remain central components of everyday clinical practice and ultrasound imaging has now become a mainstream approach, while MRI and synovial biopsies remain more research focussed approaches. But as ultrasound has changed from being a research-based approach to becoming a part of mainstream practice over the last decade or so, it is highly likely that other imaging modalities, particularly MRI will have a more dominant role in clinical practice in the future, though predicting future changes remains challenging and uncertain.

The final clinically-focussed section deals with the impact of rheumatoid arthritis on life. Disability, fatigue, problems with work and the personal and societal costs of the disease are all closely interrelated problems. Forty years have passed since the health assessment questionnaire was developed for assessing physical function in rheumatoid arthritis and in the intervening period our knowledge of the impact of joint inflammation on disability has grown exponentially. From the perspective of people with rheumatoid arthritis these issues dominate their lives, together with the high costs of the disease for patients and their families and the loss of work that results from persisting joint inflammation.

The sections on treatment are divided into non-drug approaches and drug therapies. Although each chapter focusses on a particular treatment modality – ranging from exercise to different biologics and Janus Kinase inhibitors – patients need multiple interventions given concurrently. Whilst not all patients need specific drugs such as biologics, almost everyone with rheumatoid arthritis needs to be encouraged to exercise and to engage in self-management. Analgesics, non-steroidal anti-inflammatory drugs and glucocorticoids have been used over many decades, whilst biologics and Janus Kinase inhibitors are relatively recent innovations. Nevertheless, all these approaches have a role in some patients. Disease management is an area where controversies abound. Some clinicians prefer some approaches, whilst others focus on different approaches. The use of glucocorticoids is one area where opinions vary. The same is true for combinations of conventional synthetic disease modifying drugs. Experts inevitably interpret the same clinical evidence quite differently, depending upon their experience and perspectives. Whilst it is not possible to capture all viewpoints in a single book, we have tried to highlight which areas are controversial.

The final section on management and outcomes includes chapters on prevention, targets, outcomes, guidelines and different types of register. These chapters present different facets of the overall impact of rheumatoid arthritis. They are closely inter-related. Targets and outcomes are different faces of studying the course of rheumatoid arthritis and registers help define what happens to patients over time. The growing use of information technology in medicine means registers and other uses of "big data" will become increasingly important in the years ahead. Guidelines have changed the way in which clinical practice is viewed, and the chapter on different guidelines highlights how they have developed over the years. However, it is fascinating that there is not one single guideline, but a series of different guidelines from different countries and continents, each of which have subtle and unique variations in their recommendations.

Multi-author textbooks involve collaborations between many different groups. The editors, authors of individual chapters, and the publishers all need to work together. However, inevitably the book needs a champion to drive forward these various parties. This book was fortunate to have Sylvia Warren, from Oxford University Press, oversee its development and keep all those involved focussed on producing the final text. The editors are grateful for her commitment and support during the development and production of this book; without her help and support it may well not have come to fruition.

Contents

Contributors ix
Symbols and abbreviations xi

SECTION 1
History, diagnosis, and epidemiology

1. **The history of rheumatoid arthritis** 3
   David L. Scott

2. **Diagnosis** 13
   Daniel Aletaha and Helga Radner

3. **The descriptive epidemiology of rheumatoid arthritis** 23
   James Gwinnutt and Deborah Symmons

4. **Modifiable and other risk factors for rheumatoid arthritis: A basis for prevention and better therapy** 33
   Lars Klareskog and Lars Alfredsson

SECTION 2
Pathogenesis

5. **Genetics and epigenetics of rheumatoid arthritis** 45
   Anne Barton

6. **Dysregulation of synovial fibroblasts in rheumatoid arthritis** 55
   Thomas Crowley, Jason D. Turner, Andrew Filer, Andy Clarke, and Chris Buckley

7. **Autoantibodies in rheumatoid arthritis** 65
   Tom W.J. Huizinga

8. **Dendritic cells and T cells in rheumatoid arthritis** 73
   Soi-Cheng Law, Pascale Wehr, Harriet Purvis, and Ranjeny Thomas

9. **Mechanisms of bone and cartilage destruction** 85
   Ulrike Harre and Georg Schett

10. **Cytokines and other mediators** 95
    Marina Frleta-Gilchrist and Iain B. McInnes

SECTION 3
Clinical presentation

11. **Clinical features of rheumatoid arthritis** 109
    Annette van der Helm-van Mil

12. **Pre-rheumatoid arthritis** 121
    Karim Raza, Catherine McGrath, Laurette van Boheemen, and Dirkjan van Schaardenburg

13. **Non-articular manifestations of rheumatoid arthritis** 133
    Katherine Macdonald, Jennifer Hannah, and James Galloway

14. **Comorbidity in rheumatoid arthritis** 145
    Kimme Hyrich and Sarah Skeoch

SECTION 4
Disease assessment

15. **Disease activity assessment in rheumatoid arthritis** 161
    Josef Smolen

16. **Synovial biopsies** 169
    Douglas J. Veale and Ursula Fearon

17. **Radiography in rheumatoid arthritis** 177
    Charles Peterfy, Philip G. Conaghan, and Mikkel Østergaard

18. **Ultrasound in rheumatoid arthritis** 195
    Andrew Filer, Maria Antonietta D'Agostino, and Ilfita Sahbudin

19. **Magnetic resonance imaging in rheumatoid arthritis** 207
    Mikkel Østergaard, Philip G. Conaghan, and Charles Peterfy

SECTION 5
Impact on life

20. **Patient physical function in rheumatoid arthritis** 221
    Kathryn A. Gibson and Theodore Pincus

21. **Fatigue** 251
    Emma Dures and Neil Basu

22. **Health economics of rheumatoid arthritis** 259
    David L. Scott and Allan Wailoo

23. **Rheumatoid arthritis and work** 271
    Suzanne Verstappen, Cheryl Jones, Abdullah Houssien, and James Galloway

SECTION 6
Non-drug treatments

24. **Physical activity and exercise** 285
    Lindsay M. Bearne and Christina H. Opava

25. **Foot health** 297
    Heidi J. Siddle and Anthony C. Redmond

26. **Occupational therapy** 311
    Alison Hammond, Joanne Adams, and Yeliz Prior

27. **Self-management: A patient's perspective** 321
    Marieke M.J.H. Voshaar

SECTION 7
Drug treatments

28. **Analgesics, opioids, and NSAIDs** 331
    Mark D. Russell and Nidhi Sofat

29. **Glucocorticoids** 339
    Johannes W.G. Jacobs, Marlies C. van der Goes, Johannes W.J. Bijlsma, and José A.P. da Silva

30. **Conventional disease-modifying drugs** 355
    David L. Scott

31. **Tumour necrosis factor inhibitors** 371
    Peter C. Taylor and Nehal Narayan

32. **Interleukin-6 inhibitors** 389
    Neelam Hassan and Ernest Choy

33. **B-cell therapies** 399
    Md Yuzaiful Md Yusof, Edward M. Vital, and Maya H. Buch

34. **Biosimilars** 411
    Vibeke Strand, Jeffrey Kaine, and John Isaacs

35. **Immunogenicity in response to biologic agents** 425
    Meghna Jani, John Isaacs, and Vibeke Strand

36. **The use of JAK inhibitors in the treatment of rheumatoid arthritis** 443
    Katie Bechman, James Galloway, and Peter C. Taylor

37. **Combination therapy in rheumatoid arthritis** 457
    Ben G.T. Coumbe, Elena Nikiphorou, and Tuulikki Sokka-Isler

38. **Translation of new therapies: From bench to bedside** 463
    Jeremy Sokolove

39. **Adverse events in clinical studies in rheumatoid arthritis** 471
    Mark Yates and James Galloway

SECTION 8
Management and outcomes

40. **Prevention of rheumatoid arthritis** 487
    Tom W.J. Huizinga, Annette van der Helm-van Mil, and Andrew Cope

41. **Treatment targets and remission** 495
    Kenneth F. Baker and Arthur G. Pratt

42. **Clinical outcomes** 507
    David L. Scott

43. **Clinical recommendations** 519
    Anna-Birgitte Aga, Espen A. Haavardsholm, Till Uhlig, and Tore K. Kvien

44. **European biologics registers** 535
    Angela Zink and Anja Strangfeld

45. **Voluntary patient registries** 545
    Jeff Greenberg and Sheetal Patel

Index 551

Contributors

Joanne Adams Professor of Musculoskeletal Health, Health Sciences, University of Southampton, Southampton, UK

Anna-Birgitte Aga Rheumatologist, Department of Clinical Medicine, the University of Oslo, Oslo, Norway

Daniel Aletaha Chair of Rheumatology, Medical University of Vienna, Vienna, Austria

Lars Alfredsson Senior Professor, Institute of Environmental Medicine, Karolinska Instituet, Stockholm, Sweden

Kenneth F. Baker NIHR Clinical Lecturer in Rheumatology, Institute of Cellular Medicine, Newcastle University, Newcastle, UK

Anne Barton Professor of Rheumatology, Versus Arthritis Centre for Genetics and Genomics, Manchester, UK

Neil Basu Clinical Senior Lecturer in Rheumatology, University of Glasgow, Glasgow, UK

Lindsay M. Bearne Senior Lecturer in Rheumatology, King's College London, London, UK

Katie Bechman Clinical Research Fellow, King's College London, London, UK

Johannes W.J. Bijlsma Professor of Rheumatology, Vrije Universiteit Amsterdam and Utrecht University, Amsterdam, the Netherlands

Laurette van Boheemen Visiting Fellow in Rheumatology, Reade, Amsterdam University Medical Center, Amsterdam, the Netherlands

Maya H. Buch Director of Experimental Medicine, Centre for Musculoskeletal Research, Division of Musculoskeletal & Dermatological Sciences, School of Biological Sciences, University of Manchester, UK; NIHR Manchester Biomedical Research Centre, Manchester University Foundation Trust, UK; Visiting Professor, Leeds Institute of Rheumatic and Musculoskeletal Medicine, University of Leeds, UK

Chris Buckley Kennedy Professor of Translational Rheumatology at the Universities of Birmingham and Oxford, Birmingham, UK

Ernest Choy Clinical Professor, School of Medicine, Cardiff University, Cardiff, UK

Andy Clarke Professor of Inflammation Biology, Institute of Inflammation and Aging, University of Birmingham, Birmingham, UK

Philip G. Conaghan Professor of Musculoskeletal Medicine, Leeds Institute of Rheumatic and Musculoskeletal Medicine, University of Leeds, NIHR Leeds Biomedical Research Centre, Leeds, UK

Andrew Cope Arthritis Research UK Professor of Rheumatology, King's College London and Honorary Consultant Rheumatologist, Guy's and St Thomas' Hospital, London, UK

Ben G.T. Coumbe Rheumatologist, Northwick Park Hospital, London, UK

Thomas Crowley Research Associate, Centre for Inflammation Biology and Cancer Immunology, King's College London, London, UK

Maria Antonietta D'Agostino Professor of Rheumatology, Versailles, Ile-de-France, France

Emma Dures Associate Professor in Rheumatology and Self-Management, UWE Bristol, Bristol, UK; Department of Nursing & Midwifery, UWE Bristol and Academic Rheumatology, Bristol Royal Infirmary

Ursula Fearon Professor of Molecular Rheumatology, School of Medicine, Trinity College Dublin, Dublin, Ireland

Andrew Filer Rheumatology Research Group, Institute of Inflammation and Ageing, University of Birmingham, Birmingham, UK

Marina Frleta-Gilchrist Institute of Infection, Immunity and Inflammation, University of Glasgow, Glasgow, UK

James Galloway Senior Lecturer in Rheumatology, King's College London, and Honorary Consultant Rheumatologist, King's College London, London, UK

Kathryn A. Gibson Associate Professor, South Western Sydney Clinical School, Sydney, Australia

Marlies C. van der Goes Rheumatologist, University Medical Centre Utrecht, Utrecht, the Netherlands

Jeff Greenberg Clinical Associate Professor of Medicine, NYU Grossman School of Medicine, New York, USA; Attending Rheumatologist, Overlook Medical Center Summit, USA; Chief Medical Officer, Corrona LLC, Waltham, USA

James Gwinnutt Research Associate, Division of Musculoskeletal & Dermatological Sciences, University of Manchester, Manchester, UK

Espen A. Haavardsholm Professor, Department of Clinical Medicine, the University of Oslo, Oslo, Norway

Alison Hammond Professor in Rheumatology Rehabilitation, University of Salford, Salford, UK

Jennifer Hannah Department of Rheumatology, Guys and St Thomas' NHS Foundation Trust, London, UK

Ulrike Harre Friedrich Alexander University Erlangen Nürnberg, Universitätsklinikum Erlangen, Erlangen, Germany

Neelam Hassan Musculoskeletal Research Unit, University of Bristol, Bristol, UK

Abdullah Houssien Clinical Research Fellow, King's College London, London, UK

Tom W.J. Huizinga Professor of Rheumatology, Universiteit Leiden, Leiden, the Netherlands

Kimme Hyrich Professor of Epidemiology, the Arthritis Research UK Centre for Epidemiology, University of Manchester, Manchester, UK

John Isaacs Professor of Rheumatology, Institute of Cellular Medicine, Newcastle University, Newcastle, UK

Johannes W.G. Jacobs Department of Rheumatology and Clinical Immunology, University Medical Center Utrecht, Utrecht, the Netherlands

Meghna Jani NIHR Academic Clinical Lecturer, University of Manchester, Manchester, UK

Cheryl Jones Research Fellow, University of Manchester, Manchester, UK

Jeffrey Kaine Rheumatologist, Venice Arthritis Centre, Venice, USA

Lars Klareskog Senior Professor, Department of Medicine, Karolinska Instituet, Stockholm, Sweden

Tore K. Kvien Professor of Rheumatology, University of Oslo, Oslo, Norway

Soi-Cheng Law Research Officer, Mater Research Institute, University of Queensland, Brisbane, Australia

Katherine Macdonald Clinical Research Fellow, King's College London, London, UK

Catherine McGrath Researcher, Institute of Inflammation and Ageing, University of Birmingham, Birmingham, UK

Iain B. McInnes Professor of Experimental Medicine, Institute of Infection, University of Glasgow, Glasgow, UK

Annette van der Helm-van Mil Professor in Rheumatology, Leiden University Medical Centre, Leiden, the Netherlands

Nehal Narayan Honorary Clinical Research Fellow in Rheumatology, Nuffield Department of Orthopaedics, Rheumatology, and Musculoskeletal Sciences, University of Oxford, Oxford, UK

Elena Nikiphorou Senior Research Fellow, School of Immunology and Microbial Sciences, King's College London, London, UK

Contributors

Christina H. Opava Professor of Physiotherapy, Department of Neurobiology, Care Sciences, and Society, Karolinska Institutet, Stockholm, Sweden

Mikkel Østergaard Clinical Professor, Copenhagen Center for Arthritis Research, Center for Rheumatology and Spine Diseases, Rigshospitalet, Glostrup and Department of Clinical Medicine, University of Copenhagen, Copenhagen, Denmark

Sheetal Patel Attending Rheumatologist, Overlook Medical Centre, Summit, USA

Charles Peterfy Founder, Spire Sciences, Boca Raton, USA

Theodore Pincus Former Professor of Medicine and Rheumatology, and Principle Investigator, Yazici Rheumatology Outcomes Research Unit, NYU Lagone School of Medicine, New York, USA

Arthur G. Pratt Clinical Senior Lecturer in Rheumatology, Newcastle University, and Honorary Consultant Rheumatologist, Freeman Hospital, Newcastle, UK

Yeliz Prior Senior Research Fellow, School of Health and Society, University of Salford Manchester, Salford, UK; Advanced Clinical Specialist Occupational Therapist, Rheumatology Outpatients, Leighton Hospital, Mid Cheshire NHS Foundation Trust, Crewe, UK

Harriet Purvis Post Doctoral Student, Centre for Inflammation Biology and Cancer Immunology, King's College London, London, UK

Helga Radner Division of Rheumatology, Department of Internal Medicine III, Medical University Vienna, Vienna, Austria

Karim Raza Professor of Rheumatology supported by Versus Arthritis, University of Birmingham, Birmingham, UK; and Honorary Consultant Rheumatologist, Sandwell & West Birmingham Hospitals NHS Trust, Birmingham, UK

Anthony C. Redmond Professor of Clinical Biomechanics, Leeds Institute of Rheumatic and Musculoskeletal Medicine and NIHR Leeds Biomedical Research Centre, University of Leeds, Leeds, UK

Mark D. Russell Department of Academic Rheumatology, King's College, London, UK

Ilfita Sahbudin Clinical Lecturer in Rheumatology, Institute of Inflammation and Ageing, University of Birmingham, Birmingham, UK

Dirkjan van Schaardenburg Professor of Rheumatology, University of Amsterdam, Amsterdam, the Netherlands

Georg Schett Professor and Chair of Internal Medicine III, Friedrich-Alexander-University Erlangen-Nürnberg, Universitätsklinikum Erlangen, Erlangen, Germany

David L. Scott Emeritus Professor of Rheumatology, King's College London, London, UK

Heidi J. Siddle Associate Professor and Honorary Consultant Podiatrist, Leeds Institute of Rheumatic and Musculoskeletal Medicine, University of Leeds, Leeds, UK

José A.P. da Silva Rheumatology Service, Hospital and University Centre of Coimbra Praceta, Coimbra, Portugal

Sarah Skeoch Consultant Rheumatologist, Royal National Hospital for Rheumatic Diseases, Royal United Hospitals NHS Trust, Bath, UK; and Honorary Clinical Lecturer, Centre for Epidemiology Versus Arthritis, University of Manchester, UK

Josef Smolen Professor of Internal Medicine and Chairman of the Department of Rheumatology, University of Vienna, Vienna, Austria

Nidhi Sofat Professor of Rheumatology and Consultant Rheumatologist, Institute of Infection and Immunity, St George's University of London, London, UK

Tuulikki Sokka-Isler Professor of Rheumatic Diseases, University of Eastern Finland, Joensuu and Kuopio, Finland

Jeremy Sokolove Clinical Assistant Professor, Stanford University School of Medicine, Palo Alto, USA

Ulrike Steffen Friedrich-Alexander-University Erlangen-Nürnberg, Universitätsklinikum Erlangen, Erlangen, Germany

Vibeke Strand Biopharmaceutical Consultant and Adjunct Clinical Professor, Division of Immunology and Rheumatology, Stanford University, Palo Alto, USA

Anja Strangfeld Head Pharmacoepidemiology Group, Department of Epidemiology and Health Services Research, German Rheumatism Research Centre, Berlin, Germany

Deborah Symmons Emeritus Professor, Division of Musculoskeletal and Dermatological Sciences, University of Manchester, Manchester, UK

Peter C. Taylor Norman Collisson Professor of Musculoskeletal Sciences and Fellow of St Peter's College, University of Oxford, Oxford, UK

Ranjeny Thomas Arthritis Qld Chair of Rheumatology, The University of Queensland, Queensland, Australia

Jason D. Turner Rheumatology Research Group, Institute of Inflammation and Ageing, University of Birmingham, Birmingham, UK

Till Uhlig Professor, Department of Clinical Medicine, the University of Oslo, Oslo, Norway

Douglas J. Veale Adjunct Professor, School of Medicine, University College Dublin, Ireland

Suzanne Verstappen Reader in Musculoskeletal Epidemiology, Centre for Epidemiology Versus Arthritis, Centre for Musculoskeletal Research, The University of Manchester, Manchester, UK

Edward M. Vital Associate Professor, Leeds Institute of Rheumatic and Musculoskeletal Medicine, University of Leeds, UK; NIHR Leeds Biomedical Research Centre, Leeds Teaching Hospitals NHS Trust, UK

Marieke M.J.H. Voshaar Department of Psychology, Health and Technology, University of Twente, the Netherlands

Allan Wailoo Professor of Health Economics, University of Sheffield, Sheffield, UK

Pascale Wehr The Thomas Group, The University of Queensland, Queensland, Australia

Mark Yates Clinical Research Fellow, School of Immunology and Microbial Sciences, King's College London, London, UK

Md Yuzaiful Md Yusof NIHR Academic Clinical Lecturer, Leeds Institute of Rheumatic and Musculoskeletal Medicine, University of Leeds, UK; NIHR Leeds Biomedical Research Centre, Leeds Teaching Hospitals NHS Trust, UK

Angela Zink Head Department of Epidemiology and Health Services Research, German Rheumatism Research Centre, and Charité University Medicine Berlin, Department of Rheumatology and Clinical Immunology, Berlin, Germany

Symbols and abbreviations

α	alpha
β	beta
AA	*Aggregatibacter actinomycetemcomitans*
ABT	antigen-binding test
ACD	Anaemia of chronic disease
ACE	angiotensin-converting enzyme
ACIP	Advisory Committee on Immunization Practices
ACPA	anticitrullinated protein antibody
ACR	American College of Rheumatology
ADA	antidrug antibody
ADAPT	Alzheimer's Disease Anti-Inflammatory Prevention Trial
ADCC	antibody dependent cellular cytotoxicity
ADL	activities of daily living
AE	adverse events
AHFT	Arthritis Hand Function Test
AID	activation-induced cytidine deaminase
AIMS	arthritis impact measurement scales
AMPA	anti-post-translationally modified protein antibodies
ANA	antinuclear antibodies
ANCA	Antineutrophil cytoplasm antibodies
APC	antigen-presenting cells
APIPPRA	Arthritis Prevention in the Preclinical Phase of RA with Abatacept
ARA	American Rheumatism Association
ASMP	Arthritis Self-Management Program
ATI	antibodies to infliximab
ATP	adenosine triphosphate
ATS	American Thoracic Society
ATTACH	Anti-TNF Therapy Against Congestive Heart
AUC	area under the receiver operating characteristic curve
AUC	areas under the curve
BA	biologic agents
BAD	British Association of Dermatologists
BAFF	B-cell activating factor
BASDAI	Bath Ankylosing Spondylitis Disease Activity index
BCMA	B-cell maturation antigen
BHPR	British Health Professionals in Rheumatology
BMD	bone mineral density
BMI	body mass index
BRAGGSS	Biologics in Rheumatoid Arthritis Genetics and Genomics Study Syndicate
BSR	British Society for Rheumatology
BSUFA	Biosimilar User Fees Act
BVAS	Birmingham Vasculitis Activity Score
CAD	coronary artery disease
CAMERA	Computer-Assisted Management in Early Rheumatoid Arthritis
CAT	computer-adaptive testing
CBT	cognitive-behavioural theory
CCF	Congestive cardiac failure
CCI	Charlson Comorbidity Index
CCP	cyclic citrullinated peptide
CDAI	Clinical disease activity index
CDC	complement-dependent cytotoxicity
CESD	Centers for Epidemiologic Studies Depression
CFQ	Chalder Fatigue Questionnaire
CFS	chronic fatigue syndrome
CI	confidence interval
CIA	collagen-induced arthritis
CIS	Checklist Individual Strength
CLL	Chronic lymphocytic leukaemia
CMC	carpometacarpal
CMC	chemistry, manufacturing, and controls
CMV	cytomegalovirus
CNS	central nervous system
COPD	chronic obstructive pulmonary disease
COPM	Canadian Occupational Performance Measure
CQA	critical quality attributes
CRH	corticotropin-releasing hormone
CRP	C-reactive protein
CSA	Clinically suspect arthralgia
CSA	clinically suspect arthralgia
CSF	colony-stimulating factor
CT	computed tomography
CVD	cardiovascular disease
DAD	diffuse alveolar damage
DAS	disease activity score
DIP	desquamative interstitial pneumonia
DIP	distal interphalangeal
DM	diabetes mellitus
DMARD	disease-modifying antirheumatic drug
DRESS	drug reaction with eosinophilia and systemic symptoms
DVT	Deep vein thrombosis
DXA	dual-energy X-ray absorptiometry
EBV	Epstein–Barr virus
ECM	extracellular matrix
EDAQ	Evaluation of Daily Activity Questionnaire
EHR	Electronic health records

EIRA	Epidemiological Investigation of RA		IP	inflammatory polyarthritis
ELISA	enzyme-linked immunosorbent assay		IP	interphalangeal
ELS	ectopic lymphoid-like structures		IPF	idiopathic pulmonary fibrosis
EMA	European Medicines Agency		IR	international ratio
ENT	ears, nose, and throat		IRR	incidence rate ratio
EQTL	expression quantitative trait locus		IU	international unit
ER	endoplasmic reticulum		JAK	Janus kinase
ERS	European Respiratory Society		JH	Janus homology
ESR	erythrocyte sedimentation rate		LDA	low disease activity
EULAR	European League Against Rheumatism		LDL	low density lipoprotein
EWAS	epigenome-wide association study		LIP	lymphocytic interstitial pneumonia
FA	folic acid		LLN	lower limit of normal
FACIT	Functional Assessment of Chronic Illness Therapy		LMAP	Lifestyle Management for Arthritis Programme
FASL	Fas ligand		LPS	lipopolysaccharide
FDA	Food and Drug Administration		LTE	long-term extension
FDR	first-degree relatives		MAP	mitogen-activated protein
FFI	Foot Function Index		MCID	Minimum clinically important differences
FIS	Foot Impact Scale		MCP	metacarpophalangeal
FLS	fibroblast-like synoviocytes		MCS	Mental component summary
FSS	Fatigue Severity Scale		MDBA	multibiomarker disease activity
FVC	forced vital capacity		MDHAQ	Multidimensional Health Assessment Questionnaire
GAS	Gamma activated site		MFI	Multi-Dimensional Fatigue Inventory
GAT	Grip Ability Test		MFPDQ	Manchester Foot Pain and Disability Questionnaire
GBD	Global Burden of Disease		MHC	major histocompatibility complex
GDP	Gross domestic product		MI	myocardial infarction
GDS	Geriatric Depression Scale		MIRROR	Methotrexate Inadequate Responders Randomized Study of Rituximab
GM-CSF	granulocyte-macrophage colony-stimulating factor		MMP	matrix metalloproteinase
GR	glucocorticoid receptors		MMPI	Minnesota Multiphasic Personality Inventory
GTI	Glucocorticoid Toxicity Index		MR	magnetic resonance
GWAS	genome-wide association		MRI	magnetic resonance imaging
HACA	Human antichimeric antibody		MS	multiple sclerosis
HADS	Hospital Anxiety and Depression Scale		MSD	meso scale discovery
HAQ	Health Assessment Questionnaire		MTP	metatarsophalangeal
HAQ-DI	health assessment questionnaire disability index		MTX	methotrexate
HBV	hepatitis B virus		NADPH	nicotinamide adenine dinucleotide phosphate
HCV	hepatitis C virus		NCSL	National Conference of State Legislatures
HDL	high-density lipoprotein		NGF	Nerve growth factor
HIPAA	Health Insurance Portability and Accountability Act		NHL	non-Hodgkin's lymphomas
HITECH	Health Information Technology for Economic and Clinical Health		NIH	National Institutes of Health
HLA	human leukocyte antigen		NK	natural killer
HR	hazard ratio		NMSC	non-melanoma skin cancer
HRCT	high-resolution computed tomography		NOAR	Norfolk Arthritis Register
HRQOL	health-related quality of life		NSAID	non-steroidal anti-inflammatory drug
HS	hidradenitis suppurativa		NSIP	non-specific interstitial pneumonia
HSC	haematopoietic stem cells		NYHA	New York Heart Association
HSFC	highly sensitive flow cytometry		OA	osteoarthritis
HSV	herpes simplex virus		OI	opportunistic infections
IA	inflammatory arthritis		OP	organizing pneumonia
IBD	inflammatory bowel disease		OR	odds ratio
ICC	intraclass correlation coefficient		P&F	portal-and-forceps
ICER	incremental cost-effectiveness ratio		PAD	peptidyl-arginine deiminase
ICH	International Conference on Harmonization		PAE	Paradoxical adverse events
IGA	immunoglobulin A		PAN	polyarteritis nodosa
IGG	immunoglobulin G		PASI	Psoriasis Area and Severity Index
IGM	immunoglobulin M		PB	peripheral blood
ILD	interstitial lung disease		PBMC	peripheral blood mononuclear cell
INN	International Nonproprietary Name		PCS	physical component summary

PD	power Doppler		SAVE	Stop Arthritis Very Early
PDUS	power Doppler ultrasonography		SDAI	Simplified Disease Activity Index
PE	pulmonary embolism		SE	shared epitope
PEG	polyethylene glycol		SF	synovial fluid
PET	positron emission tomography		SIE	serious infection events
PFT	pulmonary function tests		SIR	standardized incidence ratio
PIP	proximal interphalangeal		SJC	swollen joint count
PML	progressive multifocal leucoencephalopathy		SLE	systemic lupus erythematosus
PMR	polymyalgia rheumatica		SMR	standardized mortality ratio
PPV	positive predictive value		SNP	single nucleotide polymorphism
PROF	Profile of Fatigue		SPA	spondyloarthropathy
PROM	patient-reported outcome measure		SPARRA	symptoms in persons at risk of rheumatoid arthritis
PROMIS	Patient-Reported Outcomes Measurement Information System		SPECT	single-photon emission computed tomography
PSA	patients with RA, SpA, psoriatic arthritis		ST	synovial tissue
PUK	peripheral ulcerative keratitis		STAT	signal transducers and activators of transcription
QALY	quality-adjusted life years		TCR	T-cell receptor
RA	rheumatoid arthritis		TLR	Toll-like receptor
RACAT	Rheumatoid Arthritis Comparison of Active Therapies		TNF	tumour necrosis factor
RADAI	Rheumatoid arthritis disease activity index		TNFR	tumour necrosis factor receptor
RADAR	Research on adverse drug events and reports		UA	Undifferentiated arthritis
RANKL	Receptor activator of nuclear factor kappa-B ligand		UA	undifferentiated arthritis
RAPID	Routine Assessment of Patient Index Data		UC	ulcerative colitis
RB	respiratory bronchiolitis		UIP	usual interstitial pneumonia
RCT	randomized controlled trial		ULN	upper limit of normal
RDCI	Rheumatic Diseases Comorbidities Index		UPIA	undifferentiated arthritis
REMS	Regional Examination of the Musculoskeletal System		US	ultrasound
RF	rheumatoid factor		VA	Veterans Health Administration
RNA	ribonucleic acid		VAS	visual analogue scale
ROC	receiver operating characteristic		VAS	visual analogue scale
ROS	reactive oxygen species		VEGF	Vascular endothelial growth factor
RV	rheumatoid vasculitis		VFA	vertebral fractures assessment
			VIGOR	Vioxx Gastrointestinal Research

SECTION 1
History, diagnosis, and epidemiology

1   **The history of rheumatoid arthritis**   3
David L. Scott

2   **Diagnosis**   *13*
Daniel Aletaha and Helga Radner

3   **The descriptive epidemiology of rheumatoid arthritis**   *23*
James Gwinnutt and Deborah Symmons

4   **Modifiable and other risk factors for rheumatoid arthritis: A basis for prevention and better therapy**   *33*
Lars Klareskog and Lars Alfredsson

The history of rheumatoid arthritis

David L. Scott

Introduction

Our ideas about the nature and treatment of rheumatoid arthritis continually evolve. These changes reflect the ever-shifting sands of medicine. Diseases which dominated clinical medicine half a century ago, like mitral stenosis seen as a late consequence of rheumatic heart disease, have vanished. At the same time other diseases, like human immunodeficiency virus disease, have emerged and have taken prominent roles in clinical practice. It is therefore not surprising that looking backwards into the history of rheumatoid arthritis creates many challenges and uncertainties.

Many experts have provided insights into the history of rheumatoid arthritis. These include clinical leaders from past generations of rheumatologists such as Charles Short[1] and Eric Bywaters.[2] However, as our views of the past constantly shift modern insights may bring a different flavour to a well-worn subject. The history of rheumatoid arthritis has been a personal interest to me since reviewing nineteenth-century cases from London.[3] I therefore hope to provide another and potentially more up-to-date perspective of the relatively recent past.

The obvious place to start reviewing the history of rheumatoid arthritis is with the introduction of its name. This was provided by Alfred Baring Garrod in the late 1850s.[4] Clearly many patients were described with rheumatoid arthritis before it had a name and I have therefore outlined the various descriptions of the disease before Garrod named it. Finally, I have outlined what happened from the 1860s until modern times. Deciding when historical times end and the modern era begins is challenging, but the end of the 1950s, which was over 60 years ago, seems a reasonable endpoint, as during this decade the first diagnostic criteria were agreed. By 1960 there was general agreement on the name, key clinical features, frequency in the population, overall treatment options, and outcomes of treated rheumatoid arthritis. Consequently 1960 is an appropriate year to end describing the history of rheumatoid arthritis.

Naming rheumatoid arthritis

Garrod was one of the leading physicians of Victorian London. He focused much of his work on gout. His experience in the 1840s at University College Hospital led to him identifying uric acid as a key factor in gout.[5] He later became one of the leading London physicians, being knighted in 1887 and subsequently becoming Physician Extraordinary to Queen Victoria in 1890. At the time he was practising, gout was a major problem for the wealthy in London, a finding which has been attributed to the combination of lead in fine wines, which may have come from habits such as keeping port wine in containers made from lead crystal glass, and high sugar intakes linked to the dietary habits of the well off and better educated.[6]

Whether or not Garrod was the first person to use this term is open to doubt. However, as he became a physician at my own hospital, King's College Hospital, in the 1860s I have chosen to follow precedent and credit him with its first use. A review by Parish[7] certainly concluded that he had first used the term in his notebook in 1858, based on a subsequent account by his son.[8] Garrod had written 'although unwilling to add to the number of names, I cannot help expressing a desire that one might be found for this disease, not implying any necessary relation between it and either gout or rheumatism'. He published the name the next year,[4] writing 'perhaps rheumatoid arthritis would answer the object by which term I should wish to imply an inflammatory affection of the joints, not unlike rheumatism in some of its characters but differing materially from it'. Many other names had previously been used including rheumatic gout and chronic rheumatism. Although the term rheumatoid arthritis took some decades to be generally accepted, the patients seen by Garrod appear to have the same disease as we see today.

Rheumatoid arthritis before 1859

Other early nineteenth-century cases

An historical review by Fraser[9] provides a comprehensive analysis showing that the first detailed descriptions of rheumatoid arthritis were from the Pitié-Salpêtrière Hospital in Paris, which was an asylum and hospital for patients with incurable conditions. Their first reported case was in a doctoral thesis by Landré-Beauvais in 1800. Their final report was the comprehensive analysis of 41 cases described by Charcot in his doctoral thesis in 1853. Charcot noted the condition accounted for 5% of admissions to the section for cripples at the hospital. He highlighted its variable clinical course with remissions and exacerbations. He also included several drawings of patients' hands which seem typical of severe rheumatoid arthritis.

When I evaluated the medical literature published before Garrod introduced the term rheumatoid arthritis with Geoff Storey and Marie Comer we found five possible descriptions before 1800 and other more definite descriptions from after 1800.[3] While the cases reported after 1800 include some that sound typical of rheumatoid arthritis, the earlier cases before 1800 are less well characterized (Table 1.1). However, as the descriptions of most medical conditions were very different 200 years ago compared with current practice it is difficult to reach any definite conclusions.

We also reviewed nineteenth-century records from London teaching hospitals and one infirmary.[3] These show that a small number of patients were admitted to these institutions with rheumatic diseases in the 1800s. However, there were no definite diagnoses of rheumatoid arthritis until the last decade of the century when patients were recorded as being admitted for rheumatoid arthritis in 1894 and 1895 at the London hospital.

There is strong evidence that patients with rheumatoid arthritis were seen in Paris and London after 1800. There is less evidence that the disease was definitely present before 1800. Clinical practice was very different over 200 years ago and failing to find clear examples of patients with rheumatoid arthritis does not mean the disease was not present. However, my personal assessment is that the disease most likely only came to prominence in Western Europe after 1800. Based on an assessment of the same evidence Aceves-Avila et al.[10] drew the opposite conclusion and believed it is a disease of antiquity. Clearly there is no way to reach a definitive decision on when rheumatoid arthritis started.

Historical paintings

A different approach to determining the antiquity of rheumatoid arthritis has been the examination of historical paintings. In 1977 Jan Dequeker[11] evaluated the hands of people painted by the Flemish school before 1700. He thought that in five paintings there were features in the hands that resembled rheumatoid arthritis. Dequeker found no examples in the painters from the Italian Renaissance, which he attributed to these paintings being less detailed. Some years later he reported two further portraits which he considered showed features of rheumatoid arthritis.[12,13]

Other studies by Appelboom et al.[14,15] have led to the suggestion that Paul Rubens, the Antwerp-born artist who was one of greatest European baroque painters (1577 to 1640), not only painted hands suggesting rheumatoid arthritis but may also have had the condition himself.

These various papers make fascinating reading. However, their conclusions are highly speculative. I personally find them interesting but unconvincing, though my knowledge of the paintings of the great Dutch masters is minimal. Picasso is credited with the observation that 'art is the lie that enables us to realize the truth', and I believe care is needed in assessing the reality of pictorial art.

Paleopathology

Paleopathology is the study of ancient diseases in humans and animals. For rheumatoid arthritis it has usually focused on studying skeletal remains which have been undisturbed many hundreds or thousands of years. Rothschild and his colleagues have provided extensive accounts of skeletal remains showing some features of rheumatoid arthritis.[16-18] Their most detailed study involved 84 adult skeletons from the Late Archaic Culture Period, 3000 to 5000 years ago, along 19 miles of the Tennessee River in North America.[17] They found lesions in six skeletons corresponding to changes seen in contemporary rheumatoid arthritis patients. They thought the overall pattern of joint involvement in these skeletons was strikingly like that in rheumatoid arthritis and different from spondyloarthropathies.

In a subsequent study Rothschild et al.,[19] based on the evaluation of a very large number of skeletal remains across multiple sites

Table 1.1 Descriptions of early cases of possible rheumatoid arthritis

Author	Date	Description
Robert Pierce	1697	… soon after scarlet fever her first rheumatism which left her with great stiffness of the joints … later her fingers and toes have been contracted with nodes.
Sir John Floyer	1732	… was very much swelled in all her joints by a rheumatism which lasted 4 years. Fingers were contracted so close she could not move them … she responded to treatment but her left knee remained flexed.
Robert James	1745	… gout or rheumatism as some call it which 5 or 6 years had to great measure deprived him of the use of his limbs. His left hand was distorted and useless.
Rice Charleton	1774	… who for 12 months had pain in the left hip which attacked several other joints. Joints all stiff, could not be moved without pain, which after several months treatment improved.
John Wesley	1759	… knees and joints of his toes had been rendered stiff and his fingers crooked by a combination of gout and rheumatism.
Augustin Landré-Beauvais	1800	Five cases in which several joints were involved; less severe than gout but more persistent. Two post-mortems of other cases showed articular cartilage replaced by granulation tissue.
Samuel Bardsley	1807	… a man aged 60 crippled since the age of 30 … the joints strangely distorted … with a number of red nodes which may vary in size and hardness.
Joseph Spry	1822	… woman with nodosity of joints, fingers, knees, elbows, very much contracted … attacks of rheumatic gout … lived many years a deplorable object.
W Balfour	1814	… 3 years rheumatism in its most cruel form … many joints involved … little improvements after treatment.
Robert Adams	1845	Nodosity of the joints (followed for 10 years with pathology and illustrations).

Reprinted from Storey GO, Comer M, Scott DL (1994) 'Chronic arthritis before 1876: early British cases suggesting rheumatoid arthritis'. *Ann Rheum Dis*; 53: 557–60 with permission from BMJ Publishing Ltd.

Table 1.2 Archaeological sites testing positive for rheumatoid arthritis based on analysis of 931 skeletons

State/Provenance	Years before present	Number examined	Per cent positive
Ohio			
Libben	1200–850	210	4.3
Fort Ancient	1100–800	73	2.7
Kentucky			
Carlston Annis	4300–4090	138	5.1
Tennessee			
Eva	6500–6000	134	3.7
Thompson Village	650	81	2.5
Averbuch	450	89	2.2
Alabama			
Seven Mile Island	4300	129	4.6
Koger's Island	450	77	5.2

Source: data from Rothschild BM, Woods RJ, Rothschild C, Sebes JI. Geographic distribution of rheumatoid arthritis in ancient North America: implications for pathogenesis. *Semin Arthritis Rheum* 1992; 22:181–7.

suggested rheumatoid arthritis in antiquity was localized in a specific geographic region. They found no evidence of rheumatoid arthritis in 63 archaeological sites surrounding the original catchment area and also in five Old World sites. They also found evidence of spread over time, which led them to suggest that rheumatoid arthritis is a microorganism or allergen-transmitted disease. The positive findings from the work of Rothschild are shown in Table 1.2.

Other experts provide different perspectives on this area of work. Watson Buchanan considered it provided strong evidence for the antiquity of rheumatoid arthritis and also for a New World Origin.[20] Leden and Arcini[21] thought that although rheumatoid arthritis was a long-standing disease, there is some historical evidence that it was present in was also present in Stone Age Denmark and Sweden and from Roman and medieval times in other parts of Europe. Dieppe and his colleagues have simply highlighted the difficulties in diagnosing rheumatoid arthritis in skeletal remains.[22]

There are two different challenges to research to this arena. Firstly, judging whether the changes found in the bones occurred in life or after death. Secondly, deciding the likely diagnosis causing any premortem erosive changes found in the bones. While all rheumatologists can provide an informed opinion on a patient they see, very few have expertise in examining skeletal remains. These challenges make it difficult to interpret the findings in reports about rheumatoid arthritis in antiquity. Overall this is a captivating story, but its relevance remains unclear.

Clinical descriptions of rheumatoid arthritis after 1860

Late nineteenth century

In Victorian times there remained considerable doubt about exactly which patients had rheumatoid arthritis. William Ord, writing in 1880,[23] highlighted the multiplicity of synonyms for rheumatoid arthritis. He suggested it comprised persistent or progressive inflammation of one or more joints which was not rheumatic, gouty nor scrofulous in origin and which resulted in atrophic changes

in articular cartilages and articular ends of bone, and hypertrophic changes in synovial membrane and adjoining periosteum and cartilage. Clinicians at that time had difficulties in separating rheumatoid arthritis from both rheumatic fever and from arthritis associated with sexually acquired diseases, which were common in that period.[24]

Garrod was convinced that the rheumatoid arthritis had its origin in the central nervous system.[25] His analysis of over 500 cases supported his perspective. He focused on both muscle wasting and changes in tendon reflexes and sensation in a considerable number of patients. The descriptions of Garrod's patients imply not all of them had typical features of rheumatoid arthritis. Many also appeared to have additional and potentially unrelated problems. However, his assessment was reasonable for the circumstances under which he was working, though we now have quite different perspectives.

By the 1890s, descriptions of rheumatoid arthritis had become more typical of present-day patients. The rather wonderfully named Anthony Beaufort Brabazon, who was the senior physician at the Royal Mineral Water Hospital in Bath (which has always been the leading Spa hospital in England), reported experience with 100 patients seen in the hospital in the previous 2 years.[26] His patients comprised 75 women; and of the total 100 patients, 78 had involvement of the hands and feet while many had constitutional symptoms.

Twentieth century

In the first half of the twentieth century there was continued uncertainty about how to classify rheumatoid arthritis. Even by 1935 and beyond experts included a range of infective arthropathies and Still's disease in children within the broad classification of rheumatoid arthritis.[27] Consequently in large surveys of patients with chronic arthritis, such as the 1000 patients reported by Fletcher and Lewis-Faning in 1945[28] it is difficult to know how many of these patients would have met current criteria for diagnosis rheumatoid arthritis.

Two key clinical features of rheumatoid arthritis were identified in the first three decades of the twentieth century. The first of these was the nature of radiological damage. As early as 1912 Morton described loss of joint space and erosions in hand X-rays in rheumatoid arthritis.[29] In an article in the *British Medical Journal* he wrote about 'erosion of the articular ends of the phalanges', noting that 'this erosion is not a constant feature of rheumatoid arthritis any more than it is constantly absent in osteoarthritis, but the general rule holds good'. By the 1930s the value of following X-ray changes over time had been established[30] and by the 1940s there were suggestions radiological changes may occasionally be reversed.[31]

The second feature was subcutaneous nodules. In 1930 Dawson and Boots provided a detailed clinical and histological analysis of rheumatoid nodules,[32] which is similar to current perspectives. In their clinical practice in the region of 20% of patient had nodules, though this assessment was based on patients attending a specialist centre and may have therefore overestimated their frequency in patients at large.

Towards the end of the 1940s the clinical course of rheumatoid arthritis begun to be well described and broadly comparable to our present understanding of the disease. In 1948 Short and Bauer[33] reported the follow-up of a series of 300 unselected patients with rheumatoid arthritis who were consecutive admissions to the medical wards of the Massachusetts General Hospital between 1930 and 1936. Their results were based on 250 patients followed up, with 80% followed for at least 5 years. Only simple treatments were used. They found 53% had improved and that 15% were in remission. They noted that 37% of patients seen within one year of disease onset achieved remission, compared with only 5% of patients seen after one year from diagnosis. However, 46% of patients who initially improved later relapsed. There were several subsequent reports about these patients, including a detailed monograph published in 1957 (see **Figure 1.1**).[34] In this book they highlighted good initial prognostic factors including male sex, age under 40, short duration of symptoms, and initial unilateral joint involvement. An interesting footnote to this case series was published by Charles Short in 1964.[35] He noted that of the 250 patients followed up, 23 (9%) had sustained clinical remissions lasting an average of 22 years while receiving only simple supportive treatment. In 17 of these patients the onset of their

arthritis was acute; it was only gradual in six patients. Eight had had previous episodes.

Another major observational study was reported by Duthie et al. from 1955 to 1964,[36–38] though it was essentially a 1950s study. These rheumatologists studied all patients with rheumatoid arthritis admitted to the rheumatic unit in Edinburgh from 1948 to 1951. They followed 307 patients who had been admitted because they had active disease or deformities that required correction. In 1955 they reported that 60% of patients had initially improved and that during follow-up 16% progressed rapidly, 39% progressed slowly, and in 44% there were episodic remissions and exacerbations. Their final paper in 1964 summarized what had happened to 275 patients over 9 years of follow-up; 32 patients had left Scotland or were uncontactable. They found 75 had died and 77 were severely disabled; this meant over half of their patients had died or become severely disabled. Only 41 (15%) had no residual disability.

The final major observational follow-up study was by Ragan and Farringdon.[39] They retrospectively reviewed the disease course in 500 patients seen in clinics in voluntary hospitals in New York who at least two clinicians had diagnosed rheumatoid arthritis. Patients were followed for up to 16 years. When first seen, only 18% of patients were moderately or severely disabled but after 16 years the proportion increased to 55% of patients. Patients with longer disease durations when first seen, and particularly those with prolonged active disease, had worse outcomes.

Classification and epidemiology

Rheumatoid factor

Identifying rheumatoid factors and using them diagnostically developed gradually over a period of 30 years. In 1961 Charles Ragan;[40] looked back over the development of rheumatoid factor testing; he considered the first steps had been the search for infection causes of rheumatoid arthritis by Cecil et al.[41] They had believed the cause was streptococcal infection, similarly to rheumatic fever, though this perception was eventually abandoned. However, a crucial observation was that serum from patients with rheumatoid arthritis could agglutinate certain strains of streptococci.

The next step was the work of Erik Waaler.[42] He found during in routine work with complement fixation reactions, that the serum from a patient with rheumatoid arthritis inhibited the haemolysis of sheep red cells and also caused marked agglutination of them. This research was published in 1940 but had no immediate impact, which was presumed to be a consequence of the dislocation of science by the war in Europe.

In the late 1940s a technician working under Professor Rose at Columbia University was undertaking research into rickettsial diseases. She became infected herself and in the recovery phase after the infection used her own serum in tests with the Rickettsia. She found her serum agglutinated sensitized sheep red cells. As she had rheumatoid arthritis it was appreciated that this agglutination might be due to her rheumatoid arthritis. Subsequent research showed many patients with rheumatoid arthritis agglutinated in high titre sheep red cells sensitized with anti-sheep cell rabbit serum. These findings led to the development of Rose-Waaler sheep cell tests for rheumatoid factor.[43]

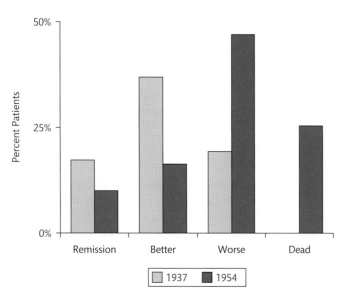

Figure 1.1 Outcomes in 293 rheumatoid arthritis patients, Short and Bauer, Harvard University Press, 1957.

Source: data from Short CL, Bauer W. (1948) 'The course of rheumatoid arthritis in patients receiving simple medical and orthopedic measures'. *N Engl J Med* 238:142–8.

There were two early modifications to sheep cell agglutination tests for rheumatoid factor. Firstly Heller and colleagues used human gamma globulin to sensitive sheep cells.[44] Secondly, Singer and Plotz used latex particles instead of sheep cells.[45] Using the latex test they found positive results in 71% of patients with rheumatoid arthritis; the test was potentially more sensitive than sheep cell agglutination.

Over the next decade testing for rheumatoid factor become routine and it was based on sheep cell, latex tests, and several variations in these approaches. Many publications had established positive rheumatoid factor tests occurred in between 70 and 90% of patients with rheumatoid arthritis. In contrast positive findings were seen in less than 5% of patients with other disorders, including conditions such as systemic lupus erythematosus that were often associated with joint manifestations.[46] At the same time the exact nature of rheumatoid factor, its role in the pathogenesis of rheumatoid arthritis and its association with other disorders remained uncertain. However, for 20 or 30 years the use of sheep cell and latex tests for rheumatoid factor was widespread and they became an accepted part of clinical practice.

Diagnostic criteria

The need for agreed criteria to classify patients with rheumatoid arthritis was shown by a North American survey of people with arthritis undertaken by Sydney Cobb and his colleagues in Pittsburgh.[47] They surveyed 10 000 people and identified 372 patients who they considered had a definite rheumatic disease but only one in eight of these patients fitted a 'classical' description of a rheumatic disease. They realized that agreed classification criteria were needed and recommended they were developed.

The next year after this publication, a committee of the American Rheumatism Association proposed diagnostic criteria for rheumatoid arthritis.[48] The criteria were based on the experiences of the committee members, the results of the Pittsburgh survey and an analysis of 332 cases provided by specialists from 19 different American centres. There were 11 criteria and a list of 19 exclusions. Patients had definite rheumatoid arthritis if they had at least 5 criteria and had joint symptoms for 6 weeks. Patients had probable rheumatoid arthritis if they had at least 3 criteria and 4 weeks of joint symptoms.

Most of the criteria remain relevant today, including joint stiffness, joint pain and swelling, symmetrical joint swelling, subcutaneous nodules, rheumatoid factor positivity, and erosions on X-ray. Three criteria—mucin tests of synovial fluid and histology of joints and nodules—have become obsolete. The exclusions remain equally valid today. They include evidence of systemic lupus erythematosus, other connective tissue diseases, and gout.

The criteria were not considered definitive. It was anticipated they would be revised over time as experience was gained using them. Some features of rheumatoid arthritis such as fatigue, though clinically important, were considered too non-specific to be part of the diagnostic criteria. The committee also proposed a further category of possible rheumatoid arthritis based on rather loose criteria. Although this was of interest, it never became widely used in clinical or epidemiologic studies as it was too broad and non-specific.

Epidemiology

As the clinical and diagnostic features of rheumatoid arthritis were recognized and agreed there was increasing interest in the frequency of the disease. Although some work was done before the Second World War, it was not until the 1950s that the epidemiology of rheumatoid arthritis was directly addressed. This was usually done by house to house surveys.

The most important of these surveys was undertaken in Leigh, a northern industrial English town. Kellgren and his colleagues[49] studied 3515 individuals over the age of 15 years, who were all questioned by a social worker in 1949 and 1950. Over 1400 said they had had some and over 1309 were examined. They found 34% of females and 31% of males had had some rheumatic complaint in the previous 5 years, and that 109 patients had a diagnosis of rheumatoid arthritis, rheumatic complaint accounting for 4.3% of females and 1.7% of males. There were substantially more patients with rheumatoid arthritis in the over 50s. Only 70 patients had rheumatoid arthritis as an active complaint.

A broadly similar population survey was undertaken by de Blecourt in the Netherlands and was reported in 1954.[50] He studied 3378 people aged over 14 from four villages in the northern Netherlands and found 621 (18%) had a rheumatic problem. There were 32 (0.8%) people with rheumatoid arthritis. The way in which rheumatoid arthritis was diagnosed was not explained in detail in this paper.

A follow-up study by Kellgren and Lawrence was published in 1956.[51] They undertook a detailed assessment combining clinical, radiological, and serological assessments in people aged 50–59 from Leigh seen in the first survey and repeated their assessments 5 years later when they were aged 55–64. The clinical features of what they termed severe rheumatoid arthritis were seen in 1.5% men and 3.0% women and were usually associated with X-ray erosions and rheumatoid factor positivity. However, many patients had features of mild inflammatory arthritis and some other patients also had some radiological erosions or positive tests for rheumatoid factor. There was therefore considerable diagnostic uncertainty about mild disease.

One other epidemiological study from the north of England, by Lawrence and Bennett,[52] described patients with benign polyarthritis identified by a community survey. They found a past history of polyarthritis in 5% of males and 7% of females in a survey of 745 people. This showed benign polyarthritis is much more frequent that severe rheumatoid arthritis.

A final North American epidemiologic study from Pittsburgh by Cobb et al.[53] involved a stratified random sample of 798 individuals over 14 years of age; 89% were interviewed and 60% examined. This was the first survey to use the agreed American Rheumatism Association criteria for definite or probable rheumatoid arthritis. They found 2.7% of the population over 14 years of age had definite or probable rheumatoid arthritis. A further 11% had possible rheumatoid arthritis. There was a marked gender difference; 0.6% of men and 4.7% of women had definite or probable rheumatoid arthritis.

Treatments

Early descriptions and symptomatic treatment

Early treatments were limited and were mainly physical therapies. These included diets, dry massage, hydrotherapy, and galvanic baths.[54] By 1909 the potential role of surgical interventions had also been highlighted by Robert Jones.[55]

Symptomatic drug treatment of rheumatic diseases salicylates and subsequently with aspirin developed from the 1870s onwards. These historical reports did not always clearly differentiate between rheumatic fever, rheumatoid arthritis, and other forms of arthritis and often used terms such as acute rheumatism. However, the use of salicylates to treat arthritis was described in the 1870s[56] and the use of aspirin after 1900.[57] They continued to be used widely into the 1940s and 1950s.[58] By 1960 rheumatoid arthritis a broader range of drug treatments was used to control pain including phenylbutazone, paracetamol, codeine, though aspirin had maintained a central role.[59] The development of a wide range of non-steroidal anti-inflammatory drugs followed on from the introduction of phenylbutazone, but most of the research in this area dates from the 1960s onwards and lies outside this historical era.

Gold and other disease-modifying drugs

The use of gold injections to treat rheumatoid arthritis was developed by Jacques Forestier in France starting in the latter part of the 1920s. By 1934 he had treated over 500 patients.[60] The rationale for using gold was that it appeared effective in tuberculosis and rheumatoid disease was considered to have some similarities with a potential infective basis. He described the benefits of weekly intramuscular injections of myocrysin, including reductions in pain, joint swelling, and the erythrocyte sedimentation rate (ESR). He found most patients improved and a minority showed substantial and sustained benefits. He noted renal, skin, and gastrointestinal adverse effects.

Many observational studies followed including large series of patients from England and North America.[61,62] These particularly highlighted the toxicity of gold including its serious haematological adverse effects, its relative effectiveness, and the particular benefits seen in patients with early disease.

The case series were followed by two trials comparing gold injections with inactive control therapy. The results of the first trial, in which 110 patients were treated and 103 patients were followed over 12 months, was reported by Fraser in 1945.[63] The second trial, the Empire Rheumatism Trial, involved 200 patients followed for 18 months.[64] Both trials provided evidence that gold injections were more effective than inactive control therapy but also gave more adverse effects. They heralded an era when gold injections were widely used though there were ongoing concerns about its substantial toxicity. Not all rheumatologists used gold but it became a standard treatment for some years into the future.

Preliminary research was also undertaken on three other disease-modifying drugs in the 1950s. These were the first stages in the development of methotrexate,[65] chloroquine,[66] and sulfasalazine.[67] The precursor drug before methotrexate, aminopterin, was given to six patients with rheumatoid arthritis by Gubner et al.[65] The drug was given daily for up to 21 days. There was evidence of improvement in most patients, which persisted for some time after treatment was stopped. There was also evidence of improvement in psoriasis, which was present in one patient. Although there was an early interest in the use of aminopterin, and then methotrexate, in psoriasis, it was several decades before the drug was developed for rheumatoid arthritis.

The use of antimalarials in rheumatoid arthritis followed earlier reports of their successful use in systemic lupus erythematosus. The first antimalarial tried with mepacrine. However, this discoloured the skin. Consequently, chloroquine was tried as a replacement.

It gave some success, though the level of benefit was modest.[66] Subsequent research focused on hydroxychloroquine, which was considered to have fewer adverse reactions.

Sulfasalazine was developed by Svartz and her colleagues in the 1930s and 1940s in an attempt to create an effective treatment for rheumatoid arthritis by combining the therapeutic properties of salicylates and sulfonamides. The use of sulfonamides reflected the perception that rheumatoid arthritis had an infective basis. Svartz had positive findings in rheumatoid arthritis patients.[67] but when it was studied by Sinclair and Duthie[68] they failed to find any positive benefits. In retrospect the reason for their failure was they only used a short-term high dose course of sulfasalazine and assessed the patients' responses a considerable time after treatment was stopped. However, their negative results meant further studies on this drug were delayed by many years.

Steroids

The discovery and introduction of steroids into clinical practice is one of the most important and fascinating historical features of rheumatoid arthritis and of rheumatology in general. There have been many detailed descriptions of the course of events leading up to the early clinical studies led by Hench and his colleagues and of the impact of this development on the pharmaceutical industry.[69-72]

Following several decades of development, a small amount of cortisone became available in the autumn of 1948 for clinical use as a result of a synthetic process developed by Merck & Co, the large American pharmaceutical company. The clinical development was led by Phillip Hench at the Mayo Clinic in North America where the first patient given cortisone. She was a 28-year-old woman with severe rheumatoid arthritis who had failed to respond conventional treatment. She received an intramuscular injection of 100 mg cortisone and this dose was continued daily for some days. The patient began to feel better by the second day, and by the third day relatively few symptoms remained. The results in this first patient led Hench and his colleagues to treat a series of patients and their experience with 14 patients was reported in the Mayo Clinic Proceedings in April 1949.[73] The patients all had moderately severe or severe rheumatoid arthritis and all showed marked improvements while receiving cortisone.

The use of cortisone rapidly extended to a range of other rheumatic diseases including arteritis, rheumatic fever, and systemic lupus erythematosus. There was also an early recognition of the many adverse events associated with steroid therapy including skin changes, euphoria, salt and water retention, and hyperglycaemia.[74] However, the impact of cortisone on the management of rheumatic diseases was so dramatic that Hench and Kendall together with Dr Tadeus Reichstein of Switzerland, who had spent his career studying adrenal hormones, were awarded the Nobel Prize for Medicine in 1950.

Soon after this early work, new and more effective steroids were synthesized, particularly metacortandralone and metacortandracin, by the Schering Corporation,[75] which were subsequently known as prednisolone and prednisone. These were not only more effective but also resulted in less salt and water retention. They were effective in rheumatoid arthritis.[76] Several other active drugs were formulated including methylprednisolone, triamcinolone, and dexamethasone. All these agents had comparable efficacy.[77]

The clinical effectiveness of cortisone, prednisone, and prednisolone was subsequently evaluated in trials undertaken by the

Medical Research Council, the Nuffield Foundation, and the Empire Rheumatism Council.[78–80] These trials followed patients for up to 3 years. They showed that prednisone and prednisolone were more effective than aspirin and cortisone and that cortisone itself had only modest benefit.

Research into the benefits of steroids in rheumatoid arthritis was accompanied by rapid increases in understanding of the range and severity of adverse events associated with treatment with their use.[81–84] However, the balance of expert opinion during the 1950s favoured the continuing use of steroids despite growing concerns about their potential risks. As there were few alternatives this was both understandable and reasonable. As effective alternatives were developed in future years the use of steroids gradually declined in ensuing years.

Conclusions

The century which passed between the naming of rheumatoid arthritis by Garrod[4] and the development of diagnostic criteria by Ropes et al.[48] saw major changes in understanding its nature and treating its symptoms. Most of the research during this time focused on what constituted rheumatoid arthritis, what happened to patients with the disease over time, and how could its symptoms be improved. Although the 1950s saw substantial improvements in the treatment of rheumatoid arthritis, none of the therapeutic approaches followed at that time are favoured today. The development of better clinical assessments and the introduction of methotrexate, other disease-modifying drugs, and biological treatments have changed the management and outcomes of rheumatoid arthritis dramatically since the 1950s. However, without some knowledge of where clinical care has come from it is difficult to assess its progress and direction of travel. For this reason, it remains useful to have some perspective on the history of rheumatoid arthritis.

REFERENCES

1. Short CL. The antiquity of rheumatoid arthritis. *Arthritis Rheum* 1974;*17*:193–205.
2. Bywaters EG. Historical aspects of the aetiology of rheumatoid arthritis. *Br J Rheumatol* 1988;*27*(Suppl 2):110–5.
3. Storey GO, Comer M, Scott DL. Chronic arthritis before 1876: early British cases suggesting rheumatoid arthritis. *Ann Rheum Dis* 1994;*53*:557–60.
4. Garrod AB. *The Nature and Treatment of Gout and Rheumatic Gout*. London, UK: Walton and Maberly, 1859.
5. Storey GD. Alfred Baring Garrod (1819–1907). *Rheumatology* 2001;*40*:1189–90.
6. Rivard C, Thomas J, Lanaspa MA, Johnson RJ. Sack and sugar, and the aetiology of gout in England between 1650 and 1900. *Rheumatology* 2013;*52*:421–6.
7. Parish LC. An historical approach to the nomenclature of rheumatoid arthritis. *Arthritis Rheum* 1963;*6*:138–58.
8. Garrod AE. *A Treatise on Rheumatism and Rheumatoid Arthritis*. Philadelphia, PA: Blakiston, 1890.
9. Fraser KJ. Anglo-French contributions to the recognition of rheumatoid arthritis. *Ann Rheum Dis* 1982;*41*:335–43.
10. Aceves-Avila FJ, Medina F, Fraga A. The antiquity of rheumatoid arthritis: a reappraisal. *J Rheumatol* 2001;*28*:751–7.
11. Dequeker J. Arthritis in Flemish paintings (1400–1700). *Br Med J* 1977;*1*:1203–5.
12. Dequeker J, Rico H. Rheumatoid arthritis-like deformities in an early 16th-century painting of the Flemish-Dutch school. *JAMA* 1992;*268*:249–51.
13. Dequeker J. Siebrandus Sixtius: evidence of rheumatoid arthritis of the robust reaction type in a seventeenth century Dutch priest. *Ann Rheum Dis* 1992;*51*:561–2.
14. Appelboom T, de Boelpaepe C, Ehrlich GE, Famaey JP. Rubens and the question of antiquity of rheumatoid arthritis. *JAMA* 1981;*245*:483–6.
15. Appelboom T. Hypothesis: Rubens—one of the first victims of an epidemic of rheumatoid arthritis that started in the 16th–17th century? *Rheumatology* 2005;*44*: 681–3.
16. Woods RJ, Rothschild BM. Population analysis of symmetrical erosive arthritis in Ohio Woodland Indians (1200 years ago). *J Rheumatol* 1988;*15*:1258–63.
17. Rothschild BM, Turner KR, DeLuca MA. Symmetrical erosive peripheral polyarthritis in the Late Archaic Period of Alabama. *Science* 1988;*241*:1498–501.
18. Rothschild BM, Woods RJ. Symmetrical erosive disease in Archaic Indians: the origin of rheumatoid arthritis in the New World? *Semin Arthritis Rheum* 1990;*19*:278–84.
19. Rothschild BM, Woods RJ, Rothschild C, Sebes JI. Geographic distribution of rheumatoid arthritis in ancient North America: implications for pathogenesis. *Semin Arthritis Rheum* 1992;*22*:181–7.
20. Buchanan WW. Rheumatoid arthritis: another New World disease? *Semin Arthritis Rheum* 1994;*23*:289–94.
21. Leden I, Arcini C. Doubts about rheumatoid arthritis as a New World disease. *Semin Arthritis Rheum* 1994;*23*:354–6.
22. Dieppe P, Loe L, Shepstone L, Watt I. What 'skeletal paleopathology' can teach us about arthritis. The contributions of the late Dr Juliet Rogers. *Reumatismo* 2006;*58*:79–84.
23. Ord WM. Address on some of the conditions included under the general term 'rheumatoid arthritis'. *Br Med J* 1880;*1*(996):155–8.
24. Storey GO, Scott DL. Arthritis associated with venereal disease in nineteenth century London. *Clin Rheumatol* 1998;*17*:500–4.
25. Garrod AB. A further contribution to the study of rheumatoid arthritis. *Med Chir Trans* 1888;*71*:265–81.
26. Brabazon AB. Analysis of 100 cases of rheumatoid arthritis treated in the Royal Mineral Water Hospital, Bath. *Br Med J* 1896;*1*(1838):723–4.
27. Hench PS, Bauer W, Fletcher AA, Ghrist D, Hall F, Preston White T. The problem of rheumatism and arthritis: review of American and English literature for 1935 (third rheumatism review). *Ann Inter Med* 1936;*10*:754–909.
28. Fletcher E, Lewis-Faning E. Chronic rheumatic diseases: with special reference to chronic arthritis a survey based on 1,000 cases. *Postgrad Med J* 1945;*21*:1–13.
29. Morton R. The X-ray diagnosis in some forms of arthritis. *BMJ* 1912;*2*(2437):481–2.
30. Morrison SL, Kuhns JG. Röntgenological changes in chronic arthritis. A correlation with clinical observation for long periods of time. *Amer J Roentgenol* 1936;*35*:645.
31. Lucchesi M, Lucchesi O. Return to normal of X-ray changes in rheumatoid arthritis case report. *Ann Rheum Dis* 1945;*5*:57–60.
32. Dawson MH, Boots RH. Subcutaneous nodules in rheumatoid (chronic infectious) arthritis. *J Am Med Assoc* 1930;*95*:1894–6.
33. Short CL, Bauer W. The course of rheumatoid arthritis in patients receiving simple medical and orthopedic measures. *N Engl J Med* 1948;*238*:142–8.

34. Short CL, Bauer W, Reynolds WE. *Rheumatoid Arthritis: A Definition of the Disease and a Clinical Description Based on a Numerical Study of 293 Patients and Controls.* Cambridge, MA: Harvard University Press, 1957.

35. Short CL. Long remissions in rheumatoid arthritis. *Medicine (Baltimore)* 1964;*43*:401–6.

36. Duthie JJ, Thompson M, Weir MM, Fletcher WB. Medical and social aspects of the treatment of rheumatoid arthritis; with special reference to factors affecting prognosis. *Ann Rheum Dis* 1955;*14*:133–49.

37. Duthie JJ, Brown PE, Knox JD, Thompson M. Course and prognosis in rheumatoid arthritis. *Ann Rheum Dis* 1957;*16*:411–24.

38. Duthie JJ, Brown PE, Truelove LH, Baragar FD, Lawrie AJ. Course and prognosis in rheumatoid arthritis. A further report. *Ann Rheum Dis* 1964;*23*:193–204.

39. Ragan C, Farrington E. The clinical features of rheumatoid arthritis: prognostic indices. *JAMA* 1962;*181*:663–7.

40. Ragan C. The history of the rheumatoid factor. *Arthritis Rheum* 1961;*4*:571–3.

41. Cecil RL, Nicholls EE, Stainsby WJ. The etiology of rheumatoid arthritis. *Am J Med Sci* 1931;*181*:12–24.

42. Waaler E. On the occurrence of a factor in human serum activating the specific agglutination of sheep blood corpuscles. *APMIS* 1940;**17**:172–88.

43. Rose NM, Ragan C, Pearce E, Lipman MO. Differential agglutination of normal and sensitized sheep erythrocytes by sera of patients with rheumatoid arthritis. *Proc Soc Exp Biol Med* 1948;*68*:1–6.

44. Heller G, Jacobson AS, Kolodny MH, Kammerer WH. The hemagglutination test for rheumatoid arthritis. II. The influence of human plasma fraction II (gamma globulin) on the reaction. *J Immunol* 1954;*72*:66–78.

45. Plotz CM, Singer JM. The latex fixation test. II. Results in rheumatoid arthritis. *Am J Med* 1956;*21*:893–6.

46. Kunkel HG. Significance of the rheumatoid factor. *Arthritis Rheum* 1958;*1*:381–3.

47. Cobb S, Merchant WR, Warren JE. An epidemiologic look at the problem of classification in the field of arthritis. *J Chronic Dis* 1955;*2*:50–4.

48. Ropes MW, Bennett GA, Cobb S, Jacox R, Jessar RA. Proposed diagnostic criteria for rheumatoid arthritis. *Bull Rheum Dis* 1956;*7*:121–4.

49. Kellgren JH, Lawrence JS, Aitken-Swan J. Rheumatic complaints in an urban population. *Ann Rheum Dis* 1953;*12*:5–15

50. de Blecourt JJ. 'Screening' of the population for rheumatic diseases. *Ann Rheum Dis* 1954;*13*:338–40.

51. Kellgren JH, Lawrence JS. Rheumatoid arthritis in a population sample. *Ann Rheum Dis* 1956;*15*:1–11.

52. Lawrence JS, Bennett PH. Benign polyarthritis. *Ann Rheum Dis* 1960;*19*:20–30.

53. Cobb S, Warren JE, Merchant WR, Thompson DJ. An estimate of the prevalence of rheumatoid arthritis. *J Chronic Dis* 1957;*5*:636–43.

54. Armstrong W. The therapeutics of rheumatoid arthritis. *Br Med J* 1896;*1846*:1197–8.

55. Jones R. An address on the surgical treatment of the rheumatoid group of joint affections. *Br Med J* 1909;*2531*:2–7.

56. [No author]. Special correspondence. *Br Med J* 1877;*2*:865.

57. Burnet J. The therapeutics of aspirin and mesotan. *Lancet* 1905;*165*:1193–6.

58. Ragan C. The general management of rheumatoid arthritis. *J Am Med Assoc* 1949;*141*:124–7.

59. Hart FD. Analgesics in rheumatic disorders. *Br Med J* 1960;*5181*:1265–6.

60. Forestier J. The treatment of rheumatoid arthritis with gold salts injections. *Lancet* 1932;*219*:441–4.

61. Hartfall SJ, Garland H G, Goldie W. Gold treatment of arthritis, a review of 900 cases. *Lancet* 1937:*784*:838.

62. Cecil, RL, Kammerer WH, DePrume FJ. Gold salts in the treatment of rheumatoid arthritis: a study of 245 cases. *Ann Intern Med* 1942;*16*:811l–827.

63. Fraser TN. Gold treatment in rheumatoid arthritis. *Ann Rheum Dis* 1945;*4*:7l–5.

64. Empire Rheumatism Council. Gold therapy in rheumatoid arthritis: report of a multicentre controlled trial. *Ann Rheum Dis* 1960;*19*:95–l19.

65. Gubner R, August S, Ginsberg V. Therapeutic suppression of tissue reactivity. II. Effect of aminopterin in rheumatoid arthritis and psoriasis. *Am J Med Sci* 1951;*22*:176–82.

66. Freedman A. Chloroquine and rheumatoid arthritis; a short-term controlled trial. *Ann Rheum Dis* 1956;*15*:251–7.

67. Svartz N. Treatment of rheumatoid arthritis with salicylazosulfapyridine. *Acta Med Scand Suppl* 1958;*341*:247–54.

68. Sinclair RJ, Duthie JJ. Salazopyrin in the treatment of rheumatoid arthritis. *Ann Rheum Dis* 1949;*8*:226–31.

69. Burns CM. The history of cortisone discovery and development. *Rheum Dis Clin North Am* 2016;*42*:1–14.

70. Benedek TG. History of the development of corticosteroid therapy. *Clin Exp Rheumatol* 2011;*29*(5 Suppl 68):S5–12.

71. Hunder GG, Matteson EL. Rheumatology practice at Mayo Clinic: the first 40 years—1920 to 1960. *Mayo Clin Proc* 2010;*85*:e17–30.

72. Hirschmann R. The cortisone era: aspects of its impact. Some contributions of the Merck Laboratories. *Steroids* 1992;*57*:579–92.

73. Hench PS, Kendall EC, Slocumb CH, Polley HF. The effect of a hormone of the adrenal cortex (17-hydroxy-11-dehydrocorticosterone; compound E) and of pituitary adrenocorticotropic hormone on rheumatoid arthritis. *Proc Staff Meet Mayo Clin* 1949;*24*:181–97.

74. Hench PS, Slocumb CH, Polley HF, Kendall EC. Effect of cortisone and pituitary adrenocorticotropic hormone (ACTH) on rheumatic diseases. *J Am Med Assoc* 1950;*144*:1327–35.

75. Herzog H, Oliveto EP. A history of significant steroid discoveries and developments originating at the Schering Corporation (USA) since 1948. *Steroids* 1992;*57*:617–23.

76. Bunim JJ, Pechet MM, Bollet AJ. Studies on metacortandralone and metacortandracin in rheumatoid arthritis; antirheumatic potency, metabolic effects, and hormonal properties. *J Am Med Assoc* 1955;*157*:311–18.

77. Neustadt DH. Corticosteroid therapy in rheumatoid arthritis; comparative study of effects of prednisone and prednisolone, methylprednisolone, triamcinolone, and dexamethasone. *J Am Med Assoc* 1959;*170*:1253–60.

78. [No author]. A comparison of prednisolone with aspirin or other analgesics in the treatment of rheumatoid arthritis. A second report by the Joint Committee of the Medical Research Council and Nuffield Foundation on Clinical Trials of Cortisone, ACTH, and other therapeutic measures in chronic rheumatic diseases. *Ann Rheum Dis* 1960;*19*:331–7.

79. [No author]. A comparison of cortisone and prednisone in treatment of rheumatoid arthritis; a report by the Joint Committee of the Medical Research Council and Nuffield Foundation on Clinical Trials of Cortisone, ACTH and other

therapeutic measures in chronic rheumatic diseases. *Br Med J* 1957;*2*:199–202.

80. Empire Rheumatism Council. Multi-centre controlled trial comparing cortisone acetate and acetyl salicylic acid in the long-term treatment of rheumatoid arthritis; results of three years' treatment. *Ann Rheum Dis* 1957;*16*:277–89.

81. Heimann WG, Freiberger RH. Avascular necrosis of the femoral and humeral heads after high-dosage corticosteroid therapy. *N Engl J Med* 1960;*263*:672–5.

82. Freiberger RH, Kammerer WH, Rivelis AL. Peptic ulcers in rheumatoid patients receiving corticosteroid therapy. *Radiology* 1958;*71*:542–7.

83. Rosenberg EF. Rheumatoid arthritis; osteoporosis and fracturer related to steroid therapy. *Acta Med Scand Suppl* 1958;*341*:211–24.

84. Bollet AJ, Black R, Bunim JJ. Major undesirable side-effects resulting from prednisolone and prednisone. *J Am Med Assoc* 1955;*158*:459–63.

2

Diagnosis

Daniel Aletaha and Helga Radner

Introduction

Rheumatoid arthritis (RA) affects approximately 1% of the adult population.[1] Currently RA is considered to be a chronic disease for which there is no cure, but remission, as a state where no active disease is present, has become an achievable goal with optimal treatment. At the same time, for the function and quality of life of patients with RA, it is crucial to recognize RA early and treat it effectively from the beginning. Both disability and the enormous costs of the disease are a function of disease activity over time. The ultimate goals are therefore to treat RA early and persistently until remission is present.

The challenge of treatment of early RA is not the lack of effective medicine, but rather the ethical and economic considerations related to risk-benefit and cost-benefit. Overtreating patients with potentially self-limiting or non-destructive disease by using disease-modifying antirheumatic drugs (DMARDs) is still often feared. The flipside of the coin is the potential undertreatment of patients with true RA, which—particularly in its early phases—can have accelerated structural consequences. This damage cannot be reversed even by optimal delayed treatment.[2,3] At the same time, prolonged use of non-steroidal anti-inflammatory drugs (NSAIDs) in patients with undifferentiated arthritis also carries significant risk of adverse events.[4] In fact, some of the DMARDs could possibly be considered safer than some of the NSAIDs, particularly if the latter are employed over longer periods of time.[5,6] With these thoughts on the table, one can draw a hypothetical risk (i.e. overtreatment or undertreatment)/benefit ratio for patients presenting with undifferentiated arthritis or arthritis that is not yet worked up. This leads to a necessary note regarding the terminology and semantics that are used: the term 'early' arthritis is used to indicate the duration of the symptom 'arthritis.' 'Undifferentiated' on the other hand, which may also be early in terms of symptom duration, is used to indicate that no specific diagnosis has yet been made. This is a challenging concept, as the lack of a specific diagnosis is related to the amount of effort that has been put into the work-up. Usually some basic work-up is deemed to have occurred, if the term 'undifferentiated' is used, otherwise typical lupus arthritis could be called undifferentiated just because the doctor had not examined the patient and noted the typical rash and Raynaud's, or ordered the immunological tests confirming high antinuclear antibodies and complement activation. In theory, however, there might also be the case of chronic undifferentiated arthritis following the aforementioned logic.

Figure 2.1 depicts the scenarios of late, delayed, and early diagnosis of RA in regard to the respective risk/benefit of subsequent treatment or lack of treatment. Scenarios are divided into two principal therapeutic options: immediate DMARD treatment for every patient with early arthritis, or DMARD treatment only upon an established diagnosis of RA. The sequence from panel A to panel C indicates that the risk/benefit ratio for either therapeutic approach improves with earlier timing of the definite diagnosis. Patients diagnosed earlier (panels B and C of **Figure 2.1**) would benefit from an earlier 'correction' of the therapeutic approach (DMARDs or symptomatic) preventing overtreatment in patients without RA, and undertreatment in those with RA, an thus improving the overall risk/benefit ratio of the therapeutic strategy.

It can be deduced that the question of whether RA should be treated before or only after establishing the definite diagnosis is secondary, but that the timing of the diagnosis in relation to the duration of symptoms is key in both approaches. DMARD institution before diagnosis may, however, be difficult for legal reasons in many countries or settings.

A few thoughts need to be considered in this context: first, the true risk of overtreatment with DMARDs in patients with undifferentiated arthritis is not yet completely clear, particularly when a diagnosis will be established within a reasonable time frame anyway; neither is the risk of prolonged symptomatic treatment (e.g. with NSAIDs), which may also be considerable. Second, early aggressive intervention in undifferentiated arthritis often leads to the challenging situation in which some patients with true RA may be prevented from eventually being diagnosed due to resolution of their symptoms, or, vice versa, some patients with self-limiting arthritis might be misdiagnosed as RA in clinical remission. Only withdrawal of therapy may reveal the underlying chronic condition, which is a diagnostic dilemma in clinical practice. Finally, in **Figure 2.1** it is assumed that the diagnostic properties of criteria will be similar at all stages of the disease, while in reality any diagnostic approach will likely be more accurate when more time has elapsed since the onset of symptoms.

All these considerations come into play when one aims to diagnose (and treat) RA early, but in fact currently no diagnostic criteria exist. Here, we discuss the principal approach to patients presenting with arthritis, looking at the potential differential diagnoses, as well as algorithms and criteria that may be helpful in eventually establishing an accurate diagnosis of RA.

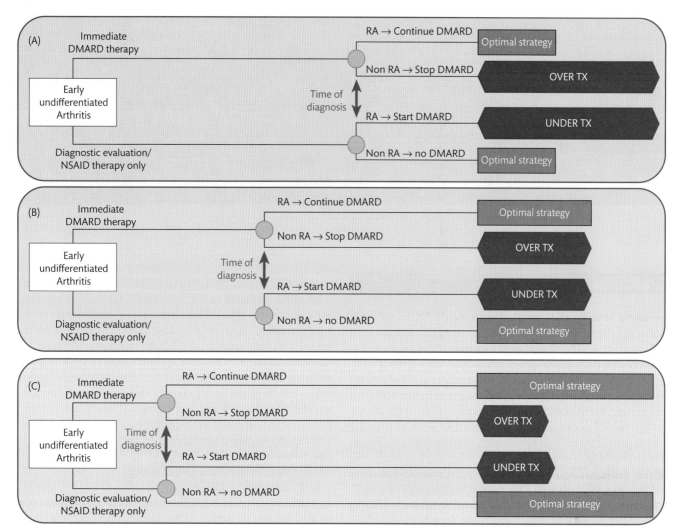

Figure 2.1 Consequences of delayed diagnosis. Three scenarios of risk/benefit are depicted for (A) late, (B) delayed, and (C) early diagnosis of definite rheumatoid arthritis (RA). Physicians face two principal therapeutic options: immediate disease-modifying antirheumatic drug (DMARD) treatment in every patient with early arthritis (top option in each panel), or DMARD treatment only upon an established diagnosis of RA (bottom option in each panel). The sequence from panel A to panel C indicates that the risk/benefit ratio for both options improves with an earlier timing of the definite diagnosis of RA.

Reprinted from Aletaha and Radner, Chapter 110: Rheumatoid Arthritis: diagnosis, in the *Oxford Textbook of Rheumatoid Arthritis* [Ed. Watts et al] (2018) with permission from Oxford University Press.

Initial evaluation of patients presenting with new-onset arthritis

The terminology for patients with recent onset arthritis is often confusing. While 'early arthritis' may be merely describe of a temporal notion, many distinguish it from 'undifferentiated arthritis'. The term 'undifferentiated' implies that some effort has already been taken to determine the type of disease underlying the 'arthritis'. This leads to the question of which steps reasonably need to be taken in order to be able to label early arthritis as 'undifferentiated'. For that purpose, an algorithm has been proposed to delineate the evaluative steps in the work-up of patients with new-onset inflammatory arthritis (**Figure 2.2**), which can either lead to a specific diagnosis or to the classification as 'undifferentiated'.[7] This includes evaluation for a history of trauma, as well as evaluating the clinical presentation of the affected joint. The major initial

distinction would be between acutely inflamed ('red hot') arthritis and other forms of arthritis. The former should arouse the suspicion of crystal-induced arthritis or septic arthritis, and although demographic and contextual factors may help to differentiate these two (e.g. age, gender, history, and lifestyle), arthrocentesis is necessary to make the specific diagnosis, as the therapeutic consequences are very different.

Synovial fluid analysis is of greatest use to distinguish between inflammatory and non-inflammatory arthropathy, usually affecting one or a few joints. Among the former are those types of inflammatory arthritis that need immediate care, particularly septic arthritis, in which the prognosis rapidly worsens with time to effective diagnosis and treatment. In fact, if the synovial fluid analysis is typical, then a confident diagnosis can be made immediately. This includes the presence of a high leucocyte count, positive Gram staining, or the presence of crystals (**Figure 2.3**). In clinical reality, the synovial fluid analysis will often not be diagnostic.

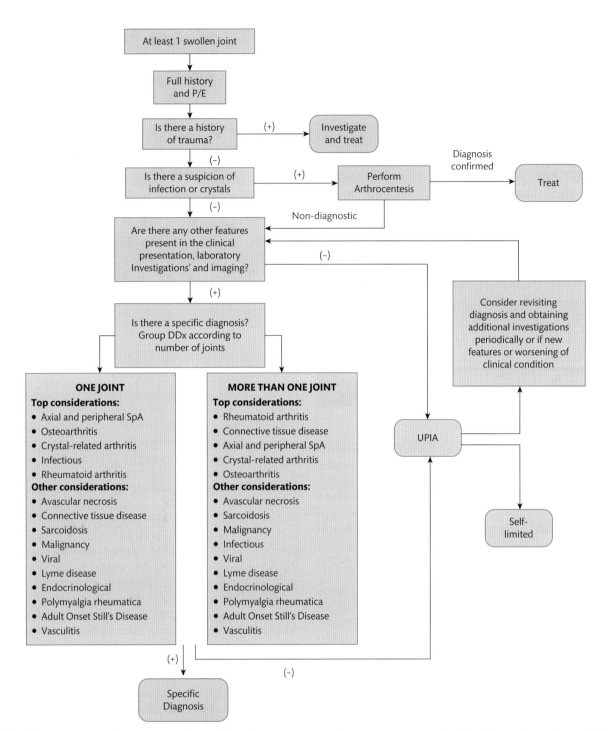

Figure 2.2 Flowchart to establishing a specific diagnosis (Dx) in new onset arthritis in at least a single swollen joint. The starting point is a full history and physical examination (P/E). After exclusion of trauma, and acute inflammatory events such as gout and septic arthritis, a specific diagnosis may be established in the presence of suggestive clinical, laboratory, or imaging features, where the differential diagnoses (DDx) differ according to the number of swollen joints involved. If no specific diagnosis can be established, the presentation may be labelled as 'undifferentiated arthritis' (in the algorithm shown as 'UPIA' for undifferentiated peripheral inflammatory arthritis). This status needs to be re-evaluated periodically, as undifferentiated arthritis may evolve into specific diagnosis over time.

Reproduced from Hazlewood G, Aletaha D, Carmona L et al. Algorithm for identification of undifferentiated peripheral inflammatory arthritis: a multinational collaboration through the 3e initiative. *J Rheumatol* Suppl. 2011; 87:54–8 with permission from *The Journal of Rheumatology*.

In general, after exclusion of crystal- or infection-related arthritis, a relatively large set of differential diagnoses is to be considered, which is different in patients with mono-, oligo-, and polyarthritis (**Figure 2.2**).[7] The most important of these are discussed in the following section (see also Chapter 12).

If no specific diagnosis can be established, the presentation can be labelled as undifferentiated arthritis. As the state of 'undifferentiated' in fact is a lack of definitive diagnosis, and hence is provisional, this state needs to be revisited periodically for evolving diagnostic hints, although the presentation may turn out to be self-limiting disease (**Figure 2.2**).

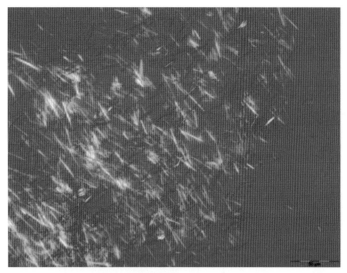 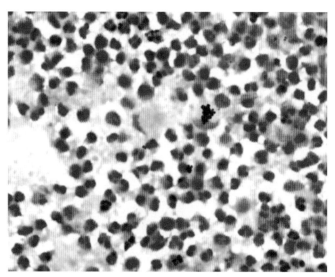

Figure 2.3 Microscopic synovial fluid analysis: (A) crystal arthritis: evidence of intracellular needle-shaped crystals; (B) septic arthritis showing positive Gram stain of cocci in typical formation; *Staphylococcus aureus*.
Courtesy of Professor Stefan Winkler, Division of Infectious Diseases, Medical University Vienna, Austria.

Important differential diagnoses of rheumatoid arthritis

Viral polyarthritis

Several types of viral infections can mimic RA by leading to typical polyarthritis of the small joints. This differs from RA in that viral polyarthritis can last from days to weeks, but is less frequently seen over the course of months, although some patients can develop a chronic arthropathy lasting for 6 months or longer.[8] A variety of viruses can lead to arthralgia, and even fewer to arthritis, the most important among the latter being the hepatitis viruses (particularly hepatitis B and C viruses—HBV and HCV), as well as parvovirus B19 and rubella.

Parvovirus B19 is the cause of erythema infectiosum (also called 'fifth disease'). It is typically a benign self-limiting disease of childhood that goes along with rash, fever, and commonly also arthritis. Less frequently, it may cause aplastic anaemia, which is a life-threatening disease. Joint involvement can impressively mimic RA by a symmetrical involvement of the small finger joints.

Patients with infectious origin of their polyarthritis may not be seronegative for rheumatoid factor, as many viral agents induce transient seropositivity.[8] Therefore determination of anticyclic citrullinated peptides (CCP) antibodies may be of more help in these circumstances, as they are less likely to be positive in diseases other than RA.[9,10] Virus-specific serological testing may be helpful to identify patients with recently acquired parvovirus infection, or to identify patients with HBV- or HCV-associated arthritis in the differential diagnosis. The treatment remains symptomatic—NSAIDs in most cases. If arthritis persists after clearance of the infection, then one might not speak of viral arthritis anymore, but the viral infection may be considered the trigger of an autoimmune disease, such as RA, in which case DMARDs may be used. Both symptomatic (NSAIDs) and disease-modifying agents are often problematic in the context of viral hepatitis.

Peripheral spondyloarthropathy

Several forms of spondyloarthropathies (SpA) are described, many of which can cause peripheral arthritis. Recently, classification criteria for peripheral SpA have been put forward,[11] which include arthritis, enthesitis, or dactylitis ('sausage digit') as important features. In combination with other typical SpA features, the diagnosis of SpA can be established as follows. If one of the three aforementioned features is present, then one of the following characteristics is sufficient for a classification: psoriasis, uveitis, inflammatory bowel disease, preceding infection (indicative of reactive arthritis), positive HLA-B27, and evidence of sacroiliitis on MRI. If two of the same features are present, then a history of inflammatory bowel disease or family history of sacroiliitis is sufficient for classification. If all three of the symptoms are present, the patient is directly classifiable.

Over and above the classification of peripheral SpA, the distribution of peripheral arthritis may help in the diagnostic process, with reactive arthritis typically affecting larger joints of the lower extremity in an asymmetric fashion.[12] Although psoriatic arthritis and RA can in most cases be distinguished based on the criteria of the classification system, the fact that RA often is also seronegative, and that joint manifestations may precede the skin manifestations in psoriatic arthritis by years,[13] may complicate the diagnostic process: a diagnosis of psoriatic arthritis can be made in patients with psoriasis who are seronegative for rheumatoid factor (RF) and antibodies directed to citrullinated peptides (ACPA); on the other hand, a diagnosis of RA may be established in psoriasis patients with a symmetric polyarthritis who are positive for rheumatoid factors or ACPA, since skin psoriasis is very common, and therefore can also simply be a comorbidity to RA. One may occasionally speak of an overlap between RA and psoriatic arthritis, if seropositive disease is present in a patient with psoriasis and radiographic changes are supportive for either diagnosis. In some patients with a symmetric inflammatory polyarthritis, the only clue to the diagnosis of psoriatic arthritis may be a family history of psoriasis.

Lyme arthritis

Lyme arthritis, a late manifestation of Lyme disease, occurs primarily in individuals who live in or travel to Lyme disease endemic areas. Lyme arthritis is characterized by intermittent or persistent inflammatory arthritis in a few large joints, especially the knee,[14] shoulder, ankle, elbow, temporomandibular joint, and wrist. Migratory arthralgias without frank arthritis may occur during early localized or early disseminated Lyme disease.

The diagnosis of Lyme arthritis may be supported by serologic testing for borrelia, which should only be done in patients presenting with undiagnosed inflammatory arthritis in endemic areas. In several respects, Lyme arthritis is different from RA as, for example, involvement of the small joints of the hands and feet is uncommon. Aside from serological testing, a positive history of erythema migrans or a tick bite may be suggestive of Lyme disease.

Sarcoid arthritis

Arthritis seen with sarcoidosis most commonly affects the ankles and knees, and less frequently, the wrist, metacarpophalangeal (MCP), and proximal interphalangeal joints. It may thus be a relevant differential diagnosis to RA in some cases. In contrast to RA, sarcoidosis can present with a variety of skin and ocular manifestations, such as erythema nodosum or uveitis, with bilateral hilar lymphadenopathy, and elevated serum concentrations of angiotensin-converting enzyme (ACE). In some cases sarcoidosis presents with the typical triad of erythema nodosum, hilar lymphadenopathy, and bilateral ankle arthritis (Löfgren's syndrome). Treatment of mild forms of sarcoid arthritis includes NSAIDs whereas more severe cases, particularly those with pulmonary involvement, require the use of glucocorticoids. A high proportion of patients with sarcoidosis have non-progressive, spontaneous remitting disease: only a small proportion require immunosuppressive agents.

Other systemic rheumatic diseases

Early RA may be difficult to distinguish from the arthritis of systemic lupus erythematosus (SLE), Sjögren's syndrome, dermatomyositis, or overlap syndromes, such as mixed connective tissue disease. In contrast with RA, these disorders are generally characterized by the presence of other systemic features such as rashes, Raynaud's syndrome, dry mouth or dry eyes, myalgia or myositis, renal or haematological abnormalities, and by various autoantibodies not seen in RA. Additionally, in connective tissue disease, particularly SLE, the values and responses of the erythrocyte sedimentation rate (ESR) and C-reactive protein (CRP) may be less well correlated with each other than in RA. Whereas both are commonly raised in RA, the CRP is often normal or only minimally elevated in patients with active SLE even when the ESR is elevated.

Polymyalgia rheumatica

Polymyalgia rheumatica (PMR) and osteoarthritis (OA, see below) are common differential diagnoses of RA in the older population. PMR is an inflammatory rheumatic disease that is typically associated with marked myalgias of the shoulder girdle and the hips, and affects individuals over the age of 50.[15] It can sometimes be mistaken for RA if the presentation includes arthritis of the small joints of the hands.[16] PMR arthritis may be distinguished from RA by the fact that it tends to be milder, more limited, often asymmetric, with rapid response of symptoms to moderate doses of glucocorticoids, the often unduly high ESR, and the seronegativity for RF and ACPA.[15] However, some cases ultimately diagnosed as RA may start with polymyalgia-like symptoms.[16]

Osteoarthritis of the hand

OA can be confused with RA in the middle-aged or older patient when the small joints of the hands are involved. However, arthritis in OA is different from RA with respect to the distribution of joint involvement, the clinical type of arthritis, and the structural and serological findings.

OA of the fingers typically affects the distal interphalangeal (DIP) joints causing the so-called Heberden's nodes in this area, as well as the carpometacarpal joint of the thumb—both joint areas are not usually involved in RA, and in fact, are therefore explicitly excluded from the current classification criteria for RA (see following text; also see Chapter 11). Joint swelling is hard and bony in OA, while it is soft in RA. Morning stiffness is typical in both OA and RA, but it is usually transient or lasts no more than a few minutes in OA, while it typically lasts more than 30–60 min in RA.

Structural investigations by conventional radiographs in OA are characterized by joint space narrowing that is asymmetric and accompanied by periarticular osteophytes, while the typical erosions of RA are not seen. OA is classically associated with the absence of RFs and ACPAs, and normal levels of acute phase reactants. However, RFs may be present, usually in low titre, consistent with the generally older age of this patient population.

Critical diagnostic features of rheumatoid arthritis

Joint pattern

Arthritis in RA is usually a polyarthritis of insidious onset,[17] affecting primarily the proximal interphalangeal (PIP), MCP, and wrist joints, as well as the ankles and the metatarsophalangeal (MTP) joints. All other joints can also be affected by RA, with the exception of the DIP joints. A monoarthritic onset of RA is less common, affecting larger joints, and usually evolves to typical polyarthritis that includes the small joints over time. Occasionally, RA may start as palindromic rheumatism, characterized by episodes of joint inflammation affecting one to several joint areas for hours to days, with intermittent periods without symptoms that may last from days to months.[18] Palindromic rheumatism may also develop into other systemic disorders, such as SLE, or resolve over time. Particularly in elderly patients, RA may evolve from an initial polymyalgia-like presentation.[16] Typically, arthritis in RA is accompanied by morning stiffness of at least 30–60 min until maximum improvement.

Serology

RFs occur in 70–80% of patients with RA. Their diagnostic utility is limited by their relatively poor specificity since they are found in

5–10% of healthy individuals, 20–30% of those with SLE, virtually all patients with mixed cryoglobulinaemia (usually caused by hepatitis C virus infections), and many other inflammatory conditions. Higher titres of RF have greater specificity for RA.[19] The prevalence of RF positivity in healthy individuals rises with age. Antibodies to citrullinated peptides/proteins (ACPA) are usually measured by enzyme-linked immunosorbent assays (ELISA) using CCP as antigen. Anti-CCP antibodies have a similar sensitivity and specificity to (particularly high levels of) RF for RA (see Chapter 7), although some argue that they may be more specific,[9,10] which is still a matter of debate. The specificity is greater in patients with higher levels of anti-CCP antibodies.

Acute phase reactants

Elevations of the ESR and/or CRP level are typically seen in inflammatory conditions such as RA. The degree of elevation of these acute phase reactants correlates with the severity of inflammation and the structural damage that will occur over time.[20] Although increased levels of acute phase reactants are not specific for RA, they are often useful for distinguishing inflammatory from non-inflammatory musculoskeletal conditions, such as OA. Therefore, elevation of acute phase reactants was also included in the 2010 classification criteria (see below and Table 2.1). On the other hand, normal acute phase reactants may also occur occasionally in untreated patients with RA.

The 2010 classification criteria for rheumatoid arthritis

The major problem for most inflammatory rheumatic diseases is that there are no diagnostic criteria (see also Chapter 11). All criteria available are classification criteria, and the major difference here is that classification criteria are developed to minimize errors at the group level (e.g. for the purpose of including most homogeneous patient populations in clinical trials of a given disease), while they inherently accept the possibility of misclassification in the individual. On the other hand, the goal of diagnostic criteria is to be correct in the individual most of the time since, as also discussed at the beginning of this chapter, the diagnosis is often linked with more or less harmful therapies. The value of a diagnostic test also depends on the *a priori* suspicion of disease ('pretest probability'). From this, it becomes clear why diagnostic criteria are scarce.

Until 2010, the classification criteria for RA in use were those by the American College of Rheumatology (ACR) dating from 1987 (see also Chapter 2).[21] These criteria have been increasingly debated in the recent past because of their lack of sensitivity in early disease, given that they were derived using mostly patients with long-standing, established RA.[22] The best example is the inclusion of erosions in these criteria as a feature for diagnosis, which over time contradicted clinical practice, which emphasized the importance of preventing structural damage instead of waiting for irreversible stigmata of RA to occur. Before the introduction of the new criteria, many rheumatologists indicated that their treatment decision was independent of fulfilment of the ACR 1987 classification criteria.[23] Rheumatoid nodules are likewise rarely

seen in early disease, and therefore even more weight is put on the remaining six variables, including erosions. In addition, new diagnostic tools, such as testing for ACPA, have emerged in recent years which tends to be at least as sensitive and specific as RF for diagnosis of RA.[10]

A joint working group of the ACR and the European League Against Rheumatism (EULAR) aimed to develop new classification criteria for RA that would replace the 1987 criteria. The work was performed between 2007 and 2010 and included a three-step approach including a data analysis phase using early arthritis cohorts, a consensus science phase, and a refinement phase. These final criteria and the detailed methodology were published in the two journals associated with the ACR and EULAR.[24–27]

As shown in Table 2.1, the 2010 criteria are made up of four domains, including the number and type of the affected joints, serology (RF and ACPA), acute phase reactants (CRP and ESR), and the duration of symptoms. For evaluation of a patient's classification, the highest category within each domain is taken, and the four scores are added together. The maximum possible score is 10, and a score of 6 or more indicates the presence of definitely classifiable RA. The details of how the various categories and domains are defined are given in the footnotes to Table 2.1. Another way to classify RA, based on the same rules, is by the tree algorithm depicted in Figure 2.4.

Inherent to classification criteria is the fact that they do not work in all individuals who can theoretically be tested. It is very important to understand the target population of the new classification criteria, that is, who they were developed to be applied to. As can be seen in the top part of Table 2.1, the target population for the criteria is well defined: the 2010 criteria may be applied to any patient who presents with at least one clinically swollen joint, for which another disease is not the most likely cause. These parameters were introduced to increase the specificity of the new criteria, and to prevent patients with, for example, gout or obvious SLE being tested with the criteria.

With imaging techniques such as MRI or ultrasonography rapidly developing, it is frequently discussed how these methods can be integrated into the new classification criteria. In this regard, it is important to make two distinctions: for the definition of the target population it is essential to have at least one clinically swollen joint. At this stage, the presence of imaging synovitis without clinical synovitis does not render a patient eligible for application of the criteria. In contrast, once clinical synovitis is confirmed, any imaging method may be used to further explore the extent of arthritis, which may increase the points achieved in the 'joint distribution' category.

The other important issue in imaging is the question about the relevance of erosions, and when to perform standard radiographic investigations. In this respect, a major objective of the new criteria was to not to bias against the diagnosis of RA in individuals who are not yet erosive. Structural joint damage is now a major (bad) outcome of RA but not a feature required for classification. Therefore, the scoring system does not give any weight to erosions, and thus does not penalize individuals without structural damage. At the same time there remains the—currently more theoretical—situation of patients with long-standing disease, who have not yet been classified, but may have become less active over

Table 2.1 2010 ACR/EULAR classification criteria for rheumatoid arthritis

- **Target population (Who should be tested?)**
- (1) Patient with *at least one joint* with definite clinical synovitis (swelling)
- Exception: patients with erosive disease typical for RA, or those with a history compatible with prior fulfilment of the 2010 criteria, or those who have previously fulfilled the 2010 criteria, should be directly classified as RA. A detailed algorithm for the use of radiographic evidence of erosions is presented in Figure 2.6.
- (2) Synovitis is **not better explained** by another disease
- In case of any doubt or uncertainty about the presence of an alternative diagnosis, the requirement of this rule is fulfilled.
- **Classification criteria for RA (score-based algorithm: add score of categories A–D)**
- A score of ≥**6/10** is needed for a definite classification of a patient with RA. Although patients with a score <6/10 are not classifiable as RA, their status can be reassessed, and the criteria might be fulfilled cumulatively over time.

(A) Joint involvement[a]

1 large[b] joint	0
2–10 large joints	1
1–3 small[c] joints (with or without involvement of large joints)	2
4–10 small joints (with or without involvement of large joints)	3
>10 joints[d] (at least one small joint)	5

(B) Serology[e] (at least one test result is needed for classification)

Negative RF *AND* negative ACPA	0
Low positive RF *OR* low positive ACPA	2
High positive RF *OR* high positive ACPA	3

(C) Acute phase reactants[f] (at least one test result is needed for classification)

Normal CRP *AND* normal ESR	0
Abnormal CRP *OR* abnormal ESR	1

(D) Duration of symptoms[g]

<6 weeks	0
≥6 weeks	1

ACPA, anticitrullinated protein/peptide antibodies; CRP, C-reactive protein; ESR, erythrocyte sedimentation rate; RF, rheumatoid factor; ULN, upper limit of normal.

[a] Joint involvement refers to any *swollen* or *tender* joint on examination, which may be confirmed by imaging evidence of synovitis. Distal interphalangeal joints (DIPs), 1st carpometacarpal (CMC) joint, and 1st metatarsophalangeal (MTP) joint are *excluded from assessment*. Categories of joint distribution are classified according to the location and number of the involved joints, with placement into the highest category possible based on the pattern of joint involvement.

[b] Large joints refer to shoulders, elbows, hips, knees, and ankles.

[c] Small joints refer to the metacarpophalangeal (MCP) joints, proximal interphalangeal (PIP) joints, metatarsophalangeal (MTP) joints 2–5, thumb interphalangeal (IP) joints, and wrists.

[d] In this category, at least one of the involved joints must be a small joint; the other joints can include any combination of large and additional small joints, as well as other joints not specifically listed elsewhere (e.g. temporomandibular, acromioclavicular, sternoclavicular, and so on).

[e] Negative refers to international unit (IU) values that are ≤ upper limit of normal (ULN) for the lab and assay; low positive refers to IU values that are >ULN but ≤3× ULN for the lab and assay; high positive refers to IU values that are >3× ULN for the lab and assay. Where RF is only available as positive or negative, a positive result should be scored as 'low positive' for RF.

[f] Normal/abnormal is determined by local laboratory standards.

[g] Duration of symptoms refers to patient self-report of the duration of signs or symptoms of synovitis (e.g. pain, swelling, tenderness) of joints that are clinically involved at the time of assessment, regardless of treatment status.

Source: data from Aletaha D et al (2004) 'Attitudes to early rheumatoid arthritis: changing patterns. Results of a survey' *Ann Rheum Dis* 63(10):1269–75 and Aletaha D et al (2010) 'Rheumatoid arthritis classification criteria: an American College of Rheumatology/European League Against Rheumatism collaborative initiative'. *Arthritis Rheum* 62(9):2569–81.

time (sometimes called 'burnt-out' disease). For these patients, an option has been introduced, which allows immediate classification by presence of typical radiographic evidence of RA. Typical erosiveness of RA has recently been defined as erosions in more than three joints.[28] This is shown in **Figure 2.5**.

Therefore, comparing the 2010 classification criteria to those developed in 1987, many aspects have remained while several have changed. The radiographic changes are not weighted into the new scoring system, while patients with long-standing unclassified disease, who do not fit the criteria, can be classified on the basis of their typical joint destruction alone. Rheumatoid nodules have completely disappeared in the new classification system, mainly due to their low prevalence, and thus low diagnostic value, in early disease. The joint distribution remains similar to the 1987 scoring system, as the weight remains on polyarthritis (which at some level inherently

includes symmetric disease) and on small joints. Serological changes were expanded from the mere use of RF to also include ACPA, and to a consideration of the antibody level (negative vs. low positive vs. high positive). Duration was introduced as a separate item in the new system, while it was integrated in the joint activity items of the 1987 criteria, and elevated acute phase response was newly introduced.

Classification vs. diagnosis of rheumatoid arthritis

The distinction between classification and diagnosis is crucial: classification criteria aim to define a homogenous disease group for clinical and epidemiological studies. To this end, they aim at differentiating a specified rheumatic disease from other diseases

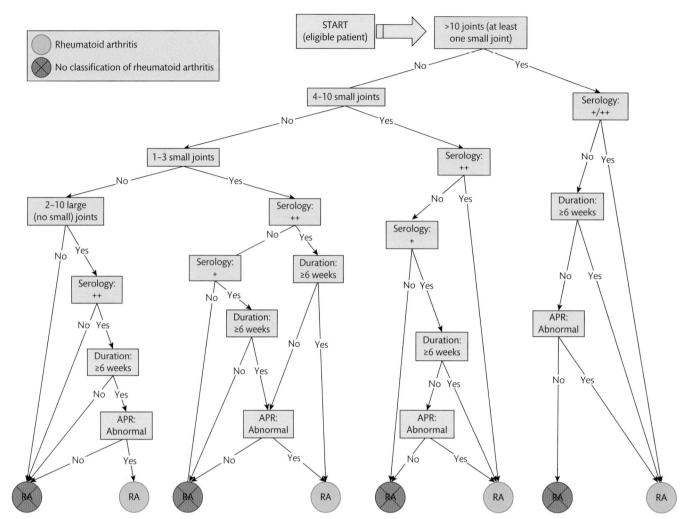

Figure 2.4 Tree algorithm to classify definite rheumatoid arthritis (green circles) or to exclude its current presence (red circles) among those who are eligible to be assessed by the new criteria. For definitions of categories (e.g. serology: +, ++, or joint regions), see footnotes to Table 2.1.

Reprinted from: 2010 rheumatoid arthritis classification criteria: an American College of Rheumatology/European League Against Rheumatism collaborative initiative. Aletaha D, Neogi T, Silman AJ, Funovits J, Felson DT, Bingham CO 3rd et al *Ann Rheum Dis*. 2010 Sep;69(9):1580–8 with permission from the BMJ Publishing Group.

(or healthy individuals). Classification criteria thus aim for a good group categorization (usually characterized by sensitivity, specificity, positive and negative predictive values, and likelihood ratios). In contrast, the clinical diagnosis aims at the correct individual categorization, to minimize misdiagnosis at the individual level.

Inherent in these concepts is the fact that classification and diagnostic criteria will not always categorize individuals into the same group (**Figure 2.6**). This leads to the issue of false-positive and false-negative classification when compared to clinical diagnosis, which is not a deficiency of any classification system, but rather a matter of fact. Since classification criteria will inevitably be applied by clinicians, for diagnostic purposes, it is important to emphasize that a clinician can at any time overrule the classification result using clinical judgement. In other words, clinicians may establish a diagnosis in unclassified patients, as well as decide not to treat classified patients for the lack of a clinical diagnosis (**Figure 2.6**).

A typical scenario for a false-positive classification by the 2010 classification criteria is a patient with osteoarthritis of the hand with one swollen PIP joint. Such a patient would score highly on the joint distribution domain (also tenderness is counted as 'joint activity') and would

likely present with a symptom duration of 6 weeks or more, and hence be classified as having RA. Vice versa, patients seronegative for RF and ACPA are prone to false-negative classification: once zero points are achieved in the serology domain, and given the fact that only one point each may be acquired from the acute phase response and the symptom duration domain, this means that patients need to show a joint distribution in the top category. In other words, this means that seronegative patients need at least 10 active joints for their disease to be classified as RA. Inherent to the label of a 'diagnosis' is the fact that some sort of therapeutic intervention usually ensues.

It is important to mention in this context that the fulfilment of the new criteria can also be achieved cumulatively, that is, through repeated assessments over time, and in case of adequate previous documentation, also retrospectively.

Conclusion

In summary, the correct diagnosis of RA still remains a challenge, and it remains the task of the rheumatologist. Because of the large

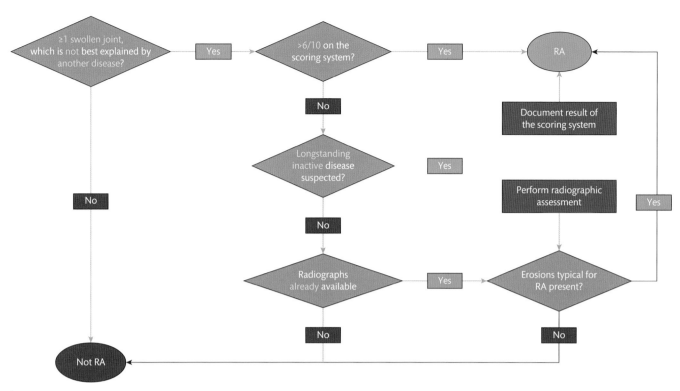

Figure 2.5 The role of radiographic examination in the 2010 ACR/EULAR classification criteria. The figure depicts an algorithm for patients who are not classifiable by the scoring system, but who are either suspected to have long-standing (unclassified) disease (decision node in the middle of the figure) or already present with radiographic damage, which may then not be ignored (decision node at the bottom). In these two instances, information from radiographs may be used and allow a direct classification of RA in case of presence of typical RA erosions. The definition of 'erosiveness typical for RA' has recently been put forward.
From the Slidekit of EULAR and ACR.

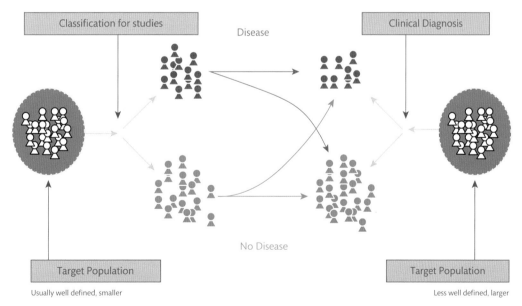

Figure 2.6 Classification vs. diagnosis. The target population for classification is usually smaller and better defined than that for diagnosis, as classification is used for study purposes. Both classification criteria and diagnostic criteria categorize individuals as diseased or not diseased. The figure implies that there might be considerable overlap between these groups. From a clinical perspective a diagnosis can be established and treatment may be initiated, even if the classification result is negative.
From the Slidekit of EULAR and ACR.

number of potential differential diagnoses, and the ability of RA to present in a very heterogeneous way, no criteria can replace the judgement and experience of the rheumatologist in this respect. Nevertheless, classification criteria may help to guide the rheumatologist in this difficult task of establishing a diagnosis, the importance of which still lies in the therapeutic implication for the patient. It is inherent to the concept of classification that it will differ from a clinical diagnosis in a potentially significant portion of individuals. As most current treatment algorithms indicate that treatment should be initiated immediately after the diagnosis of RA,[29] the rheumatologist is charged to lead and accelerate the diagnostic process by using algorithms, criteria, and other tools so as to avoid the most dangerous mistake in treatment of RA—delay.

REFERENCES

1. Kvien TK. Epidemiology and burden of illness of rheumatoid arthritis. *Pharmacoeconomics* 2004;**22**(2 Suppl.):1–12.
2. Nell VP, Machold KP, Eberl G, et al. Benefit of very early referral and very early therapy with disease-modifying anti-rheumatic drugs in patients with early rheumatoid arthritis. *Rheumatology (Oxf)* 2004;**43**(7):906–14.
3. Landewe RB, Boers M, Verhoeven AC, et al. COBRA combination therapy in patients with early rheumatoid arthritis: long-term structural benefits of a brief intervention. *Arthritis Rheum* 2002;**46**(2):347–56.
4. Bijlsma JW. Patient benefit-risk in arthritis—a rheumatologist's perspective. *Rheumatology (Oxf)* 2010;**49**(2):ii11–ii17.
5. Fries JF, Williams CA, Bloch DA. The relative toxicity of nonsteroidal antiinflammatory drugs. *Arthritis Rheum* 1991;**34**(11):1353–60.
6. Fries JF, Williams CA, Ramey D, Bloch DA. The relative toxicity of disease-modifying antirheumatic drugs. *Arthritis Rheum* 1993;**36**(3):297–306.
7. Hazlewood G, Aletaha D, Carmona L, et al. Algorithm for identification of undifferentiated peripheral inflammatory arthritis: a multinational collaboration through the 3e initiative. *J Rheumatol Suppl* 2011;**87**:54–8.
8. Moore TL. Parvovirus-associated arthritis. *Curr Opin Rheumatol* 2000;**12**(4):289–94.
9. Avouac J, Gossec L, Dougados M. Diagnostic and predictive value of anti-cyclic citrullinated protein antibodies in rheumatoid arthritis: a systematic literature review. *Ann Rheum Dis* 2006;**65**(7):845–51.
10. Nishimura K, Sugiyama D, Kogata Y, et al. Meta-analysis: diagnostic accuracy of anti-cyclic citrullinated peptide antibody and rheumatoid factor for rheumatoid arthritis. *Ann Intern Med* 2007;**146**(11):797–808.
11. Rudwaleit M, van der, HD, Landewe R, et al. The assessment of SpondyloArthritis International Society classification criteria for peripheral spondyloarthritis and for spondyloarthritis in general. *Ann Rheum Dis* 2011;**70**(1):25–31.
12. Dougados M, van der Linden, S, Juhlin R, et al. The European Spondylarthropathy Study Group preliminary criteria for the classification of spondylarthropathy. *Arthritis Rheum* 1991;**34**(10):1218–27.
13. Gladman DD, Shuckett R, Russell ML, Thorne JC, Schachter RK. Psoriatic arthritis (PSA)—an analysis of 220 patients. *Q J Med* 1987;**62**(238):127–41.
14. Steere AC, Schoen RT, Taylor E. The clinical evolution of Lyme arthritis. *Ann Intern Med* 1987;**107**(5):725–31.
15. Dasgupta B, Cimmino MA, Maradit-Kremers, H, et al. 2012 provisional classification criteria for polymyalgia rheumatica: a European League Against Rheumatism/American College of Rheumatology collaborative initiative. *Ann Rheum Dis* 2012;**71**(4):484–92.
16. Healey LA. Polymyalgia rheumatica and seronegative rheumatoid arthritis may be the same entity. *J Rheumatol* 1992;**19**(2):270–2.
17. Fleming A, Crown JM, Corbett M. Early rheumatoid disease. I. Onset. *Ann Rheum Dis* 1976;**35**(4):357–60.
18. Maksymowych WP, Suarez-Almazor, ME, Buenviaje H, et al. HLA and cytokine gene polymorphisms in relation to occurrence of palindromic rheumatism and its progression to rheumatoid arthritis. *J Rheumatol* 2002;**29**(11):2319–26.
19. Nell VPK, Machold KP, Eberl G, et al. The diagnostic and prognostic significance of autoantibodies in patients with early arthritis. *Ann Rheum Dis* 2003;**62**(Suppl. 1):OP0015.
20. van Leeuwen, MA, van Rijswijk, MH, van der Heijde, DM, et al. The acute-phase response in relation to radiographic progression in early rheumatoid arthritis: a prospective study during the first three years of the disease. *Br J Rheumatol* 1993;**32**(Suppl. 3):9–13.
21. Arnett FC, Edworthy SM, Bloch DA, et al. The American Rheumatism Association 1987 revised criteria for the classification of rheumatoid arthritis. *Arthritis Rheum* 1988;**31**(3):315–24.
22. Silman AJ, Symmons DP. Selection of study population in the development of rheumatic disease criteria: comment on the article by the American College of Rheumatology Diagnostic and Therapeutic Criteria Committee. *Arthritis Rheum* 1995;**38**(5):722–3.
23. Aletaha D, Eberl G, Nell VP, Machold KP, Smolen JS. Attitudes to early rheumatoid arthritis: changing patterns. Results of a survey. *Ann Rheum Dis* 2004;**63**(10):1269–75.
24. Aletaha D, Neogi T, Silman AJ, et al. 2010 Rheumatoid arthritis classification criteria: an American College of Rheumatology/European League Against Rheumatism collaborative initiative. *Arthritis Rheum* 2010;**62**(9):2569–81.
25. Aletaha D, Neogi T, Silman AJ, et al. 2010 rheumatoid arthritis classification criteria: an American College of Rheumatology/European League Against Rheumatism collaborative initiative. *Ann Rheum Dis* 2010;**69**(9):1580–8.
26. Funovits J, Aletaha D, Bykerk V, et al. The 2010 American College of Rheumatology/European League Against Rheumatism classification criteria for rheumatoid arthritis: methodological report phase I. *Ann Rheum Dis* 2010;**69**(9):1589–95.
27. Neogi T, Aletaha D, Silman AJ, et al. The 2010 American College of Rheumatology/European League Against Rheumatism classification criteria for rheumatoid arthritis: phase 2 methodological report. *Arthritis Rheum* 2010;**62**(9):2582–91.
28. van der Heijde, D, van der Helm-van Mil, AH, Aletaha D, et al. EULAR definition of erosive disease in light of the 2010 ACR/EULAR rheumatoid arthritis classification criteria. *Ann Rheum Dis* 2013;**72**(4):479–81.
29. Smolen JS, Landewe R, Breedveld FC, et al. EULAR recommendations for the management of rheumatoid arthritis with synthetic and biological disease-modifying antirheumatic drugs. *Ann Rheum Dis* 2010;**69**(6):964–75.

3

The descriptive epidemiology of rheumatoid arthritis

James Gwinnutt and Deborah Symmons

Introduction

The occurrence of any disease is described in terms of its incidence, prevalence, duration, and mortality. Incidence is the number of new cases occurring in the population at risk within a given time period (usually one year). Prevalence is the proportion of the population at risk which is affected by the disease at a particular point (point prevalence) or period (period prevalence) in time. Incidence and prevalence are related as follows:

Incidence × Duration = Prevalence.

The duration of disease is affected by both spontaneous resolution and death (from the disease or other cause). It is important that the numerator and the denominator of these estimates should be drawn from the same population—which is generally adults over the age of 16 or 18 years. Although rheumatoid arthritis (RA) may occur before the age of 16, it is rare and is included as a subset of juvenile idiopathic arthritis.

There are two main reasons to be interested in the occurrence, or burden, of disease within a society. The first is to provide information to those developing health policy or providing healthcare resources to that population. The second is that differences in disease occurrence—whether demographic, geographical, or temporal—can provide clues as to the aetiology of the disease.

This chapter focuses on estimates of the incidence, prevalence, and mortality of RA in adults, in particular those published over the past three decades.

Case definition

The case definition of RA used in epidemiological studies has gone a full circle in the last 60 years. Originally case definition was based on expert opinion—generally the diagnosis of a rheumatologist. However, for larger studies, it was impossible for the same rheumatologist to evaluate all possible cases and it became clear that rheumatologists did not always agree. Standardized case definitions—or classification criteria—were therefore developed to enable comparison

between studies. The first formal classification criteria were published in 1956 by a committee of the American Rheumatism Association (ARA). The criteria set comprised 11 items and 19 exclusions.[1] Three categories of RA were defined: 'definite' RA (individuals who met five or more criteria), 'probable' RA (individuals who met three or four criteria) and 'possible' RA (individuals who met another formula also published). In an attempt to improve the specificity and simplicity, the criteria were revised in 1958, adding a further category: 'classical' RA (individuals who fulfilled 7 or more of the 11 criteria).[2]

The 1987 American College of Rheumatology Classification Criteria for RA

The 1958 criteria, and a modification for epidemiological use called the Rome criteria,[3] were used for 30 years. However, during this time the construct of RA changed. Many diseases which were previously included within the RA spectrum were recognized as distinct entities (e.g. the spondyloarthropathies, calcium pyrophosphate deposition disease, polymyalgia rheumatica, and Lyme disease[4]). The distinction between 'definite' and 'classical' was not found useful and the two were usually merged. Furthermore, the long list of exclusions made it almost impossible for patients to have two concurrent inflammatory conditions. Therefore, in 1983, the ARA appointed a committee to update the criteria. This led to the formulation of the 1987 ARA (now renamed the American College of Rheumatology (ACR)) classification criteria for RA, comprised of 7 criteria (Table 3.1).[4] The criteria exist in two formats: a 'list' and a 'tree' format. The classification tree combines the 7 criteria into 8 subsets—5 of which are classified as RA. It also allows substitution for missing items—which should make it particularly useful for epidemiological studies. However, in practice, only the 'list' version was ever used. Individuals had to meet any four of the seven criteria to be classified as having RA. The 1987 classification criteria only recognize one category of RA (thus effectively combining the classical and definite categories) and there are no exclusions. Both the 1958 and the 1987 criteria were developed using the physician opinion as the 'gold standard'.

Table 3.1 The revised 1987 American College of Rheumatology Criteria

Number	Criteria
1	**Morning stiffness** Morning stiffness in and around joints, lasting at least 1 hour before maximal improvement
2	**Arthritis of three or more joint areas** Soft tissue swelling or fluid (not bony overgrowth alone) observed by a physician, present simultaneously for at least 6 weeks. The 14 possible joint areas are right or left PIP, MCP, wrist, elbow, knee, ankle, and MTP joints
3	**Arthritis of hand joints** At least one area swollen (as defined above) in a wrist, MCP, or PIP joint
4	**Symmetrical arthritis** Simultaneous involvement of the same joint areas (as defined in 2) on both sides of the body (bilateral involvement of PIPs, MCPs, or MTPs is acceptable without absolute symmetry) for at least 6 weeks
5	**Rheumatoid nodules** Subcutaneous nodules over bony prominences, or extensor surfaces, or in juxta-articular regions, observed by a physician
6	**Serum rheumatoid factor** Detected by a method positive in <5% of normal controls
7	**Radiographic changes** Radiographic changes typical of RA on postero-anterior hand and wrist radiographs, which must include erosions or unequivocal bony decalcification localized in or most marked adjacent to the involved joints (osteoarthritis changes alone do not qualify)

PIP, proximal interphalangeal joints; MCP, metacarpophalangeal joint; MTP, metatarsophalangeal joint. At least four criteria must be fulfilled for classification as RA.

Reprinted from Arnett et al (1988) The American Rheumatism Association 1987 revised criteria for the classification of rheumatoid arthritis, *Arthritis & Rheumatism* 31(3):315–24 with permission from the American College of Rheumatology.

The 1987 criteria were based on identifying RA cases with active inflammation. An adaptation was proposed by researchers at the Arthritis and Rheumatism Council Epidemiology Research Unit in Manchester, United Kingdom, which facilitated the identification of cases with currently inactive disease.[5]

Although widely used for over 20 years, the 1987 classification criteria were criticised for being poor at identifying patients with early RA. They were developed using 262 RA cases with an average disease duration of over 7 years. Several criteria only become apparent when the disease is more advanced (e.g. criteria 5 and 7). In a meta-analysis carried out in 2009, the pooled sensitivity and specificity of the criteria for early RA (<1 year disease duration) were 77% (95% confidence interval (CI) 68–84) and 77% (95% CI 68–84) respectively, against the gold standard of expert opinion.[6] In addition, as this criteria set has no exclusions, individuals were often classified as having RA when a clinician would have given a different diagnosis.

Observational research increasingly began to show the benefit of early, aggressive therapy,[7–10] yet clinical trials were not able to recruit patients early in their disease because they did not yet satisfy the 1987 criteria.[11] Furthermore, anticitrullinated protein antibody positivity had been discovered as a biomarker with high specificity for RA and was not included in the 1987 criteria.[8,12–14] The limitations of the 1987 system plus advances in the field of rheumatology prompted the development of a third set of criteria.

The 2010 ACR/EULAR classification criteria for RA

This third criteria set was published in 2010 and resulted from a collaboration between the ACR and the European League against Rheumatism (EULAR).[11] On this occasion the 'gold standard' was a physician decision to prescribe methotrexate (MTX) for inflammatory arthritis (i.e. the criteria were developed to select the same patients for whom a clinician would prescribe MTX). There are four groups of criteria with a weighted scoring system (Table 3.2). Individuals who score 6 or more (out of a maximum of 10) are classified as RA cases.

The improved sensitivity of the 2010 criteria, albeit at a loss of some specificity, has been shown in several studies. A study of 2258 patients with early arthritis recruited to the Leiden Early Arthritis cohort found that the sensitivity and specificity of the 1987 criteria were 0.61 and 0.74, respectively; and of the 2010 criteria 0.84 and 0.60 respectively, using initiation of MTX during the first year as the gold standard.[15] A similar study of 313 undiagnosed patients with joint symptoms from Keio University Hospital, Japan, reported that the sensitivity and specificity of the 2010 criteria were 0.73 and 0.71, respectively, and the sensitivity and specificity of the 1987 criteria were 0.47 and 0.93, respectively.[16]

As expected, the 2010 criteria are better than the 1987 criteria at identifying cases of early RA. In a study of patients with early inflammatory arthritis (median symptom duration = 29.6 weeks) recruited in 1990 to the Norfolk Arthritis Register (NOAR),

Table 3.2 2010 ACR/EULAR classification criteria for RA criteria

Number	Criteria	Score
1	**Joint involvement**	
	One medium to large joint	0
	Two to ten medium to large joints	1
	One to three small joints	2
	Four to ten small joints	3
	More than ten joints (with at least one small joint)	5
2	**Serology**	
	Negative RF and negative ACPA	0
	Low positive RF or low positive ACPA	2
	High positive RF or high positive ACPA	3
3	**Acute phase reactants**	
	Normal CRP and normal ESR	0
	Abnormal CRP or abnormal ESR	1
4	**Duration of symptoms**	
	Less than 6 weeks	0
	6 weeks or more	1

ACPA, anticitrullinated protein antibody; CRP, C-reactive protein; ESR, erythrocyte sedimentation rate; RF, rheumatoid factor. Small joints = metacarpophalangeal joints, interphalangeal joints, second through fifth metatarsophalangeal joints, thumb interphalangeal joints, and wrists. Large joints = shoulders, elbows, hips, knees, ankles. **A score of at least 6 must be achieved to be classified as RA.**

Data sourced from Aletaha D, Neogi T, Silman AJ et al. 2010 rheumatoid arthritis classification criteria: an American College of Rheumatology/European League Against Rheumatism collaborative initiative. *Ann Rheum Dis* 2010;69:1580–8.

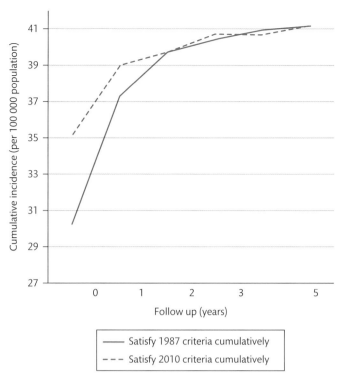

Figure 3.1 Cumulative incidence of RA in patients recruited to the Norfolk Arthritis Register in 1990 (n = 170) measured using both the 1987 and the 2010 classification criteria for RA.

Reprinted from Humphreys JH *et al* (2013) 'The incidence of rheumatoid arthritis in the UK: comparisons using the 2010 ACR/EULAR classification criteria and the 1987 ACR classification criteria. Results from the Norfolk Arthritis Register'. *Ann Rheum Dis* 72)8):1315–20 with permission from the BMJ Publishing Group.

United Kingdom (**Figure 3.1**), the age- and sex-specific IR using the 2010 criteria at baseline were similar to cumulative incidence rates using the 1987 criteria over 5 years.[17] Thus use of the 2010 criteria reduces the need for long-term follow-up to confirm classification.

However, although the 2010 criteria are of proven value in incidence studies, debate continues as to their utility in detecting prevalent cases of RA.[18] Now that the disease is treated early and aggressively, the issue of whether someone can be classified as having RA has become a grey area. Many patients on treatment have no symptoms, signs, or laboratory tests which indicate on-going inflammation. Yet epidemiologists do not want to classify a patient as having RA simply on the basis of a typical history. Ideally there needs to be documented evidence of a prior history of a combination of synovitis in the appropriate pattern of joints, raised inflammatory markers, and rheumatoid-associated autoantibodies. Furthermore, physicians are often reluctant to withdraw treatment even if the disease has resolved completely, in case the disease recurs and cannot be so easily suppressed a second time. It is therefore difficult to know whether the patient has experienced resolution of their RA (i.e. cure) or represents a case of RA in complete remission on treatment (discussed further in Chapter 41). There have been few classical studies of the prevalence of RA in the modern era because of these difficulties. Instead researchers have to focus on measuring cumulative incidence using the assumption that once a person has RA, they will always have RA.

Case definitions used for studies utilizing large healthcare databases

Many recent studies of the occurrence of RA utilize large databases; for example, the database of a national insurance system or a healthcare maintenance organization. These databases often include a physician diagnosis, laboratory results, and treatment details. However, they seldom include patient symptoms or examination findings. Once more 'classification' of RA is reliant on the diagnosis of an individual physician. Wherever possible, when the data are used for research purposes, attempts should be made to validate the physician diagnosis against a recognized criteria set in a representative sample of cases. The diagnosis will be more robust if combined with the prescription of disease-modifying antirheumatic drugs (DMARDs)—which has resonance with the gold standard for the 2010 criteria. When using epidemiological studies based on large healthcare databases, it is important to consider the eligibility criteria for belonging to that healthcare system (e.g. is it based on past occupation or age or ability to afford the cover provided?) and to remember that the data were not collected for research purposes. There may be incentives to label—or not label—an individual as having RA. For example, it may entitle the individual to free or subsidized medication; or it may facilitate or preclude their access to certain medications.

Incidence of RA in adult populations

Alamanos, Voulgari, and Drosos conducted a systematic review of incidence and prevalence studies of RA published prior to 2005 which used the 1987 classification criteria.[19] They identified 11 incidence studies (one of which actually used the 1958 criteria.[20]). We have identified two additional studies; one published from Spain[21] and the other from the United States.[22] Alamanos et al. found no incidence studies from developing countries. The methodology for the studies shown in **Table 3.3** varies substantially. Some studies are retrospective—for example, based on analysing medical records or using data from insurance systems. Others are prospective—for example, cases are identified as they present to primary or secondary care. In order to calculate incidence rates, it is essential to understand the age-sex structure of the population from which the cases are drawn and to be confident that all possible cases have been identified.

Most incidence studies using the 1987 classification criteria for RA were conducted in Northern Europe (**Table 3.3**). These studies are primarily retrospective. A study from Finland, which used the national Sickness Insurance Scheme database to identify cases of RA (supplemented with information from hospital records where necessary), estimated the annual incidence rate of RA in 1995 to be 32 per 100 000 adult population.[28] Data on the general population came from Statistics Finland. A study from France identified cases using a combination of in-patient and out-patient case-note review for the hospital rheumatology departments, private rheumatologists, and GPs; and by regional media announcements. Population data came from the national census. From these varied sources, an incidence estimate of 9 per 100 000 adults per year was calculated.[23] It seems likely that many cases may have been missed by this methodology since the estimates are substantially lower than those from other studies.

Table 3.3 Incidence estimates of RA using the 1987 RA criteria[19]

Study	Country	Annual incidence estimate (cases/100 000 adult population)		
		Total	Men	Women
Northern Europe				
Guillemin, 1994[23]	France	9	5	12
Symmons, 1994[24]	England	20	14	36
Uhlig, 1998[25]	Norway	26	14	37
Riise, 2000[26]	Norway	29	21	36
Kaipiainen-Seppänen, 2000[27]	Finland	-	24	36
Kaipiainen-Seppänen, 2001[28]	Finland	32	22	40
Soderlin, 2002[29]	Sweden	24	18	29
Savolainen, 2003[30]	Finland	36	25	46
Southern Europe				
Drosos, 1997[31]	Greece	24	12	36
Carbonell, 2008[21]	Spain	8	5	11
USA				
Doran, 2002[32]	USA	45	30	58
Myasoedova, 2010[22]	USA	41	28	53

Three of the Northern European studies used a prospective study design.[24,29,30] The NOAR aimed to identify all incident cases of inflammatory polyarthritis (which includes the subset RA) presenting to primary care in the former Norwich Health Authority Region, Norfolk, United Kingdom. Patients with two or more swollen joints for four or more weeks were referred to the research team by primary care physicians or rheumatologists. The research team then applied the 1987 criteria. Data on the population structure came from the Norfolk Family Health Services Authority. This study estimated an annual incidence of 20 cases per 100 000 adult population per year (men = 14, women = 36). The peak age of onset in the NOAR was 55–64 years for women and 65–74 for men. In the oldest age group (75+) the age specific incidence was actually higher in men (57 per 100 000) than in women (30 per 100 000).[24] In another Finnish study, based in the city of Kuopio, Savolainen et al. recruited all physicians in the local health centres, occupational health clinics, private clinics and various departments of the University Hospital and asked these centres to refer adult residents of Kuopio who had developed incident arthritis without a prior history of arthritis. The research team then applied the 1987 criteria. Population data were provided by Statistics Finland. This study estimated the annual incidence of RA, defined by the 1987 RA criteria, to be 36 per 100 000 of the adult population (men = 25, women = 46).[30]

Overall it has been suggested that the incidence of RA is lower in Southern than in Northern Europe.[19] A study conducted in Ioannina, Greece in 1995 and based on the review of hospital records reported an overall incidence of 24/100 000.[31] A study from Spain identified all patients aged over 16 seen in early arthritis units within 6 months of symptom onset. The case definition included fulfilling the 1987 ACR classification criteria within the first 6 months of follow-up.[21] Information on the denominator population was provided by the primary care practices feeding into the participating early arthritis units.

In the United States the incidence of RA has been tracked since 1955 via the Rochester Epidemiology Project based in Olmsted County, Minnesota. Doran et al. estimated the overall age and sex-adjusted annual incidence rate over four decades (1955–1995) to be 45/100 000 (women = 56; men = 30). The peak age of onset in women was 55–64 years and in men was 75–84 years. The ratio of women:men was 4:1 in the 35–44 year age group and 1.1:1 in the 75–84 year group.[32] A subsequent study, also from Olmsted County, estimated the overall age and sex-adjusted annual incidence rate for 1995–2007 as 41/100 000 (women = 53; men = 28).[22] In this time period, the peak age of onset was 65–74 years in both men and women.

Fewer studies have used the 2010 RA criteria to estimate the incidence of RA. A study from Norfolk, United Kingdom, estimated the annual incidence of RA using both the 2010 ACR/EULAR RA criteria and the 1987 ACR criteria on the same data set collected in 1990.[17] Using the 2010 criteria, 5-year cumulative incidence was estimated by taking the highest score for each parameter at any assessment over the 5 years (see Figure 3.1). For the 1987 criteria, 5-year cumulative incidence was estimated by carrying forward positive scores for a particular criterion to all future assessment. The overall age- and sex-adjusted incidence rate at baseline was 40/100 000 (women = 54; men = 25). As can be seen from Figure 3.1 the cumulative incidence using both data sets was almost identical (48/100 000 for the 2010 criteria; 44/100 000 for the 1987 criteria).[17]

A recent study from Argentina used data from a health maintenance organization that provides healthcare to 140 000 members.[33] They estimated the incidence of RA as 19 per 100 000 overall (women = 25; men = 9) for the period 2000–2015.

Time trends in incidence of RA

Doran et al. concluded that the incidence rate of RA had fallen progressively in the United States (1955–1965 = 61/100 000, 1985–1995 = 33/100 000).[32] The decline was substantially greater in women than in men—but the number of incident cases in men was small. One possible explanation is a birth cohort effect (i.e. that successive generations were successively less likely to develop RA).[34] A strong birth cohort effect has also been reported in the Pima people, a group of Native Americans living in Arizona, United States with a high prevalence of RA, in which those born in the 1880s and 1890s were more likely to be positive for rheumatoid factor (RF).[35] However, more recent research conducted in 1995–2007 in Rochester, Minnesota found a moderate rise in RA incidence to 41/100 000.[22] The increase was seen in women but not in men. These changes are likely to be attributable to changes in environmental exposures linked to the development of RA.

Kaipiainen-Seppänen and Aho reported incidence estimates for 3 years in Finland; 1980, 1985, and 1990. The incidence rate was 15% lower in 1990 compared with previous years. This fall was particularly apparent in the RF negative subgroup.[27] A small study from Japan, based on only 16 incident cases in a population of around 3000 and using the Rome criteria, found that the age-adjusted incidence rates fell from 39 per 100 000 in 1965–1975, to 24 per 100 000 in 1975–1985, and 8 per 100 000 in 1985–1996.[36]

Prevalence of RA in adult populations

RA is believed to have first been described in North America, with evidence of its existence dating back to before European settlement. To this day the highest reported prevalence is in the Native American Pima people. They have a reported prevalence of RA of 2.15% (95% CI 1.64–2.65) using the 1987 criteria.[37] The Yakima and Chippewa Native Americans also have a high prevalence of RA, but not the Blackfoot and Haida. The first reported cases of RA in Europe only date to the seventeenth century.[38] This suggests that the disease may be triggered either by an unknown infectious agent or by an environmental agent brought from the New World to the Old. Evidence of RA in Africa and Asia is more recent still. The first reported case in Africa was described in 1956.[39]

Table 3.4 lists the results of a number of prevalence studies conducted in recent times using the 1987 ACR criteria as case definition (see Table 3.4). It is challenging to compare prevalence studies directly—particularly if they do not present age- and sex-specific results. The crude overall prevalence inevitably reflects the underlying population structure. The crude prevalence will be much lower in countries with a low life expectancy than in those with a high life

Table 3.4 Prevalence estimates of RA using the 1987 RA criteria[19]

Study	Country	Prevalence estimate (% of adult population)			Population age (yrs)
		Total	Men	Women	
Northern Europe					
Hakala, 1993[40]	Finland	0.8*	0.6	1.0	≥ 16
Kvien, 1997[41]	Norway	0.4*	0.2	0.7	20–79
Power, 1999[42]	Ireland	0.5*	-	-	
Saraux, 1999[43]	France	0.5	0.2	0.8	≥ 18
Simonsson, 1999[44]	Sweden	0.5*	-	-	20–74
Riise, 2000[26]	Norway	0.4*	0.3	0.6	≥ 20
Symmons, 2002[45]	England	0.9*	0.4	1.1	≥ 16
Guillemin, 2005[46]	France	0.3	0.1	0.5	≥ 18
Southern Europe					
Drosos, 1997[31]	Greece	0.4	0.2	0.5	≥ 16
Stojanovic, 1998[47]	Yugoslavia	0.2*	0.1	0.3	≥ 20
Cimmino, 1998[48]	Italy	0.3	0.1	0.5	≥ 16
Carmona, 2002[49]	Spain	0.5*	0.2	0.8	≥ 20
Andrianakos, 2003[50]	Greece	0.7*	-	-	≥ 19
Akar, 2004[51]	Turkey	0.4*	0.2	0.8	≥ 20
Asia					
Pountain, 1991[52]	Oman	0.4*	-	-	≥ 16
Lau, 1993[53]	Hong Kong	0.4*	-	-	≥ 16
Malaviya, 1993[54]	India	0.8*	-	-	≥ 16
Dai, 2003[55]	China	0.3	0.1	0.4	≥ 16
Americas					
Gabriel, 1999[56]	USA	1.1	0.7	1.4	≥ 35
Spindler, 2002[57]	Argentina	0.2*	0.1	0.3	≥ 16
Myasodoeva, 2010[22]	USA	0.7	0.4	1.0	≥ 18

*Crude prevalence.

expectancy, even if the age- and sex-specific rates are exactly the same. This is because the prevalence of RA increases with age. For the same reasons the crude prevalence of RA (and thus the total number of cases) can be expected to rise as life expectancy increases in an individual country.

Prevalence estimates using the 1987 ACR criteria

Reported prevalence estimates in Northern Europe using the 1987 criteria range from 0.4% to 0.8%. Alamanos et al. calculated a summary prevalence estimate of 0.50% for the eight studies from Northern Europe included in their systematic review.[19] Much of the variability is probably related to study setting. A study carried out in secondary care in Tromsø, Norway, yielded a prevalence estimate of 0.4%.[26] This study was based on hospital chart review and thus assumed that all cases of RA in the community were under long-term follow-up in the rheumatology department. A population-based study conducted in 2002 in Norfolk, United Kingdom, yielded a prevalence estimate of 0.85% of the adult population. This study was based on a postal questionnaire followed by an examination of positive respondents.[45] Analysis from Olmsted County, Rochester, Minnesota suggests a prevalence of 1.1% in North Americans of European descent. The lifetime risk of RA in this population has been estimated as 3.6% for women and 1.7% for men.[58]

The prevalence of RA appears to be lower in Southern than in Northern Europe. Alamanos et al. estimated a summary prevalence of 0.35% for Southern Europe (i.e. 30% lower than in Northern Europe) in a systematic review of studies conducted prior to 2005.[19] Many of the prevalence estimates from these studies came from sampling the general population,[47–50] although a study from Greece used hospital chart review.[31] The differences in prevalence between Northern and Southern Europe could be due to differences in genetics and/or in environmental and lifestyle factors, with some studies suggesting a protective effect of the Mediterranean diet.[59–63]

There are relatively few studies from elsewhere in the world using the 1987 criteria. Generally speaking, studies from developing countries have yielded lower prevalences (around 0.2–0.4%) which may partly be attributed to lower life expectancy. A study, based on a house-to-house survey in five villages from a rural part of Northern India found a prevalence of 0.75%.[54] The peak prevalence was at age 25–29 years—much lower than in European and North American populations.

The Global Burden of Disease Study

The Global Burden of Disease (GBD) study 2000, and its update in 2010, has prompted the identification and review of studies of the prevalence of RA from around the world. The GBD study aimed to describe the mortality and morbidity from 291 major diseases, injuries, and risk factors at global, national, and regional levels. By examining trends from 1990 to 2010; and by making comparisons across populations; the GBD study facilitated understanding of the changing health challenges facing people across the world in the twenty-first century.[64] RA was one of the 291 diseases studied. The study covered 187 countries which were grouped into 21 regions

on the basis of geography and income. The musculoskeletal component of the GBD study needed a series of systematic reviews on the prevalence of each included condition. The systematic reviews aimed to identify studies in all languages and included one database which focuses on publications from Latin America, one which focuses on studies from India, and another which focuses on studies from China. A Bayesian meta-regression method was used to pool available data and to predict prevalence values for regions with no or scarce data.[65] Although the 1987 ACR classification criteria were considered the optimum case definition, the RA systematic review also included studies in which RA was diagnosed by a medical practitioner in order to maximize the number of available studies.[66] The search yielded 56 published studies from 40 countries and from 16 of the 21 regions. There were no prevalence data available from Central Asia; Australasia; Latin America, Andean; sub-Saharan Africa, Central; or sub-Saharan Africa, East. Estimates for these regions were calculated using a meta-regression tool developed by the GBD 2010 study. Table 3.5 shows the estimated prevalence of RA by region and sex.

The highest estimated prevalences are for the high-income countries of Australasia, North America, North Africa, and Western Europe and the lowest prevalences for sub-Saharan Africa, Oceania, South and East Asia, North Africa, and the Middle East. These prevalence figures are lower than those reported by individual studies because of the width of the relevant age group of the GBD project: 5–100 years.

A separate GBD publication focused on RA prevalence studies from Africa.[67] Historically, RA in Africa has been seen as a rare disease with a mild onset compared to Europe and North America.[68] Most of the evidence for this low prevalence and mild course came from studies conducted between the 1950s and 1980s.[68,69] The GBD project identified ten population-based studies, six of which were conducted in South Africa. Only two were published since 1990—and one of these was small and identified no cases.[70] Taken together these studies suggest that prevalence of RA increases with age, but that the prevalence is approximately equal in men and women in Africa.[67]

Prevalence studies using large healthcare databases

More recent studies of the prevalence of RA in Europe and North America have moved away from using population surveys, favouring the use of routinely collected medical data. In this situation the case definition is generally based on a combination of physician diagnosis and DMARD prescription. A study using hospitalization and billing data from Quebec estimated an RA prevalence of 1.0% in adults, with no adjustment for error in case definition derived from hospital and billing codes. Adjusting for the imperfect sensitivity and specificity of the case definition gave a prevalence estimate of 0.5%. Again, the estimated prevalence of RA in females (0.6%) was higher than that in males (0.4%).[71] A study using the Swedish national patient register and utilizing a case definition based around clinical diagnosis yielded a prevalence estimate of 0.8% (women = 1.1%, men = 0.4%).[72] Another Swedish study reported similar results, estimating a prevalence of RA of 0.7% (women = 0.9%, men = 0.4%) of adults using the Skåne Health Care Register, a register of every healthcare consultation in the region.[73]

Table 3.5 Global Burden of Disease Study 2010 estimates of the age-standardized prevalence of RA in the age group 5–100 years

Region	Sex	Prevalence (%)	Lower confidence limit (%)	Upper confidence limit (%)
Global	Male	0.13	0.12	0.13
	Female	0.35	0.34	0.37
Asia, central	Male	0.16	0.12	0.21
	Female	0.39	0.30	0.53
Asia, east	Male	0.08	0.08	0.09
	Female	0.24	0.22	0.27
Asia Pacific, high income	Male	0.22	0.18	0.26
	Female	0.57	0.48	0.69
Asia, south	Male	0.08	0.07	0.09
	Female	0.26	0.24	0.29
Asia, southeast	Male	0.08	0.07	0.09
	Female	0.23	0.21	0.26
Australasia	Male	0.26	0.15	0.46
	Female	0.66	0.37	1.11
Caribbean	Male	0.15	0.12	0.28
	Female	0.39	0.32	0.49
Europe, central	Male	0.15	0.12	0.18
	Female	0.41	0.31	0.52
Europe, eastern	Male	0.14	0.08	0.22
	Female	0.38	0.24	0.57
Europe, western	Male	0.24	0.21	0.28
	Female	0.63	0.55	0.75
Latin America, Andean	Male	0.15	0.10	0.22
	Female	0.39	0.25	0.59
Latin America, central	Male	0.14	0.12	0.17
	Female	0.40	0.34	0.49
Latin America, southern	Male	0.20	0.13	0.30
	Female	0.51	0.33	0.78
Latin America, tropical	Male	0.14	0.13	0.15
	Female	0.38	0.35	0.41
North Africa, Middle East	Male	0.09	0.08	0.11
	Female	0.24	0.20	0.28
North Africa, high income	Male	0.24	0.22	0.27
	Female	0.63	0.58	0.70
North America, high income	Male	0.24	0.22	0.27
	Female	0.63	0.58	0.70
Oceania	Male	0.09	0.05	0.14
	Female	0.25	0.15	0.41
Sub-Saharan Africa, central	Male	0.12	0.07	0.18
	Female	0.30	0.19	0.47
Sub-Saharan Africa, east	Male	0.11	0.08	0.14
	Female	0.29	0.23	0.37
Sub-Saharan Africa, south	Male	0.10	0.09	0.12
	Female	0.30	0.26	0.34
Sub-Saharan Africa, west	Male	0.10	0.09	0.12
	Female	0.28	0.25	0.32

Data sourced from Cross M, Smith E, Hoy D et al. 'The global burden of rheumatoid arthritis: estimates from the Global Burden of Disease 2010 study' *Ann Rheum Dis* 2014;73:1316–22.

In conclusion there is general consensus that the prevalence of RA lies between 0.5–1.0% of the adult population in Northern Europe and North America, with somewhat lower estimates from studies carried out in Southern Europe and the developing world. These differences could stem from differences in exposure to risk/protective factors between different parts of the world, different patterns in the way people access healthcare or genetic differences. The prevalence and incidence of RA is higher in women compared to men across all geographical areas, except Africa.

Mortality in patients with RA

Patients with RA are at increased risk of early mortality compared to the general population. A meta-analysis of studies published between 1966 and 2009 reported a meta-standardized mortality ratio (SMR) of 1.47 (i.e. patients with RA have a 47% increased risk of dying during a particular follow-up period compared to an age- and sex-matched sample of the general population).[74] The most recent included study was published in 1995. No decrease in SMR was seen over time—although seven of the eight included studies were started between 1980 and 1989. However, a decreasing incident mortality rate of 2.3% per year was observed, suggesting that the mortality rate in RA is falling in parallel with the falling mortality rate in the general population.

An analysis of NOAR patients recruited over the past 20 years and each followed for 7 years reported increased mortality in patients who met the 2010 EULAR/ACR RA criteria compared to the general population of Norfolk (SMR 1.22). After taking into account changes in the background rates of mortality there did not appear to be any changes in RA mortality between 1990 and 2004 (1995–1999 vs. 1990–1994: mortality rate ratio (MMR) 1.02; 2000–2004 vs. 1990–1994: MMR 1.07).[75] An analysis from Rochester, Minnesota of 822 patients with RA who had their first diagnosis between 1995 and 2000 and were followed longitudinally for a median of 11.7 years reported that RA patients had a mortality rate of 2.4 and 2.5 per 100 person-years for women and men, respectively. The mortality rate in the (age- and sex-matched) general population was 0.2 per 100 person-years in 2000 for women and 0.3 per 100 person-years for men.[76]

Most deaths in patients with RA are not attributed to the disease. Indeed a recent study found that RA was mentioned on the death certificates of only 17.7% of those in the cohort who died.[77] A study of 1429 patients with early RA from the United Kingdom, with a median follow-up of 9.1 years, reported that 31% of the excess mortality was due to cardiovascular disease, 4% due to pulmonary fibrosis and 2.3% due to lymphoma.[78] Coronary heart disease accounted for a quarter of deaths within this study. Cause specific mortality in RA is further covered in the chapter on comorbidities (Chapter 14).

Conclusion

In conclusion, the incidence and prevalence of RA varies approximately fourfold from the highest in some Native American groups to the lowest in some low- and middle-income countries in Africa, South and East Asia, and the Middle East. This may be due to genetic differences between populations or to varying environmental exposures. Since the 1950s, there is evidence first of a decline in incidence and then, in this century, a rise within the same US

population—which must be due to environmental factors. The mortality experience of patients with RA remains elevated compared to the general population—although there are few studies which have included large populations with an onset of disease in the era of early aggressive therapy and availability of biologics.

REFERENCES

1. Ropes MW, Bennett GA, Cobb S, et al. Proposed diagnostic criteria for rheumatoid arthritis; report of a study conducted by a committee of the American Rheumatism Association. *J Chronic Dis* 1957;5:630–5.
2. Ropes MW, Bennett GA, Cobb S, et al. 1958 revision of diagnostic criteria for rheumatoid arthritis. *Bull Rheum Dis* 1958;9:175–6.
3. Kellgren JH. Diagnostic criteria for population studies. *Bull Rheum Dis* 1962;13:291–2.
4. Arnett FC, Edworthy SM, Bloch DA, et al. The American Rheumatism Association 1987 revised criteria for the classification of rheumatoid arthritis. *Arthritis Rheum* 1988;31:315–24.
5. Macgregor AJ, Bamber S, Silman AJ. A comparison of the performance of different methods of disease classification for rheumatoid arthritis. Results of an analysis from a nationwide twin study. *J Rheumatol* 1994;21:1420–6.
6. Banal F, Dougados M, Combescure C, et al. Sensitivity and specificity of the American College of Rheumatology 1987 criteria for the diagnosis of rheumatoid arthritis according to disease duration: a systematic literature review and meta-analysis. *Ann Rheum Dis* 2009;68:1184–91.
7. Bukhari MA, Wiles NJ, Lunt M, et al. Influence of disease-modifying therapy on radiographic outcome in inflammatory polyarthritis at five years: results from a large observational inception study. *Arthritis Rheum* 2003;48:46–53.
8. Sokolove J, Strand V. Rheumatoid arthritis classification criteria—it's finally time to move on! *Bull NYU Hosp Jt Dis* 2010;68:232–8.
9. van der Heide A, Jacobs JW, Bijlsma JW, et al. The effectiveness of early treatment with 'second-line' antirheumatic drugs. A randomized, controlled trial. *Ann Intern Med* 1996;124:699–707.
10. van Dongen H, van Aken J, Lard LR, et al. Efficacy of methotrexate treatment in patients with probable rheumatoid arthritis: a double-blind, randomized, placebo-controlled trial. *Arthritis Rheum* 2007;56:1424–32.
11. Aletaha D, Neogi T, Silman AJ, et al. 2010 rheumatoid arthritis classification criteria: an American College of Rheumatology/European League Against Rheumatism collaborative initiative. *Ann Rheum Dis* 2010;69:1580–8.
12. Schellekens GA, Visser H, de Jong BA, et al. The diagnostic properties of rheumatoid arthritis antibodies recognizing a cyclic citrullinated peptide. *Arthritis Rheum* 2000;43:155–63.
13. Nishimura K, Sugiyama D, Kogata Y, et al. Meta-analysis: diagnostic accuracy of anti-cyclic citrullinated peptide antibody and rheumatoid factor for rheumatoid arthritis. *Ann Intern Med* 2007;146:797–808.
14. Kay J, Upchurch KS. ACR/EULAR 2010 rheumatoid arthritis classification criteria. *Rheumatology (Oxford)* 2012;51 **Suppl 6**:vi5–vi9.
15. van der Linden MP, Knevel R, Huizinga TW, et al. Classification of rheumatoid arthritis: comparison of the 1987 American

College of Rheumatology criteria and the 2010 American College of Rheumatology/European League Against Rheumatism criteria. *Arthritis Rheum* 2011;*63*:37–42.

16. Kaneko Y, Kuwana M, Kameda H, et al. Sensitivity and specificity of 2010 rheumatoid arthritis classification criteria. *Rheumatology (Oxford)* 2011;*50*:1268–74.

17. Humphreys JH, Verstappen SM, Hyrich KL, et al. The incidence of rheumatoid arthritis in the UK: comparisons using the 2010 ACR/EULAR classification criteria and the 1987 ACR classification criteria. Results from the Norfolk Arthritis Register. *Ann Rheum Dis* 2013;*72*:1315–20.

18. Humphreys JH, Verstappen SM, Scire CA, et al. How do we classify rheumatoid arthritis in established disease—can we apply the 2010 American College of Rheumatology/European League Against Rheumatism classification criteria? *J Rheumatol* 2014;*41*:2347–51.

19. Alamanos Y, Voulgari PV, Drosos AA. Incidence and prevalence of rheumatoid arthritis, based on the 1987 American College of Rheumatology criteria: a systematic review. *Semin Arthritis Rheum* 2006;*36*:182–8.

20. Chan KW, Felson DT, Yood RA, et al. Incidence of rheumatoid arthritis in central Massachusetts. *Arthritis Rheum* 1993;*36*:1691–6.

21. Carbonell J, Cobo T, Balsa A, et al. The incidence of rheumatoid arthritis in Spain: results from a nationwide primary care registry. *Rheumatology (Oxford)* 2008;*47*:1088–92.

22. Myasoedova E, Crowson CS, Kremers HM, et al. Is the incidence of rheumatoid arthritis rising?: results from Olmsted County, Minnesota, 1955–2007. *Arthritis Rheum* 2010;*62*:1576–82.

23. Guillemin F, Briancon S, Klein JM, et al. Low incidence of rheumatoid arthritis in France. *Scand J Rheumatol* 1994;*23*:264–8.

24. Symmons DP, Barrett EM, Bankhead CR, et al. The incidence of rheumatoid arthritis in the United Kingdom: results from the Norfolk Arthritis Register. *Br J Rheumatol* 1994;*33*:735–9.

25. Uhlig T, Kvien TK, Glennas A, et al. The incidence and severity of rheumatoid arthritis, results from a county register in Oslo, Norway. *J Rheumatol* 1998;*25*:1078–84.

26. Riise T, Jacobsen BK, Gran JT. Incidence and prevalence of rheumatoid arthritis in the county of Troms, northern Norway. *J Rheumatol* 2000;*27*:1386–9.

27. Kaipiainen-Seppänen O, Aho K. Incidence of chronic inflammatory joint diseases in Finland in 1995. *J Rheumatol* 2000;*27*:94–100.

28. Kaipiainen-Seppänen O, Aho K, Nikkarinen M. Regional differences in the incidence of rheumatoid arthritis in Finland in 1995. *Ann Rheum Dis* 2001;*60*:128–32.

29. Soderlin MK, Borjesson O, Kautiainen H, et al. Annual incidence of inflammatory joint diseases in a population-based study in southern Sweden. *Ann Rheum Dis* 2002;*61*:911–15.

30. Savolainen E, Kaipiainen-Seppänen O, Kroger L, et al. Total incidence and distribution of inflammatory joint diseases in a defined population: results from the Kuopio 2000 arthritis survey. *J Rheumatol* 2003;*30*:2460–8.

31. Drosos AA, Alamanos I, Voulgari PV, et al. Epidemiology of adult rheumatoid arthritis in northwest Greece 1987–1995. *J Rheumatol* 1997;*24*:2129–33.

32. Doran MF, Pond GR, Crowson CS, et al. Trends in incidence and mortality in rheumatoid arthritis in Rochester, Minnesota, over a forty-year period. *Arthritis Rheum* 2002;*46*:625–31.

33. Di WT, Vergara F, Bertiller E, et al. Incidence and prevalence of rheumatoid arthritis in a health management organization in Argentina: a 15-year study. *J Rheumatol* 2016;*43*:1306–11.

34. Silman AJ. The changing face of rheumatoid arthritis: why the decline in incidence? *Arthritis Rheum* 2002;*46*:579–81.

35. Enzer I, Dunn G, Jacobsson L, et al. An epidemiologic study of trends in prevalence of rheumatoid factor seropositivity in Pima Indians: evidence of a decline due to both secular and birth-cohort influences. *Arthritis Rheum* 2002;*46*:1729–34.

36. Shichikawa K, Inoue K, Hirota S, et al. Changes in the incidence and prevalence of rheumatoid arthritis in Kamitonda, Wakayama, Japan, 1965–1996. *Ann Rheum Dis* 1999;*58*:751–6.

37. Hirsch R, Lin JP, Scott WW Jr, et al. Rheumatoid arthritis in the Pima Indians: the intersection of epidemiologic, demographic, and genealogic data. *Arthritis Rheum* 1998;*41*:1464–9.

38. Abdel-Nasser AM, Rasker JJ, Valkenburg HA. Epidemiological and clinical aspects relating to the variability of rheumatoid arthritis. *Semin Arthritis Rheum* 1997;*27*:123–40.

39. Goodall J. Joint swelling in Africans. A review of 90 cases. *Cent Afr J Med* 1956;*2*:220–3.

40. Hakala M, Pollanen R, Nieminen P. The ARA 1987 revised criteria select patients with clinical rheumatoid arthritis from a population-based cohort of subjects with chronic rheumatic diseases registered for drug reimbursement. *J Rheumatol* 1993;*20*:1674–8.

41. Kvien TK, Glennas A, Knudsrod OG, et al. The prevalence and severity of rheumatoid arthritis in Oslo. Results from a county register and a population survey. *Scand J Rheumatol* 1997;*26*:412–18.

42. Power D, Codd M, Ivers L, et al. Prevalence of rheumatoid arthritis in Dublin, Ireland: a population-based survey. *Ir J Med Sci* 1999;*168*:197–200.

43. Saraux A, Guedes C, Allain J, et al. Prevalence of rheumatoid arthritis and spondyloarthropathy in Brittany, France. Societe de Rhumatologie de l'Ouest. *J Rheumatol* 1999;*26*:2622–7.

44. Simonsson M, Bergman S, Jacobsson LT, et al. The prevalence of rheumatoid arthritis in Sweden. *Scand J Rheumatol* 1999;*28*:340–3.

45. Symmons D, Turner G, Webb R, et al. The prevalence of rheumatoid arthritis in the United Kingdom: new estimates for a new century. *Rheumatology (Oxford)* 2002;*41*:793–800.

46. Guillemin F, Saraux A, Guggenbuhl P, et al. Prevalence of rheumatoid arthritis in France: 2001. *Ann Rheum Dis* 2005;*64*:1427–30.

47. Stojanovic R, Vlajinac H, Palic-Obradovic D, et al. Prevalence of rheumatoid arthritis in Belgrade, Yugoslavia. *Br J Rheumatol* 1998;*37*:729–32.

48. Cimmino MA, Parisi M, Moggiana G, et al. Prevalence of rheumatoid arthritis in Italy: the Chiavari Study. *Ann Rheum Dis* 1998;*57*:315–18.

49. Carmona L, Villaverde V, Hernandez-Garcia C, et al. The prevalence of rheumatoid arthritis in the general population of Spain. *Rheumatology (Oxford)* 2002;*41*:88–95.

50. Andrianakos A, Trontzas P, Christoyannis F, et al. Prevalence of rheumatic diseases in Greece: a cross-sectional population-based epidemiological study. The ESORDIG Study. *J Rheumatol* 2003;*30*:1589–601.

51. Akar S, Birlik M, Gurler O, et al. The prevalence of rheumatoid arthritis in an urban population of Izmir-Turkey. *Clin Exp Rheumatol* 2004;*22*:416–20.

52. Pountain G. The prevalence of rheumatoid arthritis in the Sultanate of Oman. *Br J Rheumatol* 1991;*30*:24–8.

53. Lau E, Symmons D, Bankhead C, et al. Low prevalence of rheumatoid arthritis in the urbanized Chinese of Hong Kong. *J Rheumatol* 1993;*20*:1133–7.

54. Malaviya AN, Kapoor SK, Singh RR, et al. Prevalence of rheumatoid arthritis in the adult Indian population. *Rheumatol Int* 1993;*13*:131–4.

55. Dai SM, Han XH, Zhao DB, et al. Prevalence of rheumatic symptoms, rheumatoid arthritis, ankylosing spondylitis, and gout in Shanghai, China: a COPCORD study. *J Rheumatol* 2003;*30*:2245–51.

56. Gabriel SE, Crowson CS, O'Fallon WM. The epidemiology of rheumatoid arthritis in Rochester, Minnesota, 1955–1985. *Arthritis Rheum* 1999;*42*:415–20.

57. Spindler A, Bellomio V, Berman A, et al. Prevalence of rheumatoid arthritis in Tucuman, Argentina. *J Rheumatol* 2002;*29*:1166–70.

58. Crowson CS, Matteson EL, Myasoedova E, et al. The lifetime risk of adult-onset rheumatoid arthritis and other inflammatory autoimmune rheumatic diseases. *Arthritis Rheum* 2011;*63*:633–9.

59. Alamanos Y, Paraskevi V, Voulgari PV, et al. Rheumatoid arthritis in Southern Europe: epidemiological, clinical, radiological and genetic considerations. *Curr Rheumatol Rev* 2005;*1*:33–6.

60. Skoldstam L, Hagfors L, Johansson G. An experimental study of a Mediterranean diet intervention for patients with rheumatoid arthritis. *Ann Rheum Dis* 2003;*62*:208–14.

61. Kremer JM, Lawrence DA, Jubiz W, et al. Dietary fish oil and olive oil supplementation in patients with rheumatoid arthritis. Clinical and immunologic effects. *Arthritis Rheum* 1990;*33*:810–20.

62. Proudman SM, James MJ, Spargo LD, et al. Fish oil in recent onset rheumatoid arthritis: a randomised, double-blind controlled trial within algorithm-based drug use. *Ann Rheum Dis* 2015;*74*:89–95.

63. Tedeschi SK, Costenbader KH. Is there a role for diet in the therapy of rheumatoid arthritis? *Curr Rheumatol Rep* 2016;*18*:23.

64. [No author]. The Global Burden of Disease Study 2010. *Lancet* 2012;*380*:2053–260.

65. Hoy DG, Smith E, Cross M, et al. The global burden of musculoskeletal conditions for 2010: an overview of methods. *Ann Rheum Dis* 2014;*73*:982–9.

66. Cross M, Smith E, Hoy D, et al. The global burden of rheumatoid arthritis: estimates from the Global Burden of Disease 2010 study. *Ann Rheum Dis* 2014;*73*:1316–22.

67. Dowman B, Campbell RM, Zgaga L, et al. Estimating the burden of rheumatoid arthritis in Africa: a systematic analysis. *J Glob Health* 2012;*2*:020406.

68. Mody GM. Rheumatoid arthritis and connective tissue disorders: sub-Saharan Africa. *Baillieres Clin Rheumatol* 1995;*9*:31–44.

69. Kalla AA, Tikly M. Rheumatoid arthritis in the developing world. *Best Pract Res Clin Rheumatol* 2003;*17*:863–75.

70. Silman AJ, Ollier W, Holligan S, et al. Absence of rheumatoid arthritis in a rural Nigerian population. *J Rheumatol* 1993;*20*:618–22.

71. Bernatsky S, Dekis A, Hudson M, et al. Rheumatoid arthritis prevalence in Quebec. *BMC Res Notes* 2014;*7*:937.

72. Neovius M, Simard JF, Askling J. Nationwide prevalence of rheumatoid arthritis and penetration of disease-modifying drugs in Sweden. *Ann Rheum Dis* 2011;*70*:624–9.

73. Englund M, Joud A, Geborek P, et al. Prevalence and incidence of rheumatoid arthritis in southern Sweden 2008 and their relation to prescribed biologics. *Rheumatology (Oxford)* 2010;*49*:1563–9.

74. Dadoun S, Zeboulon-Ktorza N, Combescure C, et al. Mortality in rheumatoid arthritis over the last fifty years: systematic review and meta-analysis. *Joint Bone Spine* 2013;*80*:29–33.

75. Humphreys JH, Warner A, Chipping J, et al. Mortality trends in patients with early rheumatoid arthritis over 20 years: results from the Norfolk Arthritis Register. *Arthritis Care Res (Hoboken)* 2014;*66*:1296–301.

76. Gonzalez A, Maradit KH, Crowson CS, et al. The widening mortality gap between rheumatoid arthritis patients and the general population. *Arthritis Rheum* 2007;*56*:3583–7.

77. Molina E, del Rincon I, Restrepo JF, et al. Mortality in rheumatoid arthritis (RA): factors associated with recording RA on death certificates. *BMC Musculoskelet Disord* 2015; *16*:277.

78. Young A, Koduri G, Batley M, et al. Mortality in rheumatoid arthritis. Increased in the early course of disease, in ischaemic heart disease and in pulmonary fibrosis. *Rheumatology (Oxford)* 2007;*46*:350–7.

4

Modifiable and other risk factors for rheumatoid arthritis: A basis for prevention and better therapy

Lars Klareskog and Lars Alfredsson

Introduction

Rheumatoid arthritis (RA) is a heterogeneous disease, consisting of distinct subsets with partly distinct aetiologies and risk factors. Such risk factors are environmental, including lifestyle-mediated and genetic, and these factors must always be considered in the context of stochastic (i.e. chance) factors. As RA is a disease where immune reactions often precede symptoms, and where symptoms that do not involve joint inflammation such as joint pain, bone loss and fatigue may precede arthritis, and where severe symptoms and comorbidities may follow after the first episode of joint inflammation, we also have to consider risk factors during these different phases of disease development.

This chapter focuses on environmental, including lifestyle, factors, and on when and how during disease development such factors are active. The chapter also describes pathogenic mechanisms that may be triggered by such risk factors. Particular emphasis is on recognition of modifiable environmental/lifestyle factors as such knowledge can be used in primary as well as secondary prevention and also to improve effects of current pharmacological treatments.

What is known about environmental/ lifestyle risk factors for RA and how has this knowledge been acquired?

Most studies on risk factors for RA have focused on risk to develop RA as defined by classification criteria at the time, so far mainly using the ACR 1987 criteria. We will first summarize such data and in subsequent sections discuss the much less complete data on risk factors active in various phases of disease. The methods that have been used to identify these risks are mainly of three categories: twin studies, cohort studies, and case-control studies. However, several of these approaches are mixed in the sense that both twin studies and case-control studies have been used to form longitudinal cohorts where information on risk factors present at an initial time point have been used to evaluate the impact of these risk factors also on the longitudinal development of disease. These different approaches all have their advantages and problems, and therefore we have chosen to describe data from all these study types to make conclusions about the role of distinct risk factors for development of RA.

Twin studies: Twin studies represent the classical way to determine the relative role of genetic factors in comparison to environmental factors and stochastic events. It is, however, much more difficult to separate the effects of environmental/lifestyle agents from chance events.

Ideally, twin studies should be 'population-based' (i.e. all twins in the population should be subject to study in order to exclude the bias that can be introduced if one twin with a certain disease is actively participating in the recruitment to the study). This difference may provide part of the explanation for the different levels of monozygotic twin concordance for disease that have been reported in various studies. Classical twin studies from Finland and the United Kingdom have indicated a monozygotic twin concordance of around 14% as compared to a dizygotic concordance of around 3.5%.[1] These figures have to some extent been challenged by more recent population-based studies in Sweden[2] and Denmark,[3] where lower monozygotic concordance rates (around 10%) for the total RA population have been reported.

As a fundamental difference in both genetic and environmental risk factors have been described for seropositive (anticitrullinated protein antibodies (ACPA) and/or rheumatoid factor (RF)) as compared to seronegative RA,[4,5] it is important to separate these two entities also in twin studies. Although numbers are still small, it appears that the monozygotic twin concordance is higher in seropositive as compared to seronegative RA[2] although different results in this respect have been reported.[6] We can conclude from these twin studies that genetic factors are important but play a smaller quantitative role as compared to environmental and stochastic factors.

Twins are in principle ideal also for the study of which environmental/lifestyle factors that are important for disease development. However, due to limited numbers of cases in available studies, only few risk factors, notably smoking, have been investigated. Here one early study from the UK twin registry was particularly informative: Out of the identified—monozygotic and RA discordant twin pairs, 13 pairs were also discordant for smoking. Notably 12 of the cases in these pairs were smokers and only one case was a non-smoker.[7] This information verifies, although in a small group, how an environmental exposure may be decisive for disease development in a genetically well-defined context.

Family studies: Whereas twin studies contain too few cases of RA to allow quantification of the influence of known versus not known genetic and environmental risk factors, large family studies that include cases with known genetic and environmental/lifestyle data can contribute with such information. Notably, one recent big family study using the Swedish multigeneration registry was able to quantify the relative contribution of yet known genetic and environmental risk factors to the 'familial heritability' of RA.[8] Notably, only approximately 25% of the familial heritability could be explained by hitherto identified genetic and environmental factors. Thus, our field is in large need for additional studies that encompass more environmental factors as well as more analyses of interactions between multiple environmental and genetic factors.

Cohort-based and case-control-based studies on environmental and lifestyle factors that contribute to or protect against onset of RA

Cohort-based and case-control-based studies on risk factors for disease complement each other and have often been used together. Cohort studies that include individuals and capture data on environment and lifestyle before onset of disease avoid biases from selective recollection of exposures. However, such studies generally suffer from relatively small numbers of individuals with the disease, and this problem is particularly obvious when RA is divided into subsets, and during efforts to identify interactions between different factors. Case-control studies suffer from risk for selection and recall biases but are able to recruit more individuals and capture more information from both cases and controls. In the rest of this section, we will present data on known risk factors for RA development, identified in both case-control and cohort settings, and divided by subsets when such data are available.

Notably, environmental and lifestyle factors and their influence on RA differ a lot between different countries, cultures, and between individuals with different genetic constitutions. Rather limited information is however available from different regions and cultures outside Europe and United States, but such information will also be commented on when available.

Overall socioeconomic and geographical factors

Socioeconomic factors, mostly measured by educational levels have a major impact on risk for RA and interact with age. Thus, low educational levels provide an overall increased risk for RA in all age groups[9] (see **Figure 4.1**).[10] When stratifying for known other risk factors, such as smoking, the effects of educational levels persist, indicating that the precise reasons for effects associated with socioeconomic differences still remain unknown. Notably, effects on risk for RA from education and income levels exist in most studies and from several countries, including the relatively egalitarian culture in Scandinavian countries.[9]

Several studies from different countries provide strong evidence that environmental factors associated with the more general life conditions play a big role. Thus, studies from African countries, for example Nigeria, have shown low prevalence of RA.[11] Interesting but quite old studies from South Africa have also indicated the migration from rural areas into towns is associated with an increased incidence and prevalence of RA.[12] Reasons for these rather large effects of environment, however, have not been clarified but differences in infections as well as presence of air pollutants may constitute such differential factors.

There is also some evidence from studies on prevalence and severity of RA in different countries with potentially higher incidence in colder climates and in Northern altitudes.[13] Such observations are very difficult to substantiate and link to defined environmental factors. There is, however, one recent report that working in a cold working environment may provide an increased risk for RA, even after correction for potentially confounding environmental/lifestyle factors.[14]

Effects of sex/gender including hormonal factors

The most predictive of all risk factors is being female, but strangely enough, we know rather little about what features of 'femaleness' constitute this risk. Presence of female sex hormones rather exert some protective role when administered in the postmenopausal age,[15] and there is also some, but not uniform evidence, that hormones taken for contraception may also have some protective effect.[16] Well established is also that disease activity in RA may diminish during pregnancy and that flares may occur after delivery whereas the effects of breastfeeding are less clear.[17] These data thus indicate major effects of sex as well as sex hormones: some data, for example in animal models for disease suggest that both macrophage and T cell reactivities maybe down-regulated by oestrogens and possibly progesterone,[18] but it is still unclear which of the fundamental factors in the immune system that cause the underlying sex difference.

Factors associated with airway exposures

Smoking is by far the most well-established risk factor for RA as summarized in a recent meta-analysis.[19] Rather high levels of smoking are needed to constitute risk and there is a clear dose-dependent increase of risk.[20,21] Other interesting features of the impact of smoking is that previous smoking infers a high risk for disease up to 20 years after cessation of smoking,[20,21] and that the effects of smoking are almost completely restricted to the seropositive (ACPA and/or RF positive) subset of the disease[4,5] (see more as follows). Notably, it has also been shown that it is the particle-containing smoke and not the nicotine that constitutes the risk factor; exposure to smoke-free, nicotine-containing tobacco such as 'snuff' is thus not associated with any increased risk for RA.[22] An interesting, so far single observation, is that also maternal exposure to smoke has been reported to increase risk for arthritis, specifically juvenile arthritis.[23]

Other airway exposures proving risk for RA are silica exposure,[24-26] exposure to solvents,[27] textile dust (in Finland and Malaysia),[28,29] and possibly high air pollution.[30-32]

(A)

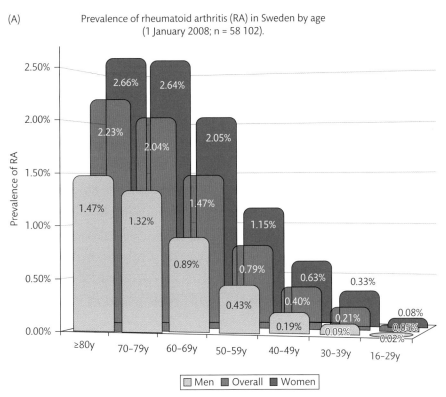

Prevalence of rheumatoid arthritis (RA) in Sweden by age
(1 January 2008; n = 58 102).

Martin Neovius et al. Ann Rheum Dis 2011;70:624–629

(B)

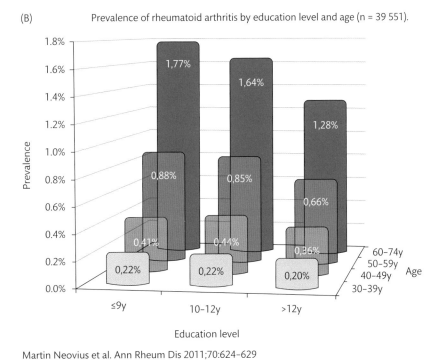

Prevalence of rheumatoid arthritis by education level and age (n = 39 551).

Martin Neovius et al. Ann Rheum Dis 2011;70:624–629

Figure 4.1 (A) Prevalence of rheumatoid arthritis, by age and sex. (B) Prevalence of rheumatoid arthritis, by education level and age (n = 39 551; This restriction is because no population statistics on education level was available for people aged ≥75 years and because people aged 18–29-year-are excluded as many may not have completed their education).

Reprinted from Neovius M. Simard J., Askling J. *et al* (2011) 'Nationwide prevalence of rheumatoid arthritis and penetration of disease-modifying drugs in Sweden'. *Annals of the Rheumatic Diseases* 70(4):624–9 with permission from the BMJ Publishing Group.

Interestingly, the most well-investigated airway exposures (i.e. silica dust exposure and cigarette smoking) constitute risk factors mainly for the seropositive subset of RA disease, and to very limited extent on the seronegative variant of RA.[2,33] Potential reasons for this restriction will be discussed next. Notably, however, other airways exposures, such as occupational exposure to textile dust (from a case-control study in Malaysia) affects both the seronegative and seropositive subsets of the disease[29] indicating that explanations provided in hypothetical form as follows on selective activation of major histocompatibility complex (MHC) class II dependent immunity against antigens modified by exposure to environmental factors in the lungs may not be the only pathogenic mechanisms involved.

Infections, including infections associated with periodontitis, and vaccinations

Infectious agents have for many years been suspected to constitute risk factors for RA. However, reproducible data linking specific infectious agents to risk for RA have been very sparse. The most solid data exist for an association between the periodontitis-associated bacterium *Porphyromonas gingivalis* and risk for RA.[34–37] Whereas the association between periodontitis and RA has been demonstrated in some studies, this has not been generally reproduced. A more reproducible finding is the association between immunity to *P. gingivalis* and seropositive RA, where the cross-reactivity between citrullinated bacterial proteins and endogenous citrullinated proteins has been well demonstrated.[34,37] These observations have led to suggestions that the autoreactivity against citrullinated proteins seen in RA may be due to classical molecular mimicry based pathogenesis. This may be true in certain instances, but the hypothesis has not yet been verified from experimental studies aimed at eliminating *P. gingivalis* and observing whether such elimination can reduce immunity to citrullinated proteins and reduce frequency or severity of seropositive RA. More recently also another bacterium associated with periodontitis, *Aggregatibacter actinomycetemcomitans* has been suggested to initiate immunity against citrullinated proteins[38] via a particular mechanism that the authors have named' hypercitrullination'. This interesting observation is, however, in need of further confirmation.

Virus infections have for many years been suspected but not proven to contribute to RA. Viruses discussed have in particular included Epstein–Barr virus (EBV), parvovirus, and cytomegalovirus (CMV). EBV-derived particles have been demonstrated in joints of RA patients, but whether the infectious contributes to disease has not been confirmed.[39] Parvovirus can cause arthritis in certain animals,[40] but in humans antibody titres against the virus have not reproducibly been linked to RA[41]; the same goes for CMV.[41] A few arboviruses, mainly Dengue and Chikungunya, have been associated with development of arthralgia as a common, but mainly relatively transient syndrome.[42,43] In more rare instances this arthralgia can develop further towards arthritis.

In summary, data are accumulating that certain bacterial infections in mucosal surfaces may trigger immunity that can contribute to RA, whereas the virus–based hypotheses have so far received less empirical support. It is possible, however, that subsets of the heterogeneous disease we call RA may be triggered by different organisms, and more work in this area is clearly warranted.

Vaccinations are another exposure where speculations have been common concerning their contribution to RA. However, the relatively few controlled and well-powered studies that have been performed in this area have so far either not been able to demonstrate any increased risk of RA after vaccinations that are most common in the populations[44] or demonstrated a limited increase of risk in certain populations.[45]

Microbiota

The idea that commensal microbes present in mucosal surfaces may contribute to RA is old, and was very actively investigated by investigators in the middle of the twentieth century, and formed as a matter of fact the basis for the introduction of the effective anti-RA drug sulfasalazine.[46] It was originally assumed that the sulphur part of this drug would modify what we today call the 'gut microbiome'. However, sulfasalazine has not been demonstrated to have any obvious effects on the microbiome, but rather displays an immunosuppressive effect. Instead, studies of the role of the microbiome waned for many years, until the development of new technologies which have allowed descriptive studies of microbiomes defined by 16S sequencing. Here, it has been well demonstrated that the microbiome in RA patients, as well as in other inflammatory diseases, display a less diverse microbiome than is the case in healthy individuals.[47] It has also been demonstrated, most clearly in animal models of arthritis, that alterations in the microbiome may have profound effects on arthritis-associated immunity and on clinical signs of arthritis.[48] It still remains unclear, however, whether changes in the microbiome are indeed causative of disease, and/or on severity of disease. This will most probably be clarified within the near future as several therapeutic studies are ongoing in the area.

A particularly interesting area in this field is the study of the microbiome in the lungs, as there is now so much evidence that link events in the lung mucosa to anticitrulline immunity and seropositive RA. Thus, also the lung microbiome of RA patients is less diverse than the lung microbiome of healthy individuals.[49] But also in this case causation remains unclear.

Dietary factors, including alcohol use

Dietary factors have for long been suspected to contribute to the development of RA, not least from the patient side, but so far, the hard data are rather scarce. Thus, the most well-established protective factors among widely used food items is oily fish[50,51] or other products with high content of omega-3 fatty acids. The most reproducible risk factor in this area is obesity.[52] A discussion has been held concerning effects of certain kinds of meat, such as red meat, but no such associations were found in the most extensive cohorts study so far.[53] There have also been a few reports that diets containing high concentrations of salt (sodium chloride) may provide a risk, in particular in smokers.[54,55] These reports require wider replication in order to be fully accepted and results be subject to implementation in healthcare.

So far, the major effects of 'food and drink studies' is associated with alcohol use, where several reports, based both on cohorts and on case-control, indicate a dose-dependent protective effect of alcohol, that appears to be due to the alcohol intake *per se*, rather than specific types of beverages.[56–60] This conclusion has also received support from protective effects of alcohol intake on arthritis in mice where addition of alcohol to the drinking water significantly reduced frequency as well as severity of the disease, by means of reduction of production of pro-inflammatory molecules by inhibition of the NF-κB signalling pathway.[61]

Other behavioural and social factors including stress, physical exercise, and strenuous work

When asking patients for their assumptions of environmental/lifestyle factors that may have triggered their disease, stressful events come up as number one, particularly in women.[62] However, no solid data do exist that such stress factors are important, and this is thus an area of need of further studies.

Another factor, often mentioned by patients, mainly men, is exposure to strenuous work situations with repeated and heavy loads. Also, such a factor (i.e. exposure of repeated strenuous loads during work) was recently reported to constitute a risk for the occurrence of RA.[63] Several of these reports still await confirmation before becoming established risk factors that may provide a basis for preventive effects.

Interactions between environmental and genetic factors in providing risk for the development of RA

As noted in the introduction, RA is a heterogeneous and complex disease, where several risk factors, environmental as well as genetic, contribute to disease and interact with each other. Nevertheless, rather few studies have been designed to systematically investigate interactions between the many environmental or lifestyle factors just described and the many genetic factors discussed in other chapters of this book. By 'interactions' we mean here the situation when risk factors being present together provide a higher risk for disease as compared with the added risk from each of these factors alone. The prime example of such interactions in RA was the demonstration of a profound interaction between smoking and the presence of certain MHC class II genes in the development of seropositive RA.[2,4,64] Notably, these two risk factors as well as the interaction between them was restricted to the ACPA/RF positive subset of disease.[2,4,64,65] Subsequently, interaction between MHC class alleles and the risk allele of *PTPN22* has been demonstrated as gene–gene interaction[66] and interaction between silica dust exposure and smoking as an environment–environment interaction.[67] Emerging data indicate that many other interactions between multiple environmental factors and multiple genetic variants exist and may explain some of the 'missing heritability' (i.e. heritability that can be defined in family studies, but where the genetic and/or environmental basis for this lack of knowledge has not yet been defined).

Effects of risk factors in different phases of the gradual development of RA

There is an increasing awareness that development of RA, in particular the seropositive form of RA, is a gradual process with several different phases being involved and a consensus group in the European League against Rheumatism (EULAR) has suggested the naming of different distinct phases in the putative development of seropositive RA.[68] Naturally, different environmental agents as well as different genetic factors may be involved in these different phases. For effort to foster prevention, it is thus important to know which factors are of importance for the ultimate disease development in the different phases that precede the active and visible joint inflammation. Unfortunately, rather little data exists in this area. So far, it appears that smoking and possibly other airway stimuli have the dominant impact in the very early stage of triggering of the autoantibody response typical for RA, whereas genetic factors may have a larger relative role in the translation from seropositivity towards clinical arthritis.[69]

Here, a new and very interesting area for research and therapy/prevention has emerged from the animal-based data that autoimmunity to citrullinated proteins/peptides (ACPAs) may indeed contribute to the development of arthralgia as well as bone loss that often precedes joint inflammation in patients with pre-existing antibodies against citrullinated and other modified antigens as well as RF.[70,71] Thus, transfer of immunoglobulin G (IgG) from seropositive RA patients, purified for reactivity against citrullinated peptides, have been shown to induce bone loss as well as joint pain after transfer to mice.[72-74] These experiments thus suggest a common mechanism between two symptoms that precede onset of seropositive arthritis (i.e. joint pain and bone loss) with the demonstration that some ACPAs are able to induce both bone loss and arthralgia after binding to osteoclasts, and inducing these cells both to erode bone and to produce pain-inducing mediators such as IL-8.[75] The results of these studies thus call for a better understanding of factors that cause production of ACPAs and RF in order to both prevent/treat the early ACPA-induced symptoms such as arthralgia and bone loss, and factors that may translate an ACPA/RF positive but not arthritic state into the chronic arthritis we call RA.

Factors that have so far been shown to be predictive for the translation from seropositivity to arthritis are on one hand the composition of the fine specificities of the ACPA response (the more specificities and higher titres, the higher risk for future development of RA), and whether also RF are present in addition to ACPAs.[76] Environmental/lifestyle factors that have been shown to influence risk of arthritis development in ACPA-positive individuals with arthralgia are primarily smoking and obesity.[77] There is an obvious need for more data in this area, as such knowledge will provide a major basis for the development of preventive programmes for the development of arthritis in individuals identified with arthralgia and simultaneous presence of ACPAs and/or RF.

Finally, environmental and lifestyle risk factors also affect the disease course and response to therapy for established arthritis and, furthermore, influence the risk for comorbidities. Such effects include negative influence of current smoking and obesity on disease course,[78-80] including numbers of erosions, as well as effects of the most common therapies. Such negative effects of smoking as well as obesity have been demonstrated for methotrexate as well as for biological TNF-blocking agents, whereas effects on other biologicals as well as of jakinibs are not yet known. Notably, however, the effects of both current smoking and of obesity on therapeutic results of methotrexate and TNF-blockade are so pronounced that these factors appear to be more important than other classical predictors of response to therapy such as presence of RF/ACPA, or erosions at onset of disease.[81] The data, although incomplete indicate that advice on lifestyle should be a mandatory component in the therapeutic strategy for patients with RA. A recent test of a web-based tool for information of risk factors to family members of patients with RA suggest that such information may be useful in increasing awareness to risk individuals of environmental/lifestyle of importance for disease development.

Use of information on environmental risk factor and gene-environment interactions to understand the aetiology and molecular pathogenesis of RA

The data summarized here describe how the presence of different mixtures of genetic and environmental/lifestyle risk factors may be involved in the development of different stages of disease and in the development of different symptoms. These data also demonstrate that different factors may contribute to different subsets of RA. Taken together, the data provide a very valuable background to any efforts trying to understand the aetiology and molecular pathologies involved in the gradual development of disease symptoms in different disease subsets. The most obvious examples of such efforts, so far, come from studies on effects of airway exposures and events in the lungs, and from studies on defined microbes present during periodontitis.

For the lungs, the recognition that smoking and later also silica exposure and textile dust exposure interact with distinct human leukocyte antigen (HLA) class alleles and do so exclusively in the ACPA-positive subsets of disease (see Figure 4.2), provided the basis for investigations of how immunity to citrullinated and other post-translationally modified autoantigens might be triggered in the lungs. Using analysis of bronchoalveolar fluids and bronchial biopsies from newly diagnosed RA patients it was demonstrated that increased citrullination caused by increased activity of citrullinating enzymes, PAD2 and PAD4, occurs after smoking,[82,83] and that both T- and B-cell activation against citrullinated antigens may occur in the lungs.[83,84] Smoking as well as exposure to silica dust and lipopolysaccharide (LPS)-containing textile dust may also cause activation of antigen-presenting cells in the lung compartment, thus providing the basis for an immune response to citrullinated antigens in individuals with HLA variants that enable such MHC

class II dependent immune reactions (see review[85]). Evidence for such events also before onset of the joint inflammation in ACPA-positive patients have also been published, further indicating that triggering of pathogenic immunity may occur in lungs preceding subsequent development of symptoms such as arthralgia and bone loss and eventually, arthritis.[86,87] The knowledge is still incomplete concerning exactly how this autoimmunity is triggered. Thus, whereas there is circumstantial evidence that T cell as well as B cell autoimmunity to citrullinated and otherwise post-translationally modified autoantigens[88,89] may be triggered in the lungs and that negative selection of such autoreactive T cells may not be complete in thymus, there is also the possibility that a primary stimulus for immune activation may come from microbes, for example, in the lung microbiome. These different options have not yet been systematically investigated, but the ongoing production of T- and B-cell clones with distinct disease-relevant specificities will enable such studies.

For the gums and periodontitis-relevant infections, properties of two such bacteria are of particular interest, i.e. *Porphyromonas gingivalis* and *Aggregatibacter actinomycetemcomitans (AA)*. In both cases, these bacteria have the capacity to both produce bacterial proteins citrullinated by the bacterial PADs,[34,38] and, at least as shown for *P. gingivalis*, to modify also self-proteins present in the same local tissue compartment as these bacteria.[34] Very interesting in these contexts is that one specific protein in *P. gingivalis*, alpha-enolase, can be citrullinated and that antibodies from RA patients have shown cross-reactivity between the citrullinated forms of this bacterial protein and several self-proteins.[34] The same goes for the AA-derived proteins where a proposed 'hypercitrullination' may provide the similar basis for autoimmunity triggered by an initial reactivity against bacterial proteins (a classical molecular mimicry situation). The epidemiology in support of the contributions of these bacteria to the anticitrulline immunity is, however, not yet as convincing as the studies indicating a role for immunity triggered in the

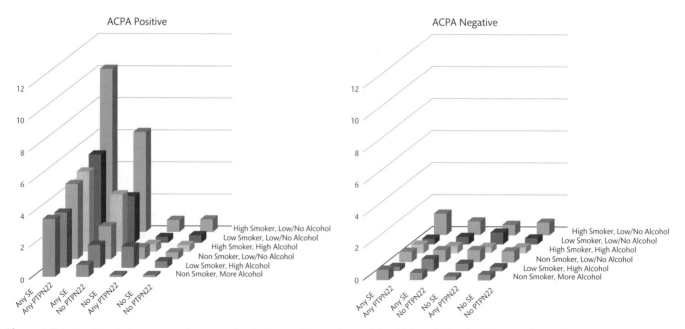

Figure 4.2 Interactions between several genes and environmental factors in providing lifetime risk for the different subsets of RA.

lungs. However, this is an active field of research where still much remains to be sorted out and where options for prevention by interference with microbes associated with periodontitis and later arthritis may be substantial.

All is not about drugs: Use of information on risk factors for prevention and to improve therapy

As already described, the many environmental components among the 'risk factors' that determine onset and disease course of RA have now been described and in some cases also quantified. This means that this information should be included in all efforts to prevent RA by public health measures as well as efforts to prevent the disease in stages where immunity has been triggered but not yet resulted in disease (see **Figure 4.3**). So far quantification of the contribution of defined environmental risk factors to the overall disease risk have been sparse, but one report has indicated that smoking would be directly responsible for around 20% of all RA cases and for one-third of seropositive cases (by population attribution).[90] These data call for strategies to communicate this information to patients and public, and in particular to individuals at high risk for RA, for example individuals with ACPAs and/or RF who have not yet developed disease.[77,91,92] Ways to publicize this information should be developed in the same way as we develop

drugs that often need modification of environment/lifestyle to have an optimal effect on the disease. Development of digital and patient-centred tools that provide visualization of environmental/lifestyle effects on disease risk and disease course represent one way towards using the information described in the present chapter in clinical practice.

Some general conclusions

The ways to understand RA and to reduce the disease burden from this disease worldwide has developed over recent years from being entirely focused on understanding and treating the inflammation in joints towards a longitudinal view of the disease where the different steps of disease development can be understood and influenced. Environmental and lifestyle factors, many of them modifiable, contribute to different phases of disease development. It is thus logical to identify and consider ways to achieve such modifications, with the same priority as we try to identify molecular mechanisms leading to disease and the subsequent development of drugs that can interfere with these pathways. The dual approach (i.e. using knowledge of molecular pathways active in different subsets of disease for selection of efficient drugs) and also knowing which environmental/lifestyle events that influence these pathways and help to modify these factors, promise to be the best way to accomplish good treatment and ultimately prevention of RA.[93]

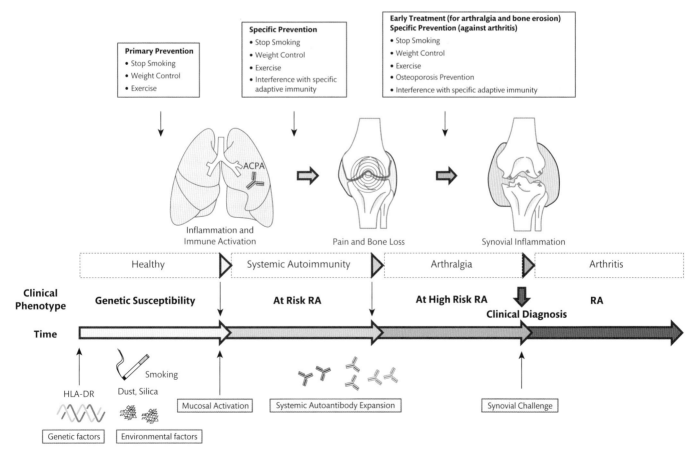

Figure 4.3 Strategies for prevention and treatment of RA using knowledge on environmental and lifestyle risk factors.

REFERENCES

1. MacGregor AJ, Snieder H, Rigby AS, et al. Characterizing the quantitative genetic contribution to rheumatoid arthritis using data from twins. *Arthritis Rheum* 2000;*43*(1):30–7.

2. Hensvold AH, Frisell T, Magnusson PK, Holmdahl R, Askling J, Catrina AI. How well do ACPA discriminate and predict RA in the general population: a study based on 12 590 population-representative Swedish twins. *Ann Rheum Dis* 2017;*76*(1):119–25.

3. Svendsen AJ, Kyvik KO, Houen G, et al. On the origin of rheumatoid arthritis: the impact of environment and genes—a population based twin study. *PLoS One* 2013;*8*(2):e57304.

4. Klareskog L, Stolt P, Lundberg K, et al. A new model for an etiology of rheumatoid arthritis: smoking may trigger HLA-DR (shared epitope)-restricted immune reactions to autoantigens modified by citrullination. *Arthritis Rheum* 2006;*54*(1):38–46.

5. van der Helm-van Mil AH, Verpoort KN, Breedveld FC, Huizinga TW, Toes RE, de Vries RR. The HLA-DRB1 shared epitope alleles are primarily a risk factor for anti-cyclic citrullinated peptide antibodies and are not an independent risk factor for development of rheumatoid arthritis. *Arthritis Rheum* 2006;*54*(4):1117–21.

6. van der Woude D, Houwing-Duistermaat JJ, Toes RE, et al. Quantitative heritability of anti-citrullinated protein antibody-positive and anti-citrullinated protein antibody-negative rheumatoid arthritis. *Arthritis Rheum* 2009;*60*(4):916–23.

7. Silman AJ, Newman J, MacGregor AJ. Cigarette smoking increases the risk of rheumatoid arthritis: results from a nationwide study of disease-discordant twins. *Arthritis Rheum* 1996;*39*:732–5.

8. Frisell T, Holmqvist M, Källberg H, Klareskog L, Alfredsson L, Askling J. Familial risks and heritability of rheumatoid arthritis: role of rheumatoid factor/anti-citrullinated protein antibody status, number and type of affected relatives, sex, and age. *Arthritis Rheum* 2013;*65*(11):2773–82.

9. Bengtsson C, Nordmark B, Klareskog L, et al. Socioeconomic status and the risk of developing rheumatoid arthritis: results from the Swedish EIRA study. *Ann Rheum Dis* 2005;*64*:1588–94.

10. Neovius M, Simard JF, Askling J; ARTIS study group. Nationwide prevalence of rheumatoid arthritis and penetration of disease-modifying drugs in Sweden. *Ann Rheum Dis* 2011;*70*(4):624–9.

11. Silman AJ, Ollier W, Holligan S, et al. Absence of rheumatoid arthritis in a rural Nigerian population. *J Rheumatol* 1993;*20*(4):618–22.

12. Abdel-Nasser AM, Rasker JJ, Valkenburg HA. Epidemiological and clinical aspects relating to the variability of rheumatoid arthritis. *Semin Arthritis Rheum* 1997;*27*(2):123–40.

13. GEO-RA Group. Latitude gradient influences the age of onset of rheumatoid arthritis: a worldwide survey. *Clin Rheumatol* 2017;*36*(3):485–97.

14. Zeng P, Bengtsson C, Klareskog L, Alfredsson L. Working in cold environment and risk of developing rheumatoid arthritis: results from the Swedish EIRA case-control study. *RMD Open* 2017;*3*(2):e000488.

15. Orellana C, Saevarsdottir S, Klareskog L, Karlson EW, Alfredsson L, Bengtsson C. Postmenopausal hormone therapy and the risk of rheumatoid arthritis: results from the Swedish EIRA population-based case-control study. *Eur J Epidemiol* 2015;*30*(5):449–57.

16. Orellana C, Saevarsdottir S, Klareskog L, Karlson EW, Alfredsson L, Bengtsson C. Oral contraceptives, breastfeeding and the risk of developing rheumatoid arthritis: results from the Swedish EIRA study. *Ann Rheum Dis* 2017;*76*(11):1845–52.

17. Wallenius M, Skomsvoll JF, Irgens LM, et al. Postpartum onset of rheumatoid arthritis and other chronic arthritides: results from a patient register linked to a medical birth registry. *Ann Rheum Dis* 2010;*69*:332–6.

18. Jochems C, Islander U, Erlandsson M, et al. Role of endogenous and exogenous female sex hormones in arthritis and osteoporosis development in B10.Q-ncf1*/* mice with collagen-induced chronic arthritis. *BMC Musculoskelet Disord* 2010;*11*:284.

19. Sugiyama D, Nishimura K, Tamaki K, et al. Impact of smoking as a risk factor for developing rheumatoid arthritis: a meta-analysis of observational studies. *Ann Rheum Dis* 2010;*69*:70–81.

20. Stolt P, Bengtsson C, Nordmark B, et al. Quantification of the influence of cigarette smoking on rheumatoid arthritis: results from a population based case-control study, using incident cases. *Ann Rheum Dis* 2003;*62*(9):835–41.

21. Costenbader KH, Feskanich D, Mandl LA, Karlson EW. Smoking intensity, duration, and cessation, and the risk of rheumatoid arthritis in women. *Am J Med* 2006;*119*:503.

22. Carlens C, Hergens MP, Grunewald J, et al. Smoking, use of moist snuff, and risk of chronic inflammatory diseases. *Am J Respir Crit Care Med* 2010;*181*(11):1217–22.

23. Jaakkola JJ, Gissler M. Maternal smoking in pregnancy as a determinant of rheumatoid arthritis and other inflammatory polyarthropathies during the first 7 years of life. *Int J Epidemiol* 2005;*34*(3):664–71.

24. Klockars M, Koskela RS, Järvinen E, Kolari PJ, Rossi A. Silica exposure and rheumatoid arthritis: a follow up study of granite workers 1940–81. *BMJ* 1987;*18*:997–1000.

25. Stolt P, Källberg H, Lundberg I, Sjögren B, Klareskog L, Alfredsson L. Silica exposure is associated with increased risk of developing rheumatoid arthritis: results from the Swedish EIRA study. *Ann Rheum Dis* 2005;*64*(4):582–6.

26. Yahya A, Bengtsson C, Larsson P, et al. Silica exposure is associated with an increased risk of developing ACPA-positive rheumatoid arthritis in an Asian population: evidence from the Malaysian MyEIRA case-control study. *Mod Rheumatol* 2014;*24*(2):271–4.

27. Lundberg I, Alfrdesson L, Plato N, Sverdrup B, Klareskog L, Klaienau S. Occupation, occupational exposures to chemnicals and rheumatological diseases: a register-based cohort study. *Scand J Rheumatol* 1994;*23*:305–10.

28. Koskela RS, Klockars M, Järvinen E. Mortality and disability among cotton mill workers. *Br J Ind Med* 1990;*47*(6):384–91.

29. Too CL, Muhamad NA, Ilar A, et al. Occupational exposure to textile dust increases the risk of rheumatoid arthritis: results from a Malaysian population-based case-control study. *Ann Rheum Dis* 2016;*75*(6):997–1002.

30. Hart JE, Laden F, Puett RC, Costenbader KH, Karlson EW. Exposure to traffic pollution and increased risk of rheumatoid arthritis. *Environ Health Perspect* 2009;*117*(7):1065–9.

31. Hart JE, Källberg H, Laden F, et al. Ambient air pollution exposures and risk of rheumatoid arthritis: results from the Swedish EIRA case-control study. *Ann Rheum Dis* 2013;*72*(6):888–94.

32. Jung CR, Hsieh HY, Hwang BF. Air pollution as a potential determinant of rheumatoid arthritis: a population-based cohort study in Taiwan. *Epidemiology* 2017;*28* Suppl 1:S54–9.

33. Stolt P, Yahya A, Bengtsson C, et al. Silica exposure among male current smokers is associated with a high risk of developing ACPA-positive rheumatoid arthritis. *Ann Rheum Dis* 2010;*69*(6):1072–6.

34. Lundberg K, Wegner N, Yucel-Lindberg T, Venables PJ. Periodontitis in RA-the citrullinated enolase connection. *Nat Rev Rheumatol* 2010;6(12):727–30.

35. Okada M, Kobayashi T, Ito S, et al. Antibody responses to periodontopathic bacteria in relation to rheumatoid arthritis in Japanese adults. *J Periodontol* 2011;82(10):1433–41.

36. Miklus TR, Thiele GM, Deane KD, et al. Porphyromonas gingivalis and disease-related autoantibodies in individuals at increased risk of rheumatoid arthritis. *Arthritis Rheum* 2012;64(11):3522–30.

37. Potemka J, Mydel P, Koziel J. The case for periodontitis in the pathogenesis of rheumatoid arthritis. *Nat Rev Rheumatol* 2017;13(10):606–20.

38. Konig MF, Abusleme L, Reinholdt J, et al. Aggregatibacter actinomycetemcomitans-induced hypercitrullination links periodontal infection to autoimmunity in rheumatoid arthritis. *Sci Transl Med* 2016;8(369):369ra176.

39. Ball RJ, Avenell A, Aucott L, Hanlon P, Vickers MA. Systematic review and meta-analysis of the sero-epidemiological association between Epstein-Barr virus and rheumatoid arthritis. *Arthritis Res Ther* 2015;17:274.

40. Takasawa N, Munakata Y, Ishii KK, et al. Human parvovirus B19 transgenic mice become susceptible to polyarthritis. *J Immunol* 2004;173(7):4675–83.

41. Sherina N, Hreggvidsdottir HS, Bengtsson C, et al. Low levels of antibodies against common viruses associate with anti-citrullinated protein antibody-positive rheumatoid arthritis; implications for disease aetiology. *Arthritis Res Ther* 2017;19(1):219.

42. Mohd Zim MA, Sam IC, Omar SF, Chan YF, AbuBakar S, Kamarulzaman A. Chikungunya infection in Malaysia: comparison with dengue infection in adults and predictors of persistent arthralgia. *J Clin Virol* 2013;56(2):141–5.

43. Amdekar S, Parashar D, Alagarasu K. Chikungunya virus-induced arthritis: role of host and viral factors in the pathogenesis. *Viral Immunol* 2017;30(10):691–702.

44. Bengtsson C, Kapetanovic MC, Källberg H, et al. Common vaccinations among adults do not increase the risk of developing rheumatoid arthritis: results from the Swedish EIRA study. *Ann Rheum Dis* 2010;69(10):1831–3.

45. Wang B, Shao X, Wang D, Xu D, Zhang JA. Vaccinations and risk of systemic lupus erythematosus and rheumatoid arthritis: a systematic review and meta-analysis. *Autoimmun Rev* 2017;16(7):756–65.

46. Svartz N. Treatment of rheumatoid arthritis with salicylazosulfapyridine. *Acta Med Scand Suppl* 1958;341:247–54.

47. Scher J, Abramson SB. The microbiome and rheumatoid arthritis. *Nat Rev Rheumatol* 2011;7(10):569–78.

48. Maeda Y, Kurakawa T, Umemoto E, et al. Dysbiosis contributes to arthritis development via activation of autoreactive T cells in the intestine. *Arthritis Rheumatol* 2016;68(11):2646–61.

49. Scher JU, Joshua V, Artacho A, et al. The lung microbiota in early rheumatoid arthritis and autoimmunity. *Microbiome* 2016;4(1):60.

50. Rosell M, Wesley AM, Rydin K, Klareskog L, Alfredsson L; EIRA study group. Dietary fish and fish oil and the risk of rheumatoid arthritis. *Epidemiology* 2009;20(6):896–901.

51. Di Giuseppe D, Crippa A, Orsini N, Wolk A. Fish consumption and risk of rheumatoid arthritis: a dose-response meta-analysis. *Arthritis Res Ther* 2014;16(5):446.

52. Feng J, Chen Q, Yu F, et al. Body mass index and risk of rheumatoid arthritis: a meta-analysis of observational studies. *Medicine (Baltimore)* 2016;95(8):e2859.

53. Benito-Garcia E, Feskanich D, Hu FB, Mandl LA, Karlson EW. Protein, iron, and meat consumption and risk for rheumatoid arthritis: a prospective cohort study. *Arthritis Res Ther* 2007;9(1):R16.

54. Sundström B, Johansson I, Rantapää-Dahlqvist S. Interaction between dietary sodium and smoking increases the risk for rheumatoid arthritis: results from a nested case-control study. *Rheumatology (Oxford)* 2015;54(3):487–93.

55. Jiang X, Sundström B, Alfredsson L, Klareskog L, Rantapää-Dahlqvist S, Bengtsson C High sodium chloride consumption enhances the effects of smoking but does not interact with SGK1 polymorphisms in the development of ACPA-positive status in patients with RA. *Ann Rheum Dis* 2016;75(5):943–6.

56. Källberg H, Jacobsen S, Bengtsson C, et al. Alcohol consumption is associated with decreased risk of rheumatoid arthritis: results from two Scandinavian case-control studies. *Ann Rheum Dis* 2009;68(2):222–7.

57. Lu B, Solomon DH, Costenbader KH, Karlson EW. Alcohol consumption and risk of incident rheumatoid arthritis in women: a prospective study. *Arthritis Rheumatol* 2014;66(8):1998–2005.

58. Huidekoper AL, van der Woude D, Knevel R, et al. Patients with early arthritis consume less alcohol than controls, regardless of the type of arthritis. *Rheumatology (Oxford)* 2013;52(9):1701–7.

59. Jin Z, Xiang C, Cai Q, Wei X, He J. Alcohol consumption as a preventive factor for developing rheumatoid arthritis: a dose-response meta-analysis of prospective studies. *Ann Rheum Dis* 2014;73(11):1962–7.

60. Scott IC, Tan R, Stahl D, Steer S, Lewis CM, Cope AP. The protective effect of alcohol on developing rheumatoid arthritis: a systematic review and meta-analysis. *Rheumatology (Oxford)* 2013;52(5):856–67.

61. Jonsson IM, Verdrengh M, Brisslert M, et al. Ethanol prevents development of destructive arthritis. *Proc Natl Acad Sci U S A* 2007;104:258–63.

62. Bergsten U, Bergman S, Fridlund B, et al. Patient´s conceptions of the cause of their rheumatoid arthritis: a qualitative study. *Musculoskeletal Care* 2009;7(4):243–55.

63. Zeng P, Klareskog L, Alfredsson L, Bengtsson C. Physical workload is associated with increased risk of rheumatoid arthritis: results from a Swedish population-based case-control study. *RMD Open* 2017;3(1):e000324.

64. Padyukov L, Silva C, Stolt P, Alfredsson L, Klareskog L. A gene-environment interaction between smoking and shared epitope genes in HLA-DR provides a high risk of seropositive rheumatoid arthritis. *Arthritis Rheum* 2004;50(10):3085–92.

65. Karlsson EW, Chang SC, Cui J, et al. Gene environment interaction between HLA-DRB1 shared epitope and heavy cigarette smoking in predicting incident rheumatoid arthritis. *Ann Rheum Dis* 2010;69(1):54–60.

66. Källberg H, Padyukov L, Plenge RM, et al. Gene-gene and gene-environment interactions involving HLA-DRB1, PTPN22, and smoking in two subsets of rheumatoid arthritis. *Am J Hum Genet* 2007;80(5):867–75.

67. Yahya A, Bengtsson C, Larsson P, et al. Silica exposure is associated with an increased risk of developing ACPA-positive rheumatoid arthritis in an Asian population: evidence from the Malaysian MyEIRA case-control study. *Mod Rheumatol* 2014 Mar;24(2):271–4.

68. Gerlag DM, Raza K, van Baarsen LG, et al. EULAR recommendations for terminology and research in individuals at risk of rheumatoid arthritis: report from the Study Group for Risk Factors for Rheumatoid Arthritis. *Ann Rheum Dis* 2012;71(5):638–41.

69. Catrina AI, Svensson CI, Malmström V, Schett G, Klareskog L. Mechanisms leading from systemic autoimmunity to

joint-specific disease in rheumatoid arthritis. *Nat Rev Rheumatol* 2017;*13*(2):79–86.

70. Stack RJ, van Tuyl LH, Sloots M, et al. Symptom complexes in patients with seropositive arthralgia and in patients newly diagnosed with rheumatoid arthritis: a qualitative exploration of symptom development. *Rheumatology (Oxford)* 2014;*53*(9):1646–53.

71. Kleyer A, Finzel S, Rech J, et al. Bone loss before the clinical onset of rheumatoid arthritis in subjects with anticitrullinated protein antibodies. *Ann Rheum Dis* 2014;*73*(5):854–60.

72. Harre U, Georgess D, Bang H, et al. Induction of osteoclastogenesis and bone loss by human autoantibodies against citrullinated vimentin. *J Clin Invest* 2012;*122*(5):1791–802.

73. Krishnamurthy A, Joshua V, Haj Hensvold A, et al. Identification of a novel chemokine-dependent molecular mechanism underlying rheumatoid arthritis-associated autoantibody-mediated bone loss. *Ann Rheum Dis* 2016 Apr;*75*(4):721–9. doi: 10.1136/annrheumdis-2015-208093. Epub 2015 Nov 26. Erratum in: *Ann Rheum Dis* 2019 Jun;*78*(6):866

74. Wigerblad G, Bas DB, Fernades-Cerqueira C, et al. Autoantibodies to citrullinated proteins induce joint pain independent of inflammation via a chemokine-dependent mechanism. *Ann Rheum Dis* 2016 Apr;*75*(4):730–8. doi: 10.1136/annrheumdis-2015-208094. Epub 2015 Nov 27. Erratum in: *Ann Rheum Dis* 2019 Jun;*78*(6):865.

75. Catrina AI, Ytterberg AJ, Reynisdottir G, Malmström V, Klareskog L. Lungs, joints and immunity against citrullinated proteins in rheumatoid arthritis. *Nat Rev Rheumatol* 2014;*10*(11):645–53.

76. Ten Brinck RM, van Steenbergen HW, van Delft MAM, et al. The risk of individual autoantibodies, autoantibody combinations and levels for arthritis development in clinically suspect arthralgia. *Rheumatology (Oxford)* 2017;*56*(12):2145–53.

77. de Hair MJ, Landewé RB, van de Sande MG, et al. Smoking and overweight determine the likelihood of developing rheumatoid arthritis. *Ann Rheum Dis* 2013;*72*(10):1654–8.

78. Saevarsdottir S, Wedrén S, Seddighzadeh M, et al. Patients with early rheumatoid arthritis who smoke are less likely to respond to treatment with methotrexate and tumor necrosis factor inhibitors: observations from the Epidemiological Investigation of Rheumatoid Arthritis and the Swedish Rheumatology Register cohorts. *Arthritis Rheum* 2011 Jan;*63*(1):26–36.

79. Lupoli R, Pizzicato P, Scalera A, et al. Impact of body weight on the achievement of minimal disease activity in patients with rheumatic diseases: a systematic review and meta-analysis. *Arthritis Res Ther* 2016;*18*(1):297.

80. Schulman E, Bartlett SJ, Schieir O, et al. Overweight, obesity, and the likelihood of achieving sustained remission in early rheumatoid arthritis: results from the Canadian Early Arthritis Cohort Study. *Arthritis Care Res (Hoboken)* 2018;*70*(8):1185–91.

81. Saevarsdottir S, Rezaei H, Geborek P, et al. Current smoking status is a strong predictor of radiographic progression in early rheumatoid arthritis: results from the SWEFOT trial. *Ann Rheum Dis* 2015;*74*(8):1509–14.

82. Makrygiannakis D, Hermansson M, Ulfgren AK, et al. Smoking increases peptidylarginine deiminase 2 enzyme expression in human lungs and increases citrullination in BAL cells. *Ann Rheum Dis* 2008;*67*(10):1488–92.

83. Reynisdottir G, Olsen H, Joshua V, et al. Signs of immune activation and local inflammation are present in the bronchial tissue of patients with untreated early rheumatoid arthritis. *Ann Rheum Dis* 2016;*75*(9):1722–7.

84. Rangel-Moreno J, Hartson L, Navarro C, Gaxiola M, Selman M, Randall TD. Inducible bronchus-associated lymphoid tissue (iBALT) in patients with pulmonary complications of rheumatoid arthritis. *J Clin Invest* 2006;*116*(12):3183–94.

85. Demoruelle MK, Solomon JJ, Fischer A, Deane KD. The lung may play a role in the pathogenesis of rheumatoid arthritis. *Int J Clin Rheumtol* 2014;*9*(3):295–309.

86. Reynisdottir G, Karimi R, Joshua V, et al. Structural changes and antibody enrichment in the lungs are early features of anti-citrullinated protein antibody-positive rheumatoid arthritis. *Arthritis Rheumatol* 2014;*66*(1):31–9.

87. Kelmenson LB, Demoruelle MK, Deane KD. The complex role of the lung in the pathogenesis and clinical outcomes of rheumatoid arthritis. *Curr Rheumatol Rep* 2016;*18*(11):69.

88. Shi J, van Veelen PA, Mahler M, et al. Carbamylation and antibodies against carbamylated proteins in autoimmunity and other pathologies. *Autoimmun Rev* 2014;*13*(3):225–30.

89. Juarez M, Bang H, Hammar F, et al. Identification of novel antiacetylated vimentin antibodies in patients with early inflammatory arthritis. *Ann Rheum Dis* 2016;*75*(6):1099–107.

90. Källberg H, Ding B, Padyukov L, et al. Smoking is a major preventable risk factor for rheumatoid arthritis: estimations of risks after various exposures to cigarette smoke. *Ann Rheum Dis* 2011;*70*(3):508–11.

91. Deane KD, Striebich CC, Holers VM. Prevention of rheumatoid arthritis: now is the time, but how to proceed? *Arthritis Rheumatol* 2017;*69*(5):873–7.

92. vanvan Steenbergen HW, da Silva JAP, Huizinga TWJ, van der Helm-van Mil AHM. Preventing progression from arthralgia to arthritis: targeting the right patients. *Nat Rev Rheumatol* 2018;*14*(1):32–41.

93. Malmström V, Catrina AI, Klareskog L. The immunopathogenesis of seropositive rheumatoid arthritis: from triggering to targeting. *Nat Rev Immunol* 2017;*17*(1):60–75.

SECTION 2
Pathogenesis

5 Genetics and epigenetics of rheumatoid arthritis 45

Anne Barton

6 Dysregulation of synovial fibroblasts in rheumatoid arthritis 55

Thomas Crowley, Jason D. Turner, Andrew Filer, Andy Clark, and Chris Buckley

7 Autoantibodies in rheumatoid arthritis 65

Tom W.J. Huizinga

8 Dendritic cells and T cells in rheumatoid arthritis 73

Soi-Cheng Law, Pascale Wehr, Harriet Purvis, and Ranjeny Thomas

9 Mechanisms of bone and cartilage destruction 85

Ulrike Harre and Georg Schett

10 Cytokines and other mediators 95

Marina Frleta-Gilchrist and Iain B. McInnes

Genetics and epigenetics of rheumatoid arthritis

Anne Barton

Evidence for a genetic component to RA susceptibility

Rheumatoid arthritis (RA) is known to have a genetic component: the evidence comes from twin and family studies as well as genetic studies themselves. First, RA is more likely to affect both individuals in a twin pair if the twins are monozygotic (assumed to be genetically identical, 15% twins concordant for RA), rather than dizygotic (share ~50% of the same genetic code, 4% twins concordant for RA). This excess concordance is evidence for a genetic contribution to disease but underestimates how much genetics contributes because the RA prevalence in twins is estimated at a single point in time; studies include twins of all ages some of whom may not yet have developed RA but who will, given time. If the study was repeated when all twin pairs were 100 years old, it is likely that more would have developed RA, because the median age at onset for RA is 55 years in the UK population.[1] This increased concordance over time is likely to be more pronounced in the identical twin pairs and so statistical methods can be used to estimate the heritability, the extent to which the disease risk in a population can be explained by genetic variation. Based on twin studies in the United Kingdom, Finland, the Netherlands and Japan the heritability of RA has been estimated to be ~60%[2-4] but estimates from other studies in twins do vary, possibly related to the smaller sample size and different ways of recruiting subjects.[5,6] In the only study to analyse the findings according to anticitrullinated protein antibody (ACPA) status, heritability estimates for ACPA-negative RA were only slightly lower than for ACPA-positive disease.[4]

Second, family studies consistently confirm that first degree relatives of patients with RA are at increased risk of developing the condition, supporting a genetic component. The most robust data comes from the Icelandic genealogical database, a population-based, computerized genealogy database used to investigate multi-generational relationships between individuals in Iceland, which represents a stable genetic population.[7] The risk ratio for developing RA in siblings of patients with RA was found to be 4.38 (3.26–5.67) with a lesser but still increased risk in second-degree relatives.

Finally, genetic studies themselves have identified genetic variants in different populations that occur consistently more frequently in DNA samples from patients with RA compared to the general population. Using genetic data from large numbers of RA cases and controls, the heritability of ACPA-positive RA has been estimated to be ~50% while in ACPA-negative RA, estimates were much lower (20%).[8] While the magnitude of the estimates of heritability vary in individual populations, overall there is largely consistent support for a genetic component to RA.

These studies also show that genetics cannot explain all the risk of RA and environmental factors are clearly important. Indeed, they confirm that RA is a complex disease where environmental factors are thought to trigger disease in genetically susceptible individuals. The disease is not caused by a single genetic defect, as in Mendelian diseases, but rather by many genetic variants, each of which confers a small risk individually. It may be that there has to be an accumulation of risk factors before the disease is triggered. In some patients who carry multiple genetic risk factors, the influence of the environment will be small whereas in others, who carry few genetic risk factors, multiple environmental factors may need to encountered before the condition is triggered (**Figure 5.1**). One way the environment could affect biology is via epigenetics. Epigenetics refers to heritable changes controlling gene activity that occur without altering genetic code; it includes DNA methylation and other modifications such as histone marks but has been extended to incorporate other factors that regulate gene activity without being strictly heritable, including non-coding RNAs such as microRNAs. Environmental factors such as smoking are known to alter the DNA methylation status of genes[9] and genetic variants could mediate their effect by altering the epigenome.

In recent years, both genetic and environmental risk factors have been investigated but, here only the findings of genetic/epigenetic studies will be considered.

Basics of genetic studies

The genome can be thought of as a book, an instruction manual, present in all cells; the same manual appears in every cell. In our alphabet, we have 26 letters but the genetic code comprises just four

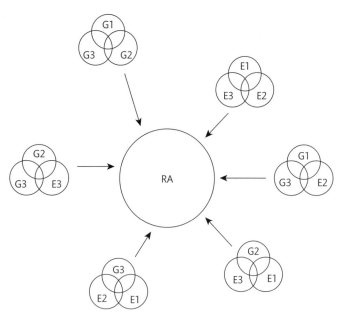

Figure 5.1 Risk of developing RA. Both genetic (G1–3) and environmental (E1–3) factors contribute to RA development, with 60% of the disease risk in the population due to genetic factors. Different combinations of genetic and environmental risk factors combine to trigger disease and several risk factors may be required before a chronic inflammatory response occurs.

base letters (nucleotides): A, G, C, and T. Different arrangements of the nucleotides in groups of three 'spell' different amino acids (akin to words in a sentence). Different combinations of amino acids make up different proteins (sentences). As with any book, typos may occur and in the genetic code, they are fairly common. Usually, a nucleotide changes from one base to another for example a C/T change and we call these single nucleotide polymorphisms (SNPs). One nucleotide is usually found more commonly in the population and is called the common allele while the alternative nucleotide is called the minor allele. Given that we have two copies of each chromosome (with the exception that men have X and Y chromosomes rather than two copies of the X chromosome), a genotype is the combination of the nucleotides present at a particular position in the genome; for example, if there is a C/T SNP present at a position, the resulting genotype could be CC, CT, or TT. The position in the genome at which the SNP is present is denoted by an 'rs' number; for example, a SNP associated with many autoimmune diseases and located within an exon of the *PTPN22* gene is denoted by rs2476601.

In terms of studying risk factors for a disease, genetic variation provides an ideal starting point for several reasons: first, one of the major advantages of genetics is that genomic DNA does not change after conception; the sequence change is present before disease onset allowing people to infer causality. Second, genetic variation can be easily, robustly, reproducibly, and reliably measured using modern genotyping platforms. Third, genetic variants that are found more frequently in patients with a disease highlight key pathways that the body cannot compensate for; there is usually a lot of redundancy in biological systems so if a genetic change is associated with disease, it means the pathway is crucial and cannot be bypassed. It should be noted that the size of the genetic effect bears no relation to the importance of the pathway in disease.

Genetic study design: While there are several study designs that could be adopted to identify genetic variants associated with disease, the simplest, most efficient, and most commonly used is the case-control design. DNA samples from unrelated cases satisfying classification criteria for disease are collected and compared with DNA from healthy or population-based controls. The potential disadvantage of case-control study designs occurs if the cases and controls are not matched for ancestry as spurious associations could occur due to population stratification. To illustrate, the gene for red hair is more common in Scotland. If all RA cases were recruited from Scotland and all controls from Devon, then the gene for red hair would appear to be associated with RA because it would be more common in RA cases than controls. This apparent association would disappear if ancestry was matched and there are now statistical methods to allow for that correction as part of standard quality control procedures in genetic studies.

It should be noted that case-control study designs are most appropriate for common disorders, particularly of late onset, like RA. This is because the genetic variants that contribute to disease risk are likely to be fairly common in the population. By contrast, Mendelian disorders are generally caused by variants that are rare in the general population but have a large effect (i.e. are sufficient to cause disease) if present. Most of those will affect reproductive ability; if the carriers cannot reproduce, the causal variant is not transmitted to the next generation and cannot become common in the general population. For Mendelian disorders, family-based linkage studies are the better design. For common diseases that occur after the fertile/reproductive years, the individual effect of each variant is fairly weak and carriers have already reproduced by the time disease occurs so the variant is established and common in the population ('common' variants or SNPs are those that occur at a frequency >1% population).

Statistical analysis: At its most basic, genetic analysis is simply counting up the number of minor alleles in a group of people without disease (control population, this gives the expected allele frequency) and in a group with disease (observed allele frequency) and comparing whether the frequencies are statistically different using a Chi-squared test. If the observed differs significantly from expected, the allele is said to be associated with disease. Given that there are approximately one million independent SNPs across the genome, using the usual p-value threshold of 0.05 would identify 50 000 SNPs that were associated at that threshold by chance alone. Therefore, in genetics, we adopt much more stringent thresholds before claiming confirmed association of a SNP with disease: $p < 5 \times 10^{-8}$ (derived using a Bonferroni correction method of 0.05/1 000 000).

Results from candidate gene and genome-wide association (GWAS) studies

The first genetic studies in RA selected genes that were thought to be strong candidates in pathogenesis and tested whether variants mapping within or close to those genes were associated with RA. That study design was used to identify the *HLA DRB1* association with RA and associations at the *PTPN22* and *STAT4* loci (reviewed in [10]). As technology advanced and costs improved, it became possible to test variants across the genome simultaneously, using genome-wide association study (GWAS) designs. These used the fact that the genome is inherited in chunks (linkage disequilibrium) so, by genotyping one SNP in a chunk, information on other SNPs in the same area can be inferred. The breakthrough study was published in *Nature* in 2007, the Wellcome Trust Case Control Consortium (WTCCC) study.[11] It tested 2000 DNA samples from each of seven common diseases, including RA, and compared with 3000 population controls. In RA, association with the *HLA DRB1* and *PTPN22* genes was confirmed but a number of other regions were also identified with suggestive evidence for association, some of which were confirmed in subsequent studies including the *TNFAIP3*, *IL2/21*, and *PRCKQ* gene regions. Meta-analysis of separate GWAS studies in RA led to more regions being identified. It quickly became apparent that many genetic variants/regions are associated with more than one autoimmune disease. Researchers in immune-mediated inflammatory diseases came together to design a genotyping array that would allow dense genotyping across those regions of the genome associated with more than one autoimmune disease.[12] By genotyping all known SNPs in 186 regions of the genome, it was possible to get a better understanding of the variants most likely to be associated with disease (fine mapping) and identify further associated regions. In RA, genotyping using Immunochip increased the number of regions associated with RA to 46.[13] The largest RA GWAS, to date, combined all previous GWAS and Immunochip data from multiple populations, including data on 30 000 RA cases and 70 000 controls and identified over 100 genetic regions associated with disease.[14]

Lessons learned/insights gained:

a. The more samples tested, the more genetic regions will be identified due to enhanced study power. The more genetic regions are identified, the more likely it is that different pathways will emerge as underpinning disease. This was exemplified by studies in Crohn's disease where >160 genes have now been identified, which fall into pathways associated with autophagy and innate mucosal defence, cytokine production, JAK/STAT signalling, and lymphocyte activation (reviewed in[15]). Preliminary attempts to place genetic loci in pathways relevant to RA have highlighted the role of immune activation and CD4+ T helper cell differentiation (Box 5.1).

b. ACPA-positive and ACPA-negative RA are probably different diseases characterized by inflammation of synovial joints. It should be noted that most GWAS have been carried out on ACPA-positive RA with fewer studies in seronegative RA. While some genetic regions are associated with both conditions (*HLA DRB1, TNFAIP3, C5orf30, STAT4, ANKRD55, BLK,* and *PTPN22*), others are uniquely associated with seronegative RA (*CLYBL, SMIM21, ANKRD55, PRL,* and *NFIA*) and may provide insight into the different pathogenesis of the diseases.[16] The studies of seronegative RA remain much smaller, and therefore less well-powered, than those in seropositive RA but it is expected that as sample sizes increase, so the number of genetic loci identified will also expand.

c. The associated variants are enriched in genes that are targets of available drugs used to treat RA. For example, a variant within the *IL6R* gene has been confirmed to be associated with RA. The variant causes increased shedding of the membrane-bound receptor to the soluble form and tocilizumab, a biologic drug used to treat RA, also acts on the IL6 pathway. Furthermore, a variant

Box 5.1 Pathways implicated in the pathogenesis of RA based on gene assignments

From the largest GWAS of RA, to date* and using https://www.genecard.org to assign function to genes.

T-cell signalling
TNFRSF14, PTPN22, CD28, CTLA4, PTPRC, TEC, CD83, TRAF6, CD5, UBASH3A, ICOSL, HLA DRB1, CD2

T-cell activation
TNFRSF9, AFF3, STAT4, TAGAP, PRKCQ, GATA3, RASGRP1, RUNX1, AIRE

Cytokine signalling
IL6R, PTPRC, IL6ST, IL20RB, IL20RA, IL21, SH2B3, TYK2, IRAK1

IL2 pathway:
IL2, IL2RA, IL2RB, PTPN2, ILF3, RUNX1

Interferon pathway
IRF4, IRF5, IRF8, IFNGR2, TYK2, RUNX1

Chemokine signalling:
CCR6, CCL19–21, CXCR5

B-cell regulation
FCRL3, FCGR2A, FCGR2B, PTPRC, REL, AFF3, RASGRP1, CLNK, CD83, BLK, ARID5B, RAG1, CD5, CXCR5, IKZF3, CD40

NK cell regulation
CD244, CD226

NFkB pathway
REL, NFKB1E, TNFAIP3, TRAF6, IRAK1

Apoptosis
CASP8, DNASE11L3

MAP Kinase pathway
SPRED2, PRKCH, RASGRP1

*Source: data from Okada Y, Wu D, Trynka G et al. Genetics of rheumatoid arthritis contributes to biology and drug discovery. *Nature* 2014;506:376–81.

mapping close to the *CTLA4* gene is also associated with RA susceptibility. The biologic drug, abatacept, is a CTLA4-Ig fusion protein that acts by blocking costimulation of T cells and is highly effective in treating RA. The implication from these findings is that other genes may be identified that could be the target against which new drugs could be developed.[14] Indeed, it is recognized that genetic evidence to support a role of a gene drug target in disease causation doubles the likelihood of the drug coming to market.[17] This could provide opportunities for drug re-purposing where drugs that are used for one condition (and are known to be safe) could be trialled in a genetically related disease.

d. Linkage disequilibrium means that if one SNP is associated with disease, many surrounding SNPs will also be associated. This has the advantage that genotyping a proportion of SNPs can provide information on many more (an advantage for GWAS genotyping). However, it creates problems in identifying which variant causes disease; that requires subsequent functional studies. If a SNP causes disease, it must have a function. In the simplest scenario, the SNP may alter the protein encoded by the gene. For example, the *IL6R* gene is associated with RA and the causal variant alters receptor shedding by altering the protein encoded by the

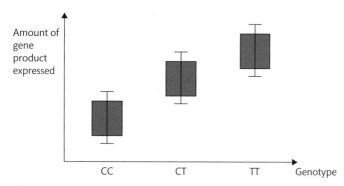

Figure 5.2 An example of an expression quantitative trait locus (eQTL). The genotype at a position in the genome correlates with the amount of gene expression and is one mechanism by which genetic changes contribute to disease causation.

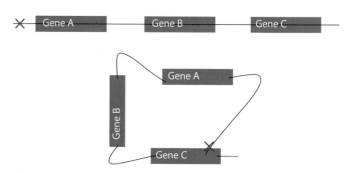

Figure 5.3 Chromosome conformation in linear versus natural folded state of DNA. The SNP associated with a disease (red cross) in the linear state would be predicted to control Gene A. However, when DNA is in its natural folded state, the SNP lies over Gene C and that is the causal gene.

gene. However, only a minority of RA-associated variants alter protein sequences. Alternatively, a SNP may act by controlling expression of a gene, that is, the expression of the gene changes according to the number of risk alleles present in which case it is called an expression quantitative trait locus (eQTL) (**Figure 5.2**). Recently, it has been recognized that the SNP may only have an effect on gene expression in certain cell types or under conditions of stimulation. For example, certain genetic variants may increase expression of a gene only in CD4+ T cells but not in CD8+ T cells or only in CD4+ T cells when those cells are stimulated by bacterial antigens that cause the cells to become activated. A SNP could also act by altering the degradation of the protein or by affecting the binding of a transcription factor. When a region of association is detected, therefore, a number of SNPs are implicated and identifying the causal variant requires further work. Fortunately, there is a wealth of information available on publicly accessible websites that can help to prioritize which variants are more likely to have a function (e.g. the UCSC Genome browser (https://genome.ucsc.edu)). DNA is usually folded and wrapped around histones and, therefore, closed when inactive. A number of histone marks indicate whether DNA is open or closed. Furthermore, enzymes that cleave DNA (DNAases), can only access open DNA. By interrogating public databases, the SNPs that map to open chromatin can be identified in different cell types. Transcription factor databases can inform whether a SNP binds to a transcription factor and whether the alternative allele alters the binding site. However, these databases only allow hypotheses to be formed about whether a variant is functional; ultimately, experimental proof is required to prove that the variant is causal. The field of functional genomics has been transformed in recent years by the discovery of genome editing technologies, the most common of which is the CRISPR/Cas9 system. Genome editing (reviewed in [18]) is a technology based on enzymes produced by bacteria that allow targeting of very specific regions of the genome to alter them. For example, the use of a dead Cas9 enzyme can repress function of a genome region, while other adaptations to the methods mean that SNPs can be deleted and even altered so the causal allele is replaced back to the non-causal variant. These technologies are constantly being refined and improved but are set to revolutionize our understanding of which variants cause disease and how.

e. Most associated variants do not lie within genes but in the regulatory regions between and around genes. Traditionally, the gene thought to be involved in disease was the nearest one to the associated SNP with a likely immune function. Indeed, in the largest RA GWAS, to date, many of the SNPs identified are assigned to more than one gene (often the closest) because it is not clear which they regulate.[14] In the natural state, DNA is folded such that regions of the genome that do not appear to lie close to each other in the linear state, can come into contact. Therefore, intergenic variants that do not appear to map close to a gene could actually lie close to and regulate a different gene when the DNA is folded (**Figure 5.3**). Methods are now available that allow this to be investigated. Studies of RA-associated SNPs have shown, for example, that variants associated with RA within an intron of *COG6*, a gene encoding a component of Golgi apparatus, actually interact with the promoter of the *FOXO1* gene, important in the survival of fibroblast-like synoviocytes in RA but mapping over 1 Mb away.[19] Obviously, this has serious implications when genes are mapped to pathways as the wrong pathways could be targeted for therapy if the incorrect gene is assigned to an associated variant.

f. The data so far indicate that CD4+ T cells appear to be the driver of RA, at least in seropositive disease. This comes from evidence that the SNP variants associated with RA are enriched in regions of the genome called enhancers, which regulate gene expression indirectly and the greatest enrichment is in enhancer regions in CD4+ T cells.[20]

A full understanding of how genetic changes cause RA will require much more work and a comprehensive analysis of the >100 variants so far associated is beyond the scope of this chapter. However, the information learned to date about some of the more important genes is outlined next.

Selected genetic regions

HLA: Since the 1960s it has been recognized that the HLA region has the largest effect on increasing risk of RA and, on average, increases the risk threefold. Variants within the *HLA-DRB1* gene have consistently been associated with RA in multiple populations. Different

SNPs encode different amino acids at different positions within the gene creating hundreds of possible versions of the protein, which is expressed at the surface of immune cells. However, due to linkage disequilibrium, there are 16 common combinations (haplotypes) that represent the majority of variation at the locus.[21] When the protein recognizes and binds a peptide, it presents it to CD4+ T cells and an immune response is mounted if the peptide is recognized as foreign. In the 1980s, it was recognized that the *HLA-DRB1* gene variants associated with RA encoded amino acids at positions 70–74 that shared a similar sequence (QKRAA or QRRAA) leading to the shared epitope hypothesis.[22] Recently, the shared epitope hypothesis has been refined with the discovery that amino acid position 11 had the greatest effect on ACPA-positive RA risk, followed by amino acid positions 71 and 74.[21] A person who carries a valine at position 11 is at 3.8-fold increased risk of ACPA-positive RA. Interestingly, this association is much stronger in smokers, indicating a gene-environment interaction.[23] Outside of the *HLA DRB1* gene, other HLA genes also confer risk of developing RA including *HLA B* (position 9) and *HLA DPB1* (also at position 9). In ACPA-negative RA, although position 11 in *HLA-DRB1* also conferred the greatest effect, a different residue (serine or leucine) was most associated and *HLA B* (position 9) was also associated with susceptibility.[24] The differences in the amino acids that confer risk even at the same position within the peptide binding groove add to the evidence that ACPA-positive and –negative RA are genetically distinct diseases.

PTPN22: A SNP encoding an arginine (R) to tryptophan (W) amino acid substitution at position 620 within the *PTPN22* gene was the second variant to be consistently and robustly associated with RA in multiple populations of Western descent.[25] Interestingly, it is not associated with RA in Eastern populations as the variant is very rare in that population. The same genetic variant is associated with almost all other autoimmune diseases although in Crohn's disease, it is the opposite allele that confers disease risk. The gene encodes a protein tyrosine phosphatase found in the cytoplasm and, in mouse models, acts as a negative regulator of T-cell activation. However, despite being identified in 2004, the mechanism by which it confers risk to RA in humans is still not clear.

TRAF1/C5: For the *HLA DRB1, PTPN22,* and *IL6R* associations referred to previously, the genetic variant associated with RA maps within an exon of the gene and alters an amino acid; hence, the gene can be confidently assigned as the causal gene for RA in that region. However, for the vast majority of RA-associated variants, the causal gene cannot yet be assigned as the associated variant lies between genes (intergenic regions), more than one of which could be the causal gene. The functional studies described previously are required to disentangle which is the causal gene in those scenarios. For example, one of the earliest GWAS studies identified association of RA with a region between two plausible candidate genes, *TRAF1* and *C5*.[26] The *TRAF1* gene encodes a protein involved in the tumour necrosis factor (TNF) inflammatory pathway while *C5* encodes a gene in the complement inflammatory pathway; interestingly, the region was investigated in a simultaneous candidate gene study as C5 had been implicated in animal models of inflammatory arthritis and also showed highly statistically significant association in that study.[27] To date, conclusive evidence to show that one but not the other gene is the causal RA gene is still not established.

6q23 locus: The 6q23 locus has been associated with several autoimmune diseases including RA, systemic lupus erythematosus, psoriasis, and multiple sclerosis but different variants associate with different diseases. In RA, the most associated variant lies between the *TNFAIP3* and *OLIG3* genes but the *IL20RA* and *TFNGR* genes also lie close by. Using the chromosome conformation studies referred to previously, this region of the genome now appears to be a master enhancer, regulating the activity of the *IL20RA, TNFAIP3,* and *IFNGR* genes together.

RA severity genes

While the identification of RA susceptibility genes can provide clues as to the pathogenesis of disease and identify targets for treatment, once patients have developed RA, genetics could potentially be useful in predicting which patients will develop more severe disease, requiring intensive early treatment. However, the identification of genetic markers of RA outcome has proved more challenging than susceptibility markers for several reasons. Firstly, there are a number of outcome measures that could be assessed and none is a perfect proxy for disease severity. The outcome measures that are used may be subjective or objective; for example, while radiographic erosions provide an objective measure of outcome, the presence of erosions may be measured at different times and using different scoring algorithms (Larsen score or Sharpe van der Heijde score) in different joints. Secondly disease outcome varies over time, often deteriorating, but that may also be affected by age and treatment effects. For example, the Health Assessment Questionnaire Disability Index (HAQ-DI) is often viewed as a surrogate for disability but HAQ scores generally improve following initial diagnosis and then deteriorate again over time. Thirdly, the statistical techniques needed to analyse the data are more advanced because the outcome measures often do not follow a normal distribution. For example, many patients will not develop erosions so there are a lot of zero values followed by a normal distribution of erosion scores in most RA patient populations and standard analysis techniques cannot be applied. Finally, it is expensive and time consuming to collect samples and data on patients and then follow them over time with regular assessments of their disease progression and outcome; hence there are few prospective cohorts of patients with good quality longitudinal data on disease outcome and sample sizes are generally modest. It is hoped that, with improvements in electronic patient records and assessments of outcome, such studies will be able to be captured in future using eHealth technology but the challenge of how to collect and store samples to accompany such research studies has not been fully solved.

Despite these challenges, a number of studies have identified genetic variants associated with outcome in RA. Of these, association with the *HLA DRB1* region is the most robustly and consistently replicated across multiple populations. For example, well-powered studies have shown that the same risk variants at positions 11/13 (the two positions are in almost complete linkage disequilibrium so a change at one position is mirrored by a change in the other), 71 and 74 that associate with disease susceptibility also correlate with erosive damage, mortality, disease activity, and HAQ score.[28,29]

Given the association of the major RA susceptibility factor with outcome, several studies have investigated non-HLA RA susceptibility genes as severity markers. Most have used radiographic damage as the severity measure as it is a more objective marker of poor outcome and correlates with disability. Association with RA susceptibility variants mapping to the *TRAF1, IL2RA*, and *IL4R* gene regions have been reported in more than one population but effect sizes are too small to prove clinically useful currently (reviewed in[30]).

Genes that influence disease severity do not necessarily have to be the same as those that associate with susceptibility and one study reported that a SNP in the *FOXO3A* gene region was associated with the disease course of several TNF-mediated conditions, including RA.[31] Carriage of the minor allele reduces the production of pro-inflammatory cytokines, including TNFα, by monocytes and was associated with a less severe disease course in RA.

Genetic factors associated with treatment response

Targeting the right treatments to the right patients would bring immediate patient benefit in RA because a number of treatment options exist and some patients will do well with each option while, in others, disease activity will remain uncontrolled leading to impaired quality of life for the patient.[32] Pharmacogenetics is the study of genetic factors in predicting treatment response but such studies in RA have been limited by the same challenges as those faced in studies of RA severity (i.e. different outcome measures encompassing both subjective and objective components; confounders such as coprescription of methotrexate, adherence and presence of antidrug antibodies, and small sample sizes, with few large prospective longitudinal cohorts with detailed information on response to therapy). Some findings have cast doubt on whether there is even a genetic component to response to TNF inhibitor (TNFi) biologic agents and few genes have been consistently associated with response. For example, association of *PDE3A-SLCO1C1* at genome-wide significance levels with TNFi response has been reported, but not replicated,[33,34] while association of the *PTPRC* gene polymorphism has been associated with TNFi response in some,[35–37] but not all studies.[38,39]

Epigenetics

Genetics cannot explain all disease liability and, while environmental factors are also very important, attention has also turned to other potential risk factors including epigenetic changes. Taking the analogy of the genome as an instruction manual, imagine the instruction manual for a car: to repair the brakes, it is not necessary to read the entire manual but just the section relating to brakes—the rest of the book can be closed. Similarly, although the entire genetic code is present in all nucleated cells, the cell does not necessarily need all the information. Thus, a liver cell needs access to genes that encode drug metabolizing genes but a hair cell does not. There are a number of epigenetic modifications that can occur to DNA but some of the best studied, to date, are described next.

DNA methylation: DNA methylation is one of the mechanisms by which genetic data that is not required by the cell is kept 'closed' because, when methylation is present, it is thought to physically obstruct the ability of transcription factors to bind to the DNA; generally, therefore, higher DNA methylation equates to lower expression levels of a gene. DNA methylation tends to occur at regions of the genome that are rich in cytosine and guanine residues, so-called CpG sites, and the amount of methylation is not an all-or-none phenomenon; rather CpG sites differ in the amount they are methylated. The pattern of methylation is reproduced when cells divide by mitosis and so DNA methylation is heritable (to daughter cells).

The amount of methylation at particular sites can be assessed across the whole genome (epigenome-wide association study (EWAS)) using high throughput array-based technology making it an attractive technology to apply to investigate disease causation or response to treatment. DNA methylation could be an independent risk factor in itself; it could provide a mechanism by which genetic changes alter gene transcription or function or, conversely, it may provide a mechanism through which environmental factors can induce changes in cellular activity without affecting the genetic code. In support of the former, widespread changes in DNA methylation have been reported in patients with RA compared with healthy controls. For example, global hypomethylation in peripheral cell subsets in RA has been reported in early RA before treatment.[40] Comparison of RA and osteoarthritis (OA) synovial fibroblasts have shown numerous differences in methylation and these are enriched on pathways relevant to the pathogenesis of RA.[41] However, whether these differences in DNA methylation are a result of disease or causal is difficult to disentangle. In type 1 diabetes, methylation changes have been observed to precede disease onset,[42] suggesting they could play a role in pathogenesis.

However, epigenetic changes could simply arise due to underlying genetic differences; twin studies potentially provide a way of separating genetic from epigenetic effects as identical twins carry the same genetic code. One study reported a statistically significant difference in DNA methylation between monozygotic but RA-discordant twins, at the *EXOSC1* gene; this finding was not replicated in a comparison of unrelated cases with RA compared with controls although it should be noted that small numbers of twins were included so the study may, therefore, have been underpowered.[43]

An alternative explanation is that methylation differences are mediators of genetic associations with disease (i.e. the methylation differences seen are due to underlying genetic changes, which act through regulating the degree of methylation at a particular site in the genome). The largest such study identified nine clusters of differentially methylated signatures in the HLA region suggesting that the genetic effect of HLA risk variants could be mediated, in part, by controlling DNA methylation.[44] Other researchers have integrated information on genetic variants and DNA methylation differences to identify genes that could be causal in RA; for example, an RA-associated genetic variant mapping to an enhancer region close to the *LBH* gene, which is involved in limb bud and heart development, was found to influence the behaviour of fibroblast-like synoviocytes by affecting the level of methylation of the enhancer and, therefore, the amount of gene transcription.[45]

DNA methylation could act as a mediator of environmental risk factors. For example, smoking has been shown to alter the methylation of numerous genes to the extent that epigenetic signatures of current, past, and never smokers have been proposed.[46] Furthermore, enrichment of differentially methylated sites was seen for regions associated with RA in current and former smokers compared with never smokers. An interaction between *HLA DRB1* and smoking in the risk of ACPA+ RA has previously been reported but a recent study found that one variant mapping to the HLA region showed higher levels of methylation in patients carrying the RA risk allele and who were current smokers but the same relationship was not seen in non-smokers.[47] This finding was replicated in a Malaysian cohort of RA cases and controls and mediation analysis suggested that DNA methylation may mediate the gene-environment interaction between HLA and smoking on the risk of developing ACPA + RA.

Interestingly, two studies have reported that methylation differences, including genes of the *HOX* family important in controlling tissue differences in embryonic development, between cells in different joints suggesting that methylation changes may affect the pattern of joint involvement.[48,49]

microRNAs: microRNAs are small non-coding RNAs, 19–25 nucleotides long while long non-coding RNAs are >200 nucleotides in length and both can reduce the translation of messenger RNA into protein or increase degradation of mRNA. Studies have confirmed overexpression of miRNA-155 and miRNA-146a in RA compared with OA in synovial tissue and PBMCs (reviewed in[50]). While the targets of miRNA-155 are unknown, in RA synovial fibroblasts, miRNA-155 overexpression was associated with reduced levels of matrix metalloproteinases while in monocytes, expression correlated with pro-inflammatory chemokine receptor expression. A recent study also suggested a key role in regulating B-cell activity in RA.[51,52] The target of miRNA-146a include IRAK1, TRAF6, and STAT1, which are all involved in regulation of pro-inflammatory pathways.

Epigenetics in treatment response

Studies have shown that DNA methylation changes with treatment. For example, methotrexate has been found to reduce methylation at the FOXP3 locus in regulatory T cells, thereby normalizing their function.[53] Hence, epigenetic changes may also provide biomarkers of treatment response. One study of 46 patients with early inflammatory arthritis who subsequently received conventional synthetic DMARD reported that pretreatment methylation status at *ADAMTSL2* and *BTN3A2* associated with response status by 6 months.[54] A study of etanercept response found that methylation at the *LRPAP1* gene in pretreatment samples correlated with response by 6 months. A genetic variant was associated with the amount of methylation present and the genetic variant also associated with treatment response in an independent group of patients treated with TNF inhibitor drugs, although the ability to predict response was too small to be clinically useful alone.[55]

Low expression of miRNA-22 combined with high expression of miRNA-886.3p was reported to be associated with a good response to adalimumab[56] but other studies have not replicated the findings.[57]

Conclusion

Understanding the genetic basis to RA can provide insight into disease mechanisms and identify targets for new or existing drug treatments. It will be important to confidently assign the associated SNPs to the genes they regulate in order to identify the pathways underlying disease in different patients and functional genomics studies are necessary to understand the mechanisms by which genes contribute to disease. Identifying genetic factors that can predict which patients will have severe disease or informing the selection

of the treatments most likely to be effective potentially has more immediate clinical benefit but those studies currently lag behind the studies of susceptibility due to issues with defining the outcome measures and the sample sizes available to test. However, precision, or personalized medicine is an aspiration for the future in the management of RA and genetic/epigenetic factors will undoubtedly be important.

REFERENCES

1. Symmons D, Turner G, Webb R, et al. The prevalence of rheumatoid arthritis in the United Kingdom: new estimates for a new century. *Rheumatology (Oxford)* 2002;41:793–800.
2. MacGregor AJ, Snieder H, Rigby AS, et al. Characterizing the quantitative genetic contribution to rheumatoid arthritis using data from twins. *Arthritis Rheum* 2000;43:30–7.
3. Terao C, Ikari K, Nakayamada S, et al. A twin study of rheumatoid arthritis in the Japanese population. *Mod Rheumatol* 2016;26:685–9.
4. van der Woude D, Houwing-Duistermaat JJ, Toes RE, et al. Quantitative heritability of anti-citrullinated protein antibody-positive and anti-citrullinated protein antibody-negative rheumatoid arthritis. *Arthritis Rheum* 2009;60:916–23.
5. Svendsen AJ, Holm NV, Kyvik K, Petersen PH, Junker P. Relative importance of genetic effects in rheumatoid arthritis: historical cohort study of Danish nationwide twin population. *BMJ* 2002;324:264–6.
6. Svendsen AJ, Kyvik KO, Houen G, et al. On the origin of rheumatoid arthritis: the impact of environment and genes—a population-based twin study. *PLoS One* 2013;8:e57304.
7. Grant SF, Thorleifsson G, Frigge ML, et al. The inheritance of rheumatoid arthritis in Iceland. *Arthritis Rheum* 2001;44:2247–54.
8. Frisell T, Holmqvist M, Kallberg H, Klareskog L, Alfredsson L, Askling J. Familial risks and heritability of rheumatoid arthritis: role of rheumatoid factor/anti-citrullinated protein antibody status, number and type of affected relatives, sex, and age. *Arthritis Rheum* 2013;65:2773–82.
9. Wilson R, Wahl S, Pfeiffer L, et al. The dynamics of smoking-related disturbed methylation: a two time-point study of methylation change in smokers, non-smokers and former smokers. *BMC Genomics* 2017;18:805.
10. Eyre S, Orozco G, Worthington J. The genetics revolution in rheumatology: large scale genomic arrays and genetic mapping. *Nat Rev Rheumatol* 2017;13:421–32.
11. Wellcome Trust Case Control Consortium. Genome-wide association study of 14,000 cases of seven common diseases and 3,000 shared controls. *Nature* 2007;447:661–78.
12. Cortes A, Brown MA. Promise and pitfalls of the Immunochip. *Arthritis Res Ther* 2011;13:101.
13. Eyre S, Bowes J, Diogo D, et al. High-density genetic mapping identifies new susceptibility loci for rheumatoid arthritis. *Nat Genet* 2012;44:1336–40.
14. Okada Y, Wu D, Trynka G, et al. Genetics of rheumatoid arthritis contributes to biology and drug discovery. *Nature* 2014;506:376–81.
15. de Lange KM, Barrett JC. Understanding inflammatory bowel disease via immunogenetics. *J Autoimmun* 2015;64:91–100.
16. Viatte S, Massey J, Bowes J, et al. Replication of associations of genetic loci outside the HLA region with susceptibility to

anti-cyclic citrullinated peptide-negative rheumatoid arthritis. *Arthritis Rheumatol* 2016;68:1603–13.

17. Nelson MR, Tipney H, Painter JL, et al. The support of human genetic evidence for approved drug indications. *Nat Genet* 2015;47:856–60.

18. Wang HX, Li M, Lee CM, et al. CRISPR/Cas9-based genome editing for disease modeling and therapy: challenges and opportunities for nonviral delivery. *Chem Rev* 2017;117:9874–906.

19. Martin P, McGovern A, Orozco G, et al. Capture Hi-C reveals novel candidate genes and complex long-range interactions with related autoimmune risk loci. *Nat Commun* 2015;6:10069.

20. Trynka G, Sandor C, Han B, et al. Chromatin marks identify critical cell types for fine mapping complex trait variants. *Nat Genet* 2013;45:124–30.

21. Raychaudhuri S, Sandor C, Stahl EA, et al. Five amino acids in three HLA proteins explain most of the association between MHC and seropositive rheumatoid arthritis. *Nat Genet* 2012;44:291–6.

22. Gregersen PK, Silver J, Winchester RJ. The shared epitope hypothesis. An approach to understanding the molecular genetics of susceptibility to rheumatoid arthritis. *Arthritis Rheum* 1987;30:1205–13.

23. Kim K, Jiang X, Cui J, et al. Interactions between amino acid-defined major histocompatibility complex class II variants and smoking in seropositive rheumatoid arthritis. *Arthritis Rheumatol* 2015;67:2611–23.

24. Han B, Diogo D, Eyre S, et al. Fine mapping seronegative and seropositive rheumatoid arthritis to shared and distinct HLA alleles by adjusting for the effects of heterogeneity. *Am J Hum Genet* 2014;94:522–32.

25. Begovich AB, Carlton VE, Honigberg LA, et al. A missense single-nucleotide polymorphism in a gene encoding a protein tyrosine phosphatase (PTPN22) is associated with rheumatoid arthritis. *Am J Hum Genet* 2004;75:330–7.

26. Plenge RM, Seielstad M, Padyukov L, et al. TRAF1-C5 as a risk locus for rheumatoid arthritis—a genome-wide study. *N Engl J Med* 2007;357:1199–209.

27. Kurreeman FA, Padyukov L, Marques RB, et al. A candidate gene approach identifies the TRAF1/C5 region as a risk factor for rheumatoid arthritis. *PLoS Med* 2007;4:e278.

28. Viatte S, Plant D, Han B, et al. Association of HLA-DRB1 haplotypes with rheumatoid arthritis severity, mortality, and treatment response. *JAMA* 2015;313:1645–56.

29. Ling SF, Viatte S, Lunt M, et al. HLA-DRB1 amino acid positions 11/13, 71, and 74 are associated with inflammation level, disease activity, and the Health Assessment Questionnaire score in patients with inflammatory polyarthritis. *Arthritis Rheumatol* 2016;68:2618–28.

30. Viatte S, Barton A. Genetics of rheumatoid arthritis susceptibility, severity, and treatment response. *Semin Immunopathol* 2017;39:395–408.

31. Lee JC, Espeli M, Anderson CA, et al. Human SNP links differential outcomes in inflammatory and infectious disease to a FOXO3-regulated pathway. *Cell* 2013;155:57–69.

32. Hyrich KL, Watson KD, Silman AJ, Symmons DP. Predictors of response to anti-TNF-alpha therapy among patients with rheumatoid arthritis: results from the British Society for Rheumatology Biologics Register. *Rheumatology (Oxford)* 2006;45:1558–65.

33. Acosta-Colman I, Palau N, Tornero J, et al. GWAS replication study confirms the association of PDE3A-SLCO1C1 with anti-TNF therapy response in rheumatoid arthritis. *Pharmacogenomics* 2013;14:727–34.

34. Smith SL, Plant D, Lee XH, et al. Previously reported PDE3A-SLCO1C1 genetic variant does not correlate with anti-TNF response in a large UK rheumatoid arthritis cohort. *Pharmacogenomics* 2016;17:715–20.

35. Cui J, Saevarsdottir S, Thomson B, et al. Rheumatoid arthritis risk allele PTPRC is also associated with response to anti-tumor necrosis factor alpha therapy. *Arthritis Rheum* 2010;62:1849–61.

36. Plant D, Prajapati R, Hyrich KL, et al. Replication of association of the PTPRC gene with response to anti-tumor necrosis factor therapy in a large UK cohort. *Arthritis Rheum* 2012;64:665–70.

37. Ferreiro-Iglesias A, Montes A, Perez-Pampin E, et al. Replication of PTPRC as genetic biomarker of response to TNF inhibitors in patients with rheumatoid arthritis. *Pharmacogenomics J* 2016;16:137–40.

38. Canhao H, Rodrigues AM, Santos MJ, et al. TRAF1/C5 but not PTPRC variants are potential predictors of rheumatoid arthritis response to anti-tumor necrosis factor therapy. *Biomed Res Int* 2015;2015:490295.

39. Zervou MI, Myrthianou E, Flouri I, et al. Lack of association of variants previously associated with anti-TNF medication response in rheumatoid arthritis patients: results from a homogeneous Greek population. *PLoS One* 2013;8:e74375.

40. de Andres MC, Perez-Pampin E, Calaza M, et al. Assessment of global DNA methylation in peripheral blood cell subpopulations of early rheumatoid arthritis before and after methotrexate. *Arthritis Res Ther* 2015;17:233.

41. Whitaker JW, Shoemaker R, Boyle DL, et al. An imprinted rheumatoid arthritis methylome signature reflects pathogenic phenotype. *Genome Med* 2013;5:40.

42. Rakyan VK, Beyan H, Down TA, et al. Identification of type 1 diabetes-associated DNA methylation variable positions that precede disease diagnosis. *PLoS Genet* 2011;7:e1002300.

43. Gomez-Cabrero D, Almgren M, Sjoholm LK, et al. High-specificity bioinformatics framework for epigenomic profiling of discordant twins reveals specific and shared markers for ACPA and ACPA-positive rheumatoid arthritis. *Genome Med* 2016;8:124.

44. Liu Y, Aryee MJ, Padyukov L, et al. Epigenome-wide association data implicate DNA methylation as an intermediary of genetic risk in rheumatoid arthritis. *Nat Biotechnol* 2013;31:142–7.

45. Hammaker D, Whitaker JW, Maeshima K, et al. LBH gene transcription regulation by the interplay of an enhancer risk allele and DNA Methylation in Rheumatoid Arthritis. *Arthritis Rheumatol* 2016;68:2637–45.

46. Joehanes R, Just AC, Marioni RE, et al. Epigenetic signatures of cigarette smoking. *Circ Cardiovasc Genet* 2016;9:436–47.

47. Meng W, Zhu Z, Jiang X, et al. DNA methylation mediates genotype and smoking interaction in the development of anti-citrullinated peptide antibody-positive rheumatoid arthritis. *Arthritis Res Ther* 2017;19:71.

48. Frank-Bertoncelj M, Trenkmann M, Klein K, et al. Epigenetically-driven anatomical diversity of synovial fibroblasts guides joint-specific fibroblast functions. *Nat Commun* 2017;8:14852.

49. Ai R, Hammaker D, Boyle DL, et al. Joint-specific DNA methylation and transcriptome signatures in rheumatoid arthritis identify distinct pathogenic processes. *Nat Commun* 2016;7:11849.

50. Ospelt C, Gay S, Klein K. Epigenetics in the pathogenesis of RA. *Semin Immunopathol* 2017;39:409–19.

51. Alivernini S, Kurowska-Stolarska M, Tolusso B, et al. MicroRNA-155 influences B-cell function through PU.1 in rheumatoid arthritis. *Nat Commun* 2016;7:12970.

52. Alivernini S, Gremese E, McSharry C, et al. MicroRNA-155-at the critical interface of innate and adaptive immunity in arthritis. *Front Immunol* 2017;8:1932.
53. Cribbs AP, Kennedy A, Penn H, et al. Methotrexate restores regulatory T cell function through demethylation of the FoxP3 upstream enhancer in patients with rheumatoid arthritis. *Arthritis Rheumatol* 2015;67:1182–92.
54. Glossop JR, Nixon NB, Emes RD, et al. DNA methylation at diagnosis is associated with response to disease-modifying drugs in early rheumatoid arthritis. *Epigenomics* 2017;9:419–28.
55. Plant D, Webster A, Nair N, et al. Differential methylation as a biomarker of response to etanercept in patients with rheumatoid arthritis. *Arthritis Rheumatol* 2016;68:1353–60.
56. Krintel SB, Dehlendorff C, Hetland ML, et al. Prediction of treatment response to adalimumab: a double-blind placebo-controlled study of circulating microRNA in patients with early rheumatoid arthritis. *Pharmacogenomics J* 2016;16:141–6.
57. Cuppen BV, Rossato M, Fritsch-Stork RD, et al. Can baseline serum microRNAs predict response to TNF-alpha inhibitors in rheumatoid arthritis? *Arthritis Res Ther* 2016;18:189.

6

Dysregulation of synovial fibroblasts in rheumatoid arthritis

Thomas Crowley, Jason D. Turner, Andrew Filer, Andy Clarke, and Chris Buckley

More than just structural elements: Inflammatory roles of synovial fibroblasts

Fibroblasts are ubiquitous stromal cells, with populations found in all organs. The traditional role of fibroblasts was thought to be mainly structural; making and modifying extracellular matrix.

It is now clear that fibroblasts are heavily involved in the immune response and perform multiple roles in inflammation.[1-4] They can respond to danger signals through the expression of Toll-like receptors (TLRs) 1, 2, 3, 4, 5, and 6, which allow fibroblasts to detect and mount a response to pathogen associated molecular patterns.[5] Fibroblasts are also capable of performing antigen presentation and phagocytosis/efferocytosis (phagocytosis of apoptotic or necrotic cells), albeit to a lesser extent than macrophages.[6,7]

A key role for fibroblasts in the joint, termed fibroblast-like synoviocytes (FLS), is to provide lubrication and support for the joint capsule. FLS produce hyaluronan, the size of which dictates the viscosity and thus the support provided by the synovial fluid.[8] Fibroblasts also provide lubricin, another mediator of joint lubrication.[9]

FLS are capable of responding to a wide variety of inflammatory mediators and of secreting a range of pro-inflammatory cytokines and chemokines such as IL-23p19, and IL-6, and also CCL2, CCL3, CCL4, CXCL8, CXCL10, and CXCL12.[10-16] The fibroblast response may therefore promote the recruitment of neutrophils, monocytes, and T lymphocytes. While this facilitates direct leukocyte recruitment, fibroblasts indirectly regulate these cells' migration into tissue by modulating the endothelial cell (EC) response to stimulation (reviewed by McGettrick[17]). In addition to the role of fibroblasts in the recruitment of cells they can also act to retain leukocytes in the tissue.

Once leukocytes reach synovial tissue, fibroblasts interact with them to provide pro-survival signals and dictate activation or differentiation via both secreted products and cell contact-dependent mechanisms.[18] FLS can also modulate the inflammatory responses of leukocytes. Examples include production of granulocyte-macrophage colony-stimulating factor (GM-CSF), which promotes survival of neutrophils and differentiation of monocytes to pro-inflammatory macrophages.[19-21] Similarly, IL-6 is a fibroblast product capable of inducing CD4+ T-cell differentiation towards Th17 cells.[22-24]

Taken together the ability of fibroblasts to produce and respond to many factors involved in the immune system indicates the degree to which they are involved in orchestrating the inflammatory response in rheumatoid arthritis (RA). This level of involvement demonstrates the importance of fibroblasts in inflammation and indicates the shift from transient to chronic inflammation in RA could be facilitated in part by synovial fibroblasts.

Aggressive fibroblasts in rheumatoid arthritis

The pathologic role of FLS in RA has been reviewed extensively.[25] Their role as initiators of, or responders to synovial inflammation is still debated after being initially proposed nearly 30 years ago.[26,27] Nevertheless, it is well recognized that they are fundamentally changed in the tissues of patients with longstanding RA undergoing arthroplasty.

Fibroblasts contribute to synovial hyperplasia

One of the characteristic traits of RA is the expansion of a thin synovial membrane into a grossly enlarged invasive structure named the pannus. FLS are a key cellular constituent of the invasive pannus tissue that actively erodes cartilage and bone in severe disease. This dominance is due to a combination of RA-FLS becoming proliferative, hyperplastic, and resistant to apoptosis.[28-30]

RA-FLS have spontaneously activated NFκB, leading to constitutively high levels of IL-6 production.[31] This may contribute to the apoptosis-resistant nature of cells involved in the development of RA, as NFκB products inhibit Fas ligand (FasL) and tumour necrosis factor alpha (TNFα) apoptosis signals in RA-FLS.[32-34] The resistance of RA-FLS to FasL induced apoptosis is mediated by several factors such as increased Bcl-2.[33] Aberrantly low IκBα may also contribute to articular damage as restoration of IκBα expression in synovial macrophages and fibroblasts had little effect on IL-10, IL-11, and

IL-1ra expression but abrogated matrix metalloproteinase (MMP) and pro-inflammatory cytokine expression.[35,36] Increased MMP expression means RA-FLS become destructive in the articular joint.[37-40]

Fibroblasts drive chronic inflammation

Interestingly, despite their role in inflammation, FLS (even in RA) produce limited quantities of TNFα and IL-1.[41-44] While they do not produce these mediators in meaningful amounts they respond strongly to them expressing several pro-inflammatory mediators such as IL-6, GM-CSF, MMPs, CXCL12, CXCL8, and CCL2 (Figure 6.1).[10,12,19,31,45,46] IL-17, a cytokine frequently implicated in the pathogenesis of RA, elicits an increase in IL-6 and CXCL8 production from RA-FLS and acts in synergy with TNFα to increase GM-CSF production.[13,19,47,48] These observations suggest that a functional 'symbiosis' between synovial macrophages that do produce IL-1 and TNFα and fibroblasts that respond to these cytokines may lie at the heart of the switch to disease persistence that underlies pathology in RA.

Two IL-6 signalling mechanisms are described: in **classical** signalling the cytokine binds directly to its membrane-bound alpha receptor subunit IL-6R, in turn coupled to its signal-transducing beta receptor subunit gp130; alternatively, ligand-binding to a soluble version of the alpha receptor subunit, sIL-6R, facilitates gp130-mediated *trans*-signalling in the absence of membrane-bound IL-6R expression.[49] RA-FLS rely on the trans-signalling mechanism, and have been shown to participate in a pro-inflammatory feedback loop in the presence of sIL-6R. Hence, sIL-6R with IL-6, but not IL-6 alone, induces secretion of receptor activator of nuclear factor kappa-B ligand (RANKL), CCL2, and IL-6 but not IL-8 and has been shown to induce RA-FLS proliferation.[50-54] Targeting trans-signalling rather than all IL-6 signalling has been shown to be effective in treating RA, suggesting an inflammatory role for trans-signalling in RA-FLS.[52,55-57]

Fibroblasts regulate leukocyte migration and survival

FLS in the RA joint play an important role in regulating leukocyte numbers through soluble mediator secretion and contact mediated mechanisms. Healthy FLS secrete chemokines but also inhibit recruitment of leukocytes by EC. However, FLS taken from the joints of patients with RA increase leukocyte adhesion to, and migration between, ECs. This difference is due to a complex interplay of IL-6 and TGFβ, in combination with other factors, during EC activation.[15] In systems lacking ECs, RA-FLS were similarly shown to increase T-cell recruitment due to their increased secretion of CXCL12, which is aberrantly expressed by FLS in RA.[10]

RA-FLS upregulate CXCL8, CCL5, and CCL8 leading to recruitment of neutrophils, monocytes, and CD4+ T cells to sites of inflammation.[10,58-60] RA-FLS preferentially recruit Th1 over Th2 polarized T lymphocytes, and predominantly use CCL5 to effect this.[14] The interaction of RA-FLS with infiltrating leukocytes also differs from that of healthy counterparts. RA-FLS can induce CD25[low] T cells to differentiate into Th17 cells rather than Tregs, establishing a pro-inflammatory feedback loop.[61]

As with their healthy counterparts RA-FLS can interact with neutrophils.[18] RA-FLS stimulated with CYR61, an extracellular matrix (ECM) protein increased in the RA synovium that is known to induce FLS proliferation, increase IL-8 production, and thus recruit neutrophils.[41] GM-CSF is higher in the RA synovium than that of controls and significantly increases neutrophil survival *in vitro*.[19] RA-FLS have also been shown to support increased survival of macrophages and T cells and modulate the macrophage response to TNFα through the up- and downregulation of pro- and anti-inflammatory gene expression.[18,61,62]

RA-FLS mediate increased survival of B cells and natural killer (NK) cells through the expression of IL-15, B-cell activating factor (BAFF), and a proliferation-inducing ligand (APRIL).[58,63-65] IL-15 engages the IL-15 receptor on NK and B cells, the expression of which on B cells is increased by BAFF stimulation, to increase survival of these cells in comparison to monoculture or coculture with osteoarthritis-fibroblast-like synoviocytes (OA-FLS) or dermal fibroblasts. Increasing the survival of infiltrating leukocytes is an important pathological feature as the combination of increased recruitment and survival maintains the presence of leukocyte infiltrates in the inflamed synovium.

Fibroblasts regulate bone and cartilage destruction

In addition to orchestrating an inappropriate immune response, RA-FLS drive other aspects of RA including inflammation-induced bone destruction. RA-FLS are capable of modulating the osteoblast/osteoclast axis through the expression of the pro-osteoclast differentiation factor RANKL.[39,40] This feature is specific to RA compared to osteoarthritis (OA) as RANKL is known to be expressed at significantly higher levels in the lining layer of the synovium in RA compared to OA and, *in vitro*, RANKL expression can be elicited in RA-FLS but not OA-FLS. Furthermore, coculturing monocytes and RA-FLS results in the differentiation of monocytes into osteoclasts.[40]

RA-FLS are potent mediators of articular cartilage damage, possessing the machinery necessary to directly degrade the collagenous tissue. In *in vitro* assays RA-FLS produce cathepsins B, D, and L and also MMP9, 1, and 3, which facilitate the damage and invasion of cartilage. When cultured RA-FLS and cartilage are implanted in a mouse with severe combined immunodeficiency (SCID) the fibroblasts continue to invade the cartilage autonomously whereas OA-FLS do not.[66-72] Furthermore, in the SCID mouse model RA-FLS are able to migrate to cartilage at sites distant from the initial site at which they were introduced, providing a potential explanation for the extended joint involvement observed clinically in RA.[73] The

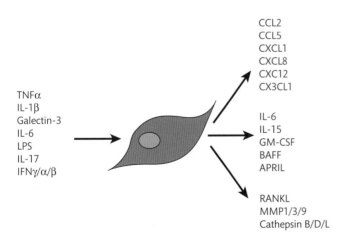

TNFα
IL-1β
Galectin-3
IL-6
LPS
IL-17
IFNγ/α/β

CCL2
CCL5
CXCL1
CXCL8
CXC12
CX3CL1

IL-6
IL-15
GM-CSF
BAFF
APRIL

RANKL
MMP1/3/9
Cathepsin B/D/L

Figure 6.1 Fibroblasts expressing pro-inflammatory mediators.

tumour suppressor gene p53 may also be involved in regulating the invasiveness of RA-FLS as increased p53 expression increases the invasiveness of normal fibroblasts and has also been demonstrated in RA-FLS that have invaded cartilage.[67,70,74,75]

Taken together the evidence that RA-FLS maintain their ability to modulate the immune system and drive bone and cartilage destruction even after removal from the joint and *in vitro* culture demonstrates the altered imprinted and aggressive phenotype of these fibroblasts and indicates epigenetic changes may occur in RA-FLS that lead to this behaviour.

The epigenetic landscape of fibroblasts in RA

The term 'epigenetic' refers to processes that influence gene expression without involving changes in nucleotide sequence. It was originally applied to long-lasting alterations of gene expression, which survived through cell division, and could even be passed from one generation to the next. Today, the term is also applied to shorter-lived mechanisms of regulation of gene expression.[76] Accumulated evidence suggests that RA-FLS have an 'imprinted' aggressive phenotype that may be mediated through disturbances in the epigenetic regulation of these cell types. There are now numerous studies demonstrating an altered epigenetic landscape, altered chromatin access, and epigenetic regulation in RA-FLS.[77–83]

Histone modifications contribute to fibroblast phenotype

At a high-level gene expression can be regulated through modification of chromatin accessibility. Repression and activation of chromatin, which regulates access to DNA of transcriptional machinery and activators, occurs at several levels. Post-translational modifications of DNA-associated histone proteins (such as acetylation, methylation, phosphorylation, and ubiquitination) can exert activating or repressive effects. For instance, histone methylation can act both as a repressive and permissive regulatory mechanism: H3K27me3 (trimethylation of histone 3 at lysine position 27) is repressive, but H3K4me3 is permissive.[84] By contrast most acetylation modifications of histones are associated with open chromatin (and active gene transcription), and is globally increased in RA compared to OA-FLS.[82] Direct modifications of the DNA (primarily methylation) at promoter sites generally represses gene expression, although methylation at other sites such as gene bodies can promote expression.[80,85,86] Aberrant profiles of such epigenetic traits have been shown to increase inflammatory mediators and curtail inhibitory aspects of RA and other chronic inflammatory diseases.[80,87,88]

The phenotypes of different arthritic disorders are often manifested in different patterns of joint involvement affecting small rather than large joints or upper limbs rather than lower, for example. Frank-Bertoncelj[89] showed that in cultured synovial fibroblasts from OA and RA, the expression of genes involved in specifying anatomical location that are patterned during embryogenesis, such as *HOX* genes, is regulated through DNA methylation and chromatin modifications. Of interest, differences in gene expression between sites resulted in the differential enrichment of disease pathways relevant to arthritis at different joints.

DNA methylation contributes to fibroblast phenotype

The DNA of FLS from RA patients is globally hypomethylated.[85,90] Further evidence from both RA and non-RA studies has shown hypomethylation at the IL6 promoter and the promoters of other pro-inflammatory cytokines.[78,79,83,87,91–93] Evidence for this hypomethylated state has been shown by the treatment of healthy synovial fibroblasts with 5-azacytidine, a demethylating agent. After three months of treatment, more than 180 genes were upregulated by at least twofold, including many genes implicated in RA pathogenesis.[90,94] While global hypomethylation is reported, it is not the case for all genes. The promoter of Death receptor three, for example, is hypermethylated in RA-FLS. This has the consequence of making RA-FLS more resistant to apoptosis.[30]

Evidence to support the hypothesis that RA-FLS are epigenetically imprinted even at the earliest stages of clinically evident disease has been demonstrated through investigation of DNA methylation in cultured fibroblasts from patients with early resolving arthritis and short or long duration RA. Karouzakis[95] found in each group a set of CpG islands, regions of DNA at which methylation occurs, which were differentially methylated and specific for each respective stage of arthritis. Investigating the differentially methylated sites highlighted pathways related to cell adhesion, cytoskeletal regulation, and antigen presentation. Importantly these findings indicate synovial fibroblasts may be important in driving persistence from the earliest stages of RA.

Micro-ribonucleic acids (RNAs) contribute to fibroblast phenotype

Other methods of gene regulation are also under scrutiny as possible methods by which RA-FLS are imprinted with an invasive phenotype. microRNAs (miRNAs), small non-coding RNA sequences that can regulate the stability and expression of multiple coding mRNA species, are one such mechanism and are also regulated by the aforementioned epigenetic mechanisms.[96] Investigations into the possible function of these molecules in the RA-FLS phenotype have recently been initiated. miR-155, miR-146a, and miR-22 are all differentially expressed between RA-FLS and OA-FLS with miR-155 and miR-146a being higher in RA-FLS than OA-FLS and miR-22 lower.[97–100] miR-155 expression is increased in RA-FLS by TNFα stimulation and downregulates the expression of MMP3 and MMP1 upon TLR or IL-1β stimulation and also inhibits JAK2/STAT3 phosphorylation in response to IL-6 stimulation. Additionally, in synovial tissue miR-155 expression is eightfold higher in RA than osteoarthritis which could reflect an attempt to restrain the chronic inflammatory state. miR-22 acts to inhibit proliferation and IL-6 production by downregulating Cry61 but is expressed at lower levels in RA than osteoarthritis synovial tissue and which may reflect the aggressive phenotype of RA-FLS.

Chronic and repeated inflammatory exposure: The concept of fibroblast memory

Throughout the instigation and perpetuation of RA, cells in the synovium receive repeated and eventually chronic stimulation by pro-inflammatory mediators. It is therefore important to understand the effect of chronic stimulation on FLS. Lee[101] reported that RA-FLS mount an unremitting response to TNFα involving continued transcription and secretion of inflammatory mediators. This was maintained for at least four days (the end of the observation period) as long as TNFα was still present. This suggests an unremitting response to pro-inflammatory mediators and perhaps a pathological inability to self-regulate. This would fit well with the 'delinquent' phenotype ascribed to them.[26] On a similar note, Dakin[102] showed that tendon fibroblasts from individuals with previous tendon injuries maintained high levels of surface markers such as podoplanin (PDPN) and CD206, both of which are known to be activation markers of fibroblasts.

An emerging concept in the RA field is that of non-lymphocytic stromal memory.[103] A commonly reported aspect of the RA natural history is periods of apparent remission followed by painful inflammatory flares. Could these represent 'remembered' inflammatory challenges which disease-phenotype cells respond to in an aggressive manner? This question fits well with the concept of tissue-resident cells learning from previous inflammatory episodes. Such concepts have indeed been demonstrated. Dakin[102] not only showed that previously injured tendon fibroblasts retain activation markers but also showed them to mount a greater inflammatory response to IL-1α *in vitro*.

Fibroblasts generate a memory response from previous inflammation

In the RA field, recent work has demonstrated that FLS have a form of inflammatory memory wherein the second response to inflammatory pressure is altered by exposure to a previous challenge. Sohn[104] demonstrated that RA-FLS secreted limited quantities of CXCL9, CXCL10, and CXCL11 in response to interferon α, β, or γ, unless previously exposed to TNFα. The 'primed' cells were capable of substantial secretions of the aforementioned chemokines upon exposure to interferons even when the TNFα was removed and an anti-TNF therapy was added for 24h as a blocking agent.

Crowley[105] demonstrated similar findings by challenging FLS twice with TNFα or IL-1α. This led to an augmented secretion of IL-6 and CCL5 but not IL-8, indicating a gene-specific form of innate immune memory. However, it should be noted that this research also demonstrated the same phenomenon in control FLS from arthralgia patients with no evidence of synovitis upon exploratory arthroscopy. This may then represent an inherent inflammatory trait in the synovium which could represent FLS as cells already on the road to aggressive inflammatory phenotypes.

The increased number of publications in this area has demonstrated the nuanced nature of innate memory in fibroblasts. Rather than challenge with endogenous mediators Klein et al examined FLS memory with repeat challenges of *E. coli* lipopolysaccharide (LPS), a TLR4 agonist. They found that expression of a select cassette of antiviral genes became refractory upon second exposure to LPS while inflammatory genes could not be abrogated. This could lead to continued pro-inflammatory secretions by the RA-FLS.[106]

The reasons for RA-FLS maintaining their inflammatory responses or remembering previous insults are still being elucidated. However, there are data demonstrating crucial roles for continued NF-κB signalling and proportionally increased or decreased chromatin access at augmented or tolerized genes, respectively.[101,102,104–106]

While in its infancy, the field of FLS response to chronic or repeated challenges is expanding. Whether this response is an inherent sign of inflammatory cells or a disease-associated pathology, it may represent a novel approach to targeting persistent synovial inflammation in the future and may provide a new approach to preventing disease flares.

Fibroblast metabolism in RA

Over the last decade it has become evident that changes in cellular metabolism are essential for differentiation and effector function of several types of leukocyte.[107–109] For example, the activation of so-called M1 inflammatory macrophages involves a profound metabolic switch, in which the function of the mitochondrial Krebs cycle is blocked at several points, and mitochondria are reprogrammed to generate reactive oxygen species. To compensate for the loss of adenosine triphosphate (ATP) generation through the Krebs cycle and coupled mitochondrial oxidative phosphorylation, activated M1 macrophages increase glycolytic metabolism, in which glucose is taken up and partially metabolized to generate lactate. This cytosolic process is inefficient in terms of ATP generation, but can be rapidly mobilized to meet cellular metabolic demands when mitochondria do not function optimally as sources of ATP. Being cytotoxic, lactate is exported from the cell by monocarboxylate transporters, in particular MCT4.[110]

As reviewed more extensively elsewhere,[111–113] alterations in the metabolic activities of synovial fibroblasts are now believed to contribute to the pathogenesis of RA. FLS from rheumatoid joints display increased glycolytic metabolism and elevated expression of genes that support this function.[114–117] Positron emission tomography (PET) scanning demonstrates increased uptake of glucose within inflamed joints,[118,119] and high levels of the glycolytic product lactate can be detected in serum, synovial fluid or tissue of patients with RA.[116,117,120,121] These findings have been ascribed to the enhanced glycolytic activity of FLS, although macrophages and other cells in the tissue are also likely to contribute to the glycolytic signature. As the pannus outgrows its blood supply, FLS are increasingly exposed to low oxygen tension. Consequent hypoxia and oxidative stress are thought to progressively impair the function of FLS mitochondria, driving an adaptive increase in glycolytic metabolism.[117,119,122] The invasive properties of FLS *in vitro* are enhanced by extracellular lactate, and impaired by blockade of glycolytic metabolism.[117,123] *In vivo*, inhibition of key glycolytic enzymes or the lactate exporter MCT4 also exerted therapeutic effects in experimental models of RA,[114,116,123] providing further evidence for a pathogenic role of glycolytic metabolism. Disruption of other processes such as choline or glutamine metabolism in FLS may also contribute to pathogenesis of RA.[124–126]

Several intriguing questions remain to be answered. Since many *in vitro* studies have been performed using FLS from patients with advanced RA, it is not yet clear at what point these cells become committed to glycolytic metabolism. Krebs cycle intermediates like succinate may accumulate when mitochondrial metabolism is impaired. In the fields of cancer and ageing, it is well recognized that these metabolites influence the epigenome and profoundly affect gene expression.[127,128] So far, possible links between metabolic disturbance and epigenetic reprogramming of FLS remain unexplored. It is not known whether the distinct FLS populations discussed just now differ in their metabolic activities in healthy or inflamed joints.

Studies including those listed here generated proof-of-principle that therapeutic effects might be exerted by manipulating metabolic pathways in FLS. However, we do not yet know whether currently used antirheumatic drugs exert significant effects at this level, or whether drugs developed to target metabolic dysregulation in cancer might have therapeutic effects on FLS.

Tropism and fibroblast subsets

As with other tissue-resident cell types, such as ECs and macrophages, fibroblasts differ in phenotype and gene expression depending on the tissue from which they are isolated. These differences may be epigenetically imprinted. For example, studies of fibroblasts from a number of tissues, have demonstrated tropism in HOX gene expression.[129,130] These positional codifiers provide geographical information to tissue-resident cell types. It is therefore unsurprising that fibroblasts of distinct anatomical locales may be stratified by HOX expression.

Synovial fibroblasts significantly differ between anatomical sites

Microarray analysis of fibroblast populations by Parsonage[131] has demonstrated variation in basal and stimulated expression of genes related to inflammatory processes. Studies by Filer et al demonstrated gene expression in dermal, synovial, and bone marrow fibroblasts is influenced by (from strongest to weakest) anatomical site of origin, serum levels in culture media, and finally, the disease status of the donor.[132]

Alongside genetic analyses, evidence abounds for altered secretory responses by fibroblasts of different anatomical sites. A range of stimuli induce distinctly different concentrations of IL-6, IL-8, GM-CSF, and mononuclear chemokines between fibroblasts of different sites.[18,133,134] Fibroblasts from tissues including joint, mouth, lung, tonsil, lymph node, skin, and lung have been shown

to vary in response to TNFα, IL-1β, Galectin-3, IL-4, IFN, wound induction, and *S. aureus* infection.[18,131,133–135]

The evidence for functional stromal heterogeneity has resulted in the hypothesis that the stroma and endothelial tissue function together to present a stromal postcode through chemokine and adhesion molecule expression that regulates the influx and subsequent retention or efflux of leukocytes in the tissue.[136] It is postulated that expression of an improper postcode leads to the retention of pro-inflammatory immune cells and the prevention anti-inflammatory/pro-resolution cells from entering diseased tissue. As an example, increased CXCL13 and CCL19 expression could lead to an increase in B lymphocyte infiltration and retention in the tissue.[137,138]

While data regarding inter-tissue variation is fascinating, it is also of interest that the variance between fibroblasts from the same site in two distinct donors is less than that found between two different sites in the same donor.[89,129] Fibroblasts within a single tissue, and indeed a single geographical area of that tissue, may therefore also vary. This illustrates the concept of fibroblast subsets (**Figure 6.2**).

Synovial fibroblasts exist as different subpopulations

As mentioned earlier the synovium is traditionally stratified into the lining and sublining layers. The fibroblasts present in these two regions differ not only in location but also in the markers they express. Lining layer cells have been shown to express markers including CD55 and VCAM-1 which sublining fibroblasts express at lower or negligible levels except in very early RA disease.[139–143] Sublining layer fibroblasts can be identified by expression of a different set of cell surface markers, including CD90 (THY1) and CD248 (Endosialin).[139,144–147] Recent single cell RNA sequencing has further divided FLS populations into CD90⁻PDPN⁺ and CD90⁺PDPN⁺ populations which are either CD34⁺ or CD34⁻.[148]

Muller-Ladner et al. showed that RA-FLS passaged *in vitro* and then transplanted into SCID mice could still degrade human cartilage in the absence of leukocytes, suggesting cell autonomous

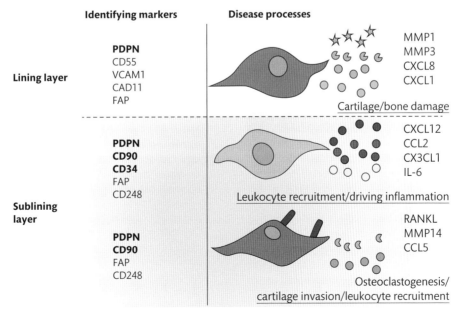

Figure 6.2 Synovial fibroblast subsets.

mechanisms drive the invasive phenotype.[67] As our understanding of FLS subsets has increased, different populations have been hypothesized to play varying roles in the progression of RA.[4,67] An example of this is the finding that the CD90+ population of sublining FLS appears to expand concurrently with sonographically measured synovial hypertrophy and increases in systemic and local inflammatory markers such as erythrocyte sedimentation rate (ESR) or CD45[+] cell influx into the synovium.[148]

Despite this inflammation-based increase in a sublining layer population, much of the invasive pathological phenotype of FLS in RA is ascribed to the lining layer. RA-FLS co-implanted with cartilage into SCID mice self-assemble into lining and sublining layers. The lining layer is PDPN+ (as in the joint) and cartilage adjacent.[67,149,150] It is this leading edge PDPN+ population that degrades cartilage and is also the first population to migrate from the primary implant site to a secondary piece of cartilage.[141] Cadherin-11 facilitates interfibroblast adhesion in the lining layer but in RA can promote cartilage invasion.[29,150-152] Its abrogation results in protection from inflammatory arthritis by stopping the lining layer becoming hyperplastic.[29] Finally, lining layer FLS expression of PDPN increases in inflamed RA tissue and is upregulated by TNF-α and IL-1β and downregulated by anti-TNF-α therapy.

This is not to say that the lining layer mediates all of the FLS contribution towards RA. Mizoguchi[148] confirmed the pro-invasive properties of the CD90[-]PDPN[+]CD34[-] lining layer by showing higher expression of MMP1 and MMP3 in this subset compared to other FLS subsets. However, using an *in vitro* assay both the CD90[+]PDPN[+]CD34[+] and CD90[+]PDPN[+]CD34[-] populations demonstrated higher invasiveness indicating the expression of degradative enzymes is not the only component dictating cartilage invasion. The CD90[+]PDPN[+]CD34[+] subset showed the highest expression of CXCL12, IL-6, CX3CL1, and CCL2 and, *in vitro*, recruited the highest number of monocytes. Surprisingly, although the CD90[+]PDPN[+]CD34[-] population had the highest expression of the osteoclastogenic factor RANKL, both the CD90[+]PDPN[+]CD34[-] and the CD90[-]PDPN[-]CD34[-] populations were similar in their *in vitro* osteoclastogenic potential and both elicited significantly more osteoclasts from monocytes than the CD90[+]PDPN[+]CD34[+] population.

Taken altogether this illustrates the growing complexity of the FLS subset field, with functions previously ascribed to the synovium in its entirety or on the basis of anatomical location now being assigned to functionally discrete subpopulations of fibroblasts.

Conclusions

The synovial fibroblast is a ubiquitous cell found throughout all joints in the body. Its shared roles across all sites has traditionally denoted an architectural cell capable of structural support and little else. However, an increasing body of evidence continues to demonstrate such a view is an oversimplification. In fields as wide-ranging as infection control, sterile inflammatory diseases, and cancer, the manifold functions of fibroblasts are now being elucidated.

The field of rheumatology has been one of the main drivers of this paradigm shift. The overwhelming adaptation of the synovial membrane into a proliferative, invasive, and destructive pannus displays the full arsenal of the immunologically competent FLS.

Many functions of FLS in healthy inflammation are represented in an exaggerated or altered form in the RA pannus. FLS appear to mount unremitting responses to inflammatory mediators and become increasingly inflammatory as the bouts of stimulation progress. Healthy FLS are capable of mounting inflammatory responses to infectious and injurious stimuli but this is amplified in the RA synovium leading to an imbalance in pro vs. anti-inflammatory mediators and thus a pro-inflammatory microenvironment.

Whether inherited or inflammation induced, the epigenetic landscape of the FLS changes in RA. This leads to increases in inflammatory secretions mentioned earlier and significantly alters gene expression to produce an apoptosis-resistant, invasive, and destructive cell.

A major step forward in the understanding of FLS biology in RA is the greater appreciation of cell subsets. FLS are an integral cell in the synovial membrane; their global depletion would cause a complete breakdown of synovial architecture. Research into the particular contributions of each subset to the pathology of RA may represent a practicable breakthrough in targeting disease persistence in RA.

REFERENCES

1. Filer A. The fibroblast as a therapeutic target in rheumatoid arthritis. *Curr Opin Pharmacol* 2013;*13*(3):413–19.
2. Juarez M, Filer A, Buckley CD. Fibroblasts as therapeutic targets in rheumatoid arthritis and cancer. *Swiss Med Wkly*, 2012;*142*:w13529.
3. Naylor AJ, Filer A, Buckley CD. The role of stromal cells in the persistence of chronic inflammation. *Clin Exp Immunol* 2013;*171*(1):30–5.
4. Turner JD, Filer A. The role of the synovial fibroblast in rheumatoid arthritis pathogenesis. *Curr Opin Rheumatol* 2015;*27*(2):175–82.
5. Ospelt C, Brentano F, Rengel Y, et al. Overexpression of Toll-like receptors 3 and 4 in synovial tissue from patients with early rheumatoid arthritis: toll-like receptor expression in early and longstanding arthritis. *Arthritis Rheum* 2008;*58*(12):3684–92.
6. Hall SE, Savill JS, Henson PM, Haslett C. Apoptotic neutrophils are phagocytosed by fibroblasts with participation of the fibroblast vitronectin receptor and involvement of a mannose/fucose-specific lectin. *J Immunol* 1994;*153*(7):3218–27.
7. Boots AM, Wimmers-Bertens AJ, Rijnders AW. Antigen-presenting capacity of rheumatoid synovial fibroblasts. *Immunology* 1994;*82*(2):268–74.
8. Wilkinson LS, Pitsillides AA, Worrall JG, Edwards JC. Light microscopic characterization of the fibroblast-like synovial intimal cell (synoviocyte). *Arthritis Rheum* 1992;*35*(10):1179–84.
9. Marcelino J, Carpten JD, Suwairi WM, et al. CACP, encoding a secreted proteoglycan, is mutated in camptodactyly-arthropathy-coxa vara-pericarditis syndrome. *Nat Genet* 1999;*23*(3):319–22.
10. Bradfield PF, Amft N, Vernon-Wilson E, et al. Rheumatoid fibroblast-like synoviocytes overexpress the chemokine stromal cell-derived factor 1 (CXCL12), which supports distinct patterns and rates of CD4+ and CD8+ T cell migration within synovial tissue. *Arthritis Rheum* 2003;*48*(9):2472–82.
11. Gitter BD, Labus JM, Lees SL, Scheetz ME. Characteristics of human synovial fibroblast activation by IL-1 beta and TNF alpha. *Immunology* 1989;*66*(2):196–200.
12. Hayashida K, Nanki T, Girschick H, Yavuz S, Ochi T, Lipsky P. Synovial stromal cells from rheumatoid arthritis patients

attract monocytes by producing MCP-1 and IL-8. *Arthritis Res* 2001;*3*(2):1–9.

13. Hwang SY, Kim JY, Kim KW, et al. IL-17 induces production of IL-6 and IL-8 in rheumatoid arthritis synovial fibroblasts via NF-kappaB- and PI3-kinase/Akt-dependent pathways. *Arthritis Res Ther* 2004;*6*(2):R120–8.

14. Shadidi KR, Aarvak T, Henriksen JE, Natvig JB, Thompson KM. The chemokines CCL5, CCL2 and CXCL12 play significant roles in the migration of Th1 cells into rheumatoid synovial tissue. *Scand J Immunol* 2003;*57*(2):192–8.

15. McGettrick HM, Smith E, Filer A, et al. Fibroblasts from different sites may promote or inhibit recruitment of flowing lymphocytes by endothelial cells. *Eur J Immunol* 2009;*39*(1):113–25.

16. Baeten D, Demetter P, Cuvelier C, et al. Comparative study of the synovial histology in rheumatoid arthritis, spondyloarthropathy, and osteoarthritis: influence of disease duration and activity. *Ann Rheum Dis* 2000;*59*(12):945–53.

17. McGettrick HM, Butler LM, Buckley CD, Rainger GE, Nash GB. Tissue stroma as a regulator of leukocyte recruitment in inflammation. *J Leukoc Biol* 2012;*91*(3):385–400.

18. Filer A, Parsonage G, Smith E, et al. Differential survival of leukocyte subsets mediated by synovial, bone marrow, and skin fibroblasts: site-specific versus activation-dependent survival of T cells and neutrophils. *Arthritis Rheum* 2006;*54*(7):2096–108.

19. Parsonage G, Filer A, Bik M, et al. Prolonged, granulocyte-macrophage colony-stimulating factor-dependent, neutrophil survival following rheumatoid synovial fibroblast activation by IL-17 and TNFalpha. *Arthritis Res Ther* 2008;*10*(2):R47.

20. Fleetwood AJ, Lawrence T, Hamilton JA, Cook AD. Granulocyte-macrophage colony-stimulating factor (CSF) and macrophage CSF-dependent macrophage phenotypes display differences in cytokine profiles and transcription factor activities: implications for CSF blockade in inflammation. *J Immunol* 2007;*178*(8):5245–52.

21. Jaguin M, Houlbert N, Fardel O, Lecureur V. Polarization profiles of human M-CSF-generated macrophages and comparison of M1-markers in classically activated macrophages from GM-CSF and M-CSF origin. *Cell Immunol* 2013;*281*(1):51–61.

22. Ivanov II, McKenzie BS, Zhou L, et al. The orphan nuclear receptor RORγt directs the differentiation program of proinflammatory IL-17+ T helper cells. *Cell* 2006;*126*(6):1121–33.

23. Okamoto H, Yamamura M, Morita Y, Harada S, Makino H, Ota Z. The synovial expression and serum levels of interleukin-6, interleukin-11, leukemia inhibitory factor, and oncostatin M in rheumatoid arthritis. *Arthritis Rheum* 1997;*40*(6):1096–105.

24. Filer A, Ward LSC, Kemble S, et al. Identification of a transitional fibroblast function in very early rheumatoid arthritis. *Ann Rheum Dis* 2017;*76*(12):2105–12.

25. Patel R, Filer A, Barone F, Buckley CD. Stroma: fertile soil for inflammation. *Best Pract Res Clin Rheumatol* 2014;*28*(4):565–76.

26. Bottini N, Firestein GS. Duality of fibroblast-like synoviocytes in RA: passive responders and imprinted aggressors. *Nat Rev Rheumatol* 2013;*9*(1):24–33.

27. Firestein GS, Zvaifler NJ. How important are T cells in chronic rheumatoid synovitis? Arthritis Rheum. 1990;*33*(6):768–73.

28. Mohr W, Beneke G, Mohing W. Proliferation of synovial lining cells and fibroblasts. *Ann Rheum Dis* 1975;*34*(3):219–24.

29. Lee DM, Kiener HP, Agarwal SK, et al. Cadherin-11 in synovial lining formation and pathology in arthritis. *Science* 2007;*315*(5814):1006–10.

30. Baier A, Meineckel I, Gay S, Pap T. Apoptosis in rheumatoid arthritis. *Curr Opin Rheumatol* 2003;*15*(3):274–9.

31. Miyazawa K, Mori A, Yamamoto K, Okudaira H. Constitutive transcription of the human interleukin-6 gene by rheumatoid synoviocytes: spontaneous activation of NF-kappaB and CBF1. *Am J Pathol* 1998;*152*(3):793–803.

32. Kobayashi T, Okamoto K, Kobata T, Hasunuma T, Sumida T, Nishioka K. Tumor necrosis factor alpha regulation of the FAS-mediated apoptosis-signaling pathway in synovial cells. *Arthritis Rheum* 1999;*42*(3):519–26.

33. Wakisaka S, Takeba S, Nagafuchi T, et al. Modulation by proinflammatory cytokines of Fas/Fas ligand-mediated apoptotic cell death of synovial cells in patients with rheumatoid arthritis (RA). *Clin Exp Immunol* 1998;*114*(1):119–28.

34. Van Antwerp DJ, Martin SJ, Verma IM, Green DR. Inhibition of TNF-induced apoptosis by NF-κB. *Trends Cell Biol* 1998;*8*(3):107–11.

35. Senftleben U, Cao Y, Xiao G, et al. Activation by IKKalpha of a second, evolutionary conserved, NF-kappa B signaling pathway. *Science* 2001;*293*(5534):1495–9.

36. Bondeson J, Foxwell B, Brennan F, Feldmann M. Defining therapeutic targets by using adenovirus: blocking NF-kappaB inhibits both inflammatory and destructive mechanisms in rheumatoid synovium but spares anti-inflammatory mediators. *Proc Natl Acad Sci U S A* 1999;*96*(10):5668–73.

37. van der Laan WH, Quax PH, Seemayer CA, et al. Cartilage degradation and invasion by rheumatoid synovial fibroblasts is inhibited by gene transfer of TIMP-1 and TIMP-3. *Gene Ther* 2003;*10*(3):234–42.

38. Xue M, McKelvey K, Shen K, et al. Endogenous MMP-9 and not MMP-2 promotes rheumatoid synovial fibroblast survival, inflammation and cartilage degradation. *Rheumatology (Oxford)* 2014;*53*(12):2270–9.

39. Kim KW, Cho ML, Lee SH, et al. Human rheumatoid synovial fibroblasts promote osteoclastogenic activity by activating RANKL via TLR-2 and TLR-4 activation. *Immunol Lett* 2007;*110*(1):54–64.

40. Kim KW, Cho ML, Oh HJ, et al. TLR-3 enhances osteoclastogenesis through upregulation of RANKL expression from fibroblast-like synoviocytes in patients with rheumatoid arthritis. *Immunol Lett* 2009;*124*(1):9–17.

41. Zhu X, Xiao L, Huo R, et al. Cyr61 is involved in neutrophil infiltration in joints by inducing IL-8 production by fibroblast-like synoviocytes in rheumatoid arthritis. *Arthritis Res Ther* 2013;*15*(6):R187.

42. Harigai M, Hara M, Kawamoto M, et al. Amplification of the synovial inflammatory response through activation of mitogen-activated protein kinases and nuclear factor kappaB using ligation of CD40 on CD14+ synovial cells from patients with rheumatoid arthritis. *Arthritis Rheum* 2004;*50*(7):2167–77.

43. Cho ML, Cho CS, Min SY, et al. Cyclosporine inhibition of vascular endothelial growth factor production in rheumatoid synovial fibroblasts. *Arthritis Rheum* 2002;*46*(5):1202–9.

44. Xiaoyan Z, Xinyi W, Li G. Pretreatment with lipopolysaccharide modulates innate immunity in corneal fibroblasts challenged with *Aspergillus fumigatus*. *Innate Immun* 2011;*17*(3):237–44.

45. Kim KW, Cho ML, Kim HR, et al. Up-regulation of stromal cell-derived factor 1 (CXCL12) production in rheumatoid synovial fibroblasts through interactions with T lymphocytes: role of interleukin-17 and CD40L-CD40 interaction. *Arthritis Rheum* 2007;*56*(4):1076–86.

46. Dayer JM, Krane SM, Russell RG, Robinson DR. Production of collagenase and prostaglandins by isolated adherent rheumatoid synovial cells. *Proc Natl Acad Sci U S A* 1976;73(3):945–9.

47. Al-Saadany HM, Hussein MS, Gaber RA, Zaytoun HA. Th-17 cells and serum IL-17 in rheumatoid arthritis patients: correlation with disease activity and severity. *The Egyptian Rheumatologist* 2016;38(1):1–7.

48. Lubberts E. The IL-23-IL-17 axis in inflammatory arthritis. *Nat Rev Rheumatol* 2015;11(7):415–29.

49. Scheller J, Chalaris A, Schmidt-Arras D, Rose-John S. The pro- and anti-inflammatory properties of the cytokine interleukin-6. *Biochim Biophys Acta* 2011;1813(5):878–88.

50. Hashizume M, Hayakawa N, Mihara M. IL-6 trans-signalling directly induces RANKL on fibroblast-like synovial cells and is involved in RANKL induction by TNF-alpha and IL-17. *Rheumatology (Oxford)* 2008;47(11):1635–40.

51. Mihara M, Moriya Y, Kishimoto T, Ohsugi Y. Interleukin-6 (IL-6) induces the proliferation of synovial fibroblastic cells in the presence of soluble IL-6 receptor. *Rheumatology* 1995;34(4):321–5.

52. Nowell MA, Richards PJ, Horiuchi S, et al. Soluble IL-6 receptor governs IL-6 activity in experimental arthritis: blockade of arthritis severity by soluble glycoprotein 130. *J Immunol* 2003;171(6):3202–9.

53. Takayanagi H, Iizuka H, Juji T, et al. Involvement of receptor activator of nuclear factor kappaB ligand/osteoclast differentiation factor in osteoclastogenesis from synoviocytes in rheumatoid arthritis. *Arthritis Rheum* 2000;43(2):259–69.

54. Hurst SM, Wilkinson TS, McLoughlin RM, et al. Il-6 and its soluble receptor orchestrate a temporal switch in the pattern of leukocyte recruitment seen during acute inflammation. *Immunity* 2001;14(6):705–14.

55. Calabrese LH, Rose-John S. IL-6 biology: implications for clinical targeting in rheumatic disease. *Nat Rev Rheumatol* 2014;10(12):720–7.

56. Atreya R, Mudter J, Finotto S, et al. Blockade of interleukin 6 trans signaling suppresses T-cell resistance against apoptosis in chronic intestinal inflammation: evidence in crohn disease and experimental colitis *in vivo*. *Nat Med* 2000;6(5):583–8.

57. Hidalgo E, Essex SJ, Yeo L, et al. The response of T cells to interleukin-6 is differentially regulated by the microenvironment of the rheumatoid synovial fluid and tissue. *Arthritis Rheum* 2011;63(11):3284–93.

58. Burger JA, Zvaifler NJ, Tsukada N, Firestein GS, Kipps TJ. Fibroblast-like synoviocytes support B-cell pseudoemperipolesis via a stromal cell-derived factor-1- and CD106 (VCAM-1)-dependent mechanism. *J Clin Invest* 2001;107(3):305–15.

59. Scaife S, Brown R, Kellie S, et al. Detection of differentially expressed genes in synovial fibroblasts by restriction fragment differential display. *Rheumatology* 2004;43(11):1346–52.

60. Pierer M, Rethage J, Seibl R, et al. Chemokine secretion of rheumatoid arthritis synovial fibroblasts stimulated by Toll-like receptor 2 ligands. *J Immunol* 2004;172(2):1256–65.

61. Komatsu N, Okamoto K, Sawa S, et al. Pathogenic conversion of Foxp3+ T cells into TH17 cells in autoimmune arthritis. *Nat Med* 2013;20:62.

62. Donlin LT, Jayatilleke A, Giannopoulou EG, Kalliolias GD, Ivashkiv LB. Modulation of TNF-induced macrophage polarization by synovial fibroblasts. *J Immunol* 2014;193(5):2373–83.

63. Benito-Miguel M, García-Carmona Y, Balsa A, et al. IL-15 expression on RA synovial fibroblasts promotes B cell survival. *PLoS One* 2012;7(7):e40620.

64. Bombardieri M, Kam NW, Brentano F, et al. A BAFF/APRIL-dependent TLR3-stimulated pathway enhances the capacity of rheumatoid synovial fibroblasts to induce AID expression and Ig class-switching in B cells. *Ann Rheum Dis* 2011;70(10):1857–65.

65. Chan A, Filer A, Parsonage G, et al. Mediation of the proinflammatory cytokine response in rheumatoid arthritis and spondylarthritis by interactions between fibroblast-like synoviocytes and natural killer cells. *Arthritis Rheum* 2008;58(3):707–17.

66. Allard SA, Maini RN, Muirden KD. Cells and matrix expressing cartilage components in fibroblastic tissue in rheumatoid pannus. *Scand J Rheumatol Suppl* 1988;76:125–9.

67. Muller-Ladner U, Kriegsmann J, Franklin BN, et al. Synovial fibroblasts of patients with rheumatoid arthritis attach to and invade normal human cartilage when engrafted into SCID mice. *Am J Pathol* 1996;149(5):1607–15.

68. Unemori EN, Hibbs MS, Amento EP. Constitutive expression of a 92-kD gelatinase (type V collagenase) by rheumatoid synovial fibroblasts and its induction in normal human fibroblasts by inflammatory cytokines. *J Clin Invest* 1991;88(5):1656–62.

69. Xue C, Takahashi M, Hasunuma T, et al. Characterisation of fibroblast-like cells in pannus lesions of patients with rheumatoid arthritis sharing properties of fibroblasts and chondrocytes. *Ann Rheum Dis* 1997;56(4):262–7.

70. Pap T, Aupperle KR, Gay S, Firestein GS, Gay RE. Invasiveness of synovial fibroblasts is regulated by p53 in the SCID mouse *in vivo* model of cartilage invasion. *Arthritis Rheum* 2001;44(3):676–81.

71. Tetlow LC, Lees M, Ogata Y, Nagase H, Woolley DE. Differential expression of gelatinase B (MMP-9) and stromelysin-1 (MMP-3) by rheumatoid synovial cells *in vitro* and *in vivo*. *Rheumatol Int* 1993;13(2):53–9.

72. Chambers M, Kirkpatrick G, Evans M, Gorski G, Foster S, Borghaei RC. IL-4 inhibition of IL-1 induced matrix metalloproteinase-3 (MMP-3) expression in human fibroblasts involves decreased AP-1 activation via negative cross-talk involving of Jun N-terminal kinase (JNK). *Exp Cell Res* 2013;319(10):1398–408.

73. Lefevre S, Knedla A, Tennie C, et al. Synovial fibroblasts spread rheumatoid arthritis to unaffected joints. *Nat Med* 2009;15(12):1414–20.

74. Inazuka M, Tahira T, Horiuchi T, et al. Analysis of p53 tumour suppressor gene somatic mutations in rheumatoid arthritis synovium. *Rheumatology* 2000;39(3):262–6.

75. Seemayer CA, Kuchen S, Neidhart M, et al. p53 in rheumatoid arthritis synovial fibroblasts at sites of invasion. *Ann Rheum Dis* 2003;62(12):1139–44.

76. Swatek KN, Komander D. Ubiquitin modifications. *Cell Res* 2016;26(4):399–422.

77. Ospelt C, Reedquist KA, Gay S, Tak PP. Inflammatory memories: is epigenetics the missing link to persistent stromal cell activation in rheumatoid arthritis? *Autoimmun Rev* 2011;10(9):519–24.

78. Wada TT, Araki Y, Sato K, et al. Aberrant histone acetylation contributes to elevated interleukin-6 production in rheumatoid arthritis synovial fibroblasts. *Biochem Biophys Res Commun* 2014;444(4):682–6.

79. Lin S, Hsieh S, Lin Y, et al. A whole genome methylation analysis of systemic lupus erythematosus: hypomethylation of the IL10 and IL1R2 promoters is associated with disease activity. *Genes Immun* 2012;13:214–20.

80. Araki Y, Tsuzuki Wada T, Aizaki Y, et al. Histone methylation and STAT-3 differentially regulate interleukin-6–induced matrix

metalloproteinase gene activation in rheumatoid arthritis synovial fibroblasts. *Arthritis Rheumatol* 2016;68(5):1111–23.

81. Armenante F, Merola M, Furia A, Palmieri M. Repression of the IL-6 Gene Is Associated with Hypermethylation. *Biochem Biophys Res Commun* 1999;258(3):644–7.

82. Kuo MH, Allis CD. Roles of histone acetyltransferases and deacetylases in gene regulation. *BioEssays* 1998;20(8):615–26.

83. Fu L, Ma C, Cong B, Li S, Chen H, Zhang J. Hypomethylation of proximal CpG motif of interleukin-10 promoter regulates its expression in human rheumatoid arthritis. *Acta Pharmacol Sin* 2011;32:1373–80.

84. Smith ZD, Meissner A. DNA methylation: roles in mammalian development. *Nat Rev Genet* 2013;14:204.

85. Nile C, Read R, Akil M, Duff G, Wilson A. Methylation status of a single CpG site in the IL6 promoter is related to IL6 messenger RNA levels and rheumatoid arthritis. *Arthritis Rheum* 2008;58:2686–93.

86. Saccani S, Pantano S, Natoli G. p38-dependent marking of inflammatory genes for increased NF-κB recruitment. *Nat Immunol* 2001;3:69.

87. Karouzakis E, Rengel Y, Jungel A, et al. DNA methylation regulates the expression of CXCL12 in rheumatoid arthritis synovial fibroblasts. *Genes Immun* 2011;12(8):643–52.

88. Pazolli E, Alspach E, Milczarek A, Prior J, Piwnica-Worms D, Stewart SA. Chromatin remodeling underlies the senescence-associated secretory phenotype of tumor stromal fibroblasts that supports cancer progression. *Cancer Res* 2012;72(9):2251–61.

89. Frank-Bertoncelj M, Trenkmann M, Klein K, et al. Epigenetically-driven anatomical diversity of synovial fibroblasts guides joint-specific fibroblast functions. *Nat Commun* 2017;8:14852.

90. Karouzakis E, Gay R, Michel B, Gay S, Neidhart M. DNA hypomethylation in rheumatoid arthritis synovial fibroblasts. *Arthritis Rheum* 2009;60:3613–22.

91. Ishida K, Kobayashi T, Ito S, et al. Interleukin-6 gene promoter methylation in rheumatoid arthritis and chronic periodontitis. *J Periodontol* 2012;83:917–25.

92. Dandrea M, Donadelli M, Costanzo C, Scarpa A, Palmieri M. MeCP2/H3meK9 are involved in IL-6 gene silencing in pancreatic adenocarcinoma cell lines. *Nucleic Acids Res* 2009;37(20):6681–90.

93. Ndlovu MN, Van Lint C, Van Wesemael K, et al. Hyperactivated NF-{kappa}B and AP-1 transcription factors promote highly accessible chromatin and constitutive transcription across the interleukin-6 gene promoter in metastatic breast cancer cells. *Mol Cell Biol* 2009;29(20):5488–504.

94. de la Rica L, Urquiza JM, Gómez-Cabrero D, et al. Identification of novel markers in rheumatoid arthritis through integrated analysis of DNA methylation and microRNA expression. *J Autoimmun* 2013;41(0):6–16.

95. Karouzakis E, Raza K, Kolling C, et al. Analysis of early changes in DNA methylation in synovial fibroblasts of RA patients before diagnosis. *Sci Rep* 2018;8(1):7370.

96. He L, Hannon GJ. MicroRNAs: small RNAs with a big role in gene regulation. *Nat Rev Genet* 2004;5(7):522–31.

97. Long L, Yu P, Liu Y, et al. Upregulated microRNA-155 expression in peripheral blood mononuclear cells and fibroblast-like synoviocytes in rheumatoid arthritis. *Clin Dev Immunol* 2013;2013:296139.

98. Stanczyk J, Pedrioli DML, Brentano F, et al. Altered expression of MicroRNA in synovial fibroblasts and synovial tissue in rheumatoid arthritis. *Arthritis Rheum* 2008;58(4):1001–9.

99. Lin J, Huo R, Xiao L, et al. A novel p53/microRNA-22/Cyr61 axis in synovial cells regulates inflammation in rheumatoid arthritis. *Arthritis Rheum* 2014;66(1):49–59.

100. Migita K, Iwanaga N, Izumi Y, et al. TNF-α-induced miR-155 regulates IL-6 signaling in rheumatoid synovial fibroblasts. *BMC Res Notes* 2017;10:403.

101. Lee A, Qiao Y, Grigoriev G, et al. Tumor necrosis factor alpha induces sustained signaling and a prolonged and unremitting inflammatory response in rheumatoid arthritis synovial fibroblasts. *Arthritis Rheum* 2013;65(4):928–38.

102. Dakin SG, Buckley CD, Al-Mossawi MH, et al. Persistent stromal fibroblast activation is present in chronic tendinopathy. *Arthritis Res Ther* 2017;19(1):16.

103. Crowley T, Buckley CD, Clark AR. Stroma: the forgotten cells of innate immune memory. *Clin Exp Immunol* 2018;193(1):24–36.

104. Sohn C, Lee A, Qiao Y, Loupasakis K, Ivashkiv LB, Kalliolias GD. Prolonged TNFα primes fibroblast-like synoviocytes in a gene-specific manner by altering chromatin. *Arthritis Rheum* 2014;67(1):86–95.

105. Crowley T, O'Neil JD, Adams H, et al. Priming in response to pro-inflammatory cytokines is a feature of adult synovial but not dermal fibroblasts. *Arthritis Res Ther* 2017;19(1):35.

106. Klein K, Frank-Bertoncelj M, Karouzakis E, et al. The epigenetic architecture at gene promoters determines cell type-specific LPS tolerance. *J Autoimmun* 2017;83:122–33.

107. Lee YS, Wollam J, Olefsky JM. An integrated view of immunometabolism. *Cell* 2018;172(1–2):22–40.

108. Buck MD, Sowell RT, Kaech SM, Pearce EL. Metabolic instruction of immunity. *Cell* 2017;169(4):570–86.

109. O'Neill LA, Kishton RJ, Rathmell J. A guide to immunometabolism for immunologists. *Nat Rev Immunol* 2016;16(9):553–65.

110. Pucino V, Bombardieri M, Pitzalis C, Mauro C. Lactate at the crossroads of metabolism, inflammation, and autoimmunity. *Eur J Immunol* 2017;47(1):14–21.

111. Falconer J, Murphy AN, Young SP, et al. Synovial cell metabolism and chronic inflammation in rheumatoid arthritis. *Arthritis Rheumatol* 2018;70(7):984–99.

112. Bustamante MF, Garcia-Carbonell R, Whisenant KD, Guma M. Fibroblast-like synoviocyte metabolism in the pathogenesis of rheumatoid arthritis. *Arthritis Res Ther* 2017;19(1):110.

113. Weyand CM, Goronzy JJ. Immunometabolism in early and late stages of rheumatoid arthritis. *Nat Rev Rheumatol* 2017;13(5):291–301.

114. McGarry T, Biniecka M, Gao W, et al. Resolution of TLR2-induced inflammation through manipulation of metabolic pathways in rheumatoid arthritis. *Sci Rep* 2017;7:43165.

115. Henderson B, Bitensky L, Chayen J. Glycolytic activity in human synovial lining cells in rheumatoid arthritis. *Ann Rheum Dis* 1979;38(1):63–7.

116. Fujii W, Kawahito Y, Nagahara H, et al. Monocarboxylate transporter 4, associated with the acidification of synovial fluid, is a novel therapeutic target for inflammatory arthritis. *Arthritis Rheumatol* 2015;67(11):2888–96.

117. Biniecka M, Canavan M, McGarry T, et al. Dysregulated bioenergetics: a key regulator of joint inflammation. *Ann Rheum Dis* 2016;75(12):2192–200.

118. Kubota K, Ito K, Morooka M, et al. FDG PET for rheumatoid arthritis: basic considerations and whole-body PET/CT. *Ann N Y Acad Sci* 2011;1228:29–38.

119. Fearon U, Canavan M, Biniecka M, Veale DJ. Hypoxia, mitochondrial dysfunction and synovial invasiveness in rheumatoid arthritis. *Nat Rev Rheumatol* 2016;*12*(7):385–97.

120. Hitchon CA, El-Gabalawy HS, Bezabeh T. Characterization of synovial tissue from arthritis patients: a proton magnetic resonance spectroscopic investigation. *Rheumatol Int* 2009;*29*(10):1205–11.

121. Young SP, Kapoor SR, Viant MR, et al. The impact of inflammation on metabolomic profiles in patients with arthritis. *Arthritis Rheum* 2013;*65*(8):2015–23.

122. Balogh E, Veale DJ, McGarry T, et al. Oxidative stress impairs energy metabolism in primary cells and synovial tissue of patients with rheumatoid arthritis. *Arthritis Res Ther* 2018;*20*(1):95.

123. Garcia-Carbonell R, Divakaruni AS, Lodi A, et al. Critical role of glucose metabolism in rheumatoid arthritis fibroblast-like synoviocytes. *Arthritis Rheumatol* 2016;*68*(7):1614–26.

124. Volchenkov R, Dung Cao M, Elgstoen KB, et al. Metabolic profiling of synovial tissue shows altered glucose and choline metabolism in rheumatoid arthritis samples. *Scand J Rheumatol* 2017;*46*(2):160–1.

125. Guma M, Sanchez-Lopez E, Lodi A, et al. Choline kinase inhibition in rheumatoid arthritis. *Ann Rheum Dis* 2015;*74*(7):1399–407.

126. Takahashi S, Saegusa J, Sendo S, et al. Glutaminase 1 plays a key role in the cell growth of fibroblast-like synoviocytes in rheumatoid arthritis. *Arthritis Res Ther* 2017;*19*(1):76.

127. Berger SL, Sassone-Corsi P. Metabolic signaling to chromatin. *Cold Spring Harb Perspect Biol* 2016;*8*(11): pii: a019463.

128. Salminen A, Kaarniranta K, Hiltunen M, Kauppinen A. Krebs cycle dysfunction shapes epigenetic landscape of chromatin: novel insights into mitochondrial regulation of aging process. *Cell Signal* 2014;*26*(7):1598–603.

129. Chang HY, Chi J-T, Dudoit S, et al. Diversity, topographic differentiation, and positional memory in human fibroblasts. *Proc Natl Acad Sci U S A* 2002;*99*(20):12877–82.

130. Rinn JL, Bondre C, Gladstone HB, Brown PO, Chang HY. Anatomic demarcation by positional variation in fibroblast gene expression programs. *PLoS Genet* 2006;*2*(7):e119.

131. Parsonage G, Falciani F, Burman A, et al. Global gene expression profiles in fibroblasts from synovial, skin and lymphoid tissue reveals distinct cytokine and chemokine expression patterns. *Thromb Haemost* 2003;*90*(4):688–97.

132. Filer A, Antczak P, Parsonage GN, et al. Stromal transcriptional profiles reveal hierarchies of anatomical site, serum response and disease and identify disease specific pathways. *PLoS One* 2015;*10*(3):e0120917.

133. Filer A, Bik M, Parsonage GN, et al. Galectin 3 induces a distinctive pattern of cytokine and chemokine production in rheumatoid synovial fibroblasts via selective signaling pathways. *Arthritis Rheum* 2009;*60*(6):1604–14.

134. Mah W, Jiang G, Olver D, et al. Human gingival fibroblasts display a non-fibrotic phenotype distinct from skin fibroblasts in three-dimensional cultures. *PLoS One* 2014;*9*(3):e90715.

135. Slany A, Meshcheryakova A, Beer A, Ankersmit HJ, Paulitschke V, Gerner C. Plasticity of fibroblasts demonstrated by tissue-specific and function-related proteome profiling. *Clin Proteomics* 2014;*11*(1):41.

136. Parsonage G, Filer AD, Haworth O, et al. A stromal address code defined by fibroblasts. *Trends Immunol* 2005;*26*(3):150–6.

137. Sellam J, Rouanet S, Hendel-Chavez H, et al. CCL19, a B cell chemokine, is related to the decrease of blood memory B cells and predicts the clinical response to rituximab in patients with rheumatoid arthritis. *Arthritis Rheum* 2013;*65*(9):2253–61.

138. Rupprecht TA, Plate A, Adam M, et al. The chemokine CXCL13 is a key regulator of B cell recruitment to the cerebrospinal fluid in acute Lyme neuroborreliosis. *J Neuroinflammation* 2009;*6*:42.

139. Bauer S, Jendro M, Wadle A, et al. Fibroblast activation protein is expressed by rheumatoid myofibroblast-like synoviocytes. *Arthritis Res Ther* 2006;*8*(6):R171.

140. Del Rey MJ, Faré R, Izquierdo E, et al. Clinicopathological correlations of podoplanin (gp38) expression in rheumatoid synovium and its potential contribution to fibroblast platelet crosstalk. *PLoS One* 2014;*9*(6):e99607.

141. Ekwall A-K, Eisler T, Anderberg C, et al. The tumour-associated glycoprotein podoplanin is expressed in fibroblast-like synoviocytes of the hyperplastic synovial lining layer in rheumatoid arthritis. *Arthritis Res Ther* 2011;*13*(2):R40.

142. Croft AP, Naylor AJ, Marshall JL, et al. Rheumatoid synovial fibroblasts differentiate into distinct subsets in the presence of cytokines and cartilage. *Arthritis Res Ther* 2016;*18*(1):270.

143. Choi IY, Karpus ON, Turner JD, et al. Stromal cell markers are differentially expressed in the synovial tissue of patients with early arthritis. *PLoS One* 2017;*12*(8):e0182751.

144. MacFadyen JR, Haworth O, Roberston D, et al. Endosialin (TEM1, CD248) is a marker of stromal fibroblasts and is not selectively expressed on tumour endothelium. *FEBS Letters* 2005;*579*(12):2569–75.

145. Maia M, de Vriese A, Janssens T, et al. CD248 and its cytoplasmic domain: a therapeutic target for arthritis. *Arthritis Rheum* 2010;*62*(12):3595–606.

146. Saalbach A, Aneregg U, Bruns M, Schnabel E, Herrmann K, Haustein UF. Novel fibroblast-specific monoclonal antibodies: properties and specificities. *J Invest Dermatol* 1996;*106*(6):1314–19.

147. Saalbach A, Kraft R, Herrmann K, Haustein UF, Aneregg U. The monoclonal antibody AS02 recognizes a protein on human fibroblasts being highly homologous to Thy-1. *Arch Dermatol Res* 1998;*290*(7):360–6.

148. Mizoguchi F, Slowikowski K, Wei K, et al. Functionally distinct disease-associated fibroblast subsets in rheumatoid arthritis. *Nat Commun* 2018;*9*(1):789.

149. Kiener HP, Lee DM, Agarwal SK, Brenner MB. Cadherin-11 induces rheumatoid arthritis fibroblast-like synoviocytes to form lining layers *in vitro*. *Am J Pathol* 2006;*168*(5):1486–99.

150. Kiener HP, Niederreiter B, Lee DM, Jimenez-Boj E, Smolen JS, Brenner MB. Cadherin 11 promotes invasive behavior of fibroblast-like synoviocytes. *Arthritis Rheum* 2009;*60*(5):1305–10.

151. Valencia X, Higgins JM, Kiener HP, et al. Cadherin-11 provides specific cellular adhesion between fibroblast-like synoviocytes. *J Exp Med* 2004;*200*(12):1673–9.

152. Assefnia S, Dakshanamurthy S, Auvil JMG, et al. Cadherin-11 in poor prognosis malignancies and rheumatoid arthritis: common target, common therapies. *Oncotarget* 2014;*5*(6):1458–74.

7

Autoantibodies in rheumatoid arthritis

Tom W.J. Huizinga

Introduction

Autoantibodies are a characteristic feature of autoimmune diseases. Although the exact pathogenetic role of autoantibodies is in general not known, they are very often useful for diagnostic purposes. Rheumatoid arthritis (RA) is a chronic autoimmune disease primarily affecting the joints. RA is a heterogeneous disease that encompasses several disease subsets with probable differences in underlying pathophysiology. Via a final common inflammatory pathway these different pathophysiological pathways might lead to a similar clinical presentation of arthritis. The best-known subdivision in RA is between autoantibody positive and autoantibody negative RA, which differ in both risk factors and clinical outcomes.[1] This chapter focuses on the role of autoantibodies in the pathophysiology of RA. First, the relation between autoantibodies and known risk factors for RA will be discussed. Thereafter, the specific characteristics of the autoantibody response and the pathogenic potential of the different autoantibodies are reviewed.

Several autoantibodies can be detected in serum of RA patients, of which rheumatoid factor (RF) and anticitrullinated protein antibodies (ACPA) are the best studied. Antibodies against additional post-translationally modified proteins have more recently been described, such as anticarbamylated protein antibodies (anti-CarP)[2] and antiacetylated protein antibodies.[3] Rheumatoid factors (antibodies to the Fc-portion of IgG) were detected more than 70 years ago. In recent years most research on the role of autoantibodies in disease pathophysiology has focused on ACPA, which are directed against citrullinated proteins. Citrullination is a reaction mediated by peptidyl-arginine deiminase (PAD) enzymes, which convert the DNA-encoded amino acid arginine into citrulline. This post-translational modification occurs under both physiological and pathological circumstances. Multiple known risk factors for RA are hypothesized to be related to the development of the immune response against citrullinated proteins and thus ACPA formation.

Risk factors

Genetic risk factors

Rheumatoid arthritis affects approximately 0.5 to 1% of the population. Ample research has been performed on risk factors for this disease. Twin studies have shown that genetic variation accounts for 50% to 60% of the risk on RA development.[4] The human leukocyte antigen (HLA)-DRB1*01,*04 and *10 alleles are the strongest genetic risk factor for RA development, in particular for ACPA-positive RA.[5] Most HLA-DRB1 alleles associated with RA share an identical amino acid sequence in the peptide-binding groove, which has been termed the shared epitope (SE).[6] The similarity in sequence has led to the hypothesis that all predisposing HLA-molecules containing the SE-sequence might present specific 'arthritogenic' peptides, which could lead to a joint-specific autoimmune reaction. Given the strong association with ACPA-positive RA, it has been postulated that peptides presented by SE-containing alleles might be citrullinated. It was indeed shown that conversion of an arginine into a citrulline at the peptide-SE interaction site significantly increased the affinity of the peptide for the major histocompatibility complex (MHC) molecule.[7] Furthermore, a study focusing on the crystal structure of the HLA-DRB1-antigen complex found that SE alleles preferentially bound citrullinated peptides, whereas other alleles bound both citrulline and arginine.[8] The high affinity of SE for citrullinated peptides could increase the amount of HLA-peptide complexes on the surface of antigen-presenting cells, thus leading to a (possible joint-specific) T-cell response.[7] However, the exact peptide-binding motifs for these SE-molecules are not known.

Other theories on the role of the SE in RA development have also been postulated, since SE alleles also have another function as a ligand for cell surface calreticulin (CRT), an innate immune receptor present on most human cells and specifically on dendritic cells. The SE-CRT interaction, which is more potent when CRT is citrullinated, is able to initiate a signal transduction cascade changing the phenotype of the dendritic cell and thereby leading to skewing of T-cell responses to the T helper 17 (Th17) subset and reduced regulatory T-cell formation.[9,10] However, the exact role of SE-CRT interaction to RA pathogenesis needs to be further investigated. The different hypotheses on the function of SE in RA are not mutually exclusive and their relative importance remains unclear.

Besides the HLA region, multiple single nucleotide polymorphisms are associated with rheumatoid arthritis.[11] Among these loci is the *PTPN22* gene, the second most potent genetic risk factor for RA development.[12] *PTPN22* encodes a protein tyrosine phosphatase, which is involved in T-cell and B-cell antigen receptor (TCR) signalling. Thus it may not be surprising that this gene is associated with multiple autoimmune diseases.[13] Recently, the *PTPN22* risk allele was also linked to hypercitrullination of peripheral blood mononuclear cells (PBMCs), a process mediated by PAD enzymes.[14] The relationship between *PTPN22* and both hypercitrullination and T- and B-cell receptor signalling offers new research opportunities to gain more insight in the complex events taking place during the preclinical phase of RA.

Smoking

Smoking is identified as an environmental risk factor for (ACPA-positive) RA. Several theories exist on how smoking might predispose to RA. Smoking leads to higher expression of the PAD2 enzyme, increasing the level of citrullination in the lung.[15] However, it is still unclear how tolerance against citrullinated proteins is broken and ACPAs are produced, since citrullination also occurs in physiological conditions. (Hyper)citrullination alone is therefore not enough to cause a break of tolerance and lead to autoimmunity. A gene–environment interaction has been reported between HLA-DR SE alleles, and, to a lesser extent, *PTPN22* and smoking. This interaction suggests an interplay between T cells (on which these genetic risk factors exert their effect) and the abundance of citrullinated antigens (influenced by smoking), leading to a break of tolerance.[16,17] Citrulline-specific T cells have been described in both SE-positive healthy individuals and in RA patients. However, the immune response in RA patients was more pro-inflammatory with a significantly higher number of cells and skewing to a T helper 1 (Th1) memory phenotype.[18,19]

The microbiome

Recently the microbiome has received attention as a possible factor in the pathophysiology of many diseases. Also, in RA a role for the oral and gut microbiome has been indicated. RA patients can be distinguished from healthy controls based on alterations and dysbiosis of the microbiome, for example regarding clostridium, lactobacillus and bifidobacteria species in the gut microbiota.[20] Alterations in the microbiome have not been found to induce arthritis, but could worsen or alleviate arthritis. It has been hypothesized that dysbiosis of the microbiome could lead to local inflammation, loss of barrier function, and bacterial translocation from mucosa to the bloodstream. Some bacterial cell wall components might molecularly mimic human autoantigens, triggering an immune response also directed against the joint.[21,20]

In this light the epidemiological association between RA and periodontitis, a bacterial-induced chronic inflammation of the gums, is intriguing. The bacterium *Porphyromonas gingivalis*, causing severe periodontitis, might provide a pathophysiological explanation for this epidemiological relation, since ACPAs can bind citrullinated alpha-enolase of *P. gingivalis*.[22] Furthermore, this microorganism expresses a PAD enzyme, providing a source of citrullinated antigens in a pro-inflammatory environment. The proteins citrullinated by bacterial PAD might evoke an immune response that is cross-reactive with self-peptides, thus causing a break of tolerance.[23] However, mammalian calcium-dependent PAD enzymes citrullinate specific arginine residues within polypeptide chains (endocitrullination), while the PAD enzyme of *P. gingivalis* modifies only C-terminal arginines.[24] Therefore, antigens citrullinated by *P. gingivalis* PAD differ significantly from citrullinated self-antigens, which renders this molecular mimicry theory subject to debate.

New insights into this matter were provided by a study, which found citrullinated peptides showing endocitrullination in gingival crevicular fluid of patients with periodontal disease. Only a single pathogen related to periodontitis, *Aggregatibacter actinomycetemcomitans* (Aa), has the potential to dysregulate citrullination by human PAD enzymes, leading to endocitrullination. Pore-forming toxin leukotoxin A (LtxA), produced by Aa, mediates this process by binding to β2 integrin (CD18) on neutrophils, leading to an influx of extracellular calcium and hypercitrullination of intracellular proteins by the cells' own calcium-dependent PAD enzymes. In RA patients the presence of anti-LtxA antibodies was significantly associated with both ACPA- and RF-positivity. Furthermore, the association between HLA SE alleles and ACPA were exclusively found in the concomitant presence of anti-LtxA-antibodies, supporting a role for LtxA and Aa in disease development. This theory on Aa-mediated hypercitrullination in human cells poses a new interesting mechanism for the generation of citrullinated autoantigens independent of molecular mimicry or citrullination by bacterial PAD enzymes.[24] Although this theory may provide evidence for the generation of autoantibodies it does not provide a theoretical framework how antibodies induce arthritis.

Autoantibodies in RA

Around 50% of recent onset RA patients harbour autoantibodies. The remission rates in autoantibody negative RA are higher than in autoantibody positive RA which results that in cohorts of prevalent long-standing RA patients with active disease up to 80% harbour autoantibodies.[1] The presence of autoantibodies has allowed the identification of subgroups of RA patients that are not only more homogenous with regard to risk factors, but also regarding the clinical disease course. RF, an autoantibody directed against the Fc-part of human IgG, was the first autoantibody system to be described in RA. The presence of RF was considered so characteristic for RA that it was included in the 1987 ACR classification criteria for RA, despite its suboptimal specificity. Several decades later the more RA-specific ACPA were discovered.[25,26] In the ACR-EULAR 2010 classification criteria for RA both RF and ACPA have been included. More recently, antibodies against other post-translationally modified proteins (i.e. carbamylated[2]) and acetylated proteins were identified.[3] Seropositive RA is associated with increased radiographic progression and joint damage,[27] while seronegative RA patients have higher inflammation parameters at presentation.[28] Furthermore, not only positivity for a single autoantibody, but rather the conjoined presence of multiple autoantibodies might be relevant for characterizing distinct phenotypes of RA patients.[29] Autoantibodies not merely provide useful information on disease outcome, but also offer insights into the development of RA. Research on the different autoantibodies and their characteristics has led to better understanding of the underlying pathophysiological processes in RA.

Anticitrullinated protein antibodies

As described earlier, citrullinated peptides are generated in response to a post-translational modification mediated by PAD enzymes. Multiple antibody isotypes including IgG, IgA, and IgM directed against these citrullinated peptides are detected in RA.[30] The presence of ACPA IgA is in line with the hypothesis that ACPA is related to smoking or microbiome dysbiosis, as IgA is related to a mucosal origin of the immune response. Synovial fluid from inflamed RA joints contains citrullinated proteins, suggesting that ACPA could bind to these antigens in the joint and possibly increase local inflammation.[31] A putative target protein of ACPA is vimentin. In collagen induced arthritis mouse models passive transfer of ACPA cannot cause synovitis, although it can worsen pre-existent synovitis.[32] Therefore it is suggested that multiple 'hits' are necessary for the development of RA. One hypothesis is that autoantibodies might specifically lead to non-resolving and chronicity of a normally temporary immune response, for example, after trauma or infection.

How might ACPA lead to inflammation? This could be mediated via binding to Fc-receptors or complement activation, which is described in more detail next. Furthermore, to answer this question, the molecular structure of ACPA and specifically their glycosylation has been studied in depth over the past years. Autoantibodies in general are glycoproteins, meaning carbohydrate chains are attached to both the Fc- and the Fab region of the antibody, which is essential for immune effector functions. The Fc-region of ACPA has a lower level of galactosylation and sialylation compared to IgG antibodies against recall antigens.[33] Less sialylation of antibodies in immune complexes can drive osteoclastogenesis in vitro and in vivo through altered FcγR signalling. Moreover, RA patients with low levels of ACPA-IgG Fc sialylation had lower bone volumes and trabecula numbers.[34] Thus, the specific Fc glycan signature of ACPA could influence their ability to contribute to disease pathophysiology.

Strikingly, the glycosylation of ACPA is not only distinct from other antibodies in the Fc-part, but ACPA also more frequently have N-linked glycans in their variable domains. The prevalence of these glycans is markedly increased and they also differ in structure, with Fab-glycans of ACPA having more galactose, sialic acid, and fucose residues compared to control IgG.[35] The high galactosylation and sialylation levels of the Fab-linked glycans are in marked contrast to the lower level of galactosylation and sialylation detected in the Fc-part of ACPA-IgG. It remains unclear how these distinct ACPA glycosylation patterns arise, but exposure of the B cell to environmental factors such as cytokines is likely to be of importance. The influence of increased Fab-glycosylation on ACPA effector functions is unknown. Since >95%% of ACPA-IgG is Fab glycosylated in contrast to 20% of normal IgG, it is speculated that Fab-glycosylation affects ACPA-specific B cells in a way that only ACPA-specific B cells which exhibit a Fab glycan are selected to survive.[35]

Anticarbamylated protein antibodies

Anticarbamylated protein (anti-CarP) antibodies also belong to the group of anti-post-translationally modified protein antibodies (AMPA) that have been described in RA. Carbamylation is a chemical reaction mediated by cyanide in which a lysine is converted into a homocitrulline. Certain conditions, for example, renal disease, smoking, and inflammation can increase cyanide levels and thus carbamylation.[36] Similar to citrullination, increased carbamylation alone does not seem to be sufficient to break tolerance and induce autoimmunity. Only 12% of patients with renal disease harbour anti-CarP antibodies compared to approximately 44% of RA patients.[37] Smoking might contribute to the break of tolerance as a recent study showed that smoking broadened the immune response against carbamylated vimentin in mouse models, but epidemiological research failed to show an association between anti-CarP and smoking

in RA patients.[38,39] The importance of smoking and other (environmental or genetic) factors necessary to break tolerance against carbamylated proteins such a fibrinogen remains to be elucidated. Although the molecular structures of homocitrulline and citrulline are very alike, ACPA and anti-CarP are distinct autoantibody classes, with anti-CarP being present in both ACPA-positive and ACPA-negative patients.[2] Moreover, anti-CarP is associated with radiographic progression in patients negative for RF and ACPA. Diagnostic classification of RA patients did not improve by adding anti-CarP testing, as RF and ACPA are already good predictors for disease.[40] Assays to test for the presence of anti-CarP most often use fetal calf serum, containing a mixture of carbamylated proteins. The exact autoantigens that anti-CarP bind in vivo remains unclear.

Antiacetylated protein antibodies

The latest addition to AMPAs in RA patients is antiacetylated protein antibodies which have been described in approximately 40% of RA patients, mainly in the ACPA-positive group. Detection rates in seronegative RA patients were comparable to patients with resolving arthritis, rendering it unlikely that these antibodies will be a new biomarker helpful for diagnosing RA.[3] However, antiacetylated protein antibodies might provide useful new insights in pathophysiology, especially in the era in which the microbiome seems to become increasingly important. Acetylation is an enzymatic process, which can be affected by bacteria, although the underlying mechanism is unclear. Therefore, antiacetylated antibodies could provide a possible new link between microbiome dysbiosis and the development of autoimmunity in RA.[3,41]

Development of the autoantibody response over time

The presence of the different autoantibodies in serum of (future) RA patients can be detected years before actual disease onset.[42-44] Most research on the details of the autoantibody response prior to clinical disease manifestation has been done on ACPA. From all RA patients 50% presents with ACPA. About 4 years before disease onset 50% of the patients that will be ACPA positive will harbour ACPA. At that time point the ACPA levels start to increase. The profile of citrullinated antigens recognized expands extensively and isotype switching occurs. These events predict RA development in patients with undifferentiated arthritis and correlate with a rise in inflammatory cytokine levels.[45-49] Also the Fc glycosylation pattern changes before disease onset. Galactosylation decreases while fucosylation increases, leading towards a more pro-inflammatory phenotype of the antibodies.[50]

There is one feature of ACPA, which strikingly differs from the normal development of antibody responses. In general, during B-cell maturation, class switching, somatic hypermutation, and affinity maturation are physiological processes occurring in germinal centres. B cells producing antibodies with sufficient avidity will proliferate, improving the efficacy of the immune response. In contrast to an immune response against recall antigens, the avidity maturation of ACPA is very limited, resulting in low-avidity antibodies.[51] This is interesting as it suggests that isotype switching and avidity maturation of ACPA are relatively uncoupled. Within ACPA-positive patients, those with lower avidity ACPA have increased joint destruction compared to patients with higher avidity ACPA, which might be mediated via a higher potency to activate complement.[52]

After the disease has become clinically apparent, the ACPA profile and phenotype remains stable over time.[45,49] The overall development of the autoantibody response over time raises many questions. For example, it is unclear which factors are involved in the maturation of the response before disease onset, and what the role of this maturation is after disease onset.

Pathogenic potential of autoantibodies

Several features of the anticitrulline immune response, such as the expansion of the ACPA repertoire before disease onset and the association of autoantibodies with radiographic progression suggest a possible role in disease pathology. In addition, B-cell depletion with rituximab is effective in RA patients, to a greater extent in ACPA and RF positive cases, arguing in favour of a role of B cells (and perhaps the autoantibodies they produce) in disease pathogenesis.[53] There are thus several lines of evidence that autoantibodies play a pathogenic role in RA. In the next section several hypotheses are discussed regarding mechanisms by which autoantibodies might lead to ongoing inflammation and RA symptoms.

Binding to Fc-receptors

In general antibodies exert an effect on other cells via Fc-receptor binding. Similar to recall antigen immune complexes (ICs), immune complexes containing ACPA and citrullinated fibrinogen are able to stimulate tumour necrosis factor (TNF) secretion via stimulation of Fcγ-receptors on macrophages.[54,55] The effector functions of the ACPA ICs can be modified by the presence of RF-IgM or RF-IgA, which boosts the Fcγ-receptor mediated immune response and increases complement activation.[56] This suggests that there may be a synergetic role of ACPA and RF in RA pathophysiology, which is supported by epidemiological studies showing that the combination of ACPA and RF is associated with higher disease activity.[57]

Complement activation

Another main effector function of antibodies is complement activation. The complement system can be activated via three pathways: the classical pathway (initiated by C1q), the alternative pathway (initiated by C3) and the lectin pathway (initiated by mannose-binding lectin (MBL)), which all lead to opsonization, formation of the membrane-attack complex and chemotaxis. In synovial fluid of RA patients complement levels are reduced, while complement cleavage products are increased, indicating enhanced complement activation. It has been shown that ACPA have the ability to recruit complement via both the classical and alternative pathways, but not via the lectin pathway.[58] Taken together, the evidence suggests that ACPA have the potential to augment the immune response in RA by both Fcγ-receptor binding and complement activation.

Neutrophil extracellular trap formation in RA

The augmented generation of neutrophil extracellular traps (NETs) is another mechanism through which ACPA and/or RF antibodies could affect disease development or persistence. NETs are composed of highly condensed chromatin and are expelled by neutrophils to trap and kill pathogens. NETosis by both circulating and synovial fluid neutrophils is enhanced in RA patients compared to healthy controls. The relation between NETosis and autoantibodies is interesting, as NETosis exposes autoantigens (i.e. citrullinated self-proteins) in a pro-inflammatory environment.[59] Therefore amplified citrullinated autoantigen exposure via NETosis might be involved in promoting autoantibody generation and production in predisposed hosts. It was shown that citrullinated peptides derived from deiminated histones, a component of NETs, are targeted by ACPAs.[60] B cells differentiated from synovial ectopic lymphoid tissue were reactive against the citrullinated histones exposed during NETosis.[61] On the other hand, ACPA can stimulate NETosis. NETs trigger inflammatory responses in synovial fibroblasts, including induction of IL-6, IL-8, chemokines, and adhesion molecules. ACPA might thus enhance local inflammation by increasing NETosis. Taken together aberrant NETosis might fuel the ongoing ACPA response and lead to a circular non-resolving pro-inflammatory immune response, by which RA is characterized.[59]

Bone erosion: Osteoclast activation

Seropositive RA is associated with increased damage to joints, which is commonly measured as radiographic progression.[62,63] It has been proposed that ACPA may directly affect osteoclasts and thereby lead to the formation of bone erosions. ACPA have indeed been described to bind to the osteoclast surface and enhance differentiation of osteoclast precursors *in vitro* and *in vivo*. Adoptive transfer of ACPA has also led to increased bone resorption in mouse models, although this process seemed to differ from the joint damage in RA.[64] Recently, a mediating effect of IL-8 in the relation between ACPA, stimulation of osteoclasts, and bone erosions was proposed. The finding that an IL-8 antagonist could prevent bone loss *in vitro* in humans and *in vivo* in mice supports the hypothesis that ACPA is directly linked to formation of bone erosions via IL-8 induction.[65] This hypothesis about ACPA and bone destruction is supported by preliminary data, but many questions, for example, regarding the epitopes on osteoclasts that ACPA bind to and the fine specificities of ACPA mediating the effect on bone erosions, have yet to be answered. It will be intriguing to see how this field will further develop.

Pain

Not only radiographic progression but also chronic pain is a significant clinical problem in RA. It was investigated whether autoantibodies might also (partly) provoke these symptoms. Mouse models injected with ACPAs were found to display lasting pain-like behaviour while no sign of inflammation was present. The injected ACPAs bound surface epitopes on osteoclasts and osteoclast precursors in mouse bone marrow, subchondral bone, and epiphyseal plate. These activated osteoclasts express CXCL1 (the mouse homologue of IL-8 described earlier), which might mediate the effect on nociception.[66] This research proposes a novel theory that the presence of autoantibodies might directly contribute to arthralgia, a symptom often present before arthritis in RA.

Final common inflammatory pathway

Just described are various scenarios about how autoantibodies could be involved in the pathogenesis of RA, but it has to be kept in mind that there is no definitive proof that these autoantibodies are in fact pathogenic. In the development of RA, a common inflammatory pathway seems to exist leading to a similar clinical presentation in patients with and without autoantibodies.

In this paragraph a very brief overview of this final common pathway is given, in which many cell types and processes are involved. Early in the development of arthritis, activation of the innate immune system leads to an influx of leukocytes into the normally sparsely populated synovial compartment via the local expression of adhesion molecules and chemokines.[67] Less complement factors and more complement cleavage products are found locally, indicating increased complement use.[68] Also, the adaptive immune system is triggered and stimulated dendritic cells as well as costimulatory molecules are found. These circumstances facilitate activation of Th1 T helper cells.[67] More recently the Th17 T helper cell phenotype has also been implicated as a key driver of synovitis, as these cells are potent producers of pro-inflammatory cytokines like IL-17A, IL-21, and TNF-α.[69] The pro-inflammatory T cells, cytokines, and ICs stimulate macrophages and fibroblast-like synoviocytes (FLS) to produce pro-inflammatory cytokines, like TNF-α, IL-1, IL-6, IL-15, and IL-23. In the RA joint FLS have proliferated and adapted a pro-inflammatory phenotype with increased expression of chemokines, adhesion molecules and matrix metalloproteinases (MMP). MMP can lead directly to cartilage destruction and chronic synovial inflammation. Cartilage can also be affected indirectly via cytokines leading to chondrocyte activation and tissue catabolism.[70] Besides cartilage also bone is subject to destruction in the joint of RA patients. Activated fibroblasts, T cells, B cells, and macrophages can upregulate expression of receptor activator of nuclear factor kappa-B (RANK) ligand, leading to osteoclastogenesis and thus bone destruction.[71] The central role of cytokines in RA synovitis is further affirmed by the successful use of monoclonal antibodies directed against these cytokines, the most well-known being anti-TNFα, in the treatment of RA. However, these therapies have the major downside that they target the immune system non-specifically, increasing the risk of infections and perhaps neoplasms. Therefore, research focusing on unravelling the precise immunopathology of RA might introduce possibilities for specific targeted therapy, which could significantly improve care for RA patients.

Conclusion

The search for autoantigens with relevance for pathogenesis, diagnosis, and prognosis of RA has led to the characterization of several interesting autoantibody system in RA. Studies investigating the role of anti-posttranslational modified protein antibodies, especially ACPA, have led to a better understanding of underlying pathophysiologic processes. Autoantibody formation is associated with both genetic and environmental risk factors for RA, like HLA-SE alleles, smoking, and microbiome dysbiosis, offering intriguing new views on the development of RA.

Acknowledgement

This chapter is based on the following review: Derksen VFAM, Huizinga TWJ, van der Woude D. The role of autoantibodies in the pathophysiology of rheumatoid arthritis. *Semin Immunopathol* 2017 Jun;39(4):437–46.

REFERENCES

1. Scott DL, Wolfe F, Huizinga TW. Rheumatoid arthritis. *Lancet* 2010;376(9746):1094–108.
2. Shi J, Knevel R, Suwannalai P, et al. Autoantibodies recognizing carbamylated proteins are present in sera of patients with rheumatoid arthritis and predict joint damage. *Proc Natl Acad Sci USA* 2011;108(42):17372–7.
3. Juarez M, Bang H, Hammar F, et al. Identification of novel antiacetylated vimentin antibodies in patients with early inflammatory arthritis. *Ann Rheum Dis* 2016;75(6):1099–107.
4. MacGregor AJ, Snieder H, Rigby AS, et al. Characterizing the quantitative genetic contribution to rheumatoid arthritis using data from twins. *Arthritis Rheum* 2000;43(1):30–7.
5. Huizinga TW, Amos CI, van der Helm-van Mil AH, et al. Refining the complex rheumatoid arthritis phenotype based on specificity of the HLA-DRB1 shared epitope for antibodies to citrullinated proteins. *Arthritis Rheum* 2005;52(11):3433–8.
6. Gregersen PK, Silver J, Winchester RJ. The shared epitope hypothesis. An approach to understanding the molecular genetics of susceptibility to rheumatoid arthritis. *Arthritis Rheum* 1987;30(11):1205–13.
7. Hill JA, Southwood S, Sette A, et al. Cutting edge: the conversion of arginine to citrulline allows for a high-affinity peptide interaction with the rheumatoid arthritis-associated HLA-DRB1*0401 MHC class II molecule. *J Immunol* 2003;171(2):538–41.
8. Scally SW, Petersen J, Law SC, et al. A molecular basis for the association of the HLA-DRB1 locus, citrullination, and rheumatoid arthritis. *J Exp Med* 2013;210(12):2569–82.
9. de Almeida DE, Ling S, Holoshitz J. New insights into the functional role of the rheumatoid arthritis shared epitope. *FEBS Lett* 2011;585(23):3619–26.
10. Ling S, Cline EN, Haug TS, et al. Citrullinated calreticulin potentiates rheumatoid arthritis shared epitope signaling. *Arthritis Rheum* 2013;65(3):618–26.
11. Diogo D, Okada Y, Plenge RM. Genome-wide association studies to advance our understanding of critical cell types and pathways in rheumatoid arthritis: recent findings and challenges. *Curr Opin Rheumatol* 2014;26(1):85–92.
12. Begovich AB, Carlton VE, Honigberg LA, et al. A missense single-nucleotide polymorphism in a gene encoding a protein tyrosine phosphatase (PTPN22) is associated with rheumatoid arthritis. *Am J Hum Genet* 2004;75(2):330–7.
13. Rieck M, Arechiga A, Onengut-Gumuscu S, et al. Genetic variation in PTPN22 corresponds to altered function of T and B lymphocytes. *J Immunol* 2007;179 (7):4704–10.
14. Chang HH, Liu GY, Dwivedi N, et al. A molecular signature of preclinical rheumatoid arthritis triggered by dysregulated PTPN22. *JCI Insight 1* 2016;1(17):e90045.
15. Makrygiannakis D, Hermansson M, Ulfgren AK, et al. Smoking increases peptidylarginine deiminase 2 enzyme expression in human lungs and increases citrullination in BAL cells. *Ann Rheum Dis* 2008;67(10):1488–92.
16. Klareskog L, Stolt P, Lundberg K, et al. A new model for an etiology of rheumatoid arthritis: smoking may trigger HLA-DR (shared epitope)-restricted immune reactions to autoantigens modified by citrullination. *Arthritis Rheum* 2006;54(1):38–46.
17. Kallberg H, Padyukov L, Plenge RM, et al. Gene-gene and gene-environment interactions involving HLA-DRB1, PTPN22, and smoking in two subsets of rheumatoid arthritis. *Am J Hum Genet* 2007;80(5):867–75.

18. Snir O, Rieck M, Gebe JA, et al. Identification and functional characterization of T cells reactive to citrullinated vimentin in HLA-DRB1*0401-positive humanized mice and rheumatoid arthritis patients. *Arthritis Rheum* 2011;*63*(10):2873–83.

19. James EA, Rieck M, Pieper J, et al. Citrulline-specific Th1 cells are increased in rheumatoid arthritis and their frequency is influenced by disease duration and therapy. *Arthritis Rheum* 2014;*66*(7):1712–22.

20. Zhang X, Zhang D, Jia H. The oral and gut microbiomes are perturbed in rheumatoid arthritis and partly normalized after treatment. *Nat Med* 2015;*21*(8):895–905.

21. Sandhya P, Danda D, Sharma D, et al. Does the buck stop with the bugs?: an overview of microbial dysbiosis in rheumatoid arthritis. *Int J Rheum Dis* 2016;*19*(1):8–20.

22. Lundberg K, Kinloch A, Fisher BA, et al. Antibodies to citrullinated alpha-enolase peptide 1 are specific for rheumatoid arthritis and cross-react with bacterial enolase. *Arthritis Rheum* 2008;*58*(10):3009–19.

23. Farquharson D, Butcher JP, Culshaw S. Periodontitis, porphyromonas, and the pathogenesis of rheumatoid arthritis. *Mucosal Immunol* 2012;*5*(2):112–20.

24. Konig MF, Abusleme L, Reinholdt J, et al. Aggregatibacter actinomycetemcomitans-induced hypercitrullination links periodontal infection to autoimmunity in rheumatoid arthritis. *Sci Transl Med* 2016;*8*(369):369ra176.

25. Schellekens GA, de Jong BA, van den Hoogen FH, et al. Citrulline is an essential constituent of antigenic determinants recognized by rheumatoid arthritis-specific autoantibodies. *J Clin Invest* 1998;*101*(1):273–81.

26. Schellekens GA, Visser H, de Jong BA, et al. The diagnostic properties of rheumatoid arthritis antibodies recognizing a cyclic citrullinated peptide. *Arthritis Rheum* 2000;*43*(1):155–63.

27. van der Helm-van Mil AH, Verpoort KN, Breedveld FC, et al. Antibodies to citrullinated proteins and differences in clinical progression of rheumatoid arthritis. *Arthritis Res Ther* 2005;*7*(5):R949–58.

28. Nordberg LB, Lillegraven S, Lie E, et al. Patients with seronegative RA have more inflammatory activity compared with patients with seropositive RA in an inception cohort of DMARD-naive patients classified according to the 2010 ACR/EULAR criteria. *Ann Rheum Dis* 2017;*76*(2):341–5.

29. Derksen VF, Ajeganova S, Trouw LA, et al. Rheumatoid arthritis phenotype at presentation differs depending on the number of autoantibodies present. *Ann Rheum Dis* 2016;*76*(4):716–20.

30. Verpoort KN, Jol-van der Zijde CM, Papendrecht-van der Voort EA, et al. Isotype distribution of anti-cyclic citrullinated peptide antibodies in undifferentiated arthritis and rheumatoid arthritis reflects an ongoing immune response. *Arthritis Rheum* 2006;*54*(12):3799–808.

31. van Beers JJ, Schwarte CM, Stammen-Vogelzangs J, et al. The rheumatoid arthritis synovial fluid citrullinome reveals novel citrullinated epitopes in apolipoprotein E, myeloid nuclear differentiation antigen, and beta-actin. *Arthritis Rheum* 2013;*65*(1):69–80.

32. Kuhn KA, Kulik L, Tomooka B, et al. Antibodies against citrullinated proteins enhance tissue injury in experimental autoimmune arthritis. *J Clin Invest* 2006;*116*(4):961–73.

33. Scherer HU, van der Woude D, Ioan-Facsinay A, et al. Glycan profiling of anti-citrullinated protein antibodies isolated from human serum and synovial fluid. *Arthritis Rheum* 2010;*62*(6):1620–9.

34. Harre U, Lang SC, Pfeifle R, et al. Glycosylation of immunoglobulin G determines osteoclast differentiation and bone loss. *Nature Commun* 2015;*6*:6651.

35. Hafkenscheid L, Bondt A, Scherer HU, et al. Structural analysis of variable domain glycosylation of anti-citrullinated protein antibodies in rheumatoid arthritis reveals the presence of highly sialylated glycans. *Mol Cell Proteomics* 2017;*16*(2):278–87.

36. Wang Z, Nicholls SJ, Rodriguez ER, et al. Protein carbamylation links inflammation, smoking, uremia and atherogenesis. *Nat Med* 2007;*13*(10):1176–84.

37. Verheul MK, van Erp SJ, van der Woude D, et al. Anti-carbamylated protein antibodies: a specific hallmark for rheumatoid arthritis. Comparison to conditions known for enhanced carbamylation; renal failure, smoking and chronic inflammation. *Ann Rheum Dis* 2016;*75*(8):1575–6.

38. Ospelt C, Bang H, Feist E, et al. Carbamylation of vimentin is inducible by smoking and represents an independent autoantigen in rheumatoid arthritis. *Ann Rheum Dis* 2017;*76*(7):1176–83.

39. Jiang X, Trouw LA, van Wesemael TJ, et al. Anti-CarP antibodies in two large cohorts of patients with rheumatoid arthritis and their relationship to genetic risk factors, cigarette smoking and other autoantibodies. *Ann Rheum Dis* 2014;*73*(10):1761–8.

40. Ajeganova S, van Steenbergen HW, Verheul MK, et al. The association between anti-carbamylated protein (anti-CarP) antibodies and radiographic progression in early rheumatoid arthritis: a study exploring replication and the added value to ACPA and rheumatoid factor. *Ann Rheum Dis* 2017;*76*(1):112–18.

41. Simon GM, Cheng J, Gordon JI. Quantitative assessment of the impact of the gut microbiota on lysine epsilon-acetylation of host proteins using gnotobiotic mice. *Proc Natl Acad Sci USA* 2012;*109*(28):11133–8.

42. Rantapaa-Dahlqvist S, de Jong BA, Berglin E, et al. Antibodies against cyclic citrullinated peptide and IgA rheumatoid factor predict the development of rheumatoid arthritis. *Arthritis Rheum* 2003;*48*(10):2741–9.

43. Nielen MM, van Schaardenburg D, Reesink HW, et al. Specific autoantibodies precede the symptoms of rheumatoid arthritis: a study of serial measurements in blood donors. *Arthritis Rheum* 2004;*50*(2):380–6.

44. Shi J, van de Stadt LA, Levarht EW, et al. Anti-carbamylated protein (anti-CarP) antibodies precede the onset of rheumatoid arthritis. *Ann Rheum Dis* 2014;*73*(4):780–3.

45. van der Woude D, Rantapaa-Dahlqvist S, Ioan-Facsinay A, et al. Epitope spreading of the anti-citrullinated protein antibody response occurs before disease onset and is associated with the disease course of early arthritis. *Ann Rheum Dis* 2010;*69*(8):1554–61.

46. van de Stadt LA, de Koning MH, van de Stadt RJ, et al. Development of the anti-citrullinated protein antibody repertoire prior to the onset of rheumatoid arthritis. *Arthritis Rheum* 2011;*63*(11):3226–33.

47. Kokkonen H, Mullazehi M, Berglin E, et al. Antibodies of IgG, IgA and IgM isotypes against cyclic citrullinated peptide precede the development of rheumatoid arthritis. *Arthritis Res Ther* 2011;*13*(1):R13.

48. Sokolove J, Bromberg R, Deane KD, et al. Autoantibody epitope spreading in the pre-clinical phase predicts progression to rheumatoid arthritis. *PloS One* 2012;*7*(5):e35296.

49. Brink M, Hansson M, Mathsson L, et al. Multiplex analyses of antibodies against citrullinated peptides in individuals prior to development of rheumatoid arthritis. *Arthritis Rheum* 2013;*65*(4):899–910.

50. Rombouts Y, Ewing E, van de Stadt LA, et al. Anti-citrullinated protein antibodies acquire a pro-inflammatory Fc glycosylation phenotype prior to the onset of rheumatoid arthritis. *Ann Rheum Dis* 2015;*74*(1):234–41.

51. Suwannalai P, van de Stadt LA, Radner H, et al. Avidity maturation of anti-citrullinated protein antibodies in rheumatoid arthritis. *Arthritis Rheum* 2012;*64*(5):1323–8.

52. Suwannalai P, Britsemmer K, Knevel R, et al. Low-avidity anticitrullinated protein antibodies (ACPA) are associated with a higher rate of joint destruction in rheumatoid arthritis. *Ann Rheum Dis* 2014;*73*(1):270–6.

53. Cambridge G, Leandro MJ, Edwards JC, et al. Serologic changes following B lymphocyte depletion therapy for rheumatoid arthritis. *Arthritis Rheum* 2003;*48*(8):2146–54.

54. Clavel C, Nogueira L, Laurent L, et al. Induction of macrophage secretion of tumor necrosis factor alpha through Fcgamma receptor IIa engagement by rheumatoid arthritis-specific autoantibodies to citrullinated proteins complexed with fibrinogen. *Arthritis Rheum* 2008;*58*(3):678–88.

55. Laurent L, Clavel C, Lemaire O, et al. Fcgamma receptor profile of monocytes and macrophages from rheumatoid arthritis patients and their response to immune complexes formed with autoantibodies to citrullinated proteins. *Ann Rheum Dis* 2011;*70*(6):1052–9.

56. Anquetil F, Clavel C, Offer G, et al. IgM and IgA rheumatoid factors purified from rheumatoid arthritis sera boost the Fc receptor- and complement-dependent effector functions of the disease-specific anti-citrullinated protein autoantibodies. *J Immunol* 2015;*194*(8):3664–74.

57. Sokolove J, Johnson DS, Lahey LJ, et al. Rheumatoid factor as a potentiator of anti-citrullinated protein antibody-mediated inflammation in rheumatoid arthritis. *Arthritis Rheum* 2014;*66*(4):813–21.

58. Trouw LA, Haisma EM, Levarht EW, et al. Anti-cyclic citrullinated peptide antibodies from rheumatoid arthritis patients activate complement via both the classical and alternative pathways. *Arthritis Rheum* 2009;*60*(7):1923–31.

59. Khandpur R, Carmona-Rivera C, Vivekanandan-Giri A, et al. NETs are a source of citrullinated autoantigens and stimulate inflammatory responses in rheumatoid arthritis. *Sci Transl Med* 2013;*5*(178):178ra140.

60. Pratesi F, Dioni I, Tommasi C, et al. Antibodies from patients with rheumatoid arthritis target citrullinated histone 4 contained in neutrophils extracellular traps. *Ann Rheum Dis* 2014;*73*(7):1414–22.

61. Corsiero E, Bombardieri M, Carlotti E, et al. Single cell cloning and recombinant monoclonal antibodies generation from RA synovial B cells reveal frequent targeting of citrullinated histones of NETs. *Ann Rheum Dis* 2016;*75*(10):1866–75.

62. Hecht C, Englbrecht M, Rech J, et al. Additive effect of anti-citrullinated protein antibodies and rheumatoid factor on bone erosions in patients with RA. *Ann Rheum Dis* 2015;*74*(12):2151–6.

63. van Steenbergen HW, Ajeganova S, Forslind K, et al. The effects of rheumatoid factor and anticitrullinated peptide antibodies on bone erosions in rheumatoid arthritis. *Ann Rheum Dis* 2015;*74*(1):e3.

64. Harre U, Georgess D, Bang H, et al. Induction of osteoclastogenesis and bone loss by human autoantibodies against citrullinated vimentin. *J Clin Invest* 2012;*12*(5):1791–802.

65. Krishnamurthy A, Joshua V, Haj Hensvold A, et al. Identification of a novel chemokine-dependent molecular mechanism underlying rheumatoid arthritis-associated autoantibody-mediated bone loss. *Ann Rheum Dis* 2016;*75*(4):721–9.

66. Wigerblad G, Bas DB, Fernades-Cerqueira C, Krishnamurthy A, et al. Autoantibodies to citrullinated proteins induce joint pain independent of inflammation via a chemokine-dependent mechanism. *Ann Rheum Dis* 2016;*75*(4):730–8.

67. McInnes IB, Schett G. The pathogenesis of rheumatoid arthritis. *N Engl J Med* 2011;*365*(23):2205–19.

68. Ballanti E, Perricone C, di Muzio G, et al. Role of the complement system in rheumatoid arthritis and psoriatic arthritis: relationship with anti-TNF inhibitors. *Autoimmun Rev* 2011;*10*(10):617–23.

69. Kuwabara T, Ishikawa F, Kondo M, et al. The role of IL-17 and related cytokines in inflammatory autoimmune diseases. *Mediators Inflamm* 2017;*2017*;3908061.

70. Firestein GS, McInnes IB. Immunopathogenesis of rheumatoid arthritis. *Immunity* 2017;*46*(2):183–96.

71. Smolen JS, Aletaha D, McInnes IB. Rheumatoid arthritis. *Lancet* 2016;*388*(10055):2023–38.

Dendritic cells and T cells in rheumatoid arthritis

Soi-Cheng Law, Pascale Wehr, Harriet Purvis, and Ranjeny Thomas

Introduction

Rheumatoid arthritis (RA) has a strong human leukocyte antigen (HLA)-class II association: patients carrying HLA-DR 'shared epitope' alleles, exhibit a high risk of seropositive RA while sero-negative RA is associated with other HLA-DR alleles, including HLA-DR3. The molecular mechanisms underpinning this association are increasingly appreciated, including the presentation of MHC class II-restricted autoantigens to autoreactive CD4+ T cells. Dendritic cells (DCs) are the key professional antigen-presenting cells for priming T-cell immunity. They also play a major role in immune tolerance. They are able to achieve this balance as a result of two main features. Firstly, DCs respond functionally to activation by microbial and damage-associated stimuli, and secondly DCs represent a family of subsets with specialized activities. Here we introduce the DC and T-cell players and their function in the immune system, then review the evidence for their involvement in the pathogenesis of RA, particularly through the presentation of antigen that triggers the differentiation of autoreactive T cells, as well as innate immune effector functions. Finally, we review the emerging field of transferring or targeting antigen-presenting DCs for immunotherapy of RA.

Dendritic cells and RA

Dendritic cells (DCs) are specialised antigen-presenting cells which link the innate and adaptive immune responses, activating and priming effector CD4+ T cells, cross-presenting antigen to CD8+ T cells, and promoting B-cell antibody production.[1] DCs also play important roles in the maintenance of immune tolerance. In RA, DCs are thought to drive the activation of self-peptide-reactive inflammatory T cells and ultimately B cells.[2–4] Multiple genetic and environmental factors affecting DC functions, including regulation, differentiation, maturation, migration, and antigen presentation, may influence the onset and progression of RA.

DC subsets

Two major functionally distinct subsets of DCs exist *in vivo*: classical/myeloid DCs (cDCs) and plasmacytoid DCs (pDCs). Both are thought to contribute to RA onset. Although several studies show that circulating peripheral blood (PB) cDCs and pDCs are lower in RA patients than in healthy controls,[5–7] DCs were found to be more abundant and more differentiated in the RA synovium.[8] Human DCs comprise several populations, including two subsets of CD1c+ DCs, which present antigen to CD4+ T cells, CD141+ cross-presenting DCs, which process protein antigen and cross present to CD4+ and CD8+ T cells; and pDCs, which potently secrete type 1 IFN.[7,9–12] A further monocyte-derived inflammatory DC (moDC) population is characterized by CD1c and CD14 coexpression.[13] CD1c+ DCs, pDCs, and moDCs are all consistently found to be enriched in the RA synovium. CCL19, 20, and 21 are abundant in RA synovium where they chemoattract DCs to perivascular lymphoid infiltrates.[14] Thymic stromal lymphopoietin (TSLP) also attracts CD1c+ cDCs to the synovium.[15] CCR6+ immature DCs localize to the lining layer of the RA synovium, similar to macrophages, while CCR7+ mature DCs are located within synovial lymphocyte infiltrates.[14] When activated by Toll-like receptor (TLR) ligands, activated T-cell CD40 ligand, or pro-inflammatory cytokines such as IL-1, granulocyte-macrophage colony-stimulating factor (GM-CSF), and tumour necrosis factor (TNF), DCs mature to produce cytokines and chemokines and to potentiate inflammatory T-cell responses. Secretion of IL-12 and IL-15 by synovial DCs induces T-cell secretion of GM-CSF, which further supports the differentiation of CD1c+ classical/myeloid DCs within the joint, and expands the number of synovial inflammatory moDCs.[16] Furthermore, IL-12 secretion is critically important for the development of T helper 1 (Th1) cells in response to synovial DC antigen presentation.

Antigen presentation by DCs in RA

During immune homeostasis in the absence of inflammatory stimuli, DCs constitutively pick up apoptotic tissue-derived self-antigens and migrate to draining lymph nodes via tissue lymphatics.

These apoptotic bodies actively promote DC regulation through stimulation of TGF-β secretion, enhancing production of CD4⁺ regulatory T cells (Treg), deletion of CD8+ T cells and maintaining immune tolerance.[17-19] Inflammatory immune responses involve recognition of inflammatory signals received from pathogen associated molecular patterns (PAMPs) or danger associated molecular patterns (DAMPs). Inflammatory information is transferred to the adaptive immune system via NF-κB and mitogen-activated protein (MAP) kinase activation, which promote MHC class II/antigen presentation, expression of costimulatory molecules, and the secretion of inflammatory cytokines.[20] In RA synovial DCs, NF-κB is overexpressed commensurate with disease activity, indicating that DCs are responsive to local inflammatory PAMPs and/or DAMPs. Potentially then, after initiation of inflammatory arthritis, synovial fibroblasts, or cartilage autoantigens such as vimentin, collagen II, and HCgp130 that should elicit tolerance, invoke effector T-cell responses are invoked.[4] Under conditions of endoplasmic reticulum (ER) stress, DCs may also present neo-epitopes, such as citrullinated antigens and chaperones, including *E. coli* dnaJ. Furthermore, cell surface calreticulin may bind pro-inflammatory ligands, such as the shared epitope sequence.[21] TLR 2, 3, 4, and 7 are all expressed in the joint synovium. Local synovial delivery of TLR agonists exacerbates arthritis, increasing costimulation and cytokine production.[4,22-25] Polymorphisms in genes such as *CD40*, *REL*, and *PTPN22* may contribute to altered DC responses to pathogens predisposing to RA onset. The autoimmune associated variant of *PTPN22* alters responses to TLR 3, 4, and 7 agonists and the fungal pathogen receptor dectin-1,[26-29] perturbing DC cytokine production and T-cell responses.

Innate immune DC functions in RA

RA synovial DCs secrete chemokines that attract pro-inflammatory immune cells including macrophages, monocytes, and neutrophils.[4,30] In addition, DC secretion of chemokines CCL3, CCL17, CXCL19, and CXCL10 induces T-cell migration to the RA synovium.[31] RA synovial fluid and tissue contain increased numbers of inflammatory Th17 and Th1 cells.[32,33] DCs contribute to their differentiation and expansion. Peripheral and synovial CD1c⁺ DCs from RA patients produce cytokines required for differentiation of Th17 (IL-1β, IL-6, and IL-23) and Th1 (IL-12).[13,31,34,35] In addition, RA synovial CD1c⁺ DCs have enhanced expression of HLA-DR and costimulatory molecules CD40, CD80 and CD86 required for T-cell activation[31] (Figure 8.1). Intra-articular CD1c⁺ (CD33⁺CD14^dim) DCs spontaneously promote T-cell proliferation and inflammatory cytokine production *in vitro* in autologous mixed lymphocyte cultures due to presentation of joint-derived or endogenous self-antigens.[8] Synovial fluid pDCs, though less potent than cDCs, also activate T cells and induce TNF secretion.[10] In addition to promoting inflammatory T-cell differentiation, RA synovial DCs can also induce Treg, at least *in vitro* (36), potentially through engagement of T-cell regulatory receptor PD-1.[36,37] DC-mediated activation and differentiation of inflammatory T-cells potentiates further immune responses within the synovium; for example Th17 cells mediate neutrophil recruitment, B-cell activation and osteoclastogenesis leading to bone resorption and cartilage degradation,[38] and Th1 cells promote macrophage activation.[39]

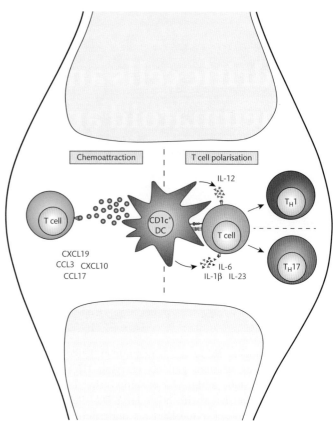

Figure 8.1 Synovial CD1c+ DC mediated T-cell chemoattraction and polarization. Intra-articular DCs secrete multiple chemokines including CCL3, CCL17, CXCL19, and CXCL10 to induce T-cell migration to the RA synovium. Synovial CD1c⁺ DCs from RA patients produce cytokines required for T-cell polarization towards Th17 (IL-1β, IL-6, and IL-23) and Th1 (IL-12) differentiation. RA synovial CD1c⁺ DCs have enhanced expression of HLA-DR and the costimulatory molecules CD40, CD80, CD86, required for T-cell activation.

T cells in RA

T-cell receptor (TCR) diversity for recognition of antigen

CD4+ and CD8+ surface TCRs recognize antigen displayed by HLA class II and class I molecules respectively. The TCR is a heterodimer comprising α and β chains, each of which is formed by somatic recombination of variable (V), diversity (D; β chain only), and junctional (J) gene segments.[40,41] In humans, the TCRα locus encodes 47 Vα and 57 Jα gene segments, while the TCRβ locus has 54 Vβ, 2Dβ and 13Jβ gene segments. Recombined gene segments are spliced together with the constant region (C) to form a functional TCRαβ complex of a single specificity.[41]

These somatic gene segment rearrangements result in combinatorial diversity (Figure 8.2)[40,41] and further random insertion/deletion of nucleotides during recombination creates junctional diversity of the highly variable complementarity-determining region 3 (CDR3).[41,42] The CDR3 region is unique to every T-cell clone, acting as a T-cell 'fingerprint', and encodes the receptor portion responsible for making the majority of TCR contacts with antigenic peptides

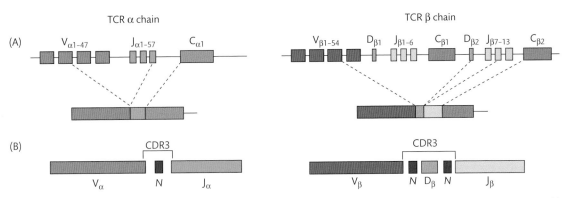

Figure 8.2 Schematic demonstrating the generation of the T-cell receptor, in addition to the complementarity-determining region 3 of both α and β chains. (A) Functional T-cell receptors (TCRs) are comprised of an α and β chain that are formed by somatic recombination of variable (V), diversity (D; β chain only), and junctional (J) gene segments. Recombined gene segments are then spliced together with the constant region (C) to form the functional TCRαβ. (B) Complementarity-determining region 3 (CDR3) is formed at the V, (D), J junction, where imprecise V, (D), J joining, and random addition of non-template encoded nucleotides (N) makes this region the most diverse component of the TCR.

presented by an HLA molecule.[43–46] The diversity in TCRs arising from combinatorial and junctional mechanisms, after thymic selection has occurred, gives rise to a predicted 2×10^7 different TCRs in the human TCR repertoire. This diverse TCR repertoire is essential for avoiding blind spots during pathogen recognition, and for distinguishing between foreign and self-antigens (Figure 8.3).[41,47]

Evidence of autoantigen and TCR selection in RA: TCR repertoire analysis

While several lines of evidence suggest antigen-specific CD4+ T cells are involved in RA pathogenesis, their identification in inflamed RA synovial tissue has been challenging. Characterization of CD4+ T cells and their antigen-specificity is crucial to understand their role in autoimmune inflammation, and to develop T-cell directed immunotherapies.

Elucidation of the TCR repertoire makes it possible to infer which T cells, if any, are expanding in response to autoantigenic stimuli in RA. TCR repertoire biases can manifest in the pre-immune

repertoire due to convergent recombination, whereby TCRs generated more easily predominate, and because of structural constraints imposed by the need for peptide recognition within particular MHC molecules.[48–53] Preferential (clonal) expansion of particular precursor T cells from the naïve repertoire in response to antigen priming can further skew the usage of particular TCR, as expanding daughter T-cell clonotypes use identical CDR3 sequences and V, D and J genes in TCR α and β chains.[41,54–57]

TCR bias in RA patients

To this end, numerous studies have examined the TCR repertoire in the synovial compartment, and PB of RA patients in an attempt to identify biased TCRα and/or β usage suggesting oligoclonal expansions, however no consensus has emerged (Table 8.1). There are many reasons why these studies failed to elucidate a common synovial TCR clonal signature, including differences in HLA haplotype of patients recruited, multiple autoantigen specificities in RA and differences in disease stage of recruited patients.

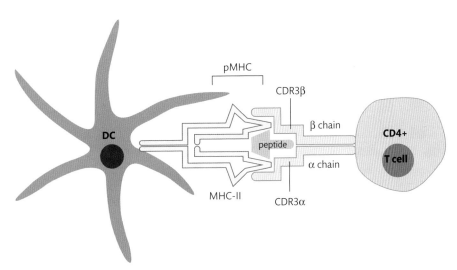

Figure 8.3 The T-cell receptor-peptide-MHC interaction. The heterodimeric T-cell receptor (TCR) on a CD4+ T-cell engages peptide displayed in the major histocompatibility complex class II (MHC-II) on dendritic cells (DC). The complementarity-determining region 3 (CDR3) is the main TCR domain in contact with the antigenic peptide.

Table 8.1 Summary of studies of TCR αβ V gene usage in RA patients

Studies	Source	TCRα/β V gene usage
Yamamoto et al. (1992)[152]	PB, ST, and SF	All Vβ genes in SF and ST relative to PB
Alam et al. (1995)[153]	PB and SM	Vβ3, Vβ17, Vβ22, and Vβ4 in SM relative to PB
Jenkins et al. (1993)[154]	PB, ST, and SF	Vβ6, Vβ15 in ST; Vβ14 in SF; Vβ1, Vβ4, Vβ5.1, Vβ10, Vβ16, Vβ19 in ST, relative to PB
Paliard et al. (1991)[155]	PB and SF	Vβ14 in SF compared to PB
Zagon et al. (1994)[156]	PB and SF	Vβ17 in PB and SF of RA patients compared to healthy controls
Cooper et al. (1994)[157]	PB and SF	Vβ2, Vβ6; Vβ13.1 and Vβ13.2 in SF compared to PB
Sottini et al. (1991)[124]	PB and SF	Vβ7 in SF compared to PB
Lunardia et al. (1992)[158]	PB and SF	Vα10, Vα15, Vα18; Vβ4, Vβ5, Vβ13 in SF compared to PB
Sun et al. (2005)[159]	PB, ST, and SF	Vβ14 and Vβ16 in ST; Vβ16 in SF, relative to PB
Fischer et al. (1996)[160]	SF	Vα17

PB, peripheral blood; ST, synovial tissue; SF, synovial fluid.

Profiling of synovial tissue TCR repertoire of recent-onset and established RA patients revealed that the repertoire of recent-onset patients was dominated by several highly expanded clones, to a significantly greater extent than observed in established RA patients.[58] These findings emphasize that T-cell clonotypes may be more readily detected in early RA patients prior to therapeutic intervention. However, the antigen-specificities of the expanded clones were not determined, and thus their contribution to RA pathogenesis is unclear.

Autoantigen-specific CD4+ T cells: Key players in RA pathogenesis

MHC class II tetramer technology represents a powerful tool to characterize antigen-specific CD4+ T cells. In the RA context, fluorescently labelled multimeric HLA-DR susceptibility molecules displaying putative autoantigenic peptides (pMHCII), which recognize specific TCR (**Figure 8.4**), have been used to interrogate autoantigenic CD4+ T cells. As the pMHCII multimers are fluorescently labelled, the (auto)antigen-specific CD4+ T cells can be identified and quantified by flow cytometry.[59,60]

Recent work identified, through tetramer staining, vimentin$_{59-71}$- and cit-vimentin$_{59-71}$-reactive CD4+ T cells in the PB of HLA-DRB1*14:02+ RA patients and anticitrullinated protein antibody (ACPA)-negative first-degree relatives (FDR).[61] These HLA-DRB1*14:02-restricted antigen-specific CD4+ T cells from RA patients and FDR displayed a differentiated memory phenotype, which was not observed among tetramer+ CD4+ T cells from healthy controls. Single-cell sorting and TCR sequencing of CD4+ T cells recognizing native and citrullinated forms of vimentin$_{59-71}$ identified repeated CDR3α and CDR3β sequences, indicating antigen-driven clonal expansion. Notably, this oligoclonal expansion was only observed in RA patients and ACPA-negative FDR, suggesting that expansion of autoantigen-specific CD4+ T cells occurs in individuals with high-risk HLA before the development of ACPA.

In ectopic lymphoid-like structures (ELS) in RA synovial tissue persistent expression of activation-induced cytidine deaminase (AID), which is crucial for somatic hypermutation and class-switch recombination of Ig genes, was noted.[62,63] Class-switched ACPA detected in these ELS, imply cognate antigen-specific CD4+ T-cell

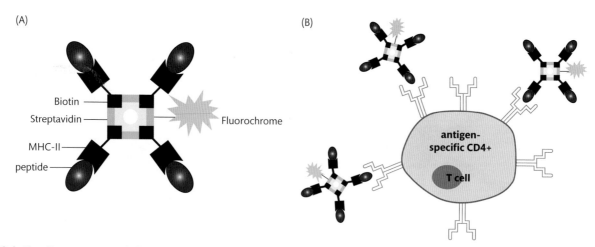

(A) Biotin / Streptavidin / MHC-II / peptide / Fluorochrome

(B) antigen-specific CD4+ T cell

Figure 8.4 Class II tetramers as tools for antigen-specific CD4+ T-cell detection. (a) Schematic depicting the structure of an MHC class II tetramer. Four identical biotinylated MHC class II molecules loaded with a candidate (auto)antigenic peptide are linked to a central streptavidin molecule. The central streptavidin is conjugated to a fluorochrome of interest. (b) Binding of fluorescently labelled class II tetramer molecules to the antigen-specific CD4+ T cell via the T-cell receptor (TCR) enables detection of antigen-specific T cells by flow cytometry.

help.[62] However, such antigen-specific CD4[+] T cells in ELS have not yet been demonstrated. Notably, RA synovial tissues displayed distinct transcriptomic clustering, including lymphoid, myeloid, two fibroblast, and mixed 'pathotypes'.[64] RA ELS of the lymphoid type were characterized by high levels of T- and B-cell gene expression, and were significantly associated with ACPA seropositivity.[64,65]

Although it has been difficult to directly link antigen-specific CD4[+] T cells in RA synovial tissue to development of specific autoantibodies, studies in humanized HLA-DR1 transgenic mouse models during collagen-induced arthritis (CIA) confirm that induced, autoantigen-specific CD4+ T cells preferentially use particular TCRβ chain V genes (TRBV), are highly clonal, and migrate to arthritic joints.[66] Interestingly, the DR1 transgene did not select for a pathogenic naïve repertoire, indicating that the biased TCR usage arose from clonal expansion due to the ability of the preferentially used TCRαβ to recognize the dominant type II collagen$_{257-274}$ epitope presented by HLA-DR1.[66] Similar to studies of RA PB T cells, autoantigen-specific CD4+ T cells generated during CIA development were shown to persist well after arthritis onset in the lymph nodes, and to maintain an activated phenotype.[67]

Thymic selection of T cells and RA

A functional immune system must be able to effectively recognize harmful pathogens but maintain tolerance to self. This is achieved by both central and peripheral tolerance. Central tolerance occurs in the thymus and is mediated by the coordinated actions of thymic cortical epithelial cells (cTEC) and medullary epithelial cells (mTEC), in conjunction with the transcription factor autoimmune regulator (AIRE).[68] Central tolerance removes T cells expressing inappropriately low or high-affinity TCR for self-peptides. Within the pool of positively selected T cells, the TCR repertoire is in fact biased towards cells with greater self-reactivity in order to yield mature T cells better able to respond to foreign antigens within the MHC context of the individual.[69] However, central tolerance is imperfect, and negative selection can be disturbed when TCR affinity for self-antigen is reduced, self-antigen is not expressed by mTEC, or mTEC numbers are reduced. Peripheral tolerance, involving active suppression by Treg and antigen-presenting cells (APC) with regulatory functions, thus plays an essential role in regulating and deleting self-reactive T cells.[70]

Dysregulated T-cell homeostasis in RA

Maintenance of the immune system relies on the continuous replenishment of the thymus with progenitor cells derived from bone marrow-derived haematopoietic stem cells (HSC). The capacity to replenish the immune system declines with age, due to thymic involution and a decline in T-cell progenitors from the HSC.[71] When balanced, HSC give rise to 90% lymphoid and 10% myeloid cells. Ageing shifts the balance towards myeloid cells, giving rise to the decline in T-cell progenitors.[72] As a result, homeostatic proliferation constitutes an important mechanism to maintain the peripheral T-cell pool. In addition, ageing alters the functional profile, whereby memory T cells progressively take up a larger proportion of the repertoire. This creates greater opportunities for cross-reactivity of T cells with self-antigens when responding to infectious antigens.[73,74]

The physiological process of immune ageing is accelerated in RA patients compared to age-matched controls, although it is not yet clear whether this is a cause or consequence of the disease. Hence,

RA patients with HLA-DRB1*04 alleles have profoundly reduced numbers of T cells carrying TCR excision circles (TREC) in individuals as young as 20–25 years of age, compared with age-matched healthy subjects. TREC serve as a marker for recent thymic emigrants.[75] Premature lymphopenia leads to compensatory proliferation of T cells and accelerates the process of T-cell senescence. The reduced TREC frequency may result from low TCR signalling capacity, further compounded by a defect in CD34[+] HSC proliferation in RA patients compared to healthy subjects, as occurs in immune ageing.[76] GM-CSF expands myeloid HSCs and inflammatory DCs in RA models, is overexpressed in RA, and shows promise as a therapeutic target.[77,78]

The conclusion that premature T-cell senescence occurs in RA was supported by studies analysing the telomeric lengths in the T-cell compartment. Telomeres are structures made up of multiple TTAGGG units located at the end of chromosomes, protecting against chromosomal instability.[71,79] Telomeres can be used as a marker for cellular division because they shorten with each division. In healthy subjects, telomeres in CD4[+] T cells are stable until 40 years of age, but thereafter start to shorten and plateau at the age of 65 years. In RA patients, nearly the entire telomeric reserve was reported to be used by age 20.[76,80] This was proposed to be due to insufficient induction of telomerase reverse transcriptase (hTERT) in naïve CD4[+] T cells and CD34[+] haematopoietic progenitor cells.[81] Furthermore, naïve RA CD4[+] T cells are prone to apoptosis, exacerbating the lymphopenic condition.[82]

Altered metabolism in RA T cells

Resting and activated T cells have distinct energy demand and metabolic programmes.[83] T cells use energy in the form of adenosine triphosphate (ATP) which can be generated from glucose, fatty acids and amino acids through glycolysis, β-oxidation, and glutaminolysis, respectively. RA patients have an altered glycolytic pathway.[84,85] Naïve CD4[+] T cells from RA patients produce lower levels of ATP and lactate than healthy control T cells, yet undergo vigorous proliferation, due to their inability to upregulate 6-phosphofructo-2-kinase/fructose-2,6-bisphosphatase 3 (PFKFB3). PFKFB3 protein levels are also low in resting naïve CD4+ T cells of RA patients, which suffer from spontaneous apoptosis. This defect is exacerbated by activation.[82]

As an adaptive mechanism, RA T cells shunt glucose towards the pentose phosphate pathway, thus increasing the level of nicotinamide adenine dinucleotide phosphate (NADPH) and diminishing intracellular reactive oxygen species (ROS). ROS play an important role in intracellular signalling. Reduced ROS levels impair T-cell differentiation and activation, as well as antigen-specific T-cell expansion and autophagy (**Figure 8.5**).[82,86-88]

CD4+ effector T-cell subsets in RA

High numbers of T cells (~50% or more of synovial cells) are detected in the inflamed synovium and are required for arthritis development in murine models.[89] RA synovium was shown to be infiltrated by CD4[+]CD45RB[dim] memory T cells with potent helper activity and diminished capacity to regulate B cells.[90] Recently, these RA synovial tissue cells were identified as PD-1[+]CXCR5[-] CD4[+] T helper cells that express factors enabling B-cell help.[91] RA patients also have an increased frequency of circulating CXCR5[+] and CCR6[+] Tfh cells and activated B cells, accompanied by higher levels of serum IL-21.[40] Together these studies indicate that T cells play an

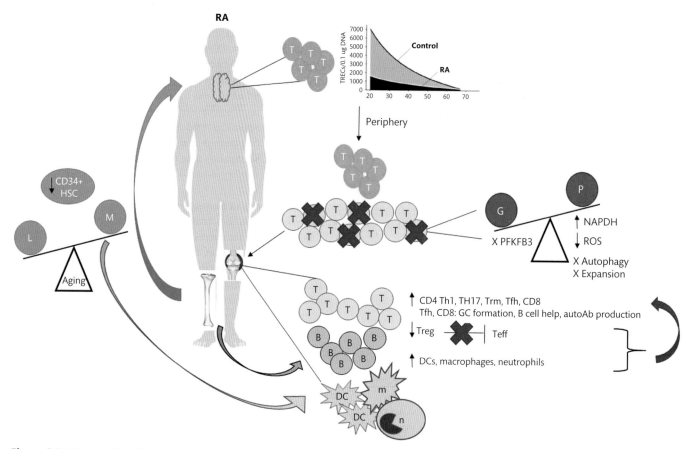

Figure 8.5 Disturbed T-cell homeostasis and autoimmunity in RA.

When balanced, CD34+ HSC give rise to 90% lymphoid (L) and 10% myeloid cells (M). Ageing shifts the balance towards myeloid cells. HLA-DRB1*04+ RA patients have profoundly reduced thymic T-cell output (TRECs)[75] (reproduced with permission). Premature lymphopenia leads to homeostatic proliferation of T cells in the periphery. The naïve T cells of RA patients are prone to apoptosis due to altered glycolytic pathway (G), and inability to upregulate PFKFB3. To compensate, RA T cells shunt glucose towards the pentose phosphate pathway (P), increasing NADPH and decreasing intracellular ROS, with impaired autophagy and survival, exacerbating the lymphopenia. Increased frequency of CD4+ Th1, Th17, Trm, Tfh, and CD8 T cells but reduced Treg observed in RA synovium. Tfh and CD8 T cells help B cells, and facilitate germinal centre formation and autoantibody production. Treg function is inhibited in the inflammatory milieu, which perpetuates joint inflammation.

active role in the production of antibodies in the synovium and perpetuate the disease.

Effector T cells, including Th1 and Th17 subsets producing pro-inflammatory cytokines such as TNF, IL-6, IFN-γ, and IL-17, have been detected in PB and synovium of RA patients.[92,93] The pathogenic role of these pro-inflammatory cytokines in RA has been demonstrated by the efficacy of treatment using biologics such as anti-TNF and anti-IL-6 receptor in RA patients.[94,95] Although IL-17 plays a key role in pathogenesis of CIA,[96,97] inhibitors of IL-17 had little impact on severity of RA, except, perhaps, in a subset of patients where IL-17 is more dominant in the pathogenesis.[98] However, synovial IL-17 contributes to bone and cartilage destruction.[99]

T-cell depleting monoclonal antibodies such as chimeric anti-CD4 and humanized anti-CD52 (CAMPATH-1H) also limited clinical efficacy. Despite profound peripheral T-cell depletion, persistent CD4+ T-cell synovial infiltration was observed in treated patients.[100] This may be due to inadequate dosing or treatment duration,[101] or resistance of synovial tissue resident memory CD4+ T cells (T_{RM}) to anti-CD4 treatment.[102–104] T_{RM} persist long-term in epithelial barrier tissues including the gastrointestinal tract, lung, and skin. T_{RM} provide rapid on-site immune protection against previously encountered pathogens, but could also contribute to persistence or flares of inflammatory synovitis when autoreactive T cells

differentiate into T_{RM} and reside in synovial tissue.[104,105] as has been shown for psoriasis.[106,107]

Regulatory T cells in RA

There are two classes of Treg identified in humans: constitutively generated thymic Treg (tTreg) and peripherally induced Treg (pTreg). The transcription factor Foxp3 is critical for CD4+ Treg development and function.[108,109] tTreg can be further delineated as resting Treg (FoxP3^{lo}CD45RA+CD25^{hi} rTreg) and activated Treg (FoxP3^{hi}CD45RA^{-}CD25^{hi} aTreg).[110] pTreg may be Foxp3+ antigen-specific cells induced in response to antigen presented by tolerogenic DCs, or Foxp3^{-} CD4+ T cells that acquire regulatory function in the periphery when exposed to antigen and tolerogenic signals. These pTreg secrete IFN-γ and IL-10 (Tr1 cells) or TGF-β.[111] Induction of pTreg represents an important mechanism for antigen-specific control of autoreactive T cells escaping selection and entering the periphery in the face of deficient central tolerance or age-related expansion of autoreactive effector-memory T-cell clones.[112]

Treg may regulate in different ways, including deletion, anergy, competition, and generation of new pTreg. For example, self-reactive T cells acquire a FR4hiCD73hi anergic phenotype in the presence of FoxP3+ Treg.[113] In RA patients, CD4+CD25+FoxP3+ Treg with high plasticity towards Th17 accumulated in inflamed synovium.[114,115]

Moreover, a subset of FoxP3+CD39+ Treg in RA synovial tissue (ST) suppressed the production of IFNγ, TNF, and IL-17F but not IL-17A.[116] PB Treg in RA patients were shown to retain suppressive capacity which was lost in synovial fluid Treg[117] and FoxP3+ Treg activated by an inflammatory cytokine milieu produced IL-17.[118] On the other hand, TNF inhibition induced a distinct population of Treg via TGF-β which enhanced regulatory function in RA.[119,120] Together these results suggest that the inflammatory cytokine milieu contributes to Treg dysfunction, which prevents efficient control of autoreactive T cells recognizing self-antigens.

CD8+ cytotoxic T cells (CTL)

While the role of CD8 T cells in RA pathogenesis is less well understood, increased central memory PB CD8 T cells,[121] increased PB and synovial fluid effector-memory T cells,[122] and elevated expression of pro-inflammatory cytokines by CD8 effector T cells in active disease have been reported.[123] Furthermore, oligoclonal CD8 memory T cells were identified in RA synovial fluid.[124-126] CD8 T cells were shown to support germinal centre formation. Together these data suggest that CD8 T cells play important roles in adaptive immunity in RA, which warrant further exploration.

Innate T cells: NKT cells

Innate T cells such as invariant natural killer T cells (iNKT) and mucosal associated invariant T cells (MAIT) provide rapid protection against foreign pathogens and bridge innate and adaptive immune responses.[127,128] Studies in antigen-induced arthritis models demonstrated a dichotomous effect of iNKT cells.[129] IFN-γ is released upon the activation of iNKT cells. In the early phase of disease, IFNγ exacerbated the severity of antigen-induced arthritis, whereas it protected later in the disease course.[130,131] While clinical and histological signs of arthritis improved when iNKT were blocked with anti-CD1d antibody,[131] activation of iNKT with exogenous α-galactosylceramide (α-GalCer) protected in an IL-10 dependent manner.[132] Similarly, circulating iNTK cells in RA patients were low and their frequency negatively correlated with DAS28. The iNKT cells also proliferated poorly in response towards α-GalCer.[133,134]

DC antigen presentation to T cells in RA

RA is characterized by the expansion of self-peptide specific effector-memory T cells and DCs are key APC for priming of naïve T-cell expansion through HLA-antigen presentation. Certain HLA alleles are associated with RA susceptibility, including HLA-DRB1*0401, *0404, *0405, and HLA-DRB1*0101.[21] RA-associated DR alleles contain amino acids with similar charge at residues 11, 13, and 71–74 within the DRβ1 binding groove, termed the shared epitope. The shared epitope influences peptide binding and T-cell recognition. Post-translational modifications, such as citrullination and carbamylation of infectious antigens and self-proteins, may be enhanced in inflammatory and stressed settings such as smoking or periodontal infection. Furthermore, neutrophils, activated during infection or inflammation, form neutrophil traps (NETs) made up of decondensed chromatin released from dying cells, which provide a source of potentially immunogenic autoantigen such as citrullinated histones.[135,136] Citrullination of self-epitopes derived from vimentin, fibrinogen, enolase, CILP, and collagen II enhances peptide binding

affinity to RA susceptibility HLA-DR allomorphs containing the shared epitope.[61,137,138] RA is also associated with single nucleotide polymorphisms (SNPs) in the MHC class II transactivator gene *MHC2TA*, which is thought to reduce the efficiency of antigen presentation both in the thymus and periphery, thus potentially altering the TCR repertoire.[139]

Citrullination of self-antigens also modulates the quality of TCR binding and signalling. For example, citrullination of aggrecan reduced T-cell proliferation, but enhanced Th17 differentiation, which was promoted by low-strength TCR signalling.[140] TCR signalling strength can also determine the severity of arthritis in murine models of RA.[141,142] In recent-onset HLA-DR shared epitope⁺ RA patients, T cells were more likely to produce IL-6 in response to cit-aggrecan than cit-vimentin or cit-fibrinogen epitopes.[59] Furthermore, while T cells recognizing cit-vimentin and cit-aggrecan circulate in both healthy controls and RA patients, these were more likely to be naïve or regulatory in healthy controls and to have an effector-memory phenotype and to display evidence of oligoclonal expansion in RA patients.[61,138] In this regard, hyperactivity of the Ras-Erk pathway was shown to prevent negative regulation of TCR signalling by the phosphatase SHP-1, leading to sustained TCR signalling in RA patients.[143] Other genetic polymorphisms associated with RA may also impact on the quality of TCR signalling and immune synapse formation. RA-associated polymorphisms in *CD28*, *CTLA4*, *PTPN22*, *PRKCQ*, and *CD247* (TCRζ) all impact TCR signalling.[142,144] Perturbations to the function of these molecules may impact on TCR signalling thresholds and therefore the ensuing immune response. Modulating the quality of interactions between DCs and T-cell is therefore an attractive therapeutic target for RA.

Antigen-specific immunotherapy targeting the DC-T-cell interaction

Current treatments for autoimmune diseases reduce inflammation, but do not cure the immune dysfunction causing disease. Tolerance-inducing antigen-specific immunotherapy would have lower toxicity and would represent a longer-term solution to controlling or preventing autoimmune disease. Such strategies would specifically target the autoimmune disease process towards RA-specific antigens presented by specific high-risk HLA-DR shared epitope gene variants and autoimmunity based on autoantibody positivity. Earlier in this chapter we discussed the role of DCs presenting RA autoantigens to T cells and that DCs with regulatory properties could promote the induction of pTreg. An important body of work demonstrated that certain subsets of DCs *in vivo*, such as CD103⁺ intestinal DCs, promote the production of pTreg.[145] Furthermore after exposure to antigen, myeloid DCs deficient in the RelB subunit of NF-κB or DCs generated in the presence of various NF-kB suppressive drugs ('tolerogenic DCs') could restore antigen-specific tolerance in primed mice or mice with antigen-induced inflammatory arthritis.[146-148] A number of shared epitope HLA-DR-restricted citrullinated autoantigenic peptides have been described in RA patients. Thus, in the first phase I proof-of-concept clinical trial of antigen-specific DC immunotherapy, HLA-DR shared epitope-positive ACPA⁺ RA patients were treated with autologous PB DCs modified with an NF-κB inhibitor and exposed to four citrullinated peptide autoantigens. Treatment was safe, and reduced both inflammation and CD4⁺ effector T cells and increased the Treg to effector T-cell ratio.[149] A trial of intra-articular tolerogenic DCs demonstrated safety,[150] and further trials are ongoing. These trials have their basis in the understanding of DC and T-cell biology in RA and begin to build a mechanistic understanding around the potential for DC-based antigen-specific immunotherapies to rebalance antigen-specific regulatory to effector T cells for future treatment of patients with and at risk of RA.[151–162]

REFERENCES

1. Merad M, Sathe P, Helft J, Miller J, Mortha A. The dendritic cell lineage: ontogeny and function of dendritic cells and their subsets in the steady state and the inflamed setting. *Annu Rev Immunol* 2013;*31*: 563–604.
2. Ganguly D, Haak S, Sisirak V, Reizis B. The role of dendritic cells in autoimmunity. *Nat Rev Immunol* 2013;*13*:566–77.
3. Lutzky V, Hannawi S, Thomas R. Cells of the synovium in rheumatoid arthritis. Dendritic cells. *Arthritis Res Ther* 2007;*9*:219.
4. Yu MB, Langridge WHR. The function of myeloid dendritic cells in rheumatoid arthritis. *Rheumatol Int* 2017;*37*:1043–51.
5. Richez C, Barnetche T, Khoryati L, et al. Tocilizumab treatment decreases circulating myeloid dendritic cells and monocytes, 2 components of the myeloid lineage. *J Rheumatol* 2012;*39*: 1192–7.
6. Jongbloed, S. L., M. C. Lebre, A. R. Fraser, et al. Enumeration and phenotypical analysis of distinct dendritic cell subsets in psoriatic arthritis and rheumatoid arthritis. *Arthritis Res Ther* 2006;*8*:R15.
7. Richez C, Schaeverbeke T, Dumoulin C, Dehais J, Moreau JF, Blanco P. Myeloid dendritic cells correlate with clinical response whereas plasmacytoid dendritic cells impact autoantibody development in rheumatoid arthritis patients treated with infliximab. *Arthritis Res Ther* 2009;*11*:R100.
8. Thomas R, Davis LS, Lipsky PE. Rheumatoid synovium is enriched in mature antigen-presenting dendritic cells. *J Immunol* 1994;*152*: 2613–23.
9. Zvaifler NJ, Steinman RM, Kaplan G., Lau LL, Rivelis M. Identification of immunostimulatory dendritic cells in the synovial effusions of patients with rheumatoid arthritis. *J Clin Invest* 1985;*76*:789–800.
10. Cavanagh LL, Boyce A, Smith L, et al. Rheumatoid arthritis synovium contains plasmacytoid dendritic cells. *Arthritis Res Ther* 2005;*7*:R230–40.
11. Van Krinks CH, Matyszak MK, Gaston JS. Characterization of plasmacytoid dendritic cells in inflammatory arthritis synovial fluid. *Rheumatology (Oxford)* 2004;*43*:453–60.
12. Villani AC, Satija R, Reynolds G, et al. Single-cell RNA-seq reveals new types of human blood dendritic cells, monocytes, and progenitors. *Science* 2017;*356*(6335):pii: eaah4573.
13. Segura E, Touzot M, Bohineust A, et al. Human inflammatory dendritic cells induce Th17 cell differentiation. *Immunity* 2013;*38*:336–48.
14. Page G, Lebecque S, Miossec P. Anatomic localization of immature and mature dendritic cells in an ectopic lymphoid organ: correlation with selective chemokine expression in rheumatoid synovium. *J Immunol* 2002;*168*:5333–41.
15. Moret FM, van der Wurff-Jacobs KM, Bijlsma JW, Lafeber FP, van Roon JA. Synovial T cell hyporesponsiveness to myeloid

16. Reynolds G, Gibbon JR, Pratt AG, et al. Synovial CD4+ T-cell-derived GM-CSF supports the differentiation of an inflammatory dendritic cell population in rheumatoid arthritis. *Ann Rheum Dis* 2016;*75*:899–907.
17. Huang FP, Platt N, Wykes M, et al. A discrete subpopulation of dendritic cells transports apoptotic intestinal epithelial cells to T cell areas of mesenteric lymph nodes. *J Exp Med* 2000;*191*:435–44.
18. Sauter B, Albert ML, Francisco L, Larsson M, Somersan S, Bhardwaj N. Consequences of cell death: exposure to necrotic tumor cells, but not primary tissue cells or apoptotic cells, induces the maturation of immunostimulatory dendritic cells. *J Exp Med* 2000;*191*:423–34.
19. Fadok VA, Bratton DL, Konowal A, Freed PW, Westcott JY, Henson PM. Macrophages that have ingested apoptotic cells *in vitro* inhibit proinflammatory cytokine production through autocrine/paracrine mechanisms involving TGF-beta, PGE2, and PAF. *J Clin Invest* 1998;*101*:890–8.
20. O'Sullivan BJ, Thomas R. CD40 Ligation conditions dendritic cell antigen-presenting function through sustained activation of NF-kappaB. *J Immunol* 2002;*168*:5491–8.
21. de Almeida DE, Ling S, Holoshitz J. New insights into the functional role of the rheumatoid arthritis shared epitope. *FEBS Lett* 2011;*585*:3619–26.
22. Duffau P, Menn-Josephy H, Cuda CM, et al. Promotion of inflammatory arthritis by interferon regulatory factor 5 in a mouse model. *Arthritis Rheumatol* 2015;*67*:3146–57.
23. Roelofs MF, Joosten LA, Abdollahi-Roodsaz S, et al. The expression of toll-like receptors 3 and 7 in rheumatoid arthritis synovium is increased and costimulation of toll-like receptors 3, 4, and 7/8 results in synergistic cytokine production by dendritic cells. *Arthritis Rheum* 2005;*52*:2313–22.
24. Abdollahi-Roodsaz S, Joosten LA, Roelofs MF, et al. Inhibition of Toll-like receptor 4 breaks the inflammatory loop in autoimmune destructive arthritis. *Arthritis Rheum* 2007;*56*:2957–67.
25. Scher JU, Sczesnak A, Longman RS, et al. Expansion of intestinal Prevotella copri correlates with enhanced susceptibility to arthritis. *Elife* 2013;*2*:e01202.
26. Wang Y, Shaked I, Stanford SM, et al. The autoimmunity-associated gene PTPN22 potentiates toll-like receptor-driven, type 1 interferon-dependent immunity. *Immunity* 2013;*39*:111–22.
27. Zhang J, Zahir N, Jiang Q, et al. The autoimmune disease-associated PTPN22 variant promotes calpain-mediated Lyp/Pep degradation associated with lymphocyte and dendritic cell hyperresponsiveness. *Nat Genet* 2011;*43*:902–7.
28. Wang Y, Ewart D, Crabtree JN, et al. PTPN22 variant R620W is associated with reduced Toll-like receptor 7-induced type I interferon in systemic lupus erythematosus. *Arthritis Rheumatol* 2015;*67*:2403–14.
29. Purvis HA, Clarke F, Jordan CK, et al. Protein tyrosine phosphatase PTPN22 regulates IL-1beta dependent Th17 responses by modulating dectin-1 signaling in mice. *Eur J Immunol* 2017;*48*(2):306–15.
30. Prevosto C, Goodall JC, Hill Gaston JS. Cytokine secretion by pathogen recognition receptor-stimulated dendritic cells in rheumatoid arthritis and ankylosing spondylitis. *J Rheumatol* 2012;*39*:1918–28.
31. Moret FM, Hack CE, van der Wurff-Jacobs KMG, et al. Intra-articular CD1c-expressing myeloid dendritic cells from

rheumatoid arthritis patients express a unique set of T cell-attracting chemokines and spontaneously induce Th1, Th17 and Th2 cell activity. *Arthritis Res Ther* 2013;15:R155.

32. Yamada H, Nakashima Y, Okazaki K, et al. Th1 but not Th17 cells predominate in the joints of patients with rheumatoid arthritis. *Ann Rheum Dis* 2008;67:1299–304.

33. Arroyo-Villa I, Bautista-Caro MB, Balsa A, et al. Frequency of Th17 CD4+ T cells in early rheumatoid arthritis: a marker of anti-CCP seropositivity. *PLoS One* 2012;7:e42189.

34. Lebre MC, Jongbloed SL, Tas SW, Smeets TJ, McInnes IB, Tak PP. Rheumatoid arthritis synovium contains two subsets of CD83-DC-LAMP- dendritic cells with distinct cytokine profiles. *Am J Pathol* 2008;172:940–50.

35. Santiago B, Izquierdo E, Rueda P, et al. CXCL12gamma isoform is expressed on endothelial and dendritic cells in rheumatoid arthritis synovium and regulates T cell activation. *Arthritis Rheum* 2012;64:409–17.

36. Estrada-Capetillo L, Hernandez-Castro B, Monsivais-Urenda A, et al. Induction of Th17 lymphocytes and Treg cells by monocyte-derived dendritic cells in patients with rheumatoid arthritis and systemic lupus erythematosus. *Clin Dev Immunol* 2013;2013:584303.

37. Moret FM, Hack CE, van der Wurff-Jacobs KM, Radstake TR, Lafeber FP, van Roon JA. Thymic stromal lymphopoietin, a novel proinflammatory mediator in rheumatoid arthritis that potently activates CD1c+ myeloid dendritic cells to attract and stimulate T cells. *Arthritis Rheumatol* 2014;66:1176–84.

38. Azizi G, Jadidi-Niaragh F, Mirshafiey A. Th17 Cells in immunopathogenesis and treatment of rheumatoid arthritis. *Int J Rheum Dis* 2013;16:243–53.

39. Hume DA. The many alternative faces of macrophage activation. *Front Immunol* 2015;6:370.

40. Lefranc MP, Giudicelli V, Ginestoux C, et al. IMGT, the international ImMunoGeneTics database. *Nucleic Acids Res* 1999;27:209–12.

41. Turner SJ, Doherty PC, McCluskey J, Rossjohn J. Structural determinants of T-cell receptor bias in immunity. *Nat Rev Immunol* 2006;6:883–94.

42. Davis MM. T cell receptor gene diversity and selection. *Annu Rev Biochem* 1990;59:475–96.

43. Davis MM, Bjorkman PJ. T-cell antigen receptor genes and T-cell recognition. *Nature* 1988;334:395–402.

44. Pannetier C, Cochet M, Darche S, Casrouge A, Zoller M, Kourilsky P. The sizes of the CDR3 hypervariable regions of the murine T-cell receptor β chains vary as a function of the recombined germ-line segments. *Proc Natl Acad Sci U S A* 1993;90:4319–23.

45. Kjer-Nielsen L, Clements CS, Purcell AW, et al. A structural basis for the selection of dominant alphabeta T cell receptors in antiviral immunity. *Immunity* 2003;18:53–64.

46. Garboczi DN, Ghosh P, Utz U, Fan QR, Biddison WE, Wiley DC. Structure of the complex between human T-cell receptor, viral peptide and HLA-A2. *Nature* 1996;384:134–41.

47. Arstila TP, Casrouge A, Baron V, Even J, Kanellopoulos J, Kourilsky P. A direct estimate of the human alphabeta T cell receptor diversity. *Science* 1999;286:958–61.

48. Venturi V, Kedzierska K, Price DA, et al. Sharing of T cell receptors in antigen-specific responses is driven by convergent recombination. *Proc Natl Acad Sci U S A* 2006;103:18691–6.

49. Venturi V, Price DA, Douek DC, Davenport MP. The molecular basis for public T-cell responses? *Nat Rev Immunol* 2008;8:231–8.

50. Gras S, Kjer-Nielsen L, Burrows SR, McCluskey J, Rossjohn J. T-cell receptor bias and immunity. *Curr Opin Immunol* 2008;20:119–25.

51. Rudolph MG, Stanfield RL, Wilson IA. How TCRs bind MHCs, peptides, and coreceptors. *Annu Rev Immunol* 2006;24:419–66.

52. La Gruta NL, Rothwell WT, Cukalac T, et al. Primary CTL response magnitude in mice is determined by the extent of naive T cell recruitment and subsequent clonal expansion. *J Clin Investig* 2010;120:1885–94.

53. Moon JJ, Chu HH, Pepper M, et al. Naive CD4(+) T cell frequency varies for different epitopes and predicts repertoire diversity and response magnitude. *Immunity* 2007;27:203–13.

54. Busch DH, Pamer EG. T cell affinity maturation by selective expansion during infection. *J Exp Med* 1999;189:701–10.

55. Day EK, Carmichael AJ, ten Berge IJ, Waller EC, Sissons JG, Wills MR. Rapid CD8+ T cell repertoire focusing and selection of high-affinity clones into memory following primary infection with a persistent human virus: human cytomegalovirus. *J Immunol* 2007;179:3203–13.

56. La Gruta NL, Thomas PG. Interrogating the relationship between naive and immune antiviral T cell repertoires. *Curr Opin Virol* 2013;3:447–51.

57. Goronzy JJ, Bartz-Bazzanella P, Hu W, Jendro MC, Walser-Kuntz DR, Weyand CM. Dominant clonotypes in the repertoire of peripheral CD4+ T cells in rheumatoid arthritis. *J Clin Investig* 1994;94:2068–76.

58. Hair DMJH, Tak PP, Doorenspleet ME, et al. Inflamed target tissue provides a specific niche for highly expanded T-cell clones in early human autoimmune disease. *Ann Rheum Dis* 2012;71:1088–93.

59. Law SC, Street S, Yu CH, et al. T-cell autoreactivity to citrullinated autoantigenic peptides in rheumatoid arthritis patients carrying HLA-DRB1 shared epitope alleles. *Arthritis Res Ther* 2012;14:R118.

60. Jansen D, Ramnoruth N, Loh KL, et al. Flow cytometric clinical immunomonitoring using peptide-MHC class II tetramers: optimization of methods and protocol development. *Front Immunol* 2018;9:8.

61. Scally SW, Law SC, Ting YT, et al. Molecular basis for increased susceptibility of Indigenous North Americans to seropositive rheumatoid arthritis. *Ann Rheum Dis* 2017;76(11):1915–23.

62. Humby F, Bombardieri M, Manzo A, et al. Ectopic lymphoid structures support ongoing production of class-switched autoantibodies in rheumatoid synovium. *PLoS Med* 2009;6:e1.

63. Muramatsu M, Kinoshita K, Fagarasan S, Yamada S, Shinkai Y, Honjo T. Class switch recombination and hypermutation require activation-induced cytidine deaminase (AID), a potential RNA editing enzyme. *Cell* 2000;102:553–63.

64. Pitzalis C, Kelly S, Humby F. New learnings on the pathophysiology of RA from synovial biopsies. *Curr Opin Rheumatol* 2013;25:334–44.

65. DiCicco M, Humby F, Kelly S, et al. O49 synovial lymphocytic aggregates associate with highly active RA and predict erosive disease progression at 12 months: results from the pathobiology of early arthritis cohort. *Rheumatology* 2016;55:i59–i59.

66. Qian Z, Latham KA, Whittington KB, Miller DC, Brand DD, Rosloniec EF. An autoantigen-specific, highly restricted T cell repertoire infiltrates the arthritic joints of mice in an HLA-DR1 humanized mouse model of autoimmune arthritis. *J Immunol* 2010;185:110–18.

67. Latham KA, Whittington KB, Zhou R, Qian Z, Rosloniec EF. Ex vivo characterization of the autoimmune T cell response in the

HLA-DR1 mouse model of collagen-induced arthritis reveals long-term activation of type II collagen-specific cells and their presence in arthritic joints. *J Immunol* 2005;*174*:3978–85.

68. Danke NA, Koelle DM, Yee C, Beheray S, Kwok WW. Autoreactive T cells in healthy individuals. *J Immunol* 2004;*172*:5967–72.

69. Mandl JN, Monteiro JP, Vrisekoop N, Germain RN. T cell-positive selection uses self-ligand binding strength to optimize repertoire recognition of foreign antigens. *Immunity* 2013;*38*:263–74.

70. Cope AP, Schulze-Koops H, Aringer M. The central role of T cells in rheumatoid arthritis. *Clin Exp Rheumatol* 2007;*25*:S4–11.

71. Lindstrom TM, Robinson WH. Rheumatoid arthritis: a role for immunosenescence? *J Am Geriatr Soc* 2010;*58*:1565–75.

72. Cho RH, Sieburg HB, Muller-Sieburg CE. A new mechanism for the aging of hematopoietic stem cells: aging changes the clonal composition of the stem cell compartment but not individual stem cells. *Blood* 2008;*111*: 5553–61.

73. Wooldridge L, Ekeruche-Makinde J, van den Berg HA, et al. A single autoimmune T cell receptor recognizes more than a million different peptides. *J Biol Chem* 2012;*287*:1168–77.

74. Koning F, Thomas R, Rossjohn J, Toes RE. Coeliac disease and rheumatoid arthritis: similar mechanisms, different antigens. *Nat Rev Rheumatol* 2015;*11*:450–61.

75. Weyand CM, Fulbright JW, Goronzy JJ. Immunosenescence, autoimmunity, and rheumatoid arthritis. *Exp Gerontol* 2003;*38*:833–41.

76. Colmegna I, Diaz-Borjon A, Fujii H, Schaefer L, Goronzy JJ, Weyand CM. Defective proliferative capacity and accelerated telomeric loss of hematopoietic progenitor cells in rheumatoid arthritis. *Arthritis Rheum* 2008;*58*:990–1000.

77. Cook AD, Turner AL, Braine EL, Pobjoy J, Lenzo JC, Hamilton JA. Regulation of systemic and local myeloid cell subpopulations by bone marrow cell-derived granulocyte-macrophage colony-stimulating factor in experimental inflammatory arthritis. *Arthritis Rheum* 2011;*63*:2340–51.

78. Avci AB, Feist E, Burmester GR. Targeting GM-CSF in rheumatoid arthritis. *Clin Exp Rheumatol* 2016;*34*:39–44.

79. Hohensinner PJ, Goronzy JJ, Weyand CM. Targets of immune regeneration in rheumatoid arthritis. *Mayo Clin Proc* 2014;*89*:563–75.

80. Koetz K, Bryl E, Spickschen K, O'Fallon WM, Goronzy JJ, Weyand CM. T cell homeostasis in patients with rheumatoid arthritis. *Proc Natl Acad Sci U S A* 2000;*97*:9203–8.

81. Fujii H, Shao L, Colmegna I, Goronzy JJ, Weyand CM. Telomerase insufficiency in rheumatoid arthritis. *Proc Natl Acad Sci U S A* 2009;*106*:4360–5.

82. Yang Z, Fujii H, Mohan SV, Goronzy JJ, Weyand CM. Phosphofructokinase deficiency impairs ATP generation, autophagy, and redox balance in rheumatoid arthritis T cells. *J Exp Med* 2013;*210*:2119–34.

83. Bental M, Deutsch C. Metabolic changes in activated T cells: an NMR study of human peripheral blood lymphocytes. *Magn Reson Med* 1993;*29*:317–26.

84. Sun L, Chai Y. Bioinformatic analysis to find small molecules related to rheumatoid arthritis. *Int J Rheum Dis* 2014;*17*:71–7.

85. Balakrishnan L, Bhattacharjee M, Ahmad S, et al. Differential proteomic analysis of synovial fluid from rheumatoid arthritis and osteoarthritis patients. *Clin Proteomics* 2014;*11*:1.

86. Sena LA, Li S, Jairaman A, et al. Mitochondria are required for antigen-specific T cell activation through reactive oxygen species signaling. *Immunity* 2013;*38*:225–36.

87. Scherz-Shouval R, Shvets E, Fass E, Shorer H, Gil L, Elazar Z. Reactive oxygen species are essential for autophagy and specifically regulate the activity of Atg4. *Embo J* 2007;*26*:1749–60.

88. Winter S, Hultqvist Hopkins M, Laulund F, Holmdahl R. A reduction in intracellular reactive oxygen species due to a mutation in NCF4 promotes autoimmune arthritis in mice. *Antioxid Redox Signal* 2016;*25*:983–96.

89. Petrow PK, Thoss K, Katenkamp D, Brauer R. Adoptive transfer of susceptibility to antigen-induced arthritis into severe combined immunodeficient (SCID) mice: role of CD4+ and CD8+ T cells. *Immunol Invest* 1996;*25*:341–53.

90. Thomas R, McIlraith M, Davis LS, Lipsky PE. Rheumatoid synovium is enriched in CD45RBdim mature memory T cells that are potent helpers for B cell differentiation. *Arthritis Rheum* 1992;*35*:1455–65.

91. Rao DA, Gurish MF, Marshall JL, et al. Pathologically expanded peripheral T helper cell subset drives B cells in rheumatoid arthritis. *Nature* 2017;*542*:110–14.

92. Miossec P. Dynamic interactions between T cells and dendritic cells and their derived cytokines/chemokines in the rheumatoid synovium. *Arthritis Res Ther* 2008;*10* Suppl 1:S2.

93. Leung BP, McInnes IB, Esfandiari E, Wei XQ, Liew FY. Combined effects of IL-12 and IL-18 on the induction of collagen-induced arthritis. *J Immunol* 2000;*164*: 6495–502.

94. Schwartzman S, Fleischmann R, Morgan GJ Jr. Do anti-TNF agents have equal efficacy in patients with rheumatoid arthritis? *Arthritis Res Ther* 2004;*6* Suppl 2:S3–11.

95. Nishimoto N, Miyasaka N, Yamamoto K, Kawai S, Takeuchi T, Azuma J. Long-term safety and efficacy of tocilizumab, an anti-IL-6 receptor monoclonal antibody, in monotherapy, in patients with rheumatoid arthritis (the STREAM study): evidence of safety and efficacy in a 5-year extension study. *Ann Rheum Dis* 2009;*68*:1580–4.

96. Hirota K, Hashimoto M, Yoshitomi H, et al. T cell self-reactivity forms a cytokine milieu for spontaneous development of IL-17+ Th cells that cause autoimmune arthritis. *J Exp Med* 2007;*204*:41–7.

97. Andersson AK, Li C, Brennan FM. Recent developments in the immunobiology of rheumatoid arthritis. *Arthritis Res Ther* 2008;*10*:204.

98. Kellner H. Targeting interleukin-17 in patients with active rheumatoid arthritis: rationale and clinical potential. *Ther Adv Musculoskelet Dis* 2013;*5*:141–52.

99. Chabaud M, Lubberts E, Joosten L, van Den Berg W, Miossec P. IL-17 derived from juxta-articular bone and synovium contributes to joint degradation in rheumatoid arthritis. *Arthritis Res* 2001;*3*:168–77.

100. Ruderman EM, Weinblatt ME, Thurmond LM, Pinkus GS, Gravallese EM. Synovial tissue response to treatment with Campath-1H. *Arthritis Rheum* 1995;*38*:254–8.

101. Choy EH, Pitzalis C, Cauli A, et al. Percentage of anti-CD4 monoclonal antibody-coated lymphocytes in the rheumatoid joint is associated with clinical improvement. Implications for the development of immunotherapeutic dosing regimens. *Arthritis Rheum* 1996;*39*:52–6.

102. Goldschmidt TJ, Andersson M, Malmstrom V, Holmdahl R. Activated type II collagen reactive T cells are not eliminated by *in vivo* anti-CD4 treatment. Implications for therapeutic approaches on autoimmune arthritis. *Immunobiology* 1992;*184*:359–71.

103. Jendro MC, Ganten T, Matteson EL, Weyand CM, Goronzy JJ. Emergence of oligoclonal T cell populations following

therapeutic T cell depletion in rheumatoid arthritis. *Arthritis Rheum* 1995;38:1242–51.

104. Henderson LA, King SL, Ameri S, et al. A161: novel 3-dimensional explant method facilitates the study of lymphocyte populations in the synovium and reveals a large population of resident memory T cells in rheumatoid arthritis. *Arthritis Rheumatol* 2014;66:S209.

105. Clark RA. Resident memory T cells in human health and disease. *Sci Transl Med* 2015;7:269rv261.

106. Boyman O, Hefti HP, Conrad C, Nickoloff BJ, Suter M, Nestle FO. Spontaneous development of psoriasis in a new animal model shows an essential role for resident T cells and tumor necrosis factor-alpha. *J Exp Med* 2004;199:731–6.

107. Cheuk S, Wiken M, Blomqvist L, Nylen S, Talme T, Stahle M, Eidsmo L. Epidermal Th22 and Tc17 cells form a localized disease memory in clinically healed psoriasis. *J Immunol* 2014;192:3111–20.

108. Hori S, Nomura T, Sakaguchi S. Control of regulatory T cell development by the transcription factor Foxp3. *Science* 2003;299:1057–61.

109. Fontenot JD, Gavin MA, Rudensky AY. Foxp3 programs the development and function of CD4+CD25+ regulatory T cells. *Nat Immunol* 2003;4:330–6.

110. Miyara M, Yoshioka Y, Kitoh A, et al. Functional delineation and differentiation dynamics of human CD4+ T cells expressing the FoxP3 transcription factor. *Immunity* 2009;30:899–911.

111. Lan Q, Fan H, Quesniaux V, Ryffel B, Liu Z, Zheng SG. Induced Foxp3(+) regulatory T cells: a potential new weapon to treat autoimmune and inflammatory diseases? *J Mol Cell Biol* 2012;4:22–8.

112. Nguyen TL, Sullivan NL, Ebel M, Teague RM, DiPaolo RJ. Antigen-specific TGF-beta-induced regulatory T cells secrete chemokines, regulate T cell trafficking, and suppress ongoing autoimmunity. *J Immunol* 2011;187:1745–53.

113. Martinez RJ, Zhang N, Thomas SR, et al. Arthritogenic self-reactive CD4+ T cells acquire an FR4hiCD73hi anergic state in the presence of Foxp3+ regulatory T cells. *J Immunol* 2012;188:170–81.

114. Mottonen M, Heikkinen J, Mustonen L, Isomaki P, Luukkainen R, Lassila O. CD4+ CD25+ T cells with the phenotypic and functional characteristics of regulatory T cells are enriched in the synovial fluid of patients with rheumatoid arthritis. *Clin Exp Immunol* 2005;140:360–7.

115. Komatsu N, Okamoto K, Sawa S, et al. Pathogenic conversion of Foxp3(+) T cells into TH17 cells in autoimmune arthritis. *Nat Med* 2014;20:62–8.

116. Herrath J, Chemin K, Albrecht I, Catrina AI, Malmstrom V. Surface expression of CD39 identifies an enriched Treg-cell subset in the rheumatic joint, which does not suppress IL-17A secretion. *Eur J Immunol* 2014;44:2979–89.

117. Wang T, Sun X, Zhao J, et al. Regulatory T cells in rheumatoid arthritis showed increased plasticity toward Th17 but retained suppressive function in peripheral blood. *Ann Rheum Dis* 2015;74:1293–301.

118. Beriou G, Costantino CM, Ashley CW, et al. IL-17-producing human peripheral regulatory T cells retain suppressive function. *Blood* 2009;113:4240–9.

119. Nie H, Zheng Y, Li R, et al. Phosphorylation of FOXP3 controls regulatory T cell function and is inhibited by TNF-alpha in rheumatoid arthritis. *Nat Med* 2013;19:322–8.

120. Nadkarni S, Mauri C, Ehrenstein MR. Anti-TNF-alpha therapy induces a distinct regulatory T cell population in patients with rheumatoid arthritis via TGF-beta. *J Exp Med* 2007;204:33–9.

121. Maldonado A, Mueller YM, Thomas P, Bojczuk P, O'Connors C, Katsikis PD. Decreased effector memory CD45RA+ CD62L– CD8+ T cells and increased central memory CD45RA– CD62L+ CD8+ T cells in peripheral blood of rheumatoid arthritis patients. *Arthritis Res Ther* 2003;5:R91–6.

122. Cho BA, Sim JH, Park JA, et al. Characterization of effector memory CD8+ T cells in the synovial fluid of rheumatoid arthritis. *J Clin Immunol* 2012;32:709–20.

123. Carvalheiro H, Duarte C, Silva-Cardoso S, da Silva JA, Souto-Carneiro MM. CD8+ T cell profiles in patients with rheumatoid arthritis and their relationship to disease activity. *Arthritis Rheumatol* 2015;67:363–71.

124. Sottini A, Imberti L, Gorla R, Cattaneo R, Primi D. Restricted expression of T cell receptor V beta but not V alpha genes in rheumatoid arthritis. *Eur J Immunol* 1991;21:461–6.

125. Masuko-Hongo K, Sekine T, Ueda S, Kobata T, Yamamoto K, Nishioka K, Kato T. Long-term persistent accumulation of CD8+ T cells in synovial fluid of rheumatoid arthritis. *Ann Rheum Dis* 1997;56:613–21.

126. Kang YM, Zhang X, Wagner UG, et al. CD8 T cells are required for the formation of ectopic germinal centers in rheumatoid synovitis. *J Exp Med* 2002;195:1325–36.

127. Gao Y, Williams AP. Role of innate T cells in anti-bacterial immunity. *Front Immunol* 2015;6:302.

128. Fergusson JR, Smith KE, Fleming VM, et al. CD161 defines a transcriptional and functional phenotype across distinct human T cell lineages. *Cell Rep* 2014;9:1075–88.

129. Drennan MB, Aspeslagh S, Elewaut D. Invariant natural killer T cells in rheumatic disease: a joint dilemma. *Nat Rev Rheumatol* 2010;6:90–8.

130. Coppieters K, Van Beneden K, Jacques P, et al. A single early activation of invariant NK T cells confers long-term protection against collagen-induced arthritis in a ligand-specific manner. *J Immunol* 2007;179:2300–9.

131. Miellot-Gafsou A, Biton J, Bourgeois E, Herbelin A, Boissier MC, Bessis N. Early activation of invariant natural killer T cells in a rheumatoid arthritis model and application to disease treatment. *Immunology* 2010;130:296–306.

132. Miellot A, Zhu R, Diem S, Boissier MC, Herbelin A, Bessis N. Activation of invariant NK T cells protects against experimental rheumatoid arthritis by an IL-10-dependent pathway. *Eur J Immunol* 2005;35:3704–13.

133. Linsen L, Thewissen M, Baeten K, et al. Peripheral blood but not synovial fluid natural killer T cells are biased towards a Th1-like phenotype in rheumatoid arthritis. *Arthritis Res Ther* 2005;7:R493–502.

134. Mansour S, Tocheva AS, Sanderson JP, et al. Structural and functional changes of the invariant nkt clonal repertoire in early rheumatoid arthritis. *J Immunol* 2015;195:5582–91.

135. Ospelt C, Bang H, Feist E, et al. Carbamylation of vimentin is inducible by smoking and represents an independent autoantigen in rheumatoid arthritis. *Ann Rheum Dis* 2017;76:1176–83.

136. Sorensen OE, Borregaard N. Neutrophil extracellular traps—the dark side of neutrophils. *J Clin Invest* 2016;126:1612–20.

137. Sidney J, Becart S, Zhou M, et al. Citrullination only infrequently impacts peptide binding to HLA class II MHC. *PLoS One* 2017;12:e0177140.

138. Scally SW, Petersen J, Law SC, et al. A molecular basis for the association of the HLA-DRB1 locus, citrullination, and rheumatoid arthritis. *J Exp Med* 2013;*210*:2569–82.

139. Swanberg M, Lidman O, Padyukov L, et al. MHC2TA is associated with differential MHC molecule expression and susceptibility to rheumatoid arthritis, multiple sclerosis and myocardial infarction. *Nat Genet* 2005;*37*:486–94.

140. Tibbitt C, Falconer J, Stoop J, van Eden W, Robinson JH, Hilkens CM. Reduced TCR-dependent activation through citrullination of a T-cell epitope enhances Th17 development by disruption of the STAT3/5 balance. *Eur J Immunol* 2016;*46*:1633–43.

141. Thomas R, Turner M, Cope AP. High avidity autoreactive T cells with a low signalling capacity through the T-cell receptor: central to rheumatoid arthritis pathogenesis? *Arthritis Res Ther* 2008;*10*:210.

142. Sakaguchi S, Benham H, Cope AP, Thomas R. T-cell receptor signaling and the pathogenesis of autoimmune arthritis: insights from mouse and man. *Immunol Cell Biol* 2012;*90*:277–87.

143. Singh K, Deshpande P, Pryshchep S, et al. ERK-dependent T cell receptor threshold calibration in rheumatoid arthritis. *J Immunol* 2009;*183*:8258–67.

144. Purvis HA, Stoop JN, Mann J, et al. Low strength T-cell activation promotes Th17 responses. *Blood* 2010;*116*(23):4829–37.

145. Coombes JL, Siddiqui KR, Arancibia-Carcamo CV, et al. A functionally specialized population of mucosal CD103+ DCs induces Foxp3+ regulatory T cells via a TGF-beta and retinoic acid-dependent mechanism. *J Exp Med* 2007;*204*:1757–64.

146. Martin E, Capini C, Duggan E, et al. Antigen-specific suppression of established arthritis in mice by dendritic cells deficient in NF-kappaB. *Arthritis Rheum* 2007;*56*:2255–66.

147. Martin E, O'Sullivan B, Low P, Thomas R. Antigen-specific suppression of a primed immune response by dendritic cells mediated by regulatory T cells secreting interleukin-10. *Immunity* 2003;*18*:155–67.

148. Stoop JN, Harry RA, von Delwig A, Isaacs JD, Robinson JH, Hilkens CM. Therapeutic effect of tolerogenic dendritic cells in established collagen-induced arthritis is associated with a reduction in Th17 responses. *Arthritis Rheum* 2010;*62*(12):3656–65.

149. Benham H, Nel HJ, Law SC, et al. Citrullinated peptide dendritic cell immunotherapy in HLA risk genotype-positive rheumatoid arthritis patients. *Sci Transl Med* 2015;*7*:290ra287.

150. Bell GM, Anderson AE, Diboll J, et al. Autologous tolerogenic dendritic cells for rheumatoid and inflammatory arthritis. *Ann Rheum Dis* 2017;*76*:227–34.

151. Thomas R. Dendritic cells and the promise of antigen-specific therapy in rheumatoid arthritis. *Arthritis Res Ther* 2013;*15*:204.

152. Yamamoto K, Sakoda H, Nakajima T, et al. Accumulation of multiple T cell clonotypes in the synovial lesions of patients with rheumatoid arthritis revealed by a novel clonality analysis. *Int Immunol* 1992;*4*:1219–23.

153. Alam A, Lule J, Coppin H, et al. T-cell receptor variable region of the beta-chain gene use in peripheral blood and multiple synovial membranes during rheumatoid arthritis. *Hum Immunol* 1995;*42*:331–9.

154. Jenkins RN, Nikaein A, Zimmermann A, Meek K, Lipsky PE. T cell receptor V beta gene bias in rheumatoid arthritis. *J Clin Investig* 1993;*92*:2688–701.

155. Paliard X, West S, Lafferty J, et al. Evidence for the effects of a superantigen in rheumatoid arthritis. *Science* 1991;*253*:325–9.

156. Zagon G, Tumang JR, Li Y, Friedman SM, Crow MK. Increased frequency of V beta 17-positive T cells in patients with rheumatoid arthritis. *Arthritis Rheum* 1994;*37*:1431–40.

157. Cooper SM, Roessner KD, Naito-Hoopes M, Howard DB, Gaur LK, Budd RC. Increased usage of V beta 2 and V beta 6 in rheumatoid synovial fluid T cells. *Arthritis Rheum* 1994;*37*:1627–36.

158. Lunardi C, Marguerie C, So AK. An altered repertoire of T cell receptor V gene expression by rheumatoid synovial fluid T lymphocytes. *Clin Exp Immunol* 1992;*90*:440–6.

159. Sun W, Nie H, Li N, et al. Skewed T-cell receptor BV14 and BV16 expression and shared CDR3 sequence and common sequence motifs in synovial T cells of rheumatoid arthritis. *Genes Immun* 2005;*6*:248–61.

160. Fischer D-C, Opalka B, Hoffmann A, Mayr W, Haubeck H-D. Limited heterogeneity of rearranged T cell receptor Vα and Vβ transcripts in synovial fluid T cells in early stages of rheumatoid arthritis. *Arthritis Rheum* 1996;*39*:454–62.

161. Woodsworth DJ, Castellarin M, Holt RA. Sequence analysis of T-cell repertoires in health and disease. *Genome Med* 2013;*5*:98.

162. Law SC, Benham H, Reid HH, Rossjohn J, Thomas R. Identification of self-antigen-specific T cells reflecting loss of tolerance in autoimmune disease underpins preventative immunotherapeutic strategies in rheumatoid arthritis. *Rheum Dis Clin N Am* 2014;*40*:735–52.

9

Mechanisms of bone and cartilage destruction

Ulrike Harre and Georg Schett

Introduction

Rheumatoid arthritis (RA) is an autoimmune disease that leads to chronic inflammation. A hallmark of RA is the manifestation of a chronic inflammatory symmetrical polyarthritis mainly affecting diarthrodial joints, which are surrounded by a joint capsule merging with the periosteum of the linked bones. The joint capsule consists of an outer layer, the so-called articular capsule, and an inner layer, the so-called synovial membrane, and is filled with synovial fluid. Under healthy conditions, the synovial membrane is formed by very few cell layers of macrophage-like synoviocytes (= type A cells) and fibroblast-like synoviocytes (= type B cells).[1] In the course of RA, joint inflammation starts with the proliferation of these synovial lining cells together with neovascularization. Secondary, large amounts of immune cells, such as neutrophil granulocytes, macrophages, B cells, and T cells invade into the synovial membrane and fluid. This process is driven by a plethora of inflammatory cytokines and autoantibodies and sustained by epigenetic changes in the fibroblast-like synoviocytes supporting further inflammation. The aim of this review is, to summarize how synovial inflammation leads to structural damage of the bone and the cartilage in patients with RA.

Bone erosion is mediated by osteoclasts

Patients with RA display three different forms of bone damage: (1) local bone erosions at the joint margins that are in direct contact with the inflamed synovium (**Figure 9.1**); (2) periarticular bone loss adjacent to the inflamed joints; and (3) systemic osteopenia or osteoporosis.[2] All three forms are mediated by an elevated osteoclast differentiation and function paired with suppressed osteoblast activity. The reasons for the enhanced osteoclast activity in RA are multifaceted and range from cellular effects to pro-inflammatory cytokines and autoantibodies.

Osteoclasts are multinucleated giant cells that differentiate by cell fusion of macrophage-like precursors. In mammals, they represent the only known cell type that resorbs bone. Bone resorption is initiated by the attachment of an osteoclast to the bone surface and the subsequent formation of a sealing zone, a ring-like filamentous actin (F-actin)–rich structure that encircles the resorption lacuna, an enclosed microcavity between the bone surface and the osteoclast. Into this compartment, the osteoclast actively releases protons via the H^+ATPase as well as a couple of proteases and phosphatases, such as cathepsin K, matrix metalloproteinase (MMP)-9 and tartrate resistant acidic phosphatase (TRAP). The acidification of the microcavity leads to the disintegration of calcium hydroxyapatite, the mineral component of bone matrix. Collagen and other proteins of the bone matrix are subsequently digested by the secreted proteases.[3,4]

Osteoclasts are important for the maintenance of bone integrity as they resorb old or damaged bone, typically at sites of transcortical microvessels, which are connected with the osteocyte canalicular network.[5] Under physiological conditions, the resorption is followed by a recruitment of osteoblasts and the formation of new bone.[6] Up to 10% of the whole bone mass is remodelled each year. In RA, osteoclast formation and activity is dramatically increased resulting in enhanced bone resorption without sufficient bone formation. The importance of increased osteoclastogenesis for bone damage is supported by the observed reduction of bone erosions in RA patients treated with antiresorptive agents that have been originally developed for the treatment of osteoporosis.[7,8] Established antiresorptive agents are bisphosphonates such as zoledronic acid that inhibits osteoclast development and function and the RANKL-blocking antibody denosumab, which reduces the progression of arthritic bone erosion but does not ameliorate joint inflammation or cartilage damage.[7–10]

Effects of synovial and infiltrated immune cells on bone erosion

Osteoclastogenesis is mainly dependent on the presence of macrophage colony-stimulating factor (M-CSF) and receptor activator of nuclear factor-kappa B ligand (RANKL). While M-CSF serves as a survival factor, RANKL is the main driver for the differentiation into osteoclasts.[11] RANKL belongs to the tumour necrosis factor (TNF) superfamily. Like TNF-α, it is composed of three

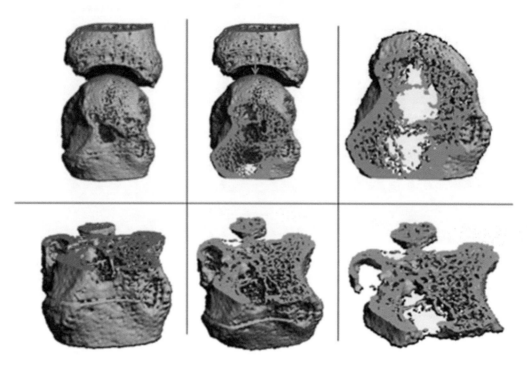

Figure 9.1 Bone erosion in rheumatoid arthritis.
High-resolution peripheral quantitative tomography scans of the metacarpal heads of a patient with rheumatoid arthritis. Upper row shows coronal sections, lower row shows transversal sections. Bone erosions appear as cortical breaks with large areas of bone resorption in the underlying peri-articular bone marrow space.

identical subunits.[12] As a type II membrane protein, RANKL exists in a membrane-bound as well as in a soluble form. The binding of RANKL to its receptor RANK on osteoclasts and their precursors initiates the activation of transcription factors like nuclear factor-kappa-B (NF-κB), c-Fos, and, most important, nuclear factor of activated T-cell c1 (NFATc1), the master regulator of osteoclastogenesis. NFATc1 enhances the expression of typical osteoclast genes, such as *TRAP*, cathepsin K, osteoclast-associated receptor (OSCAR), the vitronectin receptor, and the calcitonin receptor.[11,13]

Under physiological conditions, RANKL is mostly produced by osteoblasts and osteocytes that survey the bone status and initiate osteoclastogenesis at sites of damage. In addition to RANKL, osteoblasts release osteoprotegerin (OPG), a soluble decoy receptor for RANKL that acts as an antagonist. The ratio between RANKL and its decoy receptor OPG is an important regulator of osteoclast formation and activity. In inflamed joints, synovial cells and invading T cells increase the RANKL/OPG ratio and, thereby, the rate of osteoclastogenesis. The importance of this ratio is demonstrated by a study showing that elevated serum RANKL/OPG ratios in patients with RA correlate with a stronger progression of bone erosion.[14]

Interestingly, next to osteoclastogenesis, RANKL plays an important role in the communication between T cells and dendritic cells and is needed for the development of lymph nodes.[15] Originally, RANKL has been discovered as a factor produced by T helper cells to promote the survival of dendritic cells.[16] In the course of synovitis, numerous T cells enter the synovium and serve as an important source of RANKL for osteoclastogenesis.[13] Especially foxhead box protein 3 (Foxp3), positive T-cell-derived Th17 cells have been shown to promote osteoclastogenesis, not only by the production of RANKL, but also by the upregulation of RANKL expression in fibroblast-like synoviocytes via interleukin (IL)-17.[17]

Next to T cells, fibroblast-like synoviocytes constitute a main and probably even the major producer of RANKL in the inflamed synovium. Isolated fibroblast-like synoviocytes from the synovium of RA patients have been shown to trigger the differentiation of peripheral blood monocytes into osteoclasts in the presence of 1,25-dihydroxyvitamin D3 and M-CSF.[18] Using conditional knockout mice that lack RANKL only in T cells or fibroblast-like synoviocytes, Takayanagi et al. revealed fibroblasts as the major contributors to osteoclast-mediated bone erosion in murine arthritis models.[19] This finding is further reflected by the notion that bone resorbing osteoclasts are often found at areas that are in contact with inflamed and proliferated synovium.[18] Of note, fibroblast-like synoviocytes do not produce RANKL in the absence of inflammatory cytokines. Next to IL-17, IL-6 (in combination with the soluble IL-6 receptor) and IL-1β have been described to induce RANKL expression in fibroblast-like synoviocytes.[20]

In the course of synovitis, many activated B cells enter the synovium. A study that compared RANKL mRNA expression of leucocytes that infiltrated into the synovium of RA patients described B cells as an important source of RANKL.[21] Indeed, B cells isolated from the blood of RA patients and stimulated with anti-CD40 antibodies and phorbol myristate acetate were able to enhance osteoclastogenesis from blood monocytes.[22] However, further studies are needed to clarify the individual role of B cells in RANKL-induced osteoclastogenesis as these cells are also a major source of OPG.[23,24]

Effects of inflammatory cytokines on bone erosion

Although M-CSF and RANKL are essential for osteoclastogenesis, other cytokines can augment this process. In the last years, it became

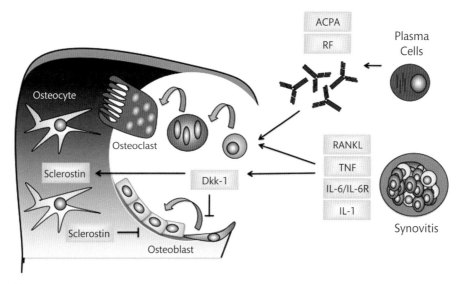

Figure 9.2 Mechanism of bone erosion.
Bone erosions form due to a local imbalance between bone resorption and bone formation. This imbalance is mediated by autoantibodies and cytokines. Plasma cells produce autoantibodies such as rheumatoid factors (RF) and anticitrullinated protein antibodies (ACPA), which directly stimulate the differentiation of bone resorbing osteoclasts. Synovitis produces pro-osteoclastogenic cytokines such as receptor activator of nuclear factor kappa B ligand (RANKL), tumour necrosis factor alpha (TNFa), complexes of interleukin-6 and its receptor (IL-6/IL-6R) and interleukin 1 (IL-1). At the same time, expression of mediators that inhibit bone formation, such as dickkopf-1 (Dkk-1) and sclerostin are increased by inflammatory cytokines

evident that several inflammatory cytokines enhance osteoclast formation and/ or activity either by direct effects on osteoclast precursors and mature osteoclasts or indirectly via the stimulation of RANKL expression by other cells in the synovium or bone. The most important cytokines triggering bone destruction in RA are TNF-α, IL-6, and IL-1 (**Figure 9.2**).

TNF-α is a key cytokine involved in joint inflammation and bone destruction in RA. In the synovium, TNF-α is mainly produced by activated macrophages and fibroblasts, but also by T cells, B cells, osteoblasts, and osteoclasts. TNF-α directly enhances osteoclastogenesis as well as survival and activity of mature osteoclasts by synergizing with RANKL and enhancing the activation of NF-κB, activator protein (AP)-1 and NFATc1, which are important transcription factors for osteoclast differentiation.[25] In addition, TNF-α induces RANKL expression in mesenchymal cells, which further triggers osteoclastogenesis.[26] Another mechanism of TNF-α-mediated bone loss might be the alteration of lineage choice of haematopoietic stem cells as systemic overexpression of TNF-α increases the number of circulating osteoclast precursor cells in murine arthritis models.[27]

Next to TNF-α, IL-6 constitutes another important cytokine involved in the pathogenesis of RA. IL-6 is mainly produced by fibroblast-like synoviocytes, macrophages, and T cells.[25] The direct effects of IL-6 on osteoclast precursors are discussed controversially, with some groups claiming stimulatory and some groups claiming inhibitory effects. *In vivo*, it seems that IL-6 mainly contributes to bone loss by the stimulation of RANKL expression in osteoblasts via activation of signal transducer and activator of transcription 3 (STAT3).[28] In a murine model of antigen-induced arthritis, IL-6 deficient mice displayed less synovitis, **osteoclast numbers and structural damage** than wild-type or TNF-α deficient mice.[29] In addition, in patients with RA, serum levels of IL-6 as well as the soluble IL-6 receptor correlate with the amount of radiographic joint destruction and systemic bone loss.[30] In accordance with these findings, the

IL-6 antagonist tocilizumab has been quite successfully used for the treatment of RA and reduces the progression of joint damage and bone erosion.[2]

In murine arthritis models, IL-1β seems to play a key role for the progression of bone destruction by altering the RANKL/OPG ratio.[31] RA patients display high levels of IL-1β in the serum and synovial fluid and polymorphism in the genes for IL-1β and its antagonist IL-1RA are associated with an increased risk to develop arthritis.[32] Furthermore, the IL-1β antagonist Anakinra, although being less efficacious than antagonists against TNF-α or IL-6 to control inflammation in patients with RA[33] has shown clear evidence for suppression of bone erosion.[34]

Effects of autoantibodies on bone erosion

Although inflammatory cytokines significantly contribute to elevated osteoclastogenesis in the course of RA, bone erosion is also driven by autoantibodies.[35] Rheumatoid factor (RF) that is directed against the constant region of immunoglobulin G (IgG) and thus leads to the formation of serum immune complexes. RF is associated with a more severe disease course of RA.[36] Autoantibodies against citrullinated proteins (ACPA) are a highly specific feature of RA. Citrullination is a post-translational modification of proteins, in which arginine residues are converted into citrulline residues. This modification is mediated by a group of enzymes called peptidylarginine deiminases (PAD) and has been found to be important for a couple of biological processes, such as apoptosis, skin keratinization, and extracellular trap formation.[36] As the transformation of arginine into citrulline alters the charge of the protein, neoepitopes can arise and lead to the development of autoantibodies as it is seen in RA. ACPA are highly specific for RA and have a strong predictive value for the progression of disease. ACPA-positive RA patients (which make about two-thirds of all RA patients) display a more aggressive disease course and more bone erosions.[37] Single B cell sequencing and the generation of monoclonal ACPA revealed that most ACPA are polyspecific and react with a variety of citrullinated proteins.[38] The synovium of RA patients contains a plethora of citrullinated peptides and proteins[39,40] that serve as antigens for ACPA resulting in the formation of immune complexes. Interestingly, the recognition of specific antigens is not associated with the severity of disease. Instead, it seems that spreading of epitope and Ig class correlates with an overall increase in ACPA levels and reflects the strength of the autoimmune response.[37]

In contrast to the RF, ACPA mainly belong to the IgG type and thereby are potent activators of Fcγ-receptors (FcγR) on immune cells. Several groups described an increase in TNF-α production in macrophages stimulated with immune complexes either directly derived from the synovial fluid of RA patients[40] or formed from serum-derived ACPA and citrullinated proteins.[41] The group of Lu et al. reported that ACPA can directly bind to citrullinated glucose-regulated protein 78 (cit-GRP78) expressed on the cell surface of macrophages and elicit the production of TNF-α.[42] As TNF-α is a potent stimulator of osteoclast differentiation and activity (see earlier section), it has long been thought that the main contribution of ACPA to bone loss is mediated via the release of pro-inflammatory cytokines.

However, in the recent years, there has been increasing evidence that ACPA also enhance bone resorption by direct interactions with osteoclasts and their precursors. We, as well as Krishnamurthy et al., demonstrated that ACPA directly bind to citrullinated proteins expressed on the cell surface of preosteoclasts.[43,44] This binding leads to an enhanced osteoclast differentiation and thereby to increased bone resorption *in vitro* as well as *in vivo*. Osteoclasts belong to the myeloid cell lineage and share several properties with macrophages.[45] Among others, they express FcγR and are therefore able to bind IgG-containing immune complexes. Recently, it has been shown that FcγR expression is even upregulated during osteoclastogenesis and that crosslinking of these receptors enhances osteoclast differentiation. Furthermore, conditional knockout mice, lacking FcγRIV specifically in osteoclasts, were partially protected from bone loss in a serum-transfer arthritis model.[46] It is therefore very likely that ACPA bound to surface proteins activate preosteoclasts via FcγR. This hypothesis is further supported by our finding, that under certain conditions also unspecific IgG complexes are able to increase osteoclastogenesis by binding to FcγR of preosteoclasts.[47] As ACPA-Fab fragments have been shown to increase osteoclastogenesis as well,[43,44] ACPA seem to directly trigger osteoclastogenesis via citrullinated proteins on the cell surface of preosteoclasts in addition to Fc receptor binding. However, the definite nature of such binding structures is still not fully clarified to date.

Of note, the Fc glycosylation of IgG is a key determinant for the effects of IgG complexes on osteoclastogenesis. IgG has one N-glycosylation site located at the asparagine-297 in the CH2 domain of the heavy chain. The attached glycan resides in the pocket between the two heavy chains and influences the binding of IgG to FcγR by altering the quaternary structure of the Fc part.[48] The Fc glycan consists of a conserved heptamer that can be extended by additional sugar residues. One of these additional sugar residues is terminal sialic acid that is present in about 20% of the IgG molecules. The presence of terminal sialic acid enables the binding of IgG to anti-inflammatory receptors like dendritic cell-specific ICAM-grabbing non-integrin (DC-SIGN) or dendritic cell immunoreceptor

(DCIR), while the absence of sialic acid seems to increase the affinity to activating FcγR.[49] Interestingly, ACPA display lower sialylation levels than random IgG[50] which might explain their strong association with bone destruction in RA patients. Indeed, we have found that a low Fc-sialylation level is needed in IgG complexes to efficiently enhance osteoclastogenesis and that the pro-osteoclastogenic capacity of ACPA is completely lost after enzymatic attachment of terminal sialic acid.[47] The importance of IgG sialylation for the manifestation of arthritis has been further demonstrated in a very recent work of Pfeifle et al. showing that, despite high collagen-specific autoantibody titres, mice lacking IL-23 are completely protected from collagen-induced arthritis because of increased IgG sialylation levels.[51] Of note, already years before the onset of arthritis, ACPA levels, epitope recognition, and isotype usage strongly increase,[52–54] but only in the last month before disease onset, the glycosylation of ACPA changes towards a more inflammatory pattern.[55]

Together, it is evident that ACPA, and most likely also the newly discovered antibodies against carbamylated proteins (anti-CarP)[56] strongly contribute to structural damage in RA. Of note, ACPA emerge up to 10 years before the onset of disease[52] and even people without synovitis display bone erosion if they are ACPA positive.[57] Hence, new concepts suggest that the initial events in the joints of patients with RA are the induction of osteoclastogenesis by autoantibodies leading to structural priming of the joints[57,58] (Figure 9.3). This process of structural priming seems to be accompanied by a widening and an increase in the numbers of so-called cortical microchannels,[58] which can be visualized in the high-resolution computed tomography scans and reflect transcortical microvessels[5,59] (Figure 9.4).

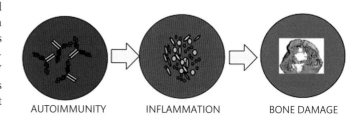

AUTOIMMUNITY   INFLAMMATION   BONE DAMAGE

AUTOIMMUNITY

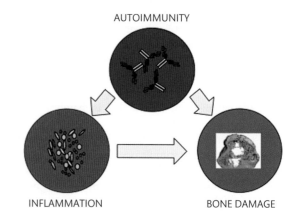

INFLAMMATION   BONE DAMAGE

Figure 9.3 Standard and new model of bone damage in rheumatoid arthritis.
Upper part: The standard model of bone damage in rheumatoid arthritis proposes that bone damage exclusively results from the degree and duration of synovial inflammation. Autoimmunity is triggering synovial inflammation. Lower part: The new model of bone damage in rheumatoid arthritis proposes that bone damage is the result from direct effects of autoimmunity as well as indirect from synovial inflammation.

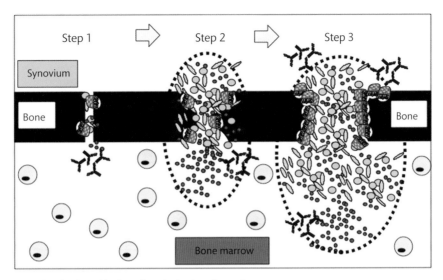

Figure 9.4 Initiation of bone erosion by the widening of cortical microchannels.
Cortical bone separates the synovial space (top) from the bone marrow space (bottom). Physiologically transcortical microvessels cross the cortical bone through cortical microchannels (also known as CoMiCs). The channels initially widen through autoantibody-mediated osteoclast differentiation and bone resorption. Once inflammation has initiated, CoMiCs further widen in their diameter by increased osteoclast-mediated bone resorption. Finally, after further widening, radiographic bone erosions develop from these channels.

Mediators of osteoblast activity

One major obstacle for the treatment of advanced RA is that established bone erosions do not repair. In clinical studies, only a small proportion of patients displayed bone regeneration.[60] In these studies, repair was strongly associated with low disease activity, which leads to the hypothesis that inflammation impairs the bone forming capacity of osteoblasts.

Osteoblasts are of mesenchymal origin and represent the only bone forming cell type in the body. They differentiate from mesenchymal stem cells via the stage of osteoprogenitor cells. The main factors driving osteoblast differentiation are *WNT*, bone morphogenic protein (BMP), insulin-like growth factor, and parathyroid hormone (PTH) that induce the expression of the key transcription factors runt-related transcription factor 2 (Runx2) and osterix.[61] During the process of bone formation, osteoblasts form the organic part of the bone matrix by the secretion of collagen, which provides bone strength as well as connecting proteins, such as osteocalcin, bone sialoprotein, or osteopontin, followed by the induction of calcification.[61,62] Some osteoblasts stay embedded in the new bone matrix and further differentiate into osteocytes.

Histological examination of synovial biopsies from RA patients revealed a shortage of mature osteoblasts at sites of focal bone erosion,[24] demonstrating that osteoblast differentiation is inhibited in inflamed joints (**Figure 9.2**). A potent inhibitor of osteoblast differentiation is the pro-inflammatory cytokine TNF-α that is abundantly expressed in the inflamed synovium. TNF-α induces the degradation of the pro-osteoblastogenic transcription factor Runx2 by upregulating the ubiquitin ligases Smurf1 and Smurf2.[63,64] In addition, TNF-α induces the expression of Dickkopf-1 (Dkk-1) by fibroblast-like synoviocytes,[65] which acts as an inhibitor of Wnt (**Figure 9.2**). In patients with RA, serum levels of DKK-1 are increased and correlate with an enhanced disease activity.[66] Treatment with a TNF-α blocker decreases the serum levels of

DKK-1.[66] In addition to the inhibition of bone formation, DKK-1 favours bone resorption by decreasing the OPG expression of osteoblasts.[67] In a murine TNF-mediated arthritis model, inhibition of DKK-1 resulted in less bone erosion and the formation of osteophytes whereas tissue inflammation was unchanged.[68] Of note, several DKK-1 single nuclear polymorphisms have been identified that are associated with increased serum DKK-1 levels and enhanced joint destruction in RA patients.[69] Together, the results demonstrate a key role of DKK-1 in the inhibition of new bone formation in RA. Furthermore, TNF-α has been found to induce the expression of BMP-3 by osteoblasts, which acts as an inhibitor of osteoblast differentiation and might contribute to local bone loss in RA.[70]

Next to TNF-α, other inflammatory cytokines like IL-1 or IL-17 have been described to inhibit osteoblast differentiation and bone formation *in vitro* as well as in murine arthritis models.[71,72]

Cartilage destruction is mediated by fibroblast-like synoviocytes

Joints are surrounded by the synovium that also serves as a connection to the adjacent musculoskeletal tissues. The synovial lining is formed by one to three layers of fibroblast-like synoviocytes interspersed with macrophage-like synoviocytes. In the adjacent sublining, fibroblast-like synoviocytes do not form a united cell structure, but are loosely embedded in an extracellular matrix. Fibroblast-like synoviocytes are mesenchymal cells and also known as type B synoviocytes or synovial fibroblasts. In the healthy synovium, they constitute about 75% of all cells. The main function of fibroblast-like synoviocytes is the secretion of components of the synovial fluid, such as lubricin and hyaluronic acid, and components of the extracellular matrix, such as heparin sulphate-linked proteoglycans, fibronectin, and a couple of collagens.[73]

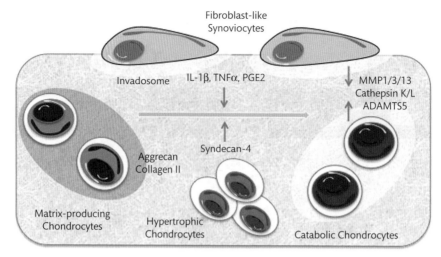

Figure 9.5 Cartilage damage in rheumatoid arthritis.

Fibroblast-like synoviocytes undergo epigenetic changes towards an inflammatory phenotype. They become invasive by the formation of invadosomes and the release of enzymes such as matrix metalloproteinases (MMPs), cathepsins and ADAMTS5 (a disintegrin and metalloproteinase with thrombospondin motifs 5). Furthermore, they release inflammatory mediators such as interleukin 1 (IL-1), tumour necrosis factor alpha (TNFa) and prostaglandin E2 (PGE2) that switch the chondrocyte phenotype from a matrix-synthetizing into a catabolic phenotype. In addition, hypertrophic chondrocytes release syndecan-4, which contributes to the catabolic phenotype of chondrocytes.

In arthritic joints, fibroblast-like synoviocytes transform into a cancer-like cell state in which they strongly proliferate, escape apoptosis, and contribute to cartilage damage.[73] Fibroblast-like synoviocytes of RA patients display altered expression and activation profiles of proto-oncogenes and tumour-suppressor genes, such as c-Fos, phosphatase and tensin homologue (PTEN) and p53.[73] As a consequence of this transformation, the synovial lining thickens up to about 10–15 cell layers. Transformed fibroblast-like synoviocytes become highly migratory and attach to or even invade into the articular cartilage. This enhanced invading capacity is mediated by the upregulation of matrix adhesion molecules. In a couple of studies, so-called invadosomes have been described that present as dot-like accumulations of F-actin enriched with integrins.[74] In contrast to other podosome-like structures, invadosomes recruit proteases that degrade the cartilage extracellular matrix, such as metalloproteinases (MMP)-1, MMP3, MMP13, cathepsins (cathepsins K and L) and aggrecanases (A disintegrin and metalloproteinase with thrombospondin motifs 5: ADAMTS5) (**Figure 9.5**). Under physiological conditions, the activity of these enzymes is controlled by the simultaneous release of tissue inhibitors of MMPs (TIMPs).[73] However, in RA this balance is strongly disturbed.

Of note, once transformed, fibroblast-like synoviocytes keep their invasive phenotype even after multiple passages in cell culture. This observation strongly suggests fibroblast-like synoviocytes to participate in the chronicity of RA. Murine transfer models showed that fibroblast-like synoviocytes isolated from RA patients or arthritic mice are able to migrate to unaffected joints when injected into naive mice and to induce synovitis.[75] This maintenance of an aggressive phenotype has been found to be due to epigenetic changes. The best-studied epigenetic mechanisms to control gene expression are DNA methylation and histone modification. DNA methylation leads to a lowered expression of the respective genes. Transformed fibroblast-like synoviocytes are significantly hypomethylated especially in genes relevant for RA, such as caspase 1 (*CASP1*), STAT3, mitogen-activated protein kinase kinase kinase 5 (*MAP3K5*), *TNF, AKT3*, CXC-motiv-chemokin 12 (*CXCL12*), and T-box transcription

factor 5 (TBX5) resulting in enhanced gene expression.[76,77] The importance of DNA methylation is reflected by the fact that treatment of normal fibroblast-like synoviocytes from patients with osteoarthritis with the demethylating drug azacitidine resulted in a phenotype similar to that of RA fibroblast-like synoviocytes.[78] Recently, even joint-specific methylation patterns of synovial fibroblasts have been described,[79] which could control their invasiveness in a site-specific fashion explaining differential cartilage destruction at the various anatomical sites in patients with RA.

The role of chondrocytes in cartilage destruction

Cartilage matrix is maintained by chondrocytes. Being the only cell type residing in the cartilage tissue, chondrocytes are not only able to build up cartilage matrix, but also to break it down. This dual ability is of need in cases of injury, when cartilage remodelling is required. Under physiological conditions, chondrocytes first degrade matrix molecules like aggrecan or collagen type II followed by the synthesis of new matrix proteins. Under chronic inflammatory conditions, the synthesis of matrix proteins is impaired, while the release of proteases is upregulated. For example, treatment with inflammatory cytokines, like IL-1 induces the upregulation of MMPs as well as ADAMTS-4 and -5 in chondrocytes, resulting in increased aggrecanolysis and reduces proteoglycan synthesis.[80] This process is reflected by a net loss of water content in the articular cartilage of RA patients, which can be depicted early by special high-resolution magnetic resonance imaging techniques (dGEMRIC)[81] (**Figure 9.6**). Furthermore, during arthritis some of the chondrocytes dedifferentiate into a hypertrophic state characterized by the expression of type X collagen. These cells are considered as kind of pacemakers of cartilage damage by producing syndecan 4, which is secreted by chondrocytes and induce the synthesis of ADAMTS5 in adjacent chondrocytes (**Figure 9.5**).[82] Hence, cartilage in RA is degraded by the dual action of fibroblast-like synoviocytes producing proteases that cleave aggrecan and the

Morphological T1 image   T2 mapping of the cartilage

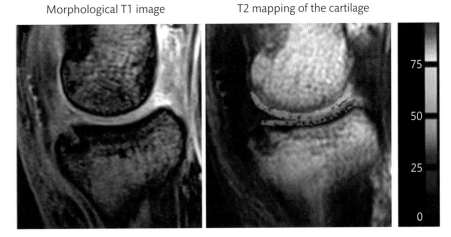

Figure 9.6 Cartilage proteoglycan loss in in rheumatoid arthritis.
High-field 3-tesla magnetic resonance imaging of the metacarpophalangeal joint of a patient with rheumatoid arthritis. The subchondral bone plate appears in black and the cartilage is light grey. Left: morphological T1 image; right: multiecho spin-echo (SE) T2 mapping showing the hydration and collagen anisotropy of the articular cartilage (higher values in milliseconds symbolized by red colour indicate lower hydration and higher anisotropy of the cartilage).

collagen backbone of the cartilage as well as chondrocytes themselves, which switch into a matrix-degrading mode, via the influence of cytokines and cartilage-borne factors syndecan-4.

Conclusion

Joint damage is a central feature of RA and characterized by the erosion of bone and cartilage. Bone erosion is caused by an enhanced osteoclast activity and aggravated by a decreased osteoblast activity. Cartilage destruction is mainly effectuated by epigenetically transformed fibroblast-like synoviocytes. The presence of autoantibodies seems to play a crucial role in the development of joint destruction. They largely contribute to synovitis by the formation of autoimmune complexes, but also directly promote bone loss by binding to osteoclast precursors. Once established, synovitis seems to become a self-perpetuating cycle driven by the interactions of autoantibodies, infiltrated immune cells, transformed fibroblast-like synoviocytes, inflammatory cytokines, and osteoclasts. Hence, an effective therapy might need to address several points of this cycle to achieve resolution of inflammation.

Acknowledgements

The authors are supported by the Deutsche Forschungsgemeinschaft (SPP1468 Immunobone and CRC 1181), the Bundesministerium für Bildung und Forschung (BMBF; METARTHROS), the Marie-Curie project Osteoimmune, the Elsbeth-Bonhoff Stiftung, and the Interdisciplinary Centre for Clinical Research of the University of Erlangen-Nuremberg.

REFERENCES

1. van de Sande MG, Baeten DL Immunopathology of synovitis: from histology to molecular pathways. *Rheumatology (Oxf)* 2016;55:599–606.

2. Zerbini CA, Clark P, Mendez-Sanchez L, et al. Biologic therapies and bone loss in rheumatoid arthritis. *Osteoporos Int* 2017;28(2):429–46.

3. Teitelbaum SL. The osteoclast and its unique cytoskeleton. *Ann N Y Acad Sci* 2011;1240:14–17.

4. Takahashi N, Udagawa N, Suda T, et al. Vitamin D endocrine system and osteoclasts. *Bonekey Rep* 2014;3:495.

5. Grueneboom A, Hawwari I, Weidner D, et al. A network of trans-cortical capillaries forms the mainstay for blood circulation in long bones. *Nat Metabol* 2019;1:236–50.

6. Nakahama K. Cellular communications in bone homeostasis and repair. *Cell Mol Life Sci* 2010;67:4001–9.

7. Cohen SB, Dore RK, Lane NE, et al. Denosumab treatment effects on structural damage, bone mineral density, and bone turnover in rheumatoid arthritis: a twelve-month, multicenter, randomized, double-blind, placebo-controlled, phase II clinical trial. *Arthritis Rheum* 2008;58:1299–309.

8. Deodhar A, Dore RK, Mandel D, Schechtman J. Denosumab-mediated increase in hand bone mineral density associated with decreased progression of bone erosion in rheumatoid arthritis patients. *Arthritis Care Res (Hoboken)* 2010;62:569–74.

9. Takeuchi T, Tanaka Y, Ishiguro N, et al. Effect of denosumab on Japanese patients with rheumatoid arthritis: a dose-response study of AMG 162 (denosumab) in patients with rheumatoid arthritis on methotrexate to validate inhibitory effect on bone erosion (DRIVE)-a 12-month, multicentre, randomised, double-blind, placebo-controlled, phase II clinical trial. *Ann Rheum Dis* 2016;75:983–90.

10. Jarrett SJ, Conaghan PG, Sloan VS, et al Preliminary evidence for a structural benefit of the new bisphosphonate zoledronic acid in early rheumatoid arthritis. *Arthritis Rheum* 2006;54:1410–4.

11. Takayanagi H. Mechanistic insight into osteoclast differentiation in osteoimmunology. *J Mol Med (Berl)* 2005;83:170–9.

12. Nelson CA, Warren JT, Wang MWH, Teitelbaum S, Fremont DH. RANKL employs distinct binding modes to engage RANK and the osteoprotegerin decoy receptor. *Structure* 2012;20:1971–82.

13. Crotti TN, Dharmapatni A, Alias E, Haynes DR. Osteoimmunology: major and costimulatory pathway expression

associated with chronic inflammatory induced bone loss. *J Immunol Res* 2015;*2015*:281287.

14. Tuyl LH, Voskuyl AE, Boers M, et al. Baseline RANKL:OPG ratio and markers of bone and cartilage degradation predict annual radiological progression over 11 years in rheumatoid arthritis. *Ann Rheum Dis* 2010;*69*:1623–8.

15. Kong YY, Yoshida H, Sarosi I, et al. OPGL is a key regulator of osteoclastogenesis, lymphocyte development and lymph-node organogenesis. *Nature* 1999;*397*:315–23.

16. Akiyama T, Shinzawa M, Akiyama N. RANKL-RANK inter-action in immune regulatory systems. *World J Orthop* 2012;*3*:142–50.

17. Sato K, Suematsu A, Okamoto K, et al. Th17 functions as an osteoclastogenic helper T cell subset that links T cell activation and bone destruction. *J Exp Med* 2006;*203*:2673–82.

18. Takayanagi H, Oda H, Yamamoto S, et al. A new mechanism of bone destruction in rheumatoid arthritis: synovial fibro-blasts induce osteoclastogenesis. *Biochem Biophys Res Commun* 1997;*240*:279–86.

19. Danks L, Komatsu N, Guerriniet MM, et al. RANKL expressed on synovial fibroblasts is primarily responsible for bone erosions during joint inflammation. *Ann Rheum Dis* 2016;*75*:1187–95.

20. Hashizume M, Hayakawa N, Mihara M. IL-6 trans-signalling directly induces RANKL on fibroblast-like synovial cells and is involved in RANKL induction by TNF-alpha and IL-17. *Rheumatology (Oxf)* 2008;*47*:1635–40.

21. Yeo L, Toellner K-M, Salmon M, et al. Cytokine mRNA profiling identifies B cells as a major source of RANKL in rheumatoid arthritis. *Ann Rheum Dis* 2011;*70*:2022–8.

22. Meednu N, Zhang H, Owen T, et al. Production of RANKL by memory B cells: a link between B cells and bone erosion in rheumatoid arthritis. *Arthritis Rheumatol* 2016;*68*:805–16.

23. Li Y, Toraldo G, Li A, et al. B cells and T cells are critical for the preservation of bone homeostasis and attainment of peak bone mass *in vivo*. *Blood* 2007;*109*:3839–48.

24. Walsh NC, Reinwald S, Manning CA, et al. Osteoblast function is compromised at sites of focal bone erosion in inflammatory arth-ritis. *J Bone Miner Res* 2009;*24*:1572–85.

25. Braun T, Zwerina J. Positive regulators of osteoclastogenesis and bone resorption in rheumatoid arthritis. *Arthritis Res Ther* 2011;*13*:235.

26. Schett G, Gravallese E. Bone erosion in rheumatoid arth-ritis: mechanisms, diagnosis and treatment. *Nat Rev Rheumatol* 2012;*8*:656–64.

27. Yao Z, Li P, Zhang Q, Schwarz E. Tumor necrosis factor-alpha increases circulating osteoclast precursor numbers by pro-moting their proliferation and differentiation in the bone marrow through up-regulation of c-Fms expression. *J Biol Chem* 2006;*281*:11846–55.

28. Mori T, Miyamoto T, Yoshida H, et al. IL-1beta and TNFalpha-initiated IL-6-STAT3 pathway is critical in mediating inflamma-tory cytokines and RANKL expression in inflammatory arthritis. *Int Immunol* 2011;*23*:701–12.

29. Wong PK, Quinn JMW, Sims NA, et al. Interleukin-6 modu-lates production of T lymphocyte-derived cytokines in antigen-induced arthritis and drives inflammation-induced osteoclastogenesis. *Arthritis Rheum* 2006;*54*:158–68.

30. Kotake S, Sato K, Kim KJ, et al. Interleukin-6 and soluble interleukin-6 receptors in the synovial fluids from rheumatoid arthritis patients are responsible for osteoclast-like cell forma-tion. *J Bone Miner Res* 1996;*11*:88–95.

31. Amarasekara DS, Yu J, Rho J, et al. Bone loss triggered by the cytokine network in inflammatory autoimmune diseases. *J Immunol Res* 2015;*2015*:832127.

32. Mateen S, Zafar A, Moin S, et al. Understanding the role of cyto-kines in the pathogenesis of rheumatoid arthritis. *Clin Chim Acta* 2016;*455*:161–71.

33. Mertens M, Singh JA. Anakinra for rheumatoid arthritis: a sys-tematic review. *J Rheumatol* 2009;*36*:1118–25.

34. Jiang Y, Genant H, Watt I, Cobby M. A multicenter, double-blind, dose-ranging, randomized, placebo-controlled study of recom-binant human interleukin-1 receptor antagonist in patients with rheumatoid arthritis: radiologic progression and correlation of Genant and Larsen scores. *Arthritis Rheum* 2000;*43*:1001–9.

35. Hecht C, Englbrecht M, Rech J, et al. Additive effect of anti-citrullinated protein antibodies and rheumatoid factor on bone erosions in patients with RA. *Ann Rheum Dis* 2015;*74*:2151–6.

36. Baka Z, Gyogy B, Geher P, et al. Citrullination under physio-logical and pathological conditions. *Joint Bone Spine* 2012;*79*:431–6.

37. Toes RE, Huizinga TJ. Update on autoantibodies to modified proteins. *Curr Opin Rheumatol* 2015;*27*:262–7.

38. Amara K, Steen J, Murray F, et al. Monoclonal IgG antibodies generated from joint-derived B cells of RA patients have a strong bias toward citrullinated autoantigen recognition. *J Exp Med* 2013;*210*:445–55.

39. Van Steendam K, Tilleman K, De Ceuleneer M, De Keyser F, Elewaut D, Deforce D. Citrullinated vimentin as an important antigen in immune complexes from synovial fluid of rheumatoid arthritis patients with antibodies against citrullinated proteins. *Arthritis Res Ther* 2010;*12*:R132.

40. Mathsson L, Lampa J, Mullazehi M, Rönnelid J. Immune complexes from rheumatoid arthritis synovial fluid induce FcgammaRIIa dependent and rheumatoid factor correlated pro-duction of tumour necrosis factor-alpha by peripheral blood mononuclear cells. *Arthritis Res Ther* 2006;*8*:R64.

41. Clavel C, Nogueira L, Laurent L, et al Induction of macrophage secretion of tumor necrosis factor alpha through Fcgamma receptor IIa engagement by rheumatoid arthritis-specific auto-antibodies to citrullinated proteins complexed with fibrinogen. *Arthritis Rheum* 2008;*58*:678–88.

42. Lu MC, Yu C-L, Yu H-C, et al. Anti-citrullinated protein anti-bodies bind surface-expressed citrullinated Grp78 on monocyte/macrophages and stimulate tumor necrosis factor alpha produc-tion. *Arthritis Rheum* 2010;*62*:1213–23.

43. Harre U, Georgess D, Banget H, et al. Induction of osteoclastogenesis and bone loss by human autoantibodies against citrullinated vimentin. *J Clin Invest* 2012;*122*:1791–802.

44. Krishnamurthy A, Joshua V, Hensvold A-H, et al Identification of a novel chemokine-dependent molecular mechanism underlying rheumatoid arthritis-associated autoantibody-mediated bone loss. *Ann Rheum Dis* 2016;*75*:721–9.

45. Harre U, Keppeler H, Ipseiz N, Derer A. Moonlighting osteoclasts as undertakers of apoptotic cells. *Autoimmunity* 2012;*45*:612–19.

46. Seeling M, Hillenhoff U, David J-F, et al Inflammatory mono-cytes and Fcgamma receptor IV on osteoclasts are critical for bone destruction during inflammatory arthritis in mice. *Proc Natl Acad Sci U S A* 2013;*110*:10729–34.

47. Harre U, Lang SC, Pfeifle R, et al. Glycosylation of immuno-globulin G determines osteoclast differentiation and bone loss. *Nat Commun* 2015;*6*:6651.

48. Arnold JN, Wormald MR, Sim RB, et al. The impact of glycosylation on the biological function and structure of human immunoglobulins. *Annu Rev Immunol* 2007;*25*:21–50.

49. Bohm S, Schwab I, Lux A, Nimmerjahnet F. The role of sialic acid as a modulator of the anti-inflammatory activity of IgG. *Semin Immunopathol* 2012;*34*:443–53.

50. Scherer HU, et al. Glycan profiling of anti-citrullinated protein antibodies isolated from human serum and synovial fluid. *Arthritis Rheum* 2010;*62*:1620–9.

51. Pfeifle R, Rothe T, Ipseiz N, et al. Regulation of autoantibody activity by the IL-23-TH17 axis determines the onset of autoimmune disease. *Nat Immunol* 2017; *18*(1):104–13.

52. van der Woude D, Rantapää-Dahlqvist S, Ioan-Facsinay A, et al. Epitope spreading of the anti-citrullinated protein antibody response occurs before disease onset and is associated with the disease course of early arthritis. *Ann Rheum Dis* 2010;*69*:1554–61.

53. Kokkonen H, Mullazehi M, Berglin E, et al. Antibodies of IgG, IgA and IgM isotypes against cyclic citrullinated peptide precede the development of rheumatoid arthritis. *Arthritis Res Ther* 2011;*13*:R13.

54. Suwannalai P, van de Stadt LA, Radner H, et al. Avidity maturation of anti-citrullinated protein antibodies in rheumatoid arthritis. *Arthritis Rheum* 2012;*64*:1323–8.

55. Rombouts Y, Ewing E, van de Stadt LA, et al. Anti-citrullinated protein antibodies acquire a pro-inflammatory Fc glycosylation phenotype prior to the onset of rheumatoid arthritis. *Ann Rheum Dis* 2015;*74*:234–41.

56. Shi J, Knevel R, Suwannalai P, et al. Autoantibodies recognizing carbamylated proteins are present in sera of patients with rheumatoid arthritis and predict joint damage. *Proc Natl Acad Sci U S A* 2011;*108*:17372–7.

57. Kleyer A, Finzel S, Rech J, et al. Bone loss before the clinical onset of rheumatoid arthritis in subjects with anticitrullinated protein antibodies. *Ann Rheum Dis* 2014;*73*:854–60.

58. Werner D, Simon D, Tascilar K, et al. Early changes of the cortical micro-channel system in the bare area of the joints of patients with rheumatoid arthritis. *Arthritis Rheumatol* 2017;*69*:1580–7.

59. Scharmga A, et al. Vascular channels in metacarpophalangeal joints: a comparative histologic and high-resolution imaging study. *Sci Rep* 2017;*7*:8966.

60. Walsh NC, Gravallese EM. Bone remodeling in rheumatic disease: a question of balance. *Immunol Rev* 2010;*233*:301–12.

61. Baum R, Gravallese EM. Bone as a target organ in rheumatic disease: impact on osteoclasts and osteoblasts. *Clin Rev Allergy Immunol* 2016;*51*:1–15.

62. Harada S, Rodan GA. Control of osteoblast function and regulation of bone mass. *Nature* 2003;*423*:349–55.

63. Gilbert L, del Prete D, Jin S, et al. Expression of the osteoblast differentiation factor RUNX2 (Cbfa1/AML3/Pebp2alpha A) is inhibited by tumor necrosis factor-alpha. *J Biol Chem* 2002;*277*:2695–701.

64. Kaneki H, Guo R, Chen D, et al. Tumor necrosis factor promotes Runx2 degradation through up-regulation of Smurf1 and Smurf2 in osteoblasts. *J Biol Chem* 2006;*281*:4326–33.

65. Yeremenko N, Zwerina K, Rigter G, et al. Tumor necrosis factor and interleukin-6 differentially regulate Dkk-1 in the inflamed arthritic joint. *Arthritis Rheumatol* 2015;*67*:2071–5.

66. Wang SY, Hu XB, Zhang W, et al. Circulating Dickkopf-1 is correlated with bone erosion and inflammation in rheumatoid arthritis. *J Rheumatol* 2011;*38*:821–7.

67. Glass DA, 2nd, Bialek P, Ahn JD, Starbuck MW. Canonical Wnt signaling in differentiated osteoblasts controls osteoclast differentiation. *Dev Cell* 2005;*8*:751–64.

68. Diarra D, Stolina M, Polzer K, Zwerina J. Dickkopf-1 is a master regulator of joint remodeling. *Nat Med* 2007;*13*:156–63.

69. de Rooy DP, Yeremenko NG, Wilson AG, et al. Genetic studies on components of the Wnt signalling pathway and the severity of joint destruction in rheumatoid arthritis. *Ann Rheum Dis* 2013;*72*:769–75.

70. Matzelle MM, Shaw AT, Baum R, et al. Inflammation in arthritis induces expression of BMP3, an inhibitor of bone formation. *Scand J Rheumatol* 2016;*45*:379–83.

71. Stashenko P, Dewhirst FE, Rooney ML, Desjardins LA. Interleukin-1 beta is a potent inhibitor of bone formation *in vitro*. *J Bone Miner Res* 1987;*2*:559–65.

72. Shaw AT, Maeda Y, Gravallese EM. IL-17A deficiency promotes periosteal bone formation in a model of inflammatory arthritis. *Arthritis Res Ther* 2016;*18*:104.

73. Neumann E, Kim S-K, Choe J-Y, et al. Rheumatoid arthritis progression mediated by activated synovial fibroblasts. *Trends Mol Med* 2010;*16*:458–68.

74. Linder S. Invadosomes at a glance. *J Cell Sci* 2009;*122*:3009–13.

75. Lefevre S, Knedla A, Tennie C, et al. Synovial fibroblasts spread rheumatoid arthritis to unaffected joints. *Nat Med* 2009;*15*:1414–20.

76. Klein K, Ospelt C, Gay S. Epigenetic contributions in the development of rheumatoid arthritis. *Arthritis Res Ther* 2012;*14*:227.

77. Karouzakis E, Raza K, Kolling C. Analysis of early changes in DNA methylation in synovial fibroblasts of RA patients before diagnosis. *Sci Rep* 2018;*8*:7370.

78. Karouzakis E, Gay RE, Michel BA, Gay S, Neidhart M. DNA hypomethylation in rheumatoid arthritis synovial fibroblasts. *Arthritis Rheum* 2009;*60*:3613–22.

79. Frank-Bertoncelj M, Trenkmann M, Klein K, et al. Epigenetically driven anatomical diversity of synovial fibroblasts guides joint-specific fibroblast functions. *Nat Comm* 2017;*8*:14852.

80. Patwari P, Gao G, Lee JH, Grodzinsky AJ, Sandy JD. Analysis of ADAMTS4 and MT4-MMP indicates that both are involved in aggrecanolysis in interleukin-1 treated bovine cartilage. *Osteoarthritis & Cartilage* 2005;*13*:269–77.

81. Herz B, Albrecht A, Englbrecht M, et al. Osteitis and synovitis, but not bone erosion, is associated with proteoglycan loss and microstructure damage in the cartilage of patients with rheumatoid arthritis. *Ann Rheum Dis* 2014;*73*:1101–6.

82. Echtermeyer F, Bertrand J, Dreier R, et al. Syndecan-4 regulates ADAMTS-5 activation and cartilage breakdown in osteoarthritis. *Nat Med* 2009;*15*:1072–6.

10

Cytokines and other mediators

Marina Frleta-Gilchrist and Iain B. McInnes

Introduction

Cytokines are small glycoprotein messengers, which are essential to the coordination of the immune system. Typically, cytokines are potent glycosylated polypeptides whose effects include regulation of pathogenic immune cell lineages as well as promoting broader tissue and metabolic processes. Discovery of the first cytokine—interleukin 1 was met with some resistance in the field, as its low concentration was considered too small to elicit a substantial biologic response. The subsequent discovery of many extended cytokine superfamilies, and the parallel elucidation of complex amplificatory cytokine signal receptor systems, mediating the capacity for cytokines to work in synergy to promote and regulate immune responses, has revolutionized our understanding of how these moieties can initiate, fine tune, and then repress inflammatory responses.

In the absence of an overarching classification system, cytokines are predominantly titled by numeric order of their discovery (currently interleukin 1 (IL-1) through IL-39), although some allude to their function (e.g. tumour necrosis factor alpha (TNFα)). Genetic sequence similarities allow recognition of cytokine superfamilies, which also share some subunits of their reciprocal receptor system. Binding of the cytokine to its receptor triggers a cascade of intracellular kinases ultimately activating or repressing downstream target genes. Current nomenclature distinguishes four families of cytokine receptors. Receptors and reciprocal binding cytokine superfamilies are illustrated in **Figure 10.1**.

Dimeric or trimeric structures of a majority of cytokine receptors allow some of the subunits to be shared between different receptors, without the loss of specificity for any given cytokine. The first superfamily of cytokines utilize type 1 receptors, proteins that are anchored to the cell membrane by a 4 alpha helical structure and contain common amino acid motif (WSXWS). By sharing of some receptor subunits, type I family of receptors serve three distinct groups of cytokines. The first group include cytokines sharing the common gamma chain of their receptor; the signature cytokine herein is IL-2—a potent T-lymphocyte survival factor. A second group comprises cytokines sharing a common β-chain in the receptor predominantly represented by a group of growth factors including macrophage survival cytokines, e.g. granulocyte macrophage colony-stimulating factor (GM-CSF). The most prominent member in the third group of cytokines is IL-6, which mediates a wide variety of inflammatory

and metabolic effects through its (membrane or soluble) receptor IL-6R and common GP130 coreceptor unit, shared with other members of this cytokine family.

Type II family of receptors are structurally similar to the type I family, with the exception of lacking a specific amino acid motif in the extracellular domain. This family of receptors bind a large superfamily of interferons (IFN), including all α and β members, interferon gamma, and a family of anti-inflammatory cytokines, such as IL-10. To make matters more complex both type I and II cytokine receptors predominantly engage Janus kinases (JAKs) and signal transducers and activators of transcription (STATs) intracellular pathways, rendering this a very arbitrary separation, especially when one considers distinct functional roles for each individual cytokine. For example, IL-6 is also termed interferon β2 (IFNβ2) for its structural similarity to IFN family of cytokines although IL-6 receptor (IL-6R) requires GP130 subunit for signalling and has no relation to family of IFN receptors. In general therefore, one should confer cytokine identity and impact on its core functional roles rather than structure or receptor specificity.

One of the largest superfamilies of cytokines is characterized by its most explored pro-inflammatory member—tumour necrosis alpha (TNFα). Other archetypal members of TNF family include receptor activator of nuclear factor kappa-B ligand (RANKL)—an essential mediator of osteoclastogenesis involved in formation of bone erosions, CD40 ligand (CD40L)—a costimulatory molecule, which mediates activation of T and B cells and the pro-apoptotic molecule FasL (CD95). Most TNF receptors are membrane bound trimeric structures, that recruit intracellular adaptor proteins such as TRAF, TRADD, RIP, and FADD to elicit signal leading to the activation of the nuclear factor kappa B (NFκB) complex, that is in turn capable of modulating broad gene expression. Some of the 27 members of TNF receptor family can be expressed in soluble form or cleaved off the membrane surface to form soluble receptors; this, in turn can have functional implications for ligating cytokine (discussed next).

Finally, one of the most diverse family of receptors are characterized by the presence of immunoglobulin binding domains—Ig-type receptors, which predominantly bind antibodies (immunoglobulins), adhesion molecules, pattern-recognition ligands, and some cytokines such as the IL-1 family; often termed 'alarmins' for their high potency in recognition and activation of early immune

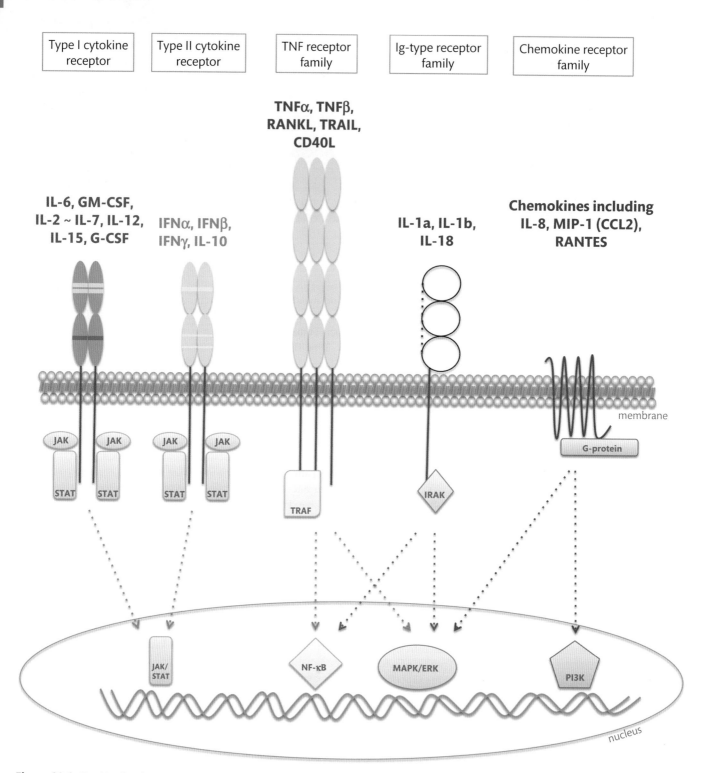

Figure 10.1 Cytokine families, receptors, and major signalling pathways.

responses. Ig-type receptors engage IRAK/MAPK/ERC to mediate downstream signalling.

Unfortunately, neither the numeric order of cytokines, nor the structural nomenclature of the receptor families, reflect individual functions of particular cytokine on cells and tissues. In contrast, a final group of immune mediators that form part of the wider cytokine family are termed chemokines that are concisely defined by their structural similarity and their function, which is to guide immune cells to the site of inflammation and control influx and efflux of leucocytes. Chemokines are crucial in maintaining homeostasis during quiescence, as well as activating and perpetuating inflammatory responses after tissue trauma/damage/insult or in the context of chronic inflammatory disease. Definitive nomenclature of chemokines and their receptors reflects the three-dimensional structure and number of C-C bridges they form. Thus, four groups are identified, including CXC, CC, CX3C, and XC chemokines. It is worth noting that some chemokines are also named as cytokines, such as IL-8 that is also known as CXCL8, an essential mediator of early inflammatory response and pain. Chemokines signal through G-protein coupled receptors and have high degree of promiscuity between receptors, ensuring translatability of message across different tissues. Intracellular signal is then translated through phosphoinositide 3-kinase (PI3K), which has been linked to the pathogenesis of RA.[1] This is also illustrated in **Figure 10.1**.

Cytokines are essential mediators of the defining features of RA as evidenced by preclinical and clinical datasets, as well as clinical trials' results. The role of cytokines in RA ranges from disturbance of homeostasis in the preclinical period, promoting the early onset of clinical synovitis through to the extension of inflammation into a chronic state and thus the development of variety of clinical and subclinical features, such as synovitis, bone erosions, but also cardiovascular risk, metabolic changes, and depression.

Relatively recently conducted genome wide studies (GWAS) in RA have implicated multiple cytokines, such as the TNF superfamily, *CTLA4* (cytotoxic T-lymphocyte antigen 4), IL-6, IL-1, IL-10, and IL-18 further anchoring the role of cytokines at the pathogenetic level. For instance, RA-associated TNF promoter polymorphisms can potentiate its expression, while IL-6 receptor polymorphism was implicated in the intensity of IL-6 signalling in RA.[2,3]

Investigating cytokine biology

Insight into the complexity of multifaceted cytokine functions required several decades of diligent research combining animal studies with *in vitro* data and extensive translational and clinical work to evaluate the full effect of cytokines on disease pathogenesis and, most importantly, once inhibited, upon patient outcomes. Initial functional studies involve recognition of the cellular source of the cytokine, definition of the stimuli regulating cytokine expression, characterization of receptor distribution, and assessment of cellular and tissue functions mediated thereafter. These studies call upon the entire range of molecular and cellular immunology and have been reviewed elsewhere.[4,5] Experimental *in vivo* models utilize neutralizing cytokine-specific antibodies or soluble receptors, modified to ensure potency and longevity in murine systems. Such agents are usually tested in so-called disease models (e.g. collagen-induced arthritis, KRN arthritis). Though helpful in defining the place of cytokines in complex systems these models do not faithfully represent true disease pathogenesis and outcomes should be interpreted with caution. A parallel animal model-based approach involves genetically modified knock-out or knock-in technology rendering cytokine or receptor deficient through embryonic stem cell manipulation or transgenic technology, enabling tissue- or cell-specific overexpression or deficiency of a particular molecule to gain more specific insight. In cases where cytokine dysfunction is lethal in the early embryonic stages, exemplified by non-viable knock-out of GP130 subunit of IL-6 receptor, conditional gene-targeting approaches can be used. This typically involves Cre recombinase, which is capable of cleaving a part of the gene upon specific stimuli, administered in the adulthood, thus circumventing embryonic lethality. *In vivo* and *in vitro* studies are now extensively aided by the discovery of CRISPR technology allowing gene editing in a simpler, yet very specific and precise manner with high efficiency (reviewed

in [6]). This technology is also being considered for therapeutic use in some genetic disorders in humans.

Translation from animal models to human biology involves *in vitro* manipulation of patient derived samples to investigate similarities and discrepancies between mouse and human pathology. Models of synovial tissue and skin explants, cell suspensions, bone, and other structural models have proved informative. At the cellular level, cascading signals, gene expression, and transcript changes, as well as cytokine expression can be evaluated by a range of methodologies (e.g. RT-PCR, microarray, RNA sequencing, immunohistochemistry, confocal analysis, western blotting). More dynamic functional assessment is supported by fluorescent cytometry, allowing identification of membrane bound cell markers alongside intracellular cytokine expression and signalling molecules. More recently, studies have evolved to capture changes in cytokine networks, by the virtue of multiple parallel measurements on a bigger scale, such as multiplex enzyme-linked immunosorbent assay (ELISA) methods or Mass Cytometry—CyTOF (reviewed in [7]). Despite an ever-expanding repertoire of scientific methodologies, there remain considerable difficulties in translating murine data into RA pathogenesis in the clinic. Thus, an integrative approach including clinical and real-life data is required to truly understand the human biology behind chronic inflammation. Therapeutic advances and single cytokine targeting modalities have enormously contributed to the understanding of function but also to discover unpredicted or previously unknown effects of certain cytokines, such as the potentially beneficial effects of anti-TNFα and anti-IL-6R treatments on cardiovascular outcomes. In this sense cytokine biology exemplifies 'bench to bedside to bench' research. Methods of cytokine biology exploration are depicted in **Figure 10.2**.

Cytokines in pre-rheumatoid arthritis

Cytokines serve to integrate various phases of the disease, with different members more prominent in early disease or transition to chronicity. The preclinical stage of RA is categorized by development of autoantibodies such as anticitrullinated protein antibody (ACPA) or rheumatoid factor (RF) and subsequent onset of arthralgia without clinical synovitis. These can precede the disease by decades.[8] Studies of synovium in preclinical serum positive individuals show relatively normal appearances until the detectable onset of the clinical symptoms.[9] On the contrary, elevated serum and plasma cytokine and chemokine concentrations can be detected some time before the full onset of local synovitis, and implicate a broad spectrum of inflammatory moieties (e.g. TNFα, IL-6, Il-1) and growth factors (GM-CSF and C-CSF).[10] One of the direct effects of IL-6 is to stimulate expression of acute phase proteins from hepatocytes and Kupffer cells, thus increasing levels of C-reactive protein (CRP) are later used for diagnostic purpose (reviewed in [4]) but may also rise prior to diagnostic classification. Interestingly, prominent changes were noticed in the potent chemokine CCL2, also known as monocyte chemoattractant protein 1 (MCP1).[11] In general, the presence of elevated serum cytokines is associated with imminent onset of the clinical features of RA in susceptible individuals and could symbolize a period of transition from generalized inflammation to local synovitis.[12]

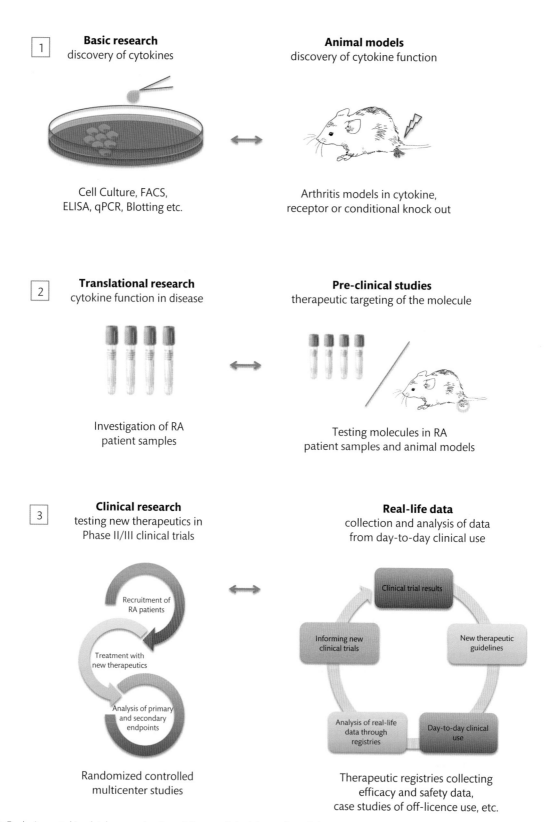

1 **Basic research**
discovery of cytokines

Cell Culture, FACS,
ELISA, qPCR, Blotting etc.

Animal models
discovery of cytokine function

Arthritis models in cytokine,
receptor or conditional knock out

2 **Translational research**
cytokine function in disease

Investigation of RA
patient samples

Pre-clinical studies
therapeutic targeting of the molecule

Testing molecules in RA
patient samples and animal models

3 **Clinical research**
testing new therapeutics in
Phase II/III clinical trials

Recruitment of
RA patients

Treatment with
new therapeutics

Analysis of primary
and secondary
endpoints

Randomized controlled
multicenter studies

Real-life data
collection and analysis of data
from day-to-day clinical use

Clinical trial results

New therapeutic
guidelines

Informing new
clinical trials

Day-to-day clinical
use

Analysis of real-life
data through
registries

Therapeutic registries collecting
efficacy and safety data,
case studies of off-licence use, etc.

Figure 10.2 Exploring cytokine biology—animal models—preclinical data—clinical data.

One such cytokine, IL-23 is implicated in direct modification of glycoprotein structure of heavy chain in Th17 cell receptor through glycosylation.[13] This 'small' conformation change is found to have significant impact on capacity for autoreactivity and expression of pro-inflammatory cytokines TNF, IL-6, and CXCL1. Formation of such autoreactive T cells then aids maturation of B cells through IL-21 and IL-22, further facilitating expression of autoantibodies and onset of clinical disease. In animal models, presence of IL-23 is critical for initiation of the disease in collagen-induced arthritis (CIA) model, but had no effect on serum transfer model where autoantibodies are already formed, confirming very early involvement of this cytokine in disease pathogenesis.[13]

Mechanisms underpinning transition to synovial inflammation and joint involvement in RA remain largely elusive (see Chapter 8), however recent studies support a role for resident articular cells during the initiation stage. Direct binding of ACPA antibodies to osteoclast cells induces the release of the chemokine IL-8 (CXCL8) that possesses potent leukocyte recruiting properties, especially neutrophils.[14] The wider role of cytokines in promoting this transition however remains largely unknown.

Cytokines and established synovitis

Through the years, our understanding of RA pathogenesis and with it the definition of the main pathogenic cells driving it has continued to evolve. Discovery of autoantibodies as a central phenomenon of seropositive RA placed the focus predominantly on B cells. However, with the onset of GWAS studies describing a substantial genetic association with major histocompatibility complex (MHC) class II molecules, focus shifted to the role of T cells, with the 'shared epitope' concept sitting central to their pathogenesis in RA (refer to Chapter 5). These pathogenetic theories share one overarching principle with cytokine biology at the heart of chronic synovial inflammation.

TNF and IL-6 are the cytokines most closely associated with chronic synovitis. Indeed, murine to human translation of cytokine targeting is clearly demonstrated in the success of TNFα and IL-6 targeting therapies.[15] TNF exhibits a persuasive in vitro profile including leukocyte activation, adhesion, migration, and regulation of endothelial function as well as angiogenesis. Other effects include direct stimulation of nociception through dorsal root ganglia and bone turnover through its family member—RANKL. In murine models, inhibition of TNF ameliorated murine CIA reducing both inflammation and articular damage. Reciprocally, anti-TNF treatment leads to depletion of the total number of synovial inflammatory cells, reduces local cytokine levels and inhibits overall recruitment to the synovium, thus confirming its dominant hierarchical position in RA.[16] Overarching effects of anti-TNF treatment extend to include rapid normalization of systemic inflammatory features such as anaemia and high platelet count, extending further to improvement in fatigue, depression, metabolism and insulin resistance in treated patients over time.[17,18] At the cellular level, anti-TNF treatment leads to abolished numbers of synovial T cells, B cells, and inflammatory macrophages, while activating and promoting proliferation of regulatory T_{REG} cells.[19] This effect appeared specific to agents targeting cytokine and binding both membrane and soluble forms, rather than to etanercept, a TNF receptor fusion protein which captures only soluble TNF. This phenomenon distinguishes the anti-inflammatory role of anti-TNF treatment mediated by blocking of TNFR1 from its secondary regulatory effect facilitated by the activation of TNFR2 on the surface of T_{reg} regulatory cells.[20] Indeed, it is accepted that adalimumab, for example, has a superior efficacy compared to etanercept in a range of autoimmune conditions.[21]

Crucial to the success of administration of anti-TNF treatment is the rapid reduction in circulating IL-6 levels, a cytokine that shares some of the synovial pro-inflammatory burden with TNF. IL-6 was initially discovered for its role in promoting T-cell (TH17)

and B-cell differentiation, before myeloid and synovial fibroblast resident cells were recognized as major producers of the cytokine in RA. In CIA murine models, deficiency of IL-6 led to markedly reduced intensity of arthritis and impaired immune responses to viral, bacterial, or parasitic infections, in a similar way to that of TNF.[22] Closer investigations revealed additional systemic features of IL-6 pathway deficiency, involving impaired wound healing, acute phase response, haematopoiesis, and glucose metabolism. In classical or cis signalling, IL-6 directly activates membrane bound IL-6R-GP130 complex and is therefore limited to the cells actively expressing IL-6R specific subunit of the receptor, such as leukocytes, megakaryocytes, and hepatocytes. Thus, classical IL-6 signalling is responsible for haematopoiesis, induction of acute systemic immune response including hyperthermia, activation of effector T cells, proliferation of B cells, and survival of antibody producing plasma cells. In contrast, broader effects of IL-6 are mediated by indirect or trans-signalling pathway where cytokine and soluble IL-6R portion form a complex capable of activating broadly expressed membrane bound GP130 subunit. IL-6 trans-signalling is implicated in perpetuating chronic inflammation by the recruitment of leucocytes and early involvement of stromal resident cells, like fibroblast-like synoviocytes (FLS), while also regulating glucose metabolism and fatigue. As with TNF, subsequent clinical trials confirmed particularly significant benefit from IL-6 pathway targeting in synovitis and elucidated additional impact on comorbid states that really defined the central role for this cytokine on pathogenesis. Head-to-head comparison of TNF and IL-6R blockade demonstrated subtle yet distinct reciprocal signatures, involving CXC13 chemokine expression and others.[23] Certainly, IL-6 pathway inhibition seems to have more profound effects on lipid metabolism than TNF, discussed later in this chapter. Summary of shared and distinct function of TNF and IL-6 are summarized in **Figure 10.3**

Complexity of synovial inflammation in active RA allows for the role of other cytokines alongside TNF and IL-6. Extensive investigation of IL-1 in animal models of arthritis held substantial promise for that cytokine as mice lacking IL-1 receptor antagonist (IL-1Ra) develop spontaneous arthritis.[24] Despite providing detailed mechanistic insights, anti-IL-1 therapies failed to translate to meaningful clinical outcomes in RA, this likely reflecting the lack of a pivotal regulatory role in human disease. IL-1 and TNF synergistically mediate many effector pathways in chronic synovitis, such as activation of prostanoid synthesis, resident chondrocytes and FLS cells,[25] but TNF occupies a critical regulatory role to which IL-1 is subservient in the context of RA. Note that the opposite is the case in inflammasome driven disorders such as gout in which IL-1 inhibition is dominant. Similarly, other promising murine and in vitro models suggesting effector roles for IL-17, B-cell activating factor (BAFF), IL-20, and IL-21 failed to deliver therapeutic benefit in established disease, though some proved successful targets in other diseases such as psoriatic arthritis that have distinct pathogenesis to RA.

Myeloid lineage and polymorphonuclear cells and cytokines in RA

The existence of distinct synovial pathotypes, including myeloid, lymphoid, or stromal rich synovial tissue types has rendered consideration of each cellular compartment ever more important.[23] Circulating monocytes, macrophages (resident as well as infiltrating populations), dendritic cells, mast cells, and neutrophils comprise

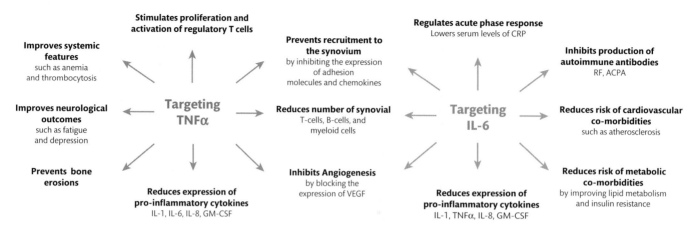

Figure 10.3 Comparative biology of TNFa and IL-6.

the majority of myeloid compartment in the synovium. Their effector functions and regulating cytokines are clearly linked to disease manifestations. More recently an emerging role for additional innate lymphoid cell lineages in tissue destruction has been characterized.[18]

In RA, monocytes and macrophages are considered major cellular drivers of cytokine production and inflammation, while inflammatory dendritic cells support activation of adaptive immune response. Macrophages serve as the principle source of TNF and IL-6 cytokines whose legion effects on disease are described earlier. In humans, definitive subpopulations of migrating monocytes include classical or 'inflammatory' cells defined by expression of surface markers CD14highCD16neg, intermediate CD14highCD16low, and non-classical CD14lowCD16high cells predominately responsible for patrolling endothelial integrity. These broad definitions are based on the investigations of equivalent murine populations expressing high or low levels of Ly6C marker.[26] Migration of myeloid cells from blood to lymph nodes or to sites of inflammation such as synovium is facilitated by chemokines.

In active diseased, circulating monocytes are primarily recruited by broadly expressed chemokine CCL2 (MCP1). Upon tissue entry, invading monocytes are guided by surrounding cytokines and growth factors to become differentiated macrophages. Exposure to activating cocktail of IL-1, IL-12, IL-23, CXCL9, CXCL10, and M-CSF or GM-CSF growth factors, as well as the contact with 'danger' signal molecules guides differentiation towards classical or inflammatory M1 type macrophages. In contrast, exposure to an anti-inflammatory cytokine IL-10 and CCL17/CCL22 chemokines predisposes towards M2 regulatory phenotype. It is now clear that synovial tissue comprises a spectrum of different macrophages with individual transcription profiles, however, abundance of TNF and IL6 expression with relative lack of IL-10 supports dominance of M1 or inflammatory cells. In synovitis, influx of large numbers of monocyte-derived macrophages is overwhelming to the underlying population of joint resident cells. Tissue resident macrophages characterized in healthy donors or during remission demonstrate quiescent cells abundant in IL-10, TGFb, and resolvins. Homeostatic resident macrophages seem unaffected by TNF targeting treatments and may be aiding resolution of inflammation through a rich repertoire of scavenging receptors.[27]

Seeking to restore balance between inflammatory and regulatory macrophage populations, attention has turned to investigation of M-CSF and GM-CSF growth factors, which play a significant role in maturation and sustenance of synovial macrophages alongside cytokines. M-CSF is a main homeostatic lineage regulator and driver of differentiation; its consistent expression is believed to regulate general macrophage numbers. In comparison, GM-CSF is produced primarily upon infectious or toxic challenge demonstrated by murine knock-out studies, in which GM-CSF dysfunction does not curtail the development of myeloid cells, but rather impairs the immune response, rendering GM-CSF more relevant in provoked immunity. The rationale for therapeutic targeting of this molecule was additionally supported by clinical finding that administration of GM-CSF to correct neutropenia in patients with RA resulted in severe disease flare.[28,29] Indeed, while blockade of M-CSF was not successful thus far in RA clinical trials, GM-CSF Receptor α targeting proved efficacious, exemplified in the use of mavrilimumab.[30]

Lastly, as one of the most abundant populations, neutrophils comprise a majority during early influx of cells in to the acutely synovitic joint. Synovial compartment neutrophils are capable of prolonged longevity and extensive expression of cytokines (TNF, IL-6) and chemokines (CXCL8) thus perpetuating immune cells recruitment to the tissue. The curious propensity for neutrophils to migrate to the fluid space and rarely reside within the synovial membrane in RA is as yet poorly understood. For this reason, their hierarchical role in pathogenesis has been debated; however, they remain a significant source of cytokine and chemokine release and via direct effects on the cartilage surface likely play a role at least in this context.

Adaptive immune cells and cytokines in RA

The role of adaptive immunity is substantial in seropositive RA defined by the presence of autoantibodies against modified self-proteins, predominantly anti-citrullinated ACPA antibodies and RF comprising a central hallmark of disease pathogenesis, in turn implicating autoreactive B cells that presumably receive T-cell help. Normal differentiation of B cells involves lengthy maturation processes in bone marrow and spleen that provides for receptor deletion and editing, rendering autoreactive clones anergic or depleted during development. Induction of tolerance requires multiple check points for the B-cell receptor but also relies on serum BAFF (B-cell activating factor, also known as B lymphocyte stimulator, BlyS) and APRIL (a proliferation-inducing ligand) for survival. Induction of central and peripheral tolerance is defective in RA, leading to accumulation of autoreactive mature naïve B cells. Links between PTPN22 poly-morphism and autoreactive B cells have been established, indicating that genetic or epigenetic changes in the bone marrow progenitors could contribute. Systemic and local support for defective B cells is evident from increased levels of BAFF, APRIL, and IL-6 in the serum and, particularly, in RA synovium. Toll-like receptor stimulation of myeloid cells, but also of resident synovial fibroblasts drive BAFF release in RA (reviewed in [5]). Unfortunately, combination targeting BAFF and April, as well as single inhibition of these factors did not show any additional benefit in the treatment of RA over the suppression of B-cell effector functions through targeting of surface CD20 molecules with rituximab. Sustained low disease activity is associated with reduced B-cell repopulation and expression of CXCL13 and CCL19 chemokines, while novel data on cellular categorization or synovium in remission is emerging (reviewed in [15]).

Activated B cells contribute to chronic inflammation beyond production of autoreactive antibodies. They are an important source of IL-6, IL-12, IL-23, and TNF in chronicity, as well as a source of RANKL supporting osteoclastogenesis in arthritic joints. Additionally, IL-6 expressing B cells were identified as an additional source supporting cross talk and maturation of naïve or follicular T cells as a critical link coordinating T-cell and B-cell activity. Profound effects on adaptive immunity were confirmed by the lack of a humoral response in IL-6−/− mice immunized with T-cell-dependant antigens.[31]

Although crucial in its own right, IL-6 relies on the surrounding milieu of cytokines to guide differentiation of naïve CD4+ T cells towards a pro-inflammatory Th17 phenotype or towards a regulatory T reg pathway. Several data support a role for the Th17 axis in RA, with the archetypal pro-inflammatory cytokine IL-17A exhibiting many effector functions, interacting and synergizing with those of TNFα and IL-6. IL-17A potentiates secretion of cytokines, such as IL-1, TNFα, IL-6, GM-CSF and potent chemokines CXCL8 (IL-8), CCL2, and CCL3, while contributing to the change of tissue architecture through remodelling of angiogenesis, and osteoclast maturation and activation. In the synovial cytokine milieu, IL-17A supports survival and activation of FLS and also of adaptive immune cells in de-novo formed 'ectopic' germinal centres. Although IL-17A levels correlate with disease activity and other clinical parameters, redundancy with other cytokines may explain the disappointing lack of therapeutic effect in RA upon IL-17 inhibition. It is possible that the role of Th17 cells is more prominent in preclinical stages of disease, such as in the initiation of autoreactive antibodies through effects of IL-23.[5,13]

Other cytokines associated with adaptive immune responses in RA include a family sharing common-γ-signalling, comprising IL-21, IL-7, and IL-15 with downstream impact on follicular T-helper cells, Th17s, and B cells, as well as dendritic cells, NK cells, and osteoclasts. Even though IL-21 is indispensable in maturation of B cells and development of plasma cells, targeting approaches in RA proved disappointing thus far. IL-7 and particularly IL-15 are also implicated in the activation and survival of a range of leukocyte subsets in RA synovium, and especially exert clear roles in driving the cross talk between macrophages and T cells (reviewed in [18,32]). The benefits ensuing from JAK3 inhibition have raised again their potential pathogenetic role.

Lastly, one of the largest cytokine groups involved in viral T-cell responses, the superfamily of type I interferons (IFNs) are easily detected and functionally active in RA. With their prime evolved function to achieve effective viral defence, members of this cytokine family have capacity to modulate the activation of many leucocyte subsets in both pro- and anti-inflammatory manner, as a substantial proportion of IFNs are primarily anti-inflammatory. The low hierarchical positioning of IFNs has rendered all therapeutic approaches either by utilizing anti-inflammatory properties or antibody mediated blockade of pro-inflammatory IFNs, inapplicable to RA clinical practice.[33] Despite this, numerous studies identify transcriptional signatures consistent with activation of interferon response elements confirming the prominent biologic activity of this superfamily of cytokines and offering new frontiers in biomarker discovery. Notably the recently introduced Jakinib drug family will directly effect IFN, GM-CSF and IL-6 pathways by virtue of inhibition of downstream intracellular JAK/STAT signalling shared among these cytokines and likely will elicit further insight into the importance or additional effect of IFN and GM-CSF blockade in comparison to mono therapeutic IL-6 pathway targeting.

Stromal cells and cytokines

Viewing stromal tissue as an inert backdrop for inflammation, orchestrated predominantly by the immune system is now a historical footnote, with a clear role for FLS cells as central players driving disease resistance now generally accepted.[34] RA FLS have a more aggressive phenotype with prolonged longevity and resistance to apoptosis, most likely sustained by epigenetic changes. This transformation includes loss of anchorage independence and loss of contact inhibition, ongoing proliferation, and potentially intrajoint trafficking, thus spreading the disease.[35] Anti-TNF treatment promotes apoptosis of activated FLSs, profoundly affecting stromal compartment, while targeting of IL-6 prevents further expression of matrix metalloproteinases 1 and 3 (matrix metalloproteinase (MMP)-1 and -3). Inhibition of these cytokines thoroughly affects expression of RANKL and curtails formation of bone erosions. Clear participation in inflammatory processes is predominantly mediated by expression of large quantities of cytokines (IL-6, IL-1), chemokines and growth factors (platelet-derived, fibroblast, and vascular endothelial growth factors, PDGF, FGF, and VEGF, respectively) released by FLS. Through the expression of tissue and angiogenic factors, FLS cells drive angiogenesis, matrix deposition, and tissue remodelling, while recruiting and maintaining leucocyte influx through expression of type I IFNs and CXCL12.[5]

Since this central role of FLS emerged, investigation of pathways that would allow targeting of a stromal compartment in RA has been a priority. Data focusing on the cancer-like properties of FLS cells identified cell-cell adhesion protein Cadherin-11 as a molecule specific to RA synovium and responsible for majority of aggressive effector functions of synoviocytes. Intriguingly, targeting Cadherin-11 in murine models ameliorates onset of arthritis with further data awaited from ongoing phase II clinical trials.[36]

Current successful cytokine therapies—anti-TNF and anti-IL6—share an overarching ability to affect each of the relevant disease compartments—myeloid, lymphoid, and stromal in a profound manner. This might provide insight as to why targeting of more cell specific cytokines, such as IL-17, failed relatively in RA, but also sustains the idea of existence of distinct disease pathotypes predominantly involving each of the above compartments.[23] Such separation could also be a feature of natural disease development exemplified by the treatment 'window of opportunity' before synovial inflammatory autonomy has fully formed.

Cytokines and articular structure

Continuous exposure of bone and cartilage to the inflammatory microenvironment of synovial tissue is a major driver of progressive disability in RA. Bone loss starts very early, and can sometimes precede clinically evident disease in seropositive individuals[37] manifest either by local bone oedema and early erosion development but also in the presence of systemic osteoporosis. In early stages, these changes may be driven by activation of bone resorbing osteoclasts upon binding of autoantibodies recognizing citrullinated vimentin and sustained by a subsequently emerging cytokine milieu. What drives pathologic bone processes in early stages of seronegative disease remains largely unknown.

It is well established *in vitro* in murine and human studies that TNF, IL-1, and IL-6 can independently and cooperatively drive formation of osteoclasts, and thus increase bone resorption directly or more likely through induction of, and cooperation with RANKL activity. This effect is sustained further by presence of M-CSF growth factor and IL-17. Multiple murine models, and more recently clinical trials have confirmed an extensive role of cytokines in promoting imbalance between osteoblasts in favour of osteoclastogenesis *in vivo*. Therapeutic targeting of IL-1 and RANKL both have protective effects on bone erosions but fail to control synovial inflammation. In turn, targeting cytokines, such as TNF and IL-6 exhibit significant bone protection effects in patients either by controlling the underlying inflammatory process or perhaps even by a direct 'inflammation independent' effect on osteoclastogenesis. Thus, patients may achieve protection from erosion in clinical trials even if judged to be clinical non-responders. Bone protection has been successful also in therapies that block intrinsic activator pathways of osteoclasts through direct blockade of RANKL or by wider inhibition of inflammatory processes, including JAK inhibitors, B-cell depletors, or through disabling osteoclast (OC) maturation processes guided by autoantibodies through costimulatory molecules, targeted by abatacept. Beneficial effects on bone turnover are expected from GM-CSF targeting, which is known to facilitate fusion of mononuclear cells and de-novo formation of osteoclasts in synovium. Recently emerging roles of new coregulators of osteoclast and osteoblast homeostasis, such as sclerostin and Dickkopf-1 (DKK) molecules suggest an intriguing possibility of bone healing, that is not yet feasible with current treatment options (Figure 10.4).[5]

Cartilage destruction is considered to arise mainly through the elaboration of MMPs from FLS, macrophages, and potentially surface interfacing neutrophils. These matrix remodelling enzymes arise as a result of cytokine stimulation—IL-1, TNF, IL-6 and IL-17 are particularly potent at inducing MMP release disproportionate to TIMP release, and thus promote chondrocyte catabolism, failed matrix synthesis, and cartilage failure over time. Hence the cartilage pannus junction described originally in pathologic descriptions of RA is likely a cytokine driven phenomenon.

Cytokines and the systemic features of RA

RA is linked with substantial comorbidities and increasingly these are a focus for therapeutic intervention. The high inflammatory burden of RA is associated with increased risk of cardiovascular and metabolic syndrome, cognitive, and neurological disorders including psychiatric disease, osteoporosis, and increased cancer rates. The role of cytokines mediating comorbidities in arthritis is reviewed next.

Cardiovascular comorbidities and metabolic syndrome

Untreated RA and perpetually raised inflammatory markers are associated with 50% increased mortality risk, predominantly due to adverse outcomes of cardiovascular disease. Raised cholesterol, high serum low-density lipoprotein (LDL-C) and low serum high-density lipoprotein (HDL-C) levels are established biomarkers for increased cardiovascular risk. Widely used blockade of cholesterol synthesis by statins thus effectively lowers LDL-C and risk of cardiovascular disease. Paradoxically, acute and chronic inflammation is associated with reduced levels of both LDL-C and HDL-C circulating lipids and increased risk of adverse cardiovascular events. This so-called 'lipid paradox' is also present in individuals with active RA (reviewed in [38]). It is possible that reduction in cholesterol and LDL-C levels precede the disease onset for up to 5 years and could be a feature of preclinical syndrome.[39]

Many risk factors including smoking, poor socioeconomic conditions, genetic predisposition, a sedentary and activity limited lifestyle, or therapeutics such as corticosteroids can be involved in elevating risk of cardiovascular comorbidity in RA. Regardless of causation, there is a strong body of evidence suggesting that vascular risk is driven at least in part by inflammatory cytokines. In contrast to murine models, administration of TNF, IL-6, or even bacterial wall lipopolysaccharide to otherwise healthy individuals demonstrates decrease in serum levels of cholesterol, LDL-C, and HDL-C lipids.[40] At the cellular level, both TNF and IL-6 promote upregulation of scavenger receptors on the surface of macrophages to facilitate uptake of oxidized LDL-C and thus promote formation of foam cells, a common feature of atherosclerotic plaques.[41]

Additionally, both cytokines increase expression of LDL-receptor and lower levels of apoB lipid carrier to increasing availability in hepatocytes. Direct evaluation of lipid profiles in RA patients with active and remising disease identified abnormally elevated LDL catabolism as primary cause for lower LDL-C levels.[42] Further exploration has particularly linked IL-6 to a hypercatabolic state, increased expression of CRP inflammatory marker and inverse correlation with serum HDL-C levels, suggesting direct effect on hepatocytes, as IL-6R expressing cells. Accordingly, abnormal lipid signatures are normalized following therapeutic IL-6 blockade regardless of any clinical response.[42] Indeed, naturally occurring single nucleotide polymorphism diminishing function of IL-6R reduces the overall risk of cardiovascular disease in carriers in the general population.[43] Inhibition of IL-6 causes more substantial changes in serum lipid levels in a head-to-head comparison study with TNF blockade.[44] Similarly the effects of IL-6 inhibition are greater than that of methotrexate and other disease-modifying antirheumatic drugs (DMARDs). Nonetheless, RA patients treated with anti-TNF treatment exhibit an average of 7% increase in HDL levels followed by 10% gradual increase in total cholesterol within 6 months of treatment (reviewed in (38)). As one would expect, inhibition of JAK signalling with new therapeutics, such as tofacitinib and baricitinib, results in similar elevation of HDL-C and total cholesterol levels. As the case with IL-6 targeting pathway, effect of Jakinibs could not be explained only by regulation of inflammation and predicts a direct effect of the JAK pathway on lipid metabolism.

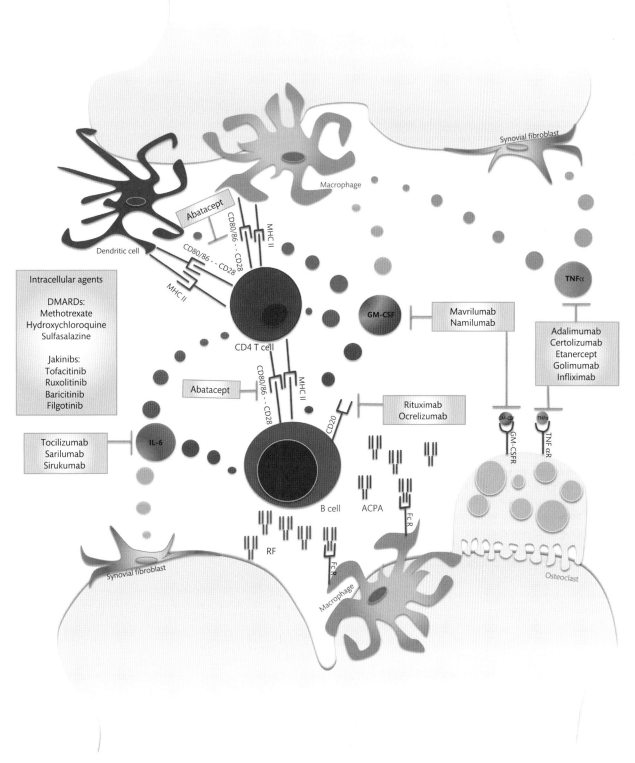

Figure 10.4 Major RA cytokines and available or tested treatments against them.

Reduction in serum lipid levels in acute systemic inflammation seen in sepsis and in chronicity, such as the case with RA, has been linked to increased mortality and higher rate of adverse events. Consequently, treatment of inflammation and correction of serum levels are expected to have beneficial long-term outcomes for patients with RA. However, causative studies investigating pathogenesis and large cohort clinical datasets are required to assess rate of prevention of chronic heart disease and adverse outcomes for RA patients.

Cognitive and neurologic comorbidities

Changes of central nervous system function in RA can vary from depressive symptoms through fatigue and cognitive dysfunction to sensitization to pain. While different underlying mechanisms can be at play, many of these features are linked to the presence of elevated levels of cytokines.

In ACPA positive disease, activation of osteoclasts drives expression of IL-8 capable of attracting leucocytes to synovial inflammation and binding to CXCR-1 and 2 chemokine receptors present on sensory neurons to induce pain. In murine models, injection of CXCL-1 causes arthralgia similar to that observed in ACPA+ mice (reviewed in [45]). These investigations would suggest a substantial role of IL-8-related pathways in preclinical arthralgia and early synovitis.

Animal models have highlighted TNF, IL-6, and IL-1β as key mediators between brain and peripheral disease. Systemic inflammation initiated by lipopolysaccharide (LPS) or by each of the cytokines separately, causes extensive behavioural changes including social withdrawal, fatigue, and cognitive dysfunction. Similarly, administration of exogenous cytokines to healthy individuals evokes depressive mood, fatigue, and sickness behaviour.[46] Similar phenomena emerged upon the treatment of people with hepatitis with type I interferons. These investigations provide some insight into the ways whereby anti-TNF and IL-6 treatments in patients with RA lead to rapid improvement in quality of life and sense of well-being even before changes in joint inflammation are noticeable. This is mediated by direct impact on serotonin transporter availability in the brain, as measured by single-photon emission computed tomography (SPECT) imaging in patients suffering from depression and RA.[47] The extent of the effect of TNF on higher neuronal functions was exemplified by clinical improvement in patients with treatment-resistant depression.[48] Functional MRI studies demonstrated additional immediate benefit of anti-TNF treatment in its capacity to dampen response to pain by direct effect on TNF and IL-1β receptors, found on neuronal and glial cells in the brain.[49] Ultimately, inhibition of underlying inflammatory pathways, including NFκB, prostaglandin, and nitric oxide synthesis ultimately leads to normalization of serotonin levels and improvement in mental and emotional functions. In comparison, IL-6R is not expressed in neuronal tissue directly, yet its coreceptor GP130 is highly present and allows unhampered access to IL-6 stimulation, with the studies investigating effect of IL-6 treatment on depressive moods, fatigue, and pain ongoing. A proportion of the debilitating effects of RA are likely due to the effects cytokines like TNF have on the brain and mood of affected patients and yet understanding of subserving pathways and promising treatments is just emerging. This is an area that requires extensive work in the near future in order to improve one of the most important outcomes for RA patients (reviewed in [50]).

Summary

Cytokines comprise a large family of mediators with defining regulatory functions at every stage of inflammation in RA. Comprehensive pathogenesis of RA clearly identifies TNF and IL-6 as dominant moieties in disease cytokine hierarchy. Treatment success in targeting these cytokines is attributed to wide spectrum of effects involving myeloid, lymphoid, and stromal compartments of disease, as well as substantial effects on comorbid states. A long and thorny path of investigations involving other cytokine families have elucidated essential specific effects, such as IL-1 and RANKL impact on osteoclastogenesis and formation of bone erosions, IL-17/IL-23 axes

effect on early evolvement of autoreactive antibodies, and the future potential of IFN signatures in search for disease biomarkers. Exploration of cytokine biology in RA has incredibly enriched our understanding of disease pathogenesis and continues to open possibilities for improving patient outcomes.

REFERENCES

1. Bartok B, Hammaker D, Firestein GS. Phosphoinositide 3-kinase δ regulates migration and invasion of synoviocytes in rheumatoid arthritis. *J Immunol* 2014;*192*(5):2063–70.
2. Fonseca JE, Cavaleiro J, Teles J, et al. Contribution for new genetic markers of rheumatoid arthritis activity and severity: sequencing of the tumor necrosis factor-alpha gene promoter. *Arthritis Res Ther* 2007;*9*(2):R37.
3. Ferreira RC, Freitag DF, Cutler AJ, et al. Functional IL6R 358Ala allele impairs classical IL-6 receptor signaling and influences risk of diverse inflammatory diseases. Gibson G, editor. *PLoS Genet* 2013;*9*(4):e1003444.
4. McInnes IB, Schett G. Cytokines in the pathogenesis of rheumatoid arthritis. *Nat Rev Immunol* 2007;*7*(6):429–42.
5. Firestein GS, McInnes IB. Immunopathogenesis of rheumatoid arthritis. *Immunity* 2017;*46*(2):183–96.
6. Lander ES. The heroes of CRISPR. *Cell* 2016;*164*(1–2):18–28.
7. Bendall SC, Nolan GP, Roederer M, Chattopadhyay PK. A deep profiler's guide to cytometry. *Trends Immunol* 2012;*33*(7):323–32.
8. Hueber W, Tomooka BH, Zhao X, et al. Proteomic analysis of secreted proteins in early rheumatoid arthritis: anti-citrulline autoreactivity is associated with up regulation of proinflammatory cytokines. *Ann Rheum Dis* 2007;*66*(6):712–19.
9. de Hair MJH, van de Sande MGH, Ramwadhdoebe TH, et al. Features of the synovium of individuals at risk of developing rheumatoid arthritis: implications for understanding preclinical rheumatoid arthritis. *Arthritis Rheumatol* 2014;*66*(3):513–22.
10. Kokkonen H, Söderström I, Rocklöv J, Hallmans G, Lejon K, Rantapää Dahlqvist S. Up-regulation of cytokines and chemokines predates the onset of rheumatoid arthritis. *Arthritis Rheum* 2010;*62*(2):383–91.
11. Rantapää-Dahlqvist S, Boman K, Tarkowski A, Hallmans G. Up regulation of monocyte chemoattractant protein-1 expression in anti-citrulline antibody and immunoglobulin M rheumatoid factor positive subjects precedes onset of inflammatory response and development of overt rheumatoid arthritis. *Ann Rheum Dis* 2006;*66*(1):121–3.
12. Deane KD, O'Donnell CI, Hueber W, et al. The number of elevated cytokines and chemokines in preclinical seropositive rheumatoid arthritis predicts time to diagnosis in an age-dependent manner. *Arthritis Rheum* 2010;*62*(11):3161–72.
13. Pfeifle R, Rothe T, Ipseiz N, et al. Regulation of autoantibody activity by the IL-23-TH17 axis determines the onset of autoimmune disease. *Nat Immunol* 2017;*18*:104–13.
14. Krishnamurthy A, Joshua V, Haj Hensvold A, et al. Identification of a novel chemokine-dependent molecular mechanism underlying rheumatoid arthritis-associated autoantibody-mediated bone loss. *Ann Rheum Dis* 2016;*75*(4):721–9.
15. McInnes IB, Schett G. Pathogenetic insights from the treatment of rheumatoid arthritis. *Lancet* 2017;*389*(10086):2328–37.
16. Williams RO, Feldmann M, Maini RN. Anti-tumor necrosis factor ameliorates joint disease in murine collagen-induced arthritis. *Proc Natl Acad Sci U S A* 1992;*89*(20):9784–8.

17. Feldmann M, Maini RN. Anti-TNF alpha therapy of rheumatoid arthritis: what have we learned? Annual Review of Immunology. *Annual Rev* 2001;*19*(1):163–96.

18. McInnes IB, Buckley CD, Isaacs JD. Cytokines in rheumatoid arthritis—shaping the immunological landscape. *Nat Rev Rheumatol* 2016;*12*(1):63–8.

19. Chen X, Oppenheim JJ. Therapy: paradoxical effects of targeting TNF signalling in the treatment of autoimmunity. *Nat Rev Rheumatol* 2016;*12*(11):625–6.

20. Nguyen DX, Ehrenstein MR. Anti-TNF drives regulatory T cell expansion by paradoxically promoting membrane TNF–TNF-RII binding in rheumatoid arthritis. *J Exp Med* 2016;*213*(7):1241–53.

21. Armuzzi A, Lionetti P, Blandizzi C, et al. anti-TNF agents as therapeutic choice in immune-mediated inflammatory diseases: focus on adalimumab. *Int J Immunopathol Pharmacol* 2014;*27*(1 Suppl):11–32.

22. Sasai M, Saeki Y, Ohshima S, et al. Delayed onset and reduced severity of collagen-induced arthritis in interleukin-6-deficient mice. *Arthritis Rheum* 1999;*42*(8):1635–43.

23. Dennis G, Holweg CT, Kummerfeld SK, et al. Synovial phenotypes in rheumatoid arthritis correlate with response to biologic therapeutics. *Arthritis Res Ther BioMed Central* 2014;*16*(2):R90.

24. Horai R, Saijo S, Tanioka H, et al. Development of chronic inflammatory arthropathy resembling rheumatoid arthritis in interleukin 1 receptor antagonist-deficient mice. *J Exp Med* 2000;*191*(2):313–20.

25. Schett G, Dayer J-M, Manger B. Interleukin-1 function and role in rheumatic disease. *Nat Rev Rheumatol* 2016;*12*(1):14–24.

26. Udalova IA, Mantovani A, Feldmann M. Macrophage heterogeneity in the context of rheumatoid arthritis. *Nat Rev Rheumatol* 2016;*12*(8):472–85.

27. Kurowska-Stolarska M, Alivernini S. Synovial tissue macrophages: friend or foe? *RMD Open* 2017;*3*(2):e000527.

28. van Nieuwenhuijze A, Koenders M, Roeleveld D, Sleeman MA, van den Berg W, Wicks IP. GM-CSF as a therapeutic target in inflammatory diseases. *Mol Immunol* 2013;*56*(4):675–82.

29. Wicks IP, Roberts AW. Targeting GM-CSF in inflammatory diseases. *Nat Rev Rheumatol* 2015;*12*(1):37–48.

30. Burmester GR, McInnes IB, Kremer J, et al. A randomised phase IIb study of mavrilimumab, a novel GM-CSF receptor alpha monoclonal antibody, in the treatment of rheumatoid arthritis. *Ann Rheum Dis* 2017;*76*(6):1020–30.

31. Barr TA, Shen P, Brown S, et al. B cell depletion therapy ameliorates autoimmune disease through ablation of IL-6-producing B cells. *J Exp Med* 2012;*209*(5):1001–10.

32. Baslund B, Tvede N, Danneskiold-Samsoe B, et al. Targeting interleukin-15 in patients with rheumatoid arthritis: a proof-of-concept study. *Arthritis Rheum* 2005;*52*(9):2686–92.

33. van Holten J. Expression of interferon in synovial tissue from patients with rheumatoid arthritis: comparison with patients with osteoarthritis and reactive arthritis. *Ann Rheum Dis* 2005;*64*(12):1780–2.

34. Buckley CD. Why does chronic inflammation persist: an unexpected role for fibroblasts. *Immunol Lett* 2011;*138*(1):12–14.

35. Lefèvre S, Knedla A, Tennie C, et al. Synovial fibroblasts spread rheumatoid arthritis to unaffected joints. *Nat Med* 2009;*15*(12):1414–20.

36. Kiener HP, Niederreiter B, Lee DM, Jimenez-Boj E, Smolen JS, Brenner MB. Cadherin 11 promotes invasive behavior of fibroblast-like synoviocytes. *Arthritis Rheum* 2009;*60*(5):1305–10.

37. Kleyer A, Finzel S, Rech J, et al. Bone loss before the clinical onset of rheumatoid arthritis in subjects with anticitrullinated protein antibodies. *Ann Rheum Dis* 2014;*73*(5):854–60.

38. Robertson J, Peters MJ, McInnes IB, Sattar N. Changes in lipid levels with inflammation and therapy in RA: a maturing paradigm. *Nat Rev Rheumatol* 2013;*9*(9):513–23.

39. Myasoedova E, Crowson CS, Kremers HM, Fitz-Gibbon PD, Therneau TM, Gabriel SE. Total cholesterol and LDL levels decrease before rheumatoid arthritis. *Ann Rheum Dis* 2010;*69*(7):1310–4.

40. Ettinger WH, Varma VK, Sorci-Thomas M, et al. Cytokines decrease apolipoprotein accumulation in medium from Hep G2 cells. *Arterioscler Thromb* 1994;*14*(1):8–13.

41. Hashizume M, Mihara M. Atherogenic effects of TNF-α and IL-6 via up-regulation of scavenger receptors. *Cytokine* 2012;*58*(3):424–30.

42. Robertson J, Porter D, Sattar N, et al. Interleukin-6 blockade raises LDL via reduced catabolism rather than via increased synthesis: a cytokine-specific mechanism for cholesterol changes in rheumatoid arthritis. *Ann Rheum Dis* 2017;*76*(11):1949–52.

43. ALLHAT Trial group. Major outcomes in moderately hypercholesterolemic, hypertensive patients randomized to pravastatin vs usual care: the Antihypertensive and Lipid-Lowering Treatment to Prevent Heart Attack Trial (ALLHAT-LLT). *JAMA* 2002;*288*(23):2998–3007.

44. Gabay C, Emery P, van Vollenhoven R, et al. Tocilizumab monotherapy versus adalimumab monotherapy for treatment of rheumatoid arthritis (ADACTA): a randomised, double-blind, controlled phase 4 trial. *Lancet* 2013;*381*(9877):1541–50.

45. Catrina AI, Svensson CI, Malmström V, Schett G, Klareskog L. Mechanisms leading from systemic autoimmunity to joint-specific disease in rheumatoid arthritis. *Nat Rev Rheumatol* 2017;*13*(2):79–86.

46. Eisenberger NI, Inagaki TK, Mashal NM, Irwin MR. Inflammation and social experience: an inflammatory challenge induces feelings of social disconnection in addition to depressed mood. *Brain Behavior and Immunity* 2010;*24*(4):558–63.

47. Cavanagh J, Paterson C, McLean J, et al. Tumour necrosis factor blockade mediates altered serotonin transporter availability in rheumatoid arthritis: a clinical, proof-of-concept study. *Ann Rheum Dis* 2010;*69*(6):1251–2.

48. Raison CL, Rutherford RE, Woolwine BJ, et al. A randomized controlled trial of the tumor necrosis factor antagonist infliximab for treatment-resistant depression. *JAMA Psychiatry* 2013;*70*(1):31.

49. Hess A, Axmann R, Rech J, et al. Blockade of TNF rapidly inhibits pain responses in the central nervous system. *Proc Natl Acad Sci* 2011;*108*(9):3731–6.

50. D'Mello C, Swain MG. Immune-to-brain communication pathways in inflammation-associated sickness and depression. *Curr Top Behav Neurosci* 2017;*31*(1):73–94.

SECTION 3
Clinical presentation

11 **Clinical features of rheumatoid arthritis** *109*
    Annette van der Helm-van Mil

12 **Pre-rheumatoid arthritis** *121*
    Karim Raza, Catherine McGrath, Laurette van Boheemen,
    and Dirkjan van Schaardenburg

13 **Non-articular manifestations of rheumatoid**
    arthritis *133*
    Katherine Macdonald, Jennifer Hannah, and James Galloway

14 **Comorbidity in rheumatoid arthritis** *145*
    Kimme Hyrich and Sarah Skeoch

11

Clinical features of rheumatoid arthritis

Annette van der Helm-van Mil

Diagnosing rheumatoid arthritis

Rheumatoid arthritis (RA) has a population prevalence of approximately 1%. It affects at least twice as many women as men and, although it can occur at any age, its peak incidence is at 50 years of age. It is a systemic disease but joint inflammation (arthritis) is the central hallmark. The characteristic feature is symmetrical polyarthritis involving hand and foot joints with a chronic, persistent course. The clinical presentation, mode of onset, and severity of the disease are very variable. Although some patients present with a very acute onset polyarthritis a gradual and insidious onset is more common. Typical articular symptoms and findings are joint pain, stiffness, and swelling. Concomitant tenosynovitis, bursitis, and carpal tunnel syndrome may also be present. Loss of energy, fatigue, weight loss, fever, and functional joint impairments frequently occur. Because of this variability in presentation, especially in the early stages of the condition, the diagnosis of RA must be based upon a combination of symptoms and signs—very often combined with investigation results—through a process of pattern recognition that demands clinical expertise.

As suggested in accompanying chapters, the recognizable phenotype of RA is likely to be the end product of diverse contributory aetiopathological pathways. With an ever-deeper understanding of these pathways, the diagnostic process may in future become more dependent on the objective measures that reflect them. However, since the pathogenesis of this heterogeneous condition remains incompletely understood, the diagnosis of RA continues to be established primarily on clinical features.

Diagnostic versus classification criteria

The distinction between diagnosis and classification is crucial. Diagnostic criteria aim to establish the correct diagnosis in the vast majority of individual patients. Because the presence of a diagnosis is generally linked with therapeutic interventions, the number of false positive or false negative diagnoses should be minimal. Classification criteria in contrast aim to define a homogeneous disease group for clinical and epidemiological studies. These criteria aim to be correct at the group level and accept misdiagnosis at the individual level. Classification criteria can lead to both false positive and false negative classifications compared to the clinical diagnosis. This risk is smallest when the classification criteria are used on top of a clinical diagnoses. Thus the target population for classification is usually smaller and better defined than that for diagnosis. However, when classification criteria are used as unqualified diagnostic criteria, there is a risk of misdiagnosing a disease among those who do not have it while overlooking it among those who do—an approach that would inevitably result in inappropriate treatment decisions. Indeed, in common with many other diseases, diagnostic criteria for RA do not exist, further emphasizing the importance of clinical experience and judgement in the process.

Classification criteria for RA

The composition of the classification criteria for RA have changed over time, as has the approach for formulating them. For the 1958 ARA-criteria, data from 332 North American cases were used; for the 1987 ACR criteria 262 patients with RA and 262 control subjects with alternative rheumatic diseases were considered. Most recently, data from 2000 European and North American cases with early arthritis (undifferentiated and rheumatoid arthritis) were used to develop the 2010 European League Against Rheumatism (EULAR)/ACR criteria. The 1958 criteria classified patients into different risk categories: classical RA (7/11 items present), definite RA (5/11 items present), probable RA (3/11 items present) and possible RA (2/11 items present) (Table 11.1). In 1987 the aim was to derive a set of criteria with fewer criteria, that was more specific than the 1958 criteria. It resulted in a set of seven items that yielded a stricter definition of RA instead of the broad spectrum of disease identified by the 1958 criteria. In 2010 the aim was to classify patients earlier in the disease course, thereby allowing the inclusion of patients at an earlier stage in clinical trials, preferably before the development of structural damage.

The 2010 ACR/EULAR criteria for RA

The 2010 criteria differ in several points from the former criteria.

- First they incorporate an entry criterion that describes the target population, stipulating that they may be applied to any patient who

Table 11.1 Classification criteria for RA

	Revised ARA 1958 criteria	Revised ACR 1987 criteria	ACR/EULAR 2010 criteria
Entry criterion	none	none	(1) Patient with at least one joint with definite clinical synovitis (swelling) (2) Synovitis is not better explained by another disease
Criteria	1. Morning stiffness 2. Swelling of a joint 3. Swelling of another joint 4. Pain on movement or tenderness in a joint 5. Symmetric swelling 6. Rheumatoid nodule 7. Rheumatoid factor 8. Radiographic changes 9. Mucin clot 10. Synovial biopsy 11. Nodule biopsy	1. morning stiffness (at least 1 hour) 2. arthritis in three or more joints 3. arthritis of hand joints (1 or more swollen joint) 4. symmetrical arthritis 5. rheumatoid nodules 6. serum rheumatoid factor 7. Radiographic changes (erosions)	*Joint involvement* 1 medium-large joint (0) 2–10 medium-large joints (1) 1–3 small joints (large joints not counted) (2) 4–10 small joints (large joints not counted) (3) >10 joints, at least one small joint (5) *RF and ACPA* Both negative (0) Low positive RF or ACPA (2) High positive RF or ACPA (3) *Acute phase reactants* Normal ESR and CRP (0) Abnormal ESR or CRP (1) Duration of symptoms < 6 weeks (0) ≥ 6 weeks (1)
Positivity	Classical RA: 7/11 Definite RA: 5/11 Probable RA: 3/11 *criteria 1–5 continue for at least 6 weeks Possible RA: 2/11 *joint symptoms at least 3 weeks	4/7 criteria present. The first four criteria must have been present for at least 6 weeks	≥6 points
Alternative classification in the absence of synovitis	–	–	Patients with erosive disease typical for RA (defined as a cortical break in at least three separate joints at any of the following sites: the proximal interphalangeal, the metacarpophalangeal, the wrist [counted as one joint] and the metatarsophalangeal joints on radiographs of both hands and feet) should be directly classified as RA).

presents with at least one clinically swollen joint for which another disease is not the most likely cause. This 'checkpoint' was introduced to increase the specificity of the new criteria, preventing their application in patients with alternative diagnoses (e.g. systemic lupus erythematosus (SLE), psoriatic arthritis).

- Second, the 2010 criteria are the first that emphasize the role of additional investigations in the classification of RA. Autoantibodies in particular are heavily weighted in these criteria: three of the required six points can be obtained in the presence of autoantibodies, and one in the presence of elevated acute phase reactants (Table 11. 1). The clinical features of symmetry and morning stiffness, present in earlier classification criteria, are by contrast no longer considered.

- Third, the results of imaging techniques such as MRI or ultrasonography may be used when applying the criteria. In this regard one important distinction must be considered: for the definition of the target population it is essential to have at least one *clinically* swollen joint; however, once clinical synovitis is confirmed, any imaging method may be used to further explore the *extent* of arthritis, which may increase the points achieved in the 'joint distribution' category.

- A final issue is that of structural damage. In order to develop criteria that are fulfilled early in disease course, the presence

of erosions was deliberately not included in the 2010 criteria. However, because patients with longstanding RA that had become less active over time (those with so-called 'burnt-out' disease) were often not classified using this approach, a EULAR definition of bony erosions 'typical' for RA was developed which, when present, enabled immediate classification of RA irrespective of the other criteria. It is defined as the presence of a radiographic erosion (defined as a cortical break) in at least three separate joints at any of the following sites: the proximal interphalangeal; the metacarpophalangeal; the wrist (counted as one joint); and the metatarsophalangeal joints on radiographs of both hands and feet.

Importantly, the fulfilment of the 2010 criteria can be achieved cumulatively (that is, through repeated assessments over time, and in case of adequate previous documentation), and also retrospectively.

What are the consequences of updated classicization criteria?

Several studies have now confirmed that 2010 criteria successfully classify RA patients earlier in their disease course than do previous algorithms[1,2] A meta-analysis evaluated the test characteristics of the 2010 criteria with different references (methotrexate [MTX] initiation, DMARD initiation or expert opinion), and pooled sensitivity and specificity for RA (defined by different reference standards) were 0.82 (95% CI 0.79–0.84) and 0.61 (0.59–0.64), suggesting that that they are more sensitive but *less specific* than the 1987 criteria.[3] Indeed, employing clinical expertise as reference, the specificity of the 2010 criteria appears rather low (48%), with up to 52% of patients not clinically considered as having RA being classifiable with the disease.[3] Thus the clinician's judgement in determining an alternative likely cause for such a patient's presentation before applying the 2010 classification is critical for avoiding RA misclassification in this scenario.

Comparison of the long-term outcome of patients classified with RA revealed that the disease outcome of patients that fulfil the 2010 criteria is milder than that of patients that fulfil the 1987 criteria.[4] This finding is in line the lower specificity of 2010 criteria; capturing patients that are 'false positives' may be the cost of earlier classification. Interestingly the converse has also been observed: many autoantibody seronegative patients with otherwise typical RA fulfilling 1987 criteria were negative for the 2010-criteria. This is a consequence of the constitution of the 2010 criteria as autoantibody-negative patients need to have more than ten involved joints to fulfil the criteria (Table 11.1). For instance, a patient that presents with clinically apparent arthritis of nine joints, symmetrically distributed at both hands, with morning stiffness and in whom the symptoms persist for more than 6 weeks, has the classic presentation of RA and fulfilled the 1987-criteria for RA. According to 2010 criteria this patient is not classified as having RA if there are no RA-related autoantibodies, even in the presence of elevated acute phase markers. By contrast, a patient presenting with just one swollen joint and no morning stiffness, but a high positive rheumatoid factor (RF) and symptoms of 6 weeks' duration despite normal acute phase markers may meet the 2010 criteria for RA classification. These two illustrations demonstrate that the 2010 criteria are weighted heavily in favour of autoantibodies over clinical features for classification purposes.

Another consequence of the revised criteria is that the general concept of RA is shifting, whereby autoantibodies are increasingly seen as the central hallmark of RA rather than its clinical presentation. Hence, some clinicians or researchers may consider patients that lack circulating anticitrullinated protein antibody (ACPA) or RF as not having RA. Although the pathogenesis of both disease subsets may be party different, this underestimates the burden of seronegative RA, which is often recognized late and has been shown to be associated with similar or even greater unmet needs than seropositive RA.[5,6]

In this context it is notable that the ability of the 2010 criteria to classify RA earlier in the disease course appears to be confined to the autoantibody-positive disease subgroup.[7] Autoantibody-negative patients in contrast failed to be classified early in up to 75% of cases.[7] Without doubt early classification of ACPA-negative RA is more challenging than that of ACPA-positive RA, and the risk of misclassification needs to be addressed. In doing so, it should be remembered that ACPA-negative patients fulfilling the 1987 criteria but who are '2010-criteria-negative' may still be classified as having RA, on grounds of having either characteristic, symmetrical small joint polyarthritis with morning stiffness, or features of longstanding disease such as erosions. However, the question of how to identify these seronegative RA patients *early*, and how to differentiate this subset from other seronegative arthritides, remains unresolved.[8,9] Novel laboratory tests (including novel autoantibodies) and/or advanced imaging modalities may be valuable here, but prognostic studies that compare which tests are most useful to apply for this purpose are awaited.

Clinical presentation in relation to disease stage

The development of novel classification criteria over time illustrates the increasingly appreciated importance of diagnosing RA early. During the last two decades the meaning of the word 'early' in this context has evolved. Whereas a diagnosis established within 2 years of symptom onset was considered early in the 1990s, an early diagnosis is now established within a few weeks of symptom onset. A systematic literature search and meta-analysis have shown that early treatment initiation is associated with less radiographic destruction, less mortality, and a higher chance of sustained, DMARD-free remission.[10] There are no randomized controlled trials supporting the concept of the window of opportunity, but based on observational studies a time period in which the disease is less 'matured' and more susceptible to disease modifying treatment, is assumed to be present.[11,12] Timelines in different studies are difficult to compare as the onset of RA is arbitrarily defined, but the first 12 weeks after symptom onset are considered to be part of this period. Therefore, EULAR recommendations on the management of early arthritis advocates that patients with suspected arthritis are referred to and seen by a rheumatologist within 6 weeks after symptom onset.[13] This recommendation has implications for the design of services for arthritis patients in both primary and in secondary care, which will be discussed later.

The clinical presentation of RA depends on the disease stage. Just as the dominant pathobiological processes shift during the course of early disease, so its clinical features evolve and become more evident as its natural history progresses. Hence diagnosing RA as early and accurately as possible poses a particular challenge to clinicians. The development of RA can be categorized in phases based on known risk factors, as outlined by the EULAR study group for risk factors for RA.[14] These same phases may also be defined from a clinical perspective, with the onset of symptoms preceding clinical arthritis heralding the first possible opportunity to recognize RA (Figure 11.1).

Arthralgia suspicious for progression to RA

The pattern of symptoms and signs (other than clinical joint swelling) that differentiates arthralgia patients who will likely progress to clinical arthritis, termed clinically suspect arthralgia (CSA), appears to be well-recognized by rheumatologists based on their clinical expertise.[15,16] A recent study revealed that <7% of arthralgia patients presenting to secondary care were identified as CSA. Importantly, the patients with CSA were 55 times as likely as other arthralgia patients to progress to RA, and the sensitivity and specificity were correspondingly high (80% and 93% respectively)[16], demonstrating the accuracy of the expert opinion of rheumatologists. Although clinical expertise is valuable for patient differentiation in daily rheumatologic practice, it may suffer from a level of subjectivity, which is problematic for clinical studies aiming to include homogenous populations. A EULAR taskforce has developed a definition of arthralgia suspicious for progression

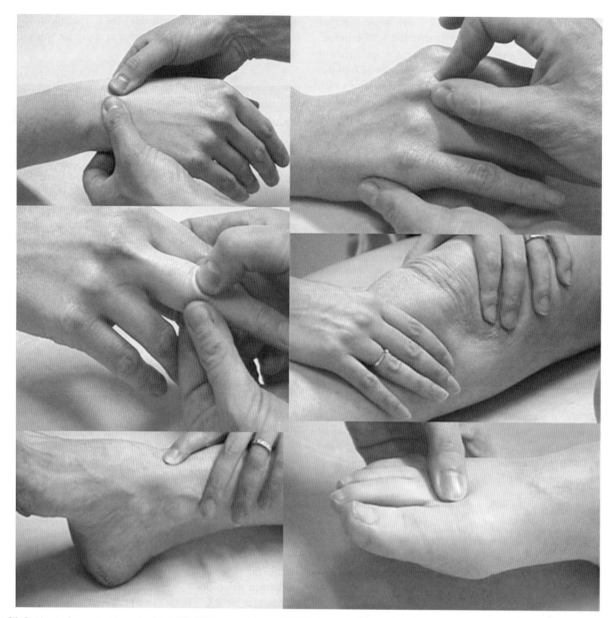

Figure 11.1 Physical examination of wrist, MCP, PIP, knee, ankle, and MTP joints in order to identify the presence of clinical arthritis.

to RA (**Figure 11.1**).[17] It consists of seven clinical parameters; five are obtained by history taking (symptom duration < 1 year, symptomatic metacarpophalangeal joints (MCPs), morning stiffness >60 minutes, most severe symptoms in the early morning, presence of a first-degree relative with RA) and two by physical examination (difficulty with making a fist, positive squeeze test of MCP joints). The definition was validated against the clinical expertise in the rheumatologic centres of the 18 participating rheumatologists and proven to be discriminative (AUC 0.92). Depending on the setting a sensitive or a specific definition can be preferred; the cut-off for a sensitive definition is three items (out of the total of seven items) present and for a specific definition the cut-off is four. The sensitive definition has also shown to be sensitivity in a longitudinal study with arthritis and RA development as outcomes (sensitivity >80%); hence the definition is also validated in longitudinal studies.[18]

Similar to the 2010-criteria, the EULAR definition of arthralgia suspicious for progression to RA has an entry criterion: it is to be used in secondary care in patients without clinical arthritis but with arthralgia in whom imminent RA is more likely than other diagnoses or other explanations. As with the 2010 classification criteria, the definition is therefore intended for use on top of the clinical expertise. It was primarily designed to allow the inclusion of (more) homogenous groups of arthralgia patients into clinical studies. Clinical features alone are insufficiently discriminative in the preclinical phase of 'symptoms', the definition needs to be combined with the results of other investigations (laboratory, imaging tests) to achieve a predictive accuracy that is acceptable for individual arthralgia patients. However, in defining a group of arthralgia patients with a clinically relevant *prior probability* of progression to RA according to Bayes' theorem, it should in turn facilitate studies appraising the additive predictive value of laboratory and/or imaging investigations for this purpose.

Arthralgia in primary care

Arthralgia is a non-specific symptom that can have many very different causes. The application of Bayes' theorem for pretest patient selection in secondary care, alluded to just now, is even more valid in primary care, where musculoskeletal symptoms are highly prevalent but progression to RA a relatively rare event. Data from 16 Dutch general practitioner (GP) practices revealed that almost one-third of the population visits a GP at least once a year with musculoskeletal symptoms. Similar numbers have been published for the United Kingdom. Inflammatory arthritis is considered by GPs as a diagnosis in only a minority of these patients, with other explanations accounting for the vast majority. Another Dutch GP study recorded an incidence of suspected arthritis of 3/1000/year.[19] Most of these patients had a monoarthritis and 60% of the patients with suspected arthritis had self-limiting symptoms and did not return after the first visit. A small proportion of patients had suspected oligo-or polyarthritis and these more often had persistent symptoms. Only a very small fraction of arthralgia patients are referred to secondary care and some studies showed that if a GP doubted on the presence of arthritis, the GP was correct in 20–40% of cases, which is accurate given the total size of the source population of patients with musculoskeletal symptoms.[20,21] Thus although musculoskeletal symptoms are very prevalent in primary care and the incidence of arthritis is low, these data support the notion that pattern recognition is also valuable for GPs to differentiate arthralgia patients. Currently there are no validated diagnostic algorithms for the identification or arthritis in primary care that might be helpful in the diagnostic process of arthritis and RA. In addition, the value in primary care of biomarkers that are commonly used in secondary care (such as autoantibodies) is relatively unexplored. Since post-test chances strongly depend on the pretest risks, adequate patient selection is also important when ordering tests in primary care, and studies exploring the discriminative value of commonly used biomarkers in primary care is urgently required.

Specific clinical features in RA

Several clinical features of RA are here described in more detail, supported by research data obtained in the secondary care setting.

Joint distribution

Arthritis is typically assessed by physical examination of joints, palpation being most important to identify soft tissue swelling caused by synovitis. The methodology of joint palpation of several joints is presented in Figure 11.2. Arthritis in typical RA is usually a polyarthritis of insidious onset, affecting primarily the proximal interphalangeal (PIP), metacarpophalangeal (MCP), and wrist joints, as well as the metatarsophalangeal (MTP) joints. All other joints can also be affected by RA, normally with the exception of the distal interphalangeal (DIP) joints. An overview of the affected joints is presented in Figure 11.3.

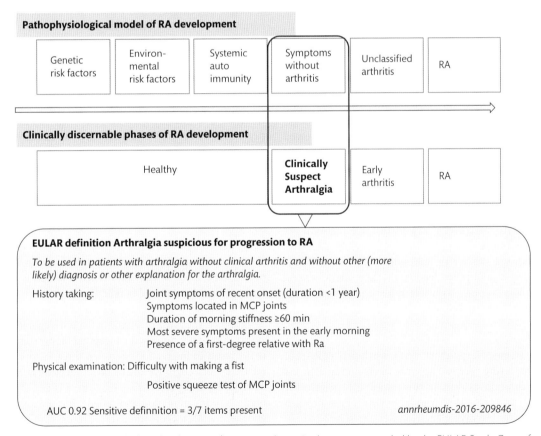

Figure 11.2 A pathophysiological model of RA development (upper panel; terminology recommended by the EULAR Study Group for Risk Factors for Rheumatoid Arthritis) mapped to the clinically discernible phases of early disease (middle panel). For identifying arthralgia patients at greatest risk of arthritis development, the EULAR definition of arthralgia suspicious for progression to RA is also provided (lower panel).

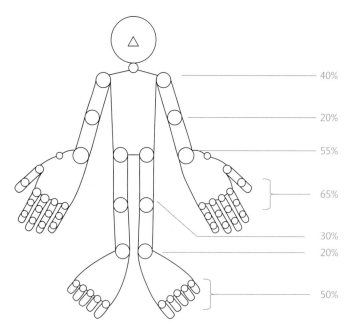

40%

20%

55%

65%

30%

20%

50%

Figure 11.3 Joint distribution frequency of synovitis in RA (% of patients).

Monoarthritis of a large joint is a less common presentation of RA and usually evolves to typical polyarthritis that includes the small joints over time. However, in very early phases RA may also present with mono- or oligoarthritis of small joints progressing to polyarthritis if left untreated. In these settings RA patients generally do not fulfil the classification criteria for RA at first presentation and may be labelled as having undifferentiated arthritis (UA). A rule for predicting risk of progression to RA during the subsequent year has been developed and internationally validated in patients with UA.[22-24] Under 2010 criteria, the vast majority of UA-patients are ACPA-negative. Neither have novel autoantibodies such as anticarbamylated autoantibodies yet proved helpful in predicting RA development among RF and ACPA seronegative patients not fulfilling the 2010-criteria. However, advanced imaging modalities have shown promise for this purpose: a large study investigating the predictive accuracy of 1.5 T MRI of hand and foot joints recently indicated that such imaging was valuable in patients presenting with oligo arthritis compared with other clinical patterns of joint involvement.[25] These data underline that the joint distribution is of interest, not only in RA, but also in patients presenting with UA.

Occasionally, RA may start as palindromic rheumatism, characterized by episodes of joint inflammation affecting one to several joint areas for hours to days, with intermittent periods without symptoms that may last from days to months.

Symmetry

The presence of a symmetric (poly) arthritis is a hallmark of RA, but can still be absent during very early phases when clinical arthritis has just become clinically evident. In this respect it is noteworthy that symmetry was part of the 1987 criteria but is no longer included in the 2010 criteria for classifying RA. Another unresolved issue is how symmetry should be defined, it can be done on individual joint level (e.g. arthritis if MCP 3 at both sides) or at joint region level (e.g. arthritis of MCPs joins at both sided but this may concern different

MCP joints). Both definitions are being used, the definition based on joint region being most common.

Morning stiffness

Morning stiffness is commonly assessed daily in the diagnostic process of arthralgia and arthritis. It is part of the 1987-criteria, but there are relatively few large-scale studies on the discriminative ability of morning stiffness. A recent study on the diagnostic value in 5202 arthralgia and arthritis patients revealed that, in arthralgia, morning stiffness ($\geq$60 minutes) was significantly associated with arthritis, but when using this symptom individually the discriminative ability, expressed using the area under the receiver operating characteristic curve (AUC), was low (0.54–0.57).[26] In patients with early arthritis, the presence of morning stiffness ($\geq$60 minutes) was associated with 2010-RA independent of other predictors and here the discriminative ability was higher (AUC in different cohorts ranging between 0.64 and 0.68). Although a duration of morning stiffness of at least 60 minutes is frequently considered characteristic for RA, a duration of $\geq$30 minutes provided the optimal discrimination for RA in early arthritis. A less frequently used method to measure morning stiffness is assessing its severity on a visual analogue scale. However, it has been reported that assessing the severity yields a higher discriminative ability for RA than assessing its presence/duration.[24,27]

The 'squeeze test'

The test involves squeezing the hand or foot across the MCP and/ or MTP joints. If this is unduly painful, it raises the suspicion of arthritis in at least one of the joints that are compressed. This test is simple to perform, rapidly done, and cheap. Also, here there is surprisingly little data on the diagnostic accuracy. Among patients with classified RA one study observed a moderate correlation between a positive squeeze test and tenderness when palpating individual joints.[28] Another study explored the squeeze test in patients with suspected arthritis. This revealed that a positive squeeze test is indeed associated with local joint inflammation but the sensitivity was low, indicating a high percentage of swollen joints with a negative squeeze test.[29] The specificity was moderate. Therefore this test, when used on its own, it is insufficient to detect early arthritis. The data also showed that the squeeze test of MCP joints performed slightly better (sensitivity 53%, specificity 82%, AUC 0.68) than that of the MTP joints (sensitivity 54%, specificity 74%, AUC 0.64).[29]

Fatigue

Fatigue is common in RA and considered as one of the most important symptoms by patients. Its prevalence in RA has been reported to be 40–80%. The importance of fatigue is illustrated by the findings that more severe fatigue is predictive for decreased physical and mental health-related quality of life, depression, and loss of work ability. The cause of fatigue in RA is thought to be multidimensional. A recently proposed conceptual model suggests that fatigue is the result of interactions between three factors: disease-process related factors, cognitive and behavioural factors (thoughts, feelings, behaviours) and personal factors. There is a relationship between markers of inflammation and fatigue, but the association is weak, and the other factors mentioned are presumed to be more important. This notion is also supported by a recent finding of improved disease outcomes thanks to the use of up-to-date treatment strategies (early treatment start and treat to target), showing less severe joint

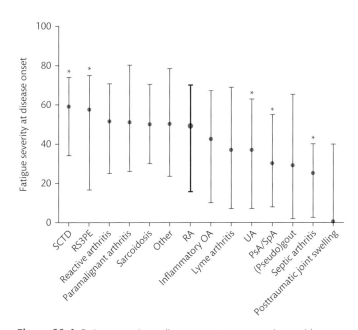

Figure 11.4 Fatigue severity at disease onset among patients with different arthritides.

Reprinted from van Steenbergen H W *et al* (2015) 'Fatigue in rheumatoid arthritis; a persistent problem: a large longitudinal study'. *RDM Open* 1:e000041 with permission from the BMJ Publishing Group.

destruction and also disappearance of the increased mortality of RA patients in recent years. However, these improved treatment strategies did not affect the severity of fatigue experienced by RA patients. Hence, fatigue in RA remains an 'unmet need'. Fatigue is not specific for RA, being common to other rheumatological diseases as illustrated in **Figure 11.4**. The severity of fatigue in RA (expressed on a visual analogue scale) is seen to be higher than that observed in patients with UA, psoriatic arthritis, spondyloarthropathy, and septic arthritis;[30] patients with systemic connective tissue diseases and RS3PE in contrast are more severely affected, however (**Figure 11.4**).[30]

Differential diagnosis

Several alternative diagnoses can be considered.

RS3PE (remitting, seronegative, symmetric synovitis with pitting oedema)

Polymyalgia rheumatica (PMR) and RS3PE are common differential diagnoses of RA in the older population. PMR is an inflammatory rheumatic disease that is typically associated with marked myalgias of the shoulder girdle and the hips, and affects individuals over the age of 50. RS3PE is especially seen at older age and is characterized by symmetric swelling of the whole hands. Both diseases (which can occur simultaneously) have a high erythrocyte sedimentation rate (ESR), are seronegative, and respond dramatically to steroid treatment.

Inflammatory osteoarthritis

Osteoarthritis (OA) can be confused with RA in the middle-aged or older patient when the small joints of the hands are involved.

However, arthritis in OA is different from RA with respect to the distribution of joint involvement. OA of the fingers typically affects the distal and proximal interphalangeal joints causing the so-called Heberden's and Bouchard's nodes. When the disease processes are active OA can have subtle or even more evident inflamed joints. Then the involved joints do not only have bony enlargements but also soft tissue swelling. Inflammatory OA can be differentiated from RA by the location, by the onset (OA mostly evolves during years), the absence of longstanding morning stiffness, the absence of elevated acute phase reactants and seronegativity. However, RFs may be present, usually in low titre, consistent with the generally older age of this patient population.

Viral polyarthritis

Several types of viral infections can mimic RA by leading to the typical polyarthritis of the small joints. This differs from RA in that viral polyarthritis is frequently self-limiting after days to weeks of arthritis. However, a small part of patients with a viral arthritis progress to a chronic arthropathy lasting for 6 months or longer. A variety of viruses can lead to arthralgia, fewer even to arthritis, the most important among the latter being the hepatitis viruses (particularly hepatitis B and C virus), as well as parvovirus B19 and rubella. Especially joint involvement of Parvovirus B19 can impressively mimic RA by a symmetrical involvement of the small finger joints.

Patients with infectious origin of their polyarthritis may not be seronegative for RF, as many viral agents induce transient seropositivity. Virus-specific serological testing may be helpful to identify patients with recently acquired parvovirus infection, or to identify patients with HBV- or HCV-associated arthritis in the differential diagnosis.

Spondyloarthropathy

Several patterns of spondyloarthropathy (SpA) are described, many of which can cause peripheral arthritis. The characteristic joint distribution seen in the different peripheral SpAs may guide the diagnostic process, such as the fact that reactive arthritis typically affects the larger joints of the lower extremity in an asymmetric fashion. A diagnosis of psoriatic arthritis can be made in patients with oligo- or poly arthritis who also have psoriasis. One may occasionally encounter overlap or diagnostic uncertainty between RA and psoriatic arthritis, especially where autoantibodies are present in a patient with psoriasis; radiographic changes may be supportive of one or other diagnosis. In some patients with a symmetric inflammatory polyarthritis, the only clue to the diagnosis of psoriatic arthritis may be a family history of psoriasis.

Lyme arthritis

Lyme arthritis, a late manifestation of Lyme disease, occurs primarily in individuals who live in or travel to Lyme disease endemic areas. Lyme arthritis is characterized by intermittent or persistent inflammatory monoarthritis in a large joint, especially the knee.

Haemochromatosis

Haemochromatosis with joint involvement is characterized by predominant degenerative changes affecting typically the second and third MCP joints, but can also cause soft tissue swelling and arthritic symptoms.

Sarcoid arthritis

Arthritis seen with sarcoidosis most commonly affects the ankles and knees, and less frequently, the wrist, metacarpophalangeal, and proximal interphalangeal joints. It may thus be a relevant differential diagnosis to RA in some cases. In contrast to RA, sarcoidosis can present with a variety of skin and ocular manifestations, such as erythema nodosum or uveitis. In some cases, sarcoidosis presents with the typical triad of erythema nodosum, hilar lymphadenopathy, and ankle arthritis (Löfgren's syndrome).

Other systemic rheumatic diseases

Early RA may be difficult to distinguish from the arthritis of SLE, Sjögren's syndrome, or overlap syndromes, such as mixed connective tissue disease. In contrast with RA, these disorders are generally characterized by the presence of other systemic features such as rashes, Raynaud's syndrome, dry mouth or dry eyes, myalgia, or myositis, renal or haematological abnormalities, and by various autoantibodies not seen in RA.

Clinical features in relation to disease subphenotypes

Palindromic rheumatism

Palindromic rheumatism is characterized by episodes of joint inflammation affecting one to several joint areas for hours to days, with intermittent periods without symptoms that may last from days to months. Palindromic rheumatism may well be ACPA-positive. In general, one-third of the patients with palindromic rheumatism develop RA over time, one-third resolves over time, and one-third remains to have a palindromic disease. Sometimes palindromic rheumatism eventually develops into other systemic disorders such as SLE. Presence of ACPA in patients with palindromic rheumatism is not always associated with progression to RA, as part of these patients continue to have a disease that comes and goes and does not result in joint destruction.

Are ACPA-positive RA and ACPA-negative RA subphenotypes?

Currently diseases in rheumatology are still being defined based on the presenting phenotype rather than on the underlying biologic mechanism. This is mainly the result of the aetiopathology being complex and multifactorial.

ACPA-positive and ACPA-negative RA appear to have distinct underlying biologic mechanisms, reflected by differences in genetic and environmental risk factors. Nonetheless there seems to be a final common pathway phenotypically recognizable as RA. Studies that compared clinical characteristics between both disease subsets found no important differences, except that the ACPA-positive patients being were on average some years younger at the time of diagnosis compared to the ACPA-negative patients.[31-33] There may be circularity here, however, as in these studies the diagnosis is verified using current classification criteria, thereby restricting inclusion to patients with a similar phenotype.

A very recent study evaluated both ACPA-positive and ACPA-negative RA patients while progressing from pre-RA (arthralgia) to clinical arthritis. It was demonstrated that at the stage of symptom onset, ACPA-negative patients had less often involvement of the feet, whereas ACPA-positive patients more often had hand and/feet or feet symptoms. In addition, at first presentation to rheumatologists, ACPA-negative patients had more often difficulty with making a fist and more tender joints than ACPA-positive patients.[32] ACPA-positive patients in contrast had a longer duration of arthralgia symptoms at their first presentation to rheumatologists, following which they developed arthritis more quickly.[32] This is most likely explained by the waxing and waning symptoms more frequently described by ACPA-positive patients, as a consequence of which they may present later in the disease phase that precedes clinical arthritis. This study was the first showing that ACPA-positive and ACPA-negative patients have also some clinical differences, present in the symptomatic phase pre-RA phase. Although consistent with the notion that ACPA-positive and ACPA-negative RA develop differently, there is at present insufficient justification for considering ACPA-positive and ACPA-negative RA to be completely different diseases.

Early recognition

Early treatment initiation is very important for an effective disease modification. It is associated with less severe radiologic joint destruction, a higher chance for achieving sustained drug-free remission and a reduction of the increased mortality risk that is traditionally associated with having a persisting inflammatory disease as RA.

Although data supporting early therapeutic intervention to improve outcomes are overwhelming, identifying RA in an early phase remains difficult. This is in part due to the clinical phenotype being less matured in early phases (posing diagnostic challenges), but it is mainly a logistic challenge. In many countries patients are first assessed by GPs, who see many patients with musculoskeletal symptoms, about one-third of the population consulting a GP for this reason per year. Despite this large burden of musculoskeletal symptoms, the occurrence of inflammatory joint disease is relatively rare and on average a GP sees only one new RA patient per year (in the developed world). Consequently, in very early disease when RA is potentially most sensitive to treatment, patients are typically seen by referring physicians who are themselves relatively inexperienced in joint examination. Providing all GPs with comprehensive training in the subtleties of small joint examination of the hands and feet may be unrealistic, and alternative simple and accurate tests to help them identify the most at-risk individuals early would be valuable. At present no such tools have been validated in primary care. Critically, however, in order to meet the EULAR recommendation for assessment of suspected inflammatory arthritis patients by rheumatologists within six weeks of symptom onset, rapid access referral pathways must also be provided. Achieving this in practice will depend on local healthcare systems but having a 'priority lane' for patients with red flag symptoms of suspected arthritis is crucial.

Features of established RA

The first part of this chapter mainly addressed clinical features of early RA. However, if suboptimally managed features of established RA may become evident. These are the very complications that prompt therapeutic intervention aims to prevent; although many of them are covered in more depth in other chapters of this text they are discussed briefly here.

Radiographic erosions

Synovitis with pannus formation may result in peri-articular bone demineralization and irreversible destruction of both cartilage and articular bone. Erosions typically develop first at the insertion region of the joint capsule, where pannus tissue starts to invade into the exposed bone structures not covered by cartilage. Thereafter erosions may enlarge. For further detail regarding these processes, which so often herald functional decline and disability, see Chapter 10.

Joint deformity

Uncontrolled inflammation results in deformities; as well as being a consequence of the structural bone damage alluded to previously, this is underpinned by tendon and soft tissue pathology. Involvement of carpal bones and MCP joints can cause ulnar drift, often in combination with radial deviation of the wrist and flexion deformities. Typical wrist deformities include volar subluxation of the hand with a visible sliding at the radiocarpal joint and radial deviation of the carpal bones. Involvement of the radioulnar joint can lead to instability and dorsal subluxation of the ulnar head with a 'piano key' phenomenon on downward pressure. The resulting instability and mechanical tension of the ulnar head can eventually cause rupture of carpal extensor tendons.

At the level of the finger joints the RA patient can have 'swan neck' deformities with hyperextension of the proximal interphalangeal (PIP) and flexion of distal interphalangeal (DIP) joints, as well as 'boutonnière' deformities with flexion of the PIP and hyperextension of DIP joints. Presence of tenosynovitis of tendon sheaths are causally related to the occurrence of these deformities. Another typical sign of established RA is atrophy of interosseous muscles of the hand mainly due to reduced use as a consequence of joint pain and stiffness.

Signs of advanced disease in the feet are clawing of the toes and dorsal dislocation of the MTP joints due to synovitis, erosions, and tenosynovitis (especially of the flexor tendons). Persistent shoulder involvement can cause erosions and destruction of the glenohumeral joint, and tendon ruptures (of tendons of the rotator cuff). Knee involvement is very common in RA, with synovitis, and with effusion especially in the suprapatellar recess. Popliteal bursitis (Baker's cyst) is associated with risk of popliteal vein compression. Rupture of a Baker's cyst can cause acute pain and inflammatory swelling of the soft tissue compartment of the lower leg and also thrombotic complications.

In the axial skeleton, RA affecting the cervical spine is important to recognize. In particular, inflammatory changes of the atlantoaxial joint (C1/C2 articulation) with destabilization and atlantoaxial dislocation represents a potentially life-threatening complication. This process is typically driven by synovitis, most commonly in the space between the transverse ligament of the atlas and the posterior part of the dens. Ventral atlantal dislocation has to be considered if the radiographic the space between the anterior dens border and atlas arch increases to 5 mm or more. Vertical dislocation of the dens can occur in conjunction with a ventral atlantal dislocation but also in isolation, leading to a rising of the dens position sometimes even passing the foramen magnum line. Erosive changes of the dens are particularly associated with the risk of dens fracture causing compression of the cervical cord and basilar invagination. This severe complication can lead to paraplegia. Therefore, appropriate imaging is strongly recommended in patients with suspected cervical involvement (pain in the neck, headache, pain with projection to shoulder and upper extremities, paraesthesiae, or numbness of upper extremities).

Extra-articular manifestations

Extra-articular disease manifestations reflect the systemic nature of RA, though are becoming infrequent thanks to improved treatment strategies; key elements are summarized here, with mode detail presented in Chapter 14.

Subcutaneous rheumatoid nodules are primarily present in seropositive patients. They present predominantly at the extensor surfaces of the upper limb, along the forearm and fingers. Occasionally they are found in internal organs, such as the lung parenchyma and myocardium, and, in some patients, the accelerated occurrence of subcutaneous nodules (e.g. of the hands) seems paradoxically pronounced during treatment with MTX.

Eye involvement includes the frequent occurrence of secondary Sjögren's syndrome as well as the rarer and mild complication of episcleritis and the potentially severe manifestation of scleritis and keratitis. Clinical symptoms are pain, vascular injection, photophobia, and visual disturbance. Often in conjunction with scleritis, the most severe eye involvement includes peripheral ulcerative keratitis (corneal 'melt'). This typically painless manifestation occurs primarily in patients with longstanding RA, and is associated with a high risk of ocular perforation and subsequent blindness.

Vasculitis is now rare and associated with disease severity and activity in RA. The most frequent manifestation is cutaneous vasculitis of small to medium-sized vessels, with clinical presentations ranging from periungual infarction through to necrosis and ulceration, predominantly of the lower legs. Furthermore, vasculitis may cause peripheral neuropathy, manifesting as either symmetrical 'glove and stocking' sensory disturbance or mononeuritis multiplex with loss of sensory and motor conduction.

Lung involvement in RA is frequent. Pleuritis might occur, as well as interstitial lung disease and nodular lung disease in association with rheumatoid nodules. Pneumonitis is also a rare but sometimes life-threatening parenchymal complication of MTX therapy, generally occurring within weeks of MTX initiation with rapidly progressive respiratory symptoms.

Secondary amyloidosis due to chronic persistent inflammation is a severe and potentially underdiagnosed condition. Deposition of amyloid A interferes especially with renal function and may lead to end stage renal failure.

REFERENCES

1. Cader MZ, Filer A, Hazlehurst J, de Pablo P, Buckley CD, Raza K. Performance of the 2010 ACR/EULAR criteria for rheumatoid arthritis: comparison with 1987 ACR criteria in a very early synovitis cohort. *Ann Rheum Dis* 2011;70(6):949–55.
2. van der Linden MP, Knevel R, Huizinga TW, van der Helm-van Mil AH. Classification of rheumatoid arthritis: comparison of the 1987 American College of Rheumatology criteria and the 2010 American College of Rheumatology/European League Against Rheumatism criteria. *Arthritis Rheum* 2011;63(1):37–42.

3. Radner H1, Neogi T, Smolen JS, Aletaha D. Performance of the 2010 ACR/EULAR classification criteria for rheumatoid arthritis: a systematic literature review. *Ann Rheum Dis* 2014;73(1):114–23.

4. Burgers LE, van Nies JA, Ho LY, de Rooy DP, Huizinga TW, van der Helm-van Mil AH. Long-term outcome of rheumatoid arthritis defined according to the 2010-classification criteria. *Ann Rheum Dis* 2014;73(2):428–32.

5. Westhoff G, Schneider M, Raspe H, et al. Advance and unmet need of health care for patients with rheumatoid arthritis in the German population—results from the German Rheumatoid Arthritis Population Survey (GRAPS). *Rheumatology (Oxf)* 2009;48(6):650–7.

6. Boer AC, Boonen A, van der Helm-van Mil AH. Is anti–citrullinated protein antibody-positive rheumatoid arthritis still a more severe disease than anti–citrullinated protein antibody–negative rheumatoid arthritis? A longitudinal cohort study in RA—patients treated from 2000 onwards. *Arthritis Care Res* 2017; doi.org/10.1002/acr.23497.

7. Boeters DM, Gaujoux-Viala C, Constantin A, van der Helm-van Mil AHM. The 2010 ACR/EULAR criteria are not sufficiently accurate in the early identification of autoantibody-negative rheumatoid arthritis: results from the Leiden EAC and ESPOIR cohorts. *Semin Arthritis Rheum* 2017;47(2):170–4.

8. de Hair MJ, Lehmann KA, van de Sande MG, Maijer KI, Gerlag DM, Tak PP. The clinical picture of rheumatoid arthritis according to the 2010 American College of Rheumatology/European League Against Rheumatism criteria: is this still the same disease? *Arthritis Rheum* 2012;64(2):389–93.

9. Ferraccioli G, Tolusso B, Fedele AL, Gremese E. Do we need to apply a T2T strategy even in ACPA-negative early rheumatoid arthritis? YES. *RMD Open* 2016;2(1):e000263.

10. van Nies JA, Krabben A, Schoones JW, Huizinga TW, Kloppenburg M, van der Helm-van Mil AH. What is the evidence for the presence of a therapeutic window of opportunity in rheumatoid arthritis? A systematic literature review. *Ann Rheum Dis* 2014;73(5):861–70.

11. van der Linden MP, le Cessie S, Raza K, et al. Long-term impact of delay in assessment of patients with early arthritis. *Arthritis Rheum* 2010;62(12):3537–46.

12. van Nies JA, Tsonaka R, Gaujoux-Viala C, Fautrel B, van der Helm-van Mil AH. Evaluating relationships between symptom duration and persistence of rheumatoid arthritis: does a window of opportunity exist? Results on the Leiden early arthritis clinic and ESPOIR cohorts. *Ann Rheum Dis* 2015;74(5):806–12.

13. Combe B, Landewe R, Daien CI, et al. 2016 update of the EULAR recommendations for the management of early arthritis. *Ann Rheum Dis* 2017;76(6):948–59.

14. Gerlag DM, Raza K, van Baarsen LG, et al. EULAR recommendations for terminology and research in individuals at risk of rheumatoid arthritis: report from the Study Group for Risk Factors for Rheumatoid Arthritis. *Ann Rheum Dis* 2012;71(5):638–41.

15. van Steenbergen HW, Mangnus L, Reijnierse M, Huizinga TW, van der Helm-van Mil AH. Clinical factors, anticitrullinated peptide antibodies and MRI-detected subclinical inflammation in relation to progression from clinically suspect arthralgia to arthritis. *Ann Rheum Dis* 2016;75(10):1824–30.

16. van Steenbergen HW, van der Helm-van Mil AH. Clinical expertise and its accuracy in differentiating arthralgia patients at risk for rheumatoid arthritis from other patients presenting with joint symptoms. *Rheumatology (Oxf)* 2016;55(6):1140–1.

17. van Steenbergen HW, Aletaha D, Beaart-van de Voorde LJ, et al. EULAR definition of arthralgia suspicious for progression to rheumatoid arthritis. *Ann Rheum Dis* 2017;76(3):491–6.

18. Burgers LE, Siljehult F, ten Brinck RM, van Steenbergen HW. Performance of the EULAR definition of arthralgia suspicious for progression to rheumatoid arthritis—a longitudinal study. *Ann Rheum Dis* 2017;76:82.

19. Knuiman C, Schers H. Het beloop van aspecifieke artritis. *Huisarts en Wetenschap*. Available at: https://www.henw.org/archief/volledig/id4565-het-beloop-van-aspecifieke-artritis.html

20. Newsum EC, de Waal MW, van Steenbergen HW, Gussekloo J, van der Helm-van Mil AH. How do general practitioners identify inflammatory arthritis? A cohort analysis of Dutch general practitioner electronic medical records. *Rheumatology (Oxf)* 2016;55(5):848–53.

21. van Nies JA, Brouwer E, van Gaalen FA, et al. Improved early identification of arthritis: evaluating the efficacy of early arthritis recognition clinics. *Ann Rheum Dis* 2013;72(8):1295–301.

22. Van der Helm-van Mil AH, le Cessie S, van Dongen H, Breedveld FC, Toes RE, Huizinga TW. A rule to predict disease outcome in patients with recent undifferentiated arthritis to guide individual treatment decisions. *Arthritis Rheum* 2007;56:433–40.

23. Van der Helm-van Mil AH, Detert J, le Cessie S, et al. Validation of a prediction rule for disease outcome in patients with recent-onset UA: moving toward individualized treatment decision-making. *Arthritis Rheum* 2008;58(8):2241–7.

24. McNally E, Keogh C, Galvin R, Fahey T. Diagnostic accuracy of a clinical prediction rule (CPR) for identifying patients with recent-onset undifferentiated arthritis who are at a high risk of developing rheumatoid arthritis: a systematic review and meta-analysis. *Semin Arthritis Rheum* 2014;43(4):498–507.

25. Nieuwenhuis WP, van Steenbergen HW, Mangnus L, et al. Evaluation of the diagnostic accuracy of hand and foot MRI for early rheumatoid arthritis. *Rheumatology (Oxf)* 2017;56:1367–77.

26. van Nies JA, Alves C, Radix-Bloemen AL, et al. Reappraisal of the diagnostic and prognostic value of morning stiffness in arthralgia and early arthritis: results from the Groningen EARC, Leiden EARC, ESPOIR, Leiden EAC and REACH. *Arthritis Res Ther* 2015;17:108.

27. Vliet Vlieland TP, Zwinderman AH, Breedveld FC, Hazes JM. Measurement of morning stiffness in rheumatoid arthritis clinical trials. *Clin Epidemiol* 1997;50(7):757–63.

28. Wiesinger T, Smolen JS, Aletaha D, et al. Compression test (Gaenslen's Squeeze Test) positivity, joint tenderness, and disease activity in patients with rheumatoid arthritis. *Arthritis Care Res* 2013;65:653–7

29. van den Bosch WB, Mangnus L, Reijnierse M, Huizinga TW, van der Helm-van Mil AH. The diagnostic accuracy of the squeeze test to identify arthritis: a cross-sectional cohort study. *Ann Rheum Dis* 2015;74(10):1886–9.

30. van Steenbergen HW, Tsonaka R, Huizinga TW, Boonen A, van der Helm-van Mil AH. Fatigue in rheumatoid arthritis; a persistent problem: a large longitudinal study. *RMD Open* 2015;1(1):e000041

31. van der Helm-van Mil AH, Verpoort KN, Breedveld FC, Toes RE, Huizinga TW. Antibodies to citrullinated proteins and differences in clinical progression of rheumatoid arthritis. *Arthritis Res Ther* 2005;*7*(5):R949–58.

32. Burgers LE, van Steenbergen HW, Ten Brinck RM, Huizinga TW, van der Helm-van Mil AH. Differences in the symptomatic phase preceding ACPA-positive and ACPA-negative RA: a longitudinal study in arthralgia during progression to clinical arthritis. Ann Rheum Dis 2017;*76*(10):1751–4.

33. Boeters DM, Mangnus L, Ajeganova S, et al. The prevalence of ACPA is lower in rheumatoid arthritis patients with an older age of onset but the composition of the ACPA response appears identical. *Arthritis Res Ther* 2017;*19*(1):115.

12

Pre-rheumatoid arthritis

Karim Raza, Catherine McGrath, Laurette van Boheemen, and Dirkjan van Schaardenburg

Introduction

Clinical manifestations of rheumatoid arthritis (RA) represent the culmination of events occurring in the months, years, or even decades before a patient is classified as having RA according to current criteria. Epidemiological risk factors likely operate from preconception, through gestation and from birth onwards, while some biomarkers are found only in the months or years before clinical arthritis is recognized. The study of the phases leading up to RA development holds the promise of a better understanding of the pathogenesis of RA and promoting the development of preventive strategies.

'Pre-RA' or 'preclinical-RA' are terms that have been widely used to describe those phases of disease before the diagnosis of RA is made, or before the disease can be formally classified as RA. Although usage of these terms vary, in our opinion preclinical-RA should specifically be reserved for individuals before the onset of clinically apparent symptoms or signs, whereas 'pre-RA' encompasses the entirety of phases leading up to the diagnosis of RA. States such as clinically suspect arthralgia (CSA) and undifferentiated arthritis all belong to the clinically apparent pre-RA stage. In patients with RA, one can look in retrospect at the pre-RA period for clues to RA disease pathogenesis thus enabling identification of putative RA risk factors. However, individuals prospectively having these same risk factors, cannot be regarded as being 'pre-RA' or having 'preclinical RA', since many of them will not go on to develop RA and we cannot yet entirely accurately predict RA development in these individuals. These persons should be termed as being 'at risk' of RA.[1] When they do develop arthritis, the disease may not be classifiable as RA even with the 2010 ACR/EULAR classification criteria for RA, which were designed to facilitate the early recognition of RA.[2] In this situation, the condition is termed 'unclassified arthritis' (UA). Some patients with UA will progress to RA at some stage, whereas others will develop an alternative diagnosis or their condition will resolve completely.

Since pre-RA encompasses all the interacting events that precede and lead to RA, it seems appropriate to present in this chapter a short overview of the **risk factors, stages, and events** occurring before the diagnosis of RA, some of which are expanded separately in other chapters. As RA pathology progresses and the disease evolves into a recognizable entity, discrete symptoms (or symptom complexes) become apparent and key structural changes can be identified with imaging techniques. A better understanding of the factors involved and their interaction will provide the opportunity to more accurately predict RA at the individual level, and to test interventions that may halt the progression to RA. Although clearly an appealing goal to strive for, possible benefits of preventive interventions must be weighed against overtreatment of persons who would never have developed RA, the side effects of treatment, and the anxiety induced in the testing of otherwise asymptomatic persons.[3]

Risk factors, prediction models, and interventions

Heritability at the population level is the proportion of phenotypic variance attributable to genetic variance and for RA is estimated to be in the range 40–60%,[4,5] including a contribution of 16% for the human leucocyte allele (HLA) susceptibility locus,[6] and the PTPN22 1858T allele as the single most important non-MHC single-gene contributor.[7] These genetic risks have been reviewed in detail in Chapter 5.

Of the lifestyle and environmental risk factors, smoking has the strongest effect (see **Figure 12.1**).[8] One of the largest studies to date linking lifestyle data with inflammatory polyarthritis (IP) is the European Prospective Investigation of Cancer, Norfolk, United Kingdom (EPIC-Norfolk), which gathered lifestyle data from 25 455 participants from 1993 to 1997.[9] In persons developing IP, diabetes mellitus was associated with increased risk of IP, while alcohol and higher social class for professional workers versus manual workers were associated with reduced risk. In women, parity for ≥2 versus no children was associated with increased risk, and increased duration of breastfeeding inversely associated with risk. Risk factors from the model were used to generate a 'risk score'. 8.4% of women had scores reflecting a >3-fold increased risk of IP over those with a score of 0. A recent review of risk factors identified traditional factors such as female sex, smoking, low education level, high birth weight, airway irritants, and comorbid conditions such as diabetes types 1 and 2 and inflammatory lung diseases.[10] Newer studies point

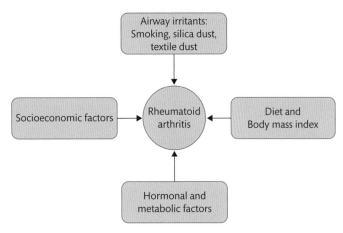

Figure 12.1 Environmental and lifestyle factors thought to be important in development of RA.

to geographic area further from the equator, obesity, high sugar consumption, low alcohol consumption,[10] and low physical activity and post-traumatic stress as risk factors for RA.[11–13]

Airway irritants: Smoking, silica dust, textile dust

The EPIC-Norfolk study calculated that smoking contributes up to 25% of the population burden of RA,[14] and in Denmark, smoking was calculated to be responsible for 33% of cases of seropositive RA.[15] The study of smoking patterns before, during, and after diagnosis of RA suggests that smoking duration rather than intensity is an important feature.[16] The increased risk for RA reaches significance from 10 pack-years after the start of smoking and increases linearly with increasing pack-years.[17] Smoking cessation reduces the risk of RA, although this may not become apparent until several years later.[17] There are no direct studies of smoking cessation interventions on RA incidence although Sparks and colleagues have reported from an ongoing proof of concept randomized controlled trial (RCT) on receiving personalized RA risk estimates in motivating RA-at-risk individuals to modify risk related behaviours.[18]

Silica and other pulmonary irritants increase the risk of RA with a synergistic interaction proposed between smoking and silica. Among ever smokers in Swedish construction workers, both silica and other inorganic dust exposure were associated with increased risk of RA, while among never smokers, neither exposure was associated with a statistically significant increased risk of RA.[19] Occupational exposure to textile dust was associated with an increased risk of developing both anticitrullinated protein antibody (ACPA)-positive and negative RA in a Malaysian female population, with the highest gene–environment interaction found between HLA-DRB1 Shared Epitope and textile dust exposure in ACPA-positive RA women (odds ratio = 39.1).[20]

These airway exposure risks offer numerous opportunities for interventions (improving indoor ventilation, use of personal protective equipment, education, and support in stopping smoking, promoting use of electric vehicles, and phasing out of diesel burning cars). Significant benefits on morbidity and mortality already

achieved in reducing air-pollution through local legislation can be seen in modelling scenarios,[21] and it might be anticipated that the widespread implementation of 'smoking bans' in public places starting since late 2000s in many countries may influence future RA incidence.[22]

Diet and body mass index

Obesity, metabolic syndrome, and type 2 diabetes mellitus are closely interlinked and the risk of RA and response to RA treatment is worse in those with high body mass index (BMI).[23,24] Obesity, in particular together with smoking, has been associated with an increased risk of RA.[23,25] In cases of established RA, dietary modifications have been shown to have a modest positive effect on disease activity, for example, with a vegan followed by vegetarian diet,[26] or with a Mediterranean diet.[27] Lower levels of omega-3 fatty acids in red blood cell membranes are associated with ACPA in first-degree relatives of patients with RA in the Studies of the Etiology of RA (SERA) cohort,[28] and the same group showed that increasing omega-3 fatty acid levels significantly decreased risk of incident arthritis in ACPA-positive subjects.[29] The Nurse's Health Study reported that a diet high in vegetables and whole grains, and low in red-processed meat, sugar, and sodium was associated with a reduced risk of RA (particularly seropositive RA) occurring at 55 years of age or younger.[30]

Vitamin D

The role of vitamin D in the pathogenesis of RA remains controversial,[31] and as with smoking, most data relate to observational studies. The COMEDRA study demonstrated that vitamin D level is inversely correlated with RA activity and with BMI,[32] and in early RA, an improved response to disease-modifying antirheumatic drugs (DMARD) therapy was seen in patients where vitamin D (and omega 3 oils) had been supplemented in the year before RA was diagnosed.[33] By contrast, a meta-analysis of the clinical repercussions on disease activity of at least 3 months of vitamin D supplementation in patients with RA did not quite reach clinical significance.[34] Further insights into the role of vitamin D may develop from the observation that there is decreased sensitivity to vitamin D in T cells from the inflamed RA joint compared to naïve T cells perhaps showing support for an earlier vitamin D 'window of opportunity'.[35] A large prospective primary interventional study involving vitamin D and omega 3 oils for several diseases is currently underway in the United States. An ancillary part of this VITamin D and OmegA-3 TriaL (VITAL; NCT 01169259) study will examine whether vitamin D or fish oil have effects upon autoimmune disease incidence and biomarkers of systemic inflammation.[36]

Other risk factors

Several other risk factors remain controversial such as periodontitis,[10] and a protective (or disease severity reducing) role for oral contraceptives.[14] In a Veterans Health Administration (VA) population of 25 million Americans, subjects with periodontal disease were 1.4 times more likely to have RA. A behavioural intervention study is also targeting dental care in at-risk individuals.[18]

Prediction models

Efforts to combine risk factors in population cohort studies has led to prediction models including genetic risk factors and smoking data, producing areas under the curve (AUC) of 0.74 to 0.80.[37,38] To more closely resemble the phenotype of patients seen in usual rheumatology practice (e.g. seropositive patients with arthralgia), clinical prediction models have been made including items such as symptoms, smoking, obesity, ACPA levels, producing AUCs from 0.67 to 0.82 (see Table 12.1). These models can help to predict RA at the individual level, but also signpost suitable patients for intervention studies.

Evolution of rheumatoid arthritis

The clinical presentation of arthritis diagnosed as RA is highly variable: it may appear dramatically as an acute polyarthritis, develop slowly after years of non-specific symptoms, perhaps at times with extended symptom-free intervals, or manifest in between these extremes. Whatever the precise picture, the symptoms are not the beginning of the disease in the biological sense. The frequent occurrence of RA-specific autoantibodies before the onset of symptoms

shows that the pathophysiological processes that underlie the clinical manifestations of RA often take place over several years.[39,40] In turn, the appearance of autoantibodies is the consequence of a break of tolerance due to a stressor or combination of stressors on the background of a predisposing genetic profile.[41]

The typical evolution of the disease recognized as RA is that a person with (a set of) genetic risk factors develops autoantibodies under environmental influences. Eventually symptoms develop; these include fatigue, pain, and stiffness in joints. Joint swelling may occur simultaneously with these other symptoms or may develop at a later time. At this stage there is clinical arthritis, but if patients do not yet fulfil the classification criteria for RA (or indeed another form of arthritis) they are referred to as having UA. The final step in the evolution to RA is typically an increase of the number of involved joints leading to the diagnosis of RA. It is clear, however, that not all patients with RA will follow this course of events. Even in those that do, the time span of the separate stages can vary largely.

As a result of the variable course of pre-RA events in individual patients, the EULAR Study Group for Risk Factors for RA has defined the various stages that a person may pass through before he or she is eventually diagnosed with RA.[42] In line with individual variability, a person does not necessarily need to progress through all the separate stages, nor do they have to occur in the order described earlier. For example, the phase of autoimmunity can be skipped or occur simultaneously with the onset of symptoms; the phases of arthralgia can be skipped with the first clinical manifestation being clinical arthritis. It is also possible that a person moves backwards through these stages. For example, a long-time smoker at risk of RA

Table 12.1 Clinical prediction models for development of rheumatoid arthritis

First author and year (ref)	Cohort; variables	Numbers	Results
van de Stadt 2013[75]	Seropositive arthralgia patients Prediction rule variables: alcohol non-use, family history, several symptoms, autoantibody status	Arthralgia: 374 (131 developed arthritis)	Prediction rule: AUC 0.82 (CI 0.75–0.89) Intermediate vs. low-risk group: HR 4.52 (CI 2.42–8.77) High vs. low risk group: HR 14.86 (CI 8.40–28)
de Hair 2013[25]	Seropositive arthralgia patients Predictive variables: smoking, BMI	Arthralgia: 55 (15 developed arthritis)	Smoking (ever vs. never) and risk of RA: HR 9.6 (CI 1.3–73) Obesity (BMI ≥25 vs. <25) and risk of RA: HR 5.6 (CI 1.3–25)
Lahiri 2014[9]	European Prospective Investigation of Cancer, UK Prediction rule variables: alcohol use, smoking, occupation, BMI, diabetes mellitus, parity	Total participants: 25 455 (184 developed IP, 138 developed RA)	Pack-years smoking in men and risk of IP: HR 1.21 (CI 1.08–1.37) Seropositive in men and risk of IP: HR 1.24 (CI 1.10–1.41) Having DM (I or II) and risk of IP: HR 2.54 (CI 1.26–5.09) Alcohol and risk of IP (per unit/day): HR 0.36 (CI 0.15–0.89) Overweight and risk of seronegative IP: HR 2.75 (CI 1.39–5.46) Parity ≥2 and risk of IP: HR 2.81 (CI 1.37–5.76) Breastfeeding and risk of IP: HR 0.66 (CI 0.46–0.94)
Rakieh 2014[108]	ACPA-positive arthralgia patients Prediction rule variables: several symptoms, high-positive ACPA, positive ultrasound power Doppler signal	Arthralgia: 100 (50 developed RA)	Power Doppler model: Harrell's C 0.67 (CI 0.59–0.74) Progression to IA: Low risk (0 points) 0% Moderate risk (1–2 points) 31% High risk (≥3 points) 62%

ACPA, anticitrullinated protein antibody; AUC, area under the receiver operating characteristic curve; BMI, body mass index; CI, confidence interval; DM, diabetes mellitus; EIRA, Epidemiological Investigation of RA; HR, hazard ratio; IA, inflammatory arthritis; IP, inflammatory polyarthritis; NHS, Nurses' Health Study; OR, odds ratio; RA, rheumatoid arthritis; VAS, visual analogue scale.

by virtue of having family members with RA may move from the stage of genetic plus environmental risk to the stage of genetic risk only after stopping smoking (albeit only 15–20 years later, after the effect of smoking has worn off).[43–45]

Shared basis of inflammatory diseases

RA can be difficult to distinguish from other inflammatory diseases in the absence of the established RA-specific ACPA and rheumatoid factor (RF). However, even though typical ACPA-positive RA is a distinct entity with characteristics such as peripheral small joint arthritis and immune reactivity to citrullinated antigens, it shares risk factors and overlaps more than expected by chance with a number of other diseases that have autoimmune or inflammatory features, including diabetes types 1 and 2, Crohn's disease, autoimmune thyroid disease, atherosclerosis, and multiple sclerosis. A combined feature of these diseases is the presence of a low-grade inflammation before the disease manifests clinically. This low-grade inflammation may be a prerequisite for, or at least a facilitator of, a breach of immune tolerance and thus a common factor underlying several autoimmune diseases.[46] RA can therefore be seen as part of a wider spectrum of inflammatory diseases promoted by an underlying pro-inflammatory life situation, wherein the genetic background of the individual influences which disease(s) will manifest in the course of a person's life.[47]

Mucosal origin of RA and translocation to the joint

Evidence suggests that the pathology of RA is initiated at mucosal surfaces, such as the gums, the lungs, and the gut. RA is associated with periodontitis, and the pathology as well as the genetic risk profile of periodontitis resembles that of RA.[48] In inflamed periodontal tissue, citrullination of proteins occurs, which can result in the production of ACPA.[49] In the saliva of RA patients and patients with periodontal disease, increased levels of immunoglobulin G (IgA)-ACPA are present, reflecting the fact that antibodies of the IgA isotype are mucous membrane-associated.[50] This was also demonstrated recently, in patients at risk of RA.[51]

RA is also associated with lung inflammation. Increased levels of parenchymal abnormalities are seen on high-resolution computed tomography (HRCT) scans of ACPA-positive RA patients,[52] and airways abnormalities such as increasing bronchial wall thickening have been detected in persons at risk of RA.[53] Biopsies of thickened bronchial tissue in the very earliest stages of untreated RA have shown inflammatory infiltrates with evidence of local ACPA production.[53,54] ACPA are also found in induced sputum specimens of first-degree relatives of RA patients without systemic autoimmunity as well as in seropositive arthralgia patients, both groups at risk of RA.[55] Local irritation by cigarette smoke, dust, and/or recurrent infections may form the basis for inflammation and ACPA production in both the mouth and the lung.

In the gut, a link between inflammation and RA has not been directly established. However, the microbiome composition of the gut appears to be altered in new-onset RA, promoting differentiation of pro-inflammatory Th-17 cells. This has specifically been linked to abundance of *Prevotella copri* in the first phase of the disease.[56]

The mechanism of translocation of the site of inflammation from the mucous membranes to the joints is not yet well understood. It has been proposed that circulating ACPA have the potential to activate osteoclasts, after which local inflammation starts in the bone/joint compartments.[57] The mechanism of extension of the ACPA-induced bone changes to the synovial membrane has to be fully elucidated but after this happens, the synovial infiltrate itself becomes a site of local ACPA production. Joint inflammation promotes citrullination of local proteins such as fibrinogen, providing the basis for binding of ACPA and the formation of immune complexes. These immune complexes also involve RF, thereby further enhancing complement-mediated inflammation. Joint inflammation can thus become self-enhancing and chronic.

Autoantibody development

The appearance of ACPA, RF, and other autoantibodies such as anticarbamylated protein antibodies (anti-CarP) is a dynamic process and coincides with an increase in low-level inflammation.[58] In general, the prevalence of positive autoantibody tests increases closer to the time of onset of clinical arthritis, approaching the prevalence of 65% found in early RA.[39,59] Maturation of the ACPA immune response includes isotypic switching from immunoglobulin A (IgA) to IgG, increase in Ig concentration, and an epitope spread to target more antigenic citrullinated sites.[60–62] In addition, the glycosylation profile of ACPA changes shortly before clinical arthritis is detected, making the ACPA molecule increasingly pro-inflammatory.[63] Autoantibodies such as anti-CarP and antiacetylated protein antibodies also appear and may appear later than ACPA.[64] RF detected in the presence of ACPA appears to have reactivity to more Ig subclasses than RF without other antibodies.[65] Complexing of ACPA Fc tails by RF in the synovium may be an important mechanism to promote inflammation and induce chronicity.[66] The presence of autoantibodies influences the risk of future arthritis in persons at risk of RA, with or without arthralgia. The mere presence of RF or low-level ACPA is not associated with increased risk, but high-level ACPA, the combination of ACPA and RF, or the presence of anti-CarP increases the risk.[64,67]

The evolution of symptoms in individuals at risk of RA

The development of systemic inflammation and systemic auto-immunity in individuals at risk of RA is often associated with, or is followed by, the onset of symptoms which progress until RA manifests. Individuals at risk of RA may go through different symptomatic stages before eventually developing RA.[68] For example, persons may be identified as having symptoms but without clinical arthritis (a phase which has also been termed 'CSA') when the rheumatologist has a high index of suspicion for the future development of RA),[69] or they may have palindromic rheumatism or UA.

In an attempt to provide clarity and consistency regarding nomenclature, a EULAR supported initiative has aimed to define CSA with a particular emphasis on symptoms which predict progression to RA. Using a combination of expert opinion and data driven approaches, seven parameters have been described as identifying a patient as having CSA (see Box 12.1).[69]

Whether patients with an inflammatory arthritis are categorized as having UA or RA depends in part on which set of RA classification criteria are applied; for example, the 2010 ACR/EULAR criteria tend to classify more patients as having RA than the 1987 ACR criteria. Consequently, the symptoms associated with inflammatory arthritis that does not meet the 2010 ACR/EULAR criteria for RA (UA 2010) could be subtly different from those associated with inflammatory arthritis that does not meet the 1987 ACR criteria for RA (UA 1987).[70–72]

Both qualitative and quantitative approaches have been used to identify symptoms in persons at risk of RA. Qualitative approaches have provided important insights into the nature of symptoms in such individuals but have their limitations. Reporting of symptoms retrospectively by RA patients is subject to recall bias.[73] Furthermore, contemporaneous symptom reporting by 'at-risk' individuals can also be problematic as not all individuals will develop RA. Ideally, a longitudinal approach would be required to assess differences across a comprehensive range of symptoms between those who eventually develop RA and those who do not—data from such studies are not yet widely available. A number of quantitative studies have explored symptoms in patients at risk of RA and related these to future RA development. A key limitation of those studies which have reported to date is that the domains across which symptom data are collected are based upon researchers' preconceptions of what symptoms are likely to be present in at-risk individuals rather than on data from qualitative studies that have captured the symptomatology of at-risk individuals. Such preconceptions are largely informed by an understanding of the symptoms associated with established RA.

Quantitative analyses have shown that common clinical manifestations in symptomatic patients prior to the development of joint swelling include symmetrical pain affecting the upper and lower extremities,[74–76] in particular the small joints of the hands.[75,76] A greater proportion of those with early morning stiffness more than 60 minutes progress to develop inflammatory arthritis at follow up.[76] A cross-sectional analysis conducted on a Dutch cohort suggested increased early morning stiffness correlates with RA development in symptomatic at-risk patients.[77] A longitudinal study of the symptomatic phase from arthralgia through progression to ACPA-positive and ACPA-negative clinical arthritis showed differences between the two groups. ACPA-negative CSA patients who eventually developed arthritis had fewer lower limb symptoms at presentation.

By contrast, those with ACPA-positive CSA developing arthritis had longer symptom duration (at presentation), fewer tender joints, and less difficulty making a fist.[78]

Predictive algorithms with demographic, clinical (including symptom related), imaging and laboratory variables have been developed for predicting the development of RA in patients with autoantibody positive arthralgia,[75] and UA.[79,80] In patients with seropositive arthralgia, symptoms of recent onset, that were intermittent, affected the upper and lower extremities and were associated with more than 1 hour of early morning stiffness, identified those more likely to progress to RA.[75] Similarly, in patients with UA, symmetrical symptoms affecting the upper and lower extremities with severe morning stiffness increased the likelihood of RA developing. The importance of symptom location has also been highlighted in a study of patients identified in primary care with non-specific musculoskeletal symptoms without clinical synovitis; those with pain in the wrists, hands, feet, and shoulders were more likely to be ACPA positive.[81]

There is a chance that some critical symptoms (that are either common and or discriminatory) in this early phase were overlooked in these quantitative studies as they were not assessed. Qualitative studies have therefore been helpful to identify the full range of musculoskeletal symptoms experienced prior to the onset of clinically apparent joint swelling. A study of patients with ACPA-positive arthralgia, and with newly diagnosed RA patients identified the following symptoms[82]:

1. **Pain** in and around the joints, sometimes preceded by tingling sensations.
2. **Joint redness, warmth, and swelling**. Some patients experience transient episodes of joint swelling, with burning sensations, warmth, and redness of the skin around their joints.
3. **Joint stiffness**. Some patients experience classical morning stiffness, while others report stiffness worse in the evenings. Stiffness duration often increases as disease progresses.
4. **Weakness**. Some patients describe transient episodes of weakness; other patients describe persistent weakness.
5. **Fatigue, sleeping difficulties, and depressive symptoms**. Extreme fatigue resulting in patients falling asleep has been reported.

At the onset, these symptoms are often migratory and transient. As symptoms progress towards RA, symptomatic episodes typically last longer before eventually persisting without episodes of resolution in between.[82]

The symptoms experienced by ACPA-positive patients are burdensome with considerable physical and psychological impact.[83,84] A recent study of patients with CSA for less than 1 year showed functional limitation as measured by the Health Assessment Questionnaire (HAQ) that were comparable to those with early arthritis.[85] In many cases, patients identified as being at risk of RA describe feeling apprehensive and anxious, not knowing if their disease would progress to RA. Such at-risk patients also describe low mood. Interestingly, many of the psychological symptoms experienced were as a result of fear of the unknown as opposed to a consequence of the physical impact of the symptoms experienced at the time. The resulting disability from physical and psychological symptoms of individuals at risk of RA can be profound.[83]

Box 12.1 EULAR symptoms describing CSA at risk of RA development

History taking
Joint symptoms of recent onset (duration <1 year)
Symptoms located in MCP joints
Duration of morning stiffness ≥60 min
Most severe symptoms present in the early morning
First-degree relative with RA

Physical examination
Difficulty making a fist
Positive squeeze test of MCP joints

Patients with palindromic rheumatism[86] represent a distinct subset of at-risk individuals and some data are available regarding the symptoms experienced by such patients. Joint swelling (which is often mono-articular) typically begins acutely and lasts hours to days, with asymptomatic periods in-between episodes.[86,87] Less common symptoms include fever accompanying episodes of arthritis, skin nodules, and warmth and a change in skin colour over the affected area.[86] Burning sensations, stiffness, and fatigue have also been described. The unpredictable nature of the attacks can cause psychological and emotional distress. In patients whose palindromic rheumatism evolves to RA, the intensity and duration of transient episodes often increase over time.[88]

Data from qualitative studies in individuals at risk of RA have been used to inform the development of a questionnaire which aims to capture the prevalence and predictive utility of these symptoms; that work is currently ongoing.[89]

Do symptoms reflect subclinical inflammation detected by imaging studies?

Symptoms in individuals at risk of RA are often considerable. Although many of these symptoms may be attributable to synovitis in those with palindromic arthritis or UA, this has not been shown unequivocally. The explanation for articular and extra-articular symptoms in patients with clinical symptoms but no clinically apparent joint swelling is even less clear. One potential explanation is the presence of subclinical synovitis or tenosynovitis and several studies have investigated this using different imaging modalities.

MRI of the symptomatic joints of the hands and feet in ACPA-positive patients without clinical arthritis revealed bone marrow oedema and synovitis at symptomatic wrist, metacarpophalangeal (MCP), PIP, and metatarsophalangeal (MTP) joints in some but not all patients.[90] Comparable findings have been reported in seronegative CSA patients.[91] A similar study from a different group looking at ACPA-positive arthralgia patients showed that the majority of patients had a RAMRIS synovitis score of at least one in at least one hand or wrist joint.[92] While subclinical synovitis may be present in many patients with CSA, some patients experience joint related symptoms in the absence of such imaging synovitis. Furthermore, such imaging synovitis can be present in heathy individuals without joint symptoms.[93] The relationship between symptoms and subclinical synovitis is thus not straightforward.

A prospective longitudinal study of CSA patients has assessed the ability of MRI-detected abnormalities to predict the development of clinically apparent inflammatory arthritis.[76] MRI-detected synovitis, bone marrow oedema, and tenosynovitis were all associated with future arthritis development. Importantly, arthritis development was unusual in the absence of subclinical synovitis.

Ultrasound has also been used to assess the presence of synovitis in individuals at risk of RA. While ultrasound evidence of synovitis (both greyscale and power Doppler) is present in ACPA-positive patients without clinical arthritis,[94] and its presence is associated with future arthritis development,[94,95] the majority of painful or tender joints in patients with autoantibody positivity and musculoskeletal symptoms do not have ultrasound evidence of synovitis.[95]

One study using positron emission tomography (PET) scanning targeting macrophages reported a positive scan of hand joints in 4 out of 29 patients, and these were predictive of future clinical arthritis.[96]

Thus, in a proportion of symptomatic patients at risk of RA, including those who are known to eventually develop RA, imaging fails to reveal subclinical synovitis. Furthermore, a study of the synovium from autoantibody positive patients showed no overt histological synovitis from knee joint synovial biopsies despite the fact that in almost half of patients the knee joint was symptomatic.[97] Consequently, histological synovitis also does not fully explain the prevalence of joint symptoms in patients with musculoskeletal symptoms and autoantibody positivity at risk of RA. Interestingly, recent data suggest that ACPA itself may play a role in the development of joint related symptoms in the absence of discernible joint inflammation with IL-8 pathways implicated.[98] Thus, while subclinical synovitis and tenosynovitis may explain some of the joint related symptoms in patients at risk of RA prior to the onset of joint swelling, and autoantibodies may play a role in the pain experience in some symptomatic autoantibody positive patients, the explanation for joint-related symptoms in all patients with arthralgia who eventually develop RA remains unclear, as do the causes of some of the extra-articular symptoms in this patient group.

Interventions for the prevention of development of RA

The number of individuals who could benefit from interventions to prevent RA is potentially large, although these individuals may not be easy to recognize. Candidates for preventive studies are at present mostly found in family members of RA patients and in persons with arthralgia with elevated RF or ACPA, or termed by a rheumatologist as having CSA. All of these, including other unrecognized individuals at risk, could benefit from health promotion on the societal level directed at diet, weight, exercise, and environmental exposures, including cigarette smoke.

We have yet to ascertain at what stage of life individual risk factors are most important. A cumulative action of genetic and environmental factors achieving a 'threshold effect' that leads to RA has been proposed.[99] Catrina and colleagues have also speculated that several different molecular events may have to act together in an (as yet to be) defined sequence to produce disease.[100] Different molecular sequences might be followed in subsets of disease such as ACPA-positive or ACPA-negative RA. There may also be a variable outcome depending on the order of environmental exposures. (See Figure 12.2.)[101]

Drug therapy interventions

An alternative to targeting lifestyle/environmental risk factors for RA is the option of pharmacological intervention in at-risk individuals (whether at-risk is defined genetically, or on the basis of RF/ACPA seropositivity with or without CSA), to see if the course of disease can be altered. There are clear data that intervention in early RA has a significant effect on the disease trajectory so there is

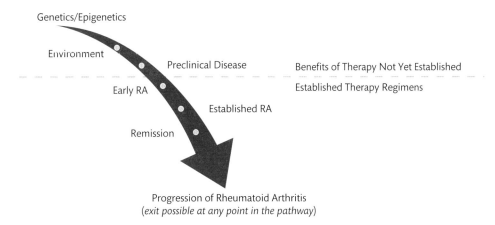

Figure 12.2 A cumulative interaction of genetic and environmental factors leading to development of RA.
Reprinted from McGrath CM and Young SP (2015). 'Lipid and Metabolic Changes in Rheumatoid Arthritis'. *Curr Rheumatol Rep* 17(9):57 with permission from Springer Nature.

a logical basis to think that earlier interventions may be even more effective in persons at risk of RA.[102–104]

Two trials in seropositive arthralgia patients have been completed. A study of intramuscular injections of dexamethasone versus placebo in HLA-DR4-positive persons with RF and/or ACPA failed to reduce these antibodies by 50% (the primary outcome measure) and had no effect on subsequent arthritis development.[105] The second, the Prevention of RA by B-cell directed therapy (PRAIRI) study assessed 82 subjects with arthralgia at high risk of RA (positive for both ACPA and RF, with C-reactive protein (CRP) levels ≥3 mg/L and/or subclinical synovitis on ultrasound or MRI of the hands).[106] This placebo-controlled trial used a single 1000 mg infusion of rituximab; 16/40 (40%) participants in the placebo group and 14/41 (34%) in the rituximab group developed RA with a delay of 12 months in the rituximab-treated group.

Several other preventive trials are currently underway and are listed in Table 12.2. The Arthritis Prevention In the Pre-clinical Phase of Rheumatoid Arthritis (APIPPRA) study, and the Abatacept Reversing Subclinical Inflammation as Measured by MRI in

ACPA-Positive Arthralgia (ARIAA) study both assess the effects of abatacept. Additional studies include 'Treat early arthralgia to reverse or limit impending exacerbation to rheumatoid arthritis' (TREAT EARLIER), using methotrexate in CSA patients with synovitis on MRI; the Strategy TO Prevent the onset of clinically apparent Rheumatoid Arthritis (STOPRA) study (treating at-risk ACPA-positive individuals, with hydroxychloroquine); and finally the STAtins to Prevent RA (STAPRA) study of atorvastatin in arthralgia patients with high-positive ACPA or ACPA plus RF.

Novel approaches to prevent RA also include administering RA-related antigens for uptake by dendritic cells and aiming for the induction immune tolerance although such studies are still in the early stages of development.[107]

To date then, limited data have been reported from drug interventions in pre-RA. The broad conclusions seem to be that the drugs tested so far may delay but do not prevent the onset of disease. However, new therapeutic approaches in the at-risk phase, combined with more accurate identification of at-risk individuals to target with these therapies may reduce the future burden of RA.

Table 12.2 Drug trials for prevention of (rheumatoid) arthritis in persons at risk

Study	Registry	Patients	Intervention	Control	Primary outcome
DEXA	Published (105)	RF and/or ACPA positive, HLA DR4 positive	Dexamethasone i.m. 100 mg 2×	Placebo	50% reduction antibody levels after 6 months (not reached)
PRAIRI	Published (106)	RF and ACPA positive, CRP >3 mg/L or synovitis on imaging	Rituximab i.v. 1000 mg 1×	Placebo	Time to occurrence of clinical arthritis
APIPPRA	ISRCTN46017566 isrctn.com	ACPA >3× ULN or ACPA plus RF, inflammatory arthralgia	Abatacept s.c. 125 mg weekly for 1 year	Placebo	Time to development of clinical synovitis or RA
ARIAA	NCT02778906 ClinicalTrials.gov	ACPA-positive arthralgia synovitis on MRI	Abatacept s.c. 125 mg weekly for 6 months	Placebo	Improvement of synovitis on MRI after 18 months
TREAT EARLIER	NTR4853 trialregister.nl	Clinically suspect arthralgia Synovitis on MRI	Methotrexate p.o. weekly for 1 year	Placebo	Clinically apparent arthritis after 2 years
STOPRA	NCT02603146 ClinicalTrials.gov	ACPA positive	Hydroxychloroquine p.o. 200–400 mg daily for 1 year	Placebo	Clinically apparent RA after 3 years
STAPRA	NTR5265 trialregister.nl	ACPA >3× ULN or ACPA plus RF	Atorvastatin p.o. 40 mg daily for 3 years	Placebo	Clinically apparent arthritis after 3 years

i.m. intramuscularly, i.v. intravenous, p.o. per os, s.c. subcutaneously

Current preventive studies target patients in different at-risk phases including patients with seronegative/seropositive CSA, with or without imaging evidence of synovitis. It is quite possible that disease mechanisms differ between these phases and that therapeutic approaches relevant to one at-risk phase may be different to approaches relevant to other at-risk phases—addressing this is a key component of the future research agenda.

The results of ongoing drug studies will hopefully inform us whether it is worthwhile to identify and treat those at risk of RA in the presynovitis stage as opposed to waiting until patients have clinically apparent arthritis. Meanwhile, counselling persons at risk to change unhealthy lifestyle factors should be actively pursued by physicians and other healthcare professionals. We will also need to address individual concerns about their perceptions of disease risk and willingness to be tested for risk of developing RA, since it is clear that not all of those at risk would necessarily wish to be identified.[3]

REFERENCES

1. Raza K, Gerlag DM. Preclinical inflammatory rheumatic diseases: an overview and relevant nomenclature. *Rheum Dis Clin North Am* 2014;40(4):569–80.
2. Aletaha D, Neogi T, Silman AJ, et al. 2010 Rheumatoid arthritis classification criteria: an American College of Rheumatology/European League Against Rheumatism collaborative initiative. *Arthritis Rheum* 2010;62(9):2569–81.
3. Stack RJ, Stoffer M, Englbrecht M, et al. Perceptions of risk and predictive testing held by the first-degree relatives of patients with rheumatoid arthritis in England, Austria and Germany: a qualitative study. *BMJ Open* 2016;6(6):e010555.
4. Yarwood A, Huizinga TW, Worthington J. The genetics of rheumatoid arthritis: risk and protection in different stages of the evolution of RA. *Rheumatology (Oxf)* 2016;55(2):199–209.
5. Frisell T, Saevarsdottir S, Askling J. Family history of rheumatoid arthritis: an old concept with new developments. *Nat Rev Rheumatol* 2016;12(6):335–43.
6. Cornelis F, Faure S, Martinez M, et al. New susceptibility locus for rheumatoid arthritis suggested by a genome-wide linkage study. *Proc Natl Acad Sci U S A* 1998;95(18):10746–50.
7. Stanford SM, Bottini N. PTPN22: the archetypal non-HLA autoimmunity gene. *Nat Rev Rheumatol* 2014;10(10):602–11.
8. Sugiyama D, Nishimura K, Tamaki K, et al. Impact of smoking as a risk factor for developing rheumatoid arthritis: a meta-analysis of observational studies. *Ann Rheum Dis* 2010;69(1):70–81.
9. Lahiri M, Luben RN, Morgan C, et al. Using lifestyle factors to identify individuals at higher risk of inflammatory polyarthritis (results from the European Prospective Investigation of Cancer-Norfolk and the Norfolk Arthritis Register--the EPIC-2-NOAR Study). *Ann Rheum Dis* 2014;73(1):219–26.
10. van Beers-Tas MH, Turk SA, van Schaardenburg D. How does established rheumatoid arthritis develop, and are there possibilities for prevention? *Best Pract Res Clin Rheumatol* 2015;29(4–5):527–42.
11. Di Giuseppe D, Bottai M, Askling J, Wolk A. Physical activity and risk of rheumatoid arthritis in women: a population-based prospective study. *Arthritis Res Ther* 2015;17:40.
12. Lee YC, Agnew-Blais J, Malspeis S, et al. Post-traumatic stress disorder and risk for incident rheumatoid arthritis. *Arthritis Care Res (Hoboken)* 2016;68(3):292–8.
13. O'Donovan A, Cohen BE, Seal KH, et al. Elevated risk for autoimmune disorders in Iraq and Afghanistan veterans with posttraumatic stress disorder. *Biol Psychiatry* 2015;77(4):365–74.
14. Lahiri M, Morgan C, Symmons DP, Bruce IN. Modifiable risk factors for RA: prevention, better than cure? *Rheumatology (Oxf)* 2012;51(3):499–512.
15. Pedersen M, Jacobsen S, Garred P, et al. Strong combined gene-environment effects in anti-cyclic citrullinated peptide-positive rheumatoid arthritis: a nationwide case-control study in Denmark. *Arthritis Rheum* 2007;56(5):1446–53.
16. Sparks JA, Karlson EW. The roles of cigarette smoking and the lung in the transitions between phases of preclinical rheumatoid arthritis. *Curr Rheumatol Rep* 2016;18(3):15.
17. Costenbader KH, Feskanich D, Mandl LA, Karlson EW. Smoking intensity, duration, and cessation, and the risk of rheumatoid arthritis in women. *Am J Med* 2006;119(6):503.e1–9.
18. Sparks JA, Iversen MD, Yu Z, et al. Disclosure of personalized rheumatoid arthritis risk using genetics, biomarkers, and lifestyle factors to motivate health behavior improvements: a randomized controlled trial. *Arthritis Care Res (Hoboken)* 2017: doi: 10.1002/acr.23411.
19. Blanc PD, Jarvholm B, Toren K. Prospective risk of rheumatologic disease associated with occupational exposure in a cohort of male construction workers. *Am J Med* 2015;128(10):1094–101.
20. Too CL, Muhamad NA, Ilar A, et al. Occupational exposure to textile dust increases the risk of rheumatoid arthritis: results from a Malaysian population-based case-control study. *Ann Rheum Dis* 2016;75(6):997–1002.
21. Archibald AT, Folberth G, Wade DC, Scott D. A world avoided: impacts of changes in anthropogenic emissions on the burden and effects of air pollutants in Europe and North America. *Faraday Discussions* 2017;200(0):475–500.
22. Hyland A, Barnoya J, Corral JE. Smoke-free air policies: past, present and future. *Tob Control* 2012;21(2):154–61.
23. Lu B, Hiraki LT, Sparks JA, et al. Being overweight or obese and risk of developing rheumatoid arthritis among women: a prospective cohort study. *Ann Rheum Dis* 2014;73(11):1914–22.
24. Levitsky A, Brismar K, Hafstrom I, et al. Obesity is a strong predictor of worse clinical outcomes and treatment responses in early rheumatoid arthritis: results from the SWEFOT trial. *RMD Open* 2017;3(2):e000458.
25. de Hair MJ, Landewe RB, van de Sande MG, et al. Smoking and overweight determine the likelihood of developing rheumatoid arthritis. *Ann Rheum Dis* 2013;72(10):1654–8.
26. Kjeldsen-Kragh J, Haugen M, Borchgrevink CF, et al. Controlled trial of fasting and one-year vegetarian diet in rheumatoid arthritis. *Lancet* 1991;338(8772):899–902.
27. Skoldstam L, Hagfors L, Johansson G. An experimental study of a Mediterranean diet intervention for patients with rheumatoid arthritis. *Ann Rheum Dis* 2003;62(3):208–14.
28. Gan RW, Young KA, Zerbe GO, et al. Lower omega-3 fatty acids are associated with the presence of anti-cyclic citrullinated peptide autoantibodies in a population at risk for future rheumatoid arthritis: a nested case-control study. *Rheumatology (Oxf)* 2016;55(2):367–76.
29. Gan RW, Bemis EA, Demoruelle MK, et al. The association between omega-3 fatty acid biomarkers and inflammatory arthritis in an anti-citrullinated protein antibody positive population. *Rheumatology (Oxf)* 2017;56(12):2229–36.

30. Hu Y, Sparks JA, Malspeis S, et al. Long-term dietary quality and risk of developing rheumatoid arthritis in women. *Ann Rheum Dis* 2017;*76*(8):1357–64.

31. Jeffery LE, Raza K, Hewison M. Vitamin D in rheumatoid arthritis-towards clinical application. *Nat Rev Rheumatol* 2016;*12*(4):201–10.

32. Cecchetti S, Tatar Z, Galan P, et al. Prevalence of vitamin D deficiency in rheumatoid arthritis and association with disease activity and cardiovascular risk factors: data from the COMEDRA study. *Clin Exp Rheumatol* 2016;*34*(6):984–90.

33. Lourdudoss C, Wolk A, Nise L, Alfredsson L, Vollenhoven RV. Are dietary vitamin D, omega-3 fatty acids and folate associated with treatment results in patients with early rheumatoid arthritis? Data from a Swedish population-based prospective study. *BMJ Open* 2017;*7*(6):e016154.

34. Franco AS, Freitas TQ, Bernardo WM, Pereira RMR. Vitamin D supplementation and disease activity in patients with immune-mediated rheumatic diseases: a systematic review and meta-analysis. *Medicine (Baltimore)* 2017;*96*(23):e7024.

35. Jeffery LE, Henley P, Marium N, et al. Decreased sensitivity to 1,25-dihydroxyvitamin D3 in T cells from the rheumatoid joint. *J Autoimmun* 2017: doi.org/10.1016/j.jaut.2017.10.001

36. Costenbader KH. Vitamin D and fish oil for autoimmune disease, inflammation and chronic knee pain. Bethesda, MD: NLoM, 2011. Available at: https://clinicaltrials.gov/ct2/show/NCT01351805

37. Sparks JA, Chen CY, Jiang X, et al. Improved performance of epidemiologic and genetic risk models for rheumatoid arthritis serologic phenotypes using family history. *Ann Rheum Dis* 2015;*74*(8):1522–9.

38. Yarwood A, Han B, Raychaudhuri S, et al. A weighted genetic risk score using all known susceptibility variants to estimate rheumatoid arthritis risk. *Ann Rheum Dis* 2015;*74*(1):170–6.

39. Nielen MM, van Schaardenburg D, Reesink HW, et al. Specific autoantibodies precede the symptoms of rheumatoid arthritis: a study of serial measurements in blood donors. *Arthritis Rheum* 2004;*50*(2):380–6.

40. Rantapaa-Dahlqvist S, de Jong BA, Berglin E, et al. Antibodies against cyclic citrullinated peptide and IgA rheumatoid factor predict the development of rheumatoid arthritis. *Arthritis Rheum* 2003;*48*(10):2741–9.

41. Catrina AI, Deane KD, Scher JU. Gene, environment, microbiome and mucosal immune tolerance in rheumatoid arthritis. *Rheumatology (Oxf)* 2016;*55*(3):391–402.

42. Gerlag DM, Raza K, van Baarsen LG, et al. EULAR recommendations for terminology and research in individuals at risk of rheumatoid arthritis: report from the Study Group for Risk Factors for Rheumatoid Arthritis. *Ann Rheum Dis* 2012;*71*(5):638–41.

43. Costenbader KH, Karlson EW. Cigarette smoking and autoimmune disease: what can we learn from epidemiology? *Lupus* 2006;*15*(11):737–45.

44. Di Giuseppe D, Orsini N, Alfredsson L, Askling J, Wolk A. Cigarette smoking and smoking cessation in relation to risk of rheumatoid arthritis in women. *Arthritis Res Ther* 2013;*15*(2):R56.

45. Di Giuseppe D, Discacciati A, Orsini N, Wolk A. Cigarette smoking and risk of rheumatoid arthritis: a dose-response meta-analysis. *Arthritis Res Ther* 2014;*16*: R61.

46. Bystrom J, Clanchy FI, Taher TE, et al. TNFalpha in the regulation of Treg and Th17 cells in rheumatoid arthritis and other autoimmune inflammatory diseases. *Cytokine* 2018;*101*:4–13.

47. Ruiz-Nunez B, Pruimboom L, Dijck-Brouwer DA, Muskiet FA. Lifestyle and nutritional imbalances associated with Western diseases: causes and consequences of chronic systemic low-grade inflammation in an evolutionary context. *J Nutr Biochem* 2013;*24*(7):1183–201.

48. Fuggle NR, Smith TO, Kaul A, Sofat N. Hand to mouth: a systematic review and meta-analysis of the association between rheumatoid arthritis and periodontitis. *Front Immunol* 2016;*7*:80.

49. Harvey GP, Fitzsimmons TR, Dhamarpatni AA, Marchant C, Haynes DR, Bartold PM. Expression of peptidylarginine deiminase-2 and -4, citrullinated proteins and anti-citrullinated protein antibodies in human gingiva. *J Periodontal Res* 2013;*48*(2):252–61.

50. Svard A, Kastbom A, Sommarin Y, Skogh T. Salivary IgA antibodies to cyclic citrullinated peptides (CCP) in rheumatoid arthritis. *Immunobiology* 2013;*218*(2):232–7.

51. Mankia K, Hunt L, Hensor E, et al. OP0246 increased prevalence of periodontal disease in anti-CCP positive individuals at risk of progression to inflammatory arthritis: a target for prevention? *Ann Rheum Dis* 2016;*75*:2–151.

52. Reynisdottir G, Karimi R, Joshua V, et al. Structural changes and antibody enrichment in the lungs are early features of anti-citrullinated protein antibody-positive rheumatoid arthritis. *Arthritis Rheumatol* 2014;*66*(1):31–9.

53. Demoruelle MK, Weisman MH, Simonian PL, et al. Brief report: airways abnormalities and rheumatoid arthritis-related autoantibodies in subjects without arthritis: early injury or initiating site of autoimmunity? *Arthritis Rheum* 2012;*64*(6):1756–61.

54. Reynisdottir G, Olsen H, Joshua V, et al. Signs of immune activation and local inflammation are present in the bronchial tissue of patients with untreated early rheumatoid arthritis. *Ann Rheum Dis* 2016;*75*(9):1722–7.

55. Willis VC, Demoruelle MK, Derber LA, et al. Sputum autoantibodies in patients with established rheumatoid arthritis and subjects at risk of future clinically apparent disease. *Arthritis Rheum* 2013;*65*(10):2545–54.

56. Scher JU, Sczesnak A, Longman RS, et al. Expansion of intestinal Prevotella copri correlates with enhanced susceptibility to arthritis. *Elife* 2013;*2*:e01202.

57. Catrina AI, Svensson CI, Malmstrom V, Schett G, Klareskog L. Mechanisms leading from systemic autoimmunity to joint-specific disease in rheumatoid arthritis. *Nat Rev Rheumatol* 2017;*13*(2):79–86.

58. Nielen MM, van Schaardenburg D, Reesink HW, et al. Simultaneous development of acute phase response and auto-antibodies in preclinical rheumatoid arthritis. *Ann Rheum Dis* 2006;*65*(4):535–7.

59. Shi J, van de Stadt LA, Levarht EW, et al. Anti-carbamylated protein (anti-CarP) antibodies precede the onset of rheumatoid arthritis. *Ann Rheum Dis* 2014;*73*(4):780–3.

60. Brink M, Verheul MK, Ronnelid J, et al. Anti-carbamylated protein antibodies in the pre-symptomatic phase of rheumatoid arthritis, their relationship with multiple anti-citrulline peptide antibodies and association with radiological damage. *Arthritis Res Ther* 2015;*17*:25.

61. van de Stadt LA, van der Horst AR, de Koning MH, et al. The extent of the anti-citrullinated protein antibody repertoire is associated with arthritis development in patients with seropositive arthralgia. *Ann Rheum Dis* 2011;*70*(1):128–33.

62. Sokolove J, Bromberg R, Deane KD, et al. Autoantibody epitope spreading in the pre-clinical phase predicts progression to rheumatoid arthritis. *PLoS One* 2012;7(5):e35296.

63. Rombouts Y, Ewing E, van de Stadt LA, et al. Anti-citrullinated protein antibodies acquire a pro-inflammatory Fc glycosylation phenotype prior to the onset of rheumatoid arthritis. *Ann Rheum Dis* 2015;74(1):234–41.

64. Shi J, van de Stadt LA, Levarht EW, et al. Anti-carbamylated protein antibodies are present in arthralgia patients and predict the development of rheumatoid arthritis. *Arthritis Rheum* 2013;65(4):911–15.

65. Falkenburg WJ, van Schaardenburg D, Ooijevaar-de Heer P, Wolbink G, Rispens T. IgG subclass specificity discriminates restricted IgM rheumatoid factor responses from more mature anti-citrullinated protein antibody-associated or isotype-switched IgA responses. *Arthritis Rheumatol* 2015;67(12):3124–34.

66. Falkenburg WJJ, van Schaardenburg D. Evolution of autoantibody responses in individuals at risk of rheumatoid arthritis. *Best Pract Res Clin Rheumatol* 2017;31(1):42–52.

67. Bos WH, Wolbink GJ, Boers M, et al. Arthritis development in patients with arthralgia is strongly associated with anti-citrullinated protein antibody status: a prospective cohort study. *Ann Rheum Dis* 2010;69(3):490–4.

68. Jutley G, Raza K, Buckley CD. New pathogenic insights into rheumatoid arthritis. *Curr Opin Rheumatol* 2015;27(3):249–55.

69. van Steenbergen HW, Aletaha D, Beaart-van de Voorde LJ, et al. EULAR definition of arthralgia suspicious for progression to rheumatoid arthritis. *Ann Rheum Dis* 2017;76(3):491–6.

70. Arnett FC, Edworthy SM, Bloch DA, McShane DJ, Fries JF, Cooper NS, et al. The American Rheumatism Association 1987 revised criteria for the classification of rheumatoid arthritis. *Arthritis Rheum* 1988;31(3):315–24.

71. Aletaha D, Neogi T, Silman AJ, et al. 2010 rheumatoid arthritis classification criteria: an American College of Rheumatology/European League Against Rheumatism collaborative initiative. *Ann Rheum Dis* 2010;69:1580–8.

72. Cader MZ, Filer A, Hazlehurst J, de Pablo P, Buckley CD, Raza K. Performance of the 2010 ACR/EULAR criteria for rheumatoid arthritis: comparison with 1987 ACR criteria in a very early synovitis cohort. *Ann Rheum Dis* 2011;70:949–55.

73. Stack RJ, Sahni M, Mallen CD, Raza K. Symptom complexes at the earliest phases of rheumatoid arthritis: a synthesis of the qualitative literature. *Arthritis Care Res (Hoboken)* 2013;65(12):1916–26.

74. Rakieh C, Nam JL, Hunt L, et al. Predicting the development of clinical arthritis in anti-CCP positive individuals with non-specific musculoskeletal symptoms: a prospective observational cohort study. *Ann Rheum Dis* 2015;74(9):1659–66.

75. van de Stadt LA, Witte BI, Bos WH, van Schaardenburg D. A prediction rule for the development of arthritis in seropositive arthralgia patients. *Ann Rheum Dis* 2013;72(12):1920–6.

76. van Steenbergen HW, Mangnus L, Reijnierse M, Huizinga TW, van der Helm-van Mil AH. Clinical factors, anticitrullinated peptide antibodies and MRI-detected subclinical inflammation in relation to progression from clinically suspect arthralgia to arthritis. *Ann Rheum Dis* 2016;75(10):1824–30.

77. van Nies JA, Alves C, Radix-Bloemen AL, et al. Reappraisal of the diagnostic and prognostic value of morning stiffness in arthralgia and early arthritis: results from the Groningen EARC, Leiden EARC, ESPOIR, Leiden EAC and REACH. *Arthritis Res Ther* 2015;17:108.

78. Burgers LE, van Steenbergen HW, ten Brinck RM, Huizinga TWJ, van der Helm-van Mil AHM. Differences in the symptomatic phase preceding ACPA-positive and ACPA-negative RA: a longitudinal study in arthralgia during progression to clinical arthritis. *Ann Rheum Dis* 2017;76(10):1751.

79. Linn-Rasker SP, van der Helm-van Mil AH, Breedveld FC, Huizinga TW. Arthritis of the large joints—in particular, the knee—at first presentation is predictive for a high level of radiological destruction of the small joints in rheumatoid arthritis. *Ann Rheum Dis* 2007;66(5):646–50.

80. van der Helm-van Mil AH, Detert J, le Cessie S, et al. Validation of a prediction rule for disease outcome in patients with recent-onset undifferentiated arthritis: moving toward individualized treatment decision-making. *Arthritis Rheum* 2008;58(8):2241–7.

81. Nam JL, Hunt L, Hensor EMA, Emery P. Enriching case selection for imminent RA: the use of anti-CCP antibodies in individuals with new non-specific musculoskeletal symptoms—a cohort study. *Ann Rheum Dis* 2016;75(8):1452.

82. Stack RJ, van Tuyl LH, Sloots M, et al. Symptom complexes in patients with seropositive arthralgia and in patients newly diagnosed with rheumatoid arthritis: a qualitative exploration of symptom development. *Rheumatology (Oxf)* 2014;53(9):1646–53.

83. van Tuyl LH, Stack RJ, Sloots M, et al. Impact of symptoms on daily life in people at risk of rheumatoid arthritis. *Musculoskeletal Care* 2016;14(3):169–73.

84. Newsum EC, van der Helm-van Mil AH, Kaptein AA. Views on clinically suspect arthralgia: a focus group study. *Clin Rheumatol* 2016;35(5):1347–52.

85. Ten Brinck RM, van Steenbergen HW, Mangnus L, et al. Functional limitations in the phase of clinically suspect arthralgia are as serious as in early clinical arthritis; a longitudinal study. *RMD Open* 2017;3(1):e000419.

86. Wajed MA, Brown DL, Currey HL. Palindromic rheumatism. Clinical and serum complement study. *Ann Rheum Dis* 1977;36(1):56–61.

87. Koskinen E, Hannonen P, Sokka T. Palindromic rheumatism: long-term outcomes of 60 patients diagnosed in 1967–84. *J Rheumatol* 2009;36(9):1873–5.

88. Latif ZP, Stack RJ, Keenan A-M, et al. A qualitative exploration of the symptoms experienced by people with palindromic rheumatism. *Rheumatology* 2016;55(suppl_1):i108–i9.

89. van Beers-Tas MH, Ter Wee MM, van Tuyl LH, et al. Initial validation and results of the Symptoms in Persons At Risk of Rheumatoid Arthritis (SPARRA) questionnaire: a EULAR project. *RMD Open* 2018 May 21;4(1):e000641.

90. Krabben A, Stomp W, van der Heijde DMFM, et al. MRI of hand and foot joints of patients with anticitrullinated peptide antibody positive arthralgia without clinical arthritis. *Ann Rheum Dis* 2013;72(9):1540.

91. van Steenbergen HW, van Nies JA, Huizinga TW, Reijnierse M, van der Helm-van Mil AH. Subclinical inflammation on MRI of hand and foot of anticitrullinated peptide antibody-negative arthralgia patients at risk for rheumatoid arthritis. *Arthritis Res Ther* 2014;16(2):R92.

92. Gent YY, Ter Wee MM, Ahmadi N, et al. Three-year clinical outcome following baseline magnetic resonance imaging in anticitrullinated protein antibody-positive arthralgia patients: an exploratory study. *Arthritis Rheumatol* 2014;66(10):2909–10.

93. Mangnus L, van Steenbergen HW, Reijnierse M, van der Helm-van Mil AH. Magnetic resonance imaging-detected features of inflammation and erosions in symptom-free persons from the general population. *Arthritis Rheumatol* 2016;68(11):2593–602.

94. Nam JL, Hensor EMA, Hunt L, Conaghan PG, Wakefield RJ, Emery P. Ultrasound findings predict progression to inflammatory arthritis in anti-CCP antibody-positive patients without clinical synovitis. *Ann Rheum Dis* 2016;*75*(12):2060.

95. van de Stadt LA, Bos WH, Meursinge Reynders M, et al. The value of ultrasonography in predicting arthritis in auto-antibody positive arthralgia patients: a prospective cohort study. *Arthritis Res Therapy* 2010;*12*(3):R98.

96. Gent YY, Voskuyl AE, Kloet RW, et al. Macrophage positron emission tomography imaging as a biomarker for preclinical rheumatoid arthritis: findings of a prospective pilot study. *Arthritis Rheum* 2012;*64*(1):62–6.

97. de Hair MJ, van de Sande MG, Ramwadhdoebe TH, et al. Features of the synovium of individuals at risk of developing rheumatoid arthritis: implications for understanding preclinical rheumatoid arthritis. *Arthritis Rheumatol* 2014;*66*(3):513–22.

98. Wigerblad G, Bas DB, Fernades-Cerqueira C, et al. Autoantibodies to citrullinated proteins induce joint pain independent of inflammation via a chemokine-dependent mechanism. *Ann Rheum Dis* 2016;*75*(4):730.

99. Edwards CJ, Cooper C. Early environmental factors and rheumatoid arthritis. *Clin Exp Immunol* 2006;*143*(1):1–5.

100. Catrina AI, Joshua V, Klareskog L, Malmstrom V. Mechanisms involved in triggering rheumatoid arthritis. *Immunol Rev* 2016;*269*(1):162–74.

101. McGrath CM, Young SP. Lipid and metabolic changes in rheumatoid arthritis. *Curr Rheumatol Rep* 2015;*17*(9):57.

102. Gwinnutt JM, Symmons DPM, MacGregor AJ, et al. Twenty-year outcome and association between early treatment and mortality and disability in an inception cohort of patients with rheumatoid arthritis: results from the Norfolk arthritis register. *Arthritis Rheumatol* 2017;*69*(8):1566–75.

103. Dumitru RB, Horton S, Hodgson R, et al. A prospective, single-centre, randomised study evaluating the clinical, imaging and immunological depth of remission achieved by very early versus delayed etanercept in patients with rheumatoid arthritis (VEDERA). *BMC Musculoskelet Disord* 2016;*17*:61.

104. Hugues B, Hilliquin S, Mitrovic S, Gossec L, Fautrel B. OP0011 Does a very early therapeutic intervention in very early arthritis/pre-rheumatoid arthritis patients prevent the onset of rheumatoid arthritis: a systematic review and metanalysis. *Ann Rheum Dis* 2017;*76*(Suppl 2):54.

105. Bos WH, Dijkmans BA, Boers M, van de Stadt RJ, van Schaardenburg D. Effect of dexamethasone on autoantibody levels and arthritis development in patients with arthralgia: a randomised trial. *Ann Rheum Dis* 2010;*69*(3):571–4.

106. Gerlag DM, Safy M, Maijer KI, et al. Effects of B-cell directed therapy on the preclinical stage of rheumatoid arthritis: the PRAIRI study. *Ann Rheum Dis* 2019 Feb;*78*(2):179–85. doi: 10.1136/annrheumdis-2017-212763. Epub 2018 Dec 1.

107. Phillips BE, Garciafigueroa Y, Trucco M, Giannoukakis N. Clinical tolerogenic dendritic cells: exploring therapeutic impact on human autoimmune disease. *Front Immunol* 2017;*8*:1279.

108. Rakieh C, Nam JL, Hunt L, et al. Predicting the development of clinical arthritis in anti-CCP positive individuals with non-specific musculoskeletal symptoms: a prospective observational cohort study. *Ann Rheum Dis* 2015;*74*(9):1659–66.

13

Non-articular manifestations of rheumatoid arthritis

Katherine Macdonald, Jennifer Hannah, and James Galloway

Introduction

Rheumatoid arthritis (RA) is a systemic disease that while primarily affecting joints, can also involve multiple organs of body including the lungs, heart, and blood vessels, bone, muscle, skin, central and peripheral nervous system, and bone marrow. In addition, RA impacts upon mental health and mood. The process by which extra-articular organs are involved is less well understood than the articular manifestations, but most effects are thought to be driven by similar immune disturbances that drive the disease of the synovium.

The 10-year cumulative incidence of any non-articular manifestation is approximately 50%, although severe manifestations are less than 10%.[1] With the changing therapeutic landscape of RA, it could be anticipated that the incidence of these manifestations would decline but with the exception of vasculitis, this does not appear to be the case as yet.[2,3] The non-articular manifestations of RA remain a common complication of the disease that account for substantial morbidity and mortality.[4]

Common risk factors for non-articular manifestations include elevated rheumatoid factor (RhF) and anticyclic citrullinated peptide (ACPA); *HLA-DRB1* gene positivity; increased age; smoking and early functional impairment.[5]

Pulmonary disease

Respiratory symptoms in RA are an important contributor to morbidity and mortality. Respiratory involvement may be attributed to pathology affecting the parenchyma, pleura, airways, or blood vessels. Rheumatoid nodules, often asymptomatic, can develop in almost any pulmonary structure, causing diagnostic uncertainty as appearances may mimic malignancy.

Most patients with RA who develop lung manifestations will do so within the first 5 years of the disease, although in a minority of people respiratory features may precede the onset of articular disease.[6,7]

Drugs used in the treatment of patients with RA can increase the risk of infection and historically have also been implicated in the development of interstitial lung disease (ILD), although this latter association is no longer considered to be causal.[8,9]

Interstitial lung disease

ILD is the most frequent pulmonary manifestation of RA. RA associated-ILD (RA-ILD) occurs more frequently in males, in contrast to the female overall predominance of RA.[10] The exact prevalence depends upon the how aggressively lung disease is screened for. For example, if all patients are screened with high-resolution computed tomography (HRCT) imaging, lung function studies, and bronchoalveolar lavage, then over half of early RA patients having detectable changes, although only around 10% patients will have symptomatic disease.[11,12]

ILD has numerous subtypes and understanding these can help connect the clinical features and prognosis. Appreciation of the ILD subtype can also inform treatment decisions.

The historic gold standard for the diagnosis of ILD is histology, however, in the absence of clinical suspicion for infection or other respiratory pathology, HRCT has become the mainstay of diagnosis for RA-ILD. The patterns of ILD observed in RA, comparing clinical features, histology, and HRCT findings are shown in Table 13.1. The most common subtype is usual interstitial pneumonia (UIP), which occurs in around 50% of cases.[13,14] This is a different from other connective tissue disorders, in which a non-specific interstitial pneumonia (NSIP) pattern is more frequently. NSIP accounts for around 25% of RA-ILD.[9,15,16]

Other patterns less commonly seen in RA include other forms of interstitial pneumonia, such as organizing pneumonia (OP), respiratory bronchiolitis (RB), lymphocytic interstitial pneumonia (LIP), desquamative interstitial pneumonia (DIP)-like patterns, and diffuse alveolar damage (DAD).

Typically, RA-ILD presents in older patients (i.e. sixth to seventh decade) and arthritis predates onset of lung disease in over 80% patients.[9] RA-ILD presents in a similar pattern as idiopathic ILD and patients experience insidious onset dyspnoea and non-productive cough.

Examination findings include bibasilar crackles, and over time signs of pulmonary hypertension can develop in RA-ILD. Clubbing is less common than in idiopathic ILD patients. There is no gold-standard diagnostic test for ILD therefore it is necessary to consider the clinical picture, alongside results from investigations such as pulmonary function tests (PFT), the 6-minute walk

Table 13.1 Patterns of RA-associated ILD (RA-ILD)

Clinical diagnosis	Pathological pattern	Radiological features	Clinical notes
Idiopathic pulmonary fibrosis (IPF)	Usual interstitial pneumonia (UIP)	Subpleural, basal predominant, reticular abnormalities with honeycombing, and traction bronchiectasis. Relative absence of ground-glass opacities.	Insidious onset. Cough common. Role of immunosuppression unclear.
Non-specific interstitial pneumonia (NSIP)	Non-specific interstitial pneumonia (NSIP)	Basilar predominant ground-glass opacities and absence of honeycombing.	Insidious onset. May be asymptomatic. Can respond to glucocorticoid/immunosuppressive therapy.
Cryptogenic organizing pneumonia (COP)	Organizing pneumonia (OP)	Multifocal patchy consolidation with subpleural and peribronchial distribution. Reverse halo sign (atoll sign) highly specific, although only seen in 20%.	Presentation similar to pneumonic illness (acute onset, fevers, cough). Can respond to glucocorticoid/immunosuppressive therapy.
Respiratory bronchiolitis interstitial lung disease (RBILD)	Respiratory bronchiolitis (RB)	Ground-glass opacification, any zone. Poorly defined centrilobular nodules may be present.	Progressive shortness of breath and chronic cough. Smoking strongly associated. RBILD and DIP have very similar histological and clinical appearances and may represent a common process. Unclear role of immunosuppression, but smoking cessation essential.
Desquamative interstitial pneumonia (DIP)	Desquamative interstitial pneumonia (DIP)	Similar to RB with ground-glass opacification. Sometimes more diffuse.	
Lymphoid interstitial pneumonia (LIP)	Lymphoid interstitial pneumonia (LIP)	Ground-glass opacification, centrilobular and subpleural nodules, no lymphadenopathy.	Form of pulmonary lymphoproliferative disease; variable disease course ranging from indolent to aggressive with potential transformation to pulmonary lymphoma. Associated with concurrent Sjogren's syndrome.
Acute interstitial pneumonia (AIP)	Diffuse alveolar damage (DAD)	Appearances similar to acute respiratory distress syndrome.	Acute presentation, productive cough, fever. Rapid deterioration common. Immunosuppression usually used, although evidence of benefit lacking.

Source: data from American Thoracic Society/European Respiratory Society International Multidisciplinary Consensus Classification of the Idiopathic Interstitial Pneumonias (2002) *Am J Respir Crit Care Med* 165(2) 277–304.

test, imaging, and bronchoscopy. PFTs typically show reduced lung volume and diffusion capacity. The 6-minute walk test may show reduced peak oxygen uptake and exercise induce hypoxaemia. Chest radiography in patients with advanced disease may demonstrate bibasilar ground-glass opacities, reticular and nodular opacities, or honeycombing. HRCT imaging is particularly useful to differentiate the category of ILD, based on patterns and distribution (see Table 13.1), and to track rate of progression and monitor response to treatment. Bronchoalveolar lavage can be of use if the clinical picture or investigations are not characteristic and may be necessary to exclude opportunistic or atypical infections, eosinophilic pneumonia, or alveolar haemorrhage. It can also have a role in investigating malignancy.

Management of RA-ILD

The decision to treat should be based on the categories of ILD, prognosis, and discussion with the patient about risks and benefits of treatment. In patients with non-progressive mild disease, the treatment focus should be as per standard RA management strategies. Impacts of Disease-modifying antirheumatic drugs (DMARDs) and biologic therapy remains uncertain, though expert consensus is to suppress systemic inflammation as much as possible. Cohort studies consistently show that ILD corresponds with RA disease severity and activity.[17] RA-ILD phenotypes which are more likely to respond to glucocorticoid and immunosuppressive treatment include OP, NSIP, and LIP.

To date, there have been no published randomized controlled trials comparing medications for the treatment of RA lung disease (although there are several on going at the time of writing). Corticosteroids (e.g. prednisolone 0.5 mg/kg) have remained the

mainstay of therapy, particularly for cases of NSIP or OP where corticosteroid treatment may lead to regression of consolidation and potential clinical improvement.[15]

Where there is evidence of progressive ILD, particularly of one of the worse prognosis phenotypes in younger patients, then there is a rationale for more aggressive treatment.

Cyclophosphamide and azathioprine were historically the agents of choice for RA-ILD,[18] although more recent trends have shifted towards the use of mycophenolate, in large part based upon the experience of these drugs in other rheumatic disease related ILD.[19,20]

Most experts consider rituximab or abatacept as first-line biologics in this setting. Rituximab is a B-cell depleting biologic that has been preferentially used by many clinicians for the treatment of RA in individuals with ILD. The rationale for using rituximab in patients with ILD was in part due to possible pulmonary toxicity with the antitumour necrosis factor (TNF) class,[8] as well as the successful use of rituximab in other systemic autoimmune diseases.[21,22] Growing evidence from observational studies has emerged more recently for the effective role of abatacept in RA-ILD.[23]

Methotrexate, a first-line agent in the treatment of RA joint disease, is known to be associated with drug-induced pneumonitis, but fortunately this is rare. However, there is no evidence that this agent leads to progression of ILD. Following 6 weeks of treatment with high-dose steroids, one research group found that treatment with methotrexate versus leflunomide or azathioprine was actually associated with an improvement in forced vital capacity (FVC) at 6 months among patients with less? fibrosis.[24] In addition, a large longitudinal cohort study saw no association between drug choice (including methotrexate) and ILD.[25] These data suggest that methotrexate use is not associated with poorer outcomes than other antirheumatic drugs.[24]

Adjuvant therapy for RA-ILD includes smoking cessation, management of gastro-oesophageal reflux disease, referral to pulmonary rehabilitation, supplemental oxygen, and vaccination against influenza and pneumococcal disease. In the absence of active RA, patients with RA lung disease who fail to respond to therapy should be considered for lung transplant. In patients with a UIP pattern, work-up for transplant should be considered early. A retrospective review of Canadian patients with advanced lung disease found no difference in outcomes between patients with RA-ILD and those with idiopathic pulmonary fibrosis (IPF) at 1 year following lung transplant, suggesting that transplant is a reasonable option for these patients.[26]

Prognosis

ILD is second only to cardiac disease as a cause of mortality in RA. In patients with RA-ILD, the five-year survival is approximately 60%.[27] Additional risk factors for mortality include advanced age, male sex, UIP pattern and extent of fibrosis on imaging or histopathology, and low gas transfer.[28] However, RA-ILD does appear to have a better prognosis when compared to similar patterns in non-connective tissue disease-associated ILD.[29]

Pleural lung disease

Patients are rarely symptomatic from pleural lung disease-associated with RA. Pleural lung disease is most common in patients with long standing RA and those with nodulosis. In post-mortem studies, over half of RA patients have some evidence of pleural disease.[30]

The classic pleural manifestation in RA is a unilateral exudative effusion.[31] The most useful test to differentiate between the different types of effusion is thoracentesis, and fluid should be sent for cell counts, protein, glucose, lactate dehydrogenase (LDH), cholesterol, microscopy, and culture and cytology. Exudative rheumatoid effusions have biochemical values consistent with the following: White cell count (WCC) <5000 /mm, fluid glucose <60 mg/dL or fluid to serum glucose ratio <0.5, pH <7.3, high pleural LDH (>700).

Rheumatoid effusions usually resolve spontaneously although therapeutic thoracentesis and corticosteroids can be considered as treatment options.[31]

In the era of biologic therapy, evidence of pleural lung disease should prompt investigation for infectious complications, notably tuberculosis which can manifest a very similar pattern of pleural disease. Tuberculoid effusions can also spontaneously regress, which may cloud the clinical picture.

Airway diseases

Cricoarytenoid arthritis, rheumatoid nodules on the vocal cords and vasculitis of the recurrent laryngeal or vagus nerve can result in upper airway obstruction.[32] Flow volume loops, HRCT, and laryngoscopy may be useful in distinguishing between these diagnoses.[33] Upper airway obstruction from cricoarytenoiditis can be life-threatening, so early involvement of ears, nose, and throat (ENT) and anaesthetic input is advised.[33]

Bronchiectasis has been reported in up to 30% of patients with RA, but is usually not clinically significant.[33] A more serious bronchiolar disease for RA patients is obliterative bronchiolitis which describes progressive concentric narrowing of membranous bronchioles

and is rare but usually fatal. Patients present acutely with cough, shortness of breath, and hypoxia. Examination reveals inspiratory crackles and classically a mid-inspiratory squeak. HRCT is useful for diagnosis, which confirms bronchial wall thickening, centrilobular emphysema, areas of low attenuation, a mosaic pattern, and bronchiectasis. Treatment consists of reviewing medication for triggers, trial of high-dose corticosteroids, and immunosuppression, though response is generally poor.[34]

Follicular bronchiolitis is hyperplasia of bronchus-associated lymphoid tissue and occurs in patients with high RhF titres. Patients present with fever, cough, dyspnoea, and may have both an obstructive and restrictive picture on PFTs. Management is aimed at treating the underlying condition and prognosis is usually good compared to obliterative bronchiolitis.[33]

Rheumatoid lung nodules

Rheumatoid nodules can occur in the lung (**Figure 13.1**) as well as elsewhere in the body. Lung rheumatoid nodules tend to occur in patients with subcutaneous rheumatoid nodules who have had the disease for a long duration. The prevalence is unclear partly because most patients are asymptomatic, and rheumatoid nodules are not visualized on chest radiography. Lung biopsy studies have demonstrated they are more common than previously thought and, in one study, were present in 13 of 40 biopsies performed.[35] They can range in size and number and are usually seen around the subpleural and interlobular septa. Histologically they resemble rheumatoid nodules seen elsewhere, and show central necrosis with palisading epithelioid cells and mononuclear cells (**Figure 13.2**).[36,37] It is important to exclude non-small cell lung cancer particularly in patients who smoke; positron emission tomography (PET) is useful in this instance. Patients are rarely symptomatic, and nodules respond to treatment for RA or resolve spontaneously.

Caplan syndrome describes RA with pneumoconiosis related to occupational dust exposure.[38] Progressive massive fibrosis can develop. The nodules can be distinguished from usual rheumatoid nodules by the layer of dust surrounding the central necrotic area. Caplan syndrome was most commonly seen among coal miners and is now thankfully rare.

Other pulmonary associations

Pulmonary hypertension can occur in patients with RA. While this is usually secondary to ILD, isolated pulmonary hypertension has also been described. Rarely pulmonary arterial hypertension related to vasculitis is seen. Studies have shown that over 20% of RA patients show asymptomatic, elevated estimated pulmonary artery pressures on echocardiogram (ECHO) even in the absence of clinically significant heart or lung disease.[39] Potentially, exertional dyspnoea symptoms go unnoticed by RA patients due to reduced mobility and exercise tolerance due to articular disease.

Venous thromboembolism risk (both deep vein thrombosis and pulmonary thromboembolism) is increased twofold in patients with RA, with the risk being highest in those with more severe extra-articular disease.[40,41]

Meta-analysis suggests that RA patients have an overall 5% increase risk of cancer compared to the general population, although how much of this is due to the disease activity, treatment, or shared risk factors (e.g. smoking) is hard to unpick.[42] Cancer risk is site specific, there appears to be a 1.5–2.5 fold increase risk in lung cancer

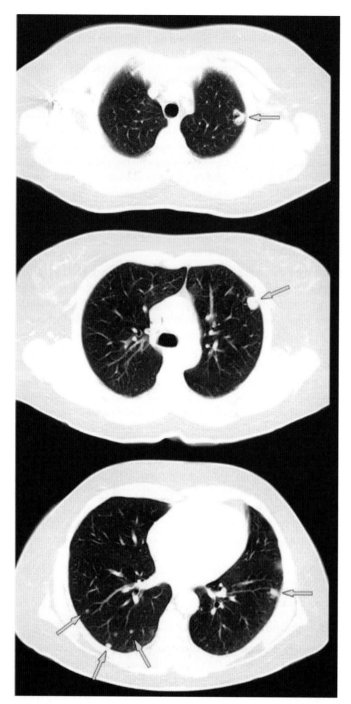

Figure 13.1 Rheumatoid lung nodules varying in size from millimetres to centimetres, mainly found on the peripheral fields of both lungs, some of them with a central cavity (arrows).

Reprinted from Andres M, Paloma V, and Romera C (2012) 'Marked improvement of lung rheumatoid nodules after treatment with tocilizumab'. *Rheumatology* 51(6) 1132–4 with permission from Oxford University Press.

and a twofold increased risk in lymphoma, but a reduced risk of breast or colorectal cancer.[43]

Infection

An important differential in a patient presenting with symptoms of lung disease is infection. With the advent of biologic therapy and immunosuppressive drugs, patients are at an increased risk of

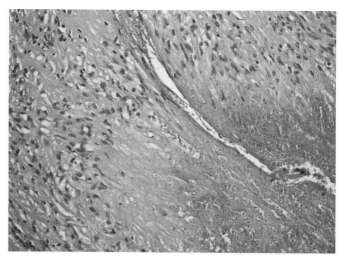

Figure 13.2 Pleural rheumatoid nodule showing granulomatous pleural inflammation, fibrinous exudate, palisading histiocytes, and scattered multinucleated giant cells.

Reprinted from Saravana, S., et al. (2003) 'Spontaneous pneumothorax: an unusual presentation of rheumatoid arthritis'. *Rheumatology* 42(11): 1415–16 with permission from Oxford University Press.

infection and wider consideration of atypical infections is required. Infection may present in conjunction with an underlying lung disease. Opportunistic infections such as *Pneumocystis jirovecii* (PCP), new and reactivated tuberculosis, non-tuberculosis mycobacterium and fungal infections (histoplasmosis, coccidioidomycosis, cryptococcosis, sporotrichosis) may present atypically. In patients on immunosuppressive agents, fever and leucocytosis may not be present, further complicating diagnosis of opportunistic infection.

Tuberculosis reactivation has been observed with all the targeted therapies, although the risk appears lowest with B-cell depletion (e.g. rituximab).[44] It is therefore advisable to screen all patients for latent tuberculosis prior to starting therapy. The incidence of PCP has similarly been reported across the breadth of targeted therapies, although the highest rate was reported for rituximab.[44] When starting aggressive immunosuppressive regimens such as cyclophosphamide, it is recommended to consider PCP prophylaxis with an agent such as co-trimoxazole. However, the risk of PCP with any of the targeted therapies (including rituximab) is well below the risk threshold to justify prophylaxis.[45] Other fungal diseases are rare, except where there are endemic species, such as coccidioidomycosis in the southwestern United States.

Drug-induced lung disease in RA

Aside from the increased risk of lung infection conferred by all immunosuppressive therapy, certain drugs used in RA are associated with lung disease. Features that may increase suspicion of drug-induced lung disease include eosinophilia in blood or bronchoalveolar lavage, rash, and improvement on withdrawing the treatment. There are case reports of leflunomide causing accelerated nodule formation.[46] Rarely pulmonary toxicity has been reported with biologic agents.[47] Sulfasalazine can be associated with a drug reaction with eosinophilia and systemic symptoms (DRESS).

Historic studies have reported methotrexate as a risk for lung fibrosis, but this is no longer thought to be the case. The original observation was due to channelling bias and confounding by indication. A meta-analysis has subsequently shown that receiving methotrexate does not increase risk of death due to lung disease or non-infectious respiratory events.[48]

Cardiovascular disease

RA can be associated with several cardiac complications and with non-cardiac vascular disease such as rheumatoid vasculitis.

Coronary artery disease (CAD)

An important extra-articular manifestation of RA is coronary artery disease (CAD). The increased risk of premature death in RA patients can be mostly attributed to CAD. CAD is not only more frequent in RA patients compared to the general population, but mortality attributable to cardiac events is also greater in RA patients. Meta-analysis of 24 studies with 111 758 patients reported CAD mortality with 59% higher frequency in RA patients compared to the general population.[49] The underlying mechanism for this is thought to be a combination of increased prevalence of traditional risk factors (particularly smoking), as well as acceleration of atherosclerosis from cytokines, inflammatory cells, coagulation abnormalities, and oxidative stress.[50]

There is a well-established lipid paradox in RA, where despite the increased cardiovascular risk, patients with active untreated RA have reduced total cholesterol (TCh), low-density lipoprotein cholesterol (LDL) and high-density lipoprotein cholesterol (HDL) levels.[51] In parallel to this, many effective treatments for RA increase lipid levels while being simultaneously associated with a reduction in cardiovascular risk.[52]

Patients present similarly to patients without RA though some studies have found that RA patients are less likely to report chest pain and present with clinically silent CAD.[53] This highlights the importance of yearly cardiovascular screening. Ensuring patients are aware of the risk of CAD and the need for adjusting modifiable risk factors is vital. Lifestyle factors such as smoking cessation, diet, and tailored exercise advice should be provided. Lipid lowering therapy and blood pressure control may be indicated. Currently there is insufficient evidence that RA is an indication in itself to initiate statins.

The most important role a rheumatologist can take in reducing CAD risk in RA is to ensure adequate control of inflammation, as there is strong evidence that reducing disease activity is associated with fewer cardiac events.[54] The caveat to this is that steroids may be detrimental.

Heart failure

Several studies have demonstrated an increased risk of both symptomatic heart failure and asymptomatic left ventricular diastolic function in RA patients compared to the general population.[55] The pathogenesis is unclear though probably involves inflammatory mediators and ischaemic heart disease. The role of antirheumatic drugs has also been recognized, in particular non-steroidal anti-inflammatory drugs (NSAIDS), chloroquine, hydroxychloroquine, and glucocorticoids. Patients with RA may already have reduced mobility and therefore do not report exertional symptoms as frequently.

The approach to management of heart failure is similar to patients without RA. In patients with New York Heart Association (NYHA) class III or IV, avoidance of anti-TNF therapies is advisable, based upon the negative outcomes observed in anti-TNF trials conducted to test the efficacy of TNF inhibition for heart failure.[56] NSAIDS and COX-2 inhibitors can also worsen pre-existing heart disease and should be avoided.

Pericarditis and myocarditis

Symptomatic pericarditis in patients with RA is uncommon although studies that have looked at ECHO findings report a higher incidence of pericarditis (Figure 13.3).[57,58] Episodes usually occur during active rheumatoid arthritis. Pericarditis causing tamponade is uncommon and alternate diagnoses, such as infection or lymphoma, should be sought. When RA is confirmed as the cause of pericardial disease, management is aimed at controlling active disease.

Myocarditis is rare, though both granulomatous and interstitial disease can occur. Again, this tends to be in the context of active disease. ECHO should be performed to look for left ventricular failure. Cardiac Magnetic resonance imaging (MRI) is becoming increasingly instrumental in diagnosis. Differentials to consider are ischaemic cardiomyopathy, drug-induced myopathy, rheumatoid nodules, and rarely amyloidosis. If the diagnosis of rheumatoid associated myocarditis is certain, a ventricular biopsy may be required. High-dose methylprednisolone can be trialled, but the role of other therapies is unclear.

Other cardiac manifestations

There are cases of rheumatoid cardiac nodules on pericardium, myocardium, and valvular structures. ECHO is useful in diagnosis. Rarely are they symptomatic but there are case reports of heart block.[59]

Rheumatoid vasculitis

Rheumatoid vasculitis (RV) is an inflammatory process of the blood vessel that can occur in patients who have had protracted, severe RA. Since the introduction of more intensive DMARD strategies and targeted therapies RV prevalence has declined significantly.[2] There are several manifestations from mild skin changes to severe systemic inflammation involving both small and medium-sized vessels the presentation of which can be similar to polyarteritis nodosa (PAN). Severe RV requires intensive immunosuppressive treatment.

The presentation varies depending on the systems involved. Classically RV was thought to present when RA was in a period of 'burn-out', although this is probably a misnomer as on ultrasound most patients have active synovitis that is not apparent on clinical examination. Figure 13.4 demonstrates some of the cutaneous manifestations which include infarcts, ulcers, purpura, and gangrene.[60] The more severe form typically presents with constitutional symptoms of fever, weight loss, and fatigue. If neuropathy does present it is usually a mononeuritis multiplex or peripheral neuropathy. Central nervous system (CNS) involvement is rare, and stroke should not be attributed to RV, though can occur. Scleritis and peripheral ulcerative keratitis are sometimes seen. Cardiac manifestations include pericarditis, myocardial infarction, and aortic incompetence but cohort studies suggest these clinical features are less common.[61]

Diagnosis of RV is ideally based on a positive tissue biopsy in the context of a very high serum RhF. Common findings of routine

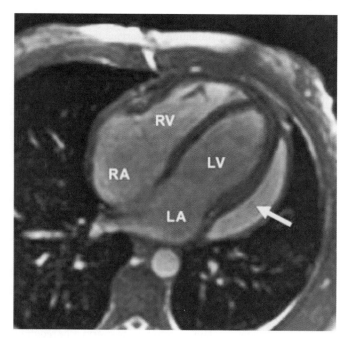

Figure 13.3 Cardiac magnetic resonance image showing constrictive pericarditis in a patient with nodular and erosive rheumatoid arthritis. Right and left ventricles (RV and LV) and right and left atria (RA and LA) are labelled. The arrow points at the pericardial effusion.

Reprinted from Aslangul, E., et al. (2005). 'Successful etanercept treatment of constrictive pericarditis complicating rheumatoid arthritis'. *Rheumatology* 44(12): 1581–3 with permission from Oxford University Press.

blood results would be a high erythrocyte sedimentation rate (ESR) and C-reactive protein (CRP), thrombocytosis, hypoalbuminaemia, and anaemia.[62] ACPA is useful as this is generally negative in other vasculitides but positive in RV. If both RhF and ACPA are negative an alternate diagnosis should be sought. PAN is histopathologically indistinguishable though two features that would indicate RV would be a history of erosive joint disease and a lack of microaneurysms. Obtaining a definitive biopsy, for example, from skin, affected nerve, muscle, kidney, or salivary gland is vital. The differentials to consider are the same as other mimics of vasculitic disease and include infective endocarditis, thromboembolic disease, lymphoma (including intravascular forms), and paraneoplastic phenomena.

Nervous system involvement

Nerve involvement may occur because of compression directly from swellings, for example synovitis, joint deformity, or pannus. Nerve involvement from RV associated neuropathy is rare and is covered earlier in this chapter.

CNS

Cervical myelopathy may result from atlantoaxial subluxation, atlantoaxial impaction, or subaxial subluxation. Joint destruction occurs due to inflammation of neurocentral joints, instability of apophyseal joints, or laxity of transfer ligament. Most commonly there is anterior movement of the atlas, but subluxation can occur in any direction and rotationally. Subluxation is typically seen in older patients with extensive erosive joint disease.[63] Anterior atlantoaxial subluxation can be detected using plain film radiographs of the cervical spine in flexion and neutral views (Figure 13.5),[64] and is considered to be present if the atlanto-dens interval is greater than 2.5 mm in women and 3 mm in men.[65]

The presenting complaint is normally pain radiating to the occiput. Slow painless sensory loss is a concerning symptom suggestive of evolving quadriparesis. Several symptoms warrant urgent attention, and this includes the sensation of the head falling forward during anterior cervical flexion, changes in consciousness level, drop attacks, loss of sphincter control, respiratory dysfunction suggestive of transient medullary dysfunction, dysarthria, dysphagia, vertigo, convulsion, hemiplegia, nystagmus, peripheral paraesthesia, Lhermitte's sign, imbalance, and hand miscoordination.[66] Examination findings will depend on the extent of cord compression and upper motor neuron signs such as increased tendon reflexes, spasticity, and extensor plantar response are concerning. Radiculopathy may result in reduced tendon reflexes. The malalignment of the atlas can sometime be palpated. MRI is useful in establishing the extent of deformity and compression although radiographic findings do not always correlate symptomatically. Progression in not inevitable though patients with signs of cord compression have a poor prognosis without surgical intervention. Other management strategies include rigid cervical collars which can protect against minor accidents that could precipitate cord compression.

Less frequent conditions involving the CNS in RA patients include rheumatoid meningitis, progressive multifocal leukoencephalopathy from JC virus (estimated to occur in 1 in 25 000 RA patients exposed to rituximab),[67] rheumatoid nodules involving the spinal cord, hyperviscosity syndrome, and ischaemic stroke.

Peripheral nervous system

Compression neuropathies are the most common neurological manifestation of RA and can arise from joint deformity, synovitic enlargement, or inflamed ligaments. Carpal tunnel syndrome and tarsal tunnel syndrome are common and present with pain and paraesthesia in the median nerve and posterior tibial nerve respectively. Posterior tibial nerve involvement causes symptoms in the sole of the foot and first, second, and third toes. Atrophy of the intrinsic foot muscles may occur. Anterior and posterior interosseous, ulnar, common peroneal, and tibial are other common sites of compression neuropathy.[68] EMG/NCS are useful though patients may have changes without symptoms. MRI and ultrasound will help evaluate the cause of compression. As in patients without RA, splinting and steroid injections may alleviate some of the symptoms and decompression should be considered if symptoms are severe.

Non-compression neuropathies

Mild distal sensory and combined sensorimotor neuropathy are uncommon. Combined sensorimotor neuropathy may be seen in the context of RV which is discussed earlier in this chapter.

Neuromuscular disorders

Muscle weakness is a frequent occurrence. Myopathy from disuse atrophy from pain is common and should be treated by managing the underlying condition, controlling the pain, and tailored exercise. Denervation atrophy in the context of mononeuritis multiplex in a RV picture may occur and muscle inflammation may be seen

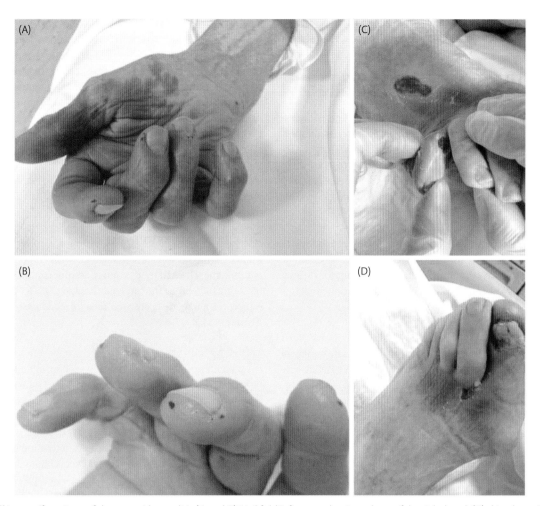

Figure 13.4 Skin manifestations of rheumatoid vasculitis (A and B) Nail fold infarcts and pointy ulcers of the right hand; (C) skin ulceration on the top of the right foot and of the fifth toe; (D) ulcer between the first and the second toe of the left foot.

Reprinted from Cammelli, D. and G. Vitiello (2016). 'A case of rheumatoid vasculitis'. Rheumatology 55(6): 1126–1126 with permission from Oxford University Press.

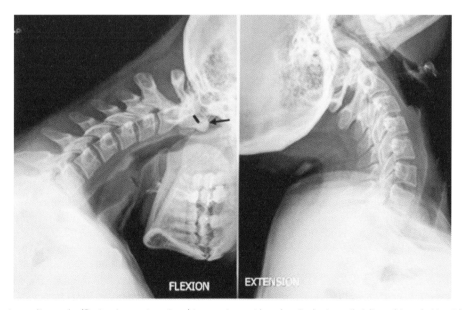

Figure 13.5 Cervical spine radiographs (flexion/extension views) in a patient with polyarticular juvenile idiopathic arthritis with anterior erosion of the odontoid process (arrow) and anterior atlantoaxial subluxation (black line) with an atlantodental interval equal to 9.3 mm

Reprinted from Elhai, M., et al. (2012). 'Radiological cervical spine involvement in young adults with polyarticular juvenile idiopathic arthritis'. *Rheumatology* 52(2): 267–75 with permission from Oxford University Press.

on biopsy. Steroid induced myopathy is an important differential to consider and typically presents with proximal muscle weakness.

Haematological abnormalities

Abnormal haematological indices are commonly encountered when managing RA patients. Both underlying inflammation and medications used in RA patients can cause minor haematological abnormalities for example mild leucocytosis and thrombocytosis are often seen with flares of disease, but more severe haematological complications can occur and physicians should be aware of these.

Anaemia

A low haemoglobin level in RA patients is most commonly due to anaemia of chronic disease, iron deficiency anaemia, or combination of the two. However, the clinician must be vigilant for rare associated haematological complications of RA such as bone marrow hypoplasia.

Anaemia of chronic disease (ACD)

ACD is typically a mild normocytic, normochromic anaemia, in which patients are asymptomatic. ACD tends to reflect RA disease activity and a study by Möller et al. found that radiographic progression increased with severity of anaemia.[69] Haematological indices typically reveal elevated serum ferritin and transferrin with low iron, although this may not be the case if there is coexisting iron deficiency anaemia. Bone marrow assessment may not be very helpful as findings are often non-specific or show haemosiderin deposition and normal cellularity. ACD should respond to control of RA. Tocilizumab, an IL-6 receptor inhibitor, has shown to be particularly effective in treating anaemias as IL-6 induces production of hepcidin, a critical regulator of iron metabolism.[70]

Iron deficiency anaemia (IDA)

IDA can occur in RA patients and should be managed similarly to the general population which involves identifying and addressing the underlying cause. Often medications such as NSAIDS are implicated and gastric protection should be considered in patients commencing NSAIDS.

Other causes of anaemia

Anaemia can develop as a side effect of medications used to treat RA patients. Macrocytic anaemia is known to be caused by methotrexate, sulfasalazine, and azathioprine. Bone marrow hypoplasia is a serious complication of RA, which can also occur because of medications such as azathioprine or cyclophosphamide.

More infrequent causes of anaemia include pure red cell aplasia. This presents with severe normocytic anaemia and a very low reticulocyte count and typically responds to immunosuppression. Haemolytic anaemia can occur in Felty's syndrome, discussed next.

Neutropenia

Felty's syndrome describes the triad of neutropenia, deforming RA, and splenomegaly that can occur in seropositive patients with longstanding disease. It is rare, with the incidence being less than 1% of RA patients.[71] Autoantibodies including Antineutrophil cytoplasmic antibodies (ANCA), Antinuclear antibodies (ANA), anti-dsDNA, antihistone antibody, and antiglucose 6 phosphate isomerase antibodies are commonly found. The mainstay of treatment for Felty's syndrome is management of the underlying RA, although there is evidence from case reports that rituximab may be of benefit.[72] It is important to exclude large granular lymphocyte leukaemia on a peripheral blood smear; immunophenotyping can distinguish between the two. Patients with large granular lymphocyte leukaemia may present with fatigue, B symptoms (fevers, night sweats, weight loss) or signs of infection, but some may be asymptomatic. RA patients with large granular lymphocyte leukaemia typically have the T-cell variant as supposed to the natural killer (NK) variant. The condition tends to be indolent with a median survival of over 10 years.[73]

Drug-induced neutropenia

Many RA medications are associated with reversible neutropenia. Among the DMARDs, the most commonly implicated agent is methotrexate. From the targeted therapies, TNF inhibitors, and IL-6 receptor antagonists are well recognized causes of drug-induced neutropenia.[74]

Lymphoproliferative disorders

RA patients are at increased risk of lymphoproliferative disorders, in particular non-Hodgkin's lymphomas (NHL) including diffuse large B-cell lymphoma.[75,76] The risk is strongly related to the cumulative burden of RA disease activity over time. Impaired T-cell function in RA may increase the risk of NHL by permitting the proliferation of oncogenic Epstein–Barr virus.[77] Apparent increased lymphoma rates seen in anti-TNF therapy may reflect channelling bias, whereby patients with the highest risk of lymphoma preferentially receive anti-TNF therapy because they will also have higher cumulative disease burden.[78]

Ocular and oral manifestations

Ocular involvement in RA patients is a relatively common occurrence.[79] Several conditions can be sight threatening, therefore early detection of these and referral to an ophthalmologist is critical. Cataracts and glaucoma can result from long-term glucocorticoid use.

Sjogren's and Sicca syndrome

Sicca syndrome describes the symptoms of keratoconjunctivitis (dry eyes) and xerostomia (dry mouth). Sjogren's syndrome describes these symptoms in the context of a positive salivary gland biopsy and positive associated autoantibodies (most commonly anti-Ro/SSA or anti-La/SSB). In the context of patients with RA this is called secondary Sjogren's syndrome, as opposed to primary when Sjogren's occurs in isolation. Both conditions are immune-mediated responses against salivary and lacrimal glands.

Patients will not necessarily present reporting dry eyes but might describe a gritty sensation, which is worse in dry or windy weather. Xerostomia might result in dysphagia and inability to eat dry food, change in taste, and poor dental hygiene. Dyspareunia and vaginal dryness can also occur as part of Sjogren's syndrome.

Examination may reveal enlarged salivary glands and this can be confirmed on ultrasound or MRI which may demonstrate glandular abnormalities. Schirmer's test is a well-tolerated investigation which involves placing a strip of filter paper in the patient's lower lid to measure tear production. A healthy subject would usually be able to produce enough moisture to spread 10 mm down the strip within 5 minutes, though the test is not particularly reliable. Histological tests are rarely required but would reveal lymphocytic infiltrate and ductal atrophy.

Symptoms of sicca does not equate to Sjogren's syndrome and other causes of dry eye should be consider including ageing, medication, sarcoid, infection, and lymphoproliferative disorders. Treatment options are supportive only, with limited evidence for effectiveness of immunomodulatory drugs. Patients should be educated in non-pharmacological management strategies including good eye and oral care. Additional artificial tears and saliva are sufficient for some patients. Alternative options include topical ciclosporin drops, pilocarpine, and punctual occlusion to prevent absorption of tears.[80] Patients with dry eyes are more susceptible to eye infections which should be treated promptly.

Episcleritis and scleritis

Episcleritis is common in RA patients and is usually self-limiting and benign, though may cause some discomfort. Vision is not affected. Scleritis manifests as severe eye pain, with pain on eye movements. It is a more sinister ocular manifestation of RA and has a poorer prognosis. RA patients that are affected tend to be older and frequently the condition it bilateral.[81] Diffuse anterior scleritis is the most common and least severe form whereas necrotizing scleritis is associated with a high risk to vision as well as significant mortality risk due to its association with systemic RV. Scleritis should be treated under the supervision of an ophthalmologist with topical immune suppression alongside systemic therapy to control the underlying RA. Scleritis can lead to visual loss due to contiguous uveitis, glaucoma, cataracts, damage to the posterior segment, and peripheral ulcerative keratitis (PUK).[81]

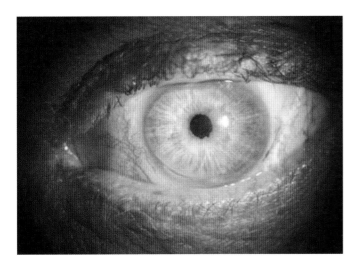

Figure 13.6 Corneal ulceration. Anterior segment photography of the left eye. Corneal ulceration is visible in the nasal inferior part of the cornea, with epithelial defect and corneal stromal thinning up to 60%.

Reprinted from Korsten, P., et al. (2017). 'Rapid healing of peripheral ulcerative keratitis in rheumatoid arthritis with prednisone, methotrexate and adalimumab combination therapy'. *Rheumatology* 56(7): 1094–1094 with permission from Oxford University Press.

Corneal disease

Corneal inflammation can lead to corneal melt which is the prelude to the serious complication of corneal perforation. PUK describes inflammation and crescent-shaped ulceration at the peripheral areas of the cornea (**Figure 13.6**).[82] In PUK high-dose systemic corticosteroids are essential and if vision is threatened pulsing with methylprednisolone is necessary. Calcineurin inhibitors, biologic therapies, and corneal transplantation are often used. Studies have previously reported a high mortality (over 50% 10-year mortality) following PUK mainly due to corresponding RV, however, these studies are mostly from the prebiologic era, so the prevalence and prognosis of PUK in recent years is less clear.[83] This condition should be managed in conjunction with an experienced ophthalmologist.

Cutaneous manifestation

Rheumatoid nodules are the most common extra-articular manifestation of RA. Rheumatoid nodules occur in seropositive patients and are associated with other extra-articular manifestations. Rheumatoid nodules are firm non-tender lumps in the subcutaneous tissue that can measure up to 5 cm. Typically, nodules occur over extensor surfaces, or areas of repetitive pressure or trauma, such as the elbow, but they can arise anywhere in the body.[84] Histology reveals central areas of necrosis surrounded by macrophages and lymphocytes. Nodulosis can occur in conjunction with geodes which are subchondral bone cysts.

Biopsy may be indicated if the diagnosis is uncertain or there is clinical suspicion a lesion could be a basal cell carcinoma. Specific treatment is rarely required though injection with glucocorticoids and local anaesthetic is sometimes used. Surgical excision can be performed if there is severe pain, compression, skin ulceration, or recurrent infections, but it is generally avoided due to the risk of recurrence.[84] Differentials include pseudo rheumatoid nodules called granuloma annulare, fibromas, sarcoidosis, xanthomastosis, ganglion, and tophi.

Other skin manifestations seen in patients with RA include: skin ulcers, which may occur due to venous stasis, arterial insufficiency, neutrophilic infiltrate, or vasculitis; neutrophilic dermatoses such as pyoderma gangrenosum, Sweet syndrome, rheumatoid neutrophilic dermatitis; manifestations of RV; medication induced skin changes; and rarely erythema elevatum diutinum, linear bands, annular lesions, urticarial eruptions, dermal papules.[85]

An increased risk of non-melanomatous skin cancers has been noted with both biological and conventional disease-modifying antirheumatic drugs compared to the general population, suggesting that monitoring for skin malignancies is important in RA.[86]

Bone

RA is a risk factor for osteoporosis which is driven by the chronic inflammatory state. Osteoporosis may be further worsened by exposure to corticosteroids. Hauser et al. identified that RA patients are at a 1.5–2-fold increase risk of osteopenia.[87] Several patterns of osteopenia have been recognized and this includes systemic, periarticular, and focal distributions the latter two being characteristic of RA. The traditional risk factors for osteopenia in the general population are relevant for RA patients.

Annual assessment of bone health should be part of routine RA care and screening tools such as fracture risk assessment tool (FRAX) score are appropriate for RA patients. Management should include lifestyle advice, optimization of vitamin D status, and bisphosphonates as indicated according to risk stratification.

Psychological manifestations

Depression and anxiety are common in RA patients. Estimates of prevalence vary with one systematic review finding one-third of patients with RA had depression.[88] Systemic inflammation may have a direct role on mood though the exact process is uncertain. Depression in RA is associated with low socioeconomic status, comorbidities, pain, and disability. Depression, in turn, is linked with worse disease activity score, poorer treatment responses, and increased RA mortality.[89,90]

Control of the RA disease activity alone seems insufficient to address the mental health impacts of RA. In a network meta-analysis exploring the impacts of biologic therapies on mental health outcomes in RA, the effect size of targeted therapies on mood was small, with no clear benefit of any one mode of action therapy over another.[91]

Conclusion

RA has a wide range of extra-articular manifestations, from asymptomatic to life-threatening. It is essential to consider RA as a systemic disease rather than just focusing on the musculoskeletal aspects.

Annual review of cardiovascular risk factors, bone health, and mental health is important to prevent future morbidity. It is vital to remain vigilant to the development of pulmonary, ocular, infectious, dermatological, or malignant complications. Controlling RA disease burden is the mainstay of management of most extra-articular manifestations, but immunomodulatory therapies come with additional specific risks which include opportunistic infections, malignancies, liver, and haematological abnormalities.

Working in close partnership with other specialties is valuable when looking after these complex patients.

REFERENCES

1. Myasoedova E, Crowson CS, Turesson C, Gabriel SE, Matteson EL. Incidence of extraarticular rheumatoid arthritis in Olmsted County, Minnesota, in 1995–2007 versus 1985–1994: a population-based study. *J Rheumatol* 2011:38(6):983–9.
2. Watts R, Mooney J, Lane S, Scott D. Rheumatoid vasculitis: becoming extinct? *Rheumatology* 2004;43(7):920–3.
3. Bartels CM, Bell CL, Shinki K, Rosenthal A, Bridges AJ. Changing trends in serious extra-articular manifestations of rheumatoid arthritis among United State veterans over 20 years. *Rheumatology* 2010;49(9):1670–5.
4. Turesson C. Extra-articular rheumatoid arthritis. *Curr Opin Rheumatol* 2013;25(3):360–6.
5. Turesson C, O'Fallon W, Crowson C, Gabriel S, Matteson E. Extra-articular disease manifestations in rheumatoid arthritis: incidence trends and risk factors over 46 years. *Ann Rheum Dis* 2003;62(8):722–7.
6. Marigliano B, Soriano A, Margiotta D, Vadacca M, Afeltra A. Lung involvement in connective tissue diseases: a comprehensive review and a focus on rheumatoid arthritis. *Autoimmun Rev* 2013;12(11):1076–84.
7. O'Dwyer DN, Armstrong ME, Cooke G, Dodd JD, Veale DJ, Donnelly SC. Rheumatoid arthritis (RA) associated interstitial lung disease (ILD). *Eur J Int Med* 2013;24(7):597–603.
8. Dixon W, Hyrich K, Watson K, Lunt M, Symmons D, Consortium BCC. Influence of anti-TNF therapy on mortality in patients with rheumatoid arthritis-associated interstitial lung disease: results from the British Society for Rheumatology Biologics Register. *Ann Rheum Dis* 2010;69(6):1086–91.
9. Kelly CA, Saravanan V, Nisar M, et al. Rheumatoid arthritis-related interstitial lung disease: associations, prognostic factors and physiological and radiological characteristics—a large multicentre UK study. *Rheumatology* 2014;53(9):1676–82.
10. de Lauretis A, Veeraraghavan S, Renzoni E. Review series: aspects of interstitial lung disease: connective tissue disease-associated interstitial lung disease: how does it differ from IPF? How should the clinical approach differ? *Chron Respir Dis* 2011;8(1):53–82.
11. Gabbay E, Tarala R, Will R, Carroll G, Adler B, Cameron D, et al. Interstitial lung disease in recent onset rheumatoid arthritis. *Am J Resp Crit Care Med* 1997;156(2):528–35.
12. Habib HM, Eisa AA, Arafat WR, Marie MA. Pulmonary involvement in early rheumatoid arthritis patients. *Clin Rheumatol* 2011;30(2):217–21.
13. Kim EJ, Elicker BM, Maldonado F, et al. Usual interstitial pneumonia in rheumatoid arthritis-associated interstitial lung disease. *Eur Resp J* 2010;35(6):1322–8.
14. Kim EJ, Collard HR, King Jr TE. Rheumatoid arthritis-associated interstitial lung disease: the relevance of histopathologic and radiographic pattern. *Chest* 2009;136(5):1397–405.
15. Hallowell RW, Horton MR. Interstitial lung disease in patients with rheumatoid arthritis: spontaneous and drug induced. *Drugs* 2014;74(4):443–50.
16. European RS, Society AT. American Thoracic Society/European Respiratory Society International Multidisciplinary Consensus Classification of the Idiopathic Interstitial Pneumonias. This joint statement of the American Thoracic Society (ATS), and the European Respiratory Society (ERS) was adopted by the ATS board of directors, June 2001 and by the ERS Executive Committee, June 2001. *Am J Resp Crit Care Med* 2002;165(2):277.
17. Bongartz T, Nannini C, Medina-Velasquez YF, et al. Incidence and mortality of interstitial lung disease in rheumatoid arthritis: a population-based study. *Arthritis Rheum* 2010;62:1583–91.
18. Roschmann RA, Rothenberg RJ. Pulmonary fibrosis in rheumatoid arthritis: a review of clinical features and therapy. *Semin Arthritis Rheum* 1987;16(3):174–85.
19. Saketkoo LA, Espinoza LR. Experience of mycophenolate mofetil in 10 patients with autoimmune-related interstitial lung disease demonstrates promising effects. *Am J Med Sci* 2009;337(5):329–35.
20. Fischer A, Brown KK, Du Bois RM, et al. Mycophenolate mofetil improves lung function in connective tissue disease-associated interstitial lung disease. *J Rheumatol* 2013:40(5):640–6.
21. Keir GJ, Maher TM, Ming D, et al. Rituximab in severe, treatment-refractory interstitial lung disease. *Respirology* 2014;19(3):353–9.
22. Md Yusof MY, Kabia A, Darby M, et al. Effect of rituximab on the progression of rheumatoid arthritis-related interstitial lung

disease: 10 years' experience at a single centre. *Rheumatology* 2017;*56*(8):1348–57.

23. Fernández-Díaz C, Loricera J, Castañeda S, et al. Abatacept in patients with rheumatoid arthritis and interstitial lung disease: a national multicenter study of 63 patients. *Semin Arthritis Rheum* 2018;*48*(1):22–7.

24. Rojas-Serrano J, González-Velásquez E, Mejía M, Sánchez-Rodríguez A, Carrillo G. Interstitial lung disease related to rheumatoid arthritis: evolution after treatment. *Reumatologia Clinica* 2012;*8*(2):68–71.

25. Koduri G, Norton S, Young A, et al. Interstitial lung disease has a poor prognosis in rheumatoid arthritis: results from an inception cohort. *Rheumatology* 2010;*49*(8):1483–9.

26. Yazdani A, Singer LG, Strand V, Gelber AC, Williams L, Mittoo S. Survival and quality of life in rheumatoid arthritis-associated interstitial lung disease after lung transplantation. *J Heart Lung Transplant* 2014;*33*(5):514–20.

27. Zamora-Legoff JA, Krause ML, Crowson CS, Ryu JH, Matteson EL. Patterns of interstitial lung disease and mortality in rheumatoid arthritis. *Rheumatology* 2016;*56*(3):344–50.

28. Assayag D, Lubin M, Lee JS, King TE, Collard HR, Ryerson CJ. Predictors of mortality in rheumatoid arthritis-related interstitial lung disease. *Respirology* 2014;*19*(4):493–500.

29. Rajasekaran A, Shovlin D, Saravanan V, Lord P, Kelly C. Interstitial lung disease in patients with rheumatoid arthritis: comparison with cryptogenic fibrosing alveolitis over 5 years. *J Rheumatol* 2006;*33*(7):1250–3.

30. Quinn DA, Mark EJ. Case 8-2002: a 56-year-old woman with a persistent left-sided pleural effusion. *N Engl J Med* 2002;*346*(11):843–50.

31. Balbir-Gurman A, Yigla M, Nahir AM, Braun-Moscovici Y. Rheumatoid pleural effusion. *Semin Arthritis Rheum* 2006:*35*(6):368–78.

32. Lofgren RH, Montgomery WW. Incidence of laryngeal involvement in rheumatoid arthritis. *N Engl J Med* 1962;*267*(4):193–5.

33. Baqir M, Ryu JH. The non-ILD pulmonary manifestations of RA. In: Fischer A, Lee JS (eds). *Lung Disease in Rheumatoid Arthritis*, pp. 163–73. Berlin, Germany: Springer, 2018.

34. Lynch JP, Weigt SS, DerHovanessian A, Fishbein MC, Gutierrez A, Belperio JA. Obliterative (constrictive) bronchiolitis. Seminars in respiratory and critical care medicine. *Semin Respir Crit Care Med* 2012;*33*(5):509–32.

35. Yousem SA, Colby TV, Carrington CB. Lung biopsy in rheumatoid arthritis. *Am Rev Resp Dis* 1985;*131*(5):770–7.

36. Ziff M. The rheumatoid nodule. *Arthritis Rheum* 1990;*33*(6):761–7.

37. Saravana S, Gillott T, Abourawi F, Peters M, Campbell A, Griffith S. Spontaneous pneumothorax: an unusual presentation of rheumatoid arthritis. *Rheumatology* 2003;*42*(11):1415–6.

38. Caplan A. Certain unusual radiological appearances in the chest of coal-miners suffering from rheumatoid arthritis. *Thorax* 1953;*8*(1):29.

39. Andres M, Vela P, Romera C. Marked improvement of lung rheumatoid nodules after treatment with tocilizumab. *Rheumatology* 2012;*51*(6):1132–4.

40. Shaw M, Collins BF, Ho LA, Raghu G. Rheumatoid arthritis-associated lung disease. *Eur Resp Rev* 2015;*24*(135):1–16.

41. van den Oever I, Sattar N, Nurmohamed M. Thromboembolic and cardiovascular risk in rheumatoid arthritis: role of the haemostatic system. *Ann Rheum Dis* 2014: *73*(6):954–7.

42. Mercer LK, Davies R, Galloway JB, et al. Risk of cancer in patients receiving non-biologic disease-modifying therapy for rheumatoid arthritis compared with the UK general population. *Rheumatology* 2012;*52*(1):91–8.

43. Smitten AL, Simon TA, Hochberg MC, Suissa S. A meta-analysis of the incidence of malignancy in adult patients with rheumatoid arthritis. *Arthritis Res Ther* 2008;*10*(2):R45.

44. Rutherford AI, Patarata E, Subesinghe S, Hyrich KL, Galloway JB. Opportunistic infections in rheumatoid arthritis patients exposed to biologic therapy: results from the British Society for Rheumatology Biologics Register for Rheumatoid Arthritis. *Rheumatology* 2018;*57*(6):997–1001.

45. Baddley J, Cantini F, Goletti D, et al. ESCMID Study Group for Infections in Compromised Hosts (ESGICH) consensus document on the safety of targeted and biological therapies: an infectious diseases perspective (soluble immune effector molecules [I]: anti-tumor necrosis factor-alpha agents). *Clin Microbiol Infect* 2018;*24*(suppl 2):S10–20.

46. Rozin A, Yigla M, Guralnik L, et al. Rheumatoid lung nodulous and osteopathy associated with leflunomide therapy. *Clin Rheumatol* 2006;*25*(3):384–8.

47. Thavarajah K, Wu P, Rhew EJ, Yeldandi AK, Kamp DW. Pulmonary complications of tumor necrosis factor-targeted therapy. *Resp Med* 2009;*103*(5):661–9.

48. Conway R, Low C, Coughlan RJ, O'Donnell MJ, Carey JJ. Methotrexate and lung disease in rheumatoid arthritis: a meta-analysis of randomized controlled trials. *Arthritis Rheum* 2014;*66*(4):803–12.

49. Aviña-Zubieta JA, Choi HK, Sadatsafavi M, Etminan M, Esdaile JM, Lacaille D. Risk of cardiovascular mortality in patients with rheumatoid arthritis: a meta-analysis of observational studies. *Arthritis Care Res* 2008;*59*(12):1690–7.

50. Crowson CS, Liao KP, Davis JM, et al. Rheumatoid arthritis and cardiovascular disease. *Am Heart J* 2013;*166*(4):622–8. e1.

51. Lazarevic MB, Vitic J, Mladenovic V, Myones BL, Skosey JL, Swedler WI. Dyslipoproteinemia in the course of active rheumatoid arthritis. *Semin Arthritis Rheum* 1992;*22*(3):172–8.

52. Low AS, Symmons DP, Lunt M, et al. Relationship between exposure to tumour necrosis factor inhibitor therapy and incidence and severity of myocardial infarction in patients with rheumatoid arthritis. *Ann Rheum Dis* 2017;*76*(4):654–60.

53. Maradit-Kremers H, Crowson CS, Nicola PJ, et al. Increased unrecognized coronary heart disease and sudden deaths in rheumatoid arthritis: a population-based cohort study. *Arthritis Rheum* 2005;*52*(2):402–11.

54. Solomon D, Reed G, Kremer J, Curtis J, Farkouh M, Harrold L, et al. Disease activity in rheumatoid arthritis and the risk of cardiovascular events. *Arthritis & rheumatology.* 2015;*67*(6):1449–55.

55. Løgstrup BB, Ellingsen T, Pedersen AB, Kjærsgaard A, Bøtker HE, Maeng M. Development of heart failure in patients with rheumatoid arthritis: a Danish population-based study. *Eur J Clin Investig* 2018;*48*(5):e12915.

56. Chung ES, Packer M, Lo KH, Fasanmade AA, Willerson JT. Randomized, double-blind, placebo-controlled, pilot trial of infliximab, a chimeric monoclonal antibody to tumor necrosis factor-α, in patients with moderate-to-severe heart failure: results of the anti-TNF Therapy Against Congestive Heart Failure (ATTACH) trial. *Circulation* 2003;*107*(25):3133–40.

57. Hara KS, Ballard DJ, Ilstrup DM, Connolly DC, Vollertsen RS. Rheumatoid pericarditis: clinical features and survival. *Medicine* 1990;*69*(2):81–91.

58. Aslangul E, Perrot S, Durand E, Mousseaux E, Le Jeunne C, Capron L. Successful etanercept treatment of constrictive pericarditis complicating rheumatoid arthritis. *Rheumatology* 2005;*44*(12):1581–3.

59. Ahern M, Lever J, Cosh J. Complete heart block in rheumatoid arthritis. *Ann Rheum Dis* 1983;*42*(4):389.

60. Cammelli D, Vitiello G. A case of rheumatoid vasculitis. *Rheumatology* 2016;*55*(6):1126–1126.

61. Ntatsaki E, Mooney J, Scott DG, Watts RA. Systemic rheumatoid vasculitis in the era of modern immunosuppressive therapy. *Rheumatology* 2013;*53*(1):145–52.

62. Turesson C, Matteson EL. Clinical features of rheumatoid arthritis: extra-articular manifestations. In: *Rheumatoid Arthritis*, pp. 62–7. Atlanta, GA: Elsevier Inc., 2009.

63. Neva MH, Isomäki P, Hannonen P, Kauppi M, Krishnan E, Sokka T. Early and extensive erosiveness in peripheral joints predicts atlantoaxial subluxations in patients with rheumatoid arthritis. *Arthritis Rheum* 2003;*48*(7):1808–13.

64. Elhai M, Wipff J, Bazeli R, et al. Radiological cervical spine involvement in young adults with polyarticular juvenile idiopathic arthritis. *Rheumatology* 2012;*52*(2):267–75.

65. Bouchaud-Chabot A, Lioté F. Cervical spine involvement in rheumatoid arthritis. A review. *Joint Bone Spine* 2002;*69*(2):141–54.

66. Gillick JL, Wainwright J, Das K. Rheumatoid arthritis and the cervical spine: a review on the role of surgery. *Int J Rheumatol* 2015;*2015*:252456.

67. Clifford DB, Ances B, Costello C, et al. Rituximab-associated progressive multifocal leukoencephalopathy in rheumatoid arthritis. *Arch Neurol* 2011;*68*(9):1156–64.

68. Nakano KK. The entrapment neuropathies of rheumatoid arthritis. *Orthop Clin N Am* 1975;*6*(3):837.

69. Möller B, Scherer A, Förger F, Villiger PM, Finckh A, Diseases SCQMPfR. Anaemia may add information to standardised disease activity assessment to predict radiographic damage in rheumatoid arthritis: a prospective cohort study. *Ann Rheum Dis* 2014;*73*(4):691–6.

70. Hashimoto M, Fujii T, Hamaguchi M, et al. Increase of hemoglobin levels by anti-IL-6 receptor antibody (Tocilizumab) in rheumatoid arthritis. *PloS One* 2014;*9*(5):e98202.

71. Sibley J, Haga M, Visram D, Mitchell D. The clinical course of Felty's syndrome compared to matched controls. *J Rheumatol* 1991;*18*(8):1163–7.

72. Heylen L, Dierickx D, Vandenberghe P, Westhovens R. Targeted therapy with rituximab in Felty's syndrome: a case report. *Open Rheumatol J* 2012;*6*:312.

73. Dhodapkar MV, Li C-Y, Lust JA, Tefferi A, Phyliky RL. Clinical spectrum of clonal proliferations of T-large granular lymphocytes: a T-cell clonopathy of undetermined significance? *Blood* 1994;*84*(5):1620–7.

74. Moots RJ, Sebba A, Rigby W, et al. Effect of tocilizumab on neutrophils in adult patients with rheumatoid arthritis: pooled analysis of data from phase 3 and 4 clinical trials. *Rheumatology* 2016;*56*(4):541–9.

75. Baecklund E, Sundström C, Ekbom A, et al. Lymphoma subtypes in patients with rheumatoid arthritis: increased proportion of diffuse large B cell lymphoma. *Arthritis Rheum* 2003;*48*(6):1543–50.

76. Baecklund E, Ekbom A, Sparén P, Feltelius N, Klareskog L. Disease activity and risk of lymphoma in patients with rheumatoid arthritis: nested case-control study. *BMJ* 1998;*317*(7152):180–1.

77. Symmons DPM. Lymphoma and rheumatoid arthritis—again. *Rheumatology* 2007;*46*(1):1–2.

78. Wolfe F, Michaud K. Lymphoma in rheumatoid arthritis: the effect of methotrexate and anti–tumor necrosis factor therapy in 18,572 patients. *Arthritis Rheum* 2004;*50*(6):1740–51.

79. Vignesh AP, Srinivasan R. Ocular manifestations of rheumatoid arthritis and their correlation with anti-cyclic citrullinated peptide antibodies. *Clin ophthalmol* 2005;*9*:393–7.

80. Thanou-Stavraki A, James JA. Primary Sjogren's syndrome: current and prospective therapies. *Semin Arthritis Rheum* 2008;*37*(5):273–92.

81. Artifoni M, Rothschild P-R, Brézin A, Guillevin L, Puéchal X. Ocular inflammatory diseases associated with rheumatoid arthritis. *Nat Rev Rheumatol* 2014;*10*(2):108.

82. Korsten P, Bahlmann D, Patschan SA. Rapid healing of peripheral ulcerative keratitis in rheumatoid arthritis with prednisone, methotrexate and adalimumab combination therapy. *Rheumatology* 2017;*56*(7):1094.

83. Watanabe R, Ishii T, Yoshida M, et al. Ulcerative keratitis in patients with rheumatoid arthritis in the modern biologic era: a series of eight cases and literature review. *Int J Rheum Dis* 2017;*20*(2):225–30.

84. Tilstra JS, Lienesch DW. Rheumatoid nodules. *Dermatol Clin* 2015;*33*(3):361–71.

85. Sayah A, English III JC. Rheumatoid arthritis: a review of the cutaneous manifestations. *J Am Acad Dermatol* 2005;*53*(2):191–209.

86. Caporali R, Crepaldi G, Codullo V, et al. 20 years of experience with tumour necrosis factor inhibitors: what have we learned? *Rheumatology* 2018;*57*(Suppl 7):vii5–vii10.

87. Hauser B, Riches PL, Wilson JF, Horne AE, Ralston SH. Prevalence and clinical prediction of osteoporosis in a contemporary cohort of patients with rheumatoid arthritis. *Rheumatology* 2014;*53*(10):1759–66.

88. Matcham F, Rayner L, Steer S, Hotopf M. The prevalence of depression in rheumatoid arthritis: a systematic review and meta-analysis. *Rheumatology* 2013;*52*(12):2136–48.

89. Matcham F, Norton S, Scott DL, Steer S, Hotopf M. Symptoms of depression and anxiety predict treatment response and long-term physical health outcomes in rheumatoid arthritis: secondary analysis of a randomized controlled trial. *Rheumatology* 2015;*55*(2):268–78.

90. Matcham F, Davies R, Hotopf M, et al. The relationship between depression and biologic treatment response in rheumatoid arthritis: an analysis of the British Society for Rheumatology Biologics Register. *Rheumatology* 2018;*57*(5):835–43.

91. Matcham F, Galloway J, Hotopf M, et al. The impact of targeted rheumatoid arthritis pharmacological treatment on mental health: a systematic review and network meta-analysis. *Arthritis Rheumatol* 2018;*70*(9):1377–91.

14

Comorbidity in rheumatoid arthritis

Kimme Hyrich and Sarah Skeoch

What is comorbidity?

Comorbidity is defined as the presence of one or more medical condition in a person at the same time as a primary disease, in this case rheumatoid arthritis (RA). Comorbid conditions are not necessarily a direct result of RA. They may be completely unrelated and occur by coincidence. They may share common genetic or environmental risk factors with RA or could be caused by RA or the treatments used in RA. Comorbidities also include conditions which occur prior to the diagnosis of RA but still have relevance as they can impact on treatment decisions, disease course, and outcomes. While RA is characterized by inflammatory arthritis there are many comorbidities recognized in RA patients that have a significant impact on life expectancy and quality.

Why is estimating comorbidity important in RA?

Presence of comorbidity in RA and in other diseases is associated with excess mortality, reduced quality of life, and higher levels of disability.[1-4] Understanding all aspects of the patient's health informs treatment decisions and allows a more individualized approach to management. At a population level, understanding the scale and type of comorbidity within the RA population informs research priorities, health service design and facilitates development of screening and surveillance strategies to reduce the incidence and impact of common or severe comorbidities. From the patient's perspective treatment decisions and communication which incorporates all aspects of their health rather than a disease or organ focused approach is important.

How is comorbidity measured in RA?

There are a number of approaches to evaluating comorbidity in RA, some of which are more relevant in a population setting, others when considering an individual patient's needs. The study of comorbidity in RA has largely focused on identifying specific conditions and studying their prevalence, impact, risk factors and relationship with RA. Different methods have been employed including surveys, cohort studies, and analysis within clinical trials. The differences in methodologies employed can lead to significant variation in estimates which must be borne in mind when synthesizing information.[5]

A second approach is to study the overall burden of comorbidities using composite measures. These measurements allow the study of the cumulative effect of comorbidities on outcomes and treatment decisions. They also facilitate patient stratification and estimation of confounding in research studies. There are more than 30 validated comorbidity indices available in the literature.[6] The most commonly used is the Charlson Comorbidity Index (CCI).[1] It includes 17 diagnoses with weighting to take account of the impact of each condition and also includes age as a factor. The CCI is not specific to RA and was originally developed in hospitalized patients with 1-year mortality as the predicted outcome. However, it has also been shown to significantly predict mortality in RA and has been used in a number of studies to evaluate the effect of comorbidity on outcomes.[2,7-9]

More recently comorbidity indices have been developed specifically for rheumatology populations. These include the Rheumatic Diseases Comorbidities Index (RDCI) and the multimorbidity index (MMI).[10] The RDCI was initially developed in patients with RA, osteoarthritis, systemic lupus erythematosus, or fibromyalgia in a US-based study using patient reported questionnaires.[2] It has also been validated for use in administrative database studies. It is a weighted index of 11 comorbidities and similar to the CCI, provides an overall value for comorbidity burden. It is predictive of mortality and a range of other outcomes including physical functioning and direct healthcare costs. When tested in RA, the RDCI performed better than the CCI for prediction of mortality and disability.[2]

The MMI was developed in a US-based RA cohort and validated within a multicentre European RA observational study.[4] The MMI is an additive count of 40 conditions that do not require weighting. It was developed to predict health related quality of life (HRQoL) rather than mortality. It was also shown to perform better than the CCI for predicting HRQoL in RA patients but its ability to predict mortality is yet to be established.[4]

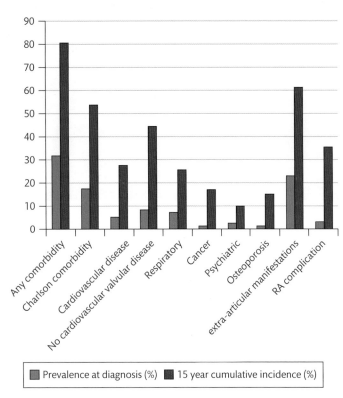

Figure 14.1 Prevalence and cumulative incidence of comorbidities in an early arthritis cohort.

Source: data from Norton S, Koduri G, Nikiphorou E et. al. 'A study of baseline prevalence and cumulative incidence of comorbidity and extra-articular manifestations in RA and their impact on outcome'. *Rheumatology (Oxford)* 2013 Jan;52(1):99–110.

What is the burden of comorbidity seen in RA?

The literature suggests that RA patients not only have a higher prevalence of comorbidities compared to non-RA controls but the impact of some comorbidities on mortality risk may be higher than is observed in patients with the same comorbidities who do not have

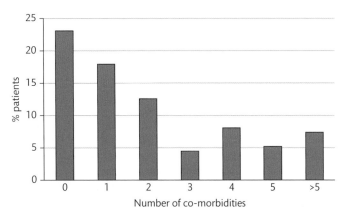

Figure 14.2 Prevalence of comorbidities observed in an international cohort of patients with established RA.

Source: data from Gron KL et al. (2014) 'The association of fatigue, comorbidity burden, disease activity, disability and gross domestic product in patients with rheumatoid arthritis. Results from 34 countries participating in the Quest-RA program'. *Clin Exp Rheumatol* 32(6):869–77.

RA.[3] Additionally, in the context of some comorbidities RA patients are less likely to undergo screening or early interventions.[11,12]

In a UK multicentre early arthritis study, 17.5% of patients had at least one item of the CCI at diagnosis (**Figure 14.1**).[3] When a wider range of comorbidities are considered, 30% to 50% of patients have one or more comorbidities at the time of RA diagnosis.[3,13] In early disease the most commonly observed comorbidities include hypertension, cardiovascular disease, osteoarthritis, respiratory disease, cancer, diabetes, and thyroid disease.[3,13]

Over time the CCI has been shown to increase in a linear fashion and 58% to 74% of patients with established RA have one or more additional medical conditions.[14] In a large international cohort of established RA, 1 in 8 patients had 5 or more comorbidities.[15] The frequency of patients with comorbidities in established RA can be seen in **Figure 14.2**. While many of the common comorbidities seen at diagnosis are also frequent in established disease, comorbidities due to complications of RA such as osteoporosis are more prevalent later in disease.[3] Importantly, studies that examine prevalence in established RA may underestimate serious life-limiting comorbidities, as patients with these conditions may not have survived to take part in research studies. It is therefore also important to consider serious comorbidities in the context of cause of death.

Figure 14.3 summarizes the common causes of death observed in a large UK cohort[16]. By far the most common cause of death in RA is cardiovascular disease (CVD), which accounted for 41%. Cancer and respiratory disease were also frequently the cause of death. While these results reflect the common causes of death seen in the general population, rates of death due to CVD, immune system malignancies, respiratory disease, and sepsis are significantly higher in RA patients compared to age and sex matched general population rates.[16]

The presence and burden of comorbidity not only has an impact on risk of death but also on quality of life and influences treatment choices and response. Presence of some comorbidities such as liver disease or infections may limit treatment choices and presence of comorbidity is associated with higher rates of adverse events while on treatment.[17] There is also evidence that the more comorbid conditions a patient has, the less likely they are to respond to therapy.[18] This association is independent of other factors including age, disability, and type of treatment.

Variations in comorbidity burden within populations

The burden and type of comorbidity is not uniform across the world. Marked geographical differences have been noted, with higher burden of comorbidy seen in patients from countries with higher GDP.[14] One international study evaluated a range of comorbidities in RA across 17 difference countries and found that prevalence of some specific comorbidities varied between counties.[19] A number of factors are likely to contribute to this variability. Firstly, differences in background prevalence rates of medical conditions along with cultural differences, socioeconomic factors, access to medical care, and treatment are likely to have a large impact. Methodological considerations also must be taken into account when comparing rates in different studies.

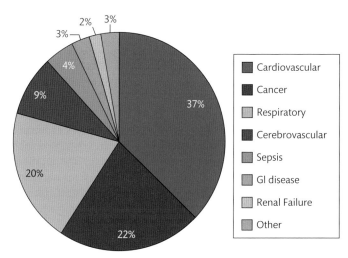

Figure 14.3 Cause of death in a UK inception cohort study.
Source: data from Young A et al. (2007) 'Mortality in rheumatoid arthritis. Increased in the early course of disease, in ischaemic heart disease and in pulmonary fibrosis'. *Rheumatology* (Oxford) 46(2):350–7.

Variations in the burden and type of comorbidity are also observed between genders. Male RA patients have a higher prevalence of comorbidity at diagnosis but females develop comorbidities at a faster rate after diagnosis. By the first decade after diagnosis women over 40 have more comorbidities than age-matched males.[3] When comparing types of comorbidities, male patients are at higher risk of developing respiratory comorbidities whereas females have a disproportionately increased risk of CVD relative to male RA patients.[3] Some comorbidities are more common in patients who have seropositive disease or more severe inflammatory burden and this will be discussed in detail in later sections.

While the study of overall comorbidity burden provides an understanding of the scale of healthcare burden in RA, in the context of service design and in individual patient assessment, an understanding of individual common and severe comorbidities is vital. Here we will discuss the specific major comorbidities further.

Cardiovascular disease

CVD it is the commonest cause of death in RA.[16] Patients are at a 50% increased risk of fatal and non-fatal CVD events (CVEs) with risk being most pronounced for myocardial infarction (MI).[20–22] This increased risk becomes apparent around 7 to 10 years after RA symptom onset and relative risk increases with disease duration[23,24] although may be earlier in patients who are rheumatoid factor positive.[23]

The clinical phenotype of cardiac disease is different in RA compared to controls. Patients have less warning symptoms prior to a significant CVE, have a higher risk of sudden cardiac death and are more likely to die within 30 days of an MI or stroke.[25] This highlights the importance of primary prevention of CVD in RA.

Shared risk factors for CVD and RA

There are a number of shared genetic and environmental risk factors for the development of CVD and RA. The HLA DRB1*01 haplotype, which is associated with increased risk of developing RA has also been implicated as a risk factor for acute MI in the general population.[26,27] Atherosclerosis, the most common underlying pathological mechanism for CVD is now accepted to be a chronic inflammatory condition.[28] A number of other genetic polymorphisms coding for regulation of inflammatory pathways are associated with susceptibility to both RA and to CVD.[29–31]

There is a well-established link between smoking and CVD and also between smoking and RA. A study based in Norfolk evaluated risk factors for the development of inflammatory arthritis.[32] Not only was the association with smoking confirmed but diabetes and obesity were also found to be associated with an increased risk of developing inflammatory arthritis, which are well known risk factors for CVD.

The role of traditional risk factors

Traditional CVD risk factors play an important role in CVD risk in RA. Selected key risk factors are summarized in Table 14.1.

Hypertension is one of the most common comorbidities seen in RA (13). Prevalence in early disease ranges from 6.2% to 7.9% and on average 2.7% of patients developed hypertension each year after RA diagnosis.[3,33] There is controversy as to whether there is an increased prevalence of hypertension in RA compared to that seen in the general population. However, on balance there is no clear increased risk in RA.[34,35] In RA, diagnosis of hypertension is associated with a twofold increased risk of a CVE.[36] No association between RA disease activity, severity, or inflammatory burden has been found with hypertension.[34] However, medications including glucocorticoids and non-steroidal anti-inflammatory drugs (NSAIDs) have been linked with increased prevalence.[37]

In early disease prevalence of diabetes is between 2.5% and 6.2%.[3,33] RA patients are 74% more likely to have diabetes compared to age and sex matched controls.[35] Patients with diabetes are more likely to develop RA and this could explain some of the increased

Table 14.1 Cardiovascular risk factors in RA patients

Risk factor	Prevalence in early RA (%)	Altered prevalence compared to general population	Risk of future CVE associated with presence of risk factor (Relative risk [95%CI])
Hypertension	18.5	No difference	2.24 [1.42, 3.06]
Hypercholesterolaemia	9.9	No difference	1.73 [1.03, 2.44]
Diabetes	6.2	Higher in RA	1.94 [1.58, 2.30]
Smoking	28	Higher in RA	1.50 [1.15, 1.84]
Obesity (BMI>30)	4.4	No difference	1.16 [1.03, 1.29]

prevalence of diabetes in RA. However, obesity and glucocorticoid use have also been shown to be associated with increased risk of diabetes in patients already diagnosed with RA.[38,39] Presence of diabetes in RA patients is associated with a 94% increased risk of future CVE compared to RA patients without diabetes.[36]

A diagnosis of RA is not associated with increased risk of hyperlipidaemia but dyslipidaemia is more prevalent.[40] In early RA, levels of total cholesterol, low density lipoprotein (LDL) and high-density lipoprotein (HDL) are all reduced. However, there is a preferential reduction of HDL leading to an adverse total cholesterol to HDL ratio (TC:HDL). There is a strong correlation between inflammation and total cholesterol and LDL levels and as RA disease activity improves TC:HDL also improves.[41] In the general population there is a log-linear relationship between total cholesterol and CVD risk. However in RA, patients with low total cholesterol are at higher risk of CVEs.[42] Despite the altered relationship between cholesterol levels and events, the diagnosis of hypercholesterolaemia in RA patients is associated with increased risk of CVD.[37,43]

The prevalence of obesity (body mass index >30) is estimated to be 4.4% in early disease with higher prevalence (16%) seen in established disease cohorts.[15] Presence of obesity is associated with 16% increased risk of CVD compared to RA patients with a BMI<30.[36] However, patients with low BMI (<20) also have a 3.45-fold increased risk of CVD compared to patients with normal BMI.[44] Patients with active disease often have rheumatoid cachexia, where there is a loss of muscle mass with relative preservation of fat. In these patients body mass index (BMI) can be normal or low but relative fat mass is high.[45,46]

As smoking is a significant risk factor for the development of RA, the prevalence of smoking is significantly higher in RA patients compared with controls.[35] Smoking is associated with a 50% increased risk of CVD in RA but the association between smoking and CVD is significantly weaker than is observed in the general population.[40] Despite this, smoking is an important modifiable risk factor with one study demonstrating a 25% reduction in the risk of CVEs for every year a patients continues smoking cessation with reduction apparent just after the first year.[47]

While traditional risk factors play an important role in CVD risk, they only account for approximately 70% of the CVD risk observed in RA.[43] A recent meta-analysis demonstrated that even on adjustment of traditional risk factors, RA patients had a 52% increased risk of MI and RA is now accepted as an independent risk factor for CVD.[48]

RA-related factors

The remaining 30% of CVD risk is attributed to RA-related factors.[43] These include presence of specific RA disease characteristics, RA-related treatments, and most importantly, chronic inflammation.

Rheumatoid factor and anticitrullinated peptide antibodies are associated with increased CVD in RA.[49,50] Presence of extra-articular manifestations and high levels of disability are also associated with increased risk.

Inflammation is now recognized as a risk factor for the development of atherosclerosis and CVD in the general population. Levels of tumour necrosis factor (TNF), IL-6, and C-reactive protein (CRP) have been shown to predict CVD death in large population studies.[29,51] Chronic inflammation is thought to be a major driver of cardiovascular risk in RA.[28] Baseline and cumulative CRP and

erythrocyte sedimentation rate (ESR) are associated with CVEs and CVD mortality in RA, independent of traditional risk factors.[23,52] Cumulative disease activity and frequency of disease flares are also predictors of events.[53,54] Inflammation leads to accelerated atherosclerosis in RA and may be associated with a more inflammatory, unstable plaque phenotype.[55,56] The risk of CVD associated with chronic inflammation is mediated both through alteration of traditional risk factors such as lipids but also though vessel wall inflammation.[42] Circulating inflammatory markers are associated with endothelial activation, arterial wall inflammation, and localized plaque inflammation in RA cohorts.[56,57] Control of inflammation is also associated with improvement in some traditional risk factors and vascular wall inflammation detected on positron emission tomography.[57,58]

Effect of treating RA on cardiovascular risk

In the last two decades there has been a paradigm shift in the treatment of RA, both in terms of new therapeutics but also in the more aggressive approach to disease control. Most studies evaluating trends in mortality over time have shown that while mortality rates are declining in RA, they are doing so in line with the general population.[59,60] Thus the excess mortality seen in RA remains.

There is evidence that improvements in disease activity are associated with reduction in CVEs and patients who go into early remission have a lower mortality risk.[4,61] Lower CVE rates have also been observed with some RA medications, such as methotrexate and certain biologics[62] compared to patients not receiving these treatments, but currently there is no evidence to suggest superiority of a single class of drug for CVD risk reduction.[63] Use of NSAIDs has been associated with higher rates of CVEs in RA, as are corticosteroids.[62] There is likely a degree of confounding as those with more severe inflammatory disease are more likely to receive steroids but even when potential confounding is taken into account, use of corticosteroids are still significantly associated with increased risk of cardiovascular mortality.

Managing cardiovascular risk in RA

There is clear evidence that cardiovascular risk factors are underdiagnosed in RA and that this has an impact of CVD event rates.[63,64] The European League Against Rheumatism (EULAR) recommends assessment of cardiovascular risk factors every 5 years, proactive management of traditional risk factors and effective control of inflammation with judicious use of steroids and anti-inflammatories.[65] It is recognized that established risk models for CVD risk underestimate risk in RA.[66] They also therefore recommend that a multiplication factor of 1.5 should be applied to risk estimates. However, in the UK, national guidelines recommend the QRISK 3 calculator which incorporates the diagnosis of RA into the risk model thus no multiplication factor is required.[48] There is evidence that use of statin therapy is as effective for lipid reduction in RA as it is in the general population and that statin use leads to lower risk of CVEs in RA.[67,68] It is unclear what levels of disease control are required to effectively reduce CVD risk in RA and this remains an area of research interest.

Increased incidence of non-ischaemic cardiac diseases is also observed in RA including pericarditis, myocarditis, and valvular disease. These are considered as extra-articular manifestation of RA and are discussed further in Chapter 14 .

Respiratory disease

Respiratory disease accounts for 15–22% of deaths in RA patients and risk of death due to respiratory disease is 2–3 times higher than in the general population.[69,70] At diagnosis 7% of patients have a concurrent respiratory disease and by 15 years 1 in 4 RA patients will have developed a new respiratory condition.[3] There are a broad range of respiratory conditions seen in RA. Common conditions include interstitial lung disease, obstructive lung disease, bronchiectasis, lung nodules, and pleural disease, the latter two being recognized extra-articular manifestations. In one study of newly diagnosed RA patients, 30% reported respiratory symptoms, 40% had reductions in gas transfer on spirometry and 67% have changes on high resolution CT (HRCT).[71] This highlights that there may be a significant subclinical burden of respiratory disease in RA.

While primary RA-related lung disease is common, respiratory infection and drug induced lung disease are also observed in RA and must be considered in the differential diagnosis in RA patients with respiratory symptoms.

Interstitial lung disease (ILD)

ILD is one of the most common respiratory complications seen in RA (3). Prevalence estimates vary depending on study design and case ascertainment and can range from 8% to 33%.[72] In an inception cohort study 1% of RA patients had RA-ILD at diagnosis and a 15-year cumulative incidence of 3.9% was observed.[3] When HRCT imaging is used in unselected RA cases 19% of patients have abnormalities consistent with ILD.[73] One-third of these patients are asymptomatic but serial imaging studies demonstrate progression in around a half of patients.[72]

In RA, the most common ILD subtype seen is usual interstitial pneumonia (UIP), accounting for 65% of RA-ILD.[74] UIP is characterized by interstitial fibrosis with honeycomb pattern seen on imaging. Other subtypes include non-specific interstitial pneumonitis which accounts for 24% of RA-ILD and other patterns including cryptogenic organizing pneumonia, mixed pattern, and diffuse alveolar damage are seen less frequently.[74,75] Few patients present with ILD at diagnosis and median time from RA diagnosis is 4.9 years.[76]

Risk factors for the development of RA-ILD include male gender, high rheumatoid factor titres, anticitrullinated protein antibody (ACPA) positivity, smoking, older age at RA diagnosis, rheumatoid nodules, and severity of joint disease.[72,74,77] Median survival after ILD diagnosis is 2.6 years.[77] A shorter survival time has been observed in those with UIP compared with other subtypes however this is partly due to confounding factors such as smoking, age, and gender.[74,78,79] One study also observed the highest mortality in patients with diffuse alveolar damage (DAD).[80] In the general population, DAD is often rapidly progressive with a high in-hospital mortality rate, thus this finding is not specific to RA. Furthermore, the low prevalence of DAD type ILD seen in RA cohort studies may reflect survival bias. Factors associated with poor prognosis include male gender, degree of transfer factor reduction, and restrictive lung defects at baseline, extent of HRCT changes at baseline and disability as measured by Health Assessment Questionnaire (HAQ) score.[76–78,81]

The effects of RA treatments on ILD

A number of frequently used RA medications have been associated with development of drug induced ILD or acute exacerbation in those with pre-existing RA-ILD.[82] Lack of standardized case definitions for drug induced ILD make it difficult to estimate its true prevalence in RA. However occurrences have been reported with a number of conventional synthetic disease-modifying antirheumatic drugs (csDMARDS) including methotrexate, leflunomide, gold, and sulfasalazine.[82] There have also been reports of the development of rapidly progressive ILD and acute severe exacerbation of pre-existing RA-ILD with anti-TNF therapy associated with a high mortality rate.[82] However, when incidence rates of ILD have been compared in those taking anti-TNF therapy or csDMARDs and also in different biologic therapies, no significant differences have been observed.[83]

Management of RA-ILD

There is a lack of evidence base for the approach to treating RA-ILD and there is no established association between control of RA disease activity and reduced incidence or progression of RA-ILD. Most recommendations are extrapolated from data in non-RA ILD and connective tissue disease related (CTD)-ILD cohorts.[72] Corticosteroids are often used in clinical practice but there is little evidence of their efficacy in RA-ILD and use is associated with increased risk of respiratory infection.[84] UIP pattern disease tends not to improve with corticosteroids and immunosuppression.[84] Subgroup analysis in one study of mycophenolate mofetil demonstrated a trend towards improvement in forced vital capacity in RA-ILD.[85] Two studies have investigated the effect on rituximab in RA-ILD progression. In one open-label study of 10 RA-ILD patients, one patient died of acute respiratory distress syndrome.[86,87] Of the 7 patients who completed treatment, 2 had improvements in gas transfer, 1 had deteriorated, and the rest remained stable. A second study evaluated RA-ILD patients treated with rituximab for active joint disease.[88] During follow-up lung function remained stable in 52% of patients, 32% had progression of ILD, and 16% had improvement in lung function.

Recently, the antifibrotic agents pirfenidone and nintedanib have been licenced for the treatment of idiopathic pulmonary fibrosis, a UIP pattern ILD which is histologically and clinically similar to the UIP subtype of RA-ILD.[89] These new agents slow the decline in lung function in idiopathic pulmonary fibrosis (IPF) patients and clinical trials are now ongoing in RA-ILD. Currently there are no established guidelines for the management of RA-ILD but patients should be managed in conjunction with respiratory physicians, have regular surveillance for progression and be offered non-pharmacological interventions including smoking cessation advice.[90] Furthermore, a high index of suspicion should be maintained for drug induced ILD and infection in new cases of suspected ILD or acute deterioration in RA-ILD. In RA-ILD patients being considered for biologic therapy Jani et al. proposed an assessment and monitoring algorithm which can be seen in **Figure 14.4**.[91]

Bronchiectasis

The reported prevalence of bronchiectasis varies widely depending on case definition. In HRCT studies in unselected RA cases, bronchiectasis is seen in 35% of patients whereas studies based on clinical diagnosis estimate prevalence at 1–5%.[71,92,93] Although no direct

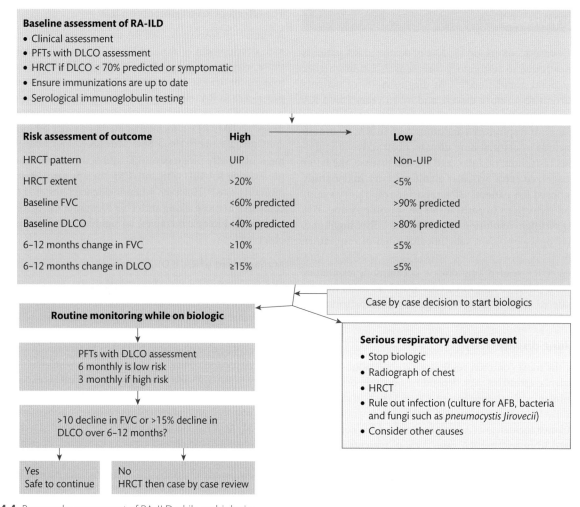

Baseline assessment of RA-ILD
- Clinical assessment
- PFTs with DLCO assessment
- HRCT if DLCO < 70% predicted or symptomatic
- Ensure immunizations are up to date
- Serological immunoglobulin testing

Risk assessment of outcome	High	Low
HRCT pattern	UIP	Non-UIP
HRCT extent	>20%	<5%
Baseline FVC	<60% predicted	>90% predicted
Baseline DLCO	<40% predicted	>80% predicted
6–12 months change in FVC	≥10%	≤5%
6–12 months change in DLCO	≥15%	≤5%

Case by case decision to start biologics

Routine monitoring while on biologic

PFTs with DLCO assessment
6 monthly is low risk
3 monthly if high risk

>10 decline in FVC or >15% decline in DLCO over 6–12 months?

Yes
Safe to continue

No
HRCT then case by case review

Serious respiratory adverse event
- Stop biologic
- Radiograph of chest
- HRCT
- Rule out infection (culture for AFB, bacteria and fungi such as *pneumocystis Jirovecii*)
- Consider other causes

Figure 14.4 Proposed management of RA-ILD while on biologics.
Reprinted from Jani M. et al (2014) 'The safety of biologic therapies in RA-associated interstitial lung disease'. *Nature Reviews Rheumatology* 10(5):284–94 with permission from Springer Nature.

comparator studies have been undertaken, prevalence is higher in RA studies than is observed in the general population.[93] There are few studies examining risk factors for bronchiectasis in RA however one study found that bronchiectasis patients were more likely to be rheumatoid factor and ACPA positive, have higher DAS28 and erosive disease.[94] There is no established association between smoking and the development of bronchiectasis in RA. In most cases bronchiectasis occurs long after RA diagnosis. However, recently the lung has been hypothesized as a site of induction of autoantibodies with significantly higher levels of APCA antibodies seen in non-RA bronchiectasis patients compared to controls, implicating bronchiectasis in the development of RA.[95]

All bronchiectasis patients are at increased risk of respiratory infection and may require prophylactic antibiotics if they suffer with frequent infections. In RA bronchiectasis patients, use of biologic therapy and evidence of microbial colonization in sputum samples are both independent risk factors for respiratory infection.[96] Five-year survival is estimated to be 87% in RA patients who have bronchiectasis and mortality is higher in RA bronchiectasis patients compared to non-RA bronchiectasis patients.[80,93] There is no established guidance specific to RA bronchiectasis, however, guidance on management of non-cystic fibrosis bronchiectasis has been published by the British Thoracic Society and should be used to guide management in RA patients.[93] These guidelines particularly recommend closer follow-up in RA-associated bronchiectasis due to the poorer prognosis. When considering DMARD therapy in RA, the frequency and severity of infections should be considered.

Chronic obstructive pulmonary disease (COPD)

At time of RA diagnosis 2% of patients already have a diagnosis of COPD and annual incidence is estimated at 0.4%.[3] COPD is twice as common in RA patients than in the general population.[97] Smoking is an important risk factor for both RA and COPD and this shared risk factor likely explains a significant proportion of the increased prevalence seen in RA. There is also a hypothesis that COPD may be implicated in the induction of auto-antibodies associated with the development of RA.[98] In one study, low titre rheumatoid factor antibodies were found in 42% of COPD patients and in a second study ACPA antibodies were found in 7.4% of COPD patients.[99,100] One study examined levels of citrullinated peptides in lung tissue and found significantly higher levels in COPD patients compared with non-COPD smokers and non-smokers.[98] The authors hypothesized that localized inflammation due to COPD may contribute to the development of ACPA antibodies, over and above the risk of smoking.

Current or previous smoking, more severe RA and male gender are all factors associated with the development of COPD in RA.[101] RA patients diagnosed with COPD were twice as likely to die during 16-year follow-up compared to RA patients without COPD, even after adjustment for other factors including smoking, age, gender, and alcohol.[101] There is no established association between disease activity or therapies and incidence of COPD in RA and no specific recommendation for its management within this population. However, smoking cessation advice, vaccination, and vigilance for respiratory infection are recommended. Similar to bronchiectasis patients, infection risk should be evaluated when considering DMARD therapy.

Cancer

When pooled international data are considered, RA patients have a 10% increased risk of developing cancer compared with the general population.[102] The risk varies between specific cancers. Standardized incidence rates of cancers in RA compared to the general population are summarized in Table 14.2. However, in a large UK study of biologic naïve patients, the risk of cancer is 28% higher than is seen in the UK general population (Table 14.2)[103]. Both in UK and international studies, rates of lymphoma, lung cancer, and melanoma are higher in RA. There are a number of shared risk factors for the development of cancer and RA including immune system dysregulation, viral infection, obesity, and smoking. Chronic immune system stimulation is thought to play a role and some immunodulatory drugs, used in RA, have also been associated with increased cancer risk.[103-105]

When anti-TNF agents were first developed there were concerns regarding increased cancer risk due to the potential antitumour effects of TNF. However, a meta-analysis of clinical trial data demonstrated no difference in rates of cancer compared to patients treated with csDMARD therapy in the short term.[106] Prospective biologics registries were set up in a number of European countries to evaluate the medium and long-term risk in anti-TNF treated patients but data so far has shown no significant increase in risk of cancer in the medium term.[65] Due to early concerns about cancer risk, initial clinical guidance suggested that anti-TNF therapy should not be used in those with a history of cancer in the prior 5 years. Therefore, the risk of recurrent or new cancers in anti-TNF treated patients with a history of cancer is

less well studied. Data from the Swedish registry demonstrated no difference in medium-term cancer risk between patients treated with anti-TNF, tocilizumab, rituximab, abatacept, and csDMARDs.[107] Registry studies are ongoing and are likely to provide important information on the long-term risk of cancer in biologic-treated patients.[108-110]

The largest excess cancer risk is observed for lymphoma. B-cell non-Hodgkin's lymphoma is the most common type of lymphoma seen in RA.[111] It accounted for 84% of all lymphomas in one large European study, of which 56% were the diffuse large B-cell subtype.[111] While Hodgkin's lymphoma is less common, the relative risk compared to the general population is higher than other types of lymphoma (three times higher). High cumulative disease activity is a significant risk factor for the development of lymphoma in RA and there is a particularly strong association with diffuse large B-cell lymphoma.[112] Other disease characteristics including Felty's syndrome, secondary Sjogren's syndrome, high ESR, and erosive disease are also associated with increased risk.[113] In the literature, rare cases of lymphoma associated with methotrexate use have been described, with spontaneous regression on drug withdrawal.[114] This may be related to higher rates of Epstein–Barr positive lymphoma in methotrexate treated patients but larger studies have not shown a significant increased risk of lymphoma with methotrexate.[104] Biologics registry data from the United Kingdom and other parts of Europe have not shown any increased risk of lymphoma in anti-TNF treated patients compared to patients on csDMARDs during medium-term follow-up.[111] Furthermore no differences in lymphoma subtypes have been seen in anti-TNF treated patients.[111]

Based on international data, RA patients are 64% more likely to develop lung cancer than age and sex matched controls.[102] However, estimates in the United Kingdom are significantly higher with a 2.4-fold increased risk being observed in a cohort of 3371 biologic naïve RA patients.[103] Higher mortality rates have also been observed in RA patients with lung cancer compared to non-RA lung cancer patients.[115] Smoking is a very strong risk factor for lung cancer and the higher prevalence of smoking seen in RA likely significantly contributes to the increased lung cancer risk seen.[90] RA smokers are 32 times more likely to die from lung cancer compared to RA non-smokers.[116] Furthermore, in the general population, ILD is associated with increased lung cancer risk thus the increased prevalence of ILD in RA may also be a contributory factor. No association between

Table 14.2 Risk of cancer in RA patients

Cancer type	International data RA compared to general population SIR [95% CI]	UK data in biologic naïve RA patients compared to general population SIR [95% CI]	UK data in anti-TNF treated patients compared to biologic naïve patients Age and sex adjusted Hazard ratio [95% CI]
All cancers	1.09 (1.06, 1.13)	1.28 (1.18, 1.58)	0.8 (0.7, 1.0)
Lymphoma	2.46 (2.05, 2.96)	3.81 (2.36, 5.82)	0.75 (0.49 to 1.15)
Lung	1.64 (1.51, 1.79)	2.39 (1.75, 3.19)	0.81 (0.56 to 1.17)
Melanoma	1.23 (1.01, 11.49)	2.05 (0.94, 3.90)	1.1 (0.8, 1.6)†
Colorectal	0.78 (0.71, 1.01)	0.96 (0.56, 1.54)	0.71 (0.41 to 1.23)
Breast	0.86 (0.72, 1.01)	1.07 (0.72, 1.52)	0.83 (0.51 to 1.35)
Cervical*	0.87 (0.72, 1.05)	0.35 (0.10, 0.90)	–
Prostate	1.15 (0.98, 1.34)	0.35 (0.11, 0.82)	–

*in UK data all female genital organ cancer rate rather than cervical cancer rate †EU registry data SIR = standardized incidence ratio; [95%CI] = 95% confidence intervals.

RA disease characteristics, inflammatory burden or medication on and lung cancer risk has been observed and rates are similar between biologic-treated and csDMARD-treated patients.[65]

Lower rates of other cancers such as colorectal cancer have been observed in RA. It is hypothesized that use of NSAIDs in RA may have a protective effect for colorectal cancer.

Management of cancer risk in RA

An international study demonstrated low rates of cancer screening in RA patients with only 52% of those eligible undergoing breast cancer screening.[11] A recent EULAR initiative has recommended routine documentation of cancer risk factors including relevant family history in all patients with RA.[117] Patients, particularly those being considered for biologic therapy, should be actively encouraged to engage in cancer screening programmes. There is currently no data to underpin recommendations of csDMARDs and biologic DMARDs in patients with precancerous conditions, but increased vigilance is recommended. Strong encouragement of smoking cessation is important and good control of disease activity may have a positive influence of cancer risk.

Infection

Infection is the fourth commonest cause of death in RA and patients are almost twice as likely to suffer or die from infection compared to age and sex matched controls, even when other risk factors such as smoking are taken into account.[118] Patients can present with less systemic response to infection often presenting without fever or raised white cell count. This can be as a result of immunosuppression or disease related immune system dysfunction. The lack of systemic upset can delay recognition and treatment of infection and may contribute to the higher rates of septicaemia seen in RA.[119] Pneumonia and soft tissue infections are the most common serious infections in RA (i.e. those which require hospitalization, intravenous antibiotics, or cause death).[119] While the joint is not a common site of infection, RA patients have a 21-fold increased risk of septic arthritis compared to the general population.[118] Septic arthritis is associated with significant mortality risk and can mimic RA flare so a high index of suspicion is always required. Patients are also at higher risk of opportunistic infections such as *Pneumocystis Jirovecii* and fungal infections, particularly when treated with biologic therapy (see also Chapter 34 on biologics).

The increased risk of infection is likely due to a combination of disease-specific factors, use of immunomodulatory drugs, shared risk factors, and other comorbidities. Disease severity and rheumatoid factor positivity are associated with increased infection risk.[119] Furthermore, RA patients are known to have impaired innate and humoral immunity. The increased prevalence of diabetes and chronic lung disease seen in RA also predispose patients to infection and could also lead to worse prognosis. Smoking is also an important and modifiable risk factor, particularly in the context of respiratory infections. One study demonstrated that patients who stopped smoking for more than 1 year were 15% less likely to develop respiratory infections within the following year.[116]

Medications used in RA are a major risk factor for infection. The use of glucocorticoids has a dose dependent association with infection risk. Patients taking less than 5 mg, 5–10 mg, or 10–20 mg are 40%, 90%, and 300% more likely to get infections, respectively compared to RA patients not taking steroids.[120] Most csDMARDs are immunosuppressant and are also associated with infection risk. Studies have not demonstrated differing risks with specific csDMARDs.[121] However, the effect of controlling disease may also have a positive influence on infection risk. The reported risk of serious infection with biologic therapy is between 10% and 80% higher than with csDMARDs.[122] The risk appears highest within the first 6 months of treatment.[123] There does not appear to be a significant difference in risk of infection between specific anti-TNF agents or indeed between different types of biologics agents.[122,124] The most common infections seen in biologic-treated patients are respiratory and soft tissue infections. Importantly there is a significant risk of tuberculosis associated with anti-TNF therapy compared to csDMARDs. Anti-TNF treated patients are also notably at higher risk of septic arthritis and opportunistic infections compared with patients on csDMARDs and this is discussed in further detail in Chapter 39.

The key principles for managing infection risk are recognizing and minimizing risk factors including smoking cessation advice and ensuring patients are vaccinated appropriately. Recent data suggests that only 20–25% of patients were vaccinated for pneumococcal and influenza infection despite national recommendation.[11] It is also important to consider infection risk when making therapeutic decisions. The need for glucocorticoids to control disease is acknowledged but judicious use for flares with quick tapering is advised to minimize risk of infection. High index of suspicion for infection, particularly in those with other comorbidities and those on biologics is important. The German biologics registry identified risk factors for serious infection and based on this developed a risk prediction tool for infection.[125] The score considers the following factors: age, history of renal or lung disease, number of previous DMARD failures and glucocorticoid use. It has been shown to predict serious infection in biologic-treated patients and is also associated with higher likelihood of admission to intensive care with infection.[126]

Osteoporosis

Osteoporosis is a common complication of RA and RA is an accepted risk factor for osteoporosis. Bone loss is observed early in the disease course.[127] Overall RA patients have a twofold increased risk of fracture compared to age and gender matched controls with the most pronounced increased risk for vertebral fracture.[128,129] The increased risk is most marked in women but is also present in men over the age of 50 years.[130] There is a strong link between inflammatory disease burden and osteoporotic fracture risk and also a well-established link with corticosteroids. Interestingly in early disease progressive joint erosions are associated with loss of bone density independent of disease activity and treatments. A number of cytokines involved in local bone loss causing erosion are also key regulators of regional bone turn. It may be that factors driving erosions may also mediate an effect on bone loss independent of inflammation.[128] Other factors associated with increased risk of fracture include age, physical inactivity, low BMI, and antibody positivity.[128]

Annual review of osteoporosis risk assessment is recommended but data suggests that assessment is undertaken in around 35% of patients.[4]

Risk assessment tools for fracture including the fracture risk assessment tool (FRAX) tool[131] incorporate RA as a risk factor in addition to glucocorticoid use. It is also recommended that in patients over the age of 70 years taking more than 7.5 mg of prednisolone per day, bone protection should be considered.[132] There is evidence that treatment with bisphosphonates or teriparatide is associated with a lower rate of fracture in RA and slows decline in bone density.[128] The effect of DMARD therapy on fracture risk is not well studied however it is likely that though better control of inflammation and lower corticosteroids requirements, they may have a positive impact on fracture risk.

Depression

Prevalence rates of depression vary depending on the methods use but self-reported rates are up to 40% in RA.[133] Prevalence is significantly higher than in the general population and depression was the most prevalent comorbidity found in one large international study of RA patients.[4] Around 1 in every 170 RA patient die as a result of suicide, 2.5 fold higher than the general population.[134] Depression is also associated with lower quality of life, adverse health outcomes and poorer treatment response in RA.[135]

A number of factors are associated with increased risk of depression including RA specific factors such as level of pain, disability, disease activity, and fatigue. Socioeconomic factors including poverty and social isolation are also important contributory factors. There is also evidence that having additional comorbidity in RA is associated with depression.[136] Inconsistent associations have been found between pro-inflammatory cytokines such as TNF and depression in RA.[137] However, there is increasing interest in the role inflammation and in particular TNF plays in depression in the general population and this is an area of active research.

There is evidence that pharmacological and non-pharmacological interventions can have a positive impact on depression in RA patients and a consequential impact on RA disease.[138] Exercise, peer support, cognitive, and behavioural interventions and internet-based interventions have all shown benefit in RA.[138]

Screening and managing comorbidity in RA

Both National and European guidelines recommend regular assessment of comorbidity however as previously discussed screening for a number of key comorbidities is underperformed in RA patients.[11] The UK National Institute for Health and Care Excellence (NICE) recommend that RA patients undergo annual assessment for comorbidities. EULAR guidance focuses on the screening and management of specific comorbidities but recommends standardized screening and recording of comorbidities, which may also help to study the scale of comorbidities across countries.[117]

REFERENCES

1. Charlson ME, Pompei P, Ales KL, MacKenzie CR. A new method of classifying prognostic comorbidity in longitudinal studies: development and validation. *J Chronic Dis* 1987;*40*(5):373–83.

2. England BR, Sayles H, Mikuls TR, Johnson DS, Michaud K. Validation of the rheumatic disease comorbidity index. *Arthritis Care Res (Hoboken)* 2015;*67*(6):865–72.

3. Norton S, Koduri G, Nikiphorou E, Dixey J, Williams P, Young A. A study of baseline prevalence and cumulative incidence of comorbidity and extra-articular manifestations in RA and their impact on outcome. *Rheumatology (Oxford)* 2013;*52*(1):99–110.

4. Radner H, Yoshida K, Mjaavatten MD, et al. Development of a multimorbidity index: impact on quality of life using a rheumatoid arthritis cohort. *Semin Arthritis Rheum* 2015;*45*(2):167–73.

5. Verstappen SM, Askling J, Berglind N, et al. Methodological challenges when comparing demographic and clinical characteristics of international observational registries. *Arthritis Care Res (Hoboken)* 2015;*67*(12):1637–45.

6. Yurkovich M, Avina-Zubieta JA, Thomas J, Gorenchtein M, Lacaille D. A systematic review identifies valid comorbidity indices derived from administrative health data. *J Clin Epidemiol* 2015;*68*(1):3–14.

7. Gabriel SE, Crowson CS, O'Fallon WM. A comparison of two comorbidity instruments in arthritis. *J Clin Epidemiol* 1999 Dec;*52*(12):1137–42.

8. Radner H, Smolen JS, Aletaha D. Comorbidity affects all domains of physical function and quality of life in patients with rheumatoid arthritis. *Rheumatology (Oxf)* 2011;*50*(2):381–8.

9. Kapetanovic MC, Lindqvist E, Nilsson JA, Geborek P, Saxne T, Eberhardt K. Development of functional impairment and disability in rheumatoid arthritis patients followed for 20 years: relation to disease activity, joint damage, and comorbidity. *Arthritis Care Res (Hoboken)* 2015;*67*(3):340–8.

10. England BR, Sayles H, Mikuls TR, Johnson DS, Michaud K. Validation of the rheumatic disease comorbidity index. *Arthritis Care Res (Hoboken)* 2015;*67*(6):865–72.

11. Dougados M, Soubrier M, Antunez A, et al. Prevalence of comorbidities in rheumatoid arthritis and evaluation of their monitoring: results of an international, cross-sectional study (COMORA). *Ann Rheum Dis* 2014;*73*(1):62–8.

12. MacLean CH, Louie R, Leake B, et al. Quality of care for patients with rheumatoid arthritis. *JAMA* 2000;*284*(8):984–92.

13. Innala L, Sjoberg C, Moller B, et al. Co-morbidity in patients with early rheumatoid arthritis—inflammation matters. *Arthritis Res Ther* 2016;*18*:33.

14. Gron KL, Ornbjerg LM, Hetland ML, et al. The association of fatigue, comorbidity burden, disease activity, disability and gross domestic product in patients with rheumatoid arthritis. Results from 34 countries participating in the Quest-RA program. *Clin Exp Rheumatol* 2014;*32*(6):869–77.

15. Gron KL, Ornbjerg LM, Hetland ML, et al. The association of fatigue, comorbidity burden, disease activity, disability and gross domestic product in patients with rheumatoid arthritis. Results from 34 countries participating in the Quest-RA program. *Clin Exp Rheumatol* 2014;*32*(6):869–77.

16. Young A et al. Mortality in rheumatoid arthritis. Increased in the early course of disease, in ischaemic heart disease and in pulmonary fibrosis. *Rheumatology* (Oxford) 2007;*46*(2):350–7.

17. Richards JS, Dowell SM, Quinones ME, Kerr GS. How to use biologic agents in patients with rheumatoid arthritis who have comorbid disease. *BMJ* 2015;*351*:h3658.

18. Ranganath VK, Maranian P, Elashoff DA, et al. Comorbidities are associated with poorer outcomes in community patients with rheumatoid arthritis. *Rheumatology (Oxf)* 2013;*52*(10):1809–17.

19. Dougados M, Soubrier M, Antunez A, et al. Prevalence of comorbidities in rheumatoid arthritis and evaluation of their monitoring: results of an international, cross-sectional study (COMORA). *Ann Rheum Dis* 2014;73(1):62–8.

20. Avina-Zubieta JA, Thomas J, Sadatsafavi M, Lehman AJ, Lacaille D. Risk of incident cardiovascular events in patients with rheumatoid arthritis: a meta-analysis of observational studies. *Ann Rheum Dis* 2012;71(9):1524–9.

21. Avina-Zubieta JA, Choi HK, Sadatsafavi M, Etminan M, Esdaile JM, Lacaille D. Risk of cardiovascular mortality in patients with rheumatoid arthritis: a meta-analysis of observational studies. *Arthritis Rheum* 2008;59(12):1690–7.

22. Schieir O, Tosevski C, Glazier RH, Hogg-Johnson S, Badley EM. Incident myocardial infarction associated with major types of arthritis in the general population: a systematic review and meta-analysis. *Ann Rheum Dis* 2017;76(8):1396–404.

23. Goodson N, Marks J, Lunt M, Symmons D. Cardiovascular admissions and mortality in an inception cohort of patients with rheumatoid arthritis with onset in the 1980s and 1990s. *Ann Rheum Dis* 2005;64(11):1595–601.

24. Radovits BJ, Fransen J, Al SS, Eijsbouts AM, van Riel PL, Laan RF. Excess mortality emerges after 10 years in an inception cohort of early rheumatoid arthritis. *Arthritis Care Res (Hoboken)* 2010;62(3):362–70.

25. Maradit-Kremers H, Crowson CS, Nicola PJ, et al. Increased unrecognized coronary heart disease and sudden deaths in rheumatoid arthritis: a population-based cohort study. *Arthritis Rheum* 2005;52(2):402–11.

26. Balandraud N, Picard C, Reviron D, et al. HLA-DRB1 genotypes and the risk of developing anti citrullinated protein antibody (ACPA) positive rheumatoid arthritis. *PLoS One* 2013;8(5):e64108.

27. Paakkanen R, Lokki ML, Seppannen M, Tierala I, Nieminen MS, Sinisalo J. Proinflammatory HLA-DRB1*01-haplotype predisposes to ST-elevation myocardial infarction. *Atherosclerosis* 2012;221(2):461–6.

28. Skeoch S, Bruce IN. Atherosclerosis in rheumatoid arthritis: is it all about inflammation? *Nat Rev Rheumatol* 2015;11(7):390–400.

29. Sarwar N, Butterworth AS, Freitag DF, et al. Interleukin-6 receptor pathways in coronary heart disease: a collaborative meta-analysis of 82 studies. *Lancet* 2012;379(9822):1205–13.

30. Nolan D, Kraus WE, Hauser E, et al. Genome-wide linkage analysis of cardiovascular disease biomarkers in a large, multigenerational family. *PLoS One* 2013;8(8):e71779.

31. Swanberg M, Lidman O, Padyukov L, et al. MHC2TA is associated with differential MHC molecule expression and susceptibility to rheumatoid arthritis, multiple sclerosis and myocardial infarction. *Nat Genet* 2005;37(5):486–94.

32. Lahiri M, Luben RN, Morgan C, et al. Using lifestyle factors to identify individuals at higher risk of inflammatory polyarthritis (results from the European Prospective Investigation of Cancer-Norfolk and the Norfolk Arthritis Register—the EPIC-2-NOAR Study). *Ann Rheum Dis* 2014;73(1):219–26.

33. Radner H, Lesperance T, Accortt NA, Solomon DH. Incidence and prevalence of cardiovascular risk factors among patients with rheumatoid arthritis, Psoriasis, or Psoriatic Arthritis. *Arthritis Care Res (Hoboken)* 2017;69(10):1510–18.

34. Panoulas VF, Metsios GS, Pace AV, et al. Hypertension in rheumatoid arthritis. *Rheumatology* 2008;47(9):1286–98.

35. Boyer JF, Gourraud PA, Cantagrel A, Davignon JL, Constantin A. Traditional cardiovascular risk factors in rheumatoid arthritis: a meta-analysis. *Joint Bone Spine* 2011;78(2):179–83.

36. Baghdadi LR, Woodman RJ, Shanahan EM, Mangoni AA. The impact of traditional cardiovascular risk factors on cardiovascular outcomes in patients with rheumatoid arthritis: a systematic review and meta-analysis. *PLoS One* 2015;10(2):e0117952.

37. Manavathongchai S, Bian A, Rho YH, et al. Inflammation and hypertension in rheumatoid arthritis. *J Rheumatol* 2013;40(11):1806–11.

38. Dubreuil M, Rho YH, Man A, et al. Diabetes incidence in psoriatic arthritis, psoriasis and rheumatoid arthritis: a UK population-based cohort study. *Rheumatology (Oxford)* 2014;53(2):346–52.

39. Movahedi M, Beauchamp ME, Abrahamowicz M, et al. Risk of incident diabetes mellitus associated with the dosage and duration of oral glucocorticoid therapy in patients with rheumatoid arthritis. *Arthritis Rheumatol* 2016;68(5):1089–98.

40. Gonzalez A, Maradit KH, Crowson CS, et al. Do cardiovascular risk factors confer the same risk for cardiovascular outcomes in rheumatoid arthritis patients as in non-rheumatoid arthritis patients? *Ann Rheum Dis* 2008;67(1):64–9.

41. Georgiadis A, Papavasiliou E, Lourida E, et al. Atherogenic lipid profile is a feature characteristic of patients with early rheumatoid arthritis: effect of early treatment—a prospective, controlled study. *Arthritis Res Ther* 2006;8(3):R82.

42. Myasoedova E, Crowson CS, Kremers HM, et al. Lipid paradox in rheumatoid arthritis: the impact of serum lipid measures and systemic inflammation on the risk of cardiovascular disease. *Ann Rheum Dis* 2011;70(3):482–7.

43. Crowson CS, Rollefstad S, Ikdahl E, et al. Impact of risk factors associated with cardiovascular outcomes in patients with rheumatoid arthritis. *Ann Rheum Dis* 2018;77(1):48–54.

44. Aubry MC, Riehle DL, Edwards WD, et al. B-Lymphocytes in plaque and adventitia of coronary arteries in two patients with rheumatoid arthritis and coronary atherosclerosis: preliminary observations. *Cardiovasc Pathol* 2004;13(4):233–6.

45. Kremers HM, Nicola PJ, Crowson CS, Ballman KV, Gabriel SE. Prognostic importance of low body mass index in relation to cardiovascular mortality in rheumatoid arthritis. *Arthritis Rheum* 2004;50(11):3450–7.

46. Giles JT, Allison M, Blumenthal RS, et al. Abdominal adiposity in rheumatoid arthritis: association with cardiometabolic risk factors and disease characteristics. *Arthritis Rheum* 2010;62(11):3173–82.

47. Joseph RM, Movahedi M, Dixon WG, Symmons DP. Risks of smoking and benefits of smoking cessation on hospitalisations for cardiovascular events and respiratory infection in patients with rheumatoid arthritis: a retrospective cohort study using the Clinical Practice Research Datalink. *RMD Open* 2017;3(2):e000506.

48. JBS3 Board. Joint British Societies' consensus recommendations for the prevention of cardiovascular disease (JBS3). *Heart* 2014;100 Suppl 2:ii1–ii67.

49. Edwards CJ, Syddall H, Goswami R, et al. The autoantibody rheumatoid factor may be an independent risk factor for ischaemic heart disease in men. *Heart* 2007;93(10):1263–7.

50. Cambridge G, Acharya J, Cooper JA, Edwards JC, Humphries SE. Antibodies to citrullinated peptides and risk of coronary heart disease. *Atherosclerosis* 2013;228(1):243–6.

51. Kaptoge S, Di AE, Pennells L, et al. C-reactive protein, fibrinogen, and cardiovascular disease prediction. *N Engl J Med* 2012;367(14):1310–20.

52. Wallberg-Jonsson S, Johansson H, Ohman ML, Rantapaa-Dahlqvist S. Extent of inflammation predicts cardiovascular

disease and overall mortality in seropositive rheumatoid arthritis. A retrospective cohort study from disease onset. *J Rheumatol* 1999;*26*(12):2562–71.

53. Innala L, Sjoberg C, Moller B, et al. Co-morbidity in patients with early rheumatoid arthritis—inflammation matters. *Arthritis Res Ther* 2016;*18*:33.

54. Myasoedova E, Chandran A, Ilhan B, et al. The role of rheumatoid arthritis (RA) flare and cumulative burden of RA severity in the risk of cardiovascular disease. *Ann Rheum Dis* 2016;*75*(3):560–5.

55. Semb AG, Rollefstad S, Provan SA, et al. Carotid plaque characteristics and disease activity in rheumatoid arthritis. *J Rheumatol* 2013;*40*(4):359–68.

56. Skeoch S, Cristinacce PL, Williams H, et al. Imaging atherosclerosis in rheumatoid arthritis: evidence for increased prevalence, altered phenotype and a link between systemic and localised plaque inflammation. *Sci Rep* 2017;*7*(1):827.

57. Maki-Petaja KM, Elkhawad M, Cheriyan J, et al. Anti-tumor necrosis factor-alpha therapy reduces aortic inflammation and stiffness in patients with rheumatoid arthritis. *Circulation* 2012;*126*(21):2473–80.

58. Robertson J, Peters MJ, McInnes IB, Sattar N. Changes in lipid levels with inflammation and therapy in RA: a maturing paradigm. *Nat Rev Rheumatol* 2013;*9*(9):513–23.

59. Humphreys JH, Warner A, Chipping J, et al. Mortality trends in patients with early rheumatoid arthritis over 20 years: results from the Norfolk Arthritis Register. *Arthritis Care Res (Hoboken)* 2014;*66*(9):1296–301.

60. Dadoun S, Zeboulon-Ktorza N, Combescure C, et al. Mortality in rheumatoid arthritis over the last fifty years: systematic review and meta-analysis. *Joint Bone Spine* 2013;*80*(1):29–33.

61. Cook MJ, Diffin J, Scire CA, et al. Predictors and outcomes of sustained, intermittent or never achieving remission in patients with recent onset inflammatory polyarthritis: results from the Norfolk Arthritis Register. *Rheumatology (Oxf)* 2016;*55*(9):1601–9.

62. Roubille C, Richer V, Starnino T, et al. Evidence-based recommendations for the management of comorbidities in rheumatoid arthritis, psoriasis, and psoriatic arthritis: expert opinion of the Canadian Dermatology-Rheumatology Comorbidity Initiative. *J Rheumatol* 2015;*42*(10):1767–80.

63. Meissner Y, Zink A, Kekow J, et al. Impact of disease activity and treatment of comorbidities on the risk of myocardial infarction in rheumatoid arthritis. *Arthritis Res Ther* 2016;*18*(1):183.

64. Tom TE, et al. Statin use in rheumatoid arthritis in relation to actual cardiovascular risk: evidence for substantial undertreatment of lipid-associated cardiovascular risk? *Ann. Rheum Dis* 2010;*69*:683–688.

65. Ramiro S, Sepriano A, Chatzidionysiou K, et al. Safety of synthetic and biological DMARDs: a systematic literature review informing the 2016 update of the EULAR recommendations for management of rheumatoid arthritis. *Ann Rheum Dis* 2017;*76*(6):1101–36.

66. Arts EEA, Popa C, den Broeder AA, et al. Performance of four current risk algorithms in predicting cardiovascular events in patients with early rheumatoid arthritis. *Ann Rheum Dis* 2015;*74*(4): 668–74.

67. Semb AG, Holme I, Kvien TK, Pedersen TR. Intensive lipid lowering in patients with rheumatoid arthritis and previous myocardial infarction: an explorative analysis from the incremental decrease in endpoints through aggressive lipid lowering trial. *Rheumatology (Oxf)* 2011;*50*(2):324–9.

68. Semb AG, Kvien TK, DeMicco DA, et al. Effect of intensive lipid-lowering therapy on cardiovascular outcome in patients with

and those without inflammatory joint disease. *Arthritis Rheum* 2012;*64*(9):2836–46.

69. Young A, Koduri G, Batley M, et al. Mortality in rheumatoid arthritis. Increased in the early course of disease, in ischaemic heart disease and in pulmonary fibrosis. *Rheumatology (Oxford)* 2007;*46*(2):350–7.

70. England BR, Sayles H, Michaud K, et al. Cause-specific mortality in male US veterans with rheumatoid arthritis. *Arthritis Care Res (Hoboken)* 2016;*68*(1):36–45.

71. Wilsher M, Voight L, Milne D, et al. Prevalence of airway and parenchymal abnormalities in newly diagnosed rheumatoid arthritis. *Respir Med* 2012;*106*(10):1441–6.

72. Doyle TJ, Lee JS, Dellaripa PF, et al. A roadmap to promote clinical and translational research in rheumatoid arthritis-associated interstitial lung disease. *Chest* 2014;*145*(3):454–63.

73. Dawson JK, Fewins HE, Desmond J, Lynch MP, Graham DR. Fibrosing alveolitis in patients with rheumatoid arthritis as assessed by high resolution computed tomography, chest radiography, and pulmonary function tests. *Thorax* 2001;*56*(8):622–7.

74. Kelly CA, Saravanan V, Nisar M, et al. Rheumatoid arthritis-related interstitial lung disease: associations, prognostic factors and physiological and radiological characteristics—a large multicentre UK study. *Rheumatology (Oxf)* 2014;*53*(9):1676–82.

75. Tsuchiya Y, Takayanagi N, Sugiura H, et al. Lung diseases directly associated with rheumatoid arthritis and their relationship to outcome. *Eur Respir J* 2011;*37*(6):1411–17.

76. Zamora-Legoff JA, Krause ML, Crowson CS, Ryu JH, Matteson EL. Progressive Decline of Lung Function in Rheumatoid Arthritis-Associated Interstitial Lung Disease. *Arthritis Rheumatol* 2017;*69*(3):542–9.

77. Bongartz T, Nannini C, Medina-Velasquez YF, et al. Incidence and mortality of interstitial lung disease in rheumatoid arthritis: a population-based study. *Arthritis Rheum* 2010;*62*(6):1583–91.

78. Kim EJ, Collard HR, King TE, Jr. Rheumatoid arthritis-associated interstitial lung disease: the relevance of histopathologic and radiographic pattern. *Chest* 2009;*136*(5):1397–405.

79. Solomon JJ, Ryu JH, Tazelaar HD, et al. Fibrosing interstitial pneumonia predicts survival in patients with rheumatoid arthritis-associated interstitial lung disease (RA-ILD). *Respir Med* 2013;*107*(8):1247–52.

80. Tsuchiya Y, Takayanagi N, Sugiura H, et al. Lung diseases directly associated with rheumatoid arthritis and their relationship to outcome. *Eur Respir J* 2011;*37*(6):1411–17.

81. Assayag D, Lubin M, Lee JS, King TE, Collard HR, Ryerson CJ. Predictors of mortality in rheumatoid arthritis-related interstitial lung disease. *Respirology* 2014;*19*(4):493–500.

82. Roubille C, Haraoui B. Interstitial lung diseases induced or exacerbated by DMARDS and biologic agents in rheumatoid arthritis: a systematic literature review. *Semin Arthritis Rheum* 2014;*43*(5):613–26.

83. Curtis JR, Sarsour K, Napalkov P, Costa LA, Schulman KL. Incidence and complications of interstitial lung disease in users of tocilizumab, rituximab, abatacept and anti-tumor necrosis factor alpha agents, a retrospective cohort study. *Arthritis Res Ther* 2015;*17*:319.

84. Yunt ZX, Solomon JJ. Lung disease in rheumatoid arthritis. *Rheum Dis Clin North Am* 2015;*41*(2):225–36.

85. Solomon JJ, Ryu JH, Tazelaar HD, et al. Fibrosing interstitial pneumonia predicts survival in patients with rheumatoid arthritis-associated interstitial lung disease (RA-ILD). *Respir Med* 2013;*107*(8):1247–52.

86. Matteson E, Bongartz T, Ryu JH, Crowson C, Hartman T, Dellaripa PF. Open-label, pilot study of the safety and clinical effects of rituximab in patients with rheumatoid arthritis-associated interstitial pneumonia. *OJRA* 2012;*2*:53–8.

87. Crowson CS, Matteson EL, Roger VL, Therneau TM, Gabriel SE. Usefulness of risk scores to estimate the risk of cardiovascular disease in patients with rheumatoid arthritis. *Am J Cardiol* 2012;*110*(3):420–4.

88. Yusof MY, Kabia A, Darby M, et al. Effect of rituximab on the progression of rheumatoid arthritis-related interstitial lung disease: 10 years' experience at a single centre. *Rheumatology (Oxf)* 2017;*56*(8):1348–57.

89. O'Riordan TG, Smith V, Raghu G. Development of novel agents for idiopathic pulmonary fibrosis: progress in target selection and clinical trial design. *Chest* 2015;*148*(4):1083–92.

90. Bluett J, Jani M, Symmons DPM. Practical management of respiratory comorbidities in patients with rheumatoid arthritis. *Rheumatol Ther* 2017;*4*(2):309–32.

91. Jani M, Hirani N, Matteson EL, Dixon WG. The safety of biologic therapies in RA-associated interstitial lung disease. *Nat Rev Rheumatol* 2014;*10*(5):284–94.

92. Aronoff A, Bywaters EG, Fearnley GR. Lung lesions in rheumatoid arthritis. *Br Med J* 1955;*2*(4933):228–32.

93. Pasteur MC, Bilton D, Hill AT. British Thoracic Society guideline for non-CF bronchiectasis. *Thorax* 2010;*65* Suppl 1:i1–58.

94. Perry E, Eggleton P, De SA, Hutchinson D, Kelly C. Increased disease activity, severity and autoantibody positivity in rheumatoid arthritis patients with co-existent bronchiectasis. *Int J Rheum Dis* 2015;*17*(1):174.

95. Quirke AM, Perry E, Cartwright A, et al. Bronchiectasis is a model for chronic bacterial infection inducing autoimmunity in rheumatoid arthritis. *Arthritis Rheumatol* 2015;*67*(9):2335–42.

96. Geri G, Dadoun S, Bui T, et al. Risk of infections in bronchiectasis during disease-modifying treatment and biologics for rheumatic diseases. *BMC Infect Dis* 2011;*11*:304.

97. Ungprasert P, Srivali N, Cheungpasitporn W, Davis Iii JM. Risk of incident chronic obstructive pulmonary disease in patients with rheumatoid arthritis: a systematic review and meta-analysis. *Joint Bone Spine* 2016;*83*(3):290–4.

98. Lugli EB, Correia RE, Fischer R, et al. Expression of citrulline and homocitrulline residues in the lungs of non-smokers and smokers: implications for autoimmunity in rheumatoid arthritis. *Arthritis Res Ther* 2015;*17*:9.

99. Yang DH, Tu CC, Wang SC, et al. Circulating anti-cyclic citrullinated peptide antibody in patients with rheumatoid arthritis and chronic obstructive pulmonary disease. *Rheumatol Int.* 2014 Jul;*34*(7):971–7.

100. Ruiz-Esquide V, Gomara MJ, Peinado VI, et al. Anti-citrullinated peptide antibodies in the serum of heavy smokers without rheumatoid arthritis. A differential effect of chronic obstructive pulmonary disease? *Clin Rheumatol* 2012 Jul;*31*(7):1047–50.

101. Nannini C, Medina-Velasquez YF, Achenbach SJ, et al. Incidence and mortality of obstructive lung disease in rheumatoid arthritis: a population-based study. *Arthritis Care Res (Hoboken)* 2013;*65*(8):1243–50.

102. Simon TA, Thompson A, Gandhi KK, Hochberg MC, Suissa S. Incidence of malignancy in adult patients with rheumatoid arthritis: a meta-analysis. *Arthritis Res Ther* 2015;*17*:212.

103. Mercer LK, Davies R, Galloway JB, et al. Risk of cancer in patients receiving non-biologic disease-modifying therapy for

104. Ertz-Archambault N, Kosiorek H, Taylor GE, et al. Association of therapy for autoimmune disease with myelodysplastic syndromes and acute myeloid leukemia. *JAMA Oncol* 2017;*3*(7):936–43.

105. Tokuhira M, Saito S, Okuyama A, et al. Clinicopathologic investigation of methotrexate-induced lymphoproliferative disorders, with a focus on regression. *Leuk Lymphoma* 2017;1–10.

106. Askling J, Fahrbach K, Nordstrom B, Ross S, Schmid CH, Symmons D. Cancer risk with tumor necrosis factor alpha (TNF) inhibitors: meta-analysis of randomized controlled trials of adalimumab, etanercept, and infliximab using patient level data. *Pharmacoepidemiol Drug Saf* 2011;*20*(2):119–30.

107. Wadstrom H, Frisell T, Askling J. Malignant neoplasms in patients with rheumatoid arthritis treated with tumor necrosis factor inhibitors, tocilizumab, abatacept, or rituximab in clinical practice: a nationwide cohort study from Sweden. *JAMA Intern Med* 2017;*177*(11):1605–12.

108. Mercer LK, Lunt M, Low AL, et al. Risk of solid cancer in patients exposed to anti-tumour necrosis factor therapy: results from the British Society for Rheumatology Biologics Register for Rheumatoid Arthritis. *Ann Rheum Dis* 2015;*74*(6):1087–93.

109. Mercer LK, Galloway JB, Lunt M, et al. Risk of lymphoma in patients exposed to antitumour necrosis factor therapy: results from the British Society for Rheumatology Biologics Register for Rheumatoid Arthritis. *Ann Rheum Dis* 2017;*76*(3):497–503.

110. Mercer LK, Askling J, Raaschou P, et al. Risk of invasive melanoma in patients with rheumatoid arthritis treated with biologics: results from a collaborative project of 11 European biologic registers. *Ann Rheum Dis* 2017;*76*(2):386–91.

111. Mercer LK, Regierer AC, Mariette X, et al. Spectrum of lymphomas across different drug treatment groups in rheumatoid arthritis: a European registries collaborative project. *Ann Rheum Dis* 2017;*76*(12):2025–30.

112. Smedby KE, Baecklund E, Askling J. Malignant lymphomas in autoimmunity and inflammation: a review of risks, risk factors, and lymphoma characteristics. *Cancer Epidemiol Biomarkers Prev* 2006;*15*(11):2069–77.

113. Baecklund E, Smedby KE, Sutton LA, Askling J, Rosenquist R. Lymphoma development in patients with autoimmune and inflammatory disorders--what are the driving forces? *Semin Cancer Biol* 2014;*24*:61–70.

114. Tokuhira M, Saito S, Okuyama A, et al. Clinicopathologic investigation of methotrexate-induced lymphoproliferative disorders, with a focus on regression. *Leuk Lymphoma* 2018;*59*(5):1143–52.

115. Abasolo L, Judez E, Descalzo MA, Gonzalez-Alvaro I, Jover JA, Carmona L. Cancer in rheumatoid arthritis: occurrence, mortality, and associated factors in a South European population. *Semin Arthritis Rheum* 2008;*37*(6):388–97.

116. Joseph RM, Movahedi M, Dixon WG, Symmons DP. Smoking-related mortality in patients with early rheumatoid arthritis: a retrospective cohort study using the clinical practice research datalink. *Arthritis Care Res (Hoboken)* 2016;*68*(11):1598–606.

117. Baillet A, Gossec L, Carmona L, et al. Points to consider for reporting, screening for and preventing selected comorbidities in chronic inflammatory rheumatic diseases in daily practice: a EULAR initiative. *Ann Rheum Dis* 2016;*75*(6):965–73.

118. Doran MF, Crowson CS, Pond GR, O'Fallon WM, Gabriel SE. Frequency of infection in patients with rheumatoid arthritis

rheumatoid arthritis compared with the UK general population. *Rheumatology (Oxf)* 2013;*52*(1):91–8.

compared with controls: a population-based study. *Arthritis Rheum* 2002;*46*(9):2287–93.

119. Doran MF, Crowson CS, Pond GR, O'Fallon WM, Gabriel SE. Predictors of infection in rheumatoid arthritis. *Arthritis Rheum* 2002 Sep;*46*(9):2294–300.

120. Dixon WG, Suissa S, Hudson M. The association between systemic glucocorticoid therapy and the risk of infection in patients with rheumatoid arthritis: systematic review and meta-analyses. *Arthritis Res Ther* 2011;*13*(4):R139.

121. Ramiro S, Gaujoux-Viala C, Nam JL, et al. Safety of synthetic and biological DMARDs: a systematic literature review informing the 2013 update of the EULAR recommendations for management of rheumatoid arthritis. *Ann Rheum Dis* 2014;*73*(3):529–35.

122. Singh JA, Cameron C, Noorbaloochi S, et al. Risk of serious infection in biological treatment of patients with rheumatoid arthritis: a systematic review and meta-analysis. *Lancet* 2015s;*386*(9990):258–65.

123. Galloway JB, Hyrich KL, Mercer LK, et al. Risk of septic arthritis in patients with rheumatoid arthritis and the effect of anti-TNF therapy: results from the British Society for Rheumatology Biologics Register. *Ann Rheum Dis* 2011;*70*(10):1810–14.

124. Ramiro S, Sepriano A, Chatzidionysiou K, et al. Safety of synthetic and biological DMARDs: a systematic literature review informing the 2016 update of the EULAR recommendations for management of rheumatoid arthritis. *Ann Rheum Dis* 2017;*76*(6):1101–36.

125. Strangfeld E, Eveslage M, Schneider M, et al. Treatment benefit or survival of the fittest: what drives the time-dependent decrease in serious infection rates under TNF inhibition and what does this imply for the individual patient? *Ann Rheum Dis* 2011 Nov; *70*(11):1914–20.

126. Pieringer H, Hintenberger R, Pohanka E, et al. RABBIT risk score and ICU admission due to infection in patients with rheumatoid arthritis. *Clin Rheumatol* 2017;*36*(11):2439–45.

127. Guler-Yuksel M, Bijsterbosch J, Goekoop-Ruiterman YP, et al. Changes in bone mineral density in patients with recent onset, active rheumatoid arthritis. *Ann Rheum Dis* 2008;*67*(6):823–8.

128. Briot K, Geusens P, Em B, Lems WF, Roux C. Inflammatory diseases and bone fragility. *Osteoporos Int* 2017;*28*(12):3301–14.

129. Brennan SL, Toomey L, Kotowicz MA, Henry MJ, Griffiths H, Pasco JA. Rheumatoid arthritis and incident fracture in women: a case-control study. *BMC Musculoskelet Disord* 2014;*15*:13.

130. Amin S, Gabriel SE, Achenbach SJ, Atkinson EJ, Melton LJ, III. Are young women and men with rheumatoid arthritis at risk for fragility fractures? A population-based study. *J Rheumatol* 2013 Oct;*40*(10):1669–76.

131. Kanis JA, Johnell O, Oden A, Johansson H, McCloskey E. FRAX and the assessment of fracture probability in men and women from the UK. *Osteoporos Int* 2008;*19*(4):385–97.

132. Compston J, Cooper A, Cooper C, et al. UK clinical guideline for the prevention and treatment of osteoporosis. *Arch Osteoporos* 2017;*12*(1):43.

133. Matcham F, Norton S, Scott DL, Steer S, Hotopf M. Symptoms of depression and anxiety predict treatment response and long-term physical health outcomes in rheumatoid arthritis: secondary analysis of a randomized controlled trial. *Rheumatology (Oxf)* 2016;*55*(2):268–78.

134. Ogdie A, Maliha S, Shin D, et al. Cause-specific mortality in patients with psoriatic arthritis and rheumatoid arthritis. *Rheumatology (Oxf)* 2017;*56*(6):907–11.

135. Cordingley L, Prajapati R, Plant D, et al. Impact of psychological factors on subjective disease activity assessments in patients with severe rheumatoid arthritis. *Arthritis Care Res (Hoboken)* 2014;*66*(6):861–8.

136. Treharne GJ, Hale ED, Lyons AC, et al. Cardiovascular disease and psychological morbidity among rheumatoid arthritis patients. *Rheumatology (Oxf)* 2005;*44*(2):241–6.

137. Iaquinta M, McCrone S. An integrative review of correlates and predictors of depression in patients with rheumatoid arthritis. *Arch Psychiatr Nurs* 2015;*29*(5):265–78.

138. Withers MH, Gonzalez LT, Karpouzas GA. Identification and treatment optimization of comorbid depression in rheumatoid arthritis. *Rheumatol Ther* 2017;*4*(2):281–91.

SECTION 4
Disease assessment

15 Disease activity assessment in rheumatoid
    arthritis *161*
    Josef Smolen

16 Synovial biopsies *169*
    Douglas J. Veale and Ursula Fearon

17 Radiography in rheumatoid arthritis *177*
    Charles Peterfy, Philip G. Conaghan, and Mikkel Østergaard

18 Ultrasound in rheumatoid arthritis *195*
    *Andrew Filer, Maria Antonietta D'Agostino,
    and Ilfita Sahbudin*

19 Magnetic resonance imaging in rheumatoid
    arthritis *207*
    Mikkel Østergaard, Philip G. Conaghan, and Charles Peterfy

Disease activity assessment in rheumatoid arthritis

Josef Smolen

Introduction

The major clinical hallmarks of rheumatoid arthritis (RA) are articular swelling, joint pain, and morning joint stiffness. They are a consequence of the pathogenetic processes eliciting synovial inflammation which include infiltration into and/or expansion of various inflammatory cell populations within the synovium and production of a variety of cytokines locally and into the circulation; among these are the pro-inflammatory cytokines tumour necrosis factor alpha (TNFα) and interleukin (IL)-6.[1] Moreover, pro-inflammatory cytokines, in particular IL-6 directly activate acute phase reactants, such as C-reactive protein (CRP) or fibrinogen, in hepatocytes, thus inducing laboratory surrogates of inflammation.[2] The presence of all these clinical and molecular abnormalities is subsumed under the term 'disease activity' which may vary in extent between and within patients.

Another hallmark of RA is the high propensity to destroy the involved joints which itself is a consequence of the inflammatory response and the high levels of pro-inflammatory cytokines[3,4]; these levels exceed those seen in other diseases.[5] Hence, synovial inflammation induces mechanisms that lead to bone and cartilage destruction by osteoclast activation and metalloproteinase production[1,6]

In itself, clinical high disease activity (i.e. high extents of pain, joint swelling and morning joint stiffness) causes physical disability, though of reversible nature, whereas joint damage, the sequel of the inflammatory response, is the major cause of irreversible disability.[7] Thus inflammation and, consequently, its clinical surrogate—disease activity, is in the centre of events, the culprit of damage and disability (Figure 15.1).

The major characteristics and variables reflecting disease activity

Assessment of disease activity is pivotal both in clinical practice and clinical trials, since it allows to reliably judge the effectiveness of treatment. The degree of disease activity impacts prognosis and influences the selection of RA medication in daily clinical life.

Many variables reflect disease activity. They span from joint swelling to patient assessment of global disease activity. A valuable variable is one that changes in response to therapy in clinical trials and clinical practice. Moreover, it is essential that the variable has criterion and construct validity by predicting important outcomes of RA, in particular disability and damage.[8,9] To this end, core set variables have been defined in the early 1990s (Table 15.1). These variables have been found to be sensitive to change and be associated with major RA outcomes.[10] They are summarized in Table 1 and relate to their association with the two major adverse outcomes of RA, damage and disability.

Individual variables

Joint assessment

Joint involvement is traditionally assessed for swelling, by clinical examination of soft tissue swelling and/or effusion, and for tenderness upon pressure.[16] Indeed, joint swelling is highly related to progression of joint damage and damage is particularly seen in those joints that are clinically swollen.[15] Moreover, joint swelling contributes more strongly to progression of damage than acute phase reactant levels.[17]

The traditional joint count involves the assessment of 68 joints for tenderness and 66 joints for swelling (Table 15.2).[18] Grading of tenderness, such as by the Ritchie index,[19] or swelling was not shown to increase reliability.[20] A simplified joint assessment, such as the 28 joint count, however, is equally reliable as extended joint counts (Figure 15.2).[21,22] The reason for not including feet and ankles in the 28 joint count relates to the fact that tenderness in the forefeet is frequently due to other reasons than arthritis and swelling of ankles and forefeet may also be confounded by oedema which is frequent in this region. This does not imply that feet are not important enough in RA to be examined; on the contrary, the feet are frequently involved and must be assessed in clinical practice, but their inclusion in joint counts does not add additional information related to short- and long-term outcomes. Some clinicians actually add the ankles and feet to form a 32-joint count, with the metatarsophalangeal (MTP) accounted for as a single joint.

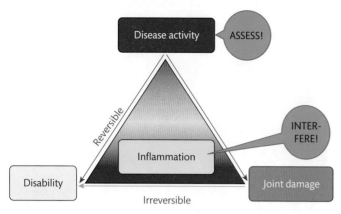

Figure 15.1 Interrelationship between inflammation, damage, and disability ('RA triad'). Inflammation leads to damage and to the reversible component of disability; damage leads to an irreversible component of total disability. Therefore, inflammation is in the centre of events and interfering effectively with inflammation by inducing clinical remission will stop progression of joint damage as well as indirectly, via halting damage, and directly prevent disability/maximize physical function. Interference with remission and control of the success of the respective therapeutic measures requires assessment of disease activity.

Source: data from Smolen et al (2018) 'Treating axial spondyloarthritis and peripheral spondyloarthritis, especially psoriatic arthritis, to target: 2017 update of recommendations by an international task force'. *Annals of the Rheumatic Diseases* 77(1):55–63.

Global assessments

Global assessments are usually performed using a visual analogue scale (VAS), i.e. a horizontal line of 100 mm with 0 meaning 'having no problem whatsoever' (e.g. no pain) and 100 reflecting a 'maximum problem' regarding the evaluated variable (e.g. maximum, unbearable pain). One can also use a numerical rating scale instead and also a 5-point Likert scale, but the traditional assessment is by a VAS. For the patient global assessment (PtGA), the usual question is, 'Considering all the ways your arthritis affects you, mark 'X' on the line for how well you are doing', with the anchors being very well and extremely bad. The other 2 assessments related to RA core set variables are physician (or evaluator or assessor) global

Table 15.1 Core set variables[']

Variable	Association with damage	Associated with impairment of physical function
Swollen joint count	+	–
Tender Joint count	–	+
Patient global assessment	–	+
Physician global assessment	+	+
Patient pain assessment	–	+
Acute phase reactants	+	–
Physical function*		–

* The European League Against Rheumatism (EULAR) regards physical function as an outcome rather than disease activity variable*.[11] the data are based on those provided in references.[12-15]

' Source: data from Felson D.T. et al (1993) 'The American College of Rheumatology preliminary core set of disease activity measures for rheumatoid arthritis clinical trials. The Committee on Outcome Measures in Rheumatoid Arthritis Clinical Trials'. *Arthritis Rheum.* 36(6):729–40.

Table 15.2 66/68 joint count. The hip joints are only assessed for pain

Characteristics of the joint score		
Swollen/tender		S/T
No. of assessed joints		68/88
Joints effectively evaluated		68/88
Graded		o
Weighted		–
Included joint regions (no. of joints on left/right side)		
DIP (4 joints)		4/4
5 joints		
	PIP/ICI: hands	5/5
	MCP	5/5
	Carpometacarpal	–
Carpus		–
Wrist		1/1
Elbow		1/1
Shoulder		1/1
5 joints		
	DIP: feet	–
	PIP/IDI: feet	5/5
	MTP	5/5
	Tarsometatarsal	–
Tarsus		1/1
Ankle		1/1
Knee		1/1
Hip		1/1
Acromioclavicular		1/1
Sternoclavicular		1/1
Temporomandibular		1/1

Source: data from 'The cooperating clinics committee of the American Rheumatism Association (1965), 'A seven-day variability study of 499 patients with peripheral rheumatoid arthritis'. *Arthritis Rheum* 8:302–34.

assessment (PhGA or EGA) and patient pain assessment by the patient (PP).

The patients relate their global assessment primarily to tender joint counts, whereas the evaluators' assessment correlates equally with tender and swollen joint counts.[23] Thus, patient assessment is primarily driven by pain and evaluator assessment by tenderness, swelling, and presumably acute phase reactants if available.

Acute phase reactants

Many proteins are elevated in the course of inflammation; they include CRP, fibrinogen, haptoglobin or serum amyloid A protein,[2] of which CRP is the most widely used and the least costly. The hepatic acute phase response is primarily induced by IL-6, and also directly or indirectly by IL-1 and TNF.[2,24] Also, an increase of the erythrocyte sedimentation rate (ESR) reflects an acute phase response, but the ESR is more complex as it depends on changes in several protein components as well as the red blood cell count. Acute phase reactant levels, especially over time, correlate well with progression of joint damage.[12–14]

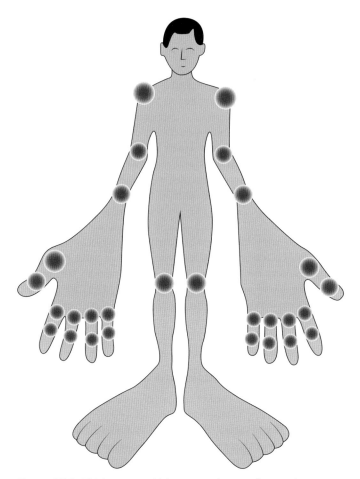

Figure 15.2 28 joint count which assesses the most frequently involved joints in RA, with the exception of ankle and foot joints that are frequently involved by other diseases.
Reprinted from Smolen JS, Aletaha D. (2010) 'The assessment of disease activity in rheumatoid arthritis'. *Clin Exp Rheumatol* 28 (Suppl 59):S18–S27 with permission from Clinical and Experimental Rheumatology Online.

Activation of the acute phase response is not specific for rheumatoid arthritis, but a general consequence of inflammation and the associated increase in pro-inflammatory cytokines. Hence, an elevation of acute phase reactant levels in RA patients must be evaluated for its cause, which is either disease activity or another type of inflammation, such as infection. Further, care must be taken to bear in mind that many RA-therapies, such as those directed at TNF, IL-6, Janus kinases, and also glucocorticoids, usually blunt the acute phase response. Therefore, an infection may not necessarily lead to increases of CRP levels or the ESR and so may be overlooked; one has to be particularly attentive to potential clinical signs and symptoms of infection other than high fever or increased levels of acute phase reactants when treating patients with these agents.

Physical function and quality of life

As indicated earlier, physical function and quality of life are not solely disease activity variables, but constitute a combination of different aspects of the disease that also comprise joint damage and even comorbidities. Indeed, within a certain range, every 10 points on the radiographic modified Sharp score equate to an irreversible disability of 0.1 on the scale of the Health Assessment Questionnaire disability index (HAQ)[25]; thus, in patients with longstanding disease and

significant joint damage, a normal HAQ cannot be reached and improvement of HAQ may be even jeopardized fully.[26] Of further note, comorbidities increase physical disability by a significant amount that is not related to disease activity, and the same is true to quality of life measures such as Short Form 36 (SF-36).[27,28] For these confounding reasons neither HAQ nor SF36 are ideal instruments for disease activity assessment; rather, they reflect overall disease outcome.

The HAQ evaluates the function of the upper and lower extremities by addressing eight categories of daily functioning, namely dressing, rising, eating, walking, hygiene, reach, grip, and usual activities. For each of these domains the difficulty is assessed on a 0–3 scale with higher levels reflecting increasing difficulty, from no difficulty (0) to inability to do (3), with some (1) and much (2) difficulty being in between. These eight categories are assessed by a total of 20 questions. A HAQ of less than 0.3 is regarded as normal, whereby normality partly depends on age.[29]

Physical function can also be assessed by the SF-36. The SF-36 measures self-reported quality of life and uses 36 questions combined into eight domains. These domains reflect different aspects of health which can be brought into physical and mental component summary scales (PCS, MCS). The SF-36 has been described elsewhere[30] and will not be addressed in detail here.

The HAQ and the SF-36 are fully patient derived and questionnaires are used for their determination.[30,31] Importantly, they are sensitive to change and, therefore, they have been included by the American College of Rheumatology (ACR) into the core set of disease activity variables. Also, in early disease they fully reflect disease activity. This is one of the reasons why a modification of the HAQ in conjunction with patient global assessment and patient pain assessment has been combined into the Routine Assessment of Patient Index Data (RAPID) 3 (see next).[32]

Composite measures of disease activity

The use of individual variables of disease activity as endpoints in clinical trials or to follow patients in clinical practice is offset by differences in their sensitivity to change as well as a variety of between and even within patient differences. This variability may relate to a disparate presentation of certain disease characteristics among patients (e.g. in some patients tenderness may be more prevalent or acute phase reactant levels higher than in others despite similar swollen joint counts), but also to distinct associations with long-term outcomes, such as joint damage and disability, as detailed earlier. Indeed, before the late 1990s, many RA clinical trials used different individual or groups of endpoints with very limited validity.[33,34] Also, the validity of single variables in relation to the major disease outcomes is poor.[9]

In contrast, the validity of composite measures that comprise several individual variables is much better,[9,35] because they capture more of the totality of RA than individual items, they level out the variability of clinical manifestations, and they reflect all important endpoints of the disease, as depicted schematically in **Figure 15.3**. This has been shown for the ACR improvement or response criteria,[36] for the original disease activity score (DAS) and its derivative using 28 joint counts (DAS28) as well as for the simplified disease activity index (SDAI) and its derivative the clinical disease activity index (CDAI; **Figure 15.3**).[37–40] These composite measures are used in clinical trials and, with the exception of the ACR response criteria, also in clinical practice; the focus here will be primarily on

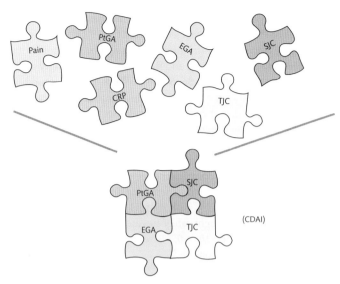

Figure 15.3 The advantage of composite measures of disease activity. Individual variables reflect just limited and somewhat disordered aspects of RA (individual jigsaw puzzle pieces), while composite measures funnel into the totality of the disease (resolution of a jigsaw puzzle). The four components depicted in the conjoined puzzle pieces reflect, as the simplest example, the clinical disease activity index (CDAI).

those used in trials and practice, even if a number of other composite measures have been developed in the past.[41]

ACR improvement criteria

In an intensive exercise that was instrumental for modern clinical trial design, Felson et al determined that a change of 20% of the core set variables, with a mandatory reduction of at least 20% in the number of tender and swollen joints plus 20% reduction in three of the other five core set variables (Table 15.1), would best distinguish active therapy from placebo.[36] Since the so called ACR20 response was felt to include patients with only minimal clinical improvement, it was subsequently expanded to 50% and 70% improvement along the same lines. These ACR50 and 70 responses were initially only used as secondary endpoints, given that the power to distinguish between active therapy and placebo decreased,[42] which was, indeed, seen in some clinical trials.[43] However, with more recent therapies

this endpoint is increasingly applied, as it relates to more powerful responses.[44,45]

While highly discriminatory in clinical trials, the ACR improvement criteria are not useful in clinical practice for several reasons. Firstly, they are categorical measures rather than continuous ones and, therefore, cannot be applied to follow actual disease activity. Secondly, they rely on a relative improvement from baseline and, therefore, the per cent improvement has different implications for patients with different disease activity levels; as an example, a patient with six swollen joints will end at three swollen joints upon 50% improvement, which may be regarded as in line with a relatively low activity state, while a patient with 30 swollen joints will still have 15 residual swollen joints upon 50% reduction, a very high level of joint involvement. Thirdly, consequently they cannot be used to define different states like low disease activity or remission, unless one targets an ACR100 or ACR90 response, the latter, again, having different meanings depending on the baseline situation. Finally, they require the assessment of seven variables (Table 15.1) which might be seen as too tedious in routine practice. For all these reasons, continuous measures of disease activity that comprise a few components appear to be more practical for clinical practice and, indeed, are widely used in daily patient care and also in clinical trials.

Continuous composite measures of disease activity

DAS and DAS28 The earliest composite measure that revolutionized disease activity assessment was developed by van der Heijde et al. almost 30 years ago.[37] The DAS was anchored at the physicians' decision to stop or start antirheumatic therapy in relation to high or low disease activity, respectively. The formula was developed by a computer program that ultimately transformed and weighted four variables: swollen and tender joint counts, patient assessment of global health (readily replaced by patient's global assessment of disease activity) and ESR. Joint counts undergo square rooting, ESR or CRP logarithmic transformation, and factoring of individual variables also occurs. However, because the DAS employed a 44 swollen joint count and the weighted Ritchie articular index for tenderness, it was seen as overly time consuming and complicated for clinical practice. Therefore, the DAS was modified to comprise the 28 tender and swollen joint counts, the DAS28.[38] The formulae for the DAS and DAS28 are shown in Table 15.3. The score has also variations with just three components (not shown).

Table 15.3 Formulae for continuous disease activity indices and ACR-EULAR remission definitions.

Index/Criterion	Formula	Cut points REM/LDA/MDA	Proposed cut points REM/LDA[46]
DAS[37,47]	$= 0.54 \times \sqrt{}$ (Ritchie) $+ 0.065 \times \sqrt{SJC44} + 0.33 \times lognat (ESR) + 0.0072 \times GH$		
DAS28-ESR[38]	$0.56 \times \sqrt{}(TJC28) + 0.28 \times \sqrt{}(SJC28) + 0.70 \times lognat (ESR) + 0.014 \times GH$[38]	2.6/3.2/5.1*	2.2/3.6**
DAS28-CRP	$= 0.56 \times \sqrt{}$ (TJC28) $+ 0.28 \times \sqrt{}(SJC28) + 0.36 \times lognat (CRP + 1) + 0.014 \times GH + 0.96$	2.6/3.2/5.1*	1.9/3.1**
SDAI	SJC28 + TJC28 + PGA + EGA + CRP[39,48]	3.3/11/26*	
CDAI	SJC28 + TJC28 + PGA + EGA[39,40,48]	2.8/10/22*	
ACR-EULAR remission[49]	Boolean: SJC, TJC, PGA, CRP Index based: SDAI Index based: CDAI	All ≤1 ≤3.3 ≤2.8	

CRP, C-reactive protein; EGA, evaluator global assessment (in cm); ESR, erythrocyte sedimentation rate; GH, global health for which patient global assessment is used (in mm); HDA, high disease activity;, MDA, moderate disease activity; PGA, patient global assessment (in cm); REM, remission; SJC, swollen joint count; TJC, tender joint count. *Above this cut point: HDA; **above this cut point: MDA.

The DAS and DAS28 were developed at a time when remission was a rare event. In the meantime, remission can be achieved in a significant proportion of patients and it turned out that patients in remission can have even many more than ten swollen joints, a situation not compatible with remission. This is due to the fact that tender joints are weighted twice as highly as swollen joints; a patient could be in deep remission in the theoretical presence of 28 swollen joints with all other elements being close to normal (Figure 15.4). Further, the ESR and CRP, despite or because of logarithmic transformation also has a big weight in the formula. Thus, a normal ESR of 20 mm contributes more points than 28 swollen joints to the DAS28 score. This becomes a problem when drugs targeting molecules that directly influence the acute phase response irrespective of clinical improvement are used. These agents include those that interfere with the IL-6 pathway which is the major stimulus of hepatic acute phase reactant production. Among these drugs are antibodies against the IL-6 receptor, against IL-6 or inhibitors of Janus kinases, since IL-6 signals via Jaks. One then arrives at the interesting situation that even though ACR20, 50, and 70 response rates are very similar, these drugs elicit much higher DAS28 remission rates than other drugs; also, within the respective studies of these molecules, DAS28 remission rates are usually higher than ACR70 rates.

There were recent proposals to lower the cut points for remission and low disease activity of the DAS28-ESR and the DAS28-CRP,[46] but even when these lower cut points are used (remission with DAS28-CRP = 1.9; and with DAS28-ESR = 2.2), there can be up to 13 residual swollen joints, and DAS28 remission rates can still exceed ACR70 rates with the above-mentioned drugs,[50] sometimes even higher than ACR50 rates,[51] a counterintuitive result, since it suggests that remission is more frequent than 70% or even 50% clinical improvement; this is neither logical nor possible, unless due to an erratic instrument.

The DAS and DAS28 are used to define the so called EULAR response criteria, namely good response, moderate response, and no response.[52] Good response is defined as a decrease in score of >1.2 and reaching a low disease activity. Moderate response is a decrease of >0.6 to 1.2 and reaching at least moderate or low disease activity. Non-response is defined as remaining in high disease activity or as having a reduction of <0.6 in other disease activity states.

SDAI and CDAI The SDAI was originally developed to provide a simple DAS that did not necessitate the use of a calculator or computer.[39] It is a simple numerical summation of the core set variables swollen joint count (SJC), tender joint count (TJC), patient and physician global assessment, and CRP (Table 15.3). Its sister, the CDAI, is calculated in the same way but without CRP[39,40]; this allows determination of disease activity even in the absence of a laboratory measure which is advantageous in many clinical settings. Both indices were validated against ACR response rates and DAS28 and both scores have construct and criterion validity by correlating well with physical function and progression of damage.[53] Aside from providing a continuous scale that allows to assess disease activity across the whole disease spectrum at any point in time, cut points for disease activity states have also been defined.[48,53] Indeed, the cut points for remission are so stringent that ACR and EULAR, in their respective research and consensus finding, use them for the definition of the ACR-EULAR index-based remission criteria, aside from a Boolean definition (Table 15.3).[54] DAS28 did not meet the stringent requirements that had been set forth by the committee, in line with the observations already described. Also, response criteria have been determined for SDAI, with 50% improvement constituting a minor, 70% a moderate, and 85% a major response.[55] A minimal clinically important change has also been determined, which—dependent on the initial score—ranges from a reduction of 12 (in high disease activity) to a reduction of 1 (in low disease activity).[56]

Scores based on patient self-assessment There exist several instruments based solely on patient self-assessments. Among these are the RADAR (Rapid Assessment of Disease Activity in Rheumatology),

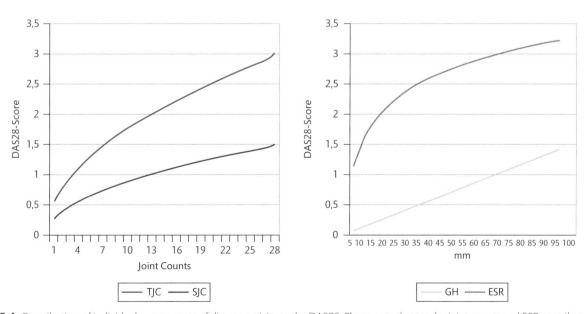

Figure 15.4 Contribution of individual components of disease activity to the DAS28. Please note that tender joint counts and ESR contribute much more points than swollen joint counts or patient global assessment due to the formula shown in Table 15.1. Likewise, the contribution of CRP in DAS28-CRP is high.

the RADAI (Rheumatoid Arthritis Disease Activity Index) and the RAPID 3 (Routine Assessment of Patient Index Data).

The RADAR comprises 2 questions on disease activity, 1 question on pain (all 3 on 100 mm VAS scales), 1 question on morning stiffness, 4 questions on physical function and an assessment of joint pain, all derived by the patients.[57] While these items are scored, there is no total index, but they serve to inform the rheumatologist.

The RADAI[58] contains 3 questions on arthritis pain and activity, 1 question on morning joint stiffness, 1 question on pain, and 8 on pre-specified joint areas. It is then summarized to provide a total index. Of note, self-assessed swollen and tender joint counts correlate well with those of trained assessors if the overall joint counts are very low, but differ dramatically in patients with higher joint counts.[59]

The RAPID3[32] is composed of 3 questions, each rated 0–10: physical function, pain, and global assessment of disease activity. The range is 0–30, but it is then transformed to a 0–10 scale.

All three self-assessment measures have been validated, are sensitive to change and RADAI and RAPID3 have defined disease activity states, including remission. However, measures that rely on questionnaires for physical function are at risk of having different ratings by patients who have early disease compared to long established disease, because with increasing joint damage impairment of physical function becomes partly irreversible (see earlier). Indeed, the European League Against Rheumatism (EULAR) and the Treat to Target (T2T) task force have only adopted scores that comprise formal joint counts in their recommendations,[60,61] and none of these scores' definition of remission has been included in the ACR-EULAR remission criteria.[54] Joints are the 'organ' that the rheumatologist has to care for and neglecting them when assessing RA and using solely patient derived questions is like a cardiologist solely relying on patient questionnaires rather than examining the heart. Moreover, formal joint counts correlate best with progression of joint damage.

Therapeutic strategy

The use of novel therapies, including biological or targeted synthetic DMARDs, is an important improvement in the opportunity to reach the best outcome for all patients. However, equally important was the development of tools to assess disease activity and of strategies for optimal benefit for patients. Tight control of disease activity with a focus on specific beneficial endpoints has dramatically changed our thinking regarding optimization of treatment for RA.[62] Further information in early and established RA has led to the treat-to-target recommendations, which have been recently updated comprising the important aspect of shared decision-making with the patients.[61] To better translate these recommendations into practice, it has been recently shown that an improvement of less than 50% in a composite index within 3 months of institutions of a new therapy is not sufficient to provide sufficient probability for reaching the treatment target of remission or low disease activity by 6 months.[63] However, if patients improve by more than 50% of, say, the CDAI (which we use in daily practice), then the likelihood of reaching low disease activity or remission is sufficiently high to warrant continuation of the same treatment. Adaptation of therapy is recommended if the treatment target is not reached within 6 months or if the improvement

of disease activity does not exceed 50% within 3 months. Thus, the combination of a strategic treatment approach using validated composite measures of disease activity and availability of a large number of therapeutic options warrants an optimal outcome for most RA patients today.

Conclusion

Disease activity assessment is pivotal when following patients with RA throughout the course of their disease, and especially when assessing improvement or deterioration upon institution of the necessary therapies.[64–66] To prevent an adverse outcome, it is essential to diagnose the disease early and to start treatment with DMARDs immediately after diagnosis. Adhering to the treat-to-target approach, which is a central strategy irrespective of the type of treatment available and the therapy applied, requires consistency in using validated composite measures of disease activity. Rather than a mere matter of using specific therapies, it is also a matter of using tools for disease activity assessment to guide therapeutic decision-making. This enables offering and achieving the best possible outcomes for RA patients.

REFERENCES

1. Smolen JS, Aletaha D, McInnes IB. Rheumatoid arthritis. *Lancet* 2016;*388*(10055):2023–38.
2. Gabay C, Kushner I. Acute-phase proteins and other systemic responses to inflammation. *N Engl J Med* 1999;*340*(6):448–54.
3. Gravallese EM. Bone destruction in arthritis. *Ann Rheum Dis* 2002;*61* (Suppl 2):ii84–6.
4. Binder NB, Puchner A, Niederreiter B, et al. Tumor necrosis factor-inhibiting therapy preferentially targets bone destruction but not synovial inflammation in a tumor necrosis factor-driven model of rheumatoid arthritis. *Arthritis Rheum* 2013;*65*(3):608–17.
5. Partsch G, Steiner G, Leeb BF, Dunky A, Broll H, Smolen JS. Highly increased levels of tumor necrosis factor-alpha and other proinflammatory cytokines in psoriatic arthritis synovial fluid. *J Rheumatol* 1997;*24*:518–23.
6. Murphy G, Lee MH. What are the roles of metalloproteinases in cartilage and bone damage? *Ann Rheum Dis* 2005;*64* Suppl 4:iv44–7.
7. Aletaha D, Smolen J, Ward MM. Measuring function in rheumatoid arthritis: identifying reversible and irreversible components. *Arthritis Rheum* 2006;*54*:2784–92.
8. Goldsmith CH, Boers M, Bombardier C, Tugwell P. Criteria for clinically important changes in outcomes: development, scoring and evaluation of rheumatoid arthritis patients and trial profiles. *J Rheumatol* 1993;*20*:561–5.
9. van der Heijde DM, Van't Hof MA, van Riel PL, van Leeuwen MA, van Rijswijk MH, van de Putte LB. Validity of single variables and composite indices for measuring disease activity in rheumatoid arthritis. *Ann Rheum Dis* 1992;*51*:177–81.
10. Felson DT, Anderson JJ, Boers M, et al. The American College of Rheumatology preliminary core set of disease activity measures for rheumatoid arthritis. The Committee on Outcome Measures in Rheumatoid Arthritis Clinical Trials. *Arthritis Rheum* 1993;*36*:729–40.

11. Smolen JS. The work of the EULAR Standing Committee on International Clinical Studies Including Therapeutic Trials. *Br J Rheumatol* 1992;*31*:219–20.

12. Van der Heijde DM, van Riel PL, van Leeuwen MA, van 't Hof MA, van Rijswijk MH, van de Putte LB. Prognostic factors for radiographic damage and physical disability in early rheumatoid arthritis. A prospective follow-up study of 147 patients. *Br J Rheumatol* 1992;*31*(8):519–25.

13. van Leeuwen MA, Van der Heijde DM, van Rijswijk MH, et al. Interrelationship of outcome measures and process variables in early rheumatoid arthritis. A comparison of radiologic damage, physical disability, joint counts, and acute phase reactants. *J Rheumatol* 1994;*21*(3):425–9.

14. Smolen JS, van der Heijde DMFM, St. Clair EW, et al. Predictors of joint damage in patients with early rheumatoid arthritis treated with high-dose methotrexate without or with concomitant infliximab. Results from the ASPIRE trial. *Arthritis Rheum* 2006;*54*:702–10.

15. Klarenbeek NB, Guler-Yuksel M, Van der Heijde DM, et al. Clinical synovitis in a particular joint is associated with progression of erosions and joint space narrowing in that same joint, but not in patients initially treated with infliximab. *Ann Rheum Dis* 2010;*69*(12):2107–13.

16. Scott DL, van Riel PC, van der Heijde DM, Studnicka-Benke A. *Assessing Disease Activity in Rheumatoid Arthritis—The EULAR Handbook of Standard Methods*. On behalf of the EULAR Standing Committee for International Clinical Studies Including Therapeutic Trials—ESCISIT (Chairman: Smolen JS). Zurich, Switzerland: EULAR, 1993.

17. Aletaha D, Alasti F, Smolen JS. Rheumatoid arthritis near remission: clinical rather than laboratory inflammation is associated with radiographic progression. *Ann Rheum Dis* 2011;*70*:1975–80.

18. The Cooperating Clinics Committee of the American Rheumatism Association. A seven-day variability study of 499 patients with peripheral rheumatoid arthritis. *Arthritis Rheum* 1965;*8*:302–34.

19. Ritchie DM, Boyle JA, McInnes JM, et al. Clinical studies with an articular index for the assessment of joint tenderness in patients with rheumatoid arthritis. *Q J Med* 1968;*37*(147):393–406.

20. Hart LE, Tugwell P, Buchanan WW, Norman GR, Grace EM, Southwell D. Grading of tenderness as a source of interrater error in the Ritchie articular index. *J Rheumatol* 1985;*12*:716–17.

21. Fuchs HA, Pincus T. Reduced joint counts in controlled clinical trials in rheumatoid arthritis. *Arthritis Rheum* 1994;*37*(4):470–5.

22. Smolen JS, Breedveld FC, Eberl G, et al. Validity and reliability of the twenty-eight-joint count for the assessment of rheumatoid arthritis activity. *Arthritis Rheum* 1995;*38*(1):38–43.

23. Aletaha D, Smolen JS. Remission of rheumatoid arthritis: should we care about definitions? *Clin Exp Rheumatol* 2006;*24*(6 Suppl 43):S045–51.

24. Kushner I. Regulation of the acute phase response by cytokines. *Perspect Biol Med* 1993;*36*(4):611–22.

25. Smolen JS, Aletaha D, Grisar JC, Stamm TA, Sharp JT. Estimation of a numerical value for joint damage-related physical disability in rheumatoid arthritis clinical trials. *Ann Rheum Dis* 2010;*69*(6):1058–64.

26. Aletaha D, Strand V, Smolen JS, Ward MM. Treatment-related improvement in physical function varies with duration of rheumatoid arthritis: a pooled analysis of clinical trial results. *Ann Rheum Dis* 2008;*67*(2):238–43.

27. Radner H, Smolen JS, Aletaha D. Impact of comorbidity on physical function in patients with rheumatoid arthritis. *Ann Rheum Dis* 2010; *69*(3):536–41.

28. Radner H, Smolen JS, Aletaha D. Comorbidity affects all domains of physical function and quality of life in patients with rheumatoid arthritis. *Rheumatology (Oxf)* 2011;*50*:381–8.

29. Vita AJ, Terry RB, Hubert HB, Fries JF. Aging, health risks, and cumulative disability. *N Engl J Med* 1998;*338*(15):1035–41.

30. Ware JE J, Sherbourne CD. The MOS 36-item short-form health survey (SF-36). I. Conceptual framework and item selection. *Med Care* 1992;*30*:473–83.

31. Fries JF, Spitz P, Kraines RG, Holman HR. Measurement of patient outcome in arthritis. *Arthritis Rheum* 1980;*23*:137–45.

32. Pincus T, Swearingen CJ, Bergman M, Yazici Y. RAPID3 (Routine Assessment of Patient Index Data 3), a rheumatoid arthritis index without formal joint counts for routine care: proposed severity categories compared to disease activity score and clinical disease activity index categories. *J Rheumatol* 2008;*35*(11):2136–47.

33. Bull BS, Westengard JC, Farr M, Bacon PA, Meyer PJ, Stuart J. Efficacy of tests used to monitor rheumatoid arthritis. *Lancet* 1989;*2*(8669):965–7.

34. Gotzsche PC. Sensitivity of effect variables in rheumatoid arthritis: a meta-analysis of 130 placebo controlled NSAID trials. *J Clin Epidemiol* 1990;*43*(12):1313–18.

35. Goldsmith CH, Smythe HA, Helewa A. Interpretation and power of a pooled index. *J Rheumatol* 1993;*20*(3):575–8.

36. Felson DT, Anderson JJ, Boers M, et al. American College of Rheumatology preliminary definition of improvement in rheumatoid arthritis. *Arthritis Rheum* 1995;*38*:727–35.

37. Van der Heijde DMFM, van't Hof M, van Riel PL, van de Putte LBA. Development of a disease activity score based on judgement in clinical practice by rheumatologists. *J Rheumatol* 1993;*20*:579–81.

38. Prevoo MLL, van't Hof MA, Kuper HH, van de Putte LBA, van Riel PLCM. Modified disease activity scores that include twenty-eight-joint counts. Development and validation in a prospective longitudinal study of patients with rheumatoid arthritis. *Arthritis Rheum* 1995;*38*:44–8.

39. Smolen JS, Breedveld FC, Schiff MH, et al. A simplified disease activity index for rheumatoid arthritis for use in clinical practice. *Rheumatology* 2003;*42*:244–57.

40. Aletaha D, Nell VPK, Stamm T, et al. Acute phase reactants add little to composite disease activity indices for rheumatoid arthritis: validation of a clinical activity score. *Arthritis Res* 2005;*7*:R796–R806.

41. Aletaha D, Smolen JS. The definition and measurement of disease modification in inflammatory rheumatic diseases. *Rheum Dis Clin North Am* 2006;*32*:9–44.

42. Felson DT, Anderson JJ, Lange ML, Wells G, La Valley MP. Should improvement in rheumatoid arthritis clinical trials be defined as fifty percent or seventy percent improvement in core set measures, rather than twenty percent? *Arthritis Rheum* 1998;*41*:1564–70.

43. Emery P, Fleischmann RM, Moreland LW, et al. Golimumab, a human anti-tumor necrosis factor alpha monoclonal antibody, injected subcutaneously every four weeks in methotrexate-naive patients with active rheumatoid arthritis: twenty-four-week results of a phase III, multicenter, randomized, double-blind, placebo-controlled study of golimumab before methotrexate as first-line therapy for early-onset rheumatoid arthritis. *Arthritis Rheum* 2009;*60*(8):2272–83.

44. Smolen JS, Weinblatt ME, Sheng S, Zhuang Y, Hsu B. Sirukumab, a human anti-interleukin-6 monoclonal antibody: a randomised, 2-part (proof-of-concept and dose-finding), phase II study in patients with active rheumatoid arthritis despite methotrexate therapy. *Ann Rheum Dis* 2014;*73*(9):1616–25.

45. Fleischmann R, Mysler E, Hall S, et al. Efficacy and safety of tofacitinib monotherapy, tofacitinib with methotrexate, and adalimumab with methotrexate in patients with rheumatoid arthritis (ORAL Strategy): a phase 3b/4, double-blind, head-to-head, randomised controlled trial. *Lancet* 2017;*390*(10093):457–68.

46. Fleischmann R, van der Heijde D, Koenig AS, et al. How much does Disease Activity Score in 28 joints ESR and CRP calculations underestimate disease activity compared with the Simplified Disease Activity Index? *Ann Rheum Dis* 2015;*74*(6):1132–7.

47. van der Heijde DMFM, Van't Hof MA, van Riel PLCM, et al. Judging disease activity in clinical practice in rheumatoid arthritis: first step in the development of a disease activity score. *Ann Rheum Dis* 1990;*49*:916–20.

48. Aletaha D, Ward MM, Machold KP, Nell VPK, Stamm T, Smolen JS. Remission and active disease in rheumatoid arthritis: defining criteria for disease activity states. *Arthritis Rheum* 2005;*52*:2625–36.

49. Felson DT, Smolen JS, Wells G, et al. American College of Rheumatology/European League Against Rheumatism provisional definition of remission in rheumatoid arthritis for clinical trials. *Ann Rheum Dis* 2011;*70*(3):404–13.

50. Schoels M, Alasti F, Smolen JS, Aletaha D. Evaluation of newly proposed remission cut-points for disease activity score in 28 joints (DAS28) in rheumatoid arthritis patients upon IL-6 pathway inhibition. *Arthritis Res Ther* 2017;*19*(1):155.

51. Emery P, Keystone E, Tony HP, et al. IL-6 receptor inhibition with tocilizumab improves treatment outcomes in patients with rheumatoid arthritis refractory to anti-tumour necrosis factor biologicals: results from a 24-week multicentre randomised placebo-controlled trial. *Ann Rheum Dis* 2008;*67*(11):1516–23.

52. Fransen J, van Riel PL. The Disease Activity Score and the EULAR response criteria. *Clin Exp Rheumatol* 2005;*23*:S93–9.

53. Aletaha D, Smolen J. The Simplified Disease Activity Index (SDAI) and the Clinical Disease Activity Index (CDAI): a review of their usefulness and validity in rheumatoid arthritis. *Clin Exp Rheumatol* 2005;*23*(Suppl 39):S100–8.

54. Felson DT, Smolen JS, Wells G, et al. American College of Rheumatology/European League Against Rheumatism provisional definition of remission in rheumatoid arthritis for clinical trials. *Ann Rheum Dis* 2011;*70*(3):404–13.

55. Aletaha D, Martinez-Avila J, Kvien TK, Smolen JS. Definition of treatment response in rheumatoid arthritis based on the simplified and the clinical disease activity index. *Ann Rheum Dis* 2012;*71*:1190–6.

56. Curtis JR, Yang S, Chen L, et al. Determining the minimally important difference in the clinical disease activity index for improvement and worsening in early rheumatoid arthritis patients. *Arthritis Care Res (Hoboken)* 2015;*67*(10):1345–53.

57. Mason JH, Anderson JJ, Meenan RF, Haralson KM, Lewis-Stevens D, Kaine JL. The rapid assessment of disease activity in rheumatology (radar) questionnaire. Validity and sensitivity to change of a patient self-report measure of joint count and clinical status. *Arthritis Rheum* 1992;*35*:156–62.

58. Stucki G, Liang MH, Stucki S, Brühlmann P, Michel BA. A self-administered rheumatoid arthritis disease activity index (RADAI) for epidemiologic research. Psychometric properties and correlation with parameters of disease activity. *Arthritis Rheum* 1995;*38*:795–8.

59. Radner H, Grisar J, Stamm T, Smolen JS, Aletaha D. Patients self-assessment of joint swelling and tenderness in rheumatoid arthritis (RA): longitudinal validity and the role of training. *Ann Rheum Dis* 2009;*68*(Suppl 3):396.

60. Smolen JS, Landewe R, Breedveld FC, et al. EULAR recommendations for the management of rheumatoid arthritis with synthetic and biological disease-modifying antirheumatic drugs. *Ann Rheum Dis* 2010;*69*(6):964–75.

61. Smolen JS, Breedveld FC, Burmester GR, et al. Treating rheumatoid arthritis to target: 2014 update of the recommendations of an international task force. *Ann Rheum Dis* 2016;*75*(1):3–15.

62. Grigor C, Capell H, Stirling A, et al. Effect of a treatment strategy of tight control for rheumatoid arthritis (the TICORA study): a single-blind randomised controlled trial. *Lancet* 2004;*364*:263–9.

63. Aletaha D, Alasti F, Smolen JS. Optimisation of a treat-to-target approach in rheumatoid arthritis: strategies for the 3-month time point. *Ann Rheum Dis* 2015;*75*(8):1479–85.

64. Smolen JS, Schols M, Braun J, et al. Treating axial spondyloarthritis and peripheral spondyloarthritis, especially psoriatic arthritis, to target: 2017 update of recommendations by an international task force. *Ann Rheum Dis* 2018;*77*(1):3–17.

65. Bakker MF, Jacobs JW, Verstappen SM, Bijlsma JW. Tight control in the treatment of rheumatoid arthritis: efficacy and feasibility. *Ann Rheum Dis* 2007;*66*(Suppl 3):iii56–0.

66. Smolen JS, Aletaha D. The assessment of disease activity in rheumatoid arthritis. *Clin Exp Rheumatol* 2010;*28*(Suppl 59):S18–S27.

16
Synovial biopsies

Douglas J. Veale and Ursula Fearon

Synovial joint structure

The non-articular surfaces of diarthrodial joints, tendons and ligaments are covered by a thin (1–3 cells in depth) connective tissue without a basement membrane, containing fibroblasts with macrophages interspersed.[1] The articular surfaces of the bones are covered by a tightly adherent cartilage, away from which the synovium is reflected; the synovial membrane, cartilage, and bone become confluent at the cartilage pannus junction. These tissues are entirely contained within the joint by a taut capsule comprised of fibrous tissues, formed by the confluence of ligaments and tendons, which provide strength and stability to the joint. The synovial joint is a dynamic structure often subject to stress and strain as a result of natural movements, weight-bearing, and occasionally trauma requiring continual reparation. Continual remodelling of the bone, cartilage and synovium within the joint is necessary, and requires a fine balance of degradative and proliferative cells that release proteolytic enzymes.

Synovial tissue inflammation

The synovium is the primary target of inflammation in rheumatoid arthritis (RA), and both the resident fibroblast-like synoviocytes (FLS) and the lining layer macrophages have been implicated in the pathogenesis of synovitis.[2] However, one of the earliest features of inflammation in synovial biopsies is new blood vessel growth or angiogenesis. The expanding and sprouting vessels throughout the sublining of the synovium allow infiltration of inflammatory cells from the systemic circulation including T and B lymphocytes, plasma cells, macrophages, neutrophils, mast cells, natural killer, and dendritic cells.

The pattern of angiogenesis appears to vary with the type of arthritis. In RA the vessels show evidence of elongation and regular branching similar to that observed in wound healing or diabetic retinopathy.[3] The new immature blood vessels are formed by endothelial sprouting and undergo a process of maturation, characterized by the recruitment and close association of pericytes with the endothelial cells.[4] The influx of inflammatory cells via the new blood vessels transforms the synovial tissue into an invading pannus, characterized by mobile FLS, that can result in direct invasion of the adjacent cartilage and bone.[5,6] In addition, although the blood supply is markedly increased in the synovial vasculature, the tissue remains profoundly hypoxic.[5] There is a close association between the level of hypoxia and inflammation: more inflamed joints, with high macroscopic synovitis scores and cellular infiltrates including CD68+ macrophages and CD3+ T cells in the sublining, are typically those with the lowest oxygen partial pressure in the synovial tissue. Specific alterations in the profile of inflammatory cells in RA synovial tissue have long been identified, and associations with the outcome of disease and its therapeutic response to both synthetic and biologic disease modifying antirheumatic drugs have been observed.[7–10] Furthermore, such tissue exhibits high expression of pro-inflammatory mediators including cytokines (e.g. IL-6, TNF, IL-1β, IFNγ), growth factors (vascular endothelial growth factor (VEGF), angiopoietins), platelet-derived growth factor (PDGF), chemokines (IL-8, MCP-1, RANTES, MIP3α/CCL20), and matrix degrading enzymes (MMP1, MMP3, MMP2,9). The role of these molecules in the initiation and propagation of synovial inflammation remains a focus of intense research efforts; although several therapeutic agents targeting them have proved useful in the clinical setting over the last two decades, identification of further potential druggable targets is probable.[11]

Ex vivo when primary synovial fluid cells are exposed to similar partial oxygen pressures as found in the inflamed joints, cell activation, proliferation, and migration are significantly increased, suggesting that hypoxia drives pathological changes in the synovial tissue.[5] Many, but not all, of the pathological features identified in RA synovium are also found in the synovial fluid. The permeability of RA synovial tissue is increased as a result of the inflammation[12] especially to large molecules, while it appears permeability to some smaller molecules is decreased (e.g. urea and glucose); this effect is due to a combination of factors such as increased cellular and vascular penetrability and resultant hyperplasia of the synovial tissue.

The synovial fluid protein levels are significantly higher in the inflamed joint compared to the normal joint. The main lubricant macromolecule—hyaluronic acid also exists in an altered form at a lower molecular weight and at a lower concentration in inflamed RA joints.[13,14]

The synovial tissue of RA patients is the primary focus for the inflammatory response and exhibits several structural, morphological, cellular, and molecular changes from healthy synovial tissue that may provide critical information regarding our knowledge and understanding of RA pathogenesis.

Synovial biopsy

The first biopsies of synovial tissue in RA are reported in the early 20th century. However it was not until the late 1950s that the first description of the histological features of synovitis, proliferative pannus formation, and cartilage damage were clearly defined in patients with long-term RA.[15] Initial studies were performed on synovial tissue samples taken at the time of surgery or post-mortem, although occasionally, biopsy samples were obtained from patients undergoing open arthroplasty for arthritis. Subsequent techniques for non-invasive biopsy of synovial tissue included percutaneous punch biopsies, needle biopsies, needle arthroscopy, and most recently imaging-guided biopsy with either a needle or forceps.[16]

Retrieving synovial tissue samples

When synovial biopsy was first performed, it was primarily to aid in the differential diagnosis of inflammatory arthritis. One of the first descriptions of synovial biopsy was reported by Forestier in 1932, he described a technique introducing a dental nerve extractor, via a large bore needle through a skin incision, into the joint.[17] A number of physicians described the use of needle biopsy of the synovium in the 1950s, all requiring a skin incision,[18,19] however, they concluded it was safe and practical as long as strict asepsis was employed. It was not until 1963 that Parker and Pearson developed a simplified 14-gauge biopsy needle that did not require a skin incision.[20] They reported a series of 125 synovial biopsies, mostly of the suprapatellar region of knee joints, all but five biopsies yielded synovial tissue for analysis and they reported no serious adverse effects. Several studies in the 1970s subsequently highlighted the usefulness of needle synovial biopsy in the research of arthritis.[21]

Arthroscopic biopsy enables the direct visualization of the synovium, in addition to obtaining synovial biopsies, the operator can select and score macroscopic inflammation of an area of synovium at the time of sampling.[22] By contrast, ultrasonography enables indirect visualization of synovial tissue to guide biopsy and by using Doppler ultrasonography can assess synovial vascularity as a measure of inflammation.[23] The Parker-Pearson needle and arthroscopic biopsy techniques have been thoroughly validated and more recently studies of ultrasound-guided biopsy procedures have also been reported and are becoming more feasible for many investigators as a research tool for proof-of-concept studies and clinical trials.[24]

Both the imaging-guided and needle arthroscopic biopsy procedures appear to be safe and well-tolerated. One large study assessed data from over 15 000 needle arthroscopic procedures performed by rheumatologists globally and reported very low complication rates—haemarthrosis 0.9%, deep vein thrombosis 0.2%, and both wound and joint infection 0.1% with a total adverse event rate of less than 0.3%.[25] A systematic review of ultrasound-guided synovial biopsies has also reported significant feasibility with very low overall adverse outcomes at rates of 0.4%.[26]

How useful are synovial biopsies?

Synovial biopsy research has advanced remarkably in the last number of decades with specific use in several important areas.

Pathogenesis of synovial inflammation in RA

It is abundantly clear from a number of studies that the cellular constituency of synovial biopsies is different from that of synovial fluid and the circulating blood.[2] This highlights the significance of synovial tissue analysis—the primary tissue involved in RA. We and others have shown that a number of cell types differ in number and state of differentiation in the RA synovium. RA synovial tissue is hyperplastic and oedematous and is characterized by the accumulation of lymphocytes, plasma cells, and macrophages, with fibroblast proliferation. However, neutrophils, mast cells, natural killer cells, and dendritic cells are also found in increased numbers in the synovial sublining.[27,28] In addition, the expression of molecular mediators may also vary between and within the main compartments, and recent evidence suggests that there may be some joint specificity also.[29-31] In a study of RA patients examining synovial biopsies obtained from two inflamed joints—one small (e.g. wrist) and one large (e.g. knee) found similar numbers of inflammatory cells in the synovial sublining tissue.[32,33] Furthermore, synovial biopsies from uninvolved knee joints appear to show similar, if slightly lower, numbers of infiltrating cells compared to joints with evidence of clinical disease.[34]

Cellular analysis

Monocyte/Macrophage cells

The CD68 macrophage marker remains the most validated cellular synovial tissue biomarker of treatment response in RA. A series of proof-of-concept studies examining the changes in synovial tissue infiltrate in patients undergoing therapy for RA have shown remarkable consistent results irrespective of treatment type.[35] In one such study the authors examined the synovial changes following prednisolone treatment for 2 weeks, this resulted in a significant reduction in the CD68+ macrophage population in the synovial sublining.[36] A short study of gold therapy was also associated with abundant changes in all areas of the synovial tissue—sublining and lining layer macrophages.[37] In studies of methotrexate[38] the reduction in CD68+ cell numbers was most pronounced in those with the highest change in the clinical measures of the American College of Rheumatology (ACR) criteria and similar changes were observed in studies of leflunomide,[39] infliximab,[40] and rituximab treatment.[41,42] It was on the basis of these data that a study was established to analyse CD68+ macrophages in the sublining of the synovial membrane as a biomarker of response across different therapeutic interventions, to definitively confirm that changes in CD68+ cell numbers correlate with changes in measures of disease activity independent of the therapy.[35] A high level of interobserver agreement was furthermore confirmed in a multicentre study of the European League Against Rheumatism (EULAR) European Synovitis Study Group confirming these findings.[43] This body of work was presented at the 2004 Outcome Measures in Rheumatology (OMERACT) conference, at which delegates voted to accept that sublining CD68 demonstrates validity, reliability and feasibility as a biomarker of disease activity and could therefore be used to assess the efficacy of novel treatments.[43] It has subsequently been used to help inform 'go/no-go' decisions for several therapies since this time. However, there are a small number of studies which found little or no change in CD68+ cells in studies of rituximab,[44] abatacept,[45] and more recently tofacitinib,[46] suggesting some possible limitations for this biomarker.

Lymphocytes

The prominent role of lymphocyte cells in the infiltrates of RA synovial tissue were first reported as biomarkers of inflammation over 20 years ago, when it was noted that after 6 months of gold therapy, T cell numbers decreased.[37] Cell staining for lymphocytes in synovium changed in response to several treatments in RA patients: methotrexate resulted in reductions of synovial T cells (CD3 and CD8) and plasma cells (CD38)[38,39]; infliximab reduced synovial T cells (CD3) in those RA patients with a clinical response (40); and prednisolone therapy for only 2 weeks reduced T cell (CD4), B cell (CD5), and plasma cell (CD38) numbers in synovial tissues of responder patients.[36] Intravenous rituximab therapy has also been shown, in several studies, to result in a partial depletion of synovial B cells, without a change in T cells.[41,42] More recently, the presence of B lymphocytes in the synovial tissue of RA patients seropositive for anticitrullinated protein antibodies (ACPA) has been shown to predict an aggressive erosive phenotype with a poor prognosis.[47]

Specific lymphocytes such as T helper 17 (Th17) cells have been reported to be overexpressed in the circulation of some RA patients, a finding that lead to the development of therapeutic monoclonal antibodies to neutralize the cytokine IL17.[48] Studies have revealed, however, limited expression of IL17 in RA synovial tissue despite an expansion of Th17 cells such that the therapeutic effect has proven somewhat disappointing.[49] Analysis of paired samples of synovial fluid and tissue from the same RA patients suggest that at the site of inflammation Th17 cells differentiate into ex-TH17 cells that produce higher levels of interferon gamma rather than IL17, which may explain why anti-IL17 therapy may be less effective in RA patients.[50]

When lymphocytes infiltrate the synovial membrane they may form a diffuse, evenly distributed infiltrate throughout the sublining tissue or aggregate in collections of cells often around blood vessels. In some cases, the aggregates appear to form mature lymphoid structures or germinal centres. It has been suggested that synovial lymphocyte aggregates predict a specific clinical pattern of disease, in particular erosive RA. Lymphocyte aggregates are described RA patient synovial tissue but no clinical phenotype has been defined.[51] Lymphocyte aggregates have also been studied in early RA, however again there was no association with an aggressive disease or poor outcome.[52] Clinical response to infliximab has been reported to be predicted by the number of lymphocyte aggregates[52,53] and increased the predictive power of a model including baseline disease activity measured by DAS28, ACPA positivity, and expression of TNF in synovial tissue. Therefore, synovial lymphoid aggregates may be useful as a biomarker of response to treatment but to date they have not been shown to represent a definitive clinical phenotype.

Fibroblasts

The synovial lining layer in RA, as already outlined, is composed of resident FLS and macrophages both of which have been implicated in the pathogenesis of RA. RA FLS first described in 1983 are of mesenchymal origin and identified by vimentin. They have been identified as key drivers of the invasive mechanisms involved in RA joint destruction.[54,55] The FLS phenotype has recently been characterized as specific to synovial tissue,[56] suggesting that they might have a dedicated function. In addition, the synovial FLS are locally invasive, glycolytic, and migrate from one site to another in an *in vivo* model.[57] Despite this finding there are no circulating biomarkers

currently available that provide a measure of FLSs invasive activity in RA.[58] Interestingly, intimal lining layer hyperplasia also appears to be controlled by local mechanisms as different joints showed no similarity in terms of the numbers of intimal macrophages or FLSs.[32] Further evidence of local mechanisms of FLS regulation within specific joints are the findings that FLSs from different joints of the same patient show distinct DNA methylation and transcriptome signatures, additionally differences in FLS function have been noted including invasiveness that might depend on positional memory.[30,31]

Whole synovial tissue explants

Analysis of specific primary cell types, as already outlined, is especially useful to delineate the precise functions of different cells in isolation, however this reveals little information about how cells function *in vivo* in the synovial tissue of a RA patients joint. To examine how the whole synovial tissue may function in response to inflammatory mediators, either stimulatory or inhibitory, an *ex vivo* whole synovial tissue explant model was established. This model maintains the synovial tissue architecture, cell–cell contact, and it spontaneously releases pro-inflammatory mediators including cytokines.[59] Cell viability of synovial tissue explants was confirmed using a calcein stain, a marker of live cells.[60] Following the *ex vivo* explant culture the biopsies were snap frozen, sectioned, and stained with haematoxylin and eosin, then examined by light microscopy to confirm that biopsy morphology was maintained.

This model has been successfully used to demonstrate that an anti-TLR2 monoclonal antibody significantly inhibits specific TLR2-induced inflammatory signals in RA synovial tissues.[60] In addition, a small molecular JAK inhibitor has been shown to significantly reduce activated signal transducer and activator of transcription (STAT) signalling and decreased spontaneous secretion of IL-6, IL-8, and MMP3 in synovial tissue explant cultures *ex vivo*.[61] This model can be utilized to examine the effect of pro-inflammatory mediators, not only on spontaneous release but also on synovial fibroblast outgrowths from explant cultures. Toll-like receptor 2 (TLR2) induces migration and invasive mechanisms in RA.[59]

Angiogenesis

New blood vessel formation is an early event in RA synovial tissue, facilitating cellular infiltration into the joint.[62-64] The new vessels develop a rich network in the synovial sublining layer. New vessels also allow delivery of nutrients and oxygen to the synovial tissue to promotes cell survival, migration, and the formation of a hyperplastic, locally invasive pannus. Angiogenesis is regulated by angiogenic growth factors and inhibitors such as VEGF a master regulator at the start of vascular morphogenesis, stimulating EC proliferation and migration.[65] Many other factors differentially expressed control vessel sprouting and maturation, such as angiopoietins 1 and 2 (Ang1 and Ang2), TGFβ, fibroblast growth factor, PDGF, TNFα, IL-8, and IL-1.[66-68] Macroscopically differential vascular patterns have been described in RA and other arthropathies.[3] In RA, synovial vascularity consists mainly of straight, regularly branching vessels that may reflect pathogenic processes. We have demonstrated that vessels are found in an immature state (without pericytes) and also mature (with pericytes) vessels.[4] Synovial vessels may therefore be constantly in flux—undergoing angiogenesis, maturation, and regression, depending on the interaction of growth factors, matrix metalloproteinases and cytokines in the microenvironment,[4,69] Thus, a dysfunctional vascular network leads to disruption of uniform blood flow in the pannus with failure to restore tissue oxygen levels resulting in an hypoxic environment. This further stimulates the synovium, maintaining a chronic, self-perpetuating, and persistent cell infiltration resulting in phenotypic changes in lining layer synoviocytes and invasion of adjacent cartilage.

Cellular bioenergetics–hypoxia and metabolism

Synovial hypoxia has been implicated in the pathogenesis of RA.[70] Reduced oxygen levels were suggested in the synovial fluid of RA patients compared to healthy controls when surrogate markers were measured.[71] Low oxygen levels were then measured directly in the tenosynovium during surgical repair of ruptured tendons in RA patients.[72] These observations suggested a paradox as synovial vascularity and blood flow was increased in patients with inflammatory arthritis, however studies indicated that the growth of an invasive synovial pannus outpaces the blood supply, resulting in hypoxia.[73,74] The role of hypoxia in the pathogenesis of RA is further supported by studies showing increased HIF1a activation in RA synovial tissue.[75,76] We used a novel Lycox probe to measure *in vivo* pO_2 levels within the RA synovium at arthroscopy to show it is profoundly hypoxic with tissue pO2 as low as 0.46%.[77] In addition, synovial pO_2 levels inversely correlated with cellular infiltration of macrophages and T cells, mitochondrial DNA mutation, oxidative damage and immature blood vessels,[4,77–79] effects of which were reversed by TNFi. Hypoxia stimulates cell invasiveness and survival, and the increased cellular demand for energy leads to a metabolic switch in favour of glycolysis.[80] Studies also show elevated lactate, succinate, and reduced glucose levels in RA synovial fluid while in the RA synovium there is increased glycolytic activity.[81–83] Furthermore, increased succinate in RA synovial fluid induces IL-1β release from macrophages an effect mediated through GPR91.[83] Previous studies have also demonstrated increased mitochondrial mutations and dysfunction in the RA synovium,[84] increased nicotinamide adenine dinucleotide phosphate (NADPH) oxidase/Nox2 in rheumatoid arthritis fibroblast-like synovial cells (RAFLS) and tissue[85,86] altered expression of *PFKFB3* in naïve CD4 T cells in RA[87] increased glycolytic mechanisms in RAFLS in response to TLR2 activation and hypoxia[59,88] and shown increased glutamine metabolism regulates RAFLS proliferation and invasive mechanisms.[89] Furthermore, treatment of RA synovial cells with glycolytic inhibitors decreases cytokine secretion, proliferation, cellular-invasion, key transcriptional pathways, and attenuates severity of inflammation in mouse models of arthritis.[90–92]

Early arthritis

Early diagnosis and treatment of RA has increasingly become an imperative since the mid-1990s. The rationale for systematic studies of clinical, histological, DNA, mRNA, and proteomic data have been established since 2002.[93] Synovial tissue analysis is progressing our understanding of early RA. Improvement in early diagnosis using clinical and serological features has been significant over the past decade, however bone erosions often develop in the first 2 years of disease.[94] Therefore, aggressive therapy introduced at the earliest possible stage is more successful than treatment commenced after damage has occurred leading to the concept of a 'window of opportunity'.[95] Indeed, one of the most useful serological biomarkers

recently identified to aid in early diagnosis is ACPA.[96] Circulating ACPA is reasonably specific (90%), however the diagnostic sensitivity in early arthritis varies widely between 40% and 70%[97] and some subjects who develop RA may never become ACPA positive. In addition, until recently the exact relationship between ACPA positive RA and synovial tissue findings have been poorly defined.

The analysis of synovial tissue from patients with early RA have, to date, revealed few molecular clues when compared to those with late disease.[98] One study has suggested that a highly expanded, synovial specific T-cell clone may be associated with the early stages of RA, underlining the importance of T lymphocytes.[99] In contrast, epigenetic characteristics of synovial FLS appear to change as the disease progresses and might be useful as a marker of early disease.[100] To find synovial tissue biomarkers for stratification of early disease a longitudinal study of 50 patients with early arthritis who had a synovial biopsy at baseline and assessment after 24 months was undertaken.[101] This study examined vascular growth factors including VEGF, angiopoietins, and their receptors—tyrosine kinase with Ig and epidermal growth factor (EGF) homology domains (TIE). Synovia from RA patients who subsequently developed bone erosion showed increased expression of the activated or phosphorylated angiopoietin receptor—TIE2, compared to those patients with self-limiting arthritis. A preliminary study of ultrasound-guided synovial tissue biopsies obtained from treatment-naïve early arthritis patients did show increased macrophage-derived chemokine CXC-chemokine ligand 4 (CXCL4; also called platelet factor 4) and CXCL7 (platelet basic protein) expression during the first phase of symptoms but not at the later phases of disease.[102] The studies of synovial tissue in early RA patients are few and small; undoubtedly more synovial tissue research is needed to enable meaningful stratification into erosive/non-erosive or persistent disease. Some studies have suggested that the presence of synovial B cells and ACPA positivity may predict chronic inflammation and response to B-cell therapies.[103,104] Amara et al., using single B cell-based cloning technology to isolate immunoglobulin genes from joint-derived B cells in RA patients with active disease, demonstrated accumulation of ACPA-producing B cells and plasma cells in the RA joint.[105] Mechanisms by which this occurs is unclear, but studies have shown increased expression of the B-cell chemoattractant chemokine ligand 13 (CXCL13) in RA synovium, associated with higher ACPA positivity and erosive disease.[106] In addition, RA patients with ACPA-hyperglycosylation has been shown to give a selective advantage to ACPA-producing B cells, further supporting the association between ACPA positivity and B-cell functionality.[107]

Seropositive arthralgia

It has been recognized for some time that circulating ACPA may predate the onset of RA by up to 10 years[108] and bone erosions have been demonstrated in ACPA positive subjects at the early stages of RA.[109] As a result of this, studies are now focused on subjects who present with arthralgia who have circulating antibodies including rheumatoid factor and ACPA.[110] Although, initial studies suggest only 30%, or less, of ACPA positive arthralgia subjects subsequently develop RA after almost 3 years.[111] It is suggested that synovial tissue analysis might provide important biomarkers to predict more accurately who will, or will not, develop RA. If synovial tissue biomarkers can be used to accurately identify those 'at risk' then the possibility of a cure for RA, or preventative therapy aimed at the restoring self-tolerance may become a reality.[112] Two small studies of synovial tissue have been performed in patients 'at risk' of developing RA and found little evidence of synovitis.[111,113] One study examined 13 patients with autoantibody positive arthralgia, knee joint biopsies showed no differences compared with healthy controls.[111] In a larger follow-up study, the authors reported a subtle infiltration of T cells in the synovium.[113] More recently, an international multicentre study has examined the gene signatures to assess the activity of the CD40-CD40L pathway at various stages of RA, including arthralgia.[110]

Interestingly, the expression of CD40L and active full-length CD40 was increased in the disease tissues, while that of a dominant-negative CD40 isoform was decreased. Gene set variation analysis revealed that CD40L-responsive genes in naïve B cells and iDC were significantly enriched in synovial tissues from arthralgia, early RA, and established RA patients.

Gene-expression profiling and novel techniques of analysis

Studies of gene-expression profiles in synovial tissue have identified changes that could represent biomarkers. Transcriptomic data might be useful clinically to create a rule-based classification to differentiate between RA and OA[114,115] examining specific cell functions in the tissue including proliferation, survival, angiogenesis, and the regulation of inflammation. Studies have demonstrated associations of gene expression and treatment responses; inflammatory genes upregulated in pretreatment biopsies may then identify responders to anti-TNF therapy.[116] In this longitudinal study of RA patients, synovial ribonucleic acid (RNA) analysis identified 38 transcripts associated with response to infliximab treatment, in patients with lymphocyte aggregates in their biopsy. Responders and non-responders to adalimumab therapy expressed different genes in a study of paired synovial tissue from RA patients after 12 weeks.[117] Two distinct families of genes were seen—those involved in regulation of the immune response and those regulating cell division. The microarray results were confirmed by synovial expression using specific antibodies demonstrating significantly higher expression of IL-7 receptor α-chain (IL-7Rα), CXCL11, IL-18, IL-18 receptor accessory protein (IL-18RAP) and the proliferation marker MKI67 in poor compared to moderate/good responders. These data confirm gene/protein expression correlations and highlight cytokine and chemokine signalling molecules as potential biomarkers of response to treatment. A study of early response to rituximab therapy demonstrated significant depletion of B cells after 8 weeks.[118] Finally, a study of paired synovial biopsies in RA patients receiving IV rituximab therapy found higher macrophage- and T-cell-associated genes in the synovial tissue of clinical responders, and increased IFNα and genes associated with matrix remodelling in the synovium of poor clinical responders.[119] The advance of new methods and technologies in synovial tissue analysis is significant, enabling faster and more detailed analyses at a molecular level. In addition, single cell analysis has provided a powerful tool for assessing individual cell functions, however, the interpretation of microarray data also raises problems as reproducibility of analysis has shown considerable variation.[120] Furthermore, array datasets may have high levels of background signals which may reduce their sensitivity to transcripts present in low numbers.[121] Future progress in identifying biomarkers, genomic and otherwise, will lead to significant results if synovial tissue analysis is included in the programme.

Conclusions

Synovial tissue represents the target tissue of RA and of many autoimmune arthritides. New, safer, and more efficient methods of obtaining synovial tissue samples are becoming more widely available and many rheumatologists are routinely learning these skills. In this chapter we have highlighted those studies that analyse the cellular and molecular characteristics of RA synovial tissue, including early disease and seropositive arthralgia subjects who may develop arthritis subsequently. We believe the results of this analysis has already advanced the field in terms of biomarkers for patient stratification, response to therapy, and discovery of novel therapeutic targets. In addition, we have reviewed the use of synovial tissue analysis as an outcome measure for clinical trials in RA. The application of recent advances in molecular technologies to synovial tissue analysis will probably lead to major benefits for patients with RA in the future.

REFERENCES

1. Veale DJ, Firestein GS. Synovium. In: Firestein GS, Budd RC, Gabriel SE, McInnes IB, O'Dell JR (eds). *Kelley and Firestein's Textbook of Rheumatology*, 10th edition, *Vol. 1*. New York, NY: Elsevier, 2017.
2. Orr C, Vieira-Sousa E, Boyle DL, et al. Synovial tissue research: a state-of-the-art review. *Nat Rev Rheumatol* 2017;*13*(8):463–75.
3. Cañete J, Parsons W, Emery P, Veale D. Distinct vascular patterns of early synovitis in psoriatic, reactive, and rheumatoid arthritis. *Arthritis Rheum* 1999;*42*(7):1481–4.
4. Kennedy A, Ng CT, Biniecka M, et al. Angiogenesis and blood vessel stability in inflammatory arthritis. *Arthritis Rheum* 2010;*62*(3):711–21.
5. Fearon U, Canavan M, Biniecka M, Veale DJ. Hypoxia, mitochondrial dysfunction and synovial invasiveness in rheumatoid arthritis. *Nat Rev Rheumatol* 2016;*12*(7):385–97.
6. Seemayer CA, Kuchen S, Kuenzler P, et al. Cartilage destruction mediated by synovial fibroblasts does not depend on proliferation in rheumatoid arthritis. *American J Pathol* 2003;*162*(5):1549–57.
7. Rooney M, Whelan A, Feighery C, Bresnihan B. Changes in lymphocyte infiltration of the synovial membrane and the clinical course of rheumatoid arthritis. *Arthritis Rheum* 1989;*32*(4):361–9.
8. Firestein GS, Paine MM, Boyle DL. Mechanisms of methotrexate action in rheumatoid arthritis. *Arthritis Rheum* 1994;*37*(2):193–200.
9. Tak PP, Van Der Lubbe PA, Cauli A, et al. Reduction of synovial inflammation after anti-CD4 monoclonal antibody treatment in early rheumatoid arthritis. *Arthritis Rheum* 1995;*38*(10):1457–65.
10. Tak PP, Taylor PC, Breedveld FC, et al. Decrease in cellularity and expression of adhesion molecules by anti–tumor necrosis factor α monoclonal antibody treatment in patients with rheumatoid arthritis. *Arthritis Rheum* 1996;*39*(7):1077–81.
11. Fearon U, Veale DJ. Key challenges in rheumatic and musculoskeletal disease translational research. *EBioMedicine* 2014;*1*(2–3):95–6.
12. Levick JR. Permeability of rheumatoid and normal human synovium to specific plasma proteins. *Arthritis Rheum* 1981;*124*(12):1550–60.

13. Dahl L, Dahl I, Engström-Laurent A, Granath K. Concentration and molecular weight of sodium hyaluronate in synovial fluid from patients with rheumatoid arthritis and other arthropathies. *Ann Rheum Dis* 1985;*44*(12):817–22.

14. Decker B, McKenzie BF, McGuckin WF, Slocumb CH. Comparative distribution of proteins and glycoproteins of serum and synovial fluid. *Arthritis Rheum* 1959;*2*(2):162–77.

15. Kulka JP. The pathogenesis of rheumatoid arthritis. *J Chronic Dis* 1959;*10*:388–402.

16. de Hair MJ, Harty L, Gerlag D, Pitzalis C, Veale D, Tak PP. Synovial tissue analysis for the discovery of diagnostic and prognostic biomarkers in patients with early arthritis. *J Rheumatol.* 2011;*38*(9):2068–72.

17. Forestier J. Instrumentation pour biopsie medicale. *Comptes Rendus des Seances–Société de Biologie et de ses Filiales* 1932;*110*:186–7.

18. Polley HF, Bickle WH, Dockerty MB. Experiences with an instrument for punch biopsy of synovial membrane. *Mayo Clin Proc* 1951;*26*:273–81.

19. Zeveley HA, French AJ, Mikkelsen WM, Duff IF. Synovial specimens obtained by knee joint punch biopsy. Histologic study in joint diseases. *Am J Med* 1956;*20*:510–19.

20. Parker RH, Pearson CM. A simplified synovial biopsy needle. *Arthritis Rheum* 1963;*6*:172–6.

21. Schumacher HR, Kitridou RC. Synovitis of recent onset. A clinicopathologic study during the first month of disease. *Arthritis Rheum* 1972;*15*(5):465–85.

22. Veale DJ. The role of arthroscopy in early arthritis. *Clin Exp Rheumatol* 1999;*17*(1):37–8.

23. Najm A, Orr C, Heymann MF, Bart G, Veale DJ, Le Goff B. Success rate and utility of ultrasound-guided synovial biopsies in clinical practice. *J Rheumatol* 2016;*43*(12):2113–19.

24. Youssef PP, Kraan M, Breedveld F, et al. Quantitative microscopic analysis of inflammation in rheumatoid arthritis synovial membrane samples selected at arthroscopy compared with samples obtained blindly by needle biopsy. *Arthritis Rheum* 1998;*41*(4):663–9.

25. Kane D, Veale D, FitzGerald O, Reece R. Survey of arthroscopy performed by rheumatologists. *Rheumatol* 2002;*41*(2):210–15.

26. Lazarou I, D'Agostino MA, Naredo E, Humby F, Filer A, Kelly SG. Ultrasound-guided synovial biopsy: a systematic review according to the OMERACT filter and recommendations for minimal reporting standards in clinical studies. *Rheumatology (Oxf)* 2015;*54*(10):1867–75.

27. Moran EM, Heydrich R, Ng CT, et al. IL-17A expression is localised to both mononuclear and polymorphonuclear synovial cell infiltrates. *PLoS One* 2011;*6*(8):e24048.

28. Tak PP, Smeets TJ, Daha MR, et al. Analysis of the synovial cell infiltrate in early rheumatoid synovial tissue in relation to local disease activity. *Arthritis Rheum* 1997;*40*(2):217–25.

29. Hui AY, McCarty WJ, Masuda K, Firestein GS, Sah RL. A systems biology approach to synovial joint lubrication in health, injury, and disease. *Syst Biol Med* 2012;*4*(1):15–37.

30. Frank-Bertoncelj M, Trenkmann M, Klein K, et al. Epigenetically driven anatomical diversity of synovial fibroblasts guides joint-specific fibroblast functions. *Nat Commun* 2017;*8*:14852.

31. Ai R, Hammaker D, Boyle DL, et al. Joint-specific DNA methylation and transcriptome signatures in rheumatoid arthritis identify distinct pathogenic processes. *Nat Commun* 2016;*7*:11849.

32. Kraan MC, Reece RJ, Smeets TJM, Veale DJ, Emery P, Tak PP. Comparison of synovial tissues from the knee joints and the small joints of rheumatoid arthritis patients: implications for pathogenesis and evaluation of treatment. *Arthritis Rheum* 2002;*46*(8):2034–8.

33. Soden M, Rooney M, Cullen A, Whelan A, Feighery C, Bresnihan B. Immunohistological features in the synovium obtained from clinically uninvolved knee joints of patients with rheumatoid arthritis. *Rheumatology* 1989;*28*(4):287–92.

34. Kraan MC, Versendaal H, Jonker M, et al. Asymptomatic synovitis precedes clinically manifest arthritis. *Arthritis Rheum* 1998;*41*(8):1481–8.

35. Haringman JJ, Gerlag DM, Zwinderman AH, et al. Synovial tissue macrophages: a sensitive biomarker for response to treatment in patients with rheumatoid arthritis. *Ann Rheum Dis* 2005;*64*(6):834–8.

36. Gerlag DM, Haringman JJ, Smeets TJM, et al. Effects of oral prednisolone on biomarkers in synovial tissue and clinical improvement in rheumatoid arthritis. *Arthritis Rheum* 2004;*50*(12):3783–91.

37. Yanni G, Nabil M, Farahat MR, Poston RN, Panayi GS. Intramuscular gold decreases cytokine expression and macrophage numbers in the rheumatoid synovial membrane. *Ann Rheum Dis* 1994;*53*(5):315–22.

38. Dolhain RJ, Tak PP, Dijkmans BA, De Kuiper P, Breedveld FC, Miltenburg AM. Methotrexate reduces inflammatory cell numbers, expression of monokines and of adhesion molecules in synovial tissue of patients with rheumatoid arthritis. *Rheumatology* 1998;*37*(5):502–8.

39. Kraan MC, Reece RJ, Barg EC, et al. Modulation of inflammation and metalloproteinase expression in synovial tissue by leflunomide and methotrexate in patients with active rheumatoid arthritis: findings in a prospective, randomized, double-blind, parallel-design clinical trial in thirty-nine patients at two centers. *Arthritis Rheum* 2000;*43*(8):1820–30.

40. Wijbrandts CA, Dijkgraaf MG, Kraan MC, et al. The clinical response to infliximab in rheumatoid arthritis is in part dependent on pretreatment tumour necrosis factor alpha expression in the synovium. *Ann Rheum Dis* 2008;*67*(8):1139–44.

41. Thurlings RM, Vos K, Wijbrandts CA, Zwinderman AH, Gerlag DM, Tak PP. Synovial tissue response to rituximab: mechanism of action and identification of biomarkers of response. *Ann Rheum Dis* 2008;*67*(7):917–25.

42. Walsh CA, Fearon U, FitzGerald O, Veale DJ, Bresnihan B. Decreased CD20 expression in rheumatoid arthritis synovium following 8 weeks of rituximab therapy. *Clin Exp Rheumatol* 2008;*26*(4):656–8.

43. Bresnihan B, Pontifex E, Thurlings RM, et al. Synovial tissue sublining CD68 expression is a biomarker of therapeutic response in rheumatoid arthritis clinical trials: consistency across centers. *J Rheumatol* 2009;*36*(8):1800–2.

44. Kavanaugh A, Rosengren S, Lee SJ, et al. Assessment of rituximab's immunomodulatory synovial effects (ARISE trial). 1: clinical and synovial biomarker results. *Ann Rheum Dis* 2008;*67*(3):402–8.

45. Buch MH, Boyle DL, Rosengren S, et al. Mode of action of abatacept in rheumatoid arthritis patients having failed tumour necrosis factor blockade: a histological, gene expression and dynamic magnetic resonance imaging pilot study. *Ann Rheum Dis* 2009;*68*(7):1220–7.

46. Boyle DL, Soma K, Hodge J, et al. The JAK inhibitor tofacitinib suppresses synovial JAK1-STAT signalling in rheumatoid arthritis. *Ann Rheum Dis* 2015;*74*(6):1311–16.

47. Orr C, Najm A, Biniecka M, McGarry T, Ng CT, Young F, Fearon U, Veale DJ. Synovial immunophenotype and anti-citrullinated peptide antibodies in rheumatoid arthritis patients: relationship to treatment response and radiologic prognosis. *Arthritis Rheumatol* 2017;*69*(11):2114–23.

48. Basdeo SA, Moran B, Cluxton D, et al. Polyfunctional, pathogenic CD161+ Th17 lineage cells are resistant to regulatory T cell-mediated suppression in the context of autoimmunity. *J Immunol* 2015;*195*(2):528–40.

49. Genovese MC, Durez P, Richards HB, et al. Efficacy and safety of secukinumab in patients with rheumatoid arthritis: a phase II, dose-finding, double-blind, randomised, placebo-controlled study. *Ann Rheum Dis* 2013;*72*(6):863–9.

50. Basdeo SA, Cluxton D, Sulaimani J, et al. Ex-Th17 (nonclassical Th1) cells are functionally distinct from classical Th1 and Th17 cells and are not constrained by regulatory T cells. *J Immunol* 2017;*198*(6):2249–59.

51. Cañete JD, Celis R, Moll C, et al. Clinical significance of synovial lymphoid neogenesis and its reversal after anti-tumour necrosis factor alpha therapy in rheumatoid arthritis. *Ann Rheum Dis* 2009;*68*(5):751–6.

52. van de Sande MG, Thurlings RM, Boumans MJ, et al. Presence of lymphocyte aggregates in the synovium of patients with early arthritis in relationship to diagnosis and outcome: is it a constant feature over time? *Ann Rheum Dis* 2011;*70*(4):700–3.

53. Klaasen R, Thurlings RM, Wijbrandts CA, et al. The relationship between synovial lymphocyte aggregates and the clinical response to infliximab in rheumatoid arthritis: a prospective study. *Arthritis Rheum* 2009;*60*(11):3217–24.

54. Fassbender HG, Simmling-Annefeld M. The potential aggressiveness of synovial tissue in rheumatoid arthritis. *Journal Pathol* 1983;*139*(3), 399–406.

55. Mor A, Abramson SB, Pillinger MH. The fibroblast-like synovial cell in rheumatoid arthritis: a key player in inflammation and joint destruction. *Clin Immunol* 2005;*115*(2):118–28.

56. Filer A, Antczak P, Parsonage GN, et al. Stromal transcriptional profiles reveal hierarchies of anatomical site, serum response and disease and identify disease specific pathways. *PLoS One* 2015;*10*(3):e0120917.

57. Lefèvre S, Knedla A, Tennie C, et al. Synovial fibroblasts spread rheumatoid arthritis to unaffected joints. *Nat Med* 2009;*15*(12):1414–20.

58. van Baarsen LG, Wijbrandts CA, Timmer TC, van der Pouw Kraan TC, Tak PP, Verweij CL. Synovial tissue heterogeneity in rheumatoid arthritis in relation to disease activity and biomarkers in peripheral blood. *Arthritis Rheum* 2010;*62*(6):1602–7.

59. McGarry T, Veale DJ, Gao W, Orr C, Fearon U, Connolly M. Toll-like receptor 2 (TLR2) induces migration and invasive mechanisms in rheumatoid arthritis. *Arthritis Res Ther* 2015;*17*:15.

60. Ultaigh SN, Saber TP, McCormick J, et al. Blockade of Toll-like receptor 2 prevents spontaneous cytokine release from rheumatoid arthritis ex vivo synovial explant cultures. *Arthritis Res Ther* 2011;*13*(1):R33.

61. Gao W, McCormick J, Connolly M, Balogh E, Veale DJ, Fearon U. Hypoxia and STAT3 signalling interactions regulate proinflammatory pathways in rheumatoid arthritis. *Ann Rheum Dis* 2015;*74*(6):1275–83.

62. Szekanecz Z, Koch AE. Endothelial cells in inflammation and angiogenesis. *Curr Drug Targets Inflamm Allergy* 2005;*4*(3):319–23.

63. Szekanecz Z, Koch AE. Mechanisms of disease: angiogenesis in inflammatory diseases. *Nat Clin Pract Rheumatol* 2007;*3*(11):635–43.

64. Kennedy A, Ng CT, Biniecka M, et al. Angiogenesis and blood vessel stability in inflammatory arthritis. *Arthritis Rheum* 2010;*62*(3):711–21.

65. Dvorak HF. Angiogenesis: update 2005. *J Thromb Haemost* 2005;*3*(8):1835–42.

66. Colville-Nash PR, Scott DL. Angiogenesis and rheumatoid arthritis: pathogenic and therapeutic implications. *Ann Rheum Dis* 1992;*51*(7):919–25.

67. Fraser A, Fearon U, Reece R, Emery P, Veale DJ. Matrix metalloproteinase 9, apoptosis, and vascular morphology in early arthritis. *Arthritis Rheum* 2001;*44*(9):2024–8.

68. Fearon U, Griosios K, Fraser A, et al. Angiopoietins, growth factors, and vascular morphology in early arthritis. *J Rheumatol* 2003;*30*(2):260–8.

69. Izquierdo E, Cañete JD, Celis R, et al. Immature blood vessels in rheumatoid synovium are selectively depleted in response to anti-TNF therapy. *PloS One* 2009;*4*(12):e8131.

70. Distler JH, Wenger RH, Gassmann M, et al. Physiologic responses to hypoxia and implications for hypoxia-inducible factors in the pathogenesis of rheumatoid arthritis. *Arthritis Rheum* 2004;*50*(1):10–23.

71. Lund-Olesen K,. Oxygen tension in synovial fluids. *Arthritis Rheum* 1970;*13*(6):769–76.

72. Sivakumar B, Akhavani MA, Winlove CP, Taylor PC, Paleolog EM, Kang N. Synovial hypoxia as a cause of tendon rupture in rheumatoid arthritis. *J Hand Surg* 2008;*33*(1):49–58.

73. Bodamyali T, Stevens CR, Billingham ME, Ohta S, Blake DR. Influence of hypoxia in inflammatory synovitis. *Ann Rheum Dis* 1998;*57*(12):703–10.

74. Stevens CR, Blake DR, Merry P, Revell PA, Levick JR. A comparative study by morphometry of the microvasculature in normal and rheumatoid synovium. *Arthritis Rheum* 1991;*34*(12):1508–13.

75. Green L, Cookson A, Bruce IN, Donn RP, Ray DW. Identification of multiple, oxygen-stable HIF1 alpha isoforms, and augmented expression of adrenomedullin in rheumatoid arthritis. *Clin Exp Rheumatol* 2013;*31*(5):672–82.

76. Li X, Wang Y, Li X, et al. Hypoxia-induced transcription factor 1α: a potent driving force behind rheumatoid arthritis. *Clin Exp Rheumatol* 2014;*32*(5):760.

77. Ng CT, Biniecka M, Kennedy A, McCormick J, Fitzgerald O, Bresnihan B. Synovial tissue hypoxia and inflammation *in vivo*. *Ann Rheum Dis* 2010;*69*(7):1389–95.

78. Biniecka M, Kennedy A, Fearon U, Ng CT, Veale DJ, O'Sullivan JN. Oxidative damage in synovial tissue is associated with *in vivo* hypoxic status in the arthritic joint. *Ann Rheumat Dis* 2010;*69*(6):1172–8.

79. Harty LC, Biniecka M, O'Sullivan J, et al. Mitochondrial mutagenesis correlates with the local inflammatory environment in arthritis. *Ann Rheum Dis* 2012;*71*(4):582–8.

80. Chang X, Wei C. Glycolysis and rheumatoid arthritis. *Int J Rheum Dis* 2011;*14*(3):217–22.

81. Henderson B, Bitensky L, Chayen J. Glycolytic activity in human synovial lining cells in rheumatoid arthritis. *Ann Rheum Dis* 1979;*38*(1):63–7.

82. Kim S, Hwang J, Xuan J, Jung YH, Cha HS, Kim KH. Global metabolite profiling of synovial fluid for the specific diagnosis of rheumatoid arthritis from other inflammatory arthritis. *PLoS One* 2014;*9*(6):e97501.

83. Littlewood-Evans A, Sarret S, Apfel V, Loesle P, Dawson J, Zhang J. GPR91 senses extracellular succinate released from inflammatory macrophages and exacerbates rheumatoid arthritis. *J Exp Med* 2016;*213*:1655–6.

84. Biniecka M, Fox E, Gao W, et al. Hypoxia induces mitochondrial mutagenesis and dysfunction in inflammatory arthritis. *Arthritis Rheum* 2011;*63*:2172–82.

85. Chi PL, Liu CJ, Lee IT, Chen YW, Hsiao LD, Yang CM. HO-1 induction by CO-RM2 attenuates TNF-α-induced cytosolic phospholipase A2 expression via inhibition of PKCα-dependent NADPH oxidase/ROS and NF-κB. *Mediators Inflamm* 2014;*2014*:279171.

86. Biniecka M, Connolly M, Gao W, et al. Redox-mediated angiogenesis in the hypoxic joint of inflammatory arthritis. *Arthritis Rheum* 2014;*66*:3300–10.

87. Yang Z, Fujii H, Mohan SV, Goronzy JJ, Weyand CM. Phosphofructokinase deficiency impairs ATP generation, autophagy, and redox balance in rheumatoid arthritis T cells. *J Exp Med* 2013;*210*:2119–34.

88. McGarry T, Biniecka M, Gao W, et al. Resolution of TLR2-induced inflammation through manipulation of metabolic pathways in rheumatoid arthritis. *Sci Rep* 2017;*7*:43165.

89. Takahashi S, Saegusa J, Sendo S, et al. Glutaminase 1 plays a key role in the cell growth of fibroblast-like synoviocytes in rheumatoid arthritis. *Arthritis Res Ther* 2017;*19*:76.

90. Yan H, Zhou HF, Hu Y, Pham CT. Suppression of experimental arthritis through AMP-activated protein kinase activation and autophagy modulation. *J Rheum Dis Treat*. 2015;*1*(1):5.

91. Son HJ, Lee J, Lee SY, et al. Metformin attenuates experimental autoimmune arthritis through reciprocal regulation of Th17/Treg balance and osteoclastogenesis. *Mediators Inflamm* 2014;*2014*:973986.

92. Biniecka M, Canavan M, McGarry T, et al. Dysregulated bioenergetics: a key regulator of joint inflammation. *Ann Rheum Dis* 2016;*75*:2192–200.

93. Scott DL. The diagnosis and prognosis of early arthritis: rationale for new prognostic criteria. *Arthritis Rheum* 2002;*46*(2):286–90.

94. van der Heijde DM. Joint erosions and patients with early rheumatoid arthritis. *Br J Rheumatol* 1995;*34* Suppl 2:74–8.

95. van de Sande MG, de Hair MJ, van der Leij C, et al. Different stages of rheumatoid arthritis: features of the synovium in the preclinical phase. *Ann Rheum Dis* 2011;*70*(5):772–7.

96. Snir O, Widhe M, Hermansson M, et al. Antibodies to several citrullinated antigens are enriched in the joints of rheumatoid arthritis patients. *Arthritis Rheum* 2010;*62*(1):44–52.

97. Lee D, Schur P. Clinical utility of the anti-CCP assay in patients with rheumatic diseases. *Ann Rheumatic Dis* 2003;*62*(9):870–4.

98. Smeets TJ1, Dolhain RJEM, Miltenburg AM, de Kuiper R, Breedveld FC, Tak PP. Poor expression of T cell-derived cytokines and activation and proliferation markers in early rheumatoid synovial tissue. *Clin Immunol Immunopathol* 1998;*88*(1):84–90.

99. Klarenbeek PL, de Hair MJ, Doorenspleet ME, et al. Inflamed target tissue provides a specific niche for highly expanded T-cell clones in early human autoimmune disease. *Ann Rheum Dis* 2012;*71*(6):1088–93.

100. Whitaker JW, Shoemaker R, Boyle DL, et al. An imprinted rheumatoid arthritis methylome signature reflects pathogenic phenotype. *Genome Med* 2013;*5*(4):40.

101. van de Sande MG, de Launay D, de Hair MJ, et al. Local synovial engagement of angiogenic TIE-2 is associated with the development of persistent erosive rheumatoid arthritis in patients with early arthritis. *Arthritis Rheum* 2013;*65*(12):3073–83.

102. Yeo L, Adlard N, Biehl M, et al. Expression of chemokines CXCL4 and CXCL7 by synovial macrophages defines an early stage of rheumatoid arthritis. *Ann Rheum Dis* 2016;*75*(4):763–71.

103. Teng YK, Verburg RJ, Verpoort KN, et al. Differential responsiveness to immunoablative therapy in refractory rheumatoid arthritis is associated with level and avidity of anti-cyclic citrullinated protein autoantibodies: a case study. *Arthritis Res Ther* 2007;*9*(5):R106.

104. Humby F, Bombardieri M, Manzo A, et al. Ectopic lymphoid structures support ongoing production of class-switched autoantibodies in rheumatoid synovium. *PLoS Med* 2009;*6*(1):e1.

105. Amara K, Steen J, Murray F, et al. Monoclonal IgG antibodies generated from joint-derived B cells of RA patients have a strong bias toward citrullinated autoantigen recognition. *J Exp Med* 2013;*210*(3):445–55.

106. Bugatti S, Manzo A, Vitolo B, et al. High expression levels of the B cell chemoattractant CXCL13 in rheumatoid synovium are a marker of severe disease. *Rheumatology (Oxf)* 2014;*53*(10):1886–95.

107. Rombouts Y, Willemze A, van Beers JJ, et al. Extensive glycosylation of ACPA-IgG variable domains modulates binding to citrullinated antigens in rheumatoid arthritis. *Ann Rheum Dis* 2016;*75*(3):578–85.

108. van de Stadt LA, de Koning MH, van de Stadt RJ, et al. Development of the anti-citrullinated protein antibody repertoire prior to the onset of rheumatoid arthritis. *Arthritis Rheum* 2011;*63*(11):3226–33.

109. Hecht C, Schett G, Finzel S. The impact of rheumatoid factor and ACPA on bone erosion in rheumatoid arthritis. *Ann Rheum Dis* 2015;*74*(1):e4.

110. Guo Y, Walsh AM, Fearon U, et al. CD40L dependent pathway is active at various stages of rheumatoid arthritis disease progression. *J Immunol* 2017;*198*(11):4490–501.

111. de Hair MJ, van de Sande MG, Ramwadhdoebe TH, et al. Features of the synovium of individuals at risk of developing rheumatoid arthritis: implications for understanding preclinical rheumatoid arthritis. *Arthritis Rheumatol* 2014;*66*(3):513–22.

112. Orr C, Vieira-Sousa E, Boyle DL, et al. Synovial tissue research: a state-of-the-art review. *Nat Rev Rheumatol* 2017;*13*(10):630.

113. Bos WH, Wolbink GJ, Boers M, et al. Arthritis development in patients with arthralgia is strongly associated with anti-citrullinated protein antibody status: a prospective cohort study. *Ann Rheum Dis* 2010;*69*(3):490–4.

114. Wang Z, Gerstein M, Snyder M. RNA-Seq: a revolutionary tool for transcriptomics. *Nat Rev Genet* 2009;*10*(1):57–63.

115. Wang LC, Zhang HY, Shao L, et al. S100A12 levels in synovial fluid may reflect clinical severity in patients with primary knee osteoarthritis. *Biomarkers* 2013;*18*(3):216–20.

116. Wijbrandts CA, Dijkgraaf MG, Kraan MC, et al. The clinical response to infliximab in rheumatoid arthritis is in part dependent on pretreatment tumour necrosis factor alpha expression in the synovium. *Ann Rheum Dis* 2008;*67*(8):1139–44.

117. Badot V, Galant C, Nzeusseu Toukap A, et al. Gene expression profiling in the synovium identifies a predictive signature of absence of response to adalimumab therapy in rheumatoid arthritis. *Arthritis Res Ther* 2009;*11*(2):R57.

118. Walsh C, Fearon U, FitzGerald O, Veale D, Bresnihan B. Decreased CD20 expression in rheumatoid arthritis synovium following 8 weeks of rituximab therapy. *Clin Exp Rheumatol* 2008;*26*(4):656.

119. Thurlings RM, Vos K, Wijbrandts CA, Zwinderman A, Gerlag DM, Tak PP. Synovial tissue response to rituximab: mechanism of action and identification of biomarkers of response. *Ann Rheum Dis* 2008;*67*(7):917–25.

120. Tan PK, Downey TJ, Spitznagel Jr EL, et al. Evaluation of gene expression measurements from commercial microarray platforms. *Nucleic Acids Res* 2003;*31*(19):5676–84.

121. Wang Z, Gerstein M, Snyder M. RNA-Seq: a revolutionary tool for transcriptomics. *Nat Rev Genet* 2009;*10*(1):57–63.

17

Radiography in rheumatoid arthritis

Charles Peterfy, Philip G. Conaghan, and Mikkel Østergaard

Introduction

The goals of imaging in clinical practice and in clinical research, regardless of the disease, are essentially the same:

1. Diagnosis and prognosis: determining which disease a patient is suffering from and how severely in order to guide treatment decisions
2. Monitoring disease progression to determine whether treatment is working and how well
3. Monitoring for complications of the disease or the treatment

The only way to determine reliably whether structural damage (bone erosion and/or articular cartilage loss) is present is with medical imaging. For most of the past century, the mainstay of imaging evaluation of rheumatoid arthritis (RA) has been conventional radiography. Radiography is inexpensive, widely available, and relatively safe. Characteristic radiographic findings are part of the American College of Rheumatology (ACR) 1987 classification criteria for RA.[1] Radiography is also a key criterion in the recent ACR/European League Against Rheumatism (EULAR) 2010 classification, in which patients displaying bone erosions typical for RA plus at least one clinically swollen joint fulfil the diagnostic criteria for RA.[2,3] Radiography can be helpful in differentiating RA from other joint conditions, such as psoriatic arthritis, osteoarthritis, and neoplasm.[4,5]

Despite the central role that this modality has played thus far, however, radiography's diagnostic power is quite limited in a number of ways, and other imaging techniques, particularly magnetic resonance imaging (MRI) and ultrasound, have proven to be more sensitive for early structural damage in RA and to correlate more closely with pathology. MRI and ultrasound are also uniquely able to identify early upstream inflammatory changes, namely synovitis and osteitis (previously called bone marrow oedema), that precede bone erosion, cartilage loss, and other structural changes, including ligament and tendon rupture, and are able to do so without exposing patients to ionizing radiation. Both MRI and ultrasound can objectively determine, often within only a couple of weeks of initiating therapy, whether or not the treatment has actually suppressed intra-articular synovitis and osteitis, at a time when placebo effects notoriously confound the reliability of clinical examination and patient-reported outcomes. Radiography, however, is unable to visualize inflammation reliably, and therefore is of little help in early

disease. MRI has further been shown to be able to determine within only a few weeks whether joint damage has also been inhibited.[6,7] In clinical trials, 6–12 months are typically needed to resolve treatment effect reliably using radiography. Despite these demonstrable advantages, however, assimilation of MRI into mainstream rheumatological practice has been slow.

The following discussion outlines the technical and interpretative principles, as well as the challenges, associated with radiographic evaluation of RA, and points to ways of dealing with some of the most common pitfalls in routine clinical practice and research.

Basic principles

X-rays are a type of electromagnetic radiation with sufficient energy to penetrate tissue. The higher the energy (keV) of the X-ray beam the greater its penetrating power. As X-rays pass through tissue, they are attenuated based on a number of factors, including tissue thickness, tissue properties (density, atomic number) and the energy of the X-ray photons. Radiographic images are produced by the X-ray photons that reach the image receptor. For plain radiography this is the film-screen cassette. For digital radiography it is either a photostimulable phosphor imaging plate in a cassette when using computed radiography or a flat panel detector when using direct radiography. Exactly how these different systems convert transmitted X-ray photons into grayscale images is beyond the scope of this discussion. However, in all cases contrast on the radiographic image is based on differences in the degree of X-ray attenuation of the different tissues exposed.

The two main mechanisms of X-ray attenuation are photoelectric absorption and Compton scattering. Photoelectric absorption actually removes X-ray photons from the image, whereas Compton scattering, as the name implies, diverts X-ray photons along random paths, creating noise, or 'film fog', that must be filtered out before reaching the radiographic receptor. This is accomplished either by placing a grid or collimator between the object and the receptor, or by separating the object and the receptor by a sufficient distance (air gap) to allow most of the scattered photons to miss the receptor (**Figure 17.1**).

For most clinical applications, Compton scattering is the principal mechanism of X-ray attenuation, and it increases with the physical

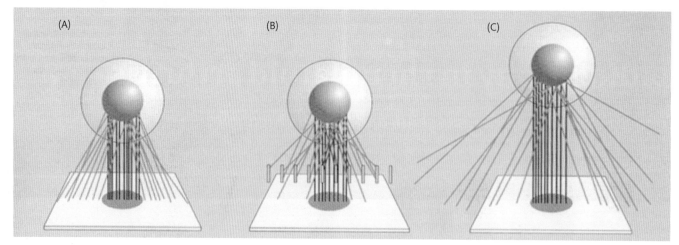

Figure 17.1 Scatter radiation. Compton interactions scatter radiation in random directions, and therefore provide little useable spatial information. This noise covers the radiographic image with a haze, or 'film fog', obscuring anatomical detail (A), and must therefore be removed. This can be accomplished by placing a grid or collimator in front of the receptor to filter out non-linear photons (B), or by allowing the scattered radiation to miss the receptor by moving the patient farther away, i.e., creating an air gap (C).

Reprinted from Peterfy CG. Imaging techniques. In: Klippel, J, Dieppe, P. (principal eds.). Rheumatology. 2nd Edition. Mosby-Wolfe, London 1998: 2.14.1–2.14.18 with permission from Elsevier.

density of the tissue. Since bone is much denser than other tissues, it is depicted with high contrast on radiographs, particularly when using low-energy X-ray photons, as photoelectric absorption becomes more pronounced at low energies. Since density among other tissues varies relatively little, soft-tissue contrast on radiographs is generally poor. Lowering beam energy can increase soft-tissue contrast, but not enough to visualize articular cartilage or discriminate synovial tissue or ligaments. Furthermore, the greater the X-ray absorption by the body, the greater is the radiation exposure. Radiographic contrast agents containing high atomic number substances, such as iodine or barium, can be useful for delineating the surfaces of articular structures during arthrography, but this applies mostly to large joints such as the knee or shoulder, and vascular perfusion is generally insufficient to discriminate among soft tissues. Additionally, these contrast materials can be toxic. Thus, they are rarely used in RA.

Radiographic detection of pathology in RA

The features of RA most reliably depicted with radiography are bone erosion and joint space narrowing. Malalignment of joints is also visible, but this is easily determined by physical examination, and thus it will not be discussed further here. Similarly, periarticular soft-tissue swelling can be seen to a variable extent with radiography, but not reliably so and not much better than by physical examination, and so this will not be discussed further either. Finally, juxta-articular osteopenia is sometimes seen in RA, but is a very unreliable finding, and its importance to the pathophysiology of the disease or its treatment is not known. Accordingly, this chapter will focus on bone erosion and joint space narrowing.

Advanced erosive disease is relatively easy to diagnose radiographically, and does not require a great deal of experience. However, detecting the earliest signs of bone erosion and differentiating them from normal vascular channels, entheseal irregularities, subarticular cysts associated with osteoarthritis or prior trauma, or other causes of cortical irregularity or focal lucency, including normal tuberosities, can be difficult (**Figures 17.2 and 17.3**),

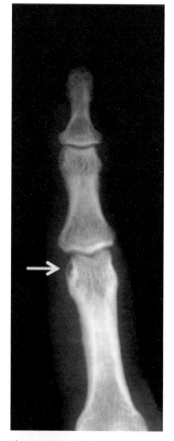
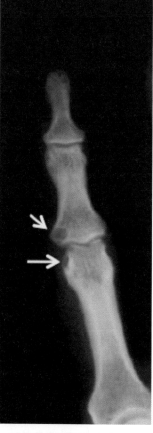

Figure 17.2 Erosions versus prominent entheseal grooves. Radiographs of the proximal interphalangeal (PIP) joint of the index finger of a patient with RA shows a focal lucency (long arrows) in the radial corner of the distal end of the proximal phalanx. This lucency does not change from baseline (left panel) to follow-up (right panel), and represents simply a prominent entheseal groove not an erosion. In contrast, the lucency (short arrow) that newly emerges on follow-up radiograph B in the radial corner of the proximal end of the middle phalanx is a true erosion.

(Images courtesy of Spire Sciences).

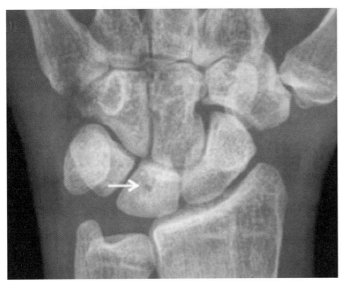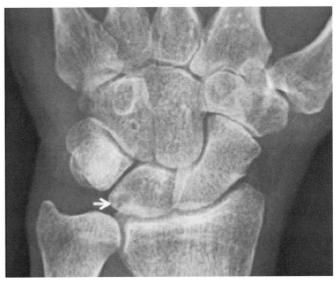

Figure 17.3 Erosion versus vascular channel. When fortuitously projected *en face*, openings for the nutrient blood vessels supplying the lunate bone through its dorsal and palmar surfaces appear as focal lucencies (long arrow) on radiographs of the wrist (left panel). When the wrist is known to belong to a patient with RA, these lucencies are often mistaken for erosions. The lunate bone shown in the right panel, also contains a focal lucency (short arrow). However, the corner location of this lesion, even though solitary in the wrist, argues more in favour of an erosion than a vascular channel. No vascular channels are visible in this lunate bone because the projection is slightly more oblique.
Images courtesy of Spire Sciences.

especially when the lesions are solitary or in elderly patients. Yet, discriminating these findings reliably is critical for establishing the erosive phenotype to determine the need for structure-modifying therapy. Accurately diagnosing early or sparse erosive disease with radiography on the basis of a single time point is particularly difficult. However, this is usually the context in which initial treatment decisions are made. Observing the behaviour of suspected bone erosions over time greatly increases diagnostic specificity and reduces false positive rates, as most findings that mimic RA erosions do not enlarge as quickly as true erosions do. Thus, observing progression of bone defects suspicious for erosion over a period of 3–6 months, for example, in a patient with other evidence of RA argues strongly in favour of true erosive disease. Non-progression, however, does

not exclude erosive disease, as fewer than 30% of patients with pre-existing active erosive RA progress within even 12 months.

One challenge to diagnosing bone erosions on the basis of a single time point is the projectional viewing perspective of conventional radiography. In contrast to tomographic techniques, such as computed tomography (CT) or MRI, which depict anatomy in individual slices, radiography projects a two-dimensional shadow of the 3D anatomy splayed out on a flat film or receptor.[3] This results in geometric distortion of the anatomy and superimposition of overlapping structures. Accordingly, only erosions along the projected edge of a bone, which is in tangent to the X-ray beam, are visible as contour defects (Figure 17.4). Erosions projected *en face* are obscured in a haystack of overlapping cortical and trabecular

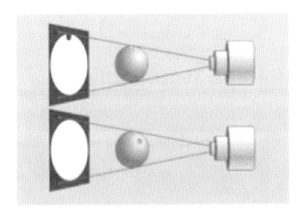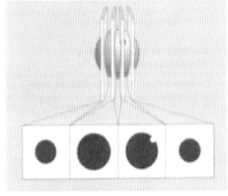

Figure 17.4 Projectional versus tomographic viewing perspective. Projectional radiography (left panel) superimposes and thus potentially obscures overlapping structures. Erosions and other contour irregularities along the edges of bones projected by tangential X-ray photons are well seen. However, erosions projected *en face*, unless extremely large, are often not visible at all. Tomographic techniques (right panel), such MRI and CT, however, depict the anatomy in individual sections, and thus can reveal projectionally occult bone erosions like holes in slices of Swiss cheese. This is one of the main reasons for MRI's superior sensitivity for bone erosions.
Reprinted from Peterfy CG. Imaging techniques. In: Klippel, J, Dieppe, P. (principal eds.). Rheumatology. 2nd Edition. Mosby-Wolfe, London 1998: 2.14.1–2.14.18 with permission from Elsevier.

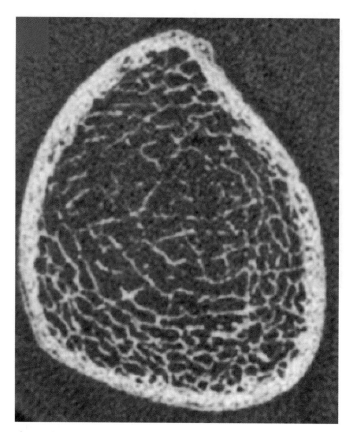

Figure 17.5 Relative distribution of cortical and trabecular bone. Axial CT through a long bone shows relative paucity of bone in the trabeculae of the medullary space compared to that in the surrounding cortex.

shadows. Rotating the anatomy relative to the X-ray beam can reveal some of these erosions by bringing them into profile, but there is a limit to the number of projections that are feasible in a radiographic examination, and there will always remain erosions that cannot be detected despite multiple views. This limitation is obviated by tomography, which can uncover such erosions, like holes in slices from a block of Swiss cheese. This is one of the reasons that MRI, CT, and to some extent ultrasonography are more sensitive for erosion than projectional radiography is.

Another limitation of radiography in detecting bone erosions has to do with the much greater concentration of bone in the cortex than in the trabeculae of the marrow space. This is illustrated in Figure 17.5. Focal lucencies on a radiograph thus reflect primarily the loss of cortical bone not trabecular bone. Most bone erosions in RA, however, are piriform in shape, with only a small opening at the cortical end, and most of the cavity within the intramedullary space (Figures 17.6 and 17. 7). Accordingly, the largest and most rapidly growing portion of the erosion (because trabecular bone is easier to erode than cortical bone is) is often radiographically occult, with the visible portion underestimating the actual size and extent of the lesion. Thus, MRI is more sensitive than radiography not only for small, early erosions, but also for most large, longstanding erosions (Figure 17.8).

Monitoring change in bone erosions is important not only diagnostically, as noted earlier, but also for evaluating disease progression and treatment response. However, because of geometric distortion and superimposition associated with projectional radiography, technical reproducibility between serially acquired radiographs is critical to accurate interpretation (Figures 17.9 and 17.10).

Projectional reproducibility is also critical for accurately monitoring joint space narrowing (JSN), as changes in patient positioning and X-ray beam angulation or centring can alter the apparent width of joint spaces. The most common manifestation of this is loss of visibility of the metatarsophalangeal (MTP) joints of the foot due to extension of the toes (Figure 17.10). Unless the cause of this is contracture or fusion (Figure 17.11), straightening the toes with tape or sandbags when radiographing the feet usually corrects the problem.

Similarly, accurate assessment of JSN longitudinally requires identical patient positioning, beam centring, and beam angulation on all serial radiographs. Figure 17.12 illustrates how changes in beam centring between examinations can affect the apparent joint space width.

Although patient positioning can vary somewhat depending on the equipment and facility set up, ideally each foot should be radiographed separately, with the foot resting flat on the cassette or receptor, with the toes straight. This can be accomplished by having the patient sit on the radiography table with the knee bent as shown in Figure 17.13. Care should be taken to keep the knee centred and not allowing it to lean to one side or the other, otherwise the foot will rotate, distorting the projectional anatomy and potentially mimicking structural change. Standardizing this positioning is thus important if serial examinations are anticipated. For other clinical indications, posteroanterior (PA) radiographs of the feet are often acquired with slight caudad angulation of the X-ray beam, as this improves visualization of the midfoot. However, for evaluating the metatarsophalangeal joints (MTP) in RA, beam angulation should be perpendicular to the cassette and centred on MTP 3.

Ideally, each hand should be imaged separately as well, with the patient seated comfortably next to the radiography table positioned at the level of the subject's shoulder. The arm should be adducted and bent 90-degrees so that the forearm lies flat on the table with the hand and wrist on the cassette palm down and the fingers and thumb together, as shown in Figure 17.14. If the table cannot be raised high enough, the subject's chair should be lowered to ensure that the forearm remains in contact with the table and wrist is not extended, as this can obscure the radiocarpal joint and even the proximal carpal row (Figure 17.15). Sandbags may be laid on the forearm to keep the arm flat against the table. The fingers and thumb should be adducted together rather than spread apart, as the former positioning is easier to reproduce, and variable abduction of the fingers can distort the joint spaces particularly of metacarpophalangeal (MCP) joints 1, 2, and 5. Serially acquired images of hands with abducted fingers also take up less monitor space, and thus are easier to view side-by-side to evaluate change. The X-ray beam is directed PA, and kept perpendicular to the cassette and centred on MCP-3.

As noted at the beginning of this discussion, however, no matter how meticulously radiographs are acquired, joint space width will always represent only an indirect and potentially inaccurate measure of cartilage thickness (Figure 17.16). This is because it assumes that the only thing separating the two articular surfaces of the joint is the articular cartilage, which of course, is not always the case. The

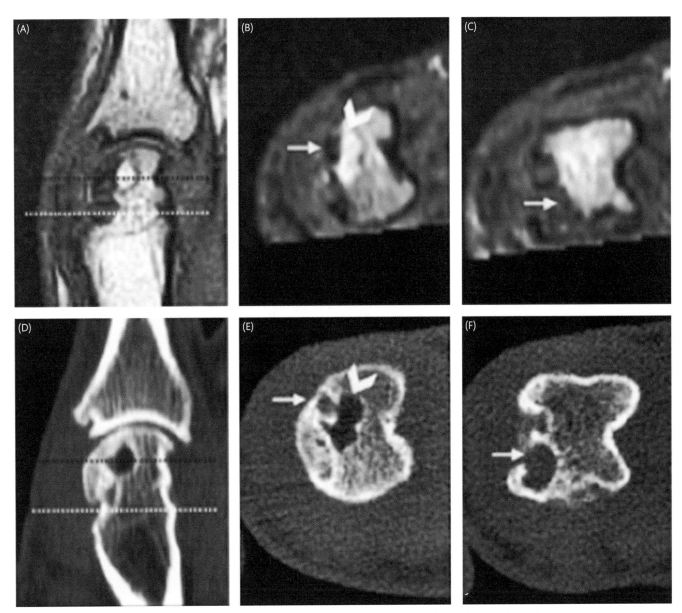

Figure 17.6 Bone erosions are mostly intramedullary. Coronal (A, D) and axial (B, C, E, F) MRI (A, B, C) and CT (D, E, F) slices through a metacarpophalangeal joint (MCP) of a patient with RA reveal not only the cortical defects (arrows) of the bone erosions depicted but the larger intramedullary components (arrowhead) of these erosions.

Reprinted from Møller Døhn U, Boonen A, Hetland ML et al. Erosive progression is minimal, but erosion healing rare, in patients with rheumatoid arthritis treated with adalimumab. A 1 year investigator-initiated follow-up study using high-resolution computed tomography as the primary outcome measure. *Ann Rheum Dis.* 2009;68(10):1585–90 with permission from the BMJ Publishing Group Ltd.

joint space also can contain joint fluid and synovial tissue, and in large joints, such as the knee, meniscal tissue. Further, if the capsular ligaments are lax or torn, or if there is significant joint effusion, even joint surfaces devoid of any articular cartilage can be widely separated.

Care should be taken to ensure that the right and left hands are accurately labelled. Image labelling can be unreliable if radiopaque markers are placed on the cassette manually. This can be problematic because if a right hand at baseline is compared to a left hand at follow-up that was erroneously labelled as right, for example, differences in the degree and distribution of abnormalities can be misinterpreted as disease progression or regression (**Figure 17.17**).

Anatomical asymmetries, when noticed, can help identify labelling errors, but these are often subtle, and many cases go unrecognized. Most clinical trials of RA have overcome this error by utilizing positioning frames with permanently embedded left-right markers designed in such a way as to make it impossible to image a hand with the wrong marker (**Figure 17.18**). Such frames are not typically used in clinical practice, however, and so the possibility of labelling errors remain.

Radiographic scoring methods

Several radiographic scoring systems have been developed for assessing RA in the hands, wrists, and feet. However, their application

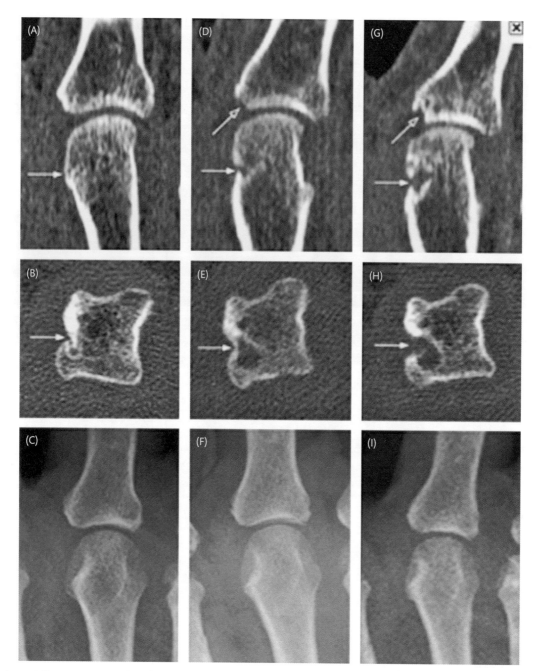

Figure 17.7 Intramedullary component of erosion progresses most rapidly. Coronal (A, D, G) and axial (B, E, H) CT and radiograph (C, F, I) of an MCP joint of a patient with RA at three successive time points from left to right. CT images show how bone erosions begin with small cortical defects (arrow), but then progress more rapidly through trabecular bone in the medullary space. The small erosion of the proximal phalanx is visible on the radiograph because it is tangential to the X-ray beam. However, the larger erosion in the metacarpal bone is not visible on the radiograph despite the large intramedullary component of this erosion.

Reprinted from Møller Døhn U, Boonen A, Hetland ML, et al. Erosive progression is minimal, but erosion healing rare, in patients with rheumatoid arthritis treated with adalimumab. A 1 year investigator-initiated follow-up study using high-resolution computed tomography as the primary outcome measure. *Ann Rheum Dis* 2009;68(10):1585–90 with permission from the BMJ Publishing Group Ltd.

has been almost exclusively in clinical research, particularly clinical trials testing putative new therapies; none are currently used in routine clinical practice. Clinical radiological reports may note the presence or absence of bone erosions, JSN, and potentially other features of RA, such as malalignment, juxta-articular osteopenia, and soft-tissue swelling, as well as which joints are affected and whether

or not there appears to have been any change on follow-up images. However, any references to severity and change are usually only subjective and not expressed in terms of any standardized scale.

Of the scoring systems that have been developed, the most widely used are versions of a composite score of aggregated ordinal scales originally described in 1971 by John Sharp.[8] In contrast to global

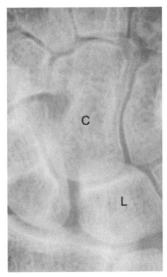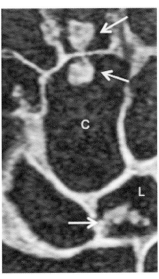

Figure 17.8 Large erosions visible on MRI can be radiographically occult. Radiograph (left panel) and MRI (right panel) of a wrist zoomed in on the capitate bone (C). The radiograph is of high quality, and shows well defined cortical and trabecular shadows, and yet, two large 'kissing' erosions (arrows) clearly visible on MRI (right panel) in the distal end of the capitate and the abutting proximal end of the third metacarpal base are completely invisible on the radiograph (left panel). Note the piriform shape of both erosions with large intramedullary components but only small cortical openings. An irregularly shaped erosion (arrow) tunnelling through the lunate bone (L) is also visible with MRI but not with radiography.
Images courtesy of Spire Sciences.

scores, such the method developed by Larsen et al.,[9] which combined the features of joint damage, the Sharp method graded bone erosion and JSN separately in multiple locations in the hands and wrists (**Figures 17.19–17.21**).

The original Sharp score evaluated most of the bones and joints (27 different locations) in the hands and wrist. In 1985 a number of joints that were infrequently involved and/or hard to read were excluded from the original scoring system, and a combination including 17 locations for erosion and 18 for JSN was proposed as optimally discriminative.[10] Genant et al.[11,12] further reduced these to 14 and 13, respectively, and added the feet. van der Heijde et al.[13] similarly reduced the number of locations to 16 and 15, respectively, and also included the feet.

These two so-called modified Sharp methods by Genant and van der Heijde differ primarily in the scales used to grade erosions, but there are also minor differences in their JSN scales and the locations scored in the hands and wrists. Both methods have been accepted by regulatory agencies as valid and have been used successfully in randomized controlled trials to gain regulatory approval of structure-modifying therapies.[14–19]

Both methods score the same locations for erosion in the hands, wrists, and feet, except that the van der Heijde–Sharp method adds the lunate bone in the wrist and separates the first carpometacarpal (CMC) joint at the base of the thumb into its two articular components (**Figures 17.22 and 17.23**).

Both methods also score erosion in the same joints of the foot (**Figure 17.24**); however, the van der Heijde–Sharp method scores the two components of each of these joints separately. This increases the maximum erosion score attainable for each joint in the foot from 5 to 10, and thus raises the ceiling of the van der Heijde–Sharp scale closer to that of the Genant–Sharp scale, but it does not add greater opportunity for detecting erosion or change in erosion, as all of these bones are also evaluated in the Genant–Sharp method. The clinical implications of erosion on one side of a joint but not the other is unknown, however since all regional scores are combined in both methods to determine total erosion scores, this does

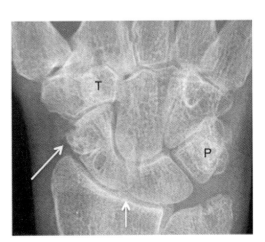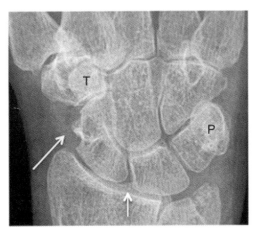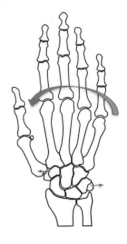

Figure 17.9 Changes in projection can mimic erosion progression. Posteroanterior (PA) radiographs of a wrist at baseline (left panel) and 24 weeks later (middle panel) show an erosion in the scaphoid bone (long arrow) that appears to enlarge over time. Close inspection shows other changes as well, including opening up of the scapholunate joint (short arrow), shift in the position of the dorsal bones, such as the trapezoid (T), radial, and/or palmar bones, such the pisiform (P), ulnarly. These projectional changes indicate relative pronation (radial rotation) of the wrist (right panel) on the follow-up radiograph. Pronation of the scaphoid bone projects towards the ulna the outer margin of the distal end of this bone that previously obscured some of the erosion on the baseline image (long arrow). This means that at least some of the apparent enlargement of the scaphoid erosion is a result of the change in projection. How much of this appearance is due to technical change rather than disease progression is difficult to say, but the example illustrates the critical importance of projectional reproducibility to accurate assessment of erosion progression. The same is true for assessing change in joint space width, as illustrated in this example by the effect of rotation on the scapholunate joint (short arrow).
Images courtesy of Spire Sciences.

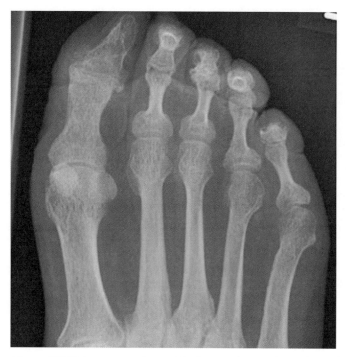
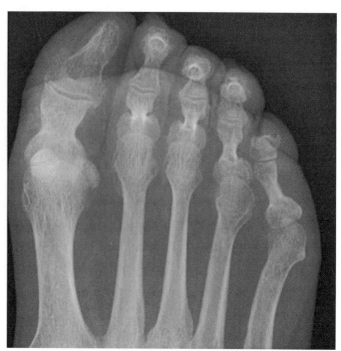

Figure 17.10 Improper patient positioning can obscure JSN. Radiographs of the forefoot with the toes properly positioned relative to the X-ray beam shows normal joint space widths of the MTP joints (left panel). When the same foot is imaged with the toes extended (right panel)—note the foreshortening of the proximal phalanges—the MTP joints are obscured and JSN cannot be assessed.
Images courtesy of Spire Sciences.

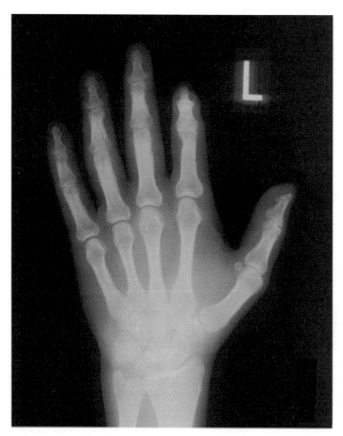
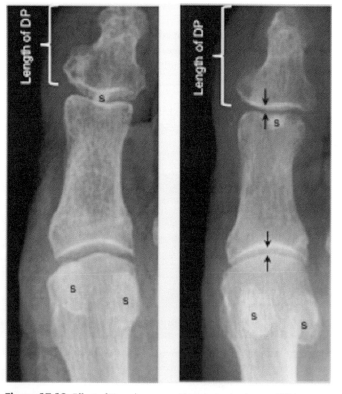

Figure 17.11 Flexion contracture can obscure JSN. The index finger on this radiograph of the hand of a patient with RA is flexed because of a contracture, and cannot be straightened. As a result, the joint spaces of PIP2 and DIP2 cannot be evaluated, and because of superimposition of the articular bones of these joints, erosions cannot be ruled out with certainty either.
Images courtesy of Spire Sciences.

Figure 17.12 Effect of X-ray beam centring on projection and JSN. Posteroanterior radiographs of a great toe at baseline (left panel) and 24 weeks later (right panel) show apparent JSN (arrows) on follow-up. However, the distal phalanx (DP) also appears longer and the sesamoid bones (s) are positioned more proximally, indicating that the projection has changed, in this case due to centring the X-ray beam more distally on the toe. Such a change in beam centring would also be expected to affect the apparent joint space width. How much of the apparent JSN is due to this change in projection rather than actual cartilage loss is difficult to say, however.
Images courtesy of Spire Sciences.

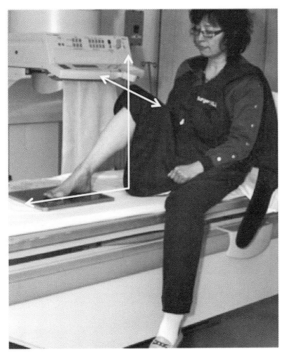
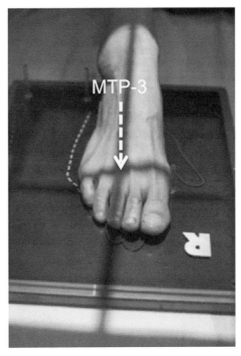

Figure 17.13 Radiography of the foot in RA. The foot should be flat with the toes straight rather than extended. Tape can be used to secure the toes if necessary. Care should be taken to ensure that the foot is not rotated between serial examinations. The X-ray beam should be perpendicular to the cassette and centred on MTP-3.

Images courtesy of Spire Sciences.

not affect discrimination of subjects or treatments on the basis of total erosion score.

The joints scored for JSN in the hands, wrists, and feet are also quite similar between the two methods (**Figures 17.23** and **17.24**).

The erosion scales differ somewhat between the methods. The Genant–Sharp method scores each location on an eight-point scale from 0 to 3.5 in increments of 0.5 (**Figure 17.25**), whereas the van

der Heijde–Sharp method uses a six-point scale with whole number values from 0 to 5 (**Figure 17.26**). Accordingly, the van der Heijde–Sharp method typically gives a larger numerical score for a given degree of erosive damage (maximum erosion score = 280) than the Genant–Sharp method does (maximum erosion score = 140), although both scales include the same number of increments (280). The JSN scale also differs for each method, but primarily with

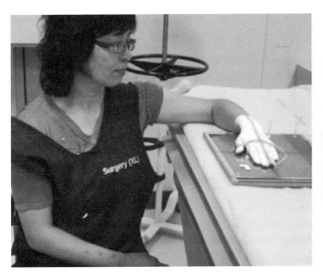
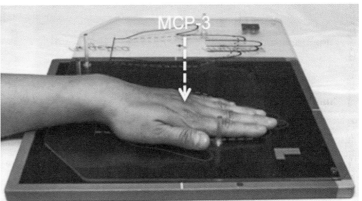

Figure 17.14 Radiography of the hand and wrist in RA. Correct positioning of the subject for hand/wrist radiography, with the arm adducted 90 degrees, the elbow bent 90 degrees, and the wrist and palm flat on the cassette. The X-ray beam is directed PA perpendicular to the cassette and centred on MCP-3. Note the use of a positioning frame with built-in Left-Right markers to avoid labelling errors.

Images courtesy of Spire Sciences.

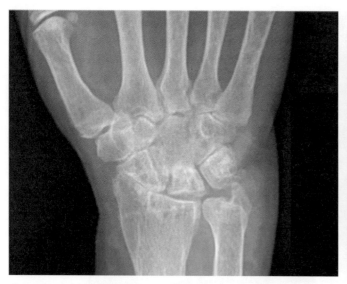
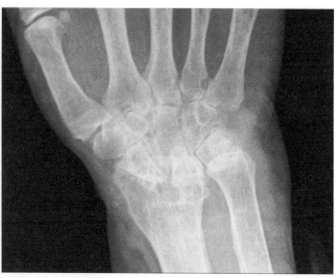

Figure 17.15 Elevation of wrist can obscure the radiocarpal joint and proximal carpal bones. Radiographs of the wrist with proper positioning (left panel) projects all the bones and joints clearly. Elevating the forearm slightly extends the wrist (right panel) and obscures the proximal carpal row, making assessment of erosions more difficult and evaluation of radiocarpal JSN impossible.
Images courtesy of Spire Sciences.

respect to the number of increments. Both range from 0 to 4, but the Genant–Sharp scale does so in nine increments of 0.5 (**Figure 17.27**), whereas the van der Heijde–Sharp scale has five whole number increments (**Figure 17.28**). As for erosion score, the van der Heijde–Sharp scale yields numerically larger values (maximum JSN score = 168) than the Genant–Sharp method does (maximum JSN score = 152), but the Genant–Sharp scale includes more increments (304 vs. 168). Finally, the Genant–Sharp total score, which

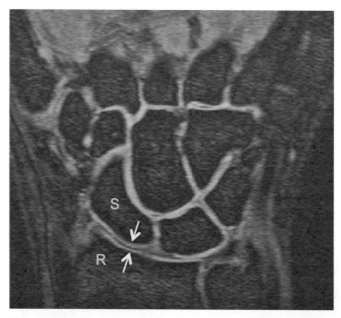
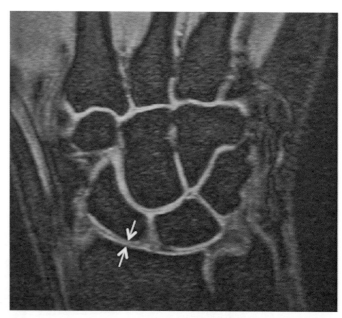

Figure 17.16 Joint space width can be an inaccurate measure of cartilage thickness. Baseline MRI of a wrist (left panel) shows the articular cortices (arrows) of the scaphoid (S) and radius (R) bones separated by high-signal hyaline cartilage lining their surfaces and low-signal joint fluid between the cartilage surfaces. The distance between the cortical surfaces (arrows) constitutes the joint space width. On follow-up MRI (right panel), this joint space width (arrows) has narrowed. However this JSN is not due to loss of articular cartilage, but rather to displacement of the intervening joint fluid. Radiographically, this would be interpreted erroneously as cartilage loss.
Reprinted from Møller Døhn U, Boonen A, Hetland ML et al. Erosive progression is minimal, but erosion healing rare, in patients with rheumatoid arthritis treated with adalimumab. A 1-year investigator-initiated follow-up study using high-resolution computed tomography as the primary outcome measure. *Ann Rheum Dis.* 2009;68(10):1585–90 with permission from the BMJ Publishing Group Ltd.

method yields larger raw values than Genant–Sharp scoring does (**Figure 17.29**), but the Genant–Sharp scale has more increments and a higher ceiling for erosions. Despite these differences, in a head-to-head comparison of the two methods[19] using a common set of radiographs of the hands, wrists, and feet of patients with RA, a common pair of readers, and scores that were normalized to the ranges of values observed with each,[20] the two methods performed similarly (**Figure 17.30**). Indeed, of all the factors affecting the accuracy of radiographic assessment of RA, the most important is reader competency not scoring method.[21] Determining whether a radiographic lucency in a bone represents a true erosion or simply a confluence of shadows mimicking an erosion, and whether an apparent change in the size of an erosion or joint space width on serial radiographs is real or due to variation in patient positioning, image projection, or film exposure requires considerable perceptual skill and experience.

Conclusion

Aside from minor study-specific modifications in some clinical trials, the Genant–Sharp and van der Heijde–Sharp scoring methods have not changed substantially over the more than two decades that the two methods have been in use. While some attempts have been made to reduce the complexity and effort needed to perform discriminative readings with such methods, most of the imaging attention in RA research over the past several years has shifted to MRI and ultrasound. These newer technologies offer broader pathophysiological information and greater sensitivity to change, and thus allow questions about drug efficacy to be answered with fewer patients, less time, and thus lower cost, than with radiography.[1,2,22,23] It is likely, therefore, that this trend towards MRI and ultrasound will increase over the next decade, and that the role of radiography, at least in clinical trials, will diminish considerably.

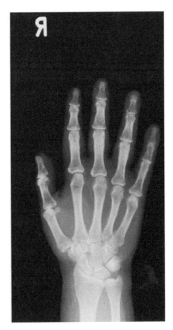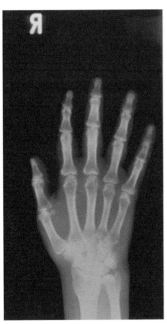

Figure 17.17 Mislabelling can result in misinterpretation of progression. Serial radiographs of a hand labelled R show greater bone erosion and JSN in the wrist of the follow-up radiograph (right panel) compared to that at baseline (left panel). However, the follow-up radiograph (right panel) is actually the left hand mislabelled as the right. In reality, there was no disease progression in this patient.
Images courtesy of Spire Sciences.

combines erosion and JSN scores, includes more increments (584) than does the van der Heijde–Sharp total score (448).

Because of the differences in the number of increments and ranges in the scales of the two methods, direct comparisons of scores generated by the Genant–Sharp and van der Heijde–Sharp methods are not meaningful. As noted earlier, the van der Heijde–Sharp

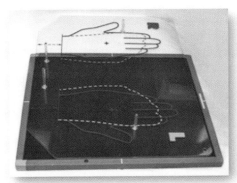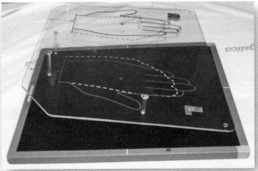

Figure 17.18 Positioning frame for ensuring accurate L–R labelling of radiographs of the hands and feet. The positioning frame has permanently fixed radiopaque R–L markers and pegs on one side preventing the frame from being used upside down. This eliminates the possibility of mislabelling.
Images courtesy of Spire Sciences.

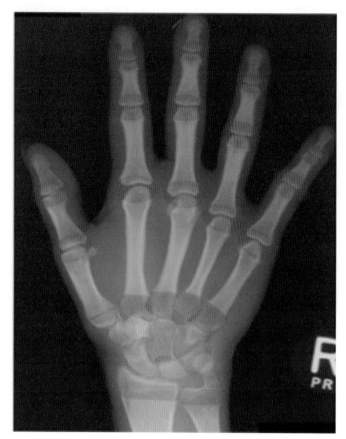 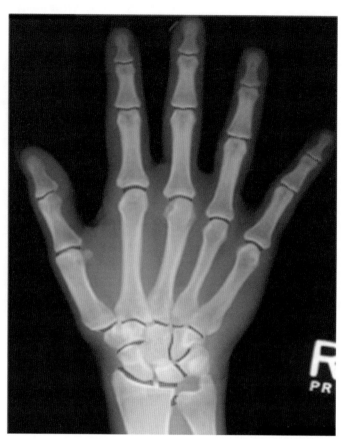

Figure 17.19 Sharp scoring locations. The original Sharp method scored 27 bones in the hand and wrist (all except the trapezoid and pisiform) for erosions (left panel), and 27 joints (all except the scaphoid-lunate, capitate-lunate, capitate-scaphoid, trapezium-trapezoid and triquetrum-pisiform) for JSN (right panel). Each location was scored using the scales outlined in Figures 17.20 and 17.21, and summed to derive a total erosion or total JSN score for that hand/wrist. Scores from bilateral hands and wrists were summed to determine the total score for the patient.
Images courtesy of Spire Sciences.

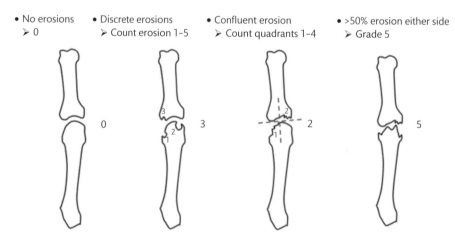

Figure 17.20 The Sharp 6-point erosion scale. Discrete erosions regardless of size are counted up to 5 per joint. If erosions are diffuse or confluent, the number of quadrants involved are counted per joint. If greater than 50% of either side of a joint is eroded, the joint is given the maximum score of 5.
Images courtesy of Spire Sciences.

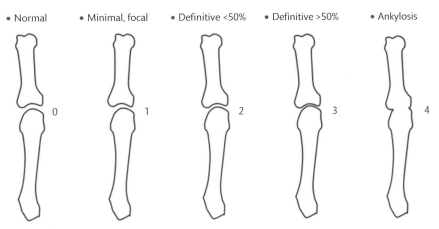

Figure 17.21 The Sharp 5-point JSN scale. Joint space width of each joint indicated in Figure 17.19B is scored from 0 to 4 as specified.
Images courtesy of Spire Sciences.

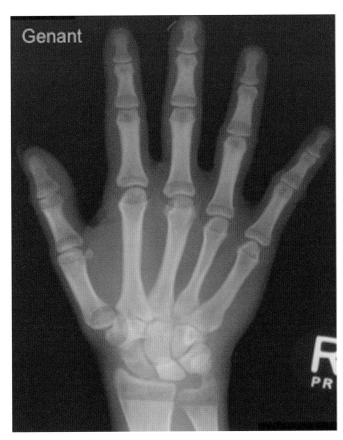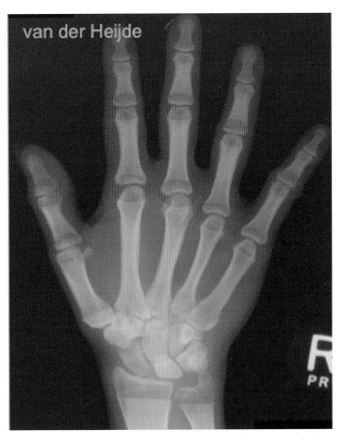

Figure 17.22 Genant–Sharp and van der Heijde–Sharp scoring locations in the hand and wrist for erosion. The locations scored for erosion with the Genant–Sharp (left panel) and van der Heijde–Sharp (right panel) methods are very similar. The van der Heijde–Sharp method includes one additional bone, the lunate (yellow), and scores the two articular bones of the CMC-1 joint separately.

Reprinted from Peterfy G, Wu C, Szechinski J et al (2011) Comparison of the Genant-modified Sharp and van der Heijde-modified Sharp scoring methods for radiographic assessment in rheumatoid arthritis *Int. J. Clin. Rheumatol.* 6(1):15–24 with permission

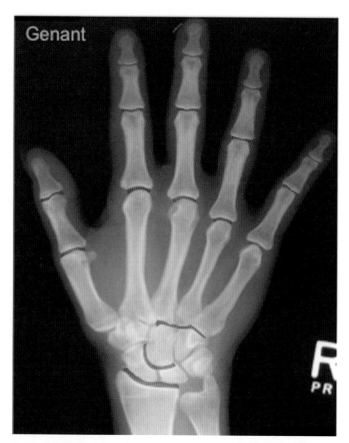 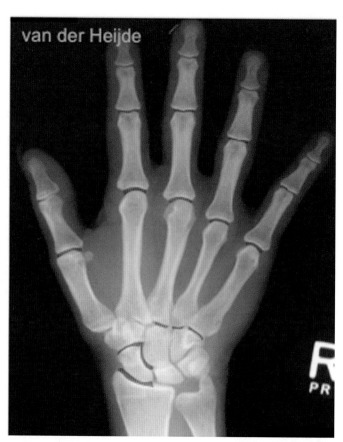

Figure 17.23 Genant–Sharp and van der Heijde–Sharp scoring locations in the hand and wrist for JSN. The locations scored for JSN with the Genant–Sharp (left panel) and van der Heijde–Sharp (right panel) methods are very similar. The van der Heijde–Sharp method adds the scaphoid-trapezium joint, excludes the first interphalangeal joint of the thumb, the capitate-lunate joint and the radius-lunate joint, and scores CMC-3, CMC-4, and CMC-5 separately rather than as a combined joint space, as is done in the Genant–Sharp method.

Reprinted from Peterfy G, Wu C, Szechinski J et al (2011) Comparison of the Genant-modified Sharp and van der Heijde-modified Sharp scoring methods for radiographic assessment in rheumatoid arthritis *Int. J. Clin. Rheumatol.* 6(1):15–24 with permission.

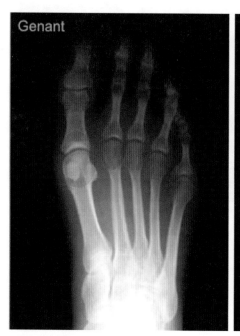 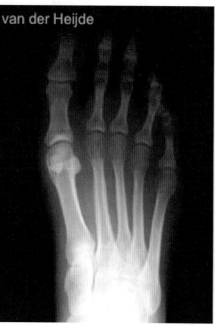 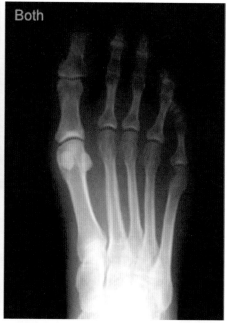

Figure 17.24 Genant–Sharp and van der Heijde–Sharp scoring locations in the forefoot. The joints scored for erosion with the Genant–Sharp (left panel) and van der Heijde–Sharp (middle panel) methods are identical, except the van der Heijde–Sharp method scores the two bones of each joint separately. The locations scored for JSN are the same for both methods (right panel).

Reprinted from Peterfy G, Wu C, Szechinski J et al (2011) Comparison of the Genant-modified Sharp and van der Heijde-modified Sharp scoring methods for radiographic assessment in rheumatoid arthritis *Int. J. Clin. Rheumatol.* 6(1):15–24 with permission.

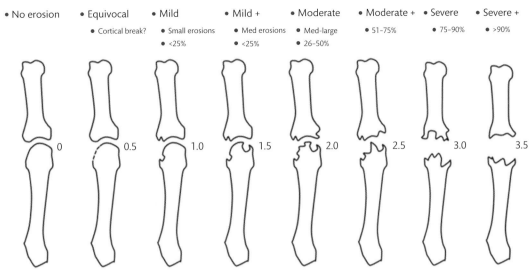

Figure 17.25 The Genant–Sharp 8-point erosion scale. The Genant–Sharp erosion scale can be regarded as three whole number grades (1 = mild, 2 = moderate, 3 = severe) based on the volume of subchondral articular bone eroded, with half grades between. Single time point evaluations usually use one of the whole number grades. The 0.5 grades are used primarily to register mild change between serially acquired images.
Courtesy of Spire Sciences.

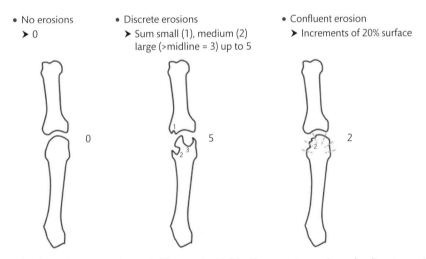

Figure 17.26 The van der Heijde–Sharp 6-point erosion scale. The van der Heijde–Sharp erosion scale grades discrete erosions as small (1), medium (2) or large (3: crossing the midline), and sums these erosions up to a maximum of 5 in each location. In the example shown there are three erosions graded 1, 2, and 3, totalling 6 yield a maximum score of 5. Superficial erosions are graded 0 to 5 in terms of the extent of the articular surface they involve in increments of 20%. In the example shown, a superficial erosion of the distal metacarpal involves 40% of the surface, giving a score of 2 for the joint.
Courtesy of Spire Sciences.

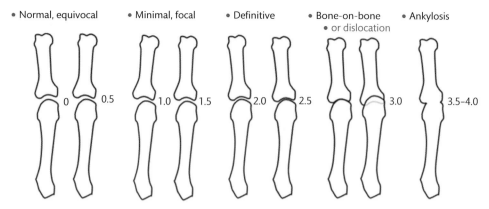

Figure 17.27 The Genant–Sharp 9-point JSN scale. The Genant–Sharp JSN scale can be regarded as four basic grades (1 = minimal/focal, 2 = definitive, 3 = severe/dislocated, 4 = fused), with half grades between each whole number grade used primarily to register mild change between serially acquired images.
Courtesy of Spire Sciences.

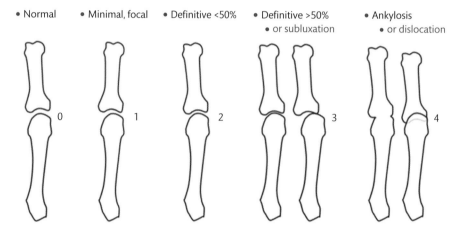

Figure 17.28 The van der Heijde–Sharp 5-point JSN scale. The van der Heijde–Sharp JSN scale is similar to the Genant–Sharp scale, but without half grades between each whole number grade.
Courtesy of Spire Sciences.

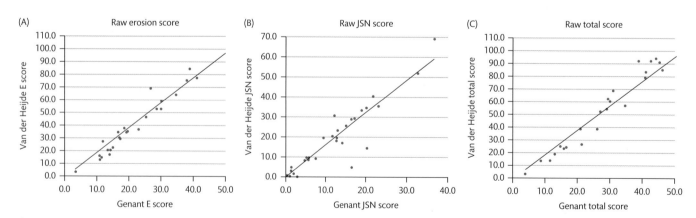

Figure 17.29 Raw van der Heijde–Sharp scores plotted against raw Genant–Sharp scores. Graphs depict erosion (A), JSN (B), and total (C) scores based on averaged values from two independent readings. Slopes of linear regression lines are 1.9, 1.6, and 1.9, respectively.
Reprinted from Peterfy G, Wu C, Szechinski J, et al (2011) Comparison of the Genant-modified Sharp and van der Heijde-modified Sharp scoring methods for radiographic assessment in rheumatoid arthritis *Int. J. Clin. Rheumatol.* 6(1):15–24 with permission.

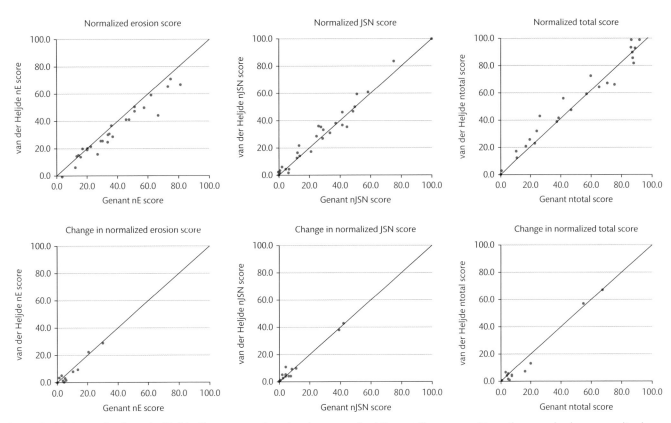

Figure 17.30 Normalized van der Heijde–Sharp scores plotted against normalized Genant–Sharp scores. Upper three graphs show normalized scores at baseline, whereas three lower graphs show scores for change from baseline at 1 year. Lines depict theoretically perfect correlation based on averaged values from the two readings. Correlation coefficients are 0.98, 0.98, 0.99, 0.95, 0.99, and 0.99, respectively. nE, normalized erosion scores; nJSN, normalized joint space narrowing scores; nTotal, normalized total scores.

Reprinted from Peterfy G, Wu C, Szechinski J et al (2011) Comparison of the Genant-modified Sharp and van der Heijde-modified Sharp scoring methods for radiographic assessment in rheumatoid arthritis *Int. J. Clin. Rheumatol.* 6(1):15–24 with permission.

REFERENCES

1. Arnett FC, Edworthy SM, Bloch DA, et al. The American Rheumatism Association 1987 revised criteria for the classification of rheumatoid arthritis. *Arthritis Rheum* 1988;*31*:315–24.
2. Aletaha D, Neogi T, Silman AJ, et al. 2010 rheumatoid arthritis classification criteria: an American College of Rheumatology/European League Against Rheumatism collaborative initiative. *Ann Rheum Dis* 2010;*69*(9):1580–8.
3. van der Heijde D, van der Helm-van Mil AH, Aletaha D, et al. EULAR definition of erosive disease in light of the 2010 ACR/EULAR rheumatoid arthritis classification criteria. *Ann Rheum Dis* 2013;*72*(4):479–81.
4. Watt I. Basic differential diagnosis of arthritis. *Eur Radiol* 1997;*7*:344–51.
5. Colebatch AN, Edwards CJ, Østergaard M, et al. EULAR recommendations for the use of imaging of the joints in the clinical management of rheumatoid arthritis. *Ann Rheum Dis* 2013;*72*(6):804–14.
6. Ranganath VK, Strand V, Peterfy CG, et al. The utility of magnetic resonance imaging for assessing structural damage in randomized controlled trials in rheumatoid arthritis: report from the imaging group of the American College of Rheumatology RA clinical trials task force. *Arthritis Rheum* 2013;*65*(10):2513–22.
7. Peterfy C, Strand V, Tian L, Østergaard M, et al. Short-term changes on MRI predict long-term changes on radiography in rheumatoid arthritis: an analysis by an OMERACT Task Force of pooled data from four randomised controlled trials. *Ann Rheum Dis* 2017;*76*(6):992–7.
8. Sharp JT, Lidsky MD, Collins LC, Moreland J. Methods of scoring the progression of radiologic changes in rheumatoid arthritis: correlation of radiologic, clinical and laboratory abnormalities. *Arthritis Rheum* 1971; *14*:706–20.
9. Larsen A, Dale K, Eek M. Radiographic evaluation of rheumatoid arthritis and related conditions by standard reference films. *Acta Radiol Diagn (Stockh)* 1977;*18*(4):481–91.
10. Sharp JT, Young DY, Bluhm GB, et al. How many joints in the hands and wrists should be included in a score of radiologic abnormalities used to assess rheumatoid arthritis? *Arthritis Rheum* 1985;*28*:1326–35.
11. Genant HK. Methods of assessing radiographic change in rheumatoid arthritis. *Am J Med* 1983;*75*(6A):35–47.
12. Genant HK, Jiang Y, Peterfy C, Lu Y, Redei J, Countryman PJ. Assessment of rheumatoid arthritis using a modified scoring method on digitized and original radiographs. *Arthritis Rheum* 1998;*41*:1583–90.
13. van der Heijde D. How to read radiographs according to the Sharp/van der Heijde method. *J Rheumatol* 2000;*27*:261–3.
14. Genant HK, Peterfy CG, Westhovens R, et al. Abatacept inhibits progression of structural damage in rheumatoid arthritis: results from the long-term extension of the AIM trial. *Ann Rheum Dis* 2008;*67*(8):1084–9.

15. Breedveld FC, Weisman MH, Kavanaugh AF, et al. The PREMIER study: a multicenter, randomized, double-blind clinical trial of combination therapy with adalimumab plus methotrexate versus methotrexate alone or adalimumab alone in patients with early, aggressive rheumatoid arthritis who had not had previous methotrexate treatment. *Arthritis Rheum* 2006;*54*(1):26–37.

16. van der Heijde D, Klareskog L, Rodriguez-Valverde V, et al. Comparison of etanercept and methotrexate, alone and combined, in the treatment of rheumatoid arthritis: two-year clinical and radiographic results from the TEMPO study, a double-blind, randomized trial. *Arthritis Rheum* 2006;*54*(4):1063–74.

17. Smolen JS, Han C, Bala C, et al. Evidence of radiographic benefit of treatment with infliximab plus methotrexate in rheumatoid arthritis patients who had no clinical improvement: a detailed subanalysis of data from the anti–tumor necrosis factor trial in rheumatoid arthritis with concomitant therapy study. *Arthritis Rheum* 2005; *52*(4):1020–30.

18. Kremer J, Genant H, Moreland L, et al. Effects of abatacept in patients with methotrexate-resistant active rheumatoid arthritis: a randomized trial. *Ann Intern Med* 2006;*144*(12):933–5.

19. Keystone E, Emery P, Peterfy CG, et al. Rituximab inhibits structural joint damage in patients with rheumatoid arthritis with an inadequate response to tumour necrosis factor inhibitor therapies. *Ann Rheum Dis* 2009;*68*(2):216–21.

20. Sharp J, Wolfe F, Lassere M, et al. Variability of precision in scoring radiographic abnormalities in rheumatoid arthritis by experienced readers. *J Rheumatol* 2004;*31*(6):1062–72.

21. Strand V, Sharp J. Radiographic data from recent randomized controlled trials in rheumatoid arthritis: what have we learned? *Arthritis Rheum* 2003;*48*(1):21–34.

22. Peterfy C, Østergaard M, Conaghan PG. MRI comes of age in RA clinical trials. *Ann Rheum Dis* 2013;*72*(6):794–6.

23. Peterfy G, Wu C, Szechinski J, et al. Comparison of the Genant-modified Sharp and van der Heijde-modified Sharp scoring methods for radiographic assessment in rheumatoid arthritis *Int J Clin Rheumatol* 2011;*6*(1):15–24.

18

Ultrasound in rheumatoid arthritis

Andrew Filer, Maria Antonietta D'Agostino, and Ilfita Sahbudin

Introduction

Ultrasound imaging is becoming increasingly popular among rheumatologists over recent years and this is further encouraged by the falling cost of ultrasound units. Ultrasound is an attractive point-of-care tool as it provides real-time image visualization to both the operator and patient, which may enhance the clinical care experience. Furthermore, it is safe, does not involve ionizing radiation, and can be easily repeated in subsequent visits. In addition, ultrasound can examine multiple regions in the same setting, unlike magnetic resonance imaging (MRI). Firstly, we summarize the principles which underpin the physics of ultrasound. Subsequently, we describe the musculoskeletal pathologies which are amenable to ultrasound examination. Lastly, we summarize the role of ultrasound according to disease area but especially in rheumatoid arthritis (RA).

Physics of ultrasound

Ultrasound systems generate images based on the use of high frequency sound waves which typically range from 1 to 20 MHz (i.e. 1–20 million vibrations per second). These sound waves are produced by the mechanical oscillations of crystals within the ultrasound transducer as a result of electrical pulses, a phenomenon known as the **piezoelectric effect**. Sound waves reflected back from the tissues in turn vibrate the same crystals, generating an electrical impulse that is recorded by the system; the probe therefore acts as both emitter and receiver. The ultrasound image generated by the system is the result of processing of emitted and received waveforms that have been modified by passing through and reflection within biological tissues.[1]

Ultrasound waves generated within the transducer propagate across the tissues, and some of these are lost through **scattering** to the surrounding tissues, while some are lost as heat energy (a process known as **attenuation**). Some ultrasound waves are deflected back as **echoes** towards the transducer. The differential in density between two adjacent tissues dictates the magnitude of intensity of the returned echo, which is then processed by the scanning machine to generate a two-dimensional ultrasound image of the region of interest. Low density tissue such as fluid effusion which is

described as **anechoic** is observed as a dark area on an ultrasound image. Ultrasound waves cannot penetrate the cortical bone surface and most ultrasound waves are reflected back as echoes towards the transducer appearing as *hyperechoic* (i.e. bright white on an ultrasound image). Low density structures such as synovial hypertrophy may appear as **hypoechoic structures (dark-grey echogenicity)**.[1] Anatomical structures with mixed density such as muscle and subcutaneous tissues appear as *isoechoic or mixed* **echogenicity** (similar to liver or thyroid parenchyma).

Given that ultrasound waves do not pass through structures such as bone, only tissues accessible by the **acoustic window** can be visualized by ultrasound scanning. **Acoustic shadowing** occurs when ultrasound waves are obstructed by a relatively high-density structure such as bone or calcification, resulting in an interruption of the ultrasound beam pathway. Structures deprived of ultrasound waves appear as a dark shadow on the corresponding ultrasound image.[1]

Higher frequency ultrasound waves have relatively short wavelengths which are easily attenuated and do not propagate into deep tissue. Therefore, high frequency transducers are suited to scan relatively superficial structures such as the small joints of the hand. Conversely, lower frequency transducers generate relatively long ultrasound wavelengths which propagate into the deeper tissues. Hence, low frequency transducers are used to visualize deeper structures such as the hip joint. The choice of transducer is critical in generating high-quality ultrasound images and largely depends on the type of joint and patient's body habitus. Table 18.1 gives a general guide on the range of ultrasound transducer in relation to the type of joint.[1]

Pathology identified by ultrasound examination

Ultrasound examination provides information about the articular bony surfaces, articular hyaline cartilage, bursae, joint recesses, tendons ligaments, and entheses. It is therefore important for the sonographer to be familiar with the appearance of normal and abnormal tissues with the ultrasound scanner and probe used.

Synovial hypertrophy appears as non-displaceable or poorly compressible hypoechoic intra-articular tissue (relative to the subcutaneous fat and interstitial tissues) but can also appear as isoechoic under some circumstances[2,3] (Figure 18.1). *Synovial* **effusion** appears as abnormal anechoic intra-articular finding that is easily displaceable by the ultrasound transducer[4] (Figure 18.2).

Table 18.1 Range of ultrasound transducer by joint

3–7 MHz	7–12 MHz	7–15 MHz	10–20 MHz
Hip	Knee	Elbow	MCP
	Shoulder	Ankle	MTP
	Hip	Knee	PIP
			DIP
			Wrist
			Ankle

Tenosynovial hypertrophy appears as abnormal hypoechoic (relative to tendon fibres) tissue within the tenosynovial sheath that is not displaceable and poorly compressible (Figure 18.3). **Tenosynovial effusion** appears as abnormal anechoic or hypoechoic (relative to tendon fibres) displaceable areas within the synovial sheath, either localized (e.g. in the synovial sheath cul-de-sacs) or surrounding the tendon (Figure 18.4).[5] **Enthesitis** appears as abnormal hypoechoic and/or thickened tendons or ligaments with loss of normal fibrillary architecture at the site of bony attachment, seen in two perpendicular planes. This may be associated with increased Doppler signal, hyperechoic foci consistent with calcification and/or bony changes, including enthesophytes, erosions, or irregularity of the bony surface.[4] **Erosion** is a cortical break or defect which may be associated with an irregular floor, seen in two perpendicular planes (Figure 18.5). **Osteophytes** are seen as step-up bony prominences at the end of the normal bone contour, or at the margin of the joint seen in two perpendicular planes, with or without acoustic shadow[6] (Figure 18.6).

While grey-scale ultrasound provides information on based on tissue acoustic impedance which is dependent on tissue density, Doppler provides information on the extent of blood flow (hyperaemia) within the region of interest (Figure 18.7). The degree of hyperaemia, shown as areas of Doppler enhancement within the synovial tissue of a joint, is closely correlated to active inflammation.[7–9]

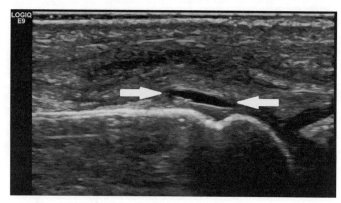

Figure 18.2 Ultrasound image shows synovial effusion with an MCP joint in longitudinal view.

Similarly, active tenosynovial inflammation (or active tenosynovitis) is indicated by the presence of peritendinous Doppler signal within the synovial sheath, excluding normal feeding vessels (i.e. vessels at the mesotenon or vinculae or vessels entering the synovial sheath from surrounding tissues) only if the tendon shows peritendinous synovial sheath tissue hypertrophy on grey scale (Figure 18.8).

Ultrasound examination cannot always distinguish between the underlying causes of imaging the pathologies just defined. For instance, synovitis caused by RA cannot be distinguished from synovitis caused by osteoarthritis using current technology. However differing patterns of involvement and pathognomic associated imaging features, for instance osteophytes in osteoarthritis (OA) or tophus in gout, can guide the diagnostic process. In addition, each of the ultrasound lesions should be observed in two perpendicular planes. As with other imaging modalities, ultrasound examination should be utilized as a part of an overall assessment; the interpretation should take into account the global picture including clinical, laboratory, and other imaging assessments.

Use of ultrasound in rheumatoid arthritis

RA is a systemic disease characterized by symmetrical polyarthritis and a tendency to erode bone and cartilage, resulting in persistent pain and significant disability. It most commonly affects peripheral joints with a predilection for small joints of the hand and foot, but the medium and large joints can also be affected. RA-associated pathologies identified by ultrasound include synovitis, tenosynovitis, effusion, bursitis, and bone erosions.

The main utility of ultrasound is based upon the overarching principle that ultrasound imaging improves the sensitivity and specificity of detecting joint and tendon inflammation compared to clinical examination. The mean detection rate of synovitis in the small joints of hand and foot using ultrasound is 2.18-fold greater than clinical examination (range: 0.55–8.96).[10]

The role of ultrasound in improving diagnostic certainty in RA and prediction of arthritis development

Ultrasound assessment may influence clinicians' clinical decisions with respect to diagnosis and planning therapy. Among newly referred patients for inflammatory arthritis, ultrasound examination

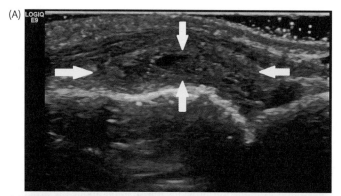

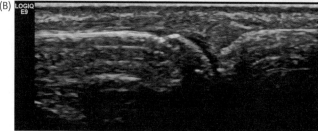

Figure 18.1 Ultrasound image of synovial hypertrophy (A) and normal appearance (B) of an MCP joint in longitudinal view.

(A)
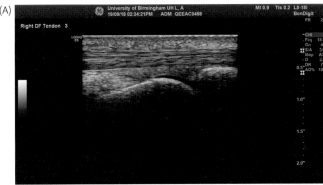

(B)
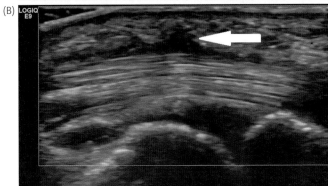

Figure 18.3 Ultrasound image shows (A) normal tendon and (B) tenosynovial hypertrophy surrounding a finger flexor tendon in an RA patient on longitudinal view.

(A)
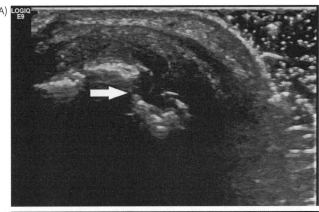

(B)
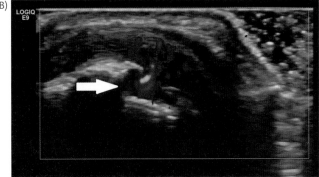

Figure 18.5 Ultrasound image shows (A) an erosion in an MCP joint of an RA patient on longitudinal view, and (B) the corresponding power Doppler (PD) image which shows PD activity within the erosion.

of small joints of the hand confirmed or changed the diagnosis in 76.3% of cases. Ultrasound assessment also influenced treatment decisions in 27% of follow-up patients.[11] Matsos and colleagues have also shown that physician certainty of specific clinical findings improved significantly following ultrasound assessment [(synovitis; (9.7% vs. 38.7%), tenosynovitis (9.7% vs. 46.8%), erosions (1.6% vs. 58.1%), and enthesitis (50.0 vs. 83.9%)]. In addition, ultrasound also influenced physicians' treatment decisions; in one study 89% of patients were planned to initiate disease-modifying antirheumatic drugs (DMARDs), but this figure fell to 48% following ultrasound assessment.[12]

Multiple studies have demonstrated the value of power Doppler in prediction of inflammatory arthritis development. In patients with

inflammatory hand symptoms for less than 12 weeks and negative autoantibodies, the presence of power Doppler increased the certainty of developing inflammatory arthritis at 12-month follow-up.[13] Similarly, Rakieh et al. reported that in a cohort of patients with new onset inflammatory symptoms and no clinical joint swelling, the presence of power Doppler (PD) enhancement on ultrasound is a risk factor to progression to inflammatory arthritis.[14]

In patients with unclassified inflammatory arthritis, the presence of PD enhancement increased the likelihood of progression to RA (odds ratio (OR) of 9.9 with one positive joint, and 48.7 if three or more positive joints. This is in the context of an OR for high titre of anticitrullinated protein antibody (ACPA) or rheumatoid factor (RF) was 10.9 in this cohort.[15] Ultrasound-detected synovitis improves the prediction of RA progression above and beyond clinical

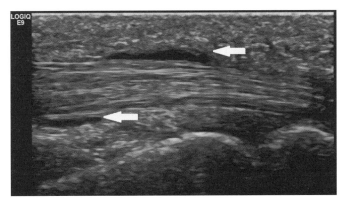

Figure 18.4 Ultrasound image illustrates tenosynovial effusion surrounding a finger flexor in an RA patient on longitudinal view.

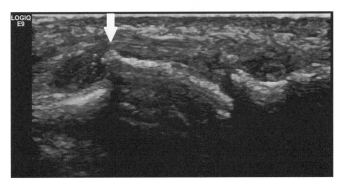

Figure 18.6 Ultrasound image shows an osteophyte at the bony margin of an MTP joint on longitudinal view.

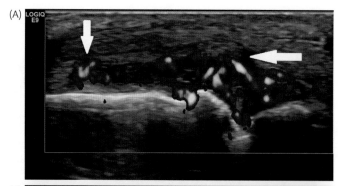

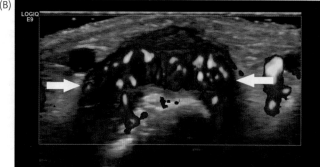

Figure 18.7 Ultrasound image shows power Doppler enhancement within the synovial hypertrophy area of an MCP joint in a patient with RA (A: longitudinal view; B: transverse view).

predictors of RA development. Filer et al. reported that the sum of Doppler grades of metacarpophalangeal (MCP) 2–3, wrists and metatarsophalangeal (MTP) 2–3 significantly improved the prediction of RA development even after taking into account clinical variables such as presence of RF and/or ACPA, inflammatory markers, and clinical joint counts. The inclusion criteria for this study were patients with at least one clinically swollen joint and symptom duration of less than 12 weeks.[16]

Although the role of ultrasound-detected joint inflammation is well-described, the value of ultrasound-detected tendon inflammation in predicting disease development is under-reported. Sahbudin and colleagues reported that ultrasound-detected digit flexor tenosynovitis predicts the development of RA even after taking into account the presence of autoantibodies and MCP joint synovitis,[17] in patients with symptom duration of less than 12 weeks and at least

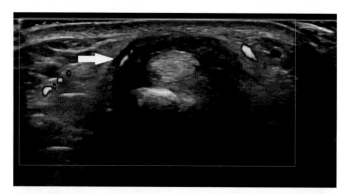

Figure 18.8 Ultrasound image shows power Doppler enhancement within the tenosynovial hypertrophy within the extensor carpi ulnaris in a patient with RA (A: longitudinal view; B: transverse view).

one clinically swollen joint. In a different study, baseline ultrasound-detected extensor carpi ulnaris tenosynovitis was a predictor of erosive progression after 1 year (OR 7.18) and 3 years (OR 3.4)] in patients with early RA.[18]

The role of ultrasound in the diagnosis of non-RA arthritides

Ultrasound features may discriminate RA from other inflammatory arthritis. Tinazzi et al. has reported that finger flexor tendon enthesopathy with enthesophyte was significantly more common in psoriatic arthritis (PsA) compared to RA and healthy subjects (p = 0.001).[19] In addition, Zabotti et al. reported that the presence of at least one extrasynovial change on hand ultrasound was significantly associated with early PsA, rather than early RA. The combination of hand ultrasound features and dotted vessels observed on nail-fold dermatoscopy increased specificity for PsA to 90.5%.[20] Ultrasound is also useful in the assessment in patients with established spondyloarthritis (SpA), particularly when discriminating from other diagnostic categories. Several studies have shown that ultrasound can differentiate SpA from RA.[21-26] In addition, ultrasound assessment is useful to discriminate PsA from non-inflammatory musculoskeletal disease such as fibromyalgia.[27-29] PD enhancement within plantar fascia enthesopathy and Achilles tendon inflammation were specific for PsA, and not for fibromyalgia patients. Importantly inflammatory changes in three or more sites had a high discriminating power between PsA and fibromyalgia.[27]

In calcium pyrophosphate disease (CPPD)-related arthritis, ultrasound can visualize hyperechogenic crystal deposition within the cartilage layer, while in gout-related arthritis crystal deposition is seen on the surface of the cartilage.[30] In osteoarthritic joints, ultrasound imaging can visualize abnormalities of articular cartilage during early disease phases, when irregularities and blurring of the cartilage margins are seen. As the disease progresses, there is loss of cartilage homogeneity and transparency. In long-standing disease, focal cartilage thinning develops which may progress to diffuse thinning and complete destruction of cartilage leading to bony denudation. Joint effusion is common in osteoarthritis and when this is present overlying the upper surface of the cartilage it may create a false impression of a normal cartilage (pseudothickening).[31] Overlying fluid must be carefully displaced to correct this artefact.

The role of ultrasound in monitoring disease activity in RA

Given that ultrasound is more sensitive than clinical examination, this imaging tool has a potential role in monitoring disease activity alongside clinical assessment. One key methodological issue to be resolved is the identification of an ultrasound scoring system that is reliable to detect meaningful changes following therapy, but also feasible to be applied in daily clinical practice.

The Outcome Measures in Rheumatology Ultrasound (OMERACT—US) Task Force, in collaboration with the European League Against Rheumatism (EULAR), has developed a composite scoring system (the EULAR-OMERACT composite power Doppler ultrasonography (PDUS) score) for joint synovitis. This scoring system, which combines grey-scale synovial hyperplasia and intrasynovial PD scores, has been shown to have good internal

---

Box 18.1 The EULAR-OMERACT synovitis scoring systems at the joint and patient levels

Joint level (for individual joints)

(A) Single components

Grey-scale inflammatory (hypoechoic) synovial hyperplasia

- Grade 0: no hypoechoic synovial hyperplasia.
- Grade 1: minimal hypoechoic synovial hyperplasia (filling the angle between the periarticular bones, without bulging over the line linking tops of the bones).
- Grade 2: hypoechoic synovial hyperplasia bulging over the line linking tops of the periarticular bones but without extension along the bone diaphysis.
- Grade 3: hypoechoic synovial hyperplasia bulging over the line linking tops of the periarticular bones and with extension to at least one of the bone diaphysis.

PD signal

- Grade 0: no flow in the hypoechoic synovial hyperplasia.
- Grade 1: up to three single spots signals or up to two confluent spots or one confluent spot plus up to two single spots.
- Grade 2: vessel signals in less than half of the area of the synovium (≤50%).
- Grade 3: vessel signals in more than half of the area of the synovium (>50%).

(B) Composite score

EULAR-OMERACT composite PDUS synovitis score

- Grade 0 (normal joint): no grey-scale-detected synovial hyperplasia and no PD signal.
- Grade 1 (minimal synovitis): grade 1 synovial hyperplasia and ≤ grade 1 PD signal.
- Grade 2 (moderate synovitis): grade 2 synovial hyperplasia and ≤ grade 2 PD signal; or grade 1 synovial hyperplasia and a grade 2 PD signal.
- Grade 3 (severe synovitis): grade 3 synovial hyperplasia and ≤ grade 3 PD signal; or grade 1 or 2 synovial hyperplasia and a grade 3 PD signal.

Patient level

Global EULAR-OMERACT synovitis score (GLOESS)

Sum of composite power Doppler ultrasound scores for all joints assessed (e.g. for MCPs 2–5, global PDUS score would range from 0 to 24).

Reproduced from D'Agostino M-A, Wakefield R., Berner-Hammer H et. al. (2016) Value of ultrasonography as a marker of early response to abatacept in patients with rheumatoid arthritis and an inadequate response to methotrexate: results from the APPRAISE study *Annals of the Rheumatic Diseases* 75:1763–9 with permission from the BMJ Publishing Group Ltd.

---

validity as well as consistent intra- and interobserver reliability. This scoring system can be applied to all peripheral joints and is consistent between machines.[32–35] Box 18.1 shows the definition of the elementary lesion of grey-scale synovial hypertrophy and PD signal, together with the composite scoring system at the joint and patient levels.

This EULAR-OMERACT composite PDUS synovitis score showed responsiveness to changes in disease activity levels in MTX-naïve patients receiving abatacept therapy as reported in the APPRAISE study.[35] In the same study, the Global EULAR-OMERACT – Synovitis Score (GLOESS) of bilateral metacarpophalangeal joints 2–5 demonstrated the rapid onset of action of abatacept as early as week 1.[35] These data indicate that ultrasound is an objective tool to monitor disease activity in patients with RA undergoing biologic treatment.

Tenosynovitis scoring has also been validated for use in clinical trials. In a multicentre trial of RA patients with ultrasound-verified tenosynovitis, the semi-quantitative tenosynovitis OMERACT scoring system showed high responsiveness to changes in disease activity levels in patients who were scheduled for treatment intensification.[36]

The role of ultrasound in treat-to-target approaches in RA

Given that ultrasound is more sensitive than clinical examination and shows potential as a disease monitoring tool. Two groups have addressed the question of whether ultrasound assessment improves outcomes in a **treat-to-target** (T2T) strategy in patients with RA. Two clinical trials have been undertaken to study the role of ultrasound within this context: TASER (Targeting Synovitis in Early Rheumatoid Arthritis)[37] and ARCTIC 'Aiming for Remission in rheumatoid arthritis: a randomized trial examining the benefit of ultrasound in a Clinical TIght Control regimen'.[38]

The TASER study tested the hypothesis that incorporating ultrasound disease activity into a T2T strategy would show superior clinical and imaging outcomes compared with a composite disease activity score strategy. RA or unclassified arthritis patients (cyclic citrullinated peptide (CCP) positive and at least three clinically swollen joints) with symptom duration less than 12 months and active disease (DAS44 >2.4) were recruited and randomized 1:1 into either a control group, in which DMARD escalation was based on DAS-28 ESR score, or intervention group, in which DMARD escalation was based on a combination of DAS28 and ultrasound findings.[37]

The ARCTIC study tested the hypothesis that a treatment strategy based on structured ultrasound assessment would improve RA outcomes, compared to a conventional strategy. The inclusion criteria for this study were patients fulfilling the RA 2010 criteria with reported disease duration of less than 2 years and require disease-modifying antirheumatic drugs. Patients were randomized 1:1 into either the ultrasound tight control or the conventional tight control group. In the ultrasound arm, therapy escalation was based on ultrasound scores while in the conventional group, therapy changes were based on the disease activity scores (DAS). The primary endpoint was the proportion of patients reaching sustained remission (DAS<1.6) at 16, 20, and 24 months, no swollen joints at 16, 20, and 24 months, and no radiographic progression between 16 and 24 months.[38]

In both studies, the ultrasound group did not show superior clinical outcomes compared to the conventional group. These results should be interpreted cautiously in the context of methodological challenges when designing clinical trials that assess the applicability of imaging technology for patients undergoing immunosuppressant therapy.[39] Firstly, the threshold of ultrasound findings that is considered to be clinically meaningful in guiding treatment escalation is currently unknown. The two studies used different ultrasound score thresholds to trigger increased therapy. Secondly, the absence of improved outcomes in the ultrasound group may be related to the 'floor' effect of current therapies in this patient population. In other words, the lack of superior outcome in the ultrasound group could be due to the limitations of therapies despite accurate levels of inflammation demonstrated by the ultrasound assessments. In addition, the absence of blinding and an open-label approach were additional limitations of these trials.[39] Although some of the methodological flaws of these studies limit the generalisability of the results, the reported outcomes from these two trials highlighted interesting points, particularly for ultrasound investigators: How many and which joint (or tendon) subtypes should be included in the assessment of disease activity level in RA patients undergoing methotrexate therapy? What is the threshold of ultrasound findings that should be considered clinically meaningful when guiding escalation therapy?[39]

The role of ultrasound in assessment of remission in RA

There is reported disparity between clinical remission and ongoing ultrasound-detected joint inflammation in RA patients. The presence of synovial hypertrophy and PD enhancement in patients with clinical remission is associated with structural progression at one year, even in asymptomatic joints.[40] In addition, the presence of ultrasound abnormalities in patients with clinical remission predicts future flare. Only 20% of patients with no PD activity at baseline had a flare compared to 42% of patients who had PD activity (p = 0.007) in a study of 94 RA patients in stable clinical remission for at least six months on either synthetic or synthetic plus biological DMARDs.[41]

Ultrasound-detected tenosynovitis is also a frequently observed in RA patients who are in clinical remission.[42] The prevalence of tenosynovitis in patients who are in clinical remission was 52.5% in a cohort of 427 RA patients recruited from 25 rheumatology centres. Interestingly, PD tenosynovitis but not PD synovitis, was associated with shorter duration of remission[42] in this RA cohort. These data highlight that subclinical joint and tendon inflammation seen on ultrasound in patients in clinical remission should be considered clinically relevant and taken into account when planning de-escalation of therapy.

The role of ultrasound in the prediction of treatment response in RA

Identifying predictors of therapy response is important, particularly when exposing patients to costly treatment which has potentially serious side effects. Given that ultrasound can assess inflammation levels accurately, Ellegaard and colleagues assessed the role of ultrasound as a predictor of treatment response. In this prospective cohort study, the presence of PD enhancement on ultrasound was the only baseline parameter to predict patients who remained on anti-TNF-α after 1 year of treatment (p = 0.024); clinical variables such as tender and swollen joint counts, CRP, DAS 28, and Health Assessment Questionnaire (HAQ) at baseline showed no significant association.[43] In this study, the fact that the patients remained on the therapy for a specified time period indicated that there was clinical effectiveness and that the drug was well-tolerated. Hence, ongoing therapy is regarded as a surrogate marker for overall effectiveness. Although US PD has been shown to predict biologic response, there is as yet no reported study that assesses US as a predictor of outcome of methotrexate therapy in inflammatory arthritis.

The role of ultrasound in the assessment and prediction of structural damage in RA

Bone erosion is a localized destructive process associated with synovitis and biomechanical factors,[44] and is also one of the components of current classification criteria for RA[45]; the presence of erosion predicts functional outcomes and further structural damage. In addition, bone erosion detected by radiograph is associated

with the development of persistent arthritis. Radiography is the classical imaging modality used to detect bone erosion. This has several advantages including accessibility, repeatability, and rapid assessment of multiple sites. However, the main limitation is false negative findings, particularly in the early phases of the disease, as radiographic erosion is only detectable after a significant amount of bone loss.[44]

Compared with computed tomography (CT) as the reference imaging modality, MRI and ultrasound have relatively high specificities (96% and 91%, respectively) in the detection of erosion within MCP 2–5 joints of RA patients.[46] However, the sensitivities for MRI and ultrasound were 68% and 42%, respectively. In the same study, the specificity of X-ray in the detection of RA bone erosions was 100%, but the sensitivity was very low (19%).

Although MRI shows higher sensitivity and accuracy compared to ultrasound, the latter is more accessible and better tolerated by patients. Micro-CT is a relatively new imaging modality that can detect bone erosions with the added advantage of higher spatial resolution and relatively minimal radiation dose (similar to exposure to X-ray of the hands). Finzel et al. reported that there was a good correlation between US and micro-CT in the detection of bone erosions (r = 0.463, p <0.0001).[47] The prevalence of ultrasound positive and micro-CT negative bone erosion was 28.6%, and these were mainly vascular bone channels of the palmar aspect of the MCP joints and also pseudo-erosions related to osteophytes.[47]

Although ultrasound can visualize a break in the bony cortical surface, it does not provide any information regarding the underlying bone structure or pathology (e.g. the presence of osteitis). MRI has the advantage of enabling the visualization of any abnormalities underneath the bony cortical layer.

Ultrasound-detected synovitis is a predictor of erosive progression. Dohn and colleagues reported that baseline power Doppler positive synovitis predicted CT measured erosive progression in a cohort of patients treated with adalimumab and methotrexate combination (baseline US PD activity RR 7.6, 95% CI 0.91–63.2, p = 0.061).[48] In a different study, baseline US-detected grey-scale synovitis was shown to predict MRI erosive progression at 1 year follow-up in a cohort of patients with early RA.[49] In addition, baseline US-detected extensor carpi ulnaris tenosynovitis is a predictor of erosive progression after 1 year (OR 7.18) and 3 years (OR 3.4) in patients with early RA.[18]

Ultrasound is also a sensitive modality for the detection of tendon damage. For instance, ultrasound was more sensitive than MRI in the detection of finger extensor tendon tears, which were later confirmed at surgery.[50] There is moderate agreement between ultrasound and MRI in the assessment of shoulder tendon pathology in patients with RA; MRI remains the reference technique for the shoulder,[51] but in general is inferior to ultrasound when dynamic assessment is required for tendon and ligament structures.

Defining the threshold of normality

One of the crucial aspects to consider when utilizing ultrasound in clinical practice and trials is defining the threshold of normality at the joint and patient level. There has been a significant improvement in ultrasound technology over the last ten years, which has led to acquisition of higher image resolution. Subsequently, ultrasound can now detect subtle lesions even in healthy individuals with no joint symptoms. In one study, Padovano et al. reported that 89% of healthy subjects (182 out of 207) had at least one ultrasound abnormality. Although this number appears high, the ultrasound findings reported were only present in 9% of the joints examined. This was mostly in the feet, particularly in the first MTP joint (33% of the positive joints). Among the type of ultrasound pathology observed, synovial effusion was the most frequent ultrasound finding (68% of the positive joints), followed by synovial hypertrophy (31%). Nevertheless, the severity of these pathology was mild (grade 1 in average), regardless of the type of ultrasound pathology. These findings indicate that the imaging boundary between normal joints (i.e. physiological changes) and those of early arthritis joints (i.e. early pathological changes) needs to be carefully studied. It is possible that a proportion of ultrasound-defined pathology observed in normal joints may be attributable to age-related changes or biomechanical factors (overuse for example). These issues highlight that it is crucial to describe the normal threshold at the joint level in each age group. This would then enable ultrasound investigators to define key thresholds to guide interventions, which includes defining ultrasound remission targets and escalation of therapy.[52]

Proposed pragmatic use of ultrasound in clinical practice for RA patients

Although there has been a rapid expansion in rheumatology ultrasound research in recent years, there are no specific guidelines on how to optimize the use of ultrasound in routine clinical practice, particularly for RA patients. Here, we summarize three algorithms based on consensus from ultrasound experts.[53]

Ultrasound to facilitate early diagnosis

There are three main areas of which ultrasound may assist in the early diagnosis: (1) to identify whether US-detected inflammation is present in at-risk patients with no clinically-apparent joint inflammation; (2) to reassess patients who do not fulfil the RA 2010 ACR/EULAR criteria on clinical examination; (3) to confirm the presence of inflammation in patients who fulfil the ACR/EULAR criteria on clinical examination, but in whom there is diagnostic uncertainty (i.e. to identify false-positive based on RA 2010 ACR/EULAR criteria). See Figure 18.9.

Assessment of treatment response

Ultrasound can detect response after therapy (between 1 week and 1 year) in patients treated with synthetic DMARDs or biological DMARDs.[53] Ultrasound biomarkers (GS and PD) are as sensitive as laboratory and clinical assessments in detecting changes of inflammation level following therapy.[35] Based on literature review and experts' opinion, patients with RA in either synthetic or biological DMARDs should undergo assessment with ultrasound at baseline and after 3–6 months of treatment to assess response. Subsequently, the therapy can be adjusted accordingly.

Figure 18.10 shows a pragmatic algorithm for the use of ultrasound in RA patients on DMARDS (synthetics or biologic): (1) to investigate non-inflammatory aetiology in patients with poor clinical response and absence of ultrasound-detected inflammatory changes; (2) to consider escalation of therapy in patients with poor clinical response and presence of ultrasound-detected inflammatory changes; (3) in patients on synthetic DMARDs to maintain or taper therapy in patients with good clinical response and presence of US

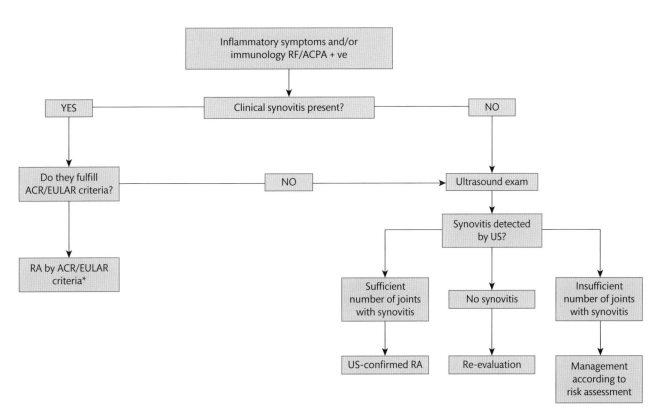

Figure 18.9 Pragmatic algorithm of the use of ultrasound in the diagnostic pathway for RA patients.

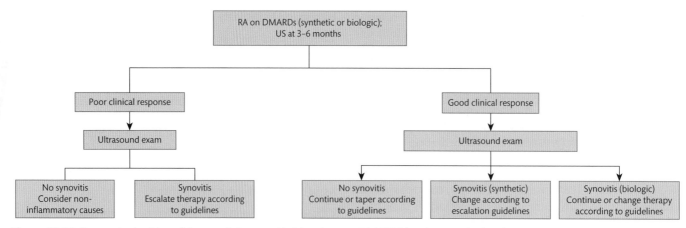

Figure 18.10 Pragmatic algorithm of the use of ultrasound in RA patients on DMARDS (synthetics or biologic).

synovitis; (4) In patients on biologic DMARDs to continue therapy as the significance of US synovitis in biologic DMARDs is unclear.[53]

To assess remission or low disease activity

Doppler signal of >1 in patients on cDMARD therapy is associated with X-ray progression[40] and GS synovitis is associated with occurrence of progression of bone erosion. The presence of PD >1 increases the risk of flare in RA patients who are in remission and PD negativity is the best predictor of continuing clinical remission.[54,55] In addition, patients with significant GS and PD US synovitis have a higher chance of relapse when stopping or reducing biologic therapy compared to those with a lower GS and PD US synovitis.[56,57]

Figure 18.11 shows a pragmatic algorithm for using ultrasound in patients with synthetic and biologic DMARDs. If the patient is clinically stable and has no US synovitis, then continue current treatment or consider tapering treatment. If US synovitis is present, then therapy escalation or change should be considered.

The role of ultrasound-guided procedures

Ultrasound-guided procedures are increasingly important in rheumatology as they have the advantage of direct visualization of the targeted region of interest. This enables the operator to avoid important structures such as nerves, tendons, ligaments, vascular structures, and bone. Ultrasound can be used to guide arthrocentesis, fluid

aspiration from joint, cysts, bursae, and tendon sheaths. In addition, ultrasound guidance can be used in needling of periarticular calcification (barbotage). The main advantages of ultrasound-guided procedures are accurate needle placement within the targeted lesion, which may improve outcomes.

Ultrasound-guided aspiration and injection

Ultrasound guidance improves the accuracy of needle placement in the small joints of the hand,[58] knee,[59] and acromioclavicular joint.[60] It also improves the accuracy of needle placement in the first or second tarsometatarsal joint compared to clinical palpation (64% vs. 25%).[61]

In a randomized controlled trial, ultrasound guidance was associated with a 43% reduction in procedural pain (p <0.001), and 26% increase in responder rate. Ultrasound also increased the rate of effusion detection by twofold and volume of aspirate by 337%.[62]

Naredo et al. reported that in a randomized study of blinded-injection vs. ultrasound-guided subacromial injection of the shoulder, shoulder pain and function were significantly higher in the ultrasound, compared to the blinded-injection group. In addition to improved outcomes, patients also reported less pain in the ultrasound-guided group in a randomized study comparing clinical landmark versus ultrasound-guided knee aspiration.[63] Ultrasound-guided procedures may also improve patients' experience of injections. A total of 88% of patients felt that their levels of worry or anxiety were better or much better as a consequence being able to

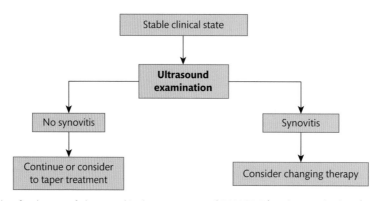

Figure 18.11 Pragmatic algorithm for the use of ultrasound in the assessment of DMARDS (synthetic or biologic).

observe the US image of the symptomatic area before and after a guided procedure. Some 92% of patients felt that observing the US images helped with the process of having an injection.[64] The effectiveness of de Quervain's tendinitis injection is based on the accuracy of steroid placement.[65] However, accuracy of needle placement does not necessarily predict treatment response in other regions. For example, the response rate of intrasheath injection of trigger finger was comparable to that of subcutaneous injection (47% vs. 50%).[66] Similarly, there is non-superiority of outcomes of conventional guidance compared to ultrasound guidance injection of plantar fasciitis,[67] and no difference in the pain and functional outcomes of indirect ultrasound-guided injection versus conventional guided injection in the acromioclavicular (AC) joints.[68]

Based on published studies, ultrasound-guided injections do not necessarily result in better clinical outcomes, depending on the procedure undertaken. However, patients' confidence in accurate needle placement during a procedure may influence the patient-reported outcomes in these studies.[64] As a pragmatic approach, ultrasound-guided injections could be considered for joints not accessible by clinical landmarks (e.g. hip and mid-tarsal joints) or joints which fail to respond to blind injection.

Ultrasound-guided synovial biopsy

Historically, synovial samples have been obtained via blind-needle biopsy and arthroscopy techniques. Although the blind-needle approach is well-tolerated, safe, and low in cost, it is limited by insufficient sampling in joints and poor-quality samples[69]; furthermore, this technique is not feasible for tissue retrieval in small joints such as the MCPs and proximal interphalangeal (PIPs). Arthroscopic biopsy techniques are considered a gold standard with the advantage of retrieving a high proportion of high-quality samples, but with significant disadvantages of expense, invasiveness, and having a significant requirement for training. It is therefore restricted to a limited number of centres.[56]

Over the last decade, techniques for synovial tissue retrieval under US-guidance have evolved, and these can be classified into two main types; the portal-and-forceps (P&F) technique or a semi-automatic guillotine-type biopsy needle (e.g. Tru-Cut or Quick-Core). These techniques are safe, well-tolerated by patients, and yield high-quality synovial samples from multiple joint sites. No complications were recorded post-procedure in 93 biopsies performed in 57 patients from five different joint types (knee, elbow, wrist, MCP, and PIP).[70] In addition, there were no differences in pain, swelling, and stiffness in those joints following biopsy. A greater ribonucleic acid (RNA) yield was associated with a high grey-scale synovitis score prebiopsy.[70] In a large comparative study (n = 524), the authors reported that all biopsy techniques (US-needle biopsy, US-guided portal and forceps, and arthroscopic-guided synovial biopsy) were safe and well-tolerated by patients.[71]

The utility of ultrasound guidance synovial biopsy is broadly related to clinical and academic purposes. In the clinical setting, synovial tissue sampling can be considered when ruling out infection, diagnosing infiltrative or granulomatous disorders, and occasionally to confirm crystal arthritis. In the academic realm, synovial tissue biopsy enables important pathophysiology studies to be performed such as understanding the mechanism of early disease phases and stratification of therapeutic response. Given the ability of US-guided biopsy techniques to retrieve high-quality samples even in

joints with minimal pathology, further research studies involving molecular analysis, gene expression studies, and next-generation sequencing can be performed.[56,63,72]

REFERENCES

1. Wakefield R, D'Agostino M. Physics of ultrasound In: Wakefield R, D'Agostino M (eds). *Essential Applications of Musculoskeletal Ultrasound in Rheumatology*, 1st edition, pp. 3–17. London, UK: Saunders Elsevier, 2010.
2. D'Agostino MA, Terslev L, Aegerter P, et al. Scoring ultrasound synovitis in rheumatoid arthritis: a EULAR-OMERACT ultrasound taskforce-Part 1: definition and development of a standardised, consensus-based scoring system. *RMD Open* 2017;3(1):e000428.
3. Terslev L, Naredo E, Aegerter P, et al. Scoring ultrasound synovitis in rheumatoid arthritis: a EULAR-OMERACT ultrasound taskforce—Part 2: reliability and application to multiple joints of a standardised consensus-based scoring system. *RMD Open* 2017;3(1):e000427.
4. Wakefield RJ, Balint PV, Szkudlarek M, et al. Musculoskeletal ultrasound including definitions for ultrasonographic pathology. *J Rheumatol* 2005;32(12):2485–7.
5. Naredo E, D'Agostino MA, Wakefield RJ, et al. Reliability of a consensus-based ultrasound score for tenosynovitis in rheumatoid arthritis. *Ann Rheum Dis* 2013;72(8):1328–34.
6. Hammer HB, Iagnocco A, Mathiessen A, et al. Global ultrasound assessment of structural lesions in osteoarthritis: a reliability study by the OMERACT ultrasonography group on scoring cartilage and osteophytes in finger joints. *Ann Rheum Dis* 2016;75(2):402–7.
7. Szkudlarek M, Court-Payen M, Strandberg C, Klarlund M, Klausen T, Ostergaard M. Power Doppler ultrasonography for assessment of synovitis in the metacarpophalangeal joints of patients with rheumatoid arthritis: a comparison with dynamic magnetic resonance imaging. *Arthritis Rheum* 2001;44(9):2018–23.
8. Terslev L, Torp-Pedersen S, Qvistgaard E, Danneskiold-Samsoe B, Bliddal H. Estimation of inflammation by Doppler ultrasound: quantitative changes after intra-articular treatment in rheumatoid arthritis. *Ann Rheum Dis* 2003;62(11):1049–53.
9. Filippucci E, Iagnocco A, Salaffi F, Cerioni A, Valesini G, Grassi W. Power Doppler sonography monitoring of synovial perfusion at the wrist joints in patients with rheumatoid arthritis treated with adalimumab. *Ann Rheum Dis* 2006;65(11):1433–7.
10. Colebatch AN, Edwards CJ, Ostergaard M, et al. EULAR recommendations for the use of imaging of the joints in the clinical management of rheumatoid arthritis. *Ann Rheum Dis* 2013;72(6):804–14.
11. Agrawal S, Bhagat SS, Dasgupta B. Improvement in diagnosis and management of musculoskeletal conditions with one-stop clinic-based ultrasonography. *Mod Rheumatol* 2009;19(1):53–6.
12. Matsos M, Harish S, Zia P, et al. Ultrasound of the hands and feet for rheumatological disorders: influence on clinical diagnostic confidence and patient management. *Skeletal Radiol* 2009;38(11):1049–54.
13. Freeston JE, Wakefield RJ, Conaghan PG, Hensor EM, Stewart SP, Emery P. A diagnostic algorithm for persistence of very early inflammatory arthritis: the utility of power Doppler ultrasound when added to conventional assessment tools. *Ann Rheum Dis* 2010;69(2):417–19.

14. Rakieh C, Nam JL, Hunt L, et al. Predicting the development of clinical arthritis in anti-CCP positive individuals with non-specific musculoskeletal symptoms: a prospective observational cohort study. *Ann Rheum Dis* 2015;74(9):1659–66.

15. Salaffi F, Ciapetti A, Gasparini S, Carotti M, Filippucci E, Grassi W. A clinical prediction rule combining routine assessment and power Doppler ultrasonography for predicting progression to rheumatoid arthritis from early-onset undifferentiated arthritis. *Clin Exp Rheumatol* 2010;28(5):686–94.

16. Filer A, de Pablo P, Allen G, et al. Utility of ultrasound joint counts in the prediction of rheumatoid arthritis in patients with very early synovitis. *Ann Rheum Dis* 2011;70(3):500–7.

17. Sahbudin I, Pickup L, Nightingale P, et al. The role of ultrasound-defined tenosynovitis and synovitis in the prediction of rheumatoid arthritis development. *Rheumatology (Oxf)* 2018: doi: 10.1093/rheumatology/key025.

18. Lillegraven S, Boyesen P, Hammer HB, et al. Tenosynovitis of the extensor carpi ulnaris tendon predicts erosive progression in early rheumatoid arthritis. *Ann Rheum Dis* 2011;70(11):2049–50.

19. Tinazzi I, McGonagle D, Zabotti A, Chessa D, Marchetta A, Macchioni P. Comprehensive evaluation of finger flexor tendon entheseal soft tissue and bone changes by ultrasound can differentiate psoriatic arthritis and rheumatoid arthritis. *Clin Exp Rheumatol* 2018;36(5):785–90.

20. Zabotti A, Errichetti E, Zuliani F, et al. Early psoriatic arthritis versus early seronegative rheumatoid arthritis: role of dermoscopy combined with ultrasonography for differential diagnosis. *J Rheumatol* 2018;45(5):648–54.

21. D'Agostino MA, Said-Nahal R, Hacquard-Bouder C, Brasseur JL, Dougados M, Breban M. Assessment of peripheral enthesitis in the spondylarthropathies by ultrasonography combined with power Doppler: a cross-sectional study. *Arthritis Rheum* 2003;48(2):523–33.

22. Fournie B, Margarit-Coll N, Champetier de Ribes TL, et al. Extrasynovial ultrasound abnormalities in the psoriatic finger. Prospective comparative power-Doppler study versus rheumatoid arthritis. *Joint Bone Spine* 2006;73(5):527–31.

23. Fiocco U, Cozzi L, Rubaltelli L, et al. Long-term sonographic follow-up of rheumatoid and psoriatic proliferative knee joint synovitis. *Br J Rheumatol.* 1996;35(2):155–63.

24. Falsetti P, Frediani B, Acciai C, et al. Ultrasonography and magnetic resonance imaging of heel fat pad inflammatory-oedematous lesions in rheumatoid arthritis. *Scand J Rheumatol* 2006;35(6):454–8.

25. Falsetti P, Frediani B, Acciai C, Baldi F, Filippou G, Marcolongo R. Heel fat pad involvement in rheumatoid arthritis and in spondyloarthropathies: an ultrasonographic study. *Scand J Rheumatol* 2004;33(5):327–31.

26. Frediani B, Falsetti P, Storri L, et al. Ultrasound and clinical evaluation of quadricipital tendon enthesitis in patients with psoriatic arthritis and rheumatoid arthritis. *Clin Rheumatol* 2002;21(4):294–8.

27. Marchesoni A, De Lucia O, Rotunno L, De Marco G, Manara M. Entheseal power Doppler ultrasonography: a compsarison of psoriatic arthritis and fibromyalgia. *J Rheumatol Suppl* 2012;89:29–31.

28. Marchesoni A, De Marco G, Merashli M, et al. The problem in differentiation between psoriatic-related polyenthesitis and fibromyalgia. *Rheumatology (Oxf)* 2018;57(1):32–40.

29. Kaeley GS, Eder L, Aydin SZ, Gutierrez M, Bakewell C. Enthesitis: a hallmark of psoriatic arthritis. *Semin Arthritis Rheum* 2018;48(1):35–43.

30. Grassi WGF, E. Crystal-associated Synovitis In: Wakefield R, D'Agostino M (eds). *Essential Applications of Musculoskeletal Ultrasound in Rheumatology*, 1st edition, pp. 187–96. London, UK: Saunders Elsevier, 2010,

31. Iagnocco A. Osteoarthritis. In: Wakefield R, D'Agostino MA (eds). *Essential Applications of Musculoskeletal Ultrasound in Rheumatology*, 1st edition, Chapter 14. London, UK: Saunders Elsevier, 2010.

32. Wakefield RJ, D'Agostino MA, Iagnocco A, et al. The OMERACT Ultrasound Group: status of current activities and research directions. *J Rheumatol* 2007;34(4):848–51.

33. Felson DT, Smolen JS, Wells G, et al. American College of Rheumatology/European League Against Rheumatism provisional definition of remission in rheumatoid arthritis for clinical trials. *Arthritis Rheum* 2011;63(3):573–86.

34. Naredo E, Rodriguez M, Campos C, et al. Validity, reproducibility, and responsiveness of a twelve-joint simplified power doppler ultrasonographic assessment of joint inflammation in rheumatoid arthritis. *Arthritis Rheum* 2008;59(4):515–22.

35. D'Agostino MA, Wakefield RJ, Berner-Hammer H, et al. Value of ultrasonography as a marker of early response to abatacept in patients with rheumatoid arthritis and an inadequate response to methotrexate: results from the APPRAISE study. *Ann Rheum Dis* 2016;75(10):1763–9.

36. Ammitzboll-Danielsen M, Ostergaard M, Naredo E, et al. The use of the OMERACT ultrasound tenosynovitis scoring system in multicenter clinical trials. *J Rheumatol* 2018;45(2):165–9.

37. Dale J, Stirling A, Zhang R, et al. Targeting ultrasound remission in early rheumatoid arthritis: the results of the TaSER study, a randomised clinical trial. *Ann Rheum Dis* 2016;75(6):1043–50.

38. Haavardsholm EA, Aga AB, Olsen IC, et al. Ultrasound in management of rheumatoid arthritis: ARCTIC randomised controlled strategy trial. *BMJ* 2016;354:i4205.

39. D'Agostino MA, Boers M, Wakefield RJ, Emery P, Conaghan PG. Is it time to revisit the role of ultrasound in rheumatoid arthritis management? *Ann Rheum Dis.* 2017;76(1):7–8.

40. Brown AK, Conaghan PG, Karim Z, et al. An explanation for the apparent dissociation between clinical remission and continued structural deterioration in rheumatoid arthritis. *Arthritis Rheum* 2008;58(10):2958–67.

41. Peluso G, Michelutti A, Bosello S, Gremese E, Tolusso B, Ferraccioli G. Clinical and ultrasonographic remission determines different chances of relapse in early and long standing rheumatoid arthritis. *Ann Rheum Dis* 2011;70(1):172–5.

42. Bellis E, Scire CA, Carrara G, et al. Ultrasound-detected tenosynovitis independently associates with patient-reported flare in patients with rheumatoid arthritis in clinical remission: results from the observational study STARTER of the Italian Society for Rheumatology. *Rheumatology (Oxf)* 2016;55(10):1826–36.

43. Ellegaard K, Christensen R, Torp-Pedersen S, et al. Ultrasound Doppler measurements predict success of treatment with anti-TNF-α drug in patients with rheumatoid arthritis: a prospective cohort study. *Rheumatology (Oxf)* 2011;50(3):506–12.

44. Wakefield R, D'Agostino M. Detection of bone erosions. In: Wakefield R, D'Agostino M (eds). *Essential Applications of Musculoskeletal Ultrasound in Rheumatology*, 1st edition, pp. 79–87. London, UK: Saunders Elsevier, 2010.

45. Arnett FC, Edworthy SM, Bloch DA, et al. The American Rheumatism Association 1987 revised criteria for the classification of rheumatoid arthritis. *Arthritis Rheum* 1988;31(3):315–24.

46. Dohn UM, Ejbjerg BJ, Court-Payen M, et al. Are bone erosions detected by magnetic resonance imaging and ultrasonography

true erosions? A comparison with computed tomography in rheumatoid arthritis metacarpophalangeal joints. *Arthritis Res Ther* 2006;*8*(4):R110.

47. Finzel S, Ohrndorf S, Englbrecht M, et al. A detailed comparative study of high-resolution ultrasound and micro-computed tomography for detection of arthritic bone erosions. *Arthritis Rheum* 2011;*63*(5):1231–6.

48. Dohn UM, Ejbjerg B, Boonen A, et al. No overall progression and occasional repair of erosions despite persistent inflammation in adalimumab-treated rheumatoid arthritis patients: results from a longitudinal comparative MRI, ultrasonography, CT and radiography study. *Ann Rheum Dis* 2011;*70*(2):252–8.

49. Boyesen P, Haavardsholm EA, van der Heijde D, et al. Prediction of MRI erosive progression: a comparison of modern imaging modalities in early rheumatoid arthritis patients. *Ann Rheum Dis* 2011;*70*(1):176–9.

50. Swen WA, Jacobs JW, Hubach PC, Klasens JH, Algra PR, Bijlsma JW. Comparison of sonography and magnetic resonance imaging for the diagnosis of partial tears of finger extensor tendons in rheumatoid arthritis. *Rheumatology (Oxf)* 2000;*39*(1):55–62.

51. Bruyn GA, Naredo E, Moller I, et al. Reliability of ultrasonography in detecting shoulder disease in patients with rheumatoid arthritis. *Ann Rheum Dis* 2009;*68*(3):357–61.

52. [No authors]. WEEKLY clinicopathological exercises: polyarteritis and vasculitis, generalized severe; acute and chronic glomerulitis; myocarditis, severe; rheumatoid arthritis; amyloidosis of kidney. *N Engl J Med* 1950;*243*(25):1003–8.

53. D'Agostino MA, Terslev L, Wakefield R, et al. Novel algorithms for the pragmatic use of ultrasound in the management of patients with rheumatoid arthritis: from diagnosis to remission. *Ann Rheum Dis* 2016;*75*(11):1902–8.

54. Saleem B, Brown AK, Quinn M, et al. Can flare be predicted in DMARD treated RA patients in remission, and is it important? A cohort study. *Ann Rheum Dis* 2012;*71*(8):1316–21.

55. Scire CA, Montecucco C, Codullo V, Epis O, Todoerti M, Caporali R. Ultrasonographic evaluation of joint involvement in early rheumatoid arthritis in clinical remission: power Doppler signal predicts short-term relapse. *Rheumatology (Oxf)* 2009;*48*(9):1092–7.

56. Lazarou I, D'Agostino MA, Naredo E, Humby F, Filer A, Kelly SG. Ultrasound-guided synovial biopsy: a systematic review according to the OMERACT filter and recommendations for minimal reporting standards in clinical studies. *Rheumatology (Oxf)* 2015;*54*(10):1867–75.

57. Iwamoto T, Ikeda K, Hosokawa J, et al. Prediction of relapse after discontinuation of biologic agents by ultrasonographic assessment in patients with rheumatoid arthritis in clinical remission: high predictive values of total gray-scale and power Doppler scores that represent residual synovial inflammation before discontinuation. *Arthritis Care Res (Hoboken)* 2014;*66*(10):1576–81.

58. Raza K, Lee CY, Pilling D, et al. Ultrasound guidance allows accurate needle placement and aspiration from small joints in patients with early inflammatory arthritis. *Rheumatology (Oxf)* 2003;*42*(8):976–9.

59. Im SH, Lee SC, Park YB, Cho SR, Kim JC. Feasibility of sonography for intra-articular injections in the knee through a medial patellar portal. *J Ultrasound Med* 2009;*28*(11):1465–70.

60. Heers G, Hedtmann A. Correlation of ultrasonographic findings to Tossy's and Rockwood's classification of acromioclavicular joint injuries. *Ultrasound Med Biol* 2005;*31*(6):725–32.

61. Khosla S, Thiele R, Baumhauer JF. Ultrasound guidance for intra-articular injections of the foot and ankle. *Foot Ankle Int* 2009;*30*(9):886–90.

62. Sibbitt WL, Jr., Peisajovich A, Michael AA, et al. Does sonographic needle guidance affect the clinical outcome of intraarticular injections? *J Rheumatol* 2009;*36*(9):1892–902.

63. Wiler JL, Costantino TG, Filippone L, Satz W. Comparison of ultrasound-guided and standard landmark techniques for knee arthrocentesis. *J Emerg Med* 2010;*39*(1):76–82.

64. Sahbudin I, Bell J, Kumar K, Raza K, Filer A. Observing real-time images during ultrasound-guided procedures improves patients' experience. *Rheumatology (Oxf)* 2016;*55*(3):585–6.

65. Zingas C, Failla JM, Van Holsbeeck M. Injection accuracy and clinical relief of de Quervain's tendinitis. *J Hand Surg Am* 1998;*23*(1):89–96.

66. Taras JS, Raphael JS, Pan WT, Movagharnia F, Sotereanos DG. Corticosteroid injections for trigger digits: is intrasheath injection necessary? *J Hand Surg Am* 1998;*23*(4):717–22.

67. Kane D, Greaney T, Shanahan M, et al. The role of ultrasonography in the diagnosis and management of idiopathic plantar fasciitis. *Rheumatology (Oxf)* 2001;*40*(9):1002–8.

68. Sabeti-Aschraf M, Ochsner A, Schueller-Weidekamm C, et al. The infiltration of the AC joint performed by one specialist: ultrasound versus palpation a prospective randomized pilot study. *Eur J Radiol* 2010;*75*(1):e37–40.

69. Humby F, Romao VC, Manzo A, et al. A multicenter retrospective analysis evaluating performance of synovial biopsy techniques in patients with inflammatory arthritis: arthroscopic versus ultrasound-guided versus blind needle biopsy. *Arthritis Rheumatol* 2018;*70*(5):702–10.

70. Kelly S, Humby F, Filer A, et al. Ultrasound-guided synovial biopsy: a safe, well-tolerated and reliable technique for obtaining high-quality synovial tissue from both large and small joints in early arthritis patients. *Ann Rheum Dis* 2015;*74*(3):611–17.

71. Just SA, Humby F, Lindegaard H, et al. Patient-reported outcomes and safety in patients undergoing synovial biopsy: comparison of ultrasound-guided needle biopsy, ultrasound-guided portal and forceps and arthroscopic-guided synovial biopsy techniques in five centres across Europe. *RMD Open* 2018;*4*(2):e000799.

72. Mizoguchi F, Slowikowski K, Wei K, et al. Functionally distinct disease-associated fibroblast subsets in rheumatoid arthritis. *Nat Commun* 2018;*9*(1):789.

19

Magnetic resonance imaging in rheumatoid arthritis

Mikkel Østergaard, Philip G. Conaghan, and Charles Peterfy

Introduction

In rheumatoid arthritis (RA), early diagnosis combined with early initiation of appropriate therapy and tight control of inflammation have been recognized as essential for optimal clinical outcomes.[1] Furthermore, conventional and targeted biological therapies have proved effective for improving signs, symptoms, and quality of life in patients and for reducing progression of structural joint damage.[2] These treatment paradigms have fuelled the need for powerful, sensitive techniques that can accurately diagnose and indicate the prognosis of patients with RA and accurately monitor the efficacy of treatment.

Conventional radiography, though able to detect structural joint damage in patients with established disease, is not sensitive in detecting early disease manifestations such as soft tissue changes and bone damage at its earliest stages.[3]

Magnetic resonance imaging (MRI) allows multiplanar tomographic imaging of the body in any plane without geometric distortions associated with projectional techniques, such as radiography, and no ionizing radiation is used. Early bone involvement and inflammatory soft tissue changes of synovitis and tenosynovitis, which are not detectable by conventional clinical, biochemical, and radiographic methods, can be directly visualized and evaluated in detail by MRI.[4] Disadvantages of MRI include relatively higher costs, longer examination times and lower availability than radiography, and, except with whole-body MRI (WBMRI), restricted anatomical coverage per session. MRI offers greater anatomical coverage than ultrasonography (US) does, because US cannot penetrate bone, and thus cannot visualize structures hidden in acoustic shadows, including the medial and lateral aspects of most of the carpal and metacarpal joints. Further, US cannot visualize inflammation within the bone marrow (i.e. osteitis), which has been shown to be highly predictive of subsequent bone erosion. MRI is able to visualize all joints in the hand and wrist and all regions of these joints, as well as osteitis. In clinical trials, the advantages of MRI compared to US are clear, due to the possibility of standardized image acquisition, centralized reading with full blinding of both image acquisition and reading. In clinical practice, US provides results immediately, and thus allows more rapid therapeutic decision making, but this requires a skilled ultrasonographer and high-end equipment in the outpatient clinic.[4]

This chapter will focus on the potential uses of MRI in the clinical management of patients with suspected or definite RA. After a section on technical aspects, it will describe the current knowledge on MRI for early detection of RA manifestations, diagnosis of RA, monitoring of disease activity and joint damage progression, and its role in determining prognosis. The usefulness in both clinical trials and routine practice will be discussed, including more novel roles such as what it can bring to the imaging of clinical remission and prior to tapering of biologics.

Technical considerations

MRI of the peripheral joints can be performed with whole-body MRI units or dedicated extremity MRI units (E-MRI). E-MRI systems expose only the extremity being imaged to the main magnetic field, and thus carry less risk of dislodging surgical implants or other metal elsewhere in the body or interfering with pacemakers or other implanted devices. E-MRI systems also obviate claustrophobia that can be a problem for some patients undergoing whole-body MRI. Some low field E-MRI units may provide similar information on synovitis and bone damage to what is obtained with high-field units,[5,6] but for some units smaller field of view, longer imaging times, and lack of certain imaging sequences (particularly spectral fat saturation (FS) at low field) may limit usefulness.[7,8]

High-resolution, T1-weighted (T1w), three-dimensional (3D) imaging sequences, obtained before and after intravenous contrast injection, and a 'water sensitive' technique, such as T2-weighted (T2w) spin echo with FS or short tau inversion recovery (STIR), constitute the standard sequences obtained in RA.[9]

For evaluating structural changes, such as bone erosion, T1-weighted images are preferred.[3,9–11] They provide good anatomical detail and have the ability to visualize tissues with high perfusion and permeability, including the inflamed synovium, after intravenous contrast injection with paramagnetic gadolinium compounds (Gd)

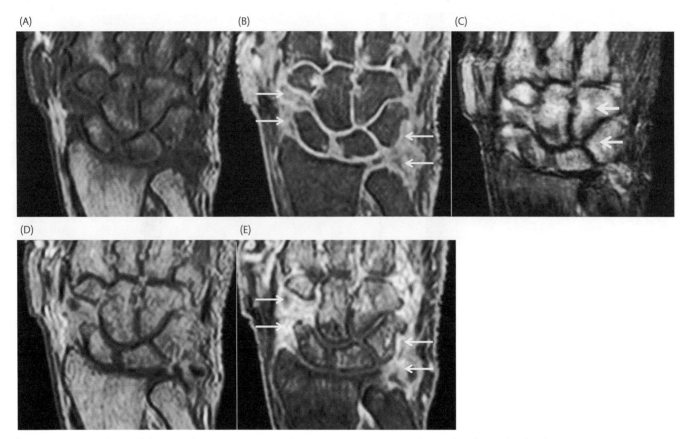

Figure 19.1 Coronal MRI of the wrist of a RA patient, acquired on 1.0 T extremity MRI unit before (A–C) and after (D–E) intravenous contrast injection, illustrating different types of sequences. T1-weighted images without (A, D) and with (B, E) fat suppression demonstrate pronounced synovitis with signal intensity increase (enhancement) on postcontrast images (D, E). The STIR sequence (C) shows bone marrow oedema in the metacarpal bases, carpal bones (hamate and triquetrum marked with thick arrows), and, less intensively, the radius.

(Figure 19.1). Intravenous contrast injection increases the sensitivity for synovitis in peripheral joints.[12] Specific sequences designed for optimal cartilage evaluation can also be applied (e.g. 3D gradient echo sequences). New MRI techniques continue to be developed, and a variety of sequences are now available for detecting free water in otherwise fatty bone marrow, indicative of inflammation—so-called bone marrow (o)edema (BME) or osteitis. These include T2w spin echo with fat saturation (T2FS) or water-excitation (T2WE) and STIR, but also T2 with water-excitation, hybrid sequences, and chemical shift–based fat-water separation, such as the Dixon technique.[13] The Dixon technique is increasingly being employed, though T2FS and STIR sequences are still most frequent, because of their high general reliability, consistency across different manufacturers and, for STIR, applicability at lower magnetic field strengths.

Whole-body MRI is promising technique that allows imaging of the entire body in one examination (i.e. simultaneous assessment of peripheral and axial joints and entheses in both RA), where it may provide an MRI-based total joint count,[14] and spondyloarthritis and psoriatic arthritis.[15–17] Improved image resolution and more validation is still needed for WBMRI imaging of the small joints of the hands and feet, before the method is ready for routine use.

Dynamic contrast-enhanced MRI (DCE-MRI) is based on the perfusion dynamics of synovial enhancement curves after contrast injection, and has been found to correlate with synovial histopathological inflammation.[18,19] Thus, DCE-MRI may allow accurate assessment of the disease activity based on a selected region of interest.[20,21] Techniques using manual segmentation to quantify pathologies such as synovial volumes have been investigated for many years,[22,23] but recent automated methods using supervised machine learning may increase the feasibility and also responsiveness when assessing RA pathologies.[24] Both methods need further validation.

MRI is very safe. It involves no ionizing radiation or risk of malignancy, with the major contraindications being claustrophobia or the presence of any metal devices including pacemakers or clips (though many of these are now made MRI safe). Adverse effects from Gd-based contrast agents are very rare, except in patients with severely impaired renal function.[25] The European Society of Urogenital Radiology (ESUR) guidelines recommend no patients should be denied a well-indicated Gd-enhanced MRI, and that agents with highest stability (lowest risk of nephrogenic systemic fibrosis) (e.g. macrocyclic Gd chelates, such as gadoterate meglumine and gadoteridol) should be used, at the lowest diagnostic dose.[25]

MRI detection of pathology in RA

The clinical value of MRI in RA relates primarily to its ability to evaluate the wrists, hands, and feet in high detail, which is also the main focus of this section. MRI is also useful for evaluating other

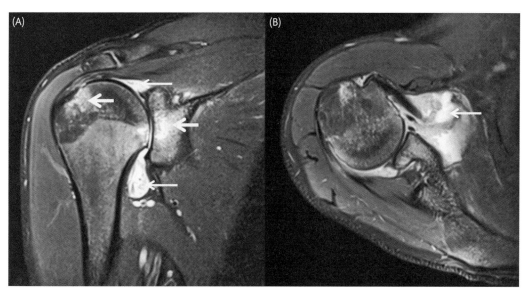

Figure 19.2 Coronal oblique (A) and axial (B) fat-suppressed T2-weighted images of a recently diagnosed RA patient show bone marrow oedema (thick arrows) and considerable amounts of joint fluid in the glenohumeral joint (arrows).

anatomical sites involved by RA, such as the knees, hips, elbows and shoulders, and the axial skeleton, particularly the cervical spine (Figure 19.2) Further, as already noted, MRI allows assessment of all the joint structures affected by RA. Definitions of key pathologies in RA and psoriatic arthritis (PsA) are provided in Table 19.1.[9,26,27]

Synovitis

Synovitis (Figures 19.1 and 19.3) is the key feature of RA. There is solid evidence from comparisons with miniarthroscopy and histopathological findings that MRI synovitis, as determined by Gd-enhanced T1-weighted MRI, reflects true synovial

inflammation.[18,19,23,28] Low-grade MRI synovitis has been reported in healthy controls without clinical signs of synovitis,[29-32] increasing with age. Since synovitis is very common in osteoarthritis (OA), including asymptomatic OA, it is not clear how many of such 'normal' joints had underlying OA. Diagnostic tests are never 100% sensitive or specific, and thus the inherent trade-off between false-negative and false-positive rates as one increases the positivity criterion for that test must be considered carefully in light of the particular role that imaging is being asked to play: (1) identifying patients for a particular treatment; (2) monitoring whether or not the treatment worked; or (3) searching for potential complications

Table 19.1 Definitions of important RA joint pathologies

Pathology	Definition	Notes
Synovitis	An area in the synovial compartment that shows above-normal postgadolinium enhancement (signal intensity increase) of a thickness greater than the width of the normal synovium	–
MRI bone erosion	A sharply marginated bone lesion, with correct juxta-articular localization and typical signal characteristics, which is visible in two planes with a cortical break seen in at least one plane	On T1-weighted images: discontinuity of the signal void of cortical bone and loss of normal high signal intensity of bone marrow fat. Rapid postgadolinium enhancement suggests presence of active, hypervascularized pannus tissue in the erosion. Other focal bone lesions and variations of normal anatomy must obviously be considered, but are generally distinguishable with associated imaging and clinical findings
MRI osteitis/bone marrow oedema	A lesion within the trabecular bone, with ill-defined margins and signal characteristics consistent with increased water content	May occur alone or surrounding an erosion. High signal intensity on T2-weigted fat saturation or STIR images, and low signal intensity on T1-weighted images
MRI joint space narrowing	Reduced joint space width compared to normal, as assessed in a slice perpendicular to the joint surface	–
MRI tenosynovitis	Peritendinous effusion and/or tenosynovial postcontrast enhancement, seen on axial sequences over ≥3 consecutive slices	High signal intensity on T2-weigted fat-saturated/STIR images. Enhancement (signal intensity increase) is judged by comparison of T1-weighted images obtained before and after i.v. gadolinium-contrast

Source: data from Østergaard M, Peterfy CG, Bird P et al. (2017) 'The OMERACT Rheumatoid Arthritis Magnetic Resonance Imaging (MRI) Scoring System: Updated Recommendations by the OMERACT MRI in Arthritis Working Group'. *J Rheumatol* 44(11):1706–12.

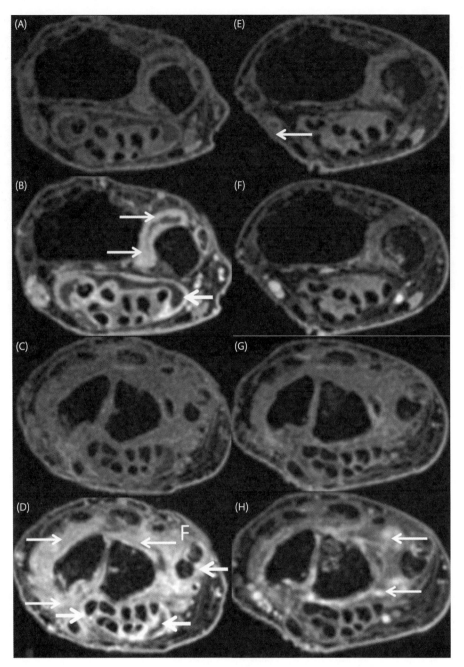

Figure 19.3 Axial fat-suppressed T1-weighted MR images before (A–D) and after (E–H) 1 year of biological therapy. Images are obtained before (A, C, E, and G) and after (B, D, F, H) intravenous injection at two different locations: through the distal radiocarpal joint (A, B, E, F) and through the proximal row of carpal bones (C, D, G, H). Considerable synovitis (short arrows) and tenosynovitis are seen at baseline while only minimal synovitis (short arrows) and no tenosynovitis is seen after treatment

of the disease or the treatment.[26,31] If trying to identify individuals at risk of RA who would benefit from closer monitoring, a high sensitivity test may be in order, whereas to identify patients for whom costly treatment with biologics would be justified, perhaps a greater degree of specificity would be needed.

Tenosynovitis

Tenosynovitis (**Figure 19.3**) is very common in RA, but may also occur in other arthritides, even very early in undifferentiated arthritis,[33] or as a consequence of overuse.[34–37] The tendon itself may appear normal, or it may be involved with thickening, irregularity and/or increased signal intensity within the tendon on T2w and STIR images (tendonitis), or with complete or incomplete tears.[34]

Bone marrow oedema

Bone marrow oedema (**Figures 19.1** and **19.2**), that is, presence of MRI-signs of increased water in the bone marrow compartment, is frequently detected in RA. When compared with histological samples obtained at surgery in RA patients, MRI BME in RA has been shown to represent inflammatory infiltrates in the bone marrow, that is, osteitis.[38,39] Whereas erosions reflect bone damage that has already occurred, BME appears to represent the link ('forerunner') from joint inflammation to bone destruction; persistent osteitis leads to trabecular bone loss and an erosion.[40–42]

Enthesitis

Enthesitis (i.e. inflammation at capsular and ligamentous insertions) is a characteristic feature in seronegative spondyloarthritides, such as PsA, but can also be seen in RA and patients without inflammatory arthritis (with presumed mechanical cause).[14,43]

Joint cartilage

Joint cartilage can be directly visualized by MRI.[44] A number of morphological and compositional MRI markers of cartilage integrity have been studied. Cartilage assessment in small joints requires high image quality and resolution, but reliable assessment systems have been developed.[45–47]

Bone erosion

Bone erosion (Figure 19.4) is detected with higher sensitivity with MRI than radiography.[36,48,49] A high level of agreement for detection

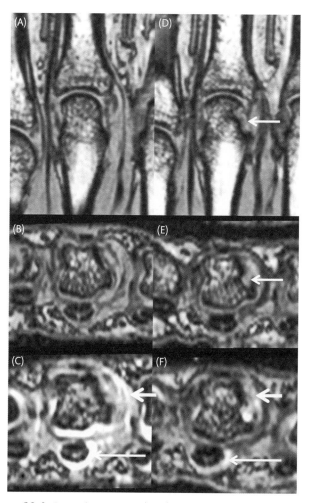

Figure 19.4 Coronal precontrast (A, D), axial precontrast (B, E), and axial postcontrast (C, F) MR images of the third metacarpophalangeal joint in an RA patient in clinical remission. At baseline (A–C), synovitis (thick arrow), and tenosynovitis (long thin arrow), but no bone erosions are seen. Four months later (D–F), a new bone erosion (thin short arrow) has developed, and synovitis and tenosynovitis have decreased, but are still present.

of bone erosions in RA wrists and metacarpophalangeal (MCP) joints between MRI and computed tomography (CT), the gold standard reference for detection of bone damage, provides evidence that MRI erosions represent true bone damage.[50,51]

Erosions are not specific for RA, as they are also frequently seen in other arthritides and erosive OA, and small erosion-like lesions can also be visualized in healthy controls (see also previous comments on OA in such patients).[31,32] To avoid overestimation, using strict definitions of bone erosion and other pathologies is essential; for example, erosions should be visible in two planes, with a cortical break visible in at least one plane to be registered, and the normal anatomy and pitfalls should be kept in mind.[26,52,53] Control groups, sequences, and reading methodology should be appropriately selected.[54]

Cervical spine involvement

Cervical spine involvement is a serious complication of RA. All joints, tendons, and ligaments of the cervical spine can be involved in RA, leading to spine instability or subluxations. Proliferating pannus from the synovial joints and anatomical malalignments can in turn lead to secondary medullary compression. The primary imaging modality is computed radiography (CR), but MRI can provide detailed information on bone and soft tissue abnormalities (e.g. the pannus tissue around the odontoid process, and this can be a valuable supplement to radiographic evaluation).[3,55,56] MRI erosions of the atlas and reduced subarachnoid space are associated with subsequent clinical neurological dysfunction,[57] and cord compression on MRI better predicts subsequent clinical deterioration than initial clinical and radiographic features.[58] The evidence-based European League Against Rheumatism (EULAR) recommendations for the use of imaging in RA clinical management state that monitoring of functional instability of the cervical spine by lateral radiograph obtained in flexion and neutral should be performed in patients with clinical suspicion of cervical involvement. When the radiographs are positive or specific neurological symptoms and signs are present, MRI should be performed.[3]

Validation for patient-important outcomes

Magnetic resonance imaging assessed hand inflammation is documented to influence the function of the hand, and is independently associated with patient-reported overall patient physical impairment (the Health Assessment Questionnaire, global assessment of disease activity and pain in early rheumatoid arthritis).[33,59,60] In late disease, but not early RA, the degree of joint damage also influences patient-reported outcomes.[61]

Diagnosis

Longitudinal studies of undifferentiated arthritis have documented an independent predictive value of MRI in the subsequent diagnosis of RA.[62,63] Presence of BME had a positive predictive value of 86.1% for subsequent development of RA,[62] and a prediction model, including clinical hand arthritis, morning stiffness, positive rheumatoid factor, and MRI bone oedema score in metatarsophalangeal and wrist joints correctly identified the development of RA or non-RA in 82% of patients.[63] Another study of undifferentiated arthritis, applying different definitions of pathologies, found high specificity but lower sensitivity of MRI tenosynovitis to differentiate patients who received a diagnosis of RA or had disease-modifying antirheumatic drugs (DMARDs) initiated versus those that did not.[64] An earlier and smaller study in pure undifferentiated arthritis showed that the combined synovitis and erosion pattern was related to the development of RA or not.[65]

In the American College of Rheumatology (ACR)/EULAR 2010 criteria for RA,[66] classification as definite RA is based on presence of definite clinical synovitis (swelling at clinical examination) in ≥1 joint, absence of an alternative diagnosis that better explains the synovitis, and achievement of a total score ≥6 (of a possible 10) from the individual scores in four domains. In the joint involvement domain, which can provide up to five points of the six needed for an RA diagnosis, MRI and US synovitis count. In other words, MRI can be used to determine the extent of joint involvement.[66–68] Synovitis/ joint inflammation as found by clinical, MRI or US examination is not specific for RA, and the ACR/EULAR criteria are classification not diagnostic criteria. In the diagnostic process of the individual patient in routine clinical practice it is important always to consider the clinical context (as with any other diagnostic test) to avoid overdiagnosis, since MRI findings are not pathognomonic. The EULAR recommendations sum this up by stating: 'When there is diagnostic doubt, CR, ultrasound or MRI can be used to improve the certainty of a diagnosis of RA above clinical criteria alone' and also 'The presence of inflammation seen with ultrasound or MRI can be used to predict the progression to clinical RA from undifferentiated inflammatory arthritis.'[3]

Monitoring disease activity and structural damage

Clinical trials and observational cohorts

To be valuable for monitoring joint inflammation and destruction, a method must reflect the disease (truth), be reproducible, and be sensitive to change. MRI allows quantitative (volumetric or, for synovitis, enhancement after intravenous contrast injection), qualitative (presence/absence) or semi-quantitative (scoring) evaluation of all RA pathologies. In observational and randomized clinical trials, semi-quantitative scoring by the OMERACT (Outcome Measures in Rheumatology) RA MRI scoring system (RAMRIS) has been the most frequently used system. It involves semi-quantitative assessment of synovitis, bone erosions, BME and, more recently, tenosynovitis and joint space narrowing in RA hands and wrists, based on consensus MRI definitions of important joint pathologies and a 'core set' of basic MRI sequences.[9,26,47,69]

Good intra- and inter-reader reliability and a high sensitivity to change has been reported, demonstrating that the OMERACT RAMRIS system, after proper training and calibration of readers, is suitable for monitoring joint inflammation and destruction in RA.[70] A EULAR-OMERACT RA MRI reference image atlas has been developed, providing a tool to enable standardized RAMRIS scoring of MR images for RA activity and damage by comparison with standard reference images.[71]

MRI allows more sensitive monitoring of inflammation (**Figure 19.3**)[72] and bone erosion (**Figure 19.4**)[73–75] than clinical and radiographic assessments. A large study of 318 methotrexate-naïve patients demonstrated that inhibition of erosive progression by biological therapy compared to placebo can be demonstrated by MRI

using half the patients and half the follow-up time when compared to CR,[75] and several randomized controlled trials have documented the superior ability of MRI to discriminate the effects of different therapies in inhibiting progressive structural bone and cartilage damage.[46,76,77] The OMERACT erosion score is closely correlated with erosion volumes estimated by MRI and CT.[78]

Due to the high responsiveness and discriminatory ability, and because MRI has demonstrated criterion validity for osteitis and synovitis with histology and construct validity for erosions when compared with CT, there has been a rapid increase in the use of MRI in RA randomized clinical trials over the past decade. A report by the imaging subcommittee of the ACR Clinical Trials Task Force[79] concluded that MRI met the OMERACT validation filter for 'truth, discrimination, and feasibility'.[80] It concluded that 'among all of the currently available imaging modalities that have been validated with supportive data, MRI best serves the purpose of achieving sensitive ascertainment of structural damage in randomized controlled trials (RCTs) while also providing objective measures of inflammatory predictors of damage'.[79] Furthermore, pooled data from four RCTs involving 1022 RA hands and wrists in early and established RA have recently been analysed. Early changes in joint damage and inflammation detected with MRI predicted changes in joint damage evident on subsequent radiographs. These findings support the validity of using MRI for both short-term studies focusing on inflammation outcomes, desirable when prolonged placebo phases are no longer justifiable in modern RA trials, and monitoring structural damage in RCTs.[81] More recently, preliminary data on quantitative volume determination of synovitis, BME and erosion based on supervised machine learning techniques involving Active Appearance Models (potentially a quantitative RAMRIS or RAMRIQ),[24] have suggested that this method may have a higher sensitivity to early treatment-induced changes in joint inflammation. As described earlier, dynamic MRI also provides quantitative outcomes though requires caution with reliability especially in multicentre studies. Whole-body MRI also shows promise as a method of assessing widespread tissue and joint involvement, though it currently requires more validation before routine clinical application.

Routine clinical practice

The EULAR recommendations state that 'US and MRI are superior to clinical examination in the detection of joint inflammation; these techniques should be considered for more accurate assessment of inflammation'.[3] MRI may be used in clinical practice to document improvement/worsening of disease activity. However important questions remain about when such imaging is needed, and when it is cost-effective. There is a lack of studies to document exactly how MRI should be used for this purpose. For instance, there is no need to do imaging to assess disease activity if the patient has obvious clinical signs of active RA and requires treatment intensification. Another important consideration is that the selection of method for providing more detailed information on the disease in the clinic depends on which expertise is present at that specific treatment centre. For instance, US can replace MRI for assessment of synovitis if an objective assessment of inflammation is needed. For assessment of inflammation in the bone (osteitis), MRI is, however, the only available modality, and it is also the best method, except for CT, for monitoring of progression of erosions.[38,39,49–51,73,82]

Predicting disease outcome

Several studies have demonstrated a predictive value of MRI-detected pathology in wrist and/or MCP joints for subsequent radiographic progression in bilateral hands, wrists, and feet. In particular BME is established as a strong independent predictor of subsequent radiographic progression in early RA.[42,83,84] Regression analyses in three-year and 5-year follow-up in two cohorts have documented that MRI bone oedema is a strong predictor of long-term (3, 5, and 11 year) radiographic progression.[85–87] Recent clinical trial data have confirmed this, and have documented that early treatment-induced changes in BME, and to some extent also synovitis, predict future radiographic progression.[88] Small studies have indicated a relationship of baseline MRI findings with long-term functional disability[89] and tendon rupture at 6 years.[90]

Thus, MRI in early RA is a useful method to predict patients with potentially worse outcomes, which may assist the clinician in the choice of treatment strategy. In agreement with this the EULAR recommendations for the use of imaging in the clinical management of RA state 'MRI bone edema is a strong independent predictor of subsequent radiographic progression in early RA and should be considered for use as a prognostic indicator'.[3] Thus, in clinical trials, presence of BME, or perhaps BME and and/or synovitis, could be used as inclusion criterion, to enrich the study population for patients with high risk of structural progression. Some studies suggest that presence of synovitis may also be used.

Utility in clinical remission

Another issue of high clinical importance is whether MRI is useful to predict the disease course in patients in clinical remission. MRI synovitis and BME are found frequently in patients in clinical remission,[91,92] These findings are significantly related to subsequent progressive structural damage.[93–95] In a cohort of routine care RA patients in sustained remission on biological disease-modifying antirheumatic drugs (bDMARDs), the bDMARD therapy was tapered according to a predefined treatment guideline. Successful tapering was independently predicted by ≤1 previous bDMARD, male gender, low baseline MRI combined inflammation score (synovitis, tenosynovitis, and bone marrow oedema) and/or combined damage score (erosion and joint space narrowing).[96] These encouraging results have already been acknowledged in

Box 19.2 MRI in RA: Areas of doubt and future research

- What is the role of MRI in clinical practice for predicting response to therapy and in defining remission in clinical practice?
- Which MRI parameters, and with which thresholds, will best guide treatment intervention?
- Should MRI form part of remission criteria?
- Will new MRI methods further improve discrimination of effective from less effective therapies in RA clinical trials?
- Will new MRI methods increase the utility and feasibility of MRI as diagnostic and monitoring tool in RA clinical practice?

international recommendations, with EULAR recommendations states that, 'MRI and US can detect inflammation that predicts subsequent joint damage, even when clinical remission is present'.[3]

The available data certainly suggest that imaging (with MRI or ultrasound) should be part of future remission criteria. It is important, however, to improve the evidence-base for incorporating modern imaging into future treat-to-target goals in RA.[97] That MRI inflammation exists where clinical detection has not found it (so-called subclinical inflammation) is beyond any doubt and documented by several studies. That such subclinical MRI/US inflammation is clinically important, in that it predicts subsequent structural damage progression *and/or* clinical flares during continued therapy *and/or* clinical flares in patients who taper/discontinue therapy, is the next step, for which there is also documentation. A study of 294 patients in clinical remission or low disease activity[95] indicates it may be possible to identify which patients will not (or at least are unlikely to) show radiographic progression. Moreover, a recent study indicates that MRI can help identifying patients in which tapering of biologics is safe.[96] However, no MRI studies have yet addressed to what extent subclinical MRI inflammation can be improved by additional treatment and whether this effort improves key endpoints, that is, whether an MRI-guided treatment strategy can improve subclinical inflammation and improve key outcomes over and above what is achieved by a strict treat-to-target therapy based on conventional clinical and biochemical examinations. However, a randomized controlled trial is ongoing.[97] The available data encourage further exploration of MRI for predicting the disease course and for evaluating disease status, including defining remission.

Conclusion

MRI is an increasingly available, sensitive technique which has documented utility in diagnosis, monitoring, and prognostication of patients with RA, and important new knowledge and technical improvements are continuously being acquired (Box 19.1). Nevertheless, there are still several questions regarding its optimal use in clinical trials and routine practice that need to be scientifically explored (Box 19.2).

Box 19.1 MRI in RA: Key recent advances

- The high sensitivity of MRI for a range of RA tissue pathologies means smaller numbers of patients will be required in clinical trials.
- Short-term changes on MRI predict long-term changes on radiography in RA, supporting the utility of MRI as a valid method for use in short-duration RCTs.
- The importance of MRI findings to patient-reported outcomes, such as functional disability and pain, has been documented.
- MRI in clinical remission has predictive value for successful tapering of bDMARDs
- New outcome techniques, including quantitative MRI techniques and whole-body MRI, offer opportunity for more responsive outcome measures.

REFERENCES

1. Combe B, Landewe R, Daien CI, et al. 2016 update of the EULAR recommendations for the management of early arthritis. *Ann Rheum Dis* 2017;76(6):948–59.

2. Smolen JS, Landewe R, Bijlsma J, et al. EULAR recommendations for the management of rheumatoid arthritis with synthetic and biological disease-modifying antirheumatic drugs: 2016 update. *Ann Rheum Dis* 2017;*76*(6):960–77.

3. Colebatch AN, Edwards CJ, Østergaard M, et al. EULAR recommendations for the use of imaging of the joints in the clinical management of rheumatoid arthritis. *Ann Rheum Dis* 2013;*72*(6):804–14.

4. Østergaard M, Pedersen SJ, Døhn UM. Imaging in rheumatoid arthritis--status and recent advances for magnetic resonance imaging, ultrasonography, computed tomography and conventional radiography. *Best Pract Res Clin Rheumatol* 2008;*22*(6):1019–44.

5. Taouli B, Zaim S, Peterfy CG, et al. Rheumatoid arthritis of the hand and wrist: comparison of three imaging techniques. *AJR Am J Roentgenol* 2004;*182*(4):937–43.

6. Ejbjerg BJ, Narvestad E, Jacobsen S, Thomsen HS, Østergaard M. Optimised, low cost, low field dedicated extremity MRI is highly specific and sensitive for synovitis and bone erosions in rheumatoid arthritis wrist and finger joints: comparison with conventional high field MRI and radiography. *Ann Rheum Dis* 2005;*64*(9):1280–7.

7. Eshed I, Krabbe S, Østergaard M, et al. Influence of field strength, coil type and image resolution on assessment of synovitis by unenhanced MRI--a comparison with contrast-enhanced MRI. *Eur Radiol* 2015;*25*(4):1059–67.

8. Krabbe S, Eshed I, Pedersen SJ, et al. Bone marrow oedema assessment by magnetic resonance imaging in rheumatoid arthritis wrist and metacarpophalangeal joints: the importance of field strength, coil type and image resolution. *Rheumatology (Oxf)* 2014;*53*(8):1446–51.

9. Østergaard M, Peterfy CG, Bird P, et al. The OMERACT rheumatoid arthritis magnetic resonance imaging (MRI) scoring system: updated recommendations by the OMERACT MRI in Arthritis Working Group. *J Rheumatol* 2017;*44*(11):1706–12.

10. Sudol-Szopinska I, Jurik AG, Eshed I, et al. Recommendations of the ESSR Arthritis Subcommittee for the Use of Magnetic Resonance Imaging in Musculoskeletal Rheumatic Diseases. *Semin Musculoskelet Radiol* 2015;*19*(4):396–411.

11. Glinatsi D, Bird P, Gandjbakhch F, et al. Validation of the OMERACT Psoriatic Arthritis Magnetic Resonance Imaging Score (PsAMRIS) for the hand and foot in a randomized placebo-controlled trial. *J Rheumatol* 2015;*42*(12):2473–9.

12. Østergaard M, Conaghan PG, O'Connor P, et al. Reducing invasiveness, duration, and cost of magnetic resonance imaging in rheumatoid arthritis by omitting intravenous contrast injection—does it change the assessment of inflammatory and destructive joint changes by the OMERACT RAMRIS? *J Rheumatol* 2009;*36*(8):1806–10.

13. Del Grande F, Santini F, Herzka DA, et al. Fat-suppression techniques for 3-T MR imaging of the musculoskeletal system. *Radiographics* 2014;*34*(1):217–33.

14. Axelsen MB, Eshed I, Duer-Jensen A, Moller JM, Pedersen SJ, Østergaard M. Whole-body MRI assessment of disease activity and structural damage in rheumatoid arthritis: first step towards an MRI joint count. *Rheumatology (Oxf)* 2014;*53*(5):845–53.

15. Weckbach S, Schewe S, Michaely HJ, Steffinger D, Reiser MF, Glaser C. Whole-body MR imaging in psoriatic arthritis: additional value for therapeutic decision making. *Eur J Radiol* 2011;*77*(1):149–55.

16. Krabbe S, Østergaard M, Eshed I, et al. Whole-body magnetic resonance imaging in axial spondyloarthritis: reduction of sacroiliac, spinal, and entheseal inflammation in a placebo-controlled trial of adalimumab. *J Rheumatol* 2018;*45*(5):621–9.

17. Østergaard M, Eshed I, Althoff CE, et al. Whole-body magnetic resonance imaging in inflammatory arthritis: systematic literature review and first steps toward standardization and an OMERACT scoring system. *J Rheumatol* 2017;*44*(11):1699–705.

18. Axelsen MB, Stoltenberg M, Poggenborg RP, et al. Dynamic gadolinium-enhanced magnetic resonance imaging allows accurate assessment of the synovial inflammatory activity in rheumatoid arthritis knee joints: a comparison with synovial histology. *Scand J Rheumatol* 2012;*41*(2):89–94.

19. Humby F, Mahto A, Ahmed M, et al. The relationship between synovial pathobiology and magnetic resonance imaging abnormalities in rheumatoid arthritis: a systematic review. *J Rheumatol* 2017;*44*(9):1311–24.

20. Boesen M, Kubassova O, Bouert R, et al. Correlation between computer-aided dynamic gadolinium-enhanced MRI assessment of inflammation and semi-quantitative synovitis and bone marrow oedema scores of the wrist in patients with rheumatoid arthritis--a cohort study. *Rheumatology (Oxf)* 2012;*51*(1):134–43.

21. Waterton JC, Ho M, Nordenmark LH, et al. Repeatability and response to therapy of dynamic contrast-enhanced magnetic resonance imaging biomarkers in rheumatoid arthritis in a large multicentre trial setting. *Eur Radiol* 2017;*27*(9):3662–8.

22. Østergaard M, Hansen M, Stoltenberg M, Lorenzen I. Quantitative assessment of the synovial membrane in the rheumatoid wrist: an easily obtained MRI score reflects the synovial volume. *Br J Rheumatol* 1996;*35*(10):965–71.

23. Østergaard M, Stoltenberg M, Løvgreen-Nielsen P, Volck B, Jensen CH, Lorenzen I. Magnetic resonance imaging-determined synovial membrane and joint effusion volumes in rheumatoid arthritis and osteoarthritis: comparison with the macroscopic and microscopic appearance of the synovium. *Arthritis Rheum* 1997;*40*(10):1856–67.

24. Conaghan PG, Østergaard M, Bowes MA, et al. Comparing the effects of tofacitinib, methotrexate and the combination, on bone marrow oedema, synovitis and bone erosion in methotrexate-naive, early active rheumatoid arthritis: results of an exploratory randomised MRI study incorporating semiquantitative and quantitative techniques. *Ann Rheum Dis* 2016;*75*(6):1024–33.

25. ESUR Contrast Media Safety Committee. *ESUR Guidelines on Nephrogenic Systemic Fibrosis. ESUR Guidelines on Contrast Media*, 9.0 ed. Vienna, Austria: ESUR Office, 2014, pp. 16–18.

26. Østergaard M, Peterfy C, Conaghan P, et al.; OMERACT Rheumatoid Arthritis Magnetic Resonance Imaging Studies. Core set of MRI acquisitions, joint pathology definitions, and the OMERACT RA-MRI scoring system. *J Rheumatol* 2003;*30*(6):1385–6.

27. Østergaard M, McQueen F, Wiell C, et al. The OMERACT Psoriatic Arthritis Magnetic Resonance Imaging Scoring System (PsAMRIS): definitions of key pathologies, suggested MRI sequences, and preliminary scoring system for PsA Hands. *J Rheumatol* 2009;*36*(8):1816–24.

28. Ostendorf B, Peters R, Dann P, et al. Magnetic resonance imaging and miniarthroscopy of metacarpophalangeal joints: sensitive detection of morphologic changes in rheumatoid arthritis. *Arthritis Rheum* 2001;*44*(11):2492–502.

29. Partik B, Rand T, Pretterklieber ML, Voracek M, Hoermann M, Helbich TH. Patterns of gadopentetate-enhanced MR imaging of radiocarpal joints of healthy subjects. *AJR Am J Roentgenol* 2002;*179*(1):193–7.

30. Tan AL, Tanner SF, Conaghan PG, et al. Role of metacarpophalangeal joint anatomic factors in the distribution of synovitis and bone erosion in early rheumatoid arthritis. *Arthritis Rheum* 2003;*48*(5):1214–22.

31. Ejbjerg B, Narvestad E, Rostrup E, et al. Magnetic resonance imaging of wrist and finger joints in healthy subjects occasionally shows changes resembling erosions and synovitis as seen in rheumatoid arthritis. *Arthritis Rheum* 2004;*50*(4):1097–106.

32. Mangnus L, Schoones JW, van der Helm-van Mil AH. What is the prevalence of MRI-detected inflammation and erosions in small joints in the general population? A collation and analysis of published data. *RMD Open* 2015;*1*(1):e000005.

33. Burgers LE, Nieuwenhuis WP, van Steenbergen HW, et al. Magnetic resonance imaging-detected inflammation is associated with functional disability in early arthritis-results of a cross-sectional study. *Rheumatology (Oxf)* 2016;*55*(12):2167–75.

34. Rubens DJ, Blebea JS, Totterman SMS, Hooper MM. Rheumatoid arthritis: evaluation of wrist extensor tendons with clinical examination versus MR imaging—a preliminary report. *Radiology* 1993;*187*:831–8.

35. Rominger MB, Bernreuter WK, Kenney PJ, Morgan SL, Blackburn WD, Alarcon GS. MR imaging of the hands in early rheumatoid arthritis: preliminary results. *Radiographics* 1993;*13*:37–46.

36. McQueen FM, Stewart N, Crabbe J, et al. Magnetic resonance imaging of the wrist in early rheumatoid arthritis reveals a high prevalence of erosion at four months after symptom onset. *Ann Rheum Dis* 1998;*57*:350–6.

37. Klarlund M, Østergaard M, Jensen KE, Madsen JL, Skjødt H, the TIRA group. Magnetic resonance imaging, radiography, and scintigraphy of the finger joints: one year follow up of patients with early arthritis. *Ann Rheum Dis* 2000;*59*(7):521–8.

38. McQueen FM, Gao A, Østergaard M, et al. High-grade MRI bone oedema is common within the surgical field in rheumatoid arthritis patients undergoing joint replacement and is associated with osteitis in subchondral bone. *Ann Rheum Dis* 2007;*66*(12):1581–7.

39. Jimenez-Boj E, Nobauer-Huhmann I, Hanslik-Schnabel B, et al. Bone erosions and bone marrow edema as defined by magnetic resonance imaging reflect true bone marrow inflammation in rheumatoid arthritis. *Arthritis Rheum* 2007;*56*(4):1118–24.

40. McQueen FM, Stewart N, Crabbe J, et al. Magnetic resonance imaging of the wrist in early rheumatoid arthritis reveals progression of erosions despite clinical improvement. *Ann Rheum Dis* 1999;*58*:156–63.

41. Conaghan PG, O'Connor P, McGonagle D, et al. Elucidation of the relationship between synovitis and bone damage: a randomized magnetic resonance imaging study of individual joints in patients with early rheumatoid arthritis. *Arthritis Rheum* 2003;*48*(1):64–71.

42. Hetland ML, Ejbjerg B, Hørslev-Petersen K, et al. MRI bone oedema is the strongest predictor of subsequent radiographic progression in early rheumatoid arthritis. Results from a 2-year randomised controlled trial (CIMESTRA). *Ann Rheum Dis* 2009;*68*(3):384–90.

43. McGonagle D, Gibbon W, Emery P. Classification of inflammatory arthritis by enthesitis. *Lancet* 1998;*352*:1137–40.

44. Peterfy CG, van Dijke CF, Lu Y, et al. Quantification of the volume of articular cartilage in the metacarpophalangeal joints of the hand: accuracy and precision of three-dimensional MR imaging. *Am J Roentgenol* 1995;*165*:371–5.

45. Peterfy CG, Olech E, DiCarlo JC, Merrill JT, Countryman PJ, Gaylis NB. Monitoring cartilage loss in the hands and wrists in rheumatoid arthritis with magnetic resonance imaging in a multi-center clinical trial: IMPRESS (NCT00425932). *Arthritis Res Ther* 2013;*15*(2):R44.

46. Peterfy C, Emery P, Tak PP, et al. MRI assessment of suppression of structural damage in patients with rheumatoid arthritis receiving rituximab: results from the randomised, placebo-controlled, double-blind RA-SCORE study. *Ann Rheum Dis* 2016;*75*(1):170–7.

47. Døhn UM, Conaghan PG, Eshed I, Boonen A, Bøyesen P, Peterfy CG, et al. The OMERACT-RAMRIS rheumatoid arthritis magnetic resonance imaging joint space narrowing score: intrareader and interreader reliability and agreement with computed tomography and conventional radiography. *J Rheumatol* 2014;*41*(2):392–7.

48. Lindegaard H, Vallø J, Hørslev-Petersen K, Junker P, Østergaard M. Low field dedicated magnetic resonance imaging in untreated rheumatoid arthritis of recent onset. *Ann Rheum Dis* 2001;*60*(8):770–6.

49. Østergaard M, Hansen M, Stoltenberg M, et al. New radiographic bone erosions in the wrists of patients with rheumatoid arthritis are detectable with magnetic resonance imaging a median of two years earlier. *Arthritis Rheum* 2003;*48*(8):2128–31.

50. Døhn UM, Ejbjerg BJ, Court-Payen, et al. Are bone erosions detected by magnetic resonance imaging and ultrasonography true erosions? A comparison with computed tomography in rheumatoid arthritis metacarpophalangeal joints. *Arthritis Res Ther* 2006;*8*(4):R110.

51. Døhn UM, Ejbjerg BJ, Hasselquist M, et al. Detection of bone erosions in rheumatoid arthritis wrist joints with magnetic resonance imaging, computed tomography and radiography. *Arthritis Res Ther* 2008;*10*(1):R25.

52. Østergaard M, Gideon P, Sørensen K, et al. Scoring of synovial membrane hypertrophy and bone erosions by MR imaging in clinically active and inactive rheumatoid arthritis of the wrist. *Scand J Rheumatol* 1995;*24*(4):212–18.

53. Conaghan P, Edmonds J, Emery P, et al. Magnetic resonance imaging in rheumatoid arthritis: summary of OMERACT activities, current status, and plans. *J Rheumatol* 2001;*28*(5):1158–62.

54. Østergaard M, Haavardsholm EA. Imaging: MRI in healthy volunteers—important to do, and do correctly. *Nat Rev Rheumatol* 2016;*12*(10):563–4.

55. Stiskal MA, Neuhold A, Szolar DH, et al. Rheumatoid arthritis of the craniocervical region by MR imaging: detection and characterization. *Am J Roentgenol* 1995;*165*:585–92.

56. Oostveen JC, Roozeboom AR, van de Laar MA, Heeres J, den Boer JA, Lindeboom SF. Functional turbo spin echo magnetic resonance imaging versus tomography for evaluating cervical spine involvement in rheumatoid arthritis. *Spine* 1998;*23*(11):1237–44.

57. Reijnierse M, Dijkmans BA, Hansen B, et al. Neurologic dysfunction in patients with rheumatoid arthritis of the cervical spine. Predictive value of clinical, radiographic and MR imaging parameters. *Eur Radiol* 2001;*11*(3):467–73.

58. Hamilton JD, Johnston RA, Madhok R, Capell HA. Factors predictive of subsequent deterioration in rheumatoid cervical myelopathy. *Rheumatology (Oxf)* 2001;*40*(7):811–15.

59. Baker JF, Conaghan PG, Emery P, Baker DG, Østergaard M. Relationship of patient-reported outcomes with MRI measures in rheumatoid arthritis. *Ann Rheum Dis* 2016;*76*(3):486–90.

60. Glinatsi D, Baker JF, Hetland ML, et al. Magnetic resonance imaging assessed inflammation in the wrist is associated with patient-reported physical impairment, global assessment of disease activity and pain in early rheumatoid arthritis: longitudinal results from two randomised controlled trials. *Ann Rheum Dis* 2017;76(10):1707–15.

61. Glinatsi D. Magnetic resonance imaging in rheumatoid arthritis: validation of tenosynovitis and joint space narrowing scoring systems and the impact of inflammation and structural damage on patient-reported outcomes (PhD thesis). Copenhagen, Denmark: University of Copenhagen 2018.

62. Tamai M, Kawakami A, Uetani M, et al. A prediction rule for disease outcome in patients with undifferentiated arthritis using magnetic resonance imaging of the wrists and finger joints and serologic autoantibodies. *Arthritis Care Res* 2009;61(6):772–8.

63. Duer-Jensen A, Hørslev-Petersen K, et al. Bone edema on magnetic resonance imaging is an independent predictor of rheumatoid arthritis development in patients with early undifferentiated arthritis. *Arthritis Rheum* 2011;63(8):2192–202.

64. Nieuwenhuis WP, van Steenbergen HW, Mangnus L, et al. Evaluation of the diagnostic accuracy of hand and foot MRI for early rheumatoid arthritis. *Rheumatology (Oxf)* 2017;56(8):1367–77.

65. Duer A, Østergaard M, Hørslev-Petersen K, Vallø J. Magnetic resonance imaging and bone scintigraphy in the differential diagnosis of unclassified arthritis. *Ann Rheum Dis* 2008;67(1):48–51.

66. Aletaha D, Neogi T, Silman AJ, et al. 2010 rheumatoid arthritis classification criteria: an American College of Rheumatology/European League Against Rheumatism collaborative initiative. *Ann Rheum Dis* 2010;69(9):1580–8.

67. Østergaard M. Clarification of the role of ultrasonography, magnetic resonance imaging and conventional radiography in the ACR/EULAR 2010 rheumatoid arthritis classification criteria—comment to the article by Aletaha et al. *Ann Rheum Dis* 2010;e-letter:Published Online 2 December 2010.

68. Aletaha D, Hawker G, Neogi T, Silman A. Re: clarification of the role of ultrasonography, magnetic resonance imaging and conventional radiography in the ACR/EULAR 2010 rheumatoid arthritis classification criteria—Reply to comment to the article by Aletaha et al. *Ann Rheum Dis* 2011;E-letter:Published online 11 January 2011.

69. Østergaard M, Bøyesen P, Eshed I, et al. Development and preliminary validation of a magnetic resonance imaging joint space narrowing score for use in rheumatoid arthritis: potential adjunct to the OMERACT RA MRI scoring system. *J Rheumatol* 2011;38(9):2045–50.

70. Haavardsholm EA, Østergaard M, Ejbjerg BJ, et al. Reliability and sensitivity to change of the OMERACT rheumatoid arthritis magnetic resonance imaging score in a multireader, longitudinal setting. *Arthritis Rheum* 2005;52(12):3860–7.

71. Østergaard M, Edmonds J, McQueen F, et al. The EULAR-OMERACT rheumatoid arthritis MRI reference image atlas. *Ann Rheum Dis* 2005;64 Suppl 1:i2–i55.

72. Haavardsholm EA, Østergaard M, Hammer HB, et al. Monitoring anti-TNF-alpha treatment in rheumatoid arthritis: responsiveness of magnetic resonance imaging and ultrasonography of the dominant wrist joint compared with conventional measures of disease activity and structural damage. *Ann Rheum Dis* 2009;68(10):1572–9.

73. Ejbjerg BJ, Vestergaard A, Jacobsen S, Thomsen HS, Østergaard M. The smallest detectable difference and sensitivity to change of magnetic resonance imaging and radiographic scoring of structural joint damage in rheumatoid arthritis finger, wrist, and toe joints: a comparison of the OMERACT rheumatoid arthritis magnetic resonance imaging score applied to different joint combinations and the Sharp/van der Heijde radiographic score. *Arthritis Rheum* 2005;52(8):2300–6.

74. Quinn MA, Conaghan PG, O'Connor PJ, et al. Very early treatment with infliximab in addition to methotrexate in early, poor-prognosis rheumatoid arthritis reduces magnetic resonance imaging evidence of synovitis and damage, with sustained benefit after infliximab withdrawal: results from a twelve-month randomized, double-blind, placebo-controlled trial. *Arthritis Rheum* 2005;52(1):27–35.

75. Østergaard M, Emery P, Conaghan PG, et al. Significant improvement in synovitis, osteitis, and bone erosion following golimumab and methotrexate combination therapy as compared with methotrexate alone: a magnetic resonance imaging study of 318 methotrexate-naive rheumatoid arthritis patients. *Arthritis Rheum* 2011;63(12):3712–22.

76. Baker JF, Conaghan PG, Emery P, Baker DG, Østergaard M. Validity of early MRI structural damage end points and potential impact on clinical trial design in rheumatoid arthritis. *Ann Rheum Dis* 2016;75(6):1114–19.

77. Peterfy C, Østergaard M, Conaghan PG. MRI comes of age in RA clinical trials. *Ann Rheum Dis* 2013;72(6):794–6.

78. Døhn UM, Ejbjerg BJ, Hasselquist M, et al. Rheumatoid arthritis bone erosion volumes on CT and MRI: reliability and correlations with erosion scores on CT, MRI and radiography. *Ann Rheum Dis* 2007;66(10):1388–92.

79. American College of Rheumatology Rheumatoid Arthritis Clinical Trials Task Force Imaging Group and Outcome Measures in Rheumatology Magnetic Resonance Imaging Inflammatory Arthritis Working Group. Review: the utility of magnetic resonance imaging for assessing structural damage in randomized controlled trials in rheumatoid arthritis. *Arthritis Rheum* 2013;65(10):2513–23.

80. Boers M, Brooks P, Strand CV, Tugwell P. The OMERACT filter for Outcome Measures in Rheumatology. *J Rheumatol* 1998;25(2):198–9.

81. Peterfy C, Strand V, Tian L, et al. Short-term changes on MRI predict long-term changes on radiography in rheumatoid arthritis: an analysis by an OMERACT Task Force of pooled data from four randomised controlled trials. *Ann Rheum Dis* 2017;76(6):992–7.

82. Døhn UM, Ejbjerg B, Boonen A, et al. No overall progression and occasional repair of erosions despite persistent inflammation in adalimumab-treated rheumatoid arthritis patients: results from a longitudinal comparative MRI, ultrasonography, CT and radiography study. *Ann Rheum Dis* 2011;70(2):252–8.

83. Haavardsholm EA, Bøyesen P, Østergaard M, Schildvold A, Kvien TK. Magnetic resonance imaging findings in 84 patients with early rheumatoid arthritis: bone marrow oedema predicts erosive progression. *Ann Rheum Dis* 2008;67(6):794–800.

84. Nieuwenhuis WP, van Steenbergen HW, Stomp W, et al. The course of bone marrow edema in early undifferentiated arthritis and rheumatoid arthritis: a longitudinal magnetic resonance imaging study at bone level. *Arthritis Rheumatol* 2016;68(5):1080–8.

85. Bøyesen P, Haavardsholm EA, Østergaard M, van der Heijde D, Sesseng S, Kvien TK. MRI in early rheumatoid arthritis: synovitis and bone marrow oedema are independent predictors of subsequent radiographic progression. *Ann Rheum Dis* 2011;70(3):428–33.

86. Hetland ML, Stengaard-Pedersen K, Junker P, et al. Radiographic progression and remission rates in early rheumatoid arthritis—MRI bone oedema and anti-CCP predicted radiographic progression in the 5-year extension of the double-blind randomised CIMESTRA trial. *Ann Rheum Dis* 2010;*69*(10):1789–95.

87. Hetland ML, Østergaard M, Stengaard-Pedersen K, et al. Anti-cyclic citrullinated peptide antibodies, 28-joint Disease Activity Score, and magnetic resonance imaging bone oedema at baseline predict 11 years' functional and radiographic outcome in early rheumatoid arthritis. *Scand J Rheumatol* 2019;*48*(1):1–8.

88. Baker JF, Østergaard M, Emery P, et al. Early MRI measures independently predict 1-year and 2-year radiographic progression in rheumatoid arthritis: secondary analysis from a large clinical trial. *Ann Rheum Dis* 2014;*73*(11):1968–74.

89. Benton N, Stewart N, Crabbe J, Robinson E, Yeoman S, McQueen F. MRI of the wrist in early rheumatoid arthritis can be used to predict functional outcome at 6 years. *Ann Rheum Dis* 2004;*63*:555–61.

90. McQueen F, Beckley V, Crabbe J, Robinson E, Yeoman S, Stewart N. Magnetic resonance imaging evidence of tendinopathy in early rheumatoid arthritis predicts tendon rupture at six years. *Arthritis Rheum* 2005;*52*(3):744–51.

91. Brown AK, Quinn MA, Karim Z, et al. Presence of significant synovitis in rheumatoid arthritis patients with disease-modifying antirheumatic drug-induced clinical remission: evidence from an imaging study may explain structural progression. *Arthritis Rheum* 2006;*54*(12):3761–73.

92. Gandjbakhch F, Conaghan PG, Ejbjerg B, et al. Synovitis and osteitis are very frequent in rheumatoid arthritis clinical remission: results from an MRI study of 294 patients in clinical remission or low disease activity state. *J Rheumatol* 2011;*38*(9):2039–44.

93. Brown AK, Conaghan PG, Karim Z, et al. An explanation for the apparent dissociation between clinical remission and continued structural deterioration in rheumatoid arthritis. *Arthritis Rheum* 2008;*58*:2958–67.

94. Gandjbakhch F, Foltz V, Mallet A, Bourgeois P, Fautrel B. Bone marrow oedema predicts structural progression in a 1-year follow-up of 85 patients with RA in remission or with low disease activity with low-field MRI. *Ann Rheum Dis* 2011;*70*(12):2159–62.

95. Gandjbakhch F, Haavardsholm EA, Conaghan PG, et al. Determining a magnetic resonance imaging inflammatory activity acceptable state without subsequent radiographic progression in rheumatoid arthritis: results from a follow-up MRI study of 254 patients in clinical remission or low disease activity. *J Rheumatol* 2014;*41*(2):398–406.

96. Brahe CH, Krabbe S, Østergaard M, et al. Dose tapering and discontinuation of biological therapy in rheumatoid arthritis patients in routine care—2-year outcomes and predictors. *Rheumatology (Oxf)* 2019;*58*(1):110–19.

97. Moller-Bisgaard S, Hørslev-Petersen K, Ejbjerg BJ, et al. Impact of a magnetic resonance imaging-guided treat-to-target strategy on disease activity and progression in patients with rheumatoid arthritis (the IMAGINE-RA trial): study protocol for a randomized controlled trial. *Trials* 2015;*16*:178.

SECTION 5
Impact on life

20 Patient physical function in rheumatoid arthritis *221*

Kathryn A. Gibson and Theodore Pincus

21 Fatigue *251*

Emma Dures and Neil Basu

22 Health economics of rheumatoid arthritis *259*

David L. Scott and Allan Wailoo

23 Rheumatoid arthritis and work *271*

Suzanne Verstappen, Cheryl Jones, Abdullah Houssien, and James Galloway

Patient physical function in rheumatoid arthritis

Kathryn A. Gibson and Theodore Pincus

Introduction

Patient physical function in rheumatoid arthritis (RA) traditionally was recorded in the medical record as 'subjective' narrative descriptions, in contrast to 'objective' laboratory tests, radiographs, and other data from high technology sources. In the absence of quantitative scores for physical function, it was suggested (accurately) in 1983 that 'clinicians may all too easily spend years writing 'doing well' in the notes of a patient who has become progressively crippled before their eyes'.[1] This view has been revised considerably over the last 30 years to recognize RA as a potentially severe disease, based on evidence of declines in physical function[2] in most patients, as well as frequent radiographic damage[3] and work disability.[4] At this time, RA is approached with an emphasis on early intervention to implement a treat-to-target strategy based on effective clinical measurement,[5] including physical function.

Of course, biomarkers and imaging data have contributed invaluably to understanding pathogenesis and development of new treatments for RA,[6,7] and possible control and even cure will emerge from basic laboratory research. However, RA biomarkers have limited clinical value to guide patient diagnosis, management, and prognosis. Tests for rheumatoid factor,[8–10] anticitrullinated protein antibodies (ACPA),[9,11] erythrocyte sedimentation rate (ESR) and C-reactive protein (CRP) are normal or negative in 30–50% of patients with RA.[9,12] All these tests are less significant in prognosis of long-term work disability and premature mortality than patient physical function assessed on a self-report questionnaire.[13]

RA differs from many other chronic diseases in the importance of information derived from the medical history and physical examination compared to laboratory tests and ancillary studies in clinical decisions concerning diagnosis and management.[14] A survey of 313 physicians (154 rheumatologists and 159 non-rheumatologists) indicated that the most prominent component of a clinical encounter in decisions concerning diagnosis and management in eight chronic diseases was vital signs in hypertension, laboratory tests in diabetes and hyperlipidaemia, and ancillary studies in lymphoma, pulmonary fibrosis, ulcerative colitis, and congestive heart failure. RA was the only one of the eight chronic conditions in which a patient history accounted for more than 50% of the information required for diagnosis and management.[14]

Self-report questionnaire scores for physical function are included in all contemporary clinical trials, required by regulatory agencies to document improvement. Ironically, only a minority of rheumatologists have adopted this practice in usual clinical care, although use appears to be increasing.[15] The only quantitative data in routine care medical records of many, if not most, patients of rheumatologists are laboratory tests, limitations of which led to the RA core data set and indices.[6,16] This chapter summarizes the scientific rationale and pragmatic advantages of patient self-report questionnaires in routine care. Four widely used patient questionnaires are presented in some detail, the Health Assessment Questionnaire (HAQ),[17] its multidimensional version MDHAQ,[18,19] short-form 36 (SF-36),[20] and Patient-Reported Outcomes Measurement Information Systems (PROMIS).[21] Further discussion concerns associations of physical function scores with other RA measures, and complexities in use and interpretation of physical function questionnaire scores in research and routine clinical care.

Overview of patient self-report questionnaires to assess physical function

Advantages of patient physical function scores as quantitative, standardized, informative 'scientific' data

Contemporary self-report questionnaire scores for physical function, as well as pain, global status, fatigue, and other patient problems are quantitative, standard, valid, and reproducible measures from a patient history, which may be regarded as providing data according to the 'scientific' method. These data often are more informative than laboratory tests and other high technology data[22,23] clinically in RA patients, in assessment, prognosis, monitoring, and outcomes. The scientific rationale to include a patient questionnaire in clinical care is supported by extensive evidence, summarized briefly here (Box 20.1).

A measure of physical function in RA is more significant than abnormal laboratory tests or radiographic scores in the prognosis of premature mortality[2,13,24–29] (Figure 20.1), confirmed in a review of all 53 RA cohorts which included prognostic variables for RA mortality[13,30] (Figure 20.2). Severe RA according to quantitative patient

Box 20.1 Scientific advantages of a self-report questionnaire measure of physical function

1 Physical function predicts mortality and work disability, at far greater significance than lab tests or X-rays.[35,37-39]

2 Physical function scores and other patient measures are as efficient as joint counts and laboratory tests to distinguish active from control treatments in clinical trials involving certolizumab, methotrexate, leflunomide, anakinra, adalimumab, abatacept, and infliximab[40-43,48,49].

3 Patient self-report scores for physical function are more reproducible than formal joint counts.[52-58]

4 Physical function and pain scores are more likely to be abnormal in new RA patients than ESR.[59]

5 Physical function scores are more informative than ESR to document incomplete responses to methotrexate with initiation of a biological agent in RA.[60]

6 An index of patient self-report scores for physical function, pain, and global assessment are correlated significantly with joint counts and laboratory tests, and indices of only patient self-report scores are correlated with traditional indices in clinical trials[44,48,49] and usual clinical care,[44,45] including categories for high, moderate, low severity and remission, as targets for a treat-to-target strategy for RA.[48,49]

7 Patient self-report physical function scores and indices are informative in patients with many rheumatic diseases beyond RA,[61] including osteo-arthritis,[61] systemic lupus erythematosus,[61,62] ankylosing spondylitis,[61,63-66] psoriatic arthritis,[61] gout,[61] vasculitis,[67] polymyalgia rheumatica,[68] and others.

Self-report physical function scores also are more significant than laboratory tests or radiographs to predict most other severe long-term outcomes of RA, including work disability,[2,4,33-35] costs,[36,37] and joint replacement surgery.[38] Radiographic progression is the only major RA outcome predicted by laboratory tests, including rheumatoid factor, elevated ESR, elevated CRP, and the shared epitope of the major histocompatibility locus.[39] However, physical function scores are far more significant than these laboratory tests (or radiographic progression) in prognosis of other severe RA outcomes.

Patient self-report questionnaire scores are as efficient as formal joint counts or laboratory tests to distinguish active from control treatments in RA clinical trials[48,49] (**Figure 20.4**). An index of scores for physical function, pain, and patient global assessment, RAPID3 (Routine Assessment of Patient Index Data),[44,45] is correlated significantly with other indices of RA disease activity such as DAS28 (disease activity score 28)[46] and CDAI (clinical disease activity index),[47] and provides similar results in clinical trials and clinical care.[44,45,48-50] RAPID3 identifies patients in categories of high, moderate, low disease severity and remission similarly to DAS28 and CDAI,[48-50] as well as ACR/EULAR (American College of Rheumatology/European League against Rheumatism) Criteria for remission.[51]

Patient self-report scores are more reproducible than formal joint counts[52-58] (**Box 20.1**), in large part because a single observer (in this case the patient) is likely more consistent than two observers (a joint count has input from both doctor and patient).[58] Physical function and pain scores are more likely to be abnormal in new RA patients than ESR,[59] and more informative than ESR to document incomplete responses to methotrexate at initiation of a biological agent in RA.[60] MDHAQ/RAPID3 identifies improvement or worsening of patient

physical function scores has been documented (30 years ago) to be associated with premature mortality in RA with 50% 5-year survival, similar to Stage IV Hodgkin's disease or three-vessel atherosclerotic cardiovascular disease[31] (**Figure 20.1**). In a normal elderly cohort in Finland, poor physical function scores are as likely to predict 5-year mortality as smoking (**Figure 20.3**).[32]

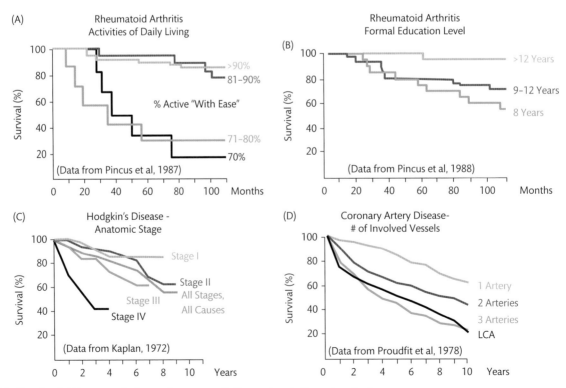

Figure 20.1 Showing 9–10-year survival according to quantitative markers in three chronic diseases

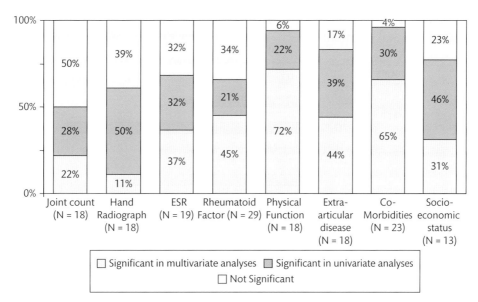

Figure 20.2 Significance of eight variables as predictors of mortality in RA in 84 published cohorts.
Source: data from Sokka T, Abelson B, and Pincus T (2008) 'Mortality in rheumatoid arthritis: 2008 update'. *Clin Exp Rheumatol* 26 (Suppl. 51):S35–S61.

status over time in patients with many rheumatic diseases beyond RA,[61] including osteoarthritis,[61] systemic lupus erythematosus,[61,62] ankylosing spondylitis,[61,63–66] psoriatic arthritis,[61] gout,[61] vasculitis,[67] polymyalgia rheumatica,[68] and others.[61] Therefore, patient self-report scores appear as 'scientific' as laboratory tests,[22] and the rationale to collect patient questionnaire data in all patients to assess their status at all routine care visits appears as strong as a rationale for routine laboratory tests[69].

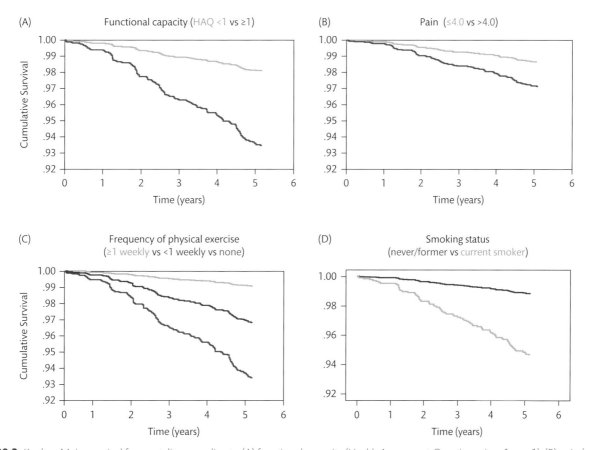

Figure 20.3 Kaplan–Meier survival for mortality according to (A) functional capacity (Health Assessment Questionnaire ≥1 vs. <1), (B) pain (>4.0 vs. ≤4.0), (C) frequency of physical exercise, and (D) smoking status, over 5 years.
Reprinted from Sokka T and Pincus T (2011) 'Poor physical function, pain and limited exercise: risk factors for premature mortality in the range of smoking or hypertension, identified on a simple patient self-report questionnaire for usual care'. *BMJ Open* 1:e000070 doi:10.1136/bmjopen-2011-000070 with permission from the BMJ Publishing Group.

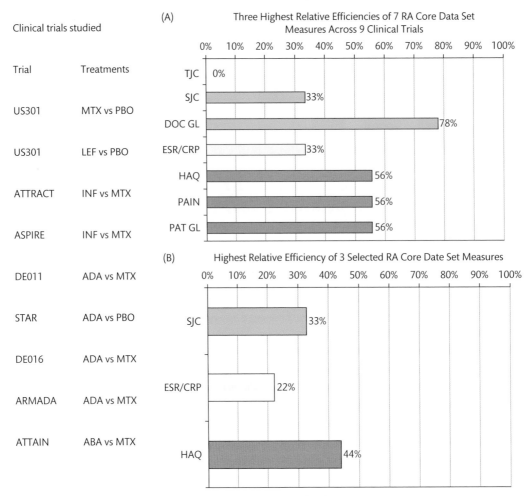

Figure 20.4 Relative efficiencies of seven core data set measures in nine RA clinical trials.

Source: Data from Pincus T, Richardson B, Strand V, Bergman MJ. Relative efficiencies of the 7 rheumatoid arthritis Core Data Set measures to distinguish active from control treatments in 9 comparisons from clinical trials of 5 agents. *Clin Exp Rheumatol* 2014;32 Suppl *85*(5):47–54.

Pragmatic advantages of routine use of patient questionnaires to assess physical function and other patient scores

Even if patient questionnaires did not provide any of the scientific advantages presented here, patient self-report questionnaires in routine care can be associated with pragmatic advantages to both health professionals and patients, particularly if a feasible questionnaire is given to the patient by the receptionist upon registration.[70] The patient does most of the work to summarize many elements of the medical history that traditionally require extensive conversation. A simple 'eyeball' review by a health professional of a completed patient questionnaire can provide information in 10–15 seconds that otherwise would require 10–15 minutes of conversation. This activity can save at least 2–3 minutes at most encounters, particularly use of a Multidimensional Health Assessment Questionnaire (MDHAQ),[18,71] which includes a self-report joint count, 60 symptom checklist, and 10 queries about recent medical history.

Completion of a questionnaire by the patient facilitates preparation of the patient for the visit, setting in effect, an 'agenda' for the encounter. Although 5–10 minutes of the patient's time and 10–15 seconds of the doctor's time are required, available information results in the saving of time through provision of factual information much

of which is negative or well-known but must be documented.[72] It must be emphasized that the patient questionnaire does not replace conversation between doctor and patient, but serves to enhance its value through focus on the primary concerns of both. Furthermore, self-report of medical history information **always** requires interpretation by a knowledgeable health professional, as is the case with a laboratory test, ultrasound, or any measure in clinical care.

Historical considerations—early quantitative assessment of patient physical function

In 1949, Steinbrocker and colleagues introduced two simple 1–4 quantitative scales to assess physical function and radiographic damage.[73] A physician-assigned global American Rheumatism Association (ARA)—now the American College of Rheumatology (ACR)—functional class on a 1–4 scale is quite robust in cross-sectional analyses of RA patients as the most representative of all available measures of clinical status,[74] including joint counts, radiographs, laboratory tests, performance measures, and patient questionnaire scores concerning physical function. However, this global measure, as any four-point scale, is severely limited to recognize potentially clinically important changes in patient function over time, as patient status may change considerably without change of

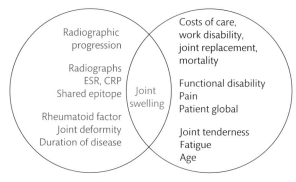

Figure 20.5 Strength of relationship between various measures used to assess RA and different disease outcomes.

the category to which a patient is assigned.[75,76] Therefore, 1–4 global scales are used infrequently at this time, other than in survey research, and have been supplanted by 0–10 scales in most clinical research and clinical care.

Performance measures of patient function in specific activities, such as grip strength,[77] walking time,[78] button test,[79] Jepsen hand function,[80,81] and others,[82] were introduced in the 1950s and 1960s. Some of these measures, notably grip strength, walking time, and button test have been termed 'rheumatology function tests'.[83] These measures were found to distinguish active from control treatments in early RA clinical trials prior to the 1980s. Performance-based measures, when available, generally are more significant than radiographs or laboratory tests in the prognosis of RA work disability and mortality (**Figure 20.5**).[2] In one study, a button test was more significant than any quantitative measure of function or laboratory test or radiographic score (including a patient questionnaire) to distinguish patients who would be alive or dead 5 years later.[74,84]

Performance measures overcome certain limitations of patient self-report questionnaires, including a need for translation of questionnaires into multiple local languages, as well as linguistic and cultural issues inherent in verbal assessments. In general, however, patient self-report questionnaire measures are as reliable, more significant in prognosis, and are far more feasible in routine care.[85,86] Performance measures are not included in the ACR core data set or widely used composite indices of patient responses to treatment and reported only in few clinical trials or routine care settings at this time. Performance measures and some early questionnaires to assess physical function continue to be used in some clinical research studies,[87] but have been supplanted largely by more feasible, short self-report questionnaires.

A more comprehensive assessment of physical function involved development of questionnaires concerning multiple activities of daily living. The earliest questionnaires involved observer judgement, as the ARA 1–4 global class. Some of these measures were not specific for arthritis,[88–90] while others were arthritis specific.[91,92] Later questionnaires were based on patient self-report, again both non-arthritis specific[93,94] and arthritis specific.[95,96] Some of these early questionnaires required 30–60 minutes to administer, and many were not adequately analysed for validity and reliability according to modern criteria.[97] Furthermore, some early questionnaires generally were oriented to patients who had considerably more functional disability than most ambulatory RA patients in recent years.[98] These early questionnaires have been supplanted in

most clinical research and clinical care by short valid and reliable questionnaires as discussed next.

Classification of patient questionnaires: Research, 'intake', and quantitative scales for routine clinical care

It appears of value to recognize that the term 'questionnaire', a patient self-report standardized form, may apply to very different types of documents, including lengthy research questionnaires, simpler clinically oriented 'intake' questionnaires for new, preoperative, and other selected patients, or brief, standardized versions for routine care (**Table 20.1**). Traditionally, the experience of many physicians with patient questionnaires has been in clinical trials and other clinical research. Research questionnaires frequently may be long and not feasible for completion by patients or review by physicians in busy clinical settings (**Table 20.1**). Indeed, in clinical trials, a clinician is directed **not** to review the questionnaire, other than for completeness; the data are forwarded to a 'data centre' for analysis after completion of the trial. The data are not collected in order to guide or have any impact on clinical care.

Long, detailed questionnaires may provide valuable data to analyse mechanisms of problems such as pain or fatigue. It is reasonable that questionnaires for research may collect far more detailed data than is suitable for questionnaires used as a part of routine care. For example, pain on a detailed Melzack pain inventory,[99] painDetect,[100–103] or FACIT (Functional Assessment of Chronic Illness Therapy)[104] provide information regarding severity of pain or fatigue as well as possible mechanisms not available from a pain or fatigue visual analogue scales (VAS) (e.g. nociceptive vs. neuropathic or central sensitization). However, it is not feasible to administer these detailed questionnaires in most clinical settings. Furthermore, a simple pain or fatigue VAS may be superior to a detailed scale to assess **changes** in pain (or fatigue and other variables) in **clinical** care.

Another type of patient questionnaire is an 'intake' questionnaire (**Table 20.1**), used to facilitate compilation of a patient medical history and demographic data in routine clinical care, generally at an initial visit or preoperatively. Information on an intake questionnaire generally is collected to be helpful in formulating narrative notes in the medical record. Very few intake questionnaires include scales designed in a standard, quantitative, protocol-driven 'scientific', format, to enhance estimates of prognosis, assess patient status over time, or analyse outcomes.

By contrast, patient questionnaires designed to guide clinical care, such as the HAQ,[17] MDHAQ,[18,19] HAQII,[105] SF36,[20] and PROMIS,[21] and others, are short—generally two sides of a single sheet of paper or electronic equivalent (**Tables 20.1 and 20.2**). The emphasis is on feasibility and clinical utility, although psychometric criteria for validity and reliability are met.

Classification of patient questionnaires: Generic, disease specific, quality of life

Patient self-report questionnaires for clinical care may be classified as 'generic' for all diseases or 'disease specific',[106] pertaining to only one or a limited number of diseases. This classification often reflects the initial purpose and the type of individuals in whom the questionnaire was developed, e.g. the HAQ was developed in patients with RA, while the SF36 was developed in normal individuals as a survey instrument for the general population. In RA, results of the

Table 20.1 Patient questionnaire measures for clinical research versus clinical care

Feature	Clinical research	New patient intake	Clinical care
Design considerations	Complex, long	Provide medical history	Patient-friendly, short, completed by patient within 5–10 min
Effect on patient visit	Adds time, interferes with flow	**Saves** time for MD and patient	**Saves** time for MD and patient
Type of questionnaire	May be 'generic', 'disease-specific', or serve other research goals	Applicable to patients with all rheumatic diseases	Applicable to patients with all rheumatic diseases
Scoring	Complex, often requires computer	Simple, may 'eyeball' results in ~30 seconds	Simple, may 'eyeball' results; scored in 10–15 seconds
Goal of data	Add to research database	Add to clinical care	Add to clinical care and to database
Focus of analysis	Groups of patients in clinical trials or observational databases	Individual patients cared for by individual physicians	Individual patients cared for by individual physicians
Data management	Send to data centre	May enter into office database to initiate patient record	Review for patient care; may enter into flow sheet to compare to previous visits
Quantitative scores	Yes	No	Yes
Entry into structured database	Yes	Usually not	Yes
Major criteria for use	Validity, reliability; assess minimal clinically important significant difference (MCID)	New patient history	Document status, medical, and medicolegal rationale for aggressive therapies
Disposition of questionnaire	Central study data centre enters into computer	Physician (or clerical staff) enters into computer	Enter into flow sheet in medical record

Table 20.2 Comparison of the Health Assessment Questionnaire (HAQ), Multidimensional Health Assessment Questionnaire (MDHAQ), SF 36, and PROMIS 29

Contents	Features	HAQ	MDHAQ	SF 36	PROMIS 29
	First report	1980	1999	1976	2004
	Patient completion	5–10 minutes	5–10 minutes	5–10 minutes	5–10 minutes
Basic items	# Activities of daily living	20 items	10 items	10 items	4 items
	Pain	10 cm VAS	21 circle VNS	2 × 5-item scales	5 items
	Patient global VAS	10 cm VAS	21 circle VNS	2 scales	No
Further items of patient status	Change in global status	No	1 week	1 year	No
	Fatigue	No	21circle VNS	1 item	4 items
Psychological items	Anxiety,	No	1 item	4 items	4 items
	Depression	No	2 items	6 items	4 items
	Sleep quality	No	1 item	No	4 items
Role items	Social role	No	No	2 items	4 items
	Work capacity	No	1 item	4 items	No
'Medical' items	Self-report painful joint count	No	0–54 scale	No	No
	Symptom checklist	No	60 symptoms	No	No
	Medical history	No	Yes	No	No
	Demographic data	No	Yes	No	No
	Social history	No	Yes	No	No
Indices	Index for clinical status	No	RAPID3	8 summaries	8 summaries
	Index for fibromyalgia	No	FAST3	No	No
	Index for adverse events	No	Yes	No	No
Additional features	Scoring templates	No	Yes	No	No
	MD scan ('eyeball')	30 seconds	10–15 seconds	10–15 seconds	10–15 seconds
	Time to score	41.8 seconds	5 seconds	?	?

'generic' SF36 and 'disease-specific' HAQ generally are similar,[107,108] although more similar for the SF 36 physical component than for other scales, reflecting the importance of limitations of physical function in patient status.[109,110]

Furthermore, derivatives of the HAQ such as the ClinHAQ[111] and MDHAQ[112] have been widely used in patients with all rheumatic diseases, indicating their 'generic' nature.[113] Almost any questionnaire to assess physical function, even the Western Ontario McMaster questionnaire (WOMAC) designed for osteoarthritis (OA),[114] appears informative in RA.[115] As noted, poor physical function based on items on a HAQ and MDHAQ was found more prognostic of mortality than smoking in elderly non-diseased individuals who were recruited as control subjects for a longitudinal study of RA patients, indicating the potential 'generic' nature of any set of queries concerning physical function.[32]

Questionnaires that query information beyond physical function are designed to address 'quality of life', including matters such as general health, work capacity, emotional health, social role, pain, global self-assessment, mental health, anxiety, depression, fatigue, and sleep quality. In general, questionnaires designed to assess more general quality of life have yielded similar results in people with rheumatic diseases to measures of physical function,[116–118] as poor physical function reduces quality of life. More detailed information is presented next concerning four commonly used questionnaires in rheumatology clinical research and clinical care, the HAQ,[17] MDHAQ,[19] SF36,[20] and PROMIS[21] (Table 20.2), recognizing space limitations to present detailed descriptions of many other valuable questionnaires.[115,117–120]

Four specific patient questionnaires to assess physical function

The Health Assessment Questionnaire (HAQ)

A major milestone in rheumatology involved reports in a 1980 issue of Arthritis and Rheumatism (now Arthritis and Rheumatology) depicting two patient-self-report questionnaires, the Health Assessment Questionnaire (HAQ)[17] (Figure 20.6, Table 20.2) and the arthritis impact measurement scales (AIMS).[120] The complete version of the HAQ includes 5 patient-centred 'd' dimensions: 'disability', pain 'discomfort', medication effects 'drugs', costs of care 'dollars' and 'death'.[17] The HAQ physical function scale, within the complete HAQ includes 20 activities of daily living (ADL), grouped into eight categories of 2 or 3 each, scored on a 0–3 scale (0 = without any difficulty, 1 = with some difficulty, 2 = with much difficulty, 3 = unable to do). The score for each section is upcoded to '2' if "use of aids or devices" or "help from another person" is reported. The physical function score is the mean 0–3 score of the highest ADL score for each of the eight categories, termed the HAQ disability index (HAQ-DI). The short, or two-page HAQ comprises only the HAQ-DI and two 0–10 cm VAS for pain and patient global assessment[17,111] thus incorporating three of seven RA core data set patient self-report measures.[121,122]

The AIMS questionnaire includes 9 scales to assess mobility, physical activity, social activity, social role, ADL, pain, depression, and anxiety, on different Likert scales with 1–4, 5, 6, or 7 options.[120] Separate scores are reported for each scale. The AIMS was designed with a multidimensional approach similar to the Short Form-36 (SF36) (see next) to assess emotional and social well-being (not in the short HAQ), in addition to physical function.[120] The AIMS has

superior psychometric properties,[123] but the HAQ proved more user-friendly and has been included in almost all RA clinical trials and many routine care sites over the last three decades.[111,124]

Several modifications of the HAQ have been developed for routine care, generally to provide additional biopsychosocial dimensions. The ClinHAQ incorporated the AIMS anxiety and depression scales.[34,125] A modified HAQ (MHAQ) with 8 ADLs, one from each HAQ category,[126] included queries about pain in ADL, patient satisfaction, and a learned helplessness scale.[127] The HAQII includes 10 ADLs, developed for a more even interval between scores according to principles known as a Rasch analysis.[105] Further revisions of the MHAQ have led to a multidimensional HAQ (MDHAQ), reported in 1999[18] and 2005,[19] and presented in detail next.

A multidimensional HAQ (MDHAQ)

The MDHAQ (Figure 20.7, Table 20.2) was developed over 25 years from 1980 to 2005 in clinical care using principles of continuous quality improvement (CQI),[128] rather than as a research activity, in contrast to all other commonly used patient questionnaires other than the ClinHAQ.[34,125] Consistent with development in a routine clinical setting, the emphasis was on feasibility and provision of clinically valuable information, saving time for the patient and physician and improving doctor–patient communication. Therefore, over the years, scales for fatigue, patient self-report painful joint count,[129] symptom checklist, and medical history information were added, as well as a four-page version which incorporates information found on a standard intake questionnaire concerning past illnesses, surgery, family history, allergies, medications, and demographic data[128,130]. In addition, the questionnaire was based on relevance to predict a clinical outcome, in the prognosis of work disability and premature mortality, analogous to a laboratory test used in clinical care.[128,130] Nonetheless, psychometric criteria for validity and reliability were met[18,19] and advances in clinical research results emerged.[131–137]

Development of the MDHAQ began with simple use of the two-page short HAQ-DI (Table 20.2) or AIMS in each patient (with any diagnosis) shortly after publication in 1980, by instructing the clinic receptionist to ask each patient to complete the questionnaire in the waiting area before seeing the doctor. It quickly became apparent that the process was feasible if **all** patients, rather than **selected** patients, were asked to complete a single questionnaire—the HAQ was preferred by patients. However, formal scoring of the HAQ in a busy clinical setting was difficult (later documented to involve about 40 seconds compared to 5 seconds for a RAPID3).[50,138] Therefore, an initial modified MHAQ was developed to include queries concerning 8 rather than 20 activities, one from each HAQ category. The MHAQ provided similar information with substantially simplified scoring,[126] while also allowing collection of additional information to improve the clinical encounter within a single page, two-sided document.

In the 1990s, clinical status of patients had improved considerably,[137] in part as a result of early treatment, wide use of methotrexate,[136] and possible secular trends toward milder disease.[139] Scores of 'zero' were found in 16% of patients on the HAQ and 31% on the MHAQ (which included 7 of the 8 activities with the lowest scores within the 8 HAQ categories as the activities most likely to be relevant to the largest number of individuals).[18] A score of zero suggested 'normal' physical function, although the patients experienced functional limitations to perform activities which were not included[18] ('floor effects'—see next). Therefore, the MDHAQ added

HEALTH ASSESSMENT QUESTIONNAIRE

Please check the response which best describes your usual abilities OVER THE PAST WEEK:

	Without ANY Difficulty	With SOME Difficulty	With MUCH Difficulty	UNABLE To Do

DRESSING & GROOMING

Are you able to:

- Dress yourself, including tying shoelaces and doing buttons? _____ 0 _____ 1 _____ 2 _____ 3
- Shampoo your hair? _____ 0 _____ 1 _____ 2 _____ 3

ARISING

Are you able to:

- Stand up from a straight chair? _____ 0 _____ 1 _____ 2 _____ 3
- Get in and out of bed? _____ 0 _____ 1 _____ 2 _____ 3

EATING

Are you able to:

- Cut your meat? _____ 0 _____ 1 _____ 2 _____ 3
- Lift a full cup or glass to your mouth? _____ 0 _____ 1 _____ 2 _____ 3
- Open a new milk carton? _____ 0 _____ 1 _____ 2 _____ 3

WALKING

Are you able to:

- Walk outdoors on flat ground? _____ 0 _____ 1 _____ 2 _____ 3
- Climb up five steps? _____ 0 _____ 1 _____ 2 _____ 3

Please check any AIDS OR DEVICES that you usually use for any of these activities:

_____ Cane   _____ Devices used for dressing (button hook, zipper pull, long-handled shoe horn, etc.)

_____ Walker   _____ Built up or special utensils

_____ Crutches   _____ Special or built up chair

_____ Wheelchair   _____ Other (Specify: _____)

Please check any categories for which you usually need HELP FROM ANOTHER PERSON:

_____ Dressing and Grooming   _____ Eating

_____ Arising   _____ Walking

Considering all the ways in which illness and health conditions may affect you at this time, please indicate below how you are doing:

VERY WELL |———————————————————————————| VERY POORLY

Figure 20.6 Health Assessment Questionnaire.

Please check the response which best describes your usual abilities OVER THE PAST WEEK:

	Without ANY Difficulty	With SOME Difficulty	With MUCH Difficulty	UNABLE To Do
HYGIENE				
Are you able to:				
- Wash and dry your body?	0	1	2	3
- Take a tub bath?	0	1	2	3
- Get on and off the toilet?	0	1	2	3
REACH				
Are you able to:				
- Reach and get down a 5 pound object (such as a bag of sugar) from just above your head?	0	1	2	3
- Bend down to pick up clothing from the floor?	0	1	2	3
GRIP				
Are you able to:				
- Open car doors?	0	1	2	3
- Open jars which have previously opened?	0	1	2	3
- Turn faucets on and off?	0	1	2	3
ACTIVITIES				
Are you able to:				
- Run errands and shop?	0	1	2	3
- Get in and out of a car?	0	1	2	3
- Do chores such as vacuuming or yard work?	0	1	2	3

Please check any AIDS OR DEVICES that you usually use for any of these activities:

_____ Raised toilet seat	_____ Bathtub bar
_____ Bathtub seat	_____ Built up or special utensils
_____ Jar opener (for jars previously opened)	_____ Special or built up chair
_____ Other (Specify: _____)	

Please check any categories for which you usually need HELP FROM ANOTHER PERSON:

_____ Hygiene	_____ Gripping and opening things
_____ Reach	_____ Errands and chores

We are also interested in learning whether or not you are affected by pain because of your illness.
How much pain have you had because of your illness IN THE PAST WEEK?

Place a vertical (I) mark on the line to indicate the severity of the pain:

NO PAIN |————————————————————————————| SEVERE PAIN

Figure 20.6 (continued)

Multi-Dimensional Health Assessment Questionnaire (MDHAQ)® (R808.21-NP2)

This questionnaire includes information not available from blood tests, X-rays, or any source other than you. Please try to answer each question, even if you do not think it is related to you at this time. Try to complete as much as you can yourself, but if you need help, please ask. <u>There are no right or wrong answers.</u>   Please answer exactly as you think or feel. Thank you.

1. Please check (√) the ONE best answer for your abilities at this time:

OVER THE LAST WEEK, were you able to:	Without ANY Difficulty	With SOME Difficulty	With MUCH Difficulty	UNABLE To Do
a. Dress yourself, including tying shoelaces and doing buttons?	0	1	2	3
b. Get in and out of bed?	0	1	2	3
c. Lift a full cup or glass to your mouth?	0	1	2	3
d. Walk outdoors on flat ground?	0	1	2	3
e. Wash and dry your entire body?	0	1	2	3
f. Bend down to pick up clothing from the floor?	0	1	2	3
g. Turn regular faucets on and off?	0	1	2	3
h. Get in and out of a car, bus, train, or airplane?	0	1	2	3
i. Walk two miles or three kilometers, if you wish?	0	1	2	3
j. Participate in recreational activities and sports as you would like, if you wish?	0	1	2	3
k. Get a good night's sleep?	0	1.1	2.2	3.3
l. Deal with feelings of anxiety or being nervous?	0	1.1	2.2	3.3
m. Deal with feelings of depression or feeling blue?	0	1.1	2.2	3.3

1.a-j FN (0-10):

1=0.3	16=5.3
2=0.7	17=5.7
3=1.0	18=6.0
4=1.3	19=6.3
5=1.7	20=6.7
6=2.0	21=7.0
7=2.3	22=7.3
8=2.7	23=7.7
9=3.0	24=8.0
10=3.3	25=8.3
11=3.7	26=8.7
12=4.0	27=9.0
13=4.3	28=9.3
14=4.7	29=9.7
15=5.0	30=10

2.PN (0-10):

2. How much pain have you had because of your condition OVER THE PAST WEEK?
   Please indicate below how severe your pain has been:

NO PAIN   ○   PAIN AS BAD AS IT COULD BE
0 0.5 1.0 1.5 2.0 2.5 3.0 3.5 4.0 4.5 5.0 5.5 6.0 6.5 7.0 7.5 8.0 8.5 9.0 9.5 10

4.PTGL (0-10):

3. Please place a check (√) in the appropriate spot to indicate the amount of pain you are having today in each of the joint areas listed below:

RAPID 3® (0-30)

	None	Mild	Moderate	Severe		None	Mild	Moderate	Severe
a. LEFT FINGERS	□ 0	□ 1	□ 2	□ 3	i. RIGHT FINGERS	□ 0	□ 1	□ 2	□ 3
b. LEFT WRIST	□ 0	□ 1	□ 2	□ 3	j. RIGHT WRIST	□ 0	□ 1	□ 2	□ 3
c. LEFT ELBOW	□ 0	□ 1	□ 2	□ 3	k. RIGHT ELBOW	□ 0	□ 1	□ 2	□ 3
d. LEFT SHOULDER	□ 0	□ 1	□ 2	□ 3	l. RIGHT SHOULDER	□ 0	□ 1	□ 2	□ 3
e. LEFT HIP	□ 0	□ 1	□ 2	□ 3	m. RIGHT HIP	□ 0	□ 1	□ 2	□ 3
f. LEFT KNEE	□ 0	□ 1	□ 2	□ 3	n. RIGHT KNEE	□ 0	□ 1	□ 2	□ 3
g. LEFT ANKLE	□ 0	□ 1	□ 2	□ 3	o. RIGHT ANKLE	□ 0	□ 1	□ 2	□ 3
h. LEFT TOES	□ 0	□ 1	□ 2	□ 3	p. RIGHT TOES	□ 0	□ 1	□ 2	□ 3
q. NECK	□ 0	□ 1	□ 2	□ 3	r. BACK	□ 0	□ 1	□ 2	□ 3

Cat:

HS = >12

MS = 6.1-12

LS = 3.1-6

R = ≤3

4. Considering all the ways in which illness and health conditions may affect you at this time, please indicate below how you are doing:

VERY WELL   ○   VERY POORLY
0 0.5 1.0 1.5 2.0 2.5 3.0 3.5 4.0 4.5 5.0 5.5 6.0 6.5 7.0 7.5 8.0 8.5 9.0 9.5 10

Figure 20.7 Multi-Dimensional Health Assessment Questionnaire (MDHAQ).

5. Please check (√) if you have experienced any of the following <u>over the last month</u>:

__Fever
__Weight gain (>10 lbs)
__Weight loss (>10 lbs)
__Feeling sickly
__Headaches
__Unusual fatigue
__Swollen glands
__Loss of appetite
__Skin rash or hives
__Unusual bruising or bleeding
__Other skin problems
__Loss of hair
__Dry eyes
__Other eye problems
__Problems with hearing
__Ringing in the ears
__Stuffy nose
__Sores in the mouth
__Dry mouth
__Problems with smell or taste

__Lump in your throat
__Cough
__Shortness of breath
__Wheezing
__Pain in the chest
__Heart pounding (palpitations)
__Trouble swallowing
__Heartburn or stomach gas
__Stomach pain or cramps
__Nausea
__Vomiting
__Constipation
__Diarrhea
__Dark or bloody stools
__Problems with urination
__Gynecological (female) problems
__Dizziness
__Losing your balance
__Muscle pain, aches, or cramps
__Muscle weakness

__Paralysis of arms or legs
__Numbness or tingling of arms or legs
__Fainting spells
__Swelling of hands
__Swelling of ankles
__Swelling in other joints
__Joint pain
__Back pain
__Neck pain
__Use of drugs not sold in stores
__Smoking cigarettes
__More than 2 alcoholic drinks per day
__Depression - feeling blue
__Anxiety - feeling nervous
__Problems with thinking
__Problems with memory
__Problems with sleeping
__Sexual problems
__Burning in sex organs
__Problems with social activities

FOR OFFICE USE ONLY

5. ROS:

[ ]

Please check (√) here if you have had none of the above over the last month: _____.

6. When you awakened in the morning OVER THE LAST WEEK, did you feel stiff? ☐ No   ☐ Yes
If "No," please go to Item 7. If "**Yes**," **please indicate the number of minutes_____, or hours _____** until you are as limber as you will be for the day.

7. How do you feel TODAY compared to ONE WEEK AGO? Please check (✓) only one.
Much **B**etter · (1),   **B**etter · (2),   the **S**ame · (3),   **W**orse · (4),   **M**uch **W**orse · (5) than one week ago

8. How often do you exercise aerobically (sweating, increased heart rate, shortness of breath) **for at least one-half hour** (30 minutes)**? Please check (✓) only one.**
☐ 3 or more times a week (3)   ☐ 1-2 times per month (1)
☐ 1-2 times per week   (2)   ☐ Do not exercise regularly (0)   ☐ Cannot exercise due to disability/ handicap (9)

9. How much of a problem has UNUSUAL fatigue or tiredness been for you OVER THE PAST WEEK?

FATIGUE IS   O O O O O O O O O O O O O O O O O O O O O   FATIGUE IS A
NO PROBLEM   0 0.5 1.0 1.5 2.0 2.5 3.0 3.5 4.0 4.5 5.0 5.5 6.0 6.5 7.0 7.5 8.0 8.5 9.0 9.5 10   MAJOR PROBLEM

10. Over the last 6 months have you had: [Please check (√)]
☐No ☐Yes An operation or new illness
☐No ☐Yes Medical emergency or stay overnight in hospital
☐No ☐Yes A fall, broken bone, or other accident or trauma
☐No ☐Yes An important new symptom or medical problem
☐No ☐Yes Side effect(s) of any medication or drug
☐No ☐Yes Smoke cigarettes regularly

☐No ☐Yes Change(s) of arthritis or other medication
☐No ☐Yes Change(s) of address
☐No ☐Yes Change(s) of marital status
☐No ☐Yes Change job or work duties, quit work, retired
☐No ☐Yes Change of medical insurance, Medicare, etc.
☐No ☐Yes Change of primary care or other doctor

Please explain any "Yes" answer below, or indicate any other health matter that affects you:

_____

_____

SEX: ☐ Female, ☐ Male **ETHNIC GROUP:** ☐ Asian, ☐ Black, ☐ Hispanic, ☐ White, ☐ Other_____

Your Occupation _____
Work Status: ☐ Full-time, ☐ Part-time, ☐ Disabled
☐ Homemaker, ☐ Self-Employed, ☐Retired,
☐ Seeking work, ☐ Other_____

Please circle the number of years of school you have completed:
1   2   3   4   5   6   7   8   9   10
11   12   13   14   15   16   17   18   19   20

Please write your   weight: _____   height: _____
pounds or kg   inches or cm

Your Name_____ Date of Birth _____   Today's Date _____

Page 2 of 2 Thank you for completing this questionnaire to help keep track of your medical care.   R808NP2

FOR OFFICE USE ONLY: I have reviewed the questionnaire responses.
Date: _____ Signature_____

Figure 20.7 (continued)

two complex activities to the physical function scale to the 8 MHAQ ADL, 'walk 2 miles or 3 kilometres', and 'participate in recreation and sports as you would like'.[18,19] The 10 activities are scored 0–3 for a 0–30 total, divided by 3 for a 0–10 physical function score, using a template on the questionnaire; this physical function scale yields scores similar to the standard HAQ-DI.[18,19]

The MDHAQ adds three mental health queries in the patient-friendly HAQ format, concerning sleep quality and capacities to deal with anxiety and depression. These items are scored 0–3.3, rather than 0–3, to provide a 0–9.9 'psychological HAQ',[18,19] which, however, is not widely used. Three VNS for pain, global assessment, and fatigue were developed in a 21-circle format, rather than a 10-cm line,[140] which facilitates photocopying and scoring for patients, doctors, and staff. RAPID three is a 0–30 composite index of 0–10 scales for physical function, pain, and patient global estimate,[45,50] which is scored in about 5 seconds (compared to 40 seconds for the HAQ-DI),[138] and is correlated significantly with the disease activity score (DAS28) and clinical disease activity index (CDAI).[13,48,50]

Additional information beyond physical function, pain, and patient global assessment, includes a 0–10 fatigue VAS,[141] morning stiffness, change in status, exercise status,[32] and demographic data including formal education level (Table 20.2). Furthermore, the MDHAQ differs from other questionnaires to assess physical function and other self-report scores with inclusion of 'medical' information based on a 0–48 patient-reported painful joint count known as a rheumatoid arthritis disease activity index (RADAI),[52] 60-symptom checklist which serves as a self-report review of systems,[142] and queries about a recent medical history (surgeries, illnesses, hospitalization, falls, and so on.). These additions were found to save time for both the physician and the patient. Documentation was also considerably improved in breadth and accuracy, including pertinent negative data that nonetheless required recording in the medical record.[143,144] MDHAQ information can facilitate focus on issues of concern to the patient and physician for higher quality visits.

The Short Form 36

The Short Form 36 (SF-36) (Figure 20.8, Table 20.2) is a 36-item patient self-report questionnaire, initially designed for survey research in the general population for health policy planning by assessment of health-related quality of life (HRQOL).[20] The SF-36 consists of eight scales grouped as four physical component summary (PCS) scores—vitality, physical functioning, bodily pain, general health perceptions, and four mental component summary (MCS) scores—physical role functioning, emotional role functioning, social role functioning, and mental health. Each domain is transformed into a 0–100 scale, assuming that each domain carries equal weight. In contrast to most other scales such as the HAQ and MDHAQ, higher scores indicate lesser disability (i.e. a score of 100 is equivalent to no disability and zero to maximum disability).

Patients with RA have lower HRQOL scores in all SF-36 domains, physical as well as mental, although physical function scores are considerably more severely affected.[109,110,118] Effects of RA on HRQOL have been found comparable or more severe than type 2 diabetes, myocardial infarction, hypertension, and chronic heart failure.[110] These data indicate the value of the SF-36 as a prototypic 'generic' questionnaire which can be informative in patients with any disease (see next), and provide comparative data concerning HRQOL. Unfortunately, comparisons of RA with other diseases remain largely unknown in the general medical and even rheumatology

communities, and the severity of RA and other rheumatic diseases tends to be underestimated by health professionals and the general public.[31]

Abbreviated variants of the SF36, including the SF-12 and SF-6D, are used commonly in health economics research to determine quality-adjusted life years in analyses of the cost-effectiveness of a health treatment.[145-147] The SF36 and variants are used in many clinical trials, and reported prominently in the medical literature. However, virtually all published data are derived from clinical trials and other clinical research studies rather than from routine clinical care.[118,147] Special software is required for scoring, unlike the HAQ and MDHAQ, limiting use in routine care, although that situation may change with availability of electronic versions.

Patient-Reported Outcomes Measurement Information System (PROMIS)

In recent years, the National Institutes of Health (NIH) Patient-Reported Outcomes Measurement Information System (PROMIS) Roadmap initiative (https://www.nihpromis.org) has been designed to develop, validate, and standardize item banks to measure patient-reported outcomes (PROs) which are relevant across common medical conditions.[21,148] The PROMIS steering committee endorsed the World Health Organization's physical, mental, and social domain framework as a high-level organizational structure under which to group multiple subdomains.

An item bank of more than 10 000 entries was constructed from existing questionnaires and literature review, leading to review and refinement to establish approximately 7000 items of relevance to the five selected domains of physical functioning, fatigue, pain, emotional distress, and social role participation. Extensive psychometric testing of the item banks resulted in a range of PROMIS measures available, free of charge as paper or electronic forms, with some of the latter incorporating computer-adaptive testing (CAT). Multiple studies have established the validity of the physical function item banks in various patient populations.[149-152]

A condensed version of PROMIS, PROMIS29 (Figure 20.9, Table 20.2), includes queries concerning anxiety, depression, sleep quality, fatigue, and social role.[23] It has been suggested that CAT is likely to outperform static tools such as the HAQ and SF36 in measurement precision and range, as well as discriminant validity,[153] although one recent study suggested that there may be large ceiling effects for some of the PROMIS 29 scales.[23] Research is ongoing to establish that the same physical function score is truly valid across various chronic disease states and to ensure that the measurement properties of the item banks are appropriate in a number of clinical trials. Although the NIH envisioned that patient self-report of physical function would be useful in clinical research, it is not yet clear that PROMIS will prove feasible to assist individual clinical practitioners in routine care in support of clinical decisions and to modify treatment plans on the basis of patient responses over time.

Physical function scores and other measures in RA

Associations of physical function scores with demographic variables

Physical function declines with advancing age in the general population and in RA. HAQ scores >0.5 were found in the Finnish general

The SF-36™ Health Survey

Instructions for Completing the Questionnaire

Please answer every question. Some questions may look like others, but each one is different. Please take the time to read and answer each question carefully by filling in the bubble that best represents your response.

EXAMPLE

This is for your review. Do not answer this question. The questionnaire begins with the section *Your Health in General* below.

For each question you will be asked to fill in a bubble in each line:

1. How strongly do you agree or disagree with each of the following statements?

	Strongly agree	Agree	Uncertain	Disagree	Strongly disagree
a) I enjoy listening to music.	○	●	○	○	○
b) I enjoy reading magazines.	●	○	○	○	○

Please begin answering the questions now.

Your Health in General

1. In general, would you say your health is:

Excellent	Very good	Good	Fair	Poor
○	○	○	○	○

2. **Compared to one year ago**, how would you rate your health in general <u>now</u>?

Much better now than one year ago	Somewhat better now than one year ago	About the same as one year ago	Somewhat worse now than one year ago	Much worse now than one year ago
○	○	○	○	○

Figure 20.8 The SF-36 Health Survey.

3. The following items are about activities you might do during a typical day. Does **your health now limit you** in these activities? If so, how much?

	Yes, Limited a lot	Yes, limited a little	No, not limited at all
a) **Vigorous activities**, such as running, lifting heavy objects, participating in strenuous sports	○	○	○
b) **Moderate activities**, such as moving a table, pushing a vacuum cleaner, bowling, or playing golf	○	○	○
c) Lifting or carrying groceries	○	○	○
d) Climbing **several** flights of stairs	○	○	○
e) Climbing **one** flight of stairs	○	○	○
f) Bending, kneeling, or stooping	○	○	○
g) Walking **more than a mile**	○	○	○
h) Walking **several blocks**	○	○	○
i) Walking **one block**	○	○	○
j) Bathing or dressing yourself	○	○	○

4. During the **past 4 weeks**, have you had any of the following problems with your work or other regular daily activities <u>as a result of your physical health</u>?

	Yes	No
a) Cut down on the **amount of time** you spent on work or other activities	○	○
b) **Accomplished less** than you would like	○	○
c) Were limited in the **kind** of work or other activities	○	○
d) Had **difficulty** performing the work or other activities (for example, it took extra time)	○	○

5. During the **past 4 weeks**, have you had any of the following problems with your work or other regular daily activities <u>as a result of any emotional problems</u> (such as feeling depressed or anxious)?

	Yes	No
a) Cut down on the **amount of time** you spent on work or other activities	○	○
b) **Accomplished less** than you would like	○	○
c) Didn't do work or other activities as **carefully** as usual	○	○

Figure 20.8 (continued)

6. During the **past 4 weeks**, to what extent has your physical health or emotional problems interfered with your normal social activities with family, friends, neighbors, or groups?

Not at all	**Slightly**	**Moderately**	**Quite a bit**	**Extremely**
○	○	○	○	○

7. How much <u>bodily</u> pain have you had during the **past 4 weeks**?

None	**Very mild**	**Mild**	**Moderate**	**Severe**	**Very severe**
○	○	○	○	○	○

8. During the **past 4 weeks**, how much did <u>pain</u> interfere with your normal work (including both work outside the home and housework)?

Not at all	**A little bit**	**Moderately**	**Quite a bit**	**Extremely**
○	○	○	○	○

9. These questions are about how you feel and how things have been with you during the **past 4 weeks**. For each question, please give the one answer that comes closest to the way you have been feeling. How much of the time during the **past 4 weeks**...

	All of the time	**Most of the time**	**A good bit of the time**	**Some of the time**	**A little of the time**	**None of the time**
a) did you feel full of pep?	○	○	○	○	○	○
b) have you been a very nervous person?	○	○	○	○	○	○
c) have you felt so down in the dumps nothing could cheer you up?	○	○	○	○	○	○
d) have you felt calm and peaceful?	○	○	○	○	○	○
e) did you have a lot of energy?	○	○	○	○	○	○
f) have you felt downhearted and blue?	○	○	○	○	○	○
g) did you feel worn out?	○	○	○	○	○	○
h) have you been a happy person?	○	○	○	○	○	○
i) did you feel tired?	○	○	○	○	○	○

10. During the **past 4 weeks**, how much of the time has your <u>physical health or emotional problems</u> interfered with your social activities (like visiting friends, relatives, etc.)?

All of the time	**Most of the time**	**Some of the time**	**A little of the time**	**None of the time**
○	○	○	○	○

11. How TRUE or FALSE is <u>each</u> of the following statements for you?

	Definitely true	**Mostly true**	**Don't know**	**Mostly false**	**Definitely false**
a) I seem to get sick a little easier than other people	○	○	○	○	○
b) I am as healthy as anybody I know	○	○	○	○	○
c) I expect my health to get worse	○	○	○	○	○
d) My health is excellent	○	○	○	○	○

THANK YOU FOR COMPLETING THIS QUESTIONNAIRE!

Figure 20.8 (continued)

PROMIS–29 Profile v1.0

Please respond to each question or statement by marking one box per row.

	Physical Function	**Without any difficulty**	**With a little difficulty**	**With some difficulty**	**With much difficulty**	**Unable to do**
1	Are you able to do chores such as vacuuming or yard work?	☐	☐	☐	☐	☐
2	Are you able to go up and down stairs at a normal pace?	☐	☐	☐	☐	☐
3	Are you able to go for a walk of at least 15 minutes?	☐	☐	☐	☐	☐
4	Are you able to run errands and shop?	☐	☐	☐	☐	☐

	Anxiety **In the past 7 days…**	**Never**	**Rarely**	**Sometimes**	**Often**	**Always**
5	I felt fearful	☐	☐	☐	☐	☐
6	I found it hard to focus on anything other than my anxiety	☐	☐	☐	☐	☐
7	My worries overwhelmed me	☐	☐	☐	☐	☐
8	I felt uneasy	☐	☐	☐	☐	☐

	Depression **In the past 7 days...**	**Never**	**Rarely**	**Sometimes**	**Often**	**Always**
9	I felt worthless	☐	☐	☐	☐	☐
10	I felt helpless	☐	☐	☐	☐	☐
11	I felt depressed	☐	☐	☐	☐	☐
12	I felt hopeless	☐	☐	☐	☐	☐

	Fatigue **During the past 7 days…**	**Not at all**	**A little bit**	**Somewhat**	**Quite a bit**	**Very much**
13	I feel fatigued	☐	☐	☐	☐	☐
14	I have trouble <u>starting</u> things because I am tired	☐	☐	☐	☐	☐

In the past 7 days…

15	How run-down did you feel on average?	☐	☐	☐	☐	☐

	In the past 7 days…	**Not at all**	**A little bit**	**Somewhat**	**Quite a bit**	**Very much**
16	How fatigued were you on average?	☐	☐	☐	☐	☐

Figure 20.9 PROMIS-29.

PROMIS–29 Profile v1.0

Sleep Disturbance
In the past 7 days...

		Very poor	Poor	Fair	Good	Very good
17	My sleep quality was.................................	☐	☐	☐	☐	☐

In the past 7 days...

		Not at all	A little bit	Somewhat	Quite a bit	Very much
18	My sleep was refreshing............................	☐	☐	☐	☐	☐
19	I had a problem with my sleep	☐	☐	☐	☐	☐
20	I had difficulty falling asleep	☐	☐	☐	☐	☐

Satisfaction with Social Role
In the past 7 days...

		Not at all	A little bit	Somewhat	Quite a bit	Very much
21	I am satisfied with how much work I can do (include work at home)	☐	☐	☐	☐	☐
22	I am satisfied with my ability to work (include work at home)...................	☐	☐	☐	☐	☐
23	I am satisfied with my ability to do regular personal and household responsibilities	☐	☐	☐	☐	☐
24	I am satisfied with my ability to perform my daily routines...................................	☐	☐	☐	☐	☐

Pain Interference
In the past 7 days...

		Not at all	A little bit	Somewhat	Quite a bit	Very much
25	How much did pain interfere with your day to day activities?.................................	☐	☐	☐	☐	☐
26	How much did pain interfere with work around the home?	☐	☐	☐	☐	☐
27	How much did pain interfere with your ability to participate in social activities?	☐	☐	☐	☐	☐
28	How much did pain interfere with your household chores?	☐	☐	☐	☐	☐

Pain Intensity
In the past 7 days...

29 | How would you rate your pain on average?...

☐ 0 No pain ☐ 1 ☐ 2 ☐ 3 ☐ 4 ☐ 5 ☐ 6 ☐ 7 ☐ 8 ☐ 9 ☐ 10 Worst imaginable pain

Figure 20.9 (continued)

population age 50–59, 60–69, and >70, respectively, in 12%, 14%, and 30% of women and 12%, 12%, and 26% of men.[154] This matter complicates interpretation of possible disease control over long periods such as 10–20 years, particularly in patients age 60 or more at baseline, as some functional decline ultimately occurs in all individuals. At the same time, it is possible that people with arthritis may interpret completion of a questionnaire in a context relative to how they were at an earlier time, and if improved, may score at lower levels than seen in the general population. It may be desirable to establish 'normal' values based on age and sex (and possibly socioeconomic status, as formal education level generally is associated with physical function scores at higher levels than age or duration of disease[142,143,155–157]) to recognize more specifically possible effects of arthritis on physical function.

Physical function scores, and all RA core data set measures, as well as almost all responses on most self-report questionnaires, suggest poorer status in females, possibly because of greater candour in acknowledging problems than in males.[158] Although females have poor physical function, which is highly significant in the prognosis of premature mortality in RA, females survive 5–10 years longer in RA and the general population. Therefore, poorer status in females may reflect in many instances primarily an ascertainment bias.

Physical function is associated with formal education level, as is the case with most measures of clinical status, including tender and swollen counts joint counts, grip strength, walking time, and ESR.[142,143] Indeed, in the only reports known to the authors in which this matter has been studied, the number of years of formal education has been found more significant than age or duration of disease as a correlate of patient status.[74,127,143,155,157] Age and duration of disease are included in almost all research reports, while education level or another more informative measure of socioeconomic status often is not included.

Associations of physical function scores with other disease measures and psychological variables

Physical function measures are correlated significantly with most other measures of RA clinical status such as the other six core data set measures[74,110,118]; indeed, all measures of clinical status in patients with RA are correlated significantly, as might be expected. However, levels of correlation of self-report of physical function with other self-report measures, including pain, fatigue, patient global assessment of status, and others, are substantially higher than with non-self-report measures, including laboratory tests, radiographs and other imaging, and joint counts.[159–161] By contrast, radiographs are correlated with ESR, CRP, ACPA, and rheumatoid factor, and each of these measures with one another, at substantially higher levels than with self-report measures (Figure 20.5), page 225.

This phenomenon extends to high correlations of self-report physical function scores with measures of psychological status, almost all of which involve self-report, including anxiety, depression,[162] poor sleep quality,[163] helplessness,[157] and others.[18] Some have suggested that associations of self-report data with psychological variables may diminish their value in clinical decisions. However, it is possible that self-report data are more informative because they reflect not only 'objective' information observed by another person, but also how the patient responds to problems, which may be critical in outcomes.

In general, there appear two clusters of measures to assess RA patient status (Figure 20.5, page 225). One involves self-report measures, including psychological measures, which are correlated with one another at considerably higher levels than with laboratory tests and radiographs. The other cluster involves laboratory and imaging measures, which are correlated with one another at considerably higher levels than with patient measures, although both clusters are correlated significantly.[160,161] As previously stated, the second cluster of 'objective' measures traditionally has been regarded as the more clinically relevant type of measure by clinicians (e.g. laboratory tests receive greater weight in revised classification criteria for RA),[164] and changes in laboratory and imaging data in clinical trials are emphasized more than changes in clinical status. Laboratory and imaging data clearly are needed to advance understanding of pathogenesis and disease course, as well as development of new medications, but it remains the case that self-report measures are substantially more significant to predict most severe clinical RA outcomes, such as work disability and premature mortality.[4,26,28,155,165]

Changes in natural history of physical function in RA over last 40 years

Historically, declines in physical function were seen throughout the course of RA in most patients,[2,3,74,165–167] associated with radiographic progression despite partial control of inflammatory activity in many patients.[3] For example, among 50 RA patients monitored over 9 years from 1973 through 1982, 47 experienced functional declines, many quite substantial.[2] In the 1980s and 1990s, widespread use of disease-modifying antirheumatic drugs (DMARDs) such as parenteral gold salts and penicillamine led to improvement in many patients, but generally over only 1 or 2 years after initiation. More than 80% of courses of gold, penicillamine, hydroxychloroquine, and azathioprine were discontinued within 2 years, due to lack of efficacy, toxicity, and/or loss of efficacy,[168,169] and functional declines resumed in what has been termed a 'J-shaped curve'.[170,171]

By the mid-1990s, progressively earlier treatment with methotrexate[136,172] led to stable physical function with no declines in many patients over long periods. For example, in the 'Behandel-Strategieën, treatment strategies' or 'BeSt' study initiated between 2000 and 2002 in the Netherlands, mean HAQ scores declined from 1.4 (of 3) to about 0.7 over the first year of treatment in each of four groups with different strategies—sequential monotherapy, step up combination therapy, initial combination with prednisone, and initial combination with infliximab—and remained stable over the next 4 years.[173]

A comparison of modified HAQ (MHAQ) scores in all 125 RA patients seen by one of the authors (TP) in 1985 versus all 150 seen in 2000, indicated mean change from 1.3–0.7 (on a 0–3 scale) 15 years later (adjusted by 0.3 points for differences between the MHAQ and HAQ scores).[137] Similarly, considerably more favourable scores were seen for radiographs and ESR,[137] providing unequivocal evidence of substantially better status of most RA patients than in earlier years, before biological agents became available in 1999.

Although low HAQ scores of 0.5 or less represent a substantial improvement from the 1980s, and scores of '0' in HAQ scores were reported in 2005 in 18% of patients with RA,[18] normal physical function with scores of '0' remain unusual in the majority of RA patients at this time. This phenomenon may be explained in part by increases in functional disability with ageing—as noted, HAQ scores >0.5 were found in 12%, 14%, and 30% of women and 12%, 12%, and 26% of men in the Finnish general population aged 50–59, 60–69, and >70, respectively, excluding individuals with severe diseases.[154] Overall, 18% (sic) of normal individuals vs. 51% of RA patients had HAQ scores >0.5.[154]

It should be recognized that usual statistical adjustments for age in regressions and other adjusted analyses may be limited to explain differences in physical function scores according to age. No difference in physical function scores might be expected in say 15 years of observation of patients between age 35 and 50 (when all scores are likely to be normal in individuals who do not have a rheumatic disease at both time points), while some decline would be anticipated when patients are studied between age 65 and 80 (when scores are likely to be abnormal even in people who have no rheumatic disease). These observations must be considered in the context of the natural history of the progression of the HAQ score over time, and may be relevant when examining analyses incorporating changes in HAQ scores over time to analyse the cost-effectiveness of biological therapies in RA.[174,175]

Complexities in use and interpretation of physical function scores

Sensitivity of physical function scores to joint damage and patient distress, in addition to inflammatory activity

Rheumatologists view themselves as physicians whose primary activity is to control inflammation in order to prevent organ damage, exemplified in the 'treat-to-target' paradigm as the standard of care for RA.[176] Clinical measurement therefore emphasizes inflammatory activity, particularly with the large increase in rheumatology clinical research directed to new agents to control inflammation. Patient self-report measures of physical function, as well as other measures in the RA core data set and indices, generally reflect inflammatory activity in patients who are selected for high levels for clinical trials. However, these measures also are sensitive to two other important problems experienced by people with RA, joint damage, and patient distress, which may be more prominent in unselected patients seen in routine clinical care.[177]

The possible impact of joint damage and patient distress can be illustrated by a patient with no inflammatory activity, indicated by no swollen joints and an ESR of 10 mm/hour, a score for physical function of 0.9/3 on a HAQ or 3/10 on an MDHAQ. Other scores of a patient with joint damage and/or distress but no inflammation might include a pain VAS of 8/10, patient global assessment VAS of 8/10, and tender joint count of 18/28. A patient with the aforementioned scores for the RA core data set measures would have a DAS28 of 5.1, CDAI of 26 (even if physician global assessment is 0/10), and RAPID3 of 19, suggesting moderate or high activity,[178–180] despite the patient having no swollen joints and a normal ESR.

Patients with high index scores but little or no inflammatory activity may present apparent anomalies for the treat-to-target approach[5] when therapy is not intensified. In one report, the basis for non-intensification were listed; joint damage and patient distress were among the most prominent reasons, along with patient choice.[181] The sensitivity of measures of physical function and RA indices to joint damage and patient distress is generally not recognized, as these quantitative data are regarded as measures strictly of inflammatory activity in clinical trials, other research, and routine care.

Quantitative measures for damage have been developed to assess patients with some rheumatic diseases, including vasculitis[182]

and SLE,[183] but not for RA. Historically, the joint count included evaluation of limited motion and deformity, which are measures of damage, in addition to swelling and tenderness.[160,184] However, limited motion and deformity are not of interest in clinical trials over 1–2 years to demonstrate efficacy of anti-inflammatory therapy, and are not assessed in clinical trial joint counts, as they are not included in the DAS28 or CDAI.

The exclusion of limited motion and deformity, unfortunately, has been extended to joint counts performed in routine care, which also generally are incorporated into DAS28 and CDAI. A quantitative estimate of limited motion and/or deformity of individual joints may be of considerable value in routine care, but these variables are assessed in very few clinical settings.

Radiographs also provide a quantitative measure of joint damage. Radiographic damage scores are correlated significantly with quantitative scores for joint limited motion and deformity, at considerably higher levels than with joint swelling, while joint tenderness is entirely independent of radiographic scores.[160] Radiographic scores are included in most recent RA clinical trials over the last three decades, and emphasized in reports of new biological agents.[185] However, quantitative radiographic assessment rarely is performed in routine care, and radiographic progression has been relatively low in most patients over the last decade. In the absence of scores for radiographs, joint deformity or joint limited motion, joint damage is recorded in the medical record at this time only as narrative descriptions, as was the case for inflammation until the 1980s.

It has been reported that HAQ scores are less sensitive to change than other core data set measures.[186–188] However, HAQ scores are as efficient as swollen joint counts or pain scores to distinguish active from control treatments in clinical trials, and more efficient than tender joint counts and ESR or CRP in most clinical trials of biological agents.[69] It may be that all RA core data set measures are affected by joint damage, but this matter has not been studied extensively.

Poor scores for physical function may also reflect patient distress, as seen in fibromyalgia and depression. Fibromyalgia (FM) is common in the general population,[189–191] and even more common in people with RA.[192,193] High HAQ and MDHAQ scores for physical function, as well scores for pain VAS, patient global VAS, and tender joint count are seen in patients with fibromyalgia.[194] Nonetheless, all core data set measures generally are interpreted as pertaining to inflammatory activity.[195,196] Damage and distress may be underestimated by many clinicians, as was physical function in the past,[1] in part based on the absence of quantitative data.

Some rheumatologists, including the authors, have added three 0–10 cm VNS subscales to the physician global assessment to assess inflammation, damage, and distress, and proportion of physician global assessment attributed to each of these three problems.[177] In settings in which the scales have been used, mean scores for damage are **higher** than for inflammation in RA patients, and mean scores for distress higher than inflammation in about 20% of patients with RA.[197] (NB The scales now termed 'RheuMetric' formerly were termed "RheumDOC") These observations may explain in part why remission according to RA core data set measures and index scores, is seen in only a minority of patients despite availability of powerful biological agents for more than 15 years.

The goal of 'no evidence of disease',[198] a term used in oncology and applied in hypertension, diabetes, and other diseases, may not be met in part because measures may reflect changes of ageing,[154] as well as joint damage and/or patient distress.[177,197] Improvement in remission rates may require changes in strategies of RA care (e.g. early arthritis clinics) beyond powerful new agents, as well as consideration of measures sensitive only to inflammation and insensitive or adjusted (through physician scores) for joint damage and/or patient distress (see next). The goal of 'no evidence of disease'[198] may require modification to 'no evidence of inflammatory activity'.

Psychometric and clinical criteria

Introduction of patient self-report information as quantitative, scientific data in clinical care was based on a new science of 'psychometrics' developed by psychiatrists and psychologists and their statistician colleagues to screen for diagnoses available only from information provided by the patient (in contrast to laboratory tests, biopsies, and so on). Early questionnaires such as the Minnesota Multiphasic Personality Inventory (MMPI),[199,200] Beck Depression Inventory,[201] and Centers for Epidemiologic Studies Depression Scale (CESD)[202] have been used widely in general clinical research and clinical care, including many reports in the rheumatology literature. Furthermore, psychometric principles have been applied to develop self-report questionnaires to develop scales for assessment of physical function, pain, fatigue, and other constructs from a patient history.[203] Analysis of validity and reliability emphasize statistical criteria so that clinicians may be assured that a questionnaire measures what it was designed to measure, is reproducible, and is amenable to testing in clinical research.[203,204]

In contrast to a psychometric approach, development of most laboratory tests used in routine care often resulted from clinical observations, many serendipitously. For example, rheumatoid factor was discovered when a positive result in a complement fixation test (a prevalent measurement method at the time) was seen in a 'control' serum. The donor of this serum fortuitously was a person with RA. Further analyses indicated that approximately 70% of patients diagnosed as having RA had a positive test, and the antibody was named 'rheumatoid factor'.[8] Rheumatoid factor was found to be a marker of more severe RA based on associations with radiographic damage,[39] and simplified approaches were developed for assessment in routine clinical care.[205]

Psychometric validity and reliability are necessary, but not necessarily sufficient, for optimal interpretation of patient self-report questionnaire data in clinical care. As with all measures in clinical medicine, including laboratory tests, interpretation by a knowledgeable physician is required. For example, a change of ESR from a normal level of 14 to an abnormal level of 64 mm/hour in an RA patient may indicate a new infection or malignancy rather than a flare of RA. Similarly, an acute increase of a physical function score may indicate an injury rather than loss of control of inflammation, and a chronic increase may result from joint damage and/or patient distress, rather than inflammatory activity. The interpretation of tests according to a simple algorithm can lead to serious errors in clinical decisions and management.

Criterion contamination

One particular complexity in interpretation of patient self-report questionnaire data involves a phenomenon known as 'criterion contamination',[206,207] which results from application of a questionnaire in different settings or people from those in which initial validation

of the questionnaire was performed. An important example involves questionnaires designed to identify and measure clinical depression, most of which were validated in young individuals who had no somatic disease. In patients with RA, responses to some items in depression questionnaires may not reflect the presence of depression, but rather of RA; for example, a response of 'false' to 'I am in just as good physical health as most of my friends' on the MMPI, 'I can work about as well as before' on the Beck Depression Inventory, or of 'true' to 'I felt that everything I did was an effort' on the CESD in a patient with RA may be simple factual comments (although they may also suggest depression) but would invariably be scored as indicating depression.

This phenomenon is known as 'criterion contamination',[206,207] and may affect interpretation of any self-report questionnaire. The interpretation that high self-report physical function reflects only inflammatory activity, and not possible joint damage or patient distress also are examples of possible criterion contamination. This phenomenon also may be seen in RA indices such as DAS28 and CDAI, which include a patient global assessment and tender joint count, and may explain in part why escalation of therapy according to 'treat to target'[5] is not implemented in up to 50% of patients with high scores.[181] Furthermore, some observers suggest that high self-report physical function scores in patients with fibromyalgia indicate that a questionnaire is 'not valid', since 'objective' observation indicates that a patient can perform an activity without difficulty but expresses 'with some difficulty' or 'much difficulty' or even 'unable to do' on a questionnaire. Certainly, interpretation in this context requires careful clinical assessment but there is some evidence that the specific pattern of response on a self-report questionnaire may assist in discrimination between inflammatory and non-inflammatory symptoms in this context.[131,208]

Floor and ceiling effects

It is optimal that a measure of physical function is sensitive over a wide range of activities from fully functional to barely ambulatory. However, scales developed primarily in severely disabled and institutionalized individuals[209] tend to have 'floor effects' when completed by individuals with moderate or mild disability, who may then be interpreted as 'normal'. By contrast, scales developed in the general population,[20] (in which modest disabilities may occur in some individuals) may have 'ceiling affects', which do not recognize moderate or severe disability.

Floor effects became more common in RA patients on the HAQ and MHAQ in the 1990s due to improved clinical status,[137] as 16% of patients had scores of '0' on the HAQ.[19] This phenomenon led to introduction of more complex activities into the MDHAQ[18,19] and HAQII.[105] PROMIS uses CAT with flexible queries to minimize floor and ceiling effects,[153] although only a few studies are available on attempts to implement PROMIS in routine care.[23]

Statistical versus clinical significance

Another consideration in interpretation of patient questionnaire data (or any medical data) is that most clinically important observations meet criteria for statistical significance (involving a probability of occurring less than 1 in 20 ($p < 0.05$) or 1 in 100 ($p < 0.001$) times by chance), but many statistically significant results according to these criteria may not be clinical important. If 100 observations are made, 5 will have a p value of ≤ 0.05 by chance, a matter that is addressed by adjustments for multiple observations.[210] Nonetheless, the fact that a phenomenon did not occur by chance does not render it clinically important, particularly when large numbers of patients are studied. A group of statisticians has cautioned against interpretation of p <0.05 as invariably of clinical value.[211]

Need for translation, cultural, and literacy considerations

One important complexity in implementation of patient questionnaires which may limit their use involves a need for translation into multiple languages. Some 'translation' is needed even within the same language, for example, the terms 'check this response' and 'miles' in the United States versus 'tick this response' and 'km' in other English-speaking countries. The four questionnaires presented in detail in this chapter, HAQ, MDHAQ, SF 36, and PROMIS, have been translated into many, but not all languages. More translations become available as questionnaires are included increasingly in clinical research and clinical care.

Cultural differences have also been noted in interpretation of responses on self-report questionnaires. For example, in one setting, scores on an MDHAQ were found to be significantly higher in patients who identified themselves as 'Hispanic' compared to patients who identified themselves as 'Asian'.[212] Clinicians are aware of differences according to ethnic groups and even between individuals within ethnic groups in interpreting information provided on an interview by the patient concerning physical function, pain, fatigue, and so on. Similarly, it is necessary that clinicians recognize possible individual and ethnic variation in interpreting results on self-report questionnaires.

Another important concern in completion and interpretation of patient self-report data involves literacy, and more specifically health literacy.[213,214] Since RA and other forms of arthritis are more common in individuals with low formal education in most cultures in which they have been studied,[215–220] and low education levels are associated with low health literacy,[213,214] it might be anticipated that some patients cannot complete self-report questionnaires or the data entered will not be accurate and informative. Indeed, almost all reports which include analyses of questionnaire responses and education level report lesser reliability (reproducibility) and correlation with other measures, such as patient vs. physician global assessment in patients of low education levels.[118,143,221–227] Some sites have cited the inability of some patients to complete questionnaires as a reason not to incorporate questionnaires into routine care in a clinical setting (Pincus, unpublished observations).

At the same time, more than 30 years of reports concerning low education levels and poor outcomes generally have been based on patient self-report questionnaire data. Almost all people who are illiterate require a 'literacy partner' to travel to a clinical setting and enrol for care. Perhaps there are a few unusual settings in which patient questionnaires would prove culturally almost impossible. In general, however, recognition of low literacy and educational level in some patients should not be used as a basis for not asking every patient to complete a self-report questionnaire at every visit. On the contrary, ultimate solutions to disparities in outcomes according to education level would appear to depend in part on further recognition and documentation through any means, the most cost-effective of which would appear patient self-report questionnaires.

Electronic versions

The growth of information technology, the internet, and computerized electronic health records (EHRs) has led to many electronic versions of patient questionnaires to assess physical function, pain, fatigue, patient global assessment, and other variables.[228] PROMIS was developed initially using CAT software[21,148] rather than paper versions, although paper versions are now available (Figure 20.6). An extensive literature indicates that, in general, most patients welcome completion of electronic questionnaires.

In one rheumatology setting, an electronic MDHAQ has been used effectively for more than a decade.[229] A Japanese electronic MDHAQ was preferred by patients over a paper version, including among elderly patients.[230] In another report, introduction of internet-based doctor–patient communication reduced doctor office spending and laboratory costs.[231] A randomized trial indicated effective introduction of self-management strategies using the internet.[232]

A review of 20 randomized controlled clinical trials which included questionnaires to assess not only physical function, but also symptoms and possible adverse events, indicated acceptability, and often preferences for electronic formats by patients and physicians, although, as in all trials, data are for groups and some expressed a preference for paper.[233,234] These trials included 12 in pulmonary diseases 6 in cancer, 6 in psychiatry, 3 in cardiovascular disease, 1 in diabetes, and none in rheumatology.[233,234] Completion of a remote questionnaire generally requires less than 10 minutes, or 2 hours for a weekly report over 12 weeks, less time than a visit to a medical care facility.

Electronic self-report questionnaires on the internet present considerable advantages to both doctors and patients, as well as to public health. An electronic format could provide the capacity for any patient to complete a questionnaire at home, within 24 hours of a visit or at random intervals to help report positive or negative changes in status, including adverse events associated with medications. Electronic capture of patient questionnaire data could allow doctors to develop flowsheets to recognize improvement or worsening in individual patients, analogous to reports of laboratory tests, which often are less informative. Electronic internet-based self-report questionnaires completed remotely could supplement and/or replace telephone conversations concerning patient status and possible early detection of adverse events associated with high-risk medications, such as biological agents, to reduce extensive costs, morbidity, and mortality.[235,236]

Availability of patient self-report questionnaire data collected prospectively in formats that allow export of group data into statistical analysis packages, could facilitate local and composite multicentre databases to analyse baseline patient questionnaire, laboratory, imaging, and medications, as well as demographic and psychosocial variables as possible prognostic markers affecting outcomes such as work disability, premature mortality, and others. Such data could raise awareness of physical function as the most significant prognostic variable for severe outcomes of work disability and premature mortality,[13] and as an important reversible risk factor for mortality in the general population, as significant as smoking.[32]

An example of use of results from an electronic MDHAQ is seen in a flowsheet depicting the course of a patient with RA. The patient was seen initially on 18 July 2014, at which time her MDHAQ physical function score was 6/10, pain VNS 10/10, patient global VNS 10/10, for a total RAPID3 of 26/30. She also reported a fatigue VNS of 10/10, 14/60 symptoms on the symptom checklist, and self-report joint count of 13/48. She had 4 swollen joints, 7 tender joints, ESR 32 mm/hour, CRP 25 mg/dL, DAS28-ESR 5.9, and CDAI 27. Treatment with low-dose prednisone, methotrexate, and etanercept led to remission. Scores on 8 June 2018 were RAPID3 0/30, fatigue VNS 0/10, 1/60 symptoms, 0/48 painful joint count, ESR was 22 mm/hour, CRP 10 mg/dL, DAS28-ESR 2.3 and CDAI 1, all indicating remission. A visit report on 2 February 2019 indicated sustained remission status.

Despite demonstration of feasibility and advantages of patient electronic entry and maintenance of self-report questionnaires, most sites that include patient questionnaires (at the time chapter is prepared in early 2019) continue to use paper versions, including clinical care of the authors. Some of the issues reflect concerns regarding privacy and security discussed in greater detail next. However, a primary barrier to use of electronic self-report questionnaires involves issues of integration into EHR. Even advanced rheumatology sites continue to have two parallel systems, the EHR, and an MDHAQ-based database.[229]

The capacity to interface software to transfer data robustly between data collection systems and the EHR has been mandated and existed for several years, but implementation requires vendor support. Many complexities may contribute to difficulties with implementation, including the priority of departments such as emergency department, intensive care unit, coronary care unit, etc. in which extensive hospital data are collected in real time compared to outpatient departments. Nonetheless, more than 90% of medical care involves outpatient medicine, in which the importance of physical function and other self-report data have substantial value in prognosis, monitoring, and outcomes, as discussed in greater detail in this chapter. Hopefully, more progress toward routine use of electronic questionnaires will be seen over the next decade.[237]

Ethical considerations

Ethical considerations have emerged in the use of patient self-report questionnaires, in both paper and electronic formats, as paper questionnaires are often scanned to be available in electronic medical records. The security of electronic medical records has been addressed through government agencies with stringent laws, such as the Health Insurance Portability and Accountability Act (HIPAA), and Health Information Technology for Economic and Clinical Health (HITECH) Act in the United States, European Data Protection Directive, and others to mandate preservation of data confidentiality, integrity, and availability for the patient. Of course, absolute protection from breaches of computer confidentiality is impossible.

In addition to the standard concerns about internet security and privacy, specific ethical concerns emerge in use of patient self-report questionnaires in routine medical care. Some concerns may emerge from patient questionnaires used primarily in psychological research which may include queries concerning detailed sensitive personal psychological matters, sexual problems, etc. However, the questionnaires presented in this chapter and other more commonly used questionnaires for rheumatology care generally do not include overly sensitive information.

Other ethical concerns concerning patient questionnaire data involve privacy of protected information—name, date of birth, medical record number, as well as possible private information—education level, income, ethnic group. Different queries may elicit different levels of concern in different cultures. These concerns can be addressed through appropriate security practices noted earlier, encryption, omitting sensitive data from questionnaires, and other measures.

It is appropriate that patients who complete a patient questionnaire are informed that the information provided has important value for direct care, and is not an adjunct which may be seen as optional, although patients always have a right to refuse to complete a questionnaire (as is the case with blood tests, imaging studies, etc.). In some settings, a formal consent may be required to complete a questionnaire, although in many settings, a clinician may ask patients to complete any questionnaire that will be used directly in clinical care, without formal consent. Formal consent may be required to compile data into reports of patient groups. Additional consents may be requested in certain settings to share de-identified data with selected research colleagues for possible multicentre analyses (while maintaining strict confidentiality), and to be contacted periodically by a data centre in the future, to monitor long-term outcomes.

Another perspective concerning ethical considerations in use of patient self-report questionnaires might suggest that it may be unethical NOT to include a patient questionnaire at each visit to assess functional status and possible other measures, not only to assess clinical status, improvement or worsening, but also clinical symptoms for clues to possible adverse events to medications. As noted earlier, patient physical function on a self-report questionnaire predicts severe clinical outcomes such as work disability and premature mortality far more significantly than any lab tests or imaging studies[13], including mortality at higher levels than smoking in the elderly non-diseased people who served as a control group for a group of RA patients[32]. Furthermore, patient questionnaire data are more reliable than joint counts[58] and more likely to document incomplete responses to methotrexate or other DMARDs than laboratory tests[60].

In more than 30 years of having every patient complete a questionnaire at every visit, little resistance of patients has been seen, although some patients may be unhappy, and this may vary in different cultures and countries. In general, however, patients are willing to share information, and in fact may be more candid to a piece of paper than to a health professional facing them, although some people may conversely withhold or falsify information in questionnaires or interviews. Since long-term information is limited, most patients are pleased to learn of an interest by health professionals in long-term outcomes, and willingly complete questionnaires in clinical settings.

Future directions—some areas for further development of physical function assessment

Incorporation of physical function assessment as a routine practice in all rheumatology care settings and training programmes

Extensive evidence supports the value of routine assessment of physical function, but the only quantitative data in the medical records of most patients with RA under care of most rheumatologists remain laboratory tests. Many possible contributory factors have been cited, including perceived concerns of clinicians of disruption of work flow with a requirement for additional physician time, lack of access to electronic tools, difficulties managing the changes in practice that may be needed to implement questionnaires, belief that such tools do not make a difference to quality of care, and lack of financial incentive or regulatory requirement.[15,228,238] However, the scientific value of assessment of physical function would appear to mandate incorporation into all routine rheumatology clinical care. Furthermore, use of self-report questionnaires in routine clinical care creates minimal issues with workflow and generally saves time for patients and doctors.[59,239]

Support for longitudinal assessment, including mortality outcomes, in rheumatic diseases

Extensive public and private support that has been available for many decades to analyse mortality outcomes in neoplastic ('tumour boards') and cardiovascular disease, but not for rheumatic diseases with similar long-term mortality. Historically, the importance of physical functional disability in increased mortality rates in RA,[13] OA,[240,241] and the general population[32] has been under-recognized, with limited public and private support to improve mortality outcomes.[242]

Poor physical function and limited exercise predict mortality in the general population at levels comparable to smoking,[32] and may be regarded as a 'potentially reversible risk factor' for premature mortality. Musculoskeletal diseases contribute significantly to the global burden of disease, which is increasing in an ageing population.[243,244] A need for research support to address improved strategies to maintain and improve physical function could improve rheumatology care and outcomes over the foreseeable future as much as research in genetics and molecular biology which dominate budgets of the NIH and other funding sources for medical research.[245,246]

Development of quantitative physician measures to assess damage and distress in clinical research and clinical care

Rheumatologists view themselves as physicians whose primary activity is to control inflammation in order to prevent organ damage, exemplified in the 'treat-to-target' paradigm as the standard of care for RA.[5,176] Clinical measurement emphasizes inflammatory activity, particularly with increasing rheumatology research involving clinical trials. However, as already noted, patient self-report measures of physical function as well as RA indices may also reflect joint damage and patient distress.[177] Measures to assess damage have been developed for assessment of patients with vasculitis[182] or SLE[183]; radiographic scores reflect damage in RA[247] and traditional joint counts (prior to dominance of clinical trials) included a measure of joint deformity which was correlated with radiographic scores.[160] At this time, quantitative clinical measurement in RA emphasizes inflammatory activity and does not address joint damage or patient distress.

The authors and a few colleagues have extended a physician/assessor global assessment VAS to 3 additional 0–10 separate physician global estimate subscales for inflammation or reversible findings, damage or irreversible findings, and distress on a RheuMetric checklist.[177,197,242] In one study, VAS scores for inflammation were highest in RA compared to other rheumatic diseases, but scores for damage are higher than, and scores for distress almost as high as for inflammation.[177] As control of inflammation becomes more prevalent, poor physical function scores may increasingly reflect damage and distress, and extension of traditional quantitative measures to reflect these changes may be of value in clinical research and care in the future.

REFERENCES

1. Smith T. Questions on clinical trials. *Br Med J (Clin Res Ed)* 1983;*287*(6392):569.
2. Pincus T, Callahan LF, Sale WG, Brooks AL, Payne LE, Vaughn WK. Severe functional declines, work disability, and increased mortality in seventy-five rheumatoid arthritis patients studied over nine years. *Arthritis Rheum* 1984;*27*(8):864–72.
3. Scott DL, Grindulis KA, Struthers GR, Coulton BL, Popert AJ, Bacon PA. Progression of radiological changes in rheumatoid arthritis. *Ann Rheum Dis* 1984;*43*(1):8–17.
4. Yelin E, Meenan R, Nevitt M, Epstein W. Work disability in rheumatoid arthritis: effects of disease, social, and work factors. *Ann Int Med* 1980;*93*(4):551–6.
5. Smolen JS, Aletaha D, Bijlsma JW, et al. Treating rheumatoid arthritis to target: recommendations of an international task force. *Ann Rheum Dis* 2010;*69*(4):631–7.
6. Pincus T, Sokka T. Laboratory tests to assess patients with rheumatoid arthritis: advantages and limitations. *Rheum Dis Clin North Am* 2009;*35*(4):731–4, vi–vii.
7. Pincus T, Gibson KA, Shmerling RH. An evidence-based approach to laboratory tests in usual care of patients with rheumatoid arthritis. *Clin Exp Rheumatol* 2014;*32*(5 Suppl 85):S-23–8.
8. Rose HM, Ragan C, Pearce E, et al. Differential agglutination of normal and sensitized sheep erythrocytes by sera of patients with rheumatoid arthritis. *Proc Soc Exp Biol Med* 1948;*68*(1):1–6.
9. Nishimura K, Sugiyama D, Kogata Y, et al. Meta-analysis: diagnostic accuracy of anti-cyclic citrullinated peptide antibody and rheumatoid factor for rheumatoid arthritis. *Ann Int Med* 2007;*146*(11):797–808.
10. Waaler E. On the occurrence of a factor in human serum activating the specific agglutination of sheep blood corpuscles. 1939. *APMIS* 2007;*115*(5):422–38; discussion 39.
11. Schellekens GA, de Jong BA, van den Hoogen FH, van de Putte LB, van Venrooij WJ. Citrulline is an essential constituent of antigenic determinants recognized by rheumatoid arthritis-specific autoantibodies. *J Clin Invest* 1998;*101*(1):273–81.
12. Sokka T, Pincus T. Erythrocyte sedimentation rate, C-reactive protein, or rheumatoid factor are normal at presentation in 35%-45% of patients with rheumatoid arthritis seen between 1980 and 2004: analyses from Finland and the United States. *J Rheumatol* 2009;*36*(7):1387–90.
13. Sokka T, Abelson B, Pincus T. Mortality in rheumatoid arthritis: 2008 update. *Clin Exp Rheumatol* 2008;*26*(5 Suppl 51):S35–61.
14. Castrejon I, McCollum L, Tanriover MD, Pincus T. Importance of patient history and physical examination in rheumatoid arthritis compared to other chronic diseases: results of a physician survey. *Arthritis Care Res (Hoboken)* 2012;*64*(8):1250–5.
15. Anderson J, Caplan L, Yazdany J, et al. Rheumatoid arthritis disease activity measures: American College of Rheumatology recommendations for use in clinical practice. *Arthritis Care Res (Hoboken)* 2012;*64*(5):640–7.

16. Goldsmith CH, Smythe HA, Helewa A. Interpretation and power of a pooled index. *J Rheumatol* 1993;20(3):575–8.

17. Fries JF, Spitz P, Kraines RG, Holman HR. Measurement of patient outcome in arthritis. *Arthritis Rheum* 1980;23(2):137–45.

18. Pincus T, Swearingen C, Wolfe F. Toward a Multidimensional Health Assessment Questionnaire (MDHAQ): assessment of advanced activities of daily living and psychological status in the patient-friendly Health Assessment Questionnaire format. *Arthritis Rheum* 1999;42(10):2220–30.

19. Pincus T, Sokka T, Kautiainen H. Further development of a physical function scale on a MDHAQ [corrected] for standard care of patients with rheumatic diseases. *J Rheumatol* 2005;32(8):1432–9.

20. Ware JE, Jr., Sherbourne CD. The MOS 36-item short-form health survey (SF-36). I. Conceptual framework and item selection. *Med Care* 1992;30(6):473–83.

21. Cella D, Yount S, Rothrock N, et al. The Patient-Reported Outcomes Measurement Information System (PROMIS): progress of an NIH roadmap cooperative group during its first two years. *Med Care* 2007;45(5 Suppl 1):S3–S11.

22. Pincus T, Castrejon I. Are patient self-report questionnaires as 'scientific' as biomarkers in 'treat-to-target' and prognosis in rheumatoid arthritis? *Curr Pharma Des* 2015;21(2):241–56.

23. Katz P, Pedro S, Michaud K. Performance of the Patient-Reported Outcomes Measurement Information System 29-item profile in rheumatoid arthritis, osteoarthritis, fibromyalgia, and systemic lupus erythematosus. *Arthritis Care Res (Hoboken)* 2017;69(9):1312–21.

24. Leigh JP, Fries JF. Mortality predictors among 263 patients with rheumatoid arthritis. *J Rheumatol* 1991;18(9):1307–12.

25. Wolfe F, Kleinheksel SM, Cathey MA, Hawley DJ, Spitz PW, Fries JF. The clinical value of the Stanford Health Assessment Questionnaire Functional Disability Index in patients with rheumatoid arthritis. *J Rheumatol* 1988;15(10):1480–8.

26. Soderlin MK, Nieminen P, Hakala M. Functional status predicts mortality in a community based rheumatoid arthritis population. *J Rheumatol* 1998;25(10):1895–9.

27. Wolfe F, Mitchell DM, Sibley JT, et al. The mortality of rheumatoid arthritis. *Arthritis Rheum* 1994;37(4):481–94.

28. Wolfe F, Michaud K, Gefeller O, Choi HK. Predicting mortality in patients with rheumatoid arthritis. *Arthritis Rheum*. 2003;48(6):1530–42.

29. Farragher TM, Lunt M, Bunn DK, Silman AJ, Symmons DP. Early functional disability predicts both all-cause and cardiovascular mortality in people with inflammatory polyarthritis: results from the Norfolk Arthritis Register. *Ann Rheum Dis* 2007;66(4):486–92.

30. Aletaha D, Landewe R, Karonitsch T, et al. Reporting disease activity in clinical trials of patients with rheumatoid arthritis: EULAR/ACR collaborative recommendations. *Arthritis Rheum* 2008;59(10):1371–7.

31. Pincus T, Callahan LF. Taking mortality in rheumatoid arthritis seriously--predictive markers, socioeconomic status and comorbidity. *J Rheumatol* 1986;13(5):841–5.

32. Sokka T, Pincus T. Poor physical function, pain and limited exercise: risk factors for premature mortality in the range of smoking or hypertension, identified on a simple patient self-report questionnaire for usual care. *BMJ Open* 2011;1(1):e000070.

33. Callahan LF, Bloch DA, Pincus T. Identification of work disability in rheumatoid arthritis: physical, radiographic and laboratory variables do not add explanatory power to demographic and functional variables. *J Clin Epidemiol* 1992;45(2):127–38.

34. Wolfe F, Hawley DJ. The long-term outcomes of rheumatoid arthritis: work disability: a prospective 18 year study of 823 patients. *J Rheumatol* 1998;25(11):2108–17.

35. Puolakka K, Kautiainen H, Mottonen T, et al. Predictors of productivity loss in early rheumatoid arthritis: a 5 year follow up study. *Ann Rheum Dis* 2005;64(1):130–3.

36. Lubeck DP, Spitz PW, Fries JF, Wolfe F, Mitchell DM, Roth SH. A multicenter study of annual health service utilization and costs in rheumatoid arthritis. *Arthritis Rheum* 1986;29(4):488–93.

37. Michaud K, Messer J, Choi HK, Wolfe F. Direct medical costs and their predictors in patients with rheumatoid arthritis: a three-year study of 7,527 patients. *Arthritis Rheum* 2003;48(10):2750–62.

38. Wolfe F, Zwillich SH. The long-term outcomes of rheumatoid arthritis: a 23-year prospective, longitudinal study of total joint replacement and its predictors in 1,600 patients with rheumatoid arthritis. *Arthritis Rheum* 1998;41(6):1072–82.

39. Olsen NJ, Callahan LF, Brooks RH, et al. Associations of HLA-DR4 with rheumatoid factor and radiographic severity in rheumatoid arthritis. *Am J Med* 1988;84(2):257–64.

40. Wells G, Li T, Maxwell L, Maclean R, Tugwell P. Responsiveness of patient-reported outcomes including fatigue, sleep quality, activity limitation, and quality of life following treatment with abatacept for rheumatoid arthritis. *Ann Rheum Dis* 2008;67(2):260–5.

41. Pincus T, Amara I, Segurado OG, Bergman M, Koch GG. Relative efficiencies of physician/assessor global estimates and patient questionnaire measures are similar to or greater than joint counts to distinguish adalimumab from control treatments in rheumatoid arthritis clinical trials. *J Rheumatol* 2008;35(2):201–5.

42. Strand V, Cohen S, Crawford B, Smolen JS, Scott DL, Leflunomide Investigators Groups. Patient-reported outcomes better discriminate active treatment from placebo in randomized controlled trials in rheumatoid arthritis. *Rheumatology (Oxf)* 2004;43(5):640–7.

43. Cohen SB, Strand V, Aguilar D, Ofman JJ. Patient-versus physician-reported outcomes in rheumatoid arthritis patients treated with recombinant interleukin-1 receptor antagonist (anakinra) therapy. *Rheumatology (Oxf)* 2004;43(6):704–11.

44. Pincus T, Yazici Y, Bergman MJ. RAPID3, an index to assess and monitor patients with rheumatoid arthritis, without formal joint counts: similar results to DAS28 and CDAI in clinical trials and clinical care. *Rheum Dis Clin North Am* 2009;35(4):773–8, viii.

45. Pincus T, Bergman MJ, Yazici Y. RAPID3-an index of physical function, pain, and global status as 'vital signs' to improve care for people with chronic rheumatic diseases. *Bull NYU Hosp Jt Dis* 2009;67(2):211–25.

46. Prevoo ML, van 't Hof MA, Kuper HH, van Leeuwen MA, van de Putte LB, van Riel PL. Modified disease activity scores that include twenty-eight-joint counts. Development and validation in a prospective longitudinal study of patients with rheumatoid arthritis. *Arthritis Rheum* 1995;38(1):44–8.

47. Aletaha D, Smolen J. The Simplified Disease Activity Index (SDAI) and the Clinical Disease Activity Index (CDAI): a review of their usefulness and validity in rheumatoid arthritis. *Clin Exp Rheumatol* 2005;23(5 Suppl 39):S100–8.

48. Pincus T, Hines P, Bergman MJ, Yazici Y, Rosenblatt LC, MacLean R. Proposed severity and response criteria for Routine Assessment of Patient Index Data (RAPID3): results for categories of disease activity and response criteria in abatacept clinical trials. *J Rheumatol* 2011;38(12):2565–71.

49. Pincus T, Furer V, Keystone E, Yazici Y, Bergman MJ, Luijtens K. RAPID3 (Routine Assessment of Patient Index Data 3) severity categories and response criteria: similar results to DAS28 (Disease Activity Score) and CDAI (Clinical Disease Activity Index) in the RAPID 1 (Rheumatoid Arthritis Prevention of Structural Damage) clinical trial of certolizumab pegol. *Arthritis Care Res (Hoboken)* 2011;63(8):1142–9.

50. Pincus T, Swearingen CJ, Bergman MJ, et al. RAPID3 (Routine Assessment of Patient Index Data) on an MDHAQ (Multidimensional Health Assessment Questionnaire): agreement with DAS28 (Disease Activity Score) and CDAI (Clinical Disease Activity Index) activity categories, scored in five versus more than ninety seconds. *Arthritis Care Res (Hoboken)* 2010;62(2):181–9.

51. Castrejon I, Dougados M, Combe B, Guillemin F, Fautrel B, Pincus T. Can remission in rheumatoid arthritis be assessed without laboratory tests or a formal joint count? possible remission criteria based on a self-report RAPID3 score and careful joint examination in the ESPOIR cohort. *J Rheumatol* 2013;40(4):386–93.

52. Yazici Y, Sokka T, Pincus T. Radiographic measures to assess patients with rheumatoid arthritis: advantages and limitations. *Rheum Dis Clin North Am* 2009;35(4):723–9, vi.

53. Hart LE, Tugwell P, Buchanan WW, Norman GR, Grace EM, Southwell D. Grading of tenderness as a source of interrater error in the Ritchie articular index. *J Rheumatol* 1985;12(4):716–17.

54. Lewis PA, O'Sullivan MM, Rumfeld WR, Coles EC, Jessop JD. Significant changes in Ritchie scores. *Br J Rheumatol* 1988;27(1):32–6.

55. Klinkhoff AV, Bellamy N, Bombardier C, et al. An experiment in reducing interobserver variability of the examination for joint tenderness. *J Rheumatol* 1988;15(3):492–4.

56. Thompson PW, Hart LE, Goldsmith CH, Spector TD, Bell MJ, Ramsden MF. Comparison of four articular indices for use in clinical trials in rheumatoid arthritis: patient, order and observer variation. *J Rheumatol* 1991;18(5):661–5.

57. Scott DL, Choy EH, Greeves A, et al. Standardising joint assessment in rheumatoid arthritis. *Clin Rheumatol* 1996;15(6):579–82.

58. Kvien TK, Mowinckel P, Heiberg T, et al. Performance of health status measures with a pen based personal digital assistant. *Ann Rheum Dis* 2005;64(10):1480–4.

59. Pincus T, Yazici Y, Castrejon I. Pragmatic and scientific advantages of MDHAQ/ RAPID3 completion by all patients at all visits in routine clinical care. *Bull NYU Hosp Jt Dis* 2012;70 (Suppl 1):30–6.

60. Pincus T. RAPID3, an index of only 3 patient self-report core data set measures, but not ESR, recognizes incomplete responses to methotrexate in usual care of patients with rheumatoid arthritis. *Bull Hosp Jt Dis (2013)* 2013;71(2):117–20.

61. Castrejon I, Bergman MJ, Pincus T. MDHAQ/RAPID3 to recognize improvement over 2 months in usual care of patients with osteoarthritis, systemic lupus erythematosus, spondyloarthropathy, and gout, as well as rheumatoid arthritis. *J Clin Rheumatol* 2013;19(4):169–74.

62. Askanase AD, Castrejon I, Pincus T. Quantitative data for care of patients with systemic lupus erythematosus in usual clinical settings: a patient Multidimensional Health Assessment Questionnaire and physician estimate of noninflammatory symptoms. *J Rheumatol* 2011;38(7):1309–16.

63. Danve A, Reddy A, Vakil-Gilani K, Garg N, Dinno A, Deodhar A. Routine Assessment of Patient Index Data 3 score (RAPID3) correlates well with Bath Ankylosing Spondylitis Disease Activity index (BASDAI) in the assessment of disease activity and monitoring progression of axial spondyloarthritis. *Clin Rheumatol* 2015;34(1):117–24.

64. Cinar M, Yilmaz S, Cinar FI, et al. A patient-reported outcome measures-based composite index (RAPID3) for the assessment of disease activity in ankylosing spondylitis. *Rheumatol Int* 2015;35(9):1575–80.

65. Michelsen B, Fiane R, Diamantopoulos AP, et al. A comparison of disease burden in rheumatoid arthritis, psoriatic arthritis and axial spondyloarthritis. *PLoS One* 2015;10(4):e0123582.

66. Park SH, Choe JY, Kim SK, Lee H, Castrejon I, Pincus T. Routine Assessment of Patient Index Data (RAPID3) and Bath Ankylosing Spondylitis Disease Activity Index (BASDAI) scores yield similar information in 85 Korean patients with ankylosing spondylitis seen in usual clinical care. *J Clin Rheumatol* 2015;21(6):300–4.

67. Annapureddy N, Elsallabi O, Baker J, Sreih AG. Patient-reported outcomes in ANCA-associated vasculitis. A comparison between Birmingham Vasculitis Activity Score and Routine Assessment of Patient Index Data 3. *Clin Rheumatol* 2015;35(2):395–400.

68. Castrejon I. The use of MDHAQ/RAPID3 in different rheumatic diseases: a review of the literature. *Bull Hosp Jt Dis (2013)* 2017;75(2):93–100.

69. Pincus T, Richardson B, Strand V, Bergman MJ. Relative efficiencies of the 7 rheumatoid arthritis Core Data Set measures to distinguish active from control treatments in 9 comparisons from clinical trials of 5 agents. *Clin Exp Rheumatol* 2014;32(Suppl 5):47–54.

70. Pincus T, Oliver AM, Bergman MJ. How to collect an MDHAQ to provide rheumatology vital signs (function, pain, global status, and RAPID3 scores) in the infrastructure of rheumatology care, including some misconceptions regarding the MDHAQ. *Rheum Dis Clin North Am* 2009;35(4):799–812, x.

71. Pincus T, Yazici Y, Bergman M. Development of a Multi-Dimensional Health Assessment Questionnaire (MDHAQ) for the infrastructure of standard clinical care. *Clin Exp Rheumatol* 2005;23(5 Suppl 39):S19–28.

72. Pincus T, Skummer PT, Grisanti MT, Castrejon I, Yazici Y. MDHAQ/RAPID3 can provide a roadmap or agenda for all rheumatology visits when the entire MDHAQ is completed at all patient visits and reviewed by the doctor before the encounter. *Bull NYU Hosp Jt Dis* 2012;70(3):177–86.

73. Steinbrocker O, Traeger CH, Batterman RC. Therapeutic criteria in rheumatoid arthritis. *J Am Med Assoc* 1949;140(8):659–62.

74. Pincus T, Callahan LF, Brooks RH, Fuchs HA, Olsen NJ, Kaye JJ. Self-report questionnaire scores in rheumatoid arthritis compared with traditional physical, radiographic, and laboratory measures. *Ann Int Med* 1989;110(4):259–66.

75. Hochberg MC, Chang RW, Dwosh I, Lindsey S, Pincus T, Wolfe F. The American College of Rheumatology 1991 revised criteria for the classification of global functional status in rheumatoid arthritis. *Arthritis Rheum* 1992;35(5):498–502.

76. Kaye JJ, Fuchs HA, Moseley JW, Nance EP, Jr., Callahan LF, Pincus T. Problems with the Steinbrocker staging system for radiographic assessment of the rheumatoid hand and wrist. *Invest Radiol* 1990;25(5):536–44.

77. Lee P, Baxter A, Dick WC, Webb J. An assessment of grip strength measurement in rheumatoid arthritis. *Scand J Rheumatol* 1974;3(1):17–23.

78. Grace EM, Gerecz EM, Kassam YB, Buchanan HM, Buchanan WW, Tugwell PS. 50-foot walking time: a critical assessment of an outcome measure in clinical therapeutic trials of antirheumatic drugs. *Br J Rheumatol* 1988;27(5):372–4.

79. Clawson DK, Souter WA, Carthum CJ, Hymen ML. Functional assessment of the rheumatoid hand. *Clin Orthop Relat Res* 1971;*77*:203–10.

80. Jebsen RH, Taylor N, Trieschmann RB, Trotter MJ, Howard LA. An objective and standardized test of hand function. *Arch Phys Med Rehabil* 1969;*50*(6):311–19.

81. Sharma S, Schumacher HR, Jr., McLellan AT. Evaluation of the Jebsen hand function test for use in patients with rheumatoid arthritis [corrected]. *Arthritis Care Res* 1994;*7*(1):16–19.

82. Poole JL. Measures of adult hand function: Arthritis Hand Function Test (AHFT), Grip Ability Test (GAT), Jebsen Test of Hand Function, and The Rheumatoid Hand Functional Disability Scale (The Duruöz Hand Index [DHI]). *Arthritis Care Res* 2003;*49*(S5):S59–S66.

83. Pincus T, Callahan LF. Rheumatology function tests: grip strength, walking time, button test and questionnaires document and predict long-term morbidity and mortality in rheumatoid arthritis. *J Rheumatol* 1992;*19*(7):1051–7.

84. Pincus T, Callahan LF, Vaughn WK. Questionnaire, walking time and button test measures of functional capacity as predictive markers for mortality in rheumatoid arthritis. *J Rheumatol.* 1987;*14*(2):240–51.

85. Pincus T, Sokka T. Quantitative measures for assessing rheumatoid arthritis in clinical trials and clinical care. *Best Pract Res Clin Rheumatol* 2003;*17*(5):753–81.

86. Callahan LF, Pincus T, Huston JW, 3rd, Brooks RH, Nance EP, Jr., Kaye JJ. Measures of activity and damage in rheumatoid arthritis: depiction of changes and prediction of mortality over five years. *Arthritis Care Res* 1997;*10*(6):381–94.

87. Loar J, Haig AJ, Yamakawa KS, Baljinnyam A. Construct validation of the Language Independent Functional Evaluation versus the Barthel Index in a Mongolian community. *Disabil Rehabil* 2011;*33*(4):319–25.

88. Katz S, Ford AB, Moskowitz RW, Jackson BA, Jaffe MW. Studies of illness in the aged: the index of ADL: a standardized measure of biological and psychosocial function. *JAMA* 1963;*185*(12):914–19.

89. Donaldson SW, Wagner CC, Gresham GE. A unified ADL evaluation form. *Arch Phys Med Rehabil* 1973;*54*(4):175–9 passim.

90. Mahoney FI, Barthel DW. Functional evaluation: the Barthel Index. *MD State Med J* 1965;*14*:61–5.

91. Lowman EW. Rehabilitation of the rheumatoid cripple; a five-year study. *Arthritis Rheum* 1958;*1*(1):38–43.

92. Kalla AA, Kotze TJ, Meyers OL, Parkyn ND. Clinical assessment of disease activity in rheumatoid arthritis: evaluation of a functional test. *Ann Rheum Dis* 1988;*47*(9):773–9.

93. Convery FR, Minteer MA, Amiel D, Connett KL. Polyarticular disability: a functional assessment. *Arch Phys Med Rehabil* 1977;*58*(11):494–9.

94. Bergner M, Bobbitt RA, Carter WB, Gilson BS. The sickness impact profile: development and final revision of a health status measure. *Med Care* 1981;*19*(8):787–805.

95. Lee P, Jasani MK, Dick WC, Buchanan WW. Evaluation of a functional index in rheumatoid arthritis. *Scand J Rheumatol* 1973;*2*(2):71–7.

96. Jette AM. Functional Status Index: reliability of a chronic disease evaluation instrument. *Arch Phys Med Rehabil* 1980;*61*(9):395–401.

97. Liang MH, Jette AM. Measuring functional ability in chronic arthritis: a critical review. *Arthritis Rheum* 1981;*24*(1):80–6.

98. Pincus T, Sokka T, Chung CP, Cawkwell G. Declines in number of tender and swollen joints in patients with rheumatoid arthritis seen in standard care in 1985 versus 2001: possible considerations for revision of inclusion criteria for clinical trials. *Ann Rheum Dis* 2006;*65*(7):878–83.

99. Melzack R. The McGill pain questionnaire: major properties and scoring methods. *Pain* 1975;*1*(3):277–99.

100. Mathieson S, Lin C. painDETECT questionnaire. *J Physiother* 2013;*59*(3):211.

101. Ahmed S, Magan T, Vargas M, Harrison A, Sofat N. Use of the painDETECT tool in rheumatoid arthritis suggests neuropathic and sensitization components in pain reporting. *J Pain Res* 2014;*7*:579–88.

102. Rifbjerg-Madsen S, Christensen AW, et al. Can the painDETECT Questionnaire score and MRI help predict treatment outcome in rheumatoid arthritis: protocol for the Frederiksberg hospital's Rheumatoid Arthritis, pain assessment and Medical Evaluation (FRAME-cohort) study. *BMJ Open* 2014;*4*(11):e006058.

103. Freynhagen R, Tolle TR, Gockel U, Baron R. The painDETECT project—far more than a screening tool on neuropathic pain. *Curr Med Res Opin* 2016;*32*(6):1033–57.

104. Webster K, Cella D, Yost K. The Functional Assessment of Chronic Illness Therapy (FACIT) Measurement System: properties, applications, and interpretation. *Health Qual Life Outcomes* 2003;*1*:79.

105. Wolfe F, Michaud K, Pincus T. Development and validation of the Health Assessment Questionnaire II: a revised version of the Health Assessment Questionnaire. *Arthritis Rheum* 2004;*50*(10):3296–305.

106. Castrejon I, Carmona L, Agrinier N, et al. The EULAR Outcome Measures Library: development and an example from a systematic review for systemic lupus erythematous instruments. *Clin Exp Rheumatol* 2015;*33*(6):910–16.

107. Tugwell P, Wells G, Strand V, et al. Clinical improvement as reflected in measures of function and health-related quality of life following treatment with leflunomide compared with methotrexate in patients with rheumatoid arthritis: sensitivity and relative efficiency to detect a treatment effect in a twelve-month, placebo-controlled trial. Leflunomide Rheumatoid Arthritis Investigators Group. *Arthritis Rheum* 2000;*43*(3):506–14.

108. Strand V, Lee EB, Fleischmann R, et al. Tofacitinib versus methotrexate in rheumatoid arthritis: patient-reported outcomes from the randomised phase III ORAL Start trial. *RMD Open* 2016;*2*(2):e000308.

109. Strand V, Crawford B, Singh J, Choy E, Smolen JS, Khanna D. Use of 'spydergrams' to present and interpret SF-36 health-related quality of life data across rheumatic diseases. *Ann Rheum Dis* 2009;*68*(12):1800–4.

110. Matcham F, Scott IC, Rayner L, et al. The impact of rheumatoid arthritis on quality-of-life assessed using the SF-36: a systematic review and meta-analysis. *Semin Arthritis Rheum* 2014;*44*(2):123–30.

111. Wolfe F, Pincus T, Fries JF. Usefulness of the HAQ in the clinic. *Ann Rheum Dis* 2001;*60*(8):811.

112. Pincus T, Askanase AD, Swearingen CJ. A Multi-Dimensional Health Assessment Questionnaire (MDHAQ) and routine assessment of patient index data (RAPID3) scores are informative in patients with all rheumatic diseases. *Rheum Dis Clin North Am* 2009;*35*(4):819–27, x.

113. Fries JF, Ramey DR. 'Arthritis specific' global health analog scales assess 'generic' health related quality-of-life in patients with rheumatoid arthritis. *J Rheumatol* 1997;*24*(9):1697–702.

114. Bellamy N, Buchanan WW, Goldsmith CH, Campbell J, Stitt LW. Validation study of WOMAC: a health status instrument

for measuring clinically important patient relevant outcomes to antirheumatic drug therapy in patients with osteoarthritis of the hip or knee. *J Rheumatol* 1988;*15*(12):1833–40.

115. Wolfe F, Kong SX. Rasch analysis of the Western Ontario MacMaster questionnaire (WOMAC) in 2205 patients with osteoarthritis, rheumatoid arthritis, and fibromyalgia. *Ann Rheum Dis* 1999;*58*(9):563–8.

116. Hurst NP, Jobanputra P, Hunter M, Lambert M, Lochhead A, Brown H. Validity of Euroqol—a generic health status instrument—in patients with rheumatoid arthritis. Economic and Health Outcomes Research Group. *Br J Rheumatol* 1994;*33*(7):655–62.

117. Linde L, Sorensen J, Ostergaard M, Horslev-Petersen K, Hetland ML. Health-related quality of life: validity, reliability, and responsiveness of SF-36, 15D, EQ-5D [corrected] RAQoL, and HAQ in patients with rheumatoid arthritis. *J Rheumatol* 2008;*35*(8):1528–37.

118. Scott IC, Ibrahim F, Lewis CM, Scott DL, Strand V. Impact of intensive treatment and remission on health-related quality of life in early and established rheumatoid arthritis. *RMD Open* 2016;*2*(2):e000270.

119. Tugwell P, Bombardier C, Buchanan WW, Goldsmith CH, Grace E, Hanna B. The MACTAR Patient Preference Disability Questionnaire—an individualized functional priority approach for assessing improvement in physical disability in clinical trials in rheumatoid arthritis. *J Rheumatol* 1987;*14*(3):446–51.

120. Meenan RF, Gertman PM, Mason JH. Measuring health status in arthritis. The arthritis impact measurement scales. *Arthritis Rheum* 1980;*23*(2):146–52.

121. Boers M, Tugwell P. The validity of pooled outcome measures (indices) in rheumatoid arthritis clinical trials. *J Rheumatol* 1993;*20*(3):568–74.

122. Felson DT, Anderson JJ, Boers M, et al. The American College of Rheumatology preliminary core set of disease activity measures for rheumatoid arthritis clinical trials. The Committee on Outcome Measures in Rheumatoid Arthritis Clinical Trials. *Arthritis Rheum* 1993;*36*(6):729–40.

123. Wolfe F, Pincus T. Standard self-report questionnaires in routine clinical and research practice--an opportunity for patients and rheumatologists. *J Rheumatol* 1991;*18*(5):643–6.

124. Pincus T, Sokka T. Quantitative clinical rheumatology: 'keep it simple, stupid': MDHAQ function, pain, global, and RAPID3 quantitative scores to improve and document the quality of rheumatologic care. *J Rheumatol* 2009;*36*(6):1099–100.

125. Wolfe F, Cathey MA. The assessment and prediction of functional disability in rheumatoid arthritis. *J Rheumatol* 1991;*18*(9):1298–306.

126. Pincus T, Summey JA, Soraci SA, Jr., Wallston KA, Hummon NP. Assessment of patient satisfaction in activities of daily living using a modified Stanford Health Assessment Questionnaire. *Arthritis Rheum* 1983;*26*(11):1346–53.

127. Nicassio PM, Wallston KA, Callahan LF, Herbert M, Pincus T. The measurement of helplessness in rheumatoid arthritis. The development of the arthritis helplessness index. *J Rheumatol* 1985;*12*(3):462–7.

128. Pincus T, Yazici Y, Bergman M, Maclean R, Harrington T. A proposed continuous quality improvement approach to assessment and management of patients with rheumatoid arthritis without formal joint counts, based on quantitative Routine Assessment of Patient Index Data (RAPID) scores on a Multidimensional Health Assessment Questionnaire (MDHAQ). *Best Pract Res Clin Rheumatol* 2007;*21*(4):789–804.

129. Stucki G, Liang MH, Stucki S, Bruhlmann P, Michel BA. A self-administered rheumatoid arthritis disease activity index (RADAI) for epidemiologic research. Psychometric properties and correlation with parameters of disease activity. *Arthritis Rheum* 1995;*38*(6):795–8.

130. Pincus T, Maclean R, Yazici Y, Harrington JT. Quantitative measurement of patient status in the regular care of patients with rheumatic diseases over 25 years as a continuous quality improvement activity, rather than traditional research. *Clin Exp Rheumatol* 2007;*25*(6 Suppl 47):69–81.

131. DeWalt DA, Reed GW, Pincus T. Further clues to recognition of patients with fibromyalgia from a simple 2-page patient Multidimensional Health Assessment Questionnaire (MDHAQ). *Clin Exp Rheumatol* 2004;*22*(4):453–61.

132. Yazici Y, Pincus T, Kautiainen H, Sokka T. Morning stiffness in patients with early rheumatoid arthritis is associated more strongly with functional disability than with joint swelling and erythrocyte sedimentation rate. *J Rheumatol* 2004;*31*(9):1723–6.

133. Pincus T, Hassett AL, Callahan LF. Clues on the MDHAQ to identify patients with fibromyalgia and similar chronic pain conditions. *Rheum Dis Clin North Am* 2009;*35*(4):865–9, xii.

134. Singh H, Gupta V, Ray S, et al. Evaluation of disease activity in rheumatoid arthritis by Routine Assessment of Patient Index Data 3 (RAPID3) and its correlation to Disease Activity Score 28 (DAS28) and Clinical Disease Activity Index (CDAI): an Indian experience. *Clin Rheumatol* 2012;*31*(12):1663–9.

135. Pincus T, Sokka T, Castrejon I, Cutolo M. Decline of mean initial prednisone dosage from 10.3 to 3.6 mg/day to treat rheumatoid arthritis between 1980 and 2004 in one clinical setting, with long-term effectiveness of dosages less than 5 mg/day. *Arthritis Care Res (Hoboken)* 2013;*65*(5):729–36.

136. Sokka T, Pincus T. Ascendancy of weekly low-dose methotrexate in usual care of rheumatoid arthritis from 1980 to 2004 at two sites in Finland and the United States. *Rheumatology (Oxf)* 2008;*47*(10):1543–7.

137. Pincus T, Sokka T, Kautiainen H. Patients seen for standard rheumatoid arthritis care have significantly better articular, radiographic, laboratory, and functional status in 2000 than in 1985. *Arthritis Rheum* 2005;*52*(4):1009–19.

138. Yazici Y, Bergman M, Pincus T. Time to score quantitative rheumatoid arthritis measures: 28-Joint Count, Disease Activity Score, Health Assessment Questionnaire (HAQ), Multidimensional HAQ (MDHAQ), and Routine Assessment of Patient Index Data (RAPID) scores. *J Rheumatol* 2008;*35*(4):603–9.

139. Silman A, Davies P, Currey HL, Evans SJ. Is rheumatoid arthritis becoming less severe? *J Chron Dis* 1983;*36*(12):891–7.

140. Pincus T, Bergman M, Sokka T, Roth J, Swearingen C, Yazici Y. Visual analog scales in formats other than a 10 centimeter horizontal line to assess pain and other clinical data. *J Rheumatol* 2008;*35*(8):1550–8.

141. Castrejon I, Nikiphorou E, Jain R, Huang A, Block JA, Pincus T. Assessment of fatigue in routine care on a Multidimensional Health Assessment Questionnaire (MDHAQ): a cross-sectional study of associations with RAPID3 and other variables in different rheumatic diseases. *Clin Exp Rheumatol* 2016;*34*(5):901–9.

142. Pincus T, Yazici Y, Bergman MJ. Beyond RAPID3—practical use of the MDHAQ to improve doctor–patient communication. *Bull NYU Hosp Jt Dis* 2010;*68*(3):223–31.

143. Callahan LF, Smith WJ, Pincus T. Self-report questionnaires in five rheumatic diseases: comparisons of health status constructs

and associations with formal education level. *Arthritis Care Res* 1989;*2*(4):122–31.

144. Callahan LF, Pincus T. Formal education level as a significant marker of clinical status in rheumatoid arthritis. *Arthritis Rheum* 1988;*31*(11):1346–57.

145. Marra CA, Woolcott JC, Kopec JA, et al. A comparison of generic, indirect utility measures (the HUI2, HUI3, SF-6D, and the EQ-5D) and disease-specific instruments (the RAQoL and the HAQ) in rheumatoid arthritis. *Soc Sci Med* 2005;*60*(7):1571–82.

146. Harrison MJ, Ahmad Y, Haque S, et al. Construct and criterion validity of the Short Form-6d utility measure in patients with systemic lupus erythematosus. *J Rheumatol* 2012;*39*(4):735–42.

147. Strand V, Sharp V, Koenig AS, et al. Comparison of health-related quality of life in rheumatoid arthritis, psoriatic arthritis and psoriasis and effects of etanercept treatment. *Ann Rheum Dis* 2012;*71*(7):1143–50.

148. Cella D, Riley W, Stone A, et al. The Patient-Reported Outcomes Measurement Information System (PROMIS) developed and tested its first wave of adult self-reported health outcome item banks: 2005–2008. *J Clin Epidemiol* 2010;*63*(11):1179–94.

149. Hung M, Hon SD, Franklin JD, et al. Psychometric properties of the PROMIS physical function item bank in patients with spinal disorders. *Spine* 2014;*39*(2):158–63.

150. Beckmann JT, Hung M, Voss MW, Crum AB, Bounsanga J, Tyser AR. Evaluation of the patient-reported outcomes measurement information system upper extremity computer adaptive test. *J Hand Surg Am* 2016;*41*(7):739–44.e4.

151. Hung M, Clegg DO, Greene T, Saltzman CL. Evaluation of the PROMIS physical function item bank in orthopaedic patients. *J Orthop Res* 2011;*29*(6):947–53.

152. Hung M, Franklin JD, Hon SD, Cheng C, Conrad J, Saltzman CL. Time for a paradigm shift with computerized adaptive testing of general physical function outcomes measurements. *Foot Ankle Int* 2014;*35*(1):1–7.

153. Rose M, Bjorner JB, Gandek B, Bruce B, Fries JF, Ware JE. The PROMIS physical function item bank was calibrated to a standardized metric and shown to improve measurement efficiency. *J Clin Epidemiol* 2014;*67*(5):516–26.

154. Sokka T, Makinen H, Hannonen P, Pincus T. Most people over age 50 in the general population do not meet ACR remission criteria or OMERACT minimal disease activity criteria for rheumatoid arthritis. *Rheumatology (Oxf)* 2007;*46*(6):1020–3.

155. Pincus T, Keysor J, Sokka T, Krishnan E, Callahan LF. Patient questionnaires and formal education level as prospective predictors of mortality over 10 years in 97% of 1416 patients with rheumatoid arthritis from 15 United States private practices. *J Rheumatol* 2004;*31*(2):229–34.

156. Callahan LF, Pincus T. Education, self-care, and outcomes of rheumatic diseases: further challenges to the 'biomedical model' paradigm. *Arthritis Care Res* 1997;*10*(5):283–8.

157. Callahan LF, Cordray DS, Wells G, Pincus T. Formal education and five-year mortality in rheumatoid arthritis: mediation by helplessness scale score. *Arthritis Care Res* 1996;*9*(6):463–72.

158. Sokka T, Toloza S, Cutolo M, et al. Women, men, and rheumatoid arthritis: analyses of disease activity, disease characteristics, and treatments in the QUEST-RA Study. *Arthritis Res Ther* 2009;*11*(1):R7.

159. Wolfe JF, Adelstein E, Sharp GC. Antinuclear antibody with distinct specificity for polymyositis. *J Clin Invest.* 1977;*59*(1):176–8.

160. Fuchs HA, Callahan LF, Kaye JJ, Brooks RH, Nance EP, Pincus T. Radiographic and joint count findings of the hand in rheumatoid arthritis. Related and unrelated findings. *Arthritis Rheum* 1988;*31*(1):44–51.

161. Pincus T, Sokka T. Quantitative measures to assess patients with rheumatic diseases: 2006 update. *Rheum Dis Clin North Am* 2006;*32*(Suppl 1):29–36.

162. Wolfe F. A reappraisal of HAQ disability in rheumatoid arthritis. *Arthritis Rheum* 2000;*43*(12):2751–61.

163. Luyster FS, Chasens ER, Wasko MC, Dunbar-Jacob J. Sleep quality and functional disability in patients with rheumatoid arthritis. *J Clin Sleep Med* 2011;*7*(1):49–55.

164. Aletaha D, Neogi T, Silman AJ, et al. 2010 rheumatoid arthritis classification criteria: an American College of Rheumatology/European League Against Rheumatism collaborative initiative. *Ann Rheum Dis* 2010;*69*(9):1580–8.

165. Pincus T, Callahan LF. What is the natural history of rheumatoid arthritis? *Rheum Dis Clin North Am.* 1993;*19*(1):123–51.

166. Scott DL, Coulton BL, Chapman JH, Bacon PA, Popert AJ. The long-term effects of treating rheumatoid arthritis. *J R Coll Physicians Lond* 1983;*17*(1):79–85.

167. Rasker JJ, Cosh JA. The natural history of rheumatoid arthritis: a fifteen year follow-up study. The prognostic significance of features noted in the first year. *Clin Rheumatol* 1984;*3*(1):11–20.

168. Wolfe F, Hawley DJ. Remission in rheumatoid arthritis. *J Rheumatol* 1985;*12*(2):245–52.

169. Pincus T, Marcum SB, Callahan LF. Long-term drug therapy for rheumatoid arthritis in seven rheumatology private practices: II. Second line drugs and prednisone. *J Rheumatol* 1992;*19*(12):1885–94.

170. Pollard L, Choy EH, Scott DL. The consequences of rheumatoid arthritis: quality of life measures in the individual patient. *Clin Exp Rheumatol* 2005;*23*(5 Suppl 39):S43–52.

171. Scott DL, Smith C, Kingsley G. Joint damage and disability in rheumatoid arthritis: an updated systematic review. *Clin Exp Rheumatol* 2003;*21*(5 Suppl 31):S20–7.

172. Pincus T, Yazici Y, Sokka T, Aletaha D, Smolen JS. Methotrexate as the 'anchor drug' for the treatment of early rheumatoid arthritis. *Clin Exp Rheumatol* 2003;*21*(5 Suppl 31):S179–85.

173. Klarenbeek NB, Guler-Yuksel M, van der Kooij SM, et al. The impact of four dynamic, goal-steered treatment strategies on the 5-year outcomes of rheumatoid arthritis patients in the BeSt study. *Ann Rheum Dis* 2011;*70*(6):1039–46.

174. Norton S, Fu B, Scott DL, et al. Health Assessment Questionnaire disability progression in early rheumatoid arthritis: systematic review and analysis of two inception cohorts. *Semin Arthritis Rheum* 2014;*44*(2):131–44.

175. Barnabe C, Sun Y, Boire G, et al. Heterogeneous disease trajectories explain variable radiographic, function and quality of life outcomes in the Canadian early arthritis cohort (CATCH). *PLoS One* 2015;*10*(8):e0135327.

176. Haraoui B, Smolen JS, Aletaha D, et al. Treating rheumatoid arthritis to target: multinational recommendations assessment questionnaire. *Ann Rheum Dis* 2011;*70*(11):1999–2002.

177. Castrejon I, Gibson KA, Block JA, Everakes SL, Jain R, Pincus T. RheuMetric: a physician checklist to record patient levels of inflammation, damage and distress as quantitative data rather than as narrative impressions. *Bull Hosp Jt Dis (2013)* 2015;*73*(3):178–84.

178. Fransen J, van Riel PL. The Disease Activity Score and the EULAR response criteria. *Rheum Dis Clin North Am* 2009;*35*(4):745–57, vii–viii.

179. Aletaha D, Smolen JS. The Simplified Disease Activity Index and Clinical Disease Activity Index to monitor patients in standard clinical care. *Rheum Dis Clin North Am* 2009;*35*(4):759–72, viii.

180. Pincus T. Can RAPID3, an index without formal joint counts or laboratory tests, serve to guide rheumatologists in tight control of rheumatoid arthritis in usual clinical care? *Bull NYU Hosp Jt Dis* 2009;*67*(3):254–66.

181. Tymms K, Zochling J, Scott J, et al. Barriers to optimal disease control for rheumatoid arthritis patients with moderate and high disease activity. *Arthritis Care Res (Hoboken)* 2014;*66*(2):190–6.

182. Luqmani RA, Bacon PA, Moots RJ, et al. Birmingham Vasculitis Activity Score (BVAS) in systemic necrotizing vasculitis. *QJM* 1994;*87*(11):671–8.

183. Gladman DD, Goldsmith CH, Urowitz MB, et al. The Systemic Lupus International Collaborating Clinics/American College of Rheumatology (SLICC/ACR) Damage Index for Systemic Lupus Erythematosus International Comparison. *J Rheumatol* 2000;*27*(2):373–6.

184. Fuchs HA, Brooks RH, Callahan LF, Pincus T. A simplified twenty-eight-joint quantitative articular index in rheumatoid arthritis. *Arthritis Rheum* 1989;*32*(5):531–7.

185. van der Heijde D, Klareskog L, Landewe R, et al. Disease remission and sustained halting of radiographic progression with combination etanercept and methotrexate in patients with rheumatoid arthritis. *Arthritis Rheum* 2007;*56*(12):3928–39.

186. Aletaha D, Smolen JS. The rheumatoid arthritis patient in the clinic: comparing more than 1,300 consecutive DMARD courses. *Rheumatology (Oxf)* 2002;*41*(12):1367–74.

187. Aletaha D, Smolen J, Ward MM. Measuring function in rheumatoid arthritis: identifying reversible and irreversible components. *Arthritis Rheum* 2006;*54*(9):2784–92.

188. Aletaha D, Alasti F, Smolen JS. Chronicity of rheumatoid arthritis affects the responsiveness of physical function, but not of disease activity measures in rheumatoid arthritis clinical trials. *Ann Rheum Dis* 2014;*74*(3):532–7.

189. Wolfe F, Brahler E, Hinz A, Hauser W. Fibromyalgia prevalence, somatic symptom reporting, and the dimensionality of polysymptomatic distress: results from a survey of the general population. *Arthritis Care & Research.* 2013;*65* (5):777–85.

190. Wolfe F, Cathey MA. Prevalence of primary and secondary fibrositis. *J Rheumatol* 1983;*10*(6):965–8.

191. Croft P, Rigby AS, Boswell R, Schollum J, Silman A. The prevalence of chronic widespread pain in the general population. *J Rheumatol* 1993;*20*(4):710–3.

192. Wolfe F, Cathey MA, Kleinheksel SM. Fibrositis (fibromyalgia) in rheumatoid arthritis. *J Rheumatol* 1984;*11*(6):814–18.

193. Clauw DJ, Katz P. The overlap between fibromyalgia and inflammatory rheumatic disease: when and why does it occur? *J Clin Rheumatol* 1995;*1*(6):335–42.

194. Pincus T, Sokka T. Can a Multi-Dimensional Health Assessment Questionnaire (MDHAQ) and Routine Assessment of Patient Index Data (RAPID) scores be informative in patients with all rheumatic diseases? *Best Pract Res Clin Rheumatol* 2007;*21*(4):733–53.

195. Sokka T, Pincus T. Most patients receiving routine care for rheumatoid arthritis in 2001 did not meet inclusion criteria for most recent clinical trials or American College of Rheumatology criteria for remission. *J Rheumatol* 2003;*30*(6):1138–46.

196. Sokka T, Pincus T. Eligibility of patients in routine care for major clinical trials of anti-tumor necrosis factor alpha agents in rheumatoid arthritis. *Arthritis Rheum* 2003;*48*(2):313–18.

197. Bergman MJ, Castrejon I, Pincus T. RHEUMDOC: a one-page RHEUMatology DOCtor form with four physician global estimates for overall status, inflammation, damage, and symptoms based on neither inflammation nor damage. *Bull Hosp Jt Dis (2013)* 2014;*72*(2):142–7.

198. Pincus T, Stein CM, Wolfe F. 'No evidence of disease' in rheumatoid arthritis using methotrexate in combination with other drugs: a contemporary goal for rheumatology care? *Clin Exp Rheumatol* 1997;*15*(6):591–6.

199. Grant Dahlstrom W, Schlager Welsh G. *An MMPI Handbook: A Guide to Use in Clinical Practice and Research.* Minneapolis, MN: University of Minnesota Press, 1964.

200. Colligan RC, Osborne D, Swenson WM, Offord KP. The aging MMPI: development of contemporary norms. *Mayo Clin Proc* 1984;*59*(6):377–90.

201. Beck AT, Ward CH, Mendelson M, Mock J, Erbaugh J. An inventory for measuring depression. *Arch Gen Psychiatry* 1961;*4*:561–71.

202. Radloff L. The CES-D Scale: a self-report depression scale for research in the general population. *Applied Psychological Measurement* 1977;*1*(3):385–401.

203. Bombardier C, Tugwell P. A methodological framework to develop and select indices for clinical trials: statistical and judgmental approaches. *J Rheumatol* 1982;*9*(5):753–7.

204. Wells G, Li T, Maxwell L, MacLean R, Tugwell P. Determining the minimal clinically important differences in activity, fatigue, and sleep quality in patients with rheumatoid arthritis. *J Rheumatol* 2007;*34*(2):280–9.

205. Plotz CM, Singer JM. The latex fixation test. I. Application to the serologic diagnosis of rheumatoid arthritis. *Am J Med* 1956;*21*(6):888–92.

206. Pincus T, Callahan LF. Depression scales in rheumatoid arthritis: criterion contamination in interpretation of patient responses. *Patient Educ Couns* 1993;*20*(2–3):133–43.

207. Pincus T, Hassett AL, Callahan LF. Criterion contamination of depression scales in patients with rheumatoid arthritis: the need for interpretation of patient questionnaires (as all clinical measures) in the context of all information about the patient. *Rheum Dis Clin North Am* 2009;*35*(4):861–4, xi–xii.

208. Callahan LF, Pincus T. A clue from a self-report questionnaire to distinguish rheumatoid arthritis from noninflammatory diffuse musculoskeletal pain. The P-VAS:D-ADL ratio. *Arthritis Rheum* 1990;*33*(9):1317–22.

209. Katz S, Downs TD, Cash HR, Grotz RC. Progress in development of the index of ADL. *Gerontologist* 1970;*10*(1):20–30.

210. Cupples LA, Heeren T, Schatzkin A, Colton T. Multiple testing of hypotheses in comparing two groups. *Ann Int Med* 1984;*100*(1):122–9.

211. Wasserstein RL, Lazar NA. The ASA's Statement on p-values: context, process, and purpose. *American Statistician* 2016;*70*(2):129–33.

212. Yazici Y, Kautiainen H, Sokka T. Differences in clinical status measures in different ethnic/racial groups with early rheumatoid arthritis: implications for interpretation of clinical trial data. *J Rheumatol* 2007;*34*(2):311–15.

213. Dewalt DA, Berkman ND, Sheridan S, Lohr KN, Pignone MP. Literacy and health outcomes: a systematic review of the literature. *J Gen Intern Med* 2004;*19*(12):1228–39.

214. Swearingen CJ, McCollum L, Daltroy LH, Pincus T, Dewalt DA, Davis TC. Screening for low literacy in a rheumatology setting: more than 10% of patients cannot read 'cartilage,' 'diagnosis,' 'rheumatologist,' or 'symptom'. *J Clin Rheumatol* 2010;*16*(8):359–64.

215. Pincus T. Formal educational level—a marker for the importance of behavioral variables in the pathogenesis, morbidity, and mortality of most diseases? *J Rheumatol* 1988;*15*(10):1457–60.

216. Callahan LF, Pincus T. Associations between clinical status questionnaire scores and formal education level in

persons with systemic lupus erythematosus. *Arthritis Rheum* 1990;*33*(3):407–11.

217. Hannan MT, Anderson JJ, Pincus T, Felson DT. Educational attainment and osteoarthritis: differential associations with radiographic changes and symptom reporting. *J Clin Epidemiol* 1992;*45*(2):139–47.

218. Sokka T, Hakkinen A, Kautiainen H, et al. Physical inactivity in patients with rheumatoid arthritis: data from twenty-one countries in a cross-sectional, international study. *Arthritis Rheum* 2008;*59*(1):42–50.

219. Bengtsson C, Nordmark B, Klareskog L, Lundberg I, Alfredsson L, Group ES. Socioeconomic status and the risk of developing rheumatoid arthritis: results from the Swedish EIRA study. *Ann Rheum Dis* 2005;*64*(11):1588–94.

220. Pedersen M, Jacobsen S, Klarlund M, Frisch M. Socioeconomic status and risk of rheumatoid arthritis: a Danish case-control study. *J Rheumatol* 2006;*33*(6):1069–74.

221. Neville C, Clarke AE, Joseph L, Belisle P, Ferland D, Fortin PR. Learning from discordance in patient and physician global assessments of systemic lupus erythematosus disease activity. *J Rheumatol* 2000;*27*(3):675–9.

222. Nicolau G, Yogui MM, Vallochi TL, Gianini RJ, Laurindo IM, Novaes GS. Sources of discrepancy in patient and physician global assessments of rheumatoid arthritis disease activity. *J Rheumatol* 2004;*31*(7):1293–6.

223. Sokka T, Hetland ML, Makinen H, et al. Remission and rheumatoid arthritis: data on patients receiving usual care in twenty-four countries. *Arthritis Rheum* 2008;*58*(9):2642–51.

224. Kim H, Jung U, Lee H, et al. Effect of formal education level on measurement of rheumatoid arthritis disease activity. *J Rheum Dis* 2015;*22*(4):231–7.

225. Lindstrom Egholm C, Krogh NS, Pincus T, Dreyer L, Ellingsen T, Glintborg B, et al. Discordance of Global Assessments by Patient and Physician Is Higher in Female than in Male Patients Regardless of the Physician's Sex: Data on Patients with Rheumatoid Arthritis, Axial Spondyloarthritis, and Psoriatic Arthritis from the DANBIO Registry. *J Rheumatol*. 2015;*42*(10):1781–5.

226. Khan NA, Spencer HJ, Abda E, et al. Determinants of discordance in patients' and physicians' rating of rheumatoid arthritis disease activity. *Arthritis Care Res (Hoboken)* 2012;*64*(2):206–14.

227. Castrejon I, Yazici Y, Samuels J, Luta G, Pincus T. Discordance of global estimates by patients and their physicians in usual care of many rheumatic diseases: association with 5 scores on a Multidimensional Health Assessment Questionnaire (MDHAQ) that are not found on the Health Assessment Questionnaire (HAQ). *Arthritis Care Res (Hoboken)* 2014;*66*(6):934–42.

228. Curtis JR, Chen L, Danila MI, Saag KG, Parham KL, Cush JJ. Routine use of quantitative disease activity measurements among us rheumatologists: implications for treat-to-target management strategies in rheumatoid arthritis. *J Rheumatol* 2018;*45*(1):40–4.

229. Newman ED, Lerch V, Billet J, Berger A, Kirchner HL. Improving the quality of care of patients with rheumatic disease using patient-centric electronic redesign software. *Arthritis Care Res (Hoboken)* 2015;*67*(4):546–53.

230. Ikeda K, Sekiguchi N, Hirai T, et al. Securely collecting multidimensional health information from patients with rheumatoid arthritis using smart device technology: beneficial effect for physicians and patients. *Musculoskeletal Care* 2018;*16*(4):494–9.

231. Baker L, Rideout J, Gertler P, Raube K. Effect of an internet-based system for doctor–patient communication on health care spending. *J Am Med Inform Assoc* 2005;*12*(5):530–6.

232. Ritter PL, Gonzalez VM, Laurent DD, Lorig KR. Measurement of pain using the visual numeric scale. *J Rheumatol* 2006;*33*(3):574–80.

233. Johansen MA, Henriksen E, Horsch A, Schuster T, Berntsen GK. Electronic symptom reporting between patient and provider for improved health care service quality: a systematic review of randomized controlled trials. Part 1: state of the art. *J Med Internet Res* 2012;*14*(5):e118.

234. Johansen MA, Berntsen GK, Schuster T, Henriksen E, Horsch A. Electronic symptom reporting between patient and provider for improved health care service quality: a systematic review of randomized controlled trials. part 2: methodological quality and effects. *J Med Internet Res* 2012;*14*(5):e126.

235. Thomsen LA, Winterstein AG, Sondergaard B, Haugbolle LS, Melander A. Systematic review of the incidence and characteristics of preventable adverse drug events in ambulatory care. *Ann Pharmacother* 2007;*41*(9):1411–26.

236. Basch E, Deal AM, Kris MG, et al. Symptom monitoring with patient-reported outcomes during routine cancer treatment: a randomized controlled trial. *J Clin Oncol* 2016;*34*(6):557–65.

237. Pincus T. Electronic Multidimensional Health Assessment Questionnaire (eMDHAQ): past, present and future of a proposed single data management system for clinical care, research, quality improvement, and monitoring of long-term outcomes. *Clin Exp Rheumatol* 2016;*34*(5 Suppl 101):S17–33.

238. Russak SM, Croft JD Jr., Furst DE, et al. The use of rheumatoid arthritis health-related quality of life patient questionnaires in clinical practice: lessons learned. *Arthritis Rheum* 2003;*49*(4):574–84.

239. Pincus T, Castrejon I. An evidence-based medical visit for patients with rheumatoid arthritis based on standard, quantitative scientific data from a patient MDHAQ and physician report. *Bull NYU Hosp Jt Dis* 2012;*70*(2):73–94.

240. Pincus T, Gibson KA, Block JA. Premature mortality: a neglected outcome in rheumatic diseases? *Arthritis Care Res (Hoboken)* 2015;*67*(8):1043–6.

241. Nuesch E, Dieppe P, Reichenbach S, Williams S, Iff S, Juni P. All cause and disease specific mortality in patients with knee or hip osteoarthritis: population-based cohort study. *BMJ* 2011;*342*:d1165.

242. Pincus T, Castrejon I, Chua J, et al. Physician visual analog scale estimates for overall global assessment, inflammation, damage, and distress to assess patients and support clinical decisions in routine rheumatology care: analysis of inter-rater reliability. *Ann Rheum Dis* 2017;*76*(Suppl 2):1466.

243. March L, Smith EU, Hoy DG, et al. Burden of disability due to musculoskeletal (MSK) disorders. *Best Pract Res Clin Rheumatol* 2014;*28*(3):353–66.

244. Ellis B, Silman A. Epidemiology: measurement matters—making musculoskeletal disease count. *Nat Rev Rheumatol* 2014;*10*(8):449–50.

245. Morris AH, Ioannidis JP. Limitations of medical research and evidence at the patient-clinician encounter scale. *Chest* 2013;*143*(4):1127–35.

246. Joyner MJ, Paneth N, Ioannidis JP. What happens when underperforming big ideas in research become entrenched? *JAMA* 2016;*316*(13):1355–6.

247. van der Heijde D, Landewe R, Klareskog L, et al. Presentation and analysis of data on radiographic outcome in clinical trials: experience from the TEMPO study. *Arthritis Rheum* 2005;*52*(1):49–60.

21

Fatigue

Emma Dures and Neil Basu

The recognition of fatigue as a patient priority

Fatigue is a common symptom in rheumatoid arthritis (RA) that can be as disabling and distressing as pain. Although the importance of fatigue to patients is now widely recognized, this is a relatively recent development over the last 15–20 years. The story of how fatigue was established as a patient priority is a compelling example of the value of collaborating with patients in shaping research agendas. A key event in bringing fatigue to the fore was the sixth Outcome Measures in Rheumatology (OMERACT) conference, held in 2002. OMERACT is a highly influential international network, comprising rheumatology experts with a range of scientific, clinical, and methodological backgrounds, aimed at improving outcome measurement in rheumatology. This includes consensus conferences every 2 years to make recommendations on core sets of measures for the major rheumatic conditions, and to reach agreement in relation to the use of standardized endpoints in randomized controlled trials and longitudinal observational studies. OMERACT 6 was the first time that patients were actively involved in the consensus process, including reviewing the American College of Rheumatology (ACR) core set for RA.[1] Until this point, rheumatology core sets had been derived by professionals, based on the research literature and expert opinion. The extent to which they captured what mattered most to patients is unknown. As a result of the collaboration with patients, agreement was reached on a research agenda to explore subjective experiences of RA, including fatigue, identified by patients as important but not encompassed within the core set of outcome measures used at that time. Subsequently, qualitative research in the United Kingdom and Sweden exploring important outcomes in RA found that, in addition to pain and mobility, fatigue was consistently mentioned by patients.[2,3] Fatigue then featured heavily at OMERACT 7 in 2004, with a clear acceptance from delegates that it was a significant symptom, experienced by the majority of patients for the majority of the time. The evidence was further considered in 2006 at OMERACT 8 when it was established that fatigue was commonly reported by patients, was often severe, could be measured, was responsive to some interventions, and provided information additional to that obtained from the commonly used outcomes. At the final OMERACT 8 plenary session, 89% of delegates endorsed the proposal that, in addition to the core set of outcome measures in widespread use, fatigue should be measured in future studies of RA whenever possible.[4] This was a major achievement for rheumatology in establishing the importance of fatigue specifically, and in recognizing the need to collaborate with patients generally.

The scale of fatigue

Fatigue has been identified by 57% of patients as the most problematic symptom of their condition.[5] Due to differences in the definitions and the instruments used to measure RA fatigue, prevalence is estimated at between 42% and 80%.[6,7] A study based on two UK cohorts found that over 80% of patients had clinically relevant fatigue (visual analogue scales (VAS) ≥20 mm) and over 50% had high levels of fatigue (VAS ≥50 mm).[8] The issue of prevalence of fatigue in RA is further complicated by the presence of comorbid rheumatic conditions. International research using the Vitality Scale of the SF-36 found that 41% of patients with RA reported severe fatigue (a score of ≤35). This rose to 49% in patients with multiple rheumatic diseases not including fibromyalgia, and up to 78% in patients with multiple rheumatic diseases including fibromyalgia.[9] These high levels of fatigue can be chronic, for example, a Dutch study using the fatigue subscale of Checklist Individual Strength (CIS) concluded that 40% of RA patients experienced persistent severe fatigue (a score of ≥35) over a 1-year period.[10]

Patient-reported outcome measures (PROMs) to measure fatigue in RA range from single item screening tools to multidimensional instruments. Among those commonly used are the Bristol Rheumatoid Arthritis Fatigue Multi-Dimensional Questionnaire (BRAF MDQ), the Chalder Fatigue Questionnaire (CFQ), the Functional Assessment Chronic Illness Therapy (Fatigue) (FACIT-F), the Multi-Dimensional Assessment of Fatigue (MAF), and the Short Form 36 Vitality Subscale (SF-36 VT), as well as a number of VAS. Some of these Patient-Reported Outcomes Measurement Information System (PROMS) capture severity of fatigue only, while others include items of severity and consequence/impact.[11]

The nature and impact of fatigue

Fatigue is a common and widespread phenomenon in the general population, defined in the *Oxford English Dictionary* as 'extreme tiredness resulting from mental or physical exertion or illness'. However, patients describe how their RA-related fatigue differs from this typically acute exhaustion. Qualitative evidence has been particularly helpful in establishing the complex, multidimensional nature of fatigue in RA, and the impact that it can have on patients' lives. While pre-RA fatigue can be attributed to circumstances such as working hard, exercise and physical activity, or lack of sleep, post-RA fatigue is experienced as unearned and unpredictable.[12] In addition to the sudden, unexplained onset of fatigue episodes, RA-related fatigue can be overwhelming and un-resolving. Patients have described a sense of 'wipe-out' and of being drained of their physical and mental energy.[13] This notion of RA fatigue as both physical and mental was investigated further when Nicklin et al., worked with patients to develop an RA-specific PROM for fatigue: the Bristol Rheumatoid Arthritis Fatigue Multi-Dimensional Scale (BRAF MDQ). Using a mix of qualitative and quantitative methods, the authors developed an underpinning conceptual framework that identified four distinct aspects: physical fatigue (e.g. levels of physical energy), cognitive fatigue (e.g. concentration and clarity of thought), living with fatigue (e.g. ability to carry out activities of daily living and social activities), and emotional fatigue (e.g. feelings of distress or upset).[14,15] Subsequently, the BRAF MDQ has been found to capture the same four aspects of fatigue in patients from France, Germany, the Netherlands, Spain, Sweden, and the United Kingdom.[16] This supports the existence of shared fatigue experiences across Europe, and the potential for tailoring treatments accordingly.

Fatigue has been identified as the consequence of RA that best differentiates between levels of health-related quality of life.[7] It is therefore not surprising that the impact of fatigue is potentially far-reaching, with patients reporting effects on their well-being, physical activities, emotions, mood, relationships, and social and family roles.[12,13,17] This impact can include feelings of frustration and shame due to an altered sense of self and the loss of valued activities that patients feel forced to give up due to their fatigue.[18] A recent survey across England with >1200 patients found that psychological distress was often attributed to the impact of pain and fatigue, with 82% of respondents reporting that would like support to manage the symptom.[19] The detrimental effects of fatigue are exacerbated by patients' perceptions that the symptom is a challenge to manage, it is not routinely addressed in clinical practice (either by patients or by rheumatology teams), and it can be ignored by professionals who do not know how to respond.[20,21]

> The dismissing of fatigue as 'part of the disease process' early after diagnosis failed to validate the real impact on all aspects of one's life, of flattening fatigue. Social, emotional, and financial. [Female, 53 years old][21]

However, the variation in fatigue and its impact should be noted. Women tend to report higher levels of fatigue than men, as well as more distress and negative emotions, and greater consequences. In particular, younger women with multiple daily roles are negatively affected by fatigue compared to older patients who might have fewer daily roles to fulfil, and who report experiencing fewer expectations and demands from other people.[22,23] In addition to the heavy individual burden imposed by fatigue, there is evidence of societal consequences. Fatigue is a significant predictor of high healthcare costs and the main reason for work disability and loss, with production losses in the United Kingdom estimated at >£2000 million.[24–27]

Our current understanding of fatigue

The heterogeneity of the mechanisms which underpin fatigue in RA represents one of the few certainties in this field. Hewlett and colleagues have proposed a dynamic conceptual model comprising three interactive domains which coherently capture the complexity of this construct (**Figure 21.1**).[28] First, biomedically orientated RA factors such as inflammation, anaemia, and cortisol response are proposed. A second domain comprises cognitive, emotional, and behavioural factors; for example, depression or dysfunctional beliefs and activities. Finally, contextual factors are emphasized. These range from managing comorbidities to occupational burdens. Critically, these factors may predict, trigger, or maintain fatigue and sometimes they may be implicated in all three processes. The specific factors implicated in fatigue are likely to vary both between and within individuals, at any one point in time.

Despite face validity of this model, a systematic review of epidemiological studies which investigated putative fatigue determinants in RA only identified elements from the cognitive, behavioural, and social domains, evidencing a dearth of associations with biomedical factors.[29] For many clinicians, the absence of a consistent relationship between peripheral inflammation and fatigue may be especially unexpected.

The biomedical community commonly assumes that fatigue in the context of inflammatory conditions such as RA is likely to be driven primarily by a low-grade perturbation within the inflammatory cascade. However, this has yet to be robustly supported in current or past literature. Epidemiological data have pointed out that rates of fatigue are similar between RA and non-inflammatory arthritides such as osteoarthritis.[30] Moreover, fatigue remains a significant symptom even among patients whose peripheral inflammation has been successfully treated. In the UK's RA biologics register, 62% of patients reporting significant pretreatment fatigue continued to report clinically relevant fatigue at 1 year despite achieving remission of their disease activity.[31] Conversely the majority of patients do report at least some important improvements in their fatigue following immunosuppression,[32] though it cannot be assumed that such improvements relate to the direct effect of peripheral inflammation. Mediation analyses, seeking to unravel the precise pathways, have actually implicated downstream reductions of pain rather than inflammation as the direct driver of fatigue reduction following biologic therapy.[33] Indeed pain appears to be one of the most consistent factors to be associated with fatigue in epidemiological research[29] which moreover appears to be centralized in nature—as observed in fibromyalgia—rather than associated with peripheral inflammation.[34]

Despite this, it would be wrong to ignore the potential role of inflammation in fatigue, especially since this concept is quite plausible to almost anyone who has experienced an infection and subsequently experienced fatigue. Traditional epidemiological studies are limited to infrequent snapshots over time and invariably measure

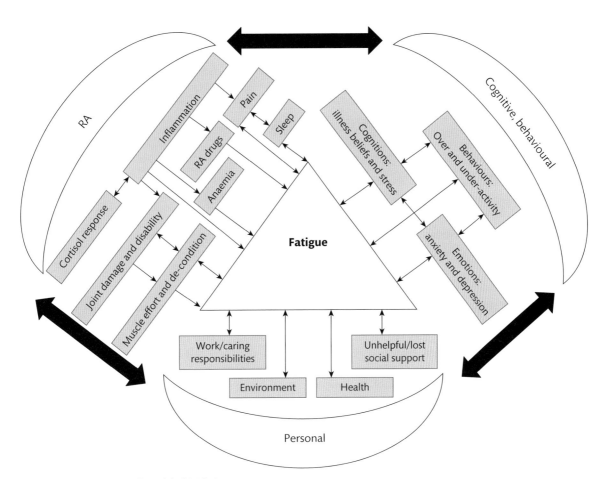

Figure 21.1 Multifaceted conceptual model of RA fatigue.
Reprinted from Hewlett S et al (2011) 'Fatigue in rheumatoid arthritis: time for a conceptual model'. *Rheumatology* 50(6):1004–6 with permission from Oxford University Press.

fatigue over a long recall period rather than the acute phenomena—which may be biologically distinct. Studies of sickness behaviour—a classical description of the subjective experience in response to an inflammatory insult—clearly includes the hallmark features of fatigue. This has been well evidenced in animal models where the injection of the cytokine stimulant lipopolysaccharide results in docile, slowed activity.[35] Indeed a similar response is observed in humans following the administration of inflammation propagating typhoid vaccine and among cancer patients receiving therapeutic interferon α (a pro-inflammatory cytokine). In the latter, approximately 80% report immediate fatigue.[35] Returning to RA, in qualitative studies and in clinical practice, patients consider fatigue exacerbations to be core to inflammatory flares.[36]

So how can we reconcile these observations with the epidemiology? One way is to accept that fatigue is not a single construct but rather a mixed state.

Borrowing heavily from the field of pain, fatigue could be considered to constitute at least two states: peripheral and centralized (Figure 21.2). Both may be underpinned by distinct biologies which demand distinct interventions (and subsequently will require investigation employing different study designs and measures). The peripheral state is more likely to be acute in nature and to include both generic and disease specific aetiologies (e.g. inflammation, peripheral pain, sleep disturbance). While the chronic state is driven by maintenance factors which may look quite similar across the chronic

disease spectrum. These include deconditioning from limited physical activity, dysfunctional coping strategies/behaviours (e.g. boom and bust), and centralized pain. Ultimately, such models are entirely hypothetical as there have been remarkably few mechanistic studies in RA fatigue, however lessons and insights can be gathered from other clinical populations where the biological study of fatigue is relatively mature.

At the genomic level, attempts to pin-point culprit markers in other conditions have been underwhelming due to small sizes, poor study designs, and the generic challenge of heterogeneity.[37,38] In this context, it has perhaps therefore been wise for the rheumatology community to not yet embark upon downstream mechanistic studies of fatigue in RA until endotypes are characterized which then enable selection of homogenous subsets. Recent efforts to cluster RA fatigue patients at a phenotypic level may facilitate this need for experimental sample homogeneity,[39] although phenotypes do not always connect with biology. This challenge should not deter future genomic based pursuits. A twin study of chronic idiopathic fatigue has indicated that fatigue heritability exceeds 50%.[40] Further, candidate gene approaches focussed on genes related to neurotransmitter and inflammation regulatory pathways have revealed some interesting findings in cancer, chronic fatigue syndrome (CFS), and other fatigued populations. These appear to implicate polymorphisms of 5-HT, rTNFa, IL1b, IL4, and IL6 genes—many of which are shared across conditions[38] and all which are potentially

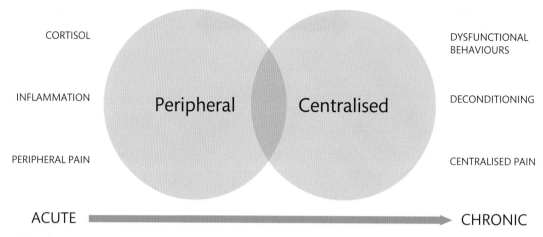

CORTISOL

INFLAMMATION

PERIPHERAL PAIN

Peripheral

Centralised

DYSFUNCTIONAL
BEHAVIOURS

DECONDITIONING

CENTRALISED PAIN

ACUTE   CHRONIC

Figure 21.2 Two basic fatigue states of RA fatigue.

relevant in RA. Further hope stems from recent advances in epigenetic analytics. A recent study in CFS reported a convergence of differentially DNA methylated sites around genes pivotal for cellular metabolism.[41] Although the challenge of heterogeneity remains a significant barrier at this –omic level, such data does inspire inspection of the downstream metabolome, where a confluence of fatigue pathways is possible.

Magnetic resonance (MR) techniques have been applied to better understand the role of skeletal muscle metabolism in the pathogenesis of fatigue among different disease populations.[42,43] In particular, 31P MR Spectroscopy (MRS) has usefully captured real time metabolic data within exercising muscle. Its application has successfully identified metabolic abnormalities in the muscles of CFS populations, where morphological abnormalities are not commonly recognized.[43,44] Furthermore, 31P MRS studies in primary biliary cirrhosis have identified associations between fatigue and mitochondrial dysfunction (as measured by abnormalities in adenosine triphosphate (ATP) metabolism).[42] Complementary to this, a recent metabolomic screen of plasma from CFS patients identified at least 20 distinct pathways, the majority representing hypometabolic states.[45] Of course there is now increasing awareness that such metabolic aberrations may actually originate from gut commensals and so providing different opportunities for future interventions. A role of the human microbiome in the pathogenesis of fatigue is very plausible given existing studies which evidence the direct impact of the microbiome on numerous brain pathways. These not only include the generation of neurotoxic metabolites, but also compounds analogous to neurotransmitters.[46] In fact there is now preliminary data suggesting a shift towards a less diverse and healthy microbiome, specifically less Firmicutes species, among patients with CFS and—of particular relevance in RA—enhanced numbers of species implicated in pro-inflammatory states (e.g. proteobacteria).[47]

Even in those populations where fatigue has been most intensely investigated, biological evidence remains sparse with minimal validation. To date, neuroimaging has been the only experimental methodology to have provided consistent mechanistic insights into fatigue across a range of conditions, reciprocating epidemiological investigations of RA-related fatigue which have identified strong associations with central factors such as cognitive dysfunctions.[29]

Although macrostructural imaging—as employed in standard clinical practice—typically fails to identify fatigue specific regions. More advanced MRI methods, such as functional, diffusion tensor (DTI), and voxel-based morphometry, are identifying potentially relevant correlates. Nonetheless, implicated brain structures remain highly heterogeneous, not only between diseases, but also for different studies within the same disease. The most common structures to be implicated are the frontal and parietal lobes, limbic system, and basal ganglia. These structures are associated with attention, memory, planning, integration of sensory information, and learning. On a theoretical level, there is strong consensus around the importance of the frontostriatal pathways. These in fact formed the basis of an original hypothesis by two neurologists, Chaudhuri and Behan, who singled out the circuitry within the basal ganglia and its connections within the frontal lobe as potentially important in chronic fatigue based on their clinical experience of managing patients with localized brain lesions.[48]

The RA research community have been slow to exploit the potential of neuroimaging to investigate fatigue, however data is now beginning to emerge. In the United Kingdom, a large (n = 54) cohort of fatigued RA patients recently underwent MRI brain multimodal scanning. Functional and structural magnetic resonance imaging correlates of fatigue in patients with rheumatoid arthritis[49] increases in the grey matter volume of the putamen (a key basal ganglia structure) were observed. This precisely aligns with existing theory but also a similar study in ankylosing spondylitis fatigue.[50] Longitudinal follow-up of the same cohort, receiving usual care, identified many changes in white matter microstructural integrity among those who reported fatigue improvement (**Figures 21.1** and **Figure 21.3**). These included apparent normalized integrity of the anterior corona radiata white matter bundles (implicated in frontal connectivity) but also others, for example, bilateral superior fronto-occipital fasciculus and fornices.[51]

Strikingly, no significant longitudinal fractional anisotropy (FA) changes were measured within those who did not report improvement on follow-up. Such diffuse findings connect with the heterogeneity that we expect from fatigue. That said, careful selection of measures is enabling the derivation of more discrete regions. As an example, connectivity analysis of functional MRI data—which seeks to select out regions of the brain which are in close functional communication in relation to a specific covariate of interest—has recently identified

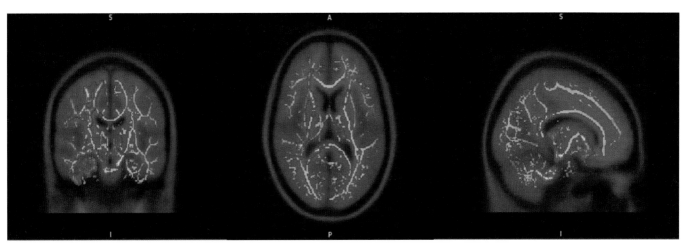

Figure 21.3 Longitudinal changes in white matter integrity showing a significant reduced white matter integrity in improver fatigue RA individuals compared to their status at baseline. Red voxels represent significant values. P maps are displayed at p <0.05, FWE corrected and overlaid on the mean FA skeleton (green), thresholded between 0.2 and 0.7 and the MNI125 T1 1 mm template using FslView open source software.

numerous connections which associate with systemic inflammation. Of these, connectivity between the dorsal attention network and frontal pole specifically and significantly related to acute fatigue (as measured by current fatigue in the scanner) but not more chronic fatigue (measured with a 4-week recall scale)[49,52]; in contrast, the recognized fibromyalgia marker of default mode network-insula was significantly related to more chronic and not acute fatigue.[53] So how do all these potentially important systems fit together? One potential model where RA peripheral inflammation may link with the central nervous system (CNS) and contribute to the generation of fatigue is via afferents of the vagus nerve—a key interface with the autonomic system.[54] Certainly, evidence of autonomic dysfunction has been commonly reported in other fatigued populations. Significant relationships between fatigue and classical autonomic symptoms, such as orthostatic intolerance or gastrointestinal and urinary dysfunctions, have been quantified using validated questionnaires in populations as diverse as Parkinson's disease[55] and Sjogren's syndrome.[56] Further, overnight aberrations in heart rate variability among CFS patients— a robust biomarker of autonomic function—appear to signal above normal sympathetic activity during these times.[57] In RA, autonomic dysfunction has been measured in approximately 60% of cases.[58] Although little is known of its relation to fatigue, it is intriguing to note recent work in RA identifying a correlation between colony-stimulating factor (CSF) pro-inflammatory cytokines and vagal tone, thus supporting the feasibility of this path.[59]

Inevitably, bioinformatics approaches will be essential to integrate and help us understand this highly complex problem. Although ultimately, it is highly unlikely that a neat, single mechanistic model will entirely explain fatigue in RA. While there is clearly substantial work to be done in order to unravel the mechanisms, this must be done carefully in parallel with stratification. We must progress from the past when for example it was not uncommon for clinicians to assume that most if not all RA patients were fatigued secondary to depression. While depression is indeed correlated with fatigue, less than 20% of fatigued RA patients are actually depressed.[31] We must anchor our future pursuits with existing conceptual models which remind us of the multidimensional nature of this construct. Future

treatments will inevitably require personalization according to the specific aetiology pathway(s) at play.

Interventions and treatments for RA-related fatigue

A systematic review of non-pharmacological interventions found moderate but significant effects of cognitive-behavioural therapy for fatigue.[60,61] This points to the benefits of addressing the psychological, social, and emotional variables that are implicated in the onset and perpetuation of fatigue, and promoting self-management of the symptom. The evidence for these non-pharmacological approaches is growing, and includes a mix of group-based and individual interventions.[62-65] Self-management interventions are typically hypothesized to work through the therapeutic mechanisms of enhancing patients' self-efficacy (the belief in their ability to achieve a desired outcome/goal) and self-determination (the motivation and competence to behave in effective and healthy ways).[66,67] This is achieved by addressing patients' illness beliefs, their coping strategies, and their acceptance of fatigue as a symptom of their RA. The interventions are often informed by cognitive-behavioural theory (CBT), an established, structured, action-orientated approach that focuses on promoting behavioural change. CBT involves looking closely at patterns of behaviour, identifying the links between the patient's thoughts, feelings and behaviours, and then working out how they are contributing to, or influencing a symptom, using a non-didactic, collaborative approach.[68] The value of addressing the impact of fatigue through increasing patients' sense of self-efficacy and autonomy in the face of a debilitating symptom is supported by evidence that learned helplessness (an individual's sense that they have little control over the events in their life and so respond passively to the problems) independently predicts disability, pain, and fatigue.[69] Qualitative evidence from patients who have taken part in a cognitive-behavioural fatigue programme has also identified the benefits of tailored goal-setting and the use of daily activity diaries to identify patterns of energy expenditure in reducing the impact of fatigue, along with a non-didactic 'guided' approach from healthcare professionals.[70]

There is also evidence for the potential of physical activity interventions to reduce fatigue in RA.[60] It is hypothesized that physical activity interventions might decrease the level and impact of RA-related fatigue through their influence on RA disease processes and other psychosocial and lifestyle factors;[71] for example, dynamic exercise programmes, such as aerobic capacity or muscle strength training, can have a positive effect on aerobic capacity. In turn, this might contribute to an improvement in fatigue through increased cardiorespiratory fitness and muscle strength. An improvement in physiological function could result in less effort required for specific tasks, thus reducing subsequent experiences of fatigue. From a psychosocial perspective, taking part in physical activity and exercise might reduce levels of anxiety and depression which might be contributing to patients' fatigue, and enhance patients' self-efficacy.[17,72] Future non-pharmacological interventions for fatigue in RA are likely to explore various modes of delivery and settings, for example guided online interventions, and interventions delivered in community settings by a range of healthcare professionals.

No current pharmacological agents are indicated for the treatment of RA-related fatigue. Indeed despite the conduct of several hundred trials of pharmacological fatigue interventions across the spectrum of chronic disease, meta-analyses have failed to evidence a substantial or safe role for any drugs.[73,74] In RA, biological agents do appear to infer a small to moderate secondary effect on fatigue.[75,76] However, recent data from the British Society for Rheumatology Biologics Register show that even among those patients reaching clinical remission, most continue to experience fatigue.[31,73,74] One reason for these modest responses may be the likely inability for existing disease-modifying antirheumatic drug (DMARD) and biologic agents to cross the blood–brain barrier. If fatigue is mediated by central inflammation then drugs such minocycline—known to have a role in microglial inactivation as well as attenuation of peripheral inflammation—maybe more efficacious.[35]

Given the putative role of the basal ganglia in existing conceptual models, along with the close alignment between fatigue and poor motivation among RA patients,[12] there is a biological rationale for why enhancement of neural dopamine may alleviate fatigue. However, although never tested in RA, drugs such as modafinil and amantadine have failed to deliver reliable fatigue effects in neurological conditions.[77,78] Otherwise, psychostimulants such as methylphenidate may have a role in palliative care patients but their adverse risk profile discourages their use in chronic disorders.[79]

This shortage of pharmacological options re-emphasizes the need to better understand mechanisms. In actuality, future solutions may well be found in alternative approaches, such transcranial direct-current brain stimulation (which may modulate fatigue specific neural correlates unveiled by neuroimaging) or dietary interventions (informed by a greater knowledge of the microbiome).

Conclusions

Patients with rheumatoid arthritis have identified fatigue as a multidimensional symptom that is a challenge to manage. Healthcare professionals increasingly recognize the scale and nature of the symptom, yet it is not routinely addressed in clinical practice.

On a positive note, evidence is accumulating that a range of non-pharmacological interventions might help alleviate fatigue and certainly reduce the impact on patients' daily lives. It is however clear that much more needs to be learnt about the pathophysiology of this patient priority—and only then can we begin to test interventions which come close to curing this problem.

REFERENCES

1. Kirwan J, Heiberg T, Hewlett S, et al. Outcomes from the Patient Perspective Workshop at OMERACT 6. *J Rheumatol* 2003;*30*(4):868–72.
2. Carr A, Hewlett S, Hughes R, et al. Rheumatology outcomes: the patient's perspective. *J Rheumatol* 2003;*30*(4):880–3.
3. Ahlmen M, Nordenskiold U, Archenholtz B, et al. Rheumatology outcomes: the patient's perspective. A multicentre focus group interview study of Swedish rheumatoid arthritis patients. *Rheumatology (Oxf)* 2005;*44*(1):105–10.
4. Kirwan JR, Minnock P, Adebajo A, et al. Patient perspective: fatigue as a recommended patient centered outcome measure in rheumatoid arthritis. *J Rheumatol* 2007;*34*(5):1174–7.
5. Stebbings S, Treharne GJ. Fatigue in rheumatic disease: an overview. *Int J Clin Rheumatol* 2010;*5*(4):487–502.
6. Suurmeijer TP, Waltz M, Moum T, et al. Quality of life profiles in the first years of rheumatoid arthritis: results from the EURIDISS longitudinal study. *Arthritis Rheum* 2001;*45*(2):111–21.
7. Rupp I, Boshuizen HC, Jacobi CE, Dinant HJ, van den Bos GA. Impact of fatigue on health-related quality of life in rheumatoid arthritis. *Arthritis Rheum* 2004;*51*(4):578–85.
8. Pollard LC, Choy EH, Gonzalez J, Khoshaba B, Scott DL. Fatigue in rheumatoid arthritis reflects pain, not disease activity. *Rheumatology (Oxf)* 2006;*45*(7):885–9.
9. Overman CL, Kool MB, Da Silva JA, Geenen R. The prevalence of severe fatigue in rheumatic diseases: an international study. *Clin Rheumatol* 2016;*35*(2):409–15.
10. Repping-Wuts H, Fransen J, van Achterberg T, Bleijenberg G, van Riel P. Persistent severe fatigue in patients with rheumatoid arthritis. *J Clin Nurs* 2007;*16*(11c):377–83.
11. Hewlett S, Dures E, Almeida C. Measures of fatigue: Bristol Rheumatoid Arthritis Fatigue Multi-Dimensional Questionnaire (BRAF MDQ), Bristol Rheumatoid Arthritis Fatigue Numerical Rating Scales (BRAF NRS) for severity, effect, and coping, Chalder Fatigue Questionnaire (CFQ), Checklist Individual Strength (CIS20R and CIS8R), Fatigue Severity Scale (FSS), Functional Assessment Chronic Illness Therapy (Fatigue) (FACIT-F), Multi-Dimensional Assessment of Fatigue (MAF), Multi-Dimensional Fatigue Inventory (MFI), Pediatric Quality Of Life (PedsQL) Multi-Dimensional Fatigue Scale, Profile of Fatigue (ProF), Short Form 36 Vitality Subscale (SF-36 VT), and Visual Analog Scales (VAS). *Arthritis Care Res* 2011;*63*(Suppl 11):S263–86.
12. Hewlett S, Cockshott Z, Byron M, et al. Patients' perceptions of fatigue in rheumatoid arthritis: overwhelming, uncontrollable, ignored. *Arthritis Rheum* 2005;*53*(5):697–702.
13. Repping-Wuts H, Uitterhoeve R, van Riel P, van Achterberg T. Fatigue as experienced by patients with rheumatoid arthritis (RA): a qualitative study. *Int J Nurs Stud* 2008;*45*(7):995–1002.
14. Nicklin J, Cramp F, Kirwan J, Urban M, Hewlett S. Collaboration with patients in the design of patient-reported outcome measures: capturing the experience of fatigue in rheumatoid arthritis. *Arthritis Care Res* 2010;*62*(11):1552–8.

15. Nicklin J, Cramp F, Kirwan J, Greenwood R, Urban M, Hewlett S. Measuring fatigue in rheumatoid arthritis: a cross-sectional study to evaluate the Bristol Rheumatoid Arthritis Fatigue Multi-Dimensional questionnaire, visual analog scales, and numerical rating scales. *Arthritis Care Res* 2010;*62*(11):1559–68.

16. Hewlett S, Kirwan J, Bode C, et al. The revised Bristol rheumatoid arthritis fatigue measures and the rheumatoid arthritis impact of disease scale: validation in six countries. *Rheumatology (Oxf)* 2018:*57*(2):300–8.

17. Matcham F, Ali S, Hotopf M, Chalder T. Psychological correlates of fatigue in rheumatoid arthritis: a systematic review. *Clin Psychol Rev* 2015;*39*(Suppl. C):16–29.

18. Feldthusen C, Bjork M, Forsblad-d'Elia H, Mannerkorpi K. Perception, consequences, communication, and strategies for handling fatigue in persons with rheumatoid arthritis of working age--a focus group study. *Clin Rheumatol* 2013;*32*(5):557–66.

19. Dures E, Almeida C, Caesley J, et al. Patient preferences for psychological support in inflammatory arthritis: a multicentre survey. *Ann Rheum Dis* 2016;*75*(1):142–7.

20. Repping-Wuts H, Hewlett S, van Riel P, van Achterberg T. Fatigue in patients with rheumatoid arthritis: British and Dutch nurses' knowledge, attitudes and management. *J Adv Nurs* 2009;*65*(4):901–11.

21. Dures E, Fraser I, Almeida C, et al. Patients' perspectives on the psychological impact of inflammatory arthritis and meeting the associated support needs: open-ended responses in a multi-centre survey. *Musculoskeletal Care* 2017;*15*(3):175–85.

22. Nikolaus S, Bode C, Taal E, van de Laar MA. Four different patterns of fatigue in rheumatoid arthritis patients: results of a Q-sort study. *Rheumatology (Oxf)* 2010;*49*(11):2191–9.

23. Feldthusen C, Grimby-Ekman A, Forsblad-d'Elia H, Jacobsson L, Mannerkorpi K. Seasonal variations in fatigue in persons with rheumatoid arthritis: a longitudinal study. *BMC Musculoskelet Disord* 2016;*17*:59.

24. Michaud K, Messer J, Choi HK, Wolfe F. Direct medical costs and their predictors in patients with rheumatoid arthritis: a three-year study of 7,527 patients. *Arthritis Rheum* 2003;*48*(10):2750–62.

25. Lacaille D, White MA, Backman CL, Gignac MA. Problems faced at work due to inflammatory arthritis: new insights gained from understanding patients' perspective. *Arthritis Rheum* 2007;*57*(7):1269–79.

26. Burton W, Morrison A, Maclean R, Ruderman E. Systematic review of studies of productivity loss due to rheumatoid arthritis. *Occup Med (Lond)* 2006;*56*(1):18–27.

27. Lundkvist J, Kastang F, Kobelt G. The burden of rheumatoid arthritis and access to treatment: health burden and costs. *Eur J Health Econ* 2008;*8*(Suppl 2):S49–60.

28. Hewlett S, Chalder T, Choy E, et al. Fatigue in rheumatoid arthritis: time for a conceptual model. *Rheumatology (Oxf)* 2011;*50*(6):1004–6.

29. Nikolaus S, Bode C, Taal E, van de Laar MA. Fatigue and factors related to fatigue in rheumatoid arthritis: a systematic review. *Arthritis Care Res* 2013;*65*(7):1128–46.

30. Bergman MJ, Shahouri SH, Shaver TS, et al. Is fatigue an inflammatory variable in rheumatoid arthritis (RA)? Analyses of fatigue in RA, osteoarthritis, and fibromyalgia. *J Rheumatol* 2009;*36*(12):2788–94.

31. Druce KL, Bhattacharya Y, Jones GT, Macfarlane GJ, Basu N. Most patients who reach disease remission following anti-TNF therapy continue to report fatigue: results from the British

Society for Rheumatology Biologics Register for Rheumatoid Arthritis. *Rheumatology (Oxf)* 2016;*55*(10):1786–90.

32. Druce KL, Jones GT, Macfarlane GJ, Basu N. Patients receiving anti-TNF therapies experience clinically important improvements in RA-related fatigue: results from the British Society for Rheumatology Biologics Register for Rheumatoid Arthritis. *Rheumatology (Oxf)* 2015;*54*(6):964–71.

33. Druce KL, Jones GT, Macfarlane GJ, Basu N. Determining pathways to improvements in fatigue in rheumatoid arthritis: results from the british society for rheumatology biologics register for rheumatoid arthritis. *Arthritis Rheumatol* 2015;*67*(9):2303–10.

34. Druce KL, Jones GT, Macfarlane GJ, Basu N. Examining changes in central and peripheral pain as mediates of fatigue improvement: results from the British Society for Rheumatology biologics register for rheumatoid arthritis. *Arthritis Care Res* 2016;*68*(7):922–6.

35. Dantzer R, Heijnen CJ, Kavelaars A, Laye S, Capuron L. The neuroimmune basis of fatigue. *Trends Neurosci* 2014;*37*(1):39–46.

36. Hewlett S, Sanderson T, May J, et al. 'I'm hurting, I want to kill myself': rheumatoid arthritis flare is more than a high joint count--an international patient perspective on flare where medical help is sought. *Rheumatology (Oxf)* 2012;*51*(1):69–76.

37. Landmark-Hoyvik H, Reinertsen KV, Loge JH, et al. The genetics and epigenetics of fatigue. *PM R* 2010;*2*(5):456–65.

38. Wang T, Yin J, Miller AH, Xiao C. A systematic review of the association between fatigue and genetic polymorphisms. *Brain Behav Immun* 2017;*62*:230–44.

39. Basu N, Jones GT, Macfarlane GJ, Druce KL. Identification and validation of clinically relevant clusters of severe fatigue in rheumatoid arthritis. *Psychosom Med* 2017;*79*(9):1051–8.

40. Buchwald D, Herrell R, Ashton S, et al. A twin study of chronic fatigue. *Psychosom Med* 2001;*63*(6):936–43.

41. de Vega WC, Herrera S, Vernon SD, McGowan PO. Epigenetic modifications and glucocorticoid sensitivity in myalgic encephalomyelitis/chronic fatigue syndrome (ME/CFS). *BMC Med Genomics* 2017;*10*(1):11.

42. Hollingsworth KG, Newton JL, Taylor R, et al. Pilot study of peripheral muscle function in primary biliary cirrhosis: potential implications for fatigue pathogenesis. *Clin Gastroenterol Hepatol* 2008;*6*(9):1041–8.

43. He J, Hollingsworth KG, Newton JL, Blamire AM. Cerebral vascular control is associated with skeletal muscle pH in chronic fatigue syndrome patients both at rest and during dynamic stimulation. *NeuroImage Clin* 2013;*2*:168–73.

44. Jones DE, Hollingsworth KG, Taylor R, Blamire AM, Newton JL. Abnormalities in pH handling by peripheral muscle and potential regulation by the autonomic nervous system in chronic fatigue syndrome. *J Int Med* 2010;*267*(4):394–401.

45. Naviaux RK, Naviaux JC, Li K, et al. Metabolic features of chronic fatigue syndrome. *Proc Natl Acad Sci U S A* 2016;*113*(37):E5472–80.

46. Flight MH. Neurodevelopmental disorders: the gut-microbiome-brain connection. *Nat Rev Drug Discov* 2014;*13*(2):104.

47. Giloteaux L, Goodrich JK, Walters WA, Levine SM, Ley RE, Hanson MR. Reduced diversity and altered composition of the gut microbiome in individuals with myalgic encephalomyelitis/chronic fatigue syndrome. *Microbiome* 2016;*4*(1):30.

48. Chaudhuri A, Behan PO. Fatigue and basal ganglia. *J Neurol Sci* 2000;*179*(S1–2):34–42.

49. Basu, N, Kaplan, CM, Ichesco, E, et al. Functional and structural magnetic resonance imaging correlates of fatigue in patients with

rheumatoid arthritis. *Rheumatology*, 2019. doi:10.1093/rheumatology/kez132 (Early Online Publication).

50. Wu Q, Inman RD, Davis KD. Fatigue in ankylosing spondylitis is associated with the brain networks of sensory salience and attention. *Arthritis Rheumatol* 2014;66(2):295–303.

51. Basu N, Alsyedalhashem M, D'Allesandro M, Murray AD, Clauw DJ, Waiter GD. Brain white matter integrity: a future biomarker for rheumatoid arthritis related fatigue? *Arthritis Rheumatol* 2015;67.

52. Schrepf A, Cummiford C, Ichesco E, et al. The neural correlates of inflammation in RA: a multi-modal MRI study. *Arthritis Rheumatol* 2017;69.

53. Basu N, Kaplan CM, Ichesco E, et al. Neurobiological features of fibromyalgia are also present among rheumatoid arthritis patients. *Arthritis Rheumatol* 2018;70(7):1000–100.

54. Dantzer R, O'Connor JC, Freund GG, Johnson RW, Kelley KW. From inflammation to sickness and depression: when the immune system subjugates the brain. *Nat Rev Neurosci* 2008;9(1):46–56.

55. Chou KL, Gilman S, Bohnen NI. Association between autonomic dysfunction and fatigue in Parkinson disease. *J Neurol Sci* 2017;377:190–2.

56. Mandl T, Hammar O, Theander E, Wollmer P, Ohlsson B. Autonomic nervous dysfunction development in patients with primary Sjogren's syndrome: a follow-up study. *Rheumatology (Oxf)* 2010;49(6):1101–6.

57. Boneva RS, Decker MJ, Maloney EM, et al. Higher heart rate and reduced heart rate variability persist during sleep in chronic fatigue syndrome: a population-based study. *Auton Neurosci* 2007;137(1–2):94–101.

58. Adlan AM, Lip GY, Paton JF, Kitas GD, Fisher JP. Autonomic function and rheumatoid arthritis: a systematic review. *Semin Arthritis Rheum* 2014;44(3):283–304.

59. Kosek E, Altawil R, Kadetoff D, et al. Evidence of different mediators of central inflammation in dysfunctional and inflammatory pain--interleukin-8 in fibromyalgia and interleukin-1 beta in rheumatoid arthritis. *J Neuroimmunol* 2015;280:49–55.

60. Cramp F, Hewlett S, Almeida C, et al. Non-pharmacological interventions for fatigue in rheumatoid arthritis. *Cochrane Database Syst Rev* 2013(8):CD008322.

61. Katz P, Margaretten M, Gregorich S, Trupin L. Physical activity to reduce fatigue in rheumatoid arthritis: a randomized, controlled trial. *Arthritis Care Res* 2018;70(1):1–10.

62. Hewlett S, Ambler N, Almeida C, et al. Self-management of fatigue in rheumatoid arthritis: a randomised controlled trial of group cognitive-behavioural therapy. *Ann Rheum Dis* 2011;70(6):1060–7.

63. Evers AW, Kraaimaat FW, van Riel PL, de Jong AJ. Tailored cognitive-behavioral therapy in early rheumatoid arthritis for patients at risk: a randomized controlled trial. *Pain* 2002;100(1–2):141–53.

64. Riemsma RP, Kirwan JR, Taal E, Rasker JJ. Patient education for adults with rheumatoid arthritis. *Cochrane Database Syst Rev* 2002(3):CD003688.

65. Hammond A, Bryan J, Hardy A. Effects of a modular behavioural arthritis education programme: a pragmatic parallel-group randomized controlled trial. *Rheumatology (Oxf)* 2008;47(11):1712–18.

66. Bandura A. Social cognitive theory: an agentic perspective. *Annu Rev Psychol* 2001;52:1–26.

67. Ng JY, Ntoumanis N, Thogersen-Ntoumani C, et al. Self-determination theory applied to health contexts: a meta-analysis. *Perspect Psychol Sci* 2012;7(4):325–40.

68. Dures E, Hewlett S. Cognitive-behavioural approaches to self-management in rheumatic disease. *Nat Rev Rheumatol* 2012;8(9):553–9.

69. Camacho EM, Verstappen SM, Chipping J, Symmons DP. Learned helplessness predicts functional disability, pain and fatigue in patients with recent-onset inflammatory polyarthritis. *Rheumatology (Oxf)* 2013;52(7):1233–8.

70. Dures E, Kitchen K, Almeida C, et al. 'They didn't tell us, they made us work it out ourselves': patient perspectives of a cognitive-behavioral program for rheumatoid arthritis fatigue. *Arthritis Care Res* 2012;64(4):494–501.

71. Salmon VE, Hewlett S, Walsh NE, Kirwan JR, Cramp F. Physical activity interventions for fatigue in rheumatoid arthritis: a systematic review. *Phys Therapy Rev* 2017;22(1–2):12–22.

72. Reinseth L, Uhlig T, Kjeken I, Koksvik HS, Skomsvoll JF, Espnes GA. Performance in leisure-time physical activities and self-efficacy in females with rheumatoid arthritis. *Scand J Occup Ther* 2011;18(3):210–18.

73. Chan R. Cochrane review summary for cancer nursing: drug therapy for the management of cancer-related fatigue. *Cancer Nurs* 2011;34(3):250–1.

74. Elbers RG, Verhoef J, van Wegen EE, Berendse HW, Kwakkel G. Interventions for fatigue in Parkinson's disease. *Cochrane Database Syst Rev* 2015(10):CD010925.

75. Almeida C, Choy EH, Hewlett S, et al. Biologic interventions for fatigue in rheumatoid arthritis. *Cochrane Database Syst Rev* 2016(6):CD008334.

76. Chauffier K, Salliot C, Berenbaum F, Sellam J. Effect of biotherapies on fatigue in rheumatoid arthritis: a systematic review of the literature and meta-analysis. *Rheumatology (Oxf)* 2012;51(1):60–8.

77. Sheng P, Hou L, Wang X, et al. Efficacy of modafinil on fatigue and excessive daytime sleepiness associated with neurological disorders: a systematic review and meta-analysis. *PLoS One* 2013;8(12):e81802.

78. Pucci E, Branas P, D'Amico R, Giuliani G, Solari A, Taus C. Amantadine for fatigue in multiple sclerosis. *Cochrane Database Syst Rev* 2007(1):CD002818.

79. Mucke M, Mochamat, Cuhls H, et al. Pharmacological treatments for fatigue associated with palliative care: executive summary of a Cochrane Collaboration systematic review. *J Cachexia Sarcopenia Muscle* 2016;7(1):23–7.

22

Health economics of rheumatoid arthritis

David L. Scott and Allan Wailoo

Summary

Cost of illness studies show rheumatoid arthritis (RA) has high costs for patients, for healthcare funders, and for society as a whole. Historically indirect costs exceeded direct costs and the costs of drugs were relatively low. Over the last 20–30 years inpatient care reduced by over 90%, outpatient care has changed little, disability pensions and sick days have fallen, and drug costs have risen 20-fold, mainly due to the use of biologics. The cost-effectiveness of established and new treatments is usually assessed using quality-adjusted life years (QALYs). In some studies, QALYs are calculated from patient responses to questionnaires like the EuroQoL EQ-5D. But in many studies, no such instruments were included and analysts therefore have to rely on estimating the relationship between measures that were included, like functional disability, and the utility-based measures that allow the calculation of QALYs. As the impact of new treatment requires understanding the natural history of treated RA from the perspective of changes in costs and QALYs over time, simulation models have been developed that synthesize the short-term effectiveness data from clinical trials with longer-term observational studies. These models are used to estimate the cost-effectiveness of new treatments compared with historic comparators. Studies show that conventional disease-modifying drugs given as monotherapy or in combinations are usually cost-effective. Biologics are far more expensive, and their cost-effectiveness lies close to the margin of what healthcare funders are prepared to pay. Less expensive biosimilars and tapering biologics after patients have responded may increase the cost-effectiveness of these drugs.

Introduction

RA, like other long-term conditions, can lead to substantial economic burdens for patients with the disease, their family members, society as a whole, and health services in particular. In this chapter we review the different ways of assessing these costs and their implications for decisions about treatment.

The high costs of RA reflect the significant economic consequences of many long-term conditions. These costs have been known for a long time and there are a large number of examples of the economic impacts of long-term disorders and comorbidities. One study by Meerding et al.[1] evaluated the demands on healthcare resources in the Netherlands caused by different types of illnesses and how these varied with age. Healthcare costs rose slowly throughout adult life and increased exponentially after age 50. Leading causes of high healthcare costs were mental retardation, musculoskeletal diseases and particularly joint diseases, and dementia. Another study by Charlson et al.[2] found in a primary care cohort that healthcare costs rose markedly in patients with multiple comorbidities. These general examples help put the economic costs of RA into perspective.

The economic issues in RA span three inter-related areas. The first of these is cost of illness studies, which look at costs from the perspectives of the patient, the patient's family, and society in general. The second is how to assess the economic impacts of treating RA. These costs are usually considered from the perspective of healthcare payers, who are usually either governments or health insurers. The final area is the costs of treatment. When low cost treatments are used for short periods of time there is little incentive to study these treatment costs in any detail. However, when high cost treatments are given for prolonged periods of time, as has happened with biologics in RA, there is considerable interest in the field. This chapter considers each of these areas in turn.

Cost of illness studies

Types of study

The studies span a range of approaches and viewpoints. The first source of variation is their perspective in assessing costs. Some studies evaluate societal perspectives, which take into account all costs irrespective of who pays and therefore include direct and indirect costs; others focus on the payer's perspective and therefore mainly assess direct medical costs.

Studies also differ in the populations they examine, which can be population based or specific samples defined by their disease onset or severity or where they are seen. Another source of variation is what information is collected about costs. Some studies collect all health cost data, without reference to RA; others only collect costs clearly related to the management of RA, though these differences can sometimes be difficult to define. Data about costs can also be collected in different ways. Some studies involve collecting data in a top down approach using national data sources; others use medical records and patient-provided information. In addition, data can be collected prospectively or retrospectively. Given these many differences it is inevitable that the findings vary substantially across different studies.

Studies before 2000

The earliest studies were relatively simple. An early investigation reported in 1978 by Meenan et al.[3] examined the annual costs of disease in 50 patients with severe RA. Their direct medical costs were three times the national average. Indirect costs, mainly due to lost income, were at least three times the direct medical costs. They found that 58% of the patients sustained major psychosocial losses, with uncovered income losses the greatest economic burden for individuals with established RA.

A few years later Stone[4] evaluated the lifetime economic costs of RA in a cohort of patients whose disease started in 1977. This study found the value of the lifetime economic costs of RA was in the region of $20 412/case in 1977 dollars, which was nearly as great as that for stroke and coronary heart disease. A subsequent more detailed study by Gabriel et al.[5] modelled costs using data from Minnesota. They calculated the median lifetime incremental costs of RA range from about $60 000 to $120 000. The incremental costs were higher for younger individuals compared to older individuals.

By 2000 sufficient research had been published for Cooper to undertake a systematic review of the field.[6] She identified 14 studies from 1978 to 1998; 9 were based in rheumatology clinics and 5 in the community. Costs calculated by the various studies varied substantially across all the categories used. The mean annual direct costs due to RA were US$5720 (using 1996 dollars). Mean costs for outpatient visits US$1855 and for inpatient stays were US$4944. Indirect costs, when assessed, were usually calculated as annual number of days absent from work and these ranged from 3 to 30 days per year. Mean annual indirect cost due to RA were US$5822. Although it was widely believed indirect costs substantially exceeded direct costs, the evidence for this assessment was incomplete, though several studies showed they were larger.

Another systematic review from 2000 by Pugner et al.[7] made international comparisons of the costs of RA based on findings in 12 studies, some of which were the same as those reviewed by Cooper.[6] This international comparative review found the mean annual expenditure (in 1998 US dollars) was $5054 for direct medical costs and $8726 for $12 210 indirect costs. It also calculated that the median annual cost for each one million of the population was $122M.

Early disease

Until 2000 studies mainly focused on hospital patients with established RA. However, the growing focus on treating RA early led to more studies in this area. One of the first to examine the costs of early inflammatory arthritis, by Cooper et al.[8] involved patients in the community-based Norfolk Arthritis Register. They estimated the health service and non-health service costs and their predictors in patients with early inflammatory polyarthritis. Their 6-month prospective longitudinal study assessed costs in a random sample of 133 patients who had enrolled in the register between 1994 and 1999. The mean 6-month total cost was estimated at £2800 per person. About 14% was health service costs; the remainder was non-health-service costs. Costs were higher in patients with lower health status and with rheumatoid factor positivity.

At about the same time Merkesdal et al.[9] evaluated indirect costs in the first 3 years of RA. They investigated 133 consecutive gainfully employed outpatients with early RA in a prospective multicentre observational study. The mean annual indirect costs were $11 750. During follow-up the costs of sick leave reduced and indirect costs fell by 21%.

In 2004 Hallert et al.[10] published the first of a triad of studies which evaluated both direct and indirect costs in early disease. The first study showed they were both high in the early phases of the disease. Costs were assessed in 297 patients with recent onset RA who were followed over 12 months. Indirect costs were more than double the direct costs. During the first year of their disease 63% of patients experienced work disability; these patients formed a 'high-indirect-cost group'. Direct costs spanned ambulatory healthcare (76%), hospital admission (12%), and medication (9%).

Hallert et al.[11] then reported the 3-year results in these patients. Indirect costs continued to exceed direct costs throughout the 3-year period. Although most patients showed clinical improvements, 15% had sustained high or moderate disease activity. In the first year, average direct costs were €3704; they fell to €2652 in the third year. All costs decreased, except those for medication and surgery. Average indirect costs were €8871 in the first year and remained essentially unchanged. Almost 50% were on sick leave or early retirement when the study started. Although sick leave decreased this was offset by increased early retirements.

The third study in the sequence reported 6-year findings.[12] The mean total cost/patient was €14 768 in year 1; this increased to €18 438 in year 6. Outpatient visits and hospitalization decreased, but costs for surgery increased from €92/patient year 1 to €444 year 6. Drugs increased from €429/patient to €2214/patient; this increase was mainly due to introduction of biologics. In the first year, drugs accounted for 10% of direct costs; this increased to 49% by the sixth year. Sick leave decreased during the first years, but disability pensions increased, resulting in unchanged indirect costs. Over the following years, disability pensions increased further and indirect costs increased from €10 284 in the first year to €13 874 by the sixth year.

Nikiphorou et al.[13] reported a longer-term follow-up of the Norfolk register patients 10 years after the initial study. A representative sample of 101 patients with inflammatory arthritis from the 1999 cohort provided complete data over another 6-month period. By this time, they had had arthritis for 10–15 years and their mean disease duration was 14 years. Mean direct medical cost per patient over the 6-month period was £1496 (inflated for 2013 prices); this cost compared with £582 (inflated to 2013) prices per patient ten years earlier. The increase in cost was mainly due to the use of biologics; these biologic costs accounted for 51% of the overall direct costs. Other components of the direct costs included primary care (11%), hospital outpatient (19%), and day care (12%) and inpatient stays (4%). The English and Swedish studies highlight the way spending on biologics has changed the nature of direct medical costs; biologics given to a minority of patients had become major drivers of medical costs.

Registers

Several Scandinavian registers have been used to assess the costs of RA.

Kvamme et al.[14] compared the costs of RA with other forms of inflammatory arthritis in patients in the Norwegian disease-modifying antirheumatic drug register during four 6-month periods after starting treatment with synthetic and biologic drugs in 1152 patients with RA and smaller numbers of patients with ankylosing spondylitis and psoriatic arthritis. The total 2-year costs across diagnoses were similar for patients receiving synthetic disease-modifying drugs. With biologic treatments RA patients had the highest mean costs of €121 900. The largest cost component across all diagnoses and treatment types was productivity loss, followed by the cost of drugs for biologic treatments and the cost of in-hospital care for synthetic disease-modifying drug therapy.

Kalkan et al.[15] assessed the total socioeconomic impact of RA in Sweden during the period 1990–2010 and examined changes in costs during this period. It was chosen to cover the decade before and after biologic drugs were introduced. Sweden has a tax-financed health insurance system allowing all residents sick leave benefits when they are unable to work. After reaching a payment level for outpatient visits of about €100 annually, healthcare is subsequently free of charge. Similarly, all prescribed drugs, including biologic drugs, are free of charge after a payment level of about €200. There were no formal restrictions on the prescription of biologic drugs in Sweden from 1999 to 2010 and their use was among the highest in Europe. During the 20-year period, inpatient care reduced by over 90% while outpatient care was unchanged at about 90 000 visits annually. Disability pensions were reduced by about a third and sick days by about half. These reductions in costs were offset by substantial increases in annual drug costs from under €10 million to almost €200 million. This meant that drug costs increased from 3% to 33% of total costs between 1990 and 2010. Consequently, the portion of total costs accounting for by indirect costs of RA fell from 75% in 1990 to just over half in 2010. These changes are shown in Figure 22.1.

Another Swedish register study from Eriksson et al.[16] took a different approach. They evaluated a cohort of prevalent patients with RA in 2010 from the national register. The patients were followed throughout the year. They were contrasted with matched general population comparators. The annual cost for hospital care, drugs, and productivity losses in prevalent working age patients with RA was in the region of €23 000; one-quarter was accounted for by healthcare costs, and three-quarters by productivity losses. These costs were two or three times higher than in the general population, corresponding to an annual cost of €15 000 attributable to RA. In patients treated with biologic drugs, the cost in the 18–64 years group and the ≥65 year's group were 4 and 6–7 times, respectively, the corresponding costs in the general population.

Broadly similar findings come from German centres between 2001 and 2011.[17] An analysis of the National Database of the German Collaborative Arthritis Centres, which assess about 3400 patients each year, showed considerable increases in direct costs. These rose from €4914 to €8206 in patients aged 18–64, and from €4100 to €6221 in those aged 65 years or more. This was mainly due to increases in prescribing biologic agents. In the under 65s they rose from 6% to 31% of patients and in the over 65s from 3% to 19%. There were decreasing costs for inpatient treatment indirect costs due to sick leave and work disability. Overall costs rose by about €2500–€2900 for patients under 65 and about €2100 for retired patients. The rise in drug costs has plateaued from 2009 and, as a consequence, no further major increases in total costs are anticipated in the foreseeable future.

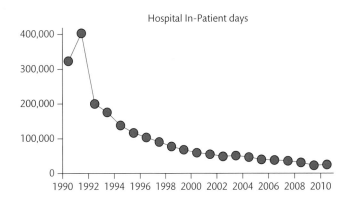

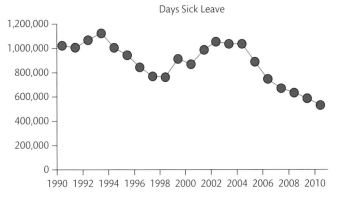

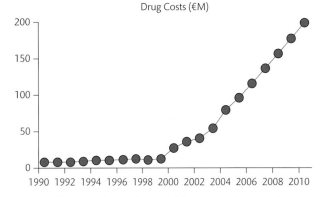

Figure 22.1 Changes in hospital care, sick leave, and drug costs in Sweden 1990–2010.
Source: data from Kalkan A et al (2014) 'Costs of rheumatoid arthritis during the period 1990–2010: a register-based cost-of-illness study in Sweden'. *Rheumatology* 53(1):153–60.

Recent studies

The most detailed information comes from a systematic review by Hresko et al.[18] They focused on studies of the direct medical costs associated with RA patients in the United States since biologics were introduced. They evaluated 12 studies; their quality varied and only one-third of them were of high quality. The total direct medical costs for all RA patients, using any treatment regimen were in the region of $12 500 per year. For patients receiving biologics the costs increased to about $36 000 per year; RA care costs were over half of the annual direct medical costs in these patients. The medical costs of RA were broadly similar to those of other long-term conditions.

There is marked geographic variation in the current cost of illness for RA depending on the arrangements for healthcare in different places. For example, the medical costs are relatively low in

China[19] but high in Australia,[20] where there is substantial biologic prescribing. Where biologics are readily available their use has expanded to about one-third of patients. The overall consequences are that direct healthcare costs have increased but socioeconomic costs have fallen. The widespread use of intensive treatments using conventional drugs appears beneficial on total costs; overall the balance of evidence is that the nature of costs has changed but the total costs have been relatively stable.[21]

Assessing when treatment is cost-effective

Historical background

The main costs of treating RA have gradually shifted over time from inpatient care towards biologic drugs. Due to their high costs, biologic drugs have been natural candidates for studies of cost-effectiveness. However, earlier studies in rheumatoid arthritis started with an interest in the cost-effectiveness of inpatient care. A trial by Helewa et al. in the 1980s[22] showed inpatient care was more expensive than outpatient management but that it resulted in sustained long-term benefits. The authors argued that it was therefore likely to be beneficial. However, they did not measure the economic benefits in a systematic way and so its overall impact was uncertain.

Another early focus was preventing deaths from upper gastrointestinal tract bleeding due to non-steroidal anti-inflammatory drugs, which may be prevented by the prophylactic use of misoprostol. Edelson et al.[23] estimated the direct medical costs, years of life lost, and therefore the cost-effectiveness of misoprostol. This study was based on an analysis of a number of published studies and involved estimations of the risks of gastrointestinal bleeding and the impact of misoprostol in different groups of patients. In some groups, such as patients with RA, the drug was cost-effective but in most patients it was not. Nowadays drugs like omeprazole are used to prevent such bleeding and these studies are historical. However, these types of studies demonstrated the feasibility of assessing cost-effectiveness, the importance of life years saved as an outcome measure, and the relevance of results for clinicians and other decision makers.

In the 1980s one new drug evaluated was auranofin, an oral gold treatment. One small trial by Thompson et al.[24] evaluated its potential benefit. However, it cost more than control treatment and was of marginal benefit, meaning that it was unlikely to be cost-effective. However, the trial was used by others to make a more general case for health economic studies to be used when assessing new treatments.[25]

Using quality-adjusted life years

By the 1990s more effective disease-modifying strategies had been identified and their cost-effectiveness was starting to be evaluated. During this decade there was a growing emphasis on using QALYs as the measure of treatment benefit. The QALY is a compound measure of benefit that combines concerns for both the quality and the quantity of life lived. One QALY represents one year in perfect health. Each year of life spent at less than full health is valued at less than 1 QALY. The fundamental principle of the QALY as a measure is that comparisons can be made across different diseases, patients, and health technologies in a consistent manner. This approach is sometimes referred to as cost utility analysis because the estimate of

how far below 1 a particular impaired health state should be ranked is determined by reference to the preferences ('utilities') of individual patients or members of the public. The QALY based approach was adopted more widely in the 1990s and was promoted by both rheumatologists and health economists.[26,27] While not without its critics, the approach is probably the most widespread form of economic evaluation at the current time.

In the 1990s these concepts became widely accepted for assessing the economic impacts of treating RA.[28] As effective disease-modifying strategies were developed it became important to also demonstrate they were cost-effective. For example, the combination of methotrexate, sulfasalazine, and short-term steroids, termed the COBRA regimen, was more effective than sulfasalazine alone in early RA. It was also more cost-effective. It cost less in combined outpatient care, inpatient care, and non-healthcare and utility scores favoured combined treatment.[29]

Estimating QALYs

In practice, QALYs tend to be calculated from so-called generic preference-based outcome measures. Instruments such as SF-6D and the EQ-5D, comprise a descriptive system where respondents indicate the degree of impairment in defined aspects of health and a set of utility values associated with all the health states of the descriptive system based on the preferences of samples of the general population.

The EQ-5D has been widely used to assess health-related quality of life across its five dimensions which comprise mobility, self-care, usual activities, pain and discomfort, and anxiety and depression. The standard version of the EQ-5D has here levels for each of the five health dimensions (no problems, some problems, extreme problems), resulting in 243 different health states.[30] A newer version that has five levels (EQ-5D-5L) has been produced. Tariffs from general population samples are available for many different countries.

Using disability assessments to estimate QALYs

Only a minority of observational studies and clinical trials in RA record generic, preference-based measures such as the EQ-5D. The situation is slowly changing as the requirements of reimbursement agencies filters down into clinical study design. But this evidence gap often exists making the estimation of QALYs more challenging and uncertain.

Most studies record disability assessments, and in particular they measure the Health Assessment Questionnaire (HAQ). Analysts have therefore attempted to bridge this evidence gap by estimating utility scores from the responses patients give to the HAQ instrument. This requires a separate data set where patients have completed both HAQ and a utility instrument, like EQ-5D. One example by Bansback et al.[31] used study data from two groups of RA patients in the United Kingdom and Canada in whom data had been collected on HAQ, EQ-5D, and Short Form 36 (SF-36), which was converted into the preference-based SF-6D. Using regression analyses they developed a model to predict SF-6D and EQ-5D across the range of HAQ scores. These types of conversion have been criticised for a variety of reasons. One particular problem is that utility measures have very complex distributions: utility is limited above at 1, below at the worst health state that can be described by the instrument, have gaps in the distribution and tend to be multimodal. These challenges are important because they lead to biased estimates of health utility, undervaluing the benefits of clinically effective health technologies, making them appear less cost-effective than they truly are.

These challenges have led to the development and application of more complex but appropriate statistical methods. For example, Hernández et al.[32] have developed a bespoke, mixture model approach to directly estimate EQ-5D from HAQ, pain and age using a large observational database with over 100 000 assessments from RA patients. Their approach improves the fit over the entire range of EQ-5D and thereby allows a robust method for linking data on clinical effectiveness into economic models to assess the cost per QALY of treatments for RA.

Long-term studies

A crucial requirement for assessing the impact of new treatment is to understand the natural history of treated disease over the long term, well beyond the timeframe measured in clinical trials. Kobelt et al.[33] took this approach in decision models using data from two cohorts of patients with early RA followed up since disease onset, which was up to 15 years. One study of 183 patients was from Sweden and the other study of 916 patients was from England. Disease progression over 10 years was modelled as annual transitions between disease states, defined by HAQ scores. Costs and utilities associated with different HAQ levels were derived from data in cohort studies and cross-sectional surveys. They found that, as RA progresses, costs increase, and quality of life decreases. In Sweden total annual costs ranged between $4900 and $33 000 dollars per patient. In England they ranged between $4900 and $14 600 dollars. As disability levels rose QALYs decreased, as shown in **Table 22.1**. This summarizes expected average 10-year costs and utilities for patients starting in different disease states at baseline. For comparison, a group of healthy people of similar age and sex distribution would have about 6.1 QALYs per person over the same period of time. Subsequent work by Kobelt and her colleagues[34] developed a more complex model based on five functional states defined by HAQ status, each one of which was divided by patients having high and low overall status based on their visual analogue scores. This showed that patients at the same HAQ levels with high visual analogue scores had consistently lower utilities than patients with low visual analogue scores.

Sheffield RA health economic model

When assessing the economic impact of treatments two separate issues need to be considered. The first one is relatively simple; costs and benefits during the study period. For effective low-cost treatments this may be all that is required. The second one is more complex; costs and benefits beyond the study period. For high cost treatments this is usually an essential undertaking as they are unlikely to be cost-effective over the short-term and, because they have disease-modifying claims, differences in both costs and benefits are likely to occur well beyond the follow-up period for a clinical trial. Indeed, differences for patients over their entire lifetimes could be expected. Failure to incorporate these long-term differences seriously underestimates the cost-effectiveness of such health technologies. To achieve this second goal, economic models are used. These synthesize data from a variety of sources, including the relevant clinical trials, in order to estimate cost-effectiveness. The Sheffield model from Tosh et al.[35] is widely used for this purpose. It uses an independent patient simulation to estimate the total costs and QALYs of treatment strategies. It generates a simulated patient with a set of baseline characteristics including age, gender, HAQ score, disease duration, and previous therapies. It allows different patient subpopulations, such as early RA and patients who have previously taken disease-modifying drugs to be evaluated. It considers patients' HAQ score at 6-monthly intervals for their whole lifetime so that a full sequence of treatments can be considered. **Figure 22.2** shows the HAQ profile for a simulated patient. HAQ scores change over time and with different treatments. The Sheffield RA model requires three key pieces of data: the initial effectiveness of a treatment; the change over time in a patient's HAQ while on treatment; and the length of time a patient will spend on treatment. Generally, the model used data from clinical trials together with observational studies, which provide long-term information.

Decision making using cost-effectiveness analysis

Treatments do not exist in a vacuum. The concept of cost-effectiveness is comparative. It asks, what is the difference in costs and the difference in health benefits between the technology of interest and comparator treatments, of which there may be several.

The incremental cost-effectiveness ratio (ICER) is the difference in costs divided by the difference in health benefit, usually measured in QALYs.

One treatment needs to be compared with another. One way to do this is through a cost-effectiveness analysis. These compare the effectiveness of two or possibly more treatments in relation to their

Table 22.1 Expected costs and QALYs for patients starting at different HAQ levels: comparison of Sweden and England

HAQ Score	Sweden		England	
	Mean US dollars	Mean QALY	Mean US dollars	Mean QALY
<0.6	54 614	5.48	26 603	5.59
0.6–1.1	73 343	5.21	35 703	5.24
1.1–1.6	91 713	4.93	40 170	4.9
1.6–2.1	112 300	4.54	46 403	4.68
2.1–2.6	127 171	4.24	53 748	4.26
>2.6	120 759	4.37	58 316	4.05

Source: data from 33. Kobelt G, et al (2002) 'Modeling the progression of rheumatoid arthritis: a two-country model to estimate costs and consequences of rheumatoid arthritis'. *Arthritis Rheum* 46: 2310–9.

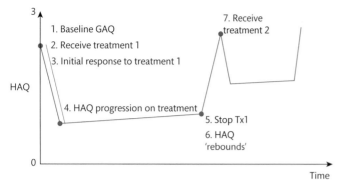

Figure 22.2 Potential HAQ profile for a patient simulated in the Sheffield model.

The patient has a simulated baseline HAQ. After receiving the first treatment there is an improvement (decrease) in their HAQ score. While on treatment, their HAQ level worsens over time, until a point comes when the treatment is stopped and their HAQ rebounds. The patient begins a second therapy that is less effective than the first in terms of the response gained and the time spent on treatment.

Reprinted from Tosh J, et al (2011) 'The Sheffield rheumatoid arthritis health economic model'. *Rheumatology* 50 Suppl 4: 26–31 with permission from Oxford University Press.

different costs. An ideal new treatment would be more effective and would cost less overall. Such a difference could be due to the costs of the treatment itself or because using it reduces other direct health costs. In general, new treatments are more effective but also cost more. In this situation healthcare funders try to balance the extra costs with the greater number of QALYs achieved. In England, the National Institute for Health and Care Excellence (NICE) provides recommendations on many new drug treatments. It uses a threshold range of £20 000 to £30 000 per QALY gained in its considerations of cost-effectiveness.

Overview

Combining methods to calculate QALYs in patients with RA with models of the progression of the disease over years enables health economists to assess the cost-effectiveness of treatments during the trial and also beyond the period of the trial. As the approaches taken vary, with different experts taking different approaches, there is considerable diversity in the calculations. Such variation is to be expected and needs to be taken into account when assessing the outputs of any economic evaluation.

Cost-effectiveness of different treatments

Leflunomide

One of the new drugs introduced in the last 20 years was leflunomide, a conventional disease-modifying antirheumatic drug. There was some interest in its cost-effectiveness, though as its costs were modest, it was not evaluated in detail. Kobelt et al.[36] assessed its benefits using a Markov model which constructed health states defined by HAQ scores. Compared to sulfasalazine there was evidence that costs were lower with leflunomide and QALYs were increased indicating it was cost-effective in this comparison. Findings against methotrexate varied in different trials and so no definitive conclusions could be drawn.

A more detailed assessment of the value of leflunomide as part of the strategy of using disease-modifying drugs by Schädlich et al.[37]

used a 3-year simulation model adapted to the German healthcare system after secondary analysis of relevant publications and data. This analysis found that after 3 years, adding leflunomide was less costly and more effective than the strategy excluding leflunomide when total costs, both direct and indirect costs, were considered.

Combinations of conventional disease-modifying drugs

The use of different combinations of conventional disease-modifying drugs, with or without steroids, has been a major research focus in the last two decades. The cost-effectiveness of different combination treatment approach in early RA was assessed by Tosh et al.[38] They included 13 studies in the review; 19 treatment arms included combination treatment strategies, and 10 trial arms considered monotherapy. Mixed treatment comparison methods estimated the relative effectiveness of the different strategies. A mathematical model was developed to compare the long-term costs and benefits of the alternative strategies, combining data from a variety of sources. Using a threshold of £20 000 per QALY, strategies most likely to be cost-effective were combination therapy with downward titration and triple combination therapy. Other approaches to combination therapy were less beneficial.

Subsequent analysis of another intensive combination therapy trial by Wailoo et al.[39] examined the benefit of triple therapy with methotrexate, ciclosporin, and short-term steroids in early RA. Two-year costs for each treatment strategy showed primary care costs were negligible across all groups. Drug and hospital costs were lowest with triple therapy, which was also the most effective; it dominated all other strategies.

However, not all studies of combination therapy showed it is effective. A 3-year trial of symptom control delivered by shared care compared with aggressive treatment delivered in hospital in patients with established RA was analysed by Davies et al.[40] They found mean cost per person was £4540 with shared care and £4440 with aggressive treatment. Mean QALYs per person for 3 years were 1.67 with shared care compared with 1.60 with aggressive treatment. There was little economic benefit from intensive treatment in most patients in this trial; however, the main reason for this finding is that the intensive treatment strategy was relatively clinically ineffective.

Biologics

Tumour necrosis factor inhibitors, interleukin 6 inhibitors, and biologics which influence T-cell and B-cell function are all effective in RA. However, they are also expensive. They are therefore natural contenders for cost-effectiveness analysis as decision makers seek to ensure that their limited budgets are used in the most efficient way.

The first substantial research in this area started in the early 2000s. Choi et al.[41] undertook a cost-effectiveness analysis of six treatment options for patients with methotrexate-resistant RA. The found that methotrexate therapy in methotrexate-naïve RA cost $1100 per ACR 20 outcome compared with no second-line agent. They also found that methotrexate continuation, ciclosporin and methotrexate combined, and etanercept monotherapy cost more, but either were not more clinically efficacious or were not cost-effective. The least expensive option, triple therapy, cost 1.3 times more per patient with ACR 20 response than methotrexate therapy for treatment-naive RA. The most effective approach, combining etanercept with methotrexate, cost 38 times more per patient with ACR 20 outcome ($4600/ACR

20). They concluded that if 15 mg/week methotrexate is considered cost-effective for achieving ACR 20 in methotrexate-naïve RA, then it was likely triple therapy was also cost-effective in methotrexate-resistant RA. Whether etanercept with methotrexate is cost-effective depends on whether $42 600/ACR 20 over a 6-month period is considered acceptable.

Wong et al.[42] made another early contribution. They projected the 54-week results from a trial of infliximab, one of the first tumour necrosis factor inhibitors to be used, into lifetime economic and clinical outcomes using a simulation model. Each infliximab infusion would cost $1393. When compared with methotrexate alone, 54 weeks of infliximab plus methotrexate decreased the likelihood of having advanced disability from 23% to 11%. This change projected to a lifetime marginal cost-effectiveness ratio of $30 500 per discounted QALY gained, considering only direct medical costs. They consequently concluded infliximab plus methotrexate was cost-effective.

At about the same time Jobanputra et al.[43] completed a more detailed assessment of two tumour necrosis factor inhibitors, etanercept and infliximab, after the failure of two previous disease-modifying drugs. They based their assessments on an analysis of six separate trials. Using a simulation model to evaluate changes in quality of life they found the biologics had a base-case ICER of £83 000 per QALY for etanercept and approximately £115 000 per QALY for infliximab. These figures reduced to £72 000 per QALY for etanercept, and £95 000 for infliximab when they were used last in the sequence of drugs. These substantial differences between the conclusions of experts reviewing broadly similar clinical trial data has persisted for almost 20 years. Some experts find biologics are cost-effective for RA and others find they are not.

Two systematic reviews summarize much of the research base about the cost-effectiveness of biologics. The first by van der Velde et al.[44] evaluated 18 different economic studies published from 2000 to 2007. The number of comparisons within each study ranged from 1 to 20 and overall there were 116 different comparisons. There was extensive heterogeneity between the studies. They included early and late RA, moderate and severe RA, and also refractory disease. Seventeen studies used model-based analytic approaches. One empirical economic evaluation used observational data. Most modelling studies used trial data to estimate patients' short-term responses to biologics and disease-modifying drugs and one used registry data. As long-term efficacy data was unavailable evaluations with longer time horizons modelled trial data with observational data to extrapolate the short-term effects of treatment. Patients who failed methotrexate combination therapy or sequential administration of disease-modifying drugs were reported in most detail. Out of 35 evaluations (**Figure 22.3**) biologics were only cost-effective in one study at an ICER of $50 000/QALY (Canadian Dollars) and at $100 000/QALY in another 14. In most cases the ratios were substantially higher. In methotrexate-naïve patients biologics were never cost-effective.

Another systematic review published in 2015 by Joensuu et al.[45] assessed studies until 2013. It included 41 cost utility analyses. When considering only direct costs, the ICER of tumour necrosis factor inhibitors varied from 39 000 to €1 273 000 € per QALY gained compared with conventional disease-modifying drugs in methotrexate-naïve patients. When patients had inadequate responses to methotrexate and other disease-modifying drugs the ratios ranged between 12 000 and 708 000 €/QALY. Rituximab was the most cost-effective alternative compared to other biologics among the patients with an insufficient response to tumour necrosis factor inhibitors.

Since these systematic reviews were published several new studies have been published. Stevenson et al.[46] evaluated biologics in an English setting. Using an economic model which assessed the cost-effectiveness of different drugs a systematic literature review and network meta-analysis established their relative clinical effectiveness.

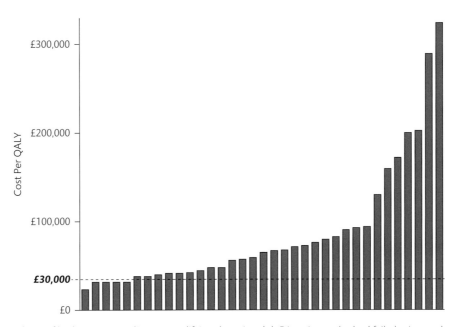

Figure 22.3 Cost utility analyses of biologics versus disease-modifying drugs in adult RA patients who had failed prior methotrexate combination therapy or sequential administration of disease-modifying drugs. Showing incremental cost-effectiveness ratios per QALY in 2009 pounds.

Source: data from van der Velde G, et al (2011) 'Cost-effectiveness of biologic response modifiers compared to disease-modifying antirheumatic drugs for rheumatoid arthritis: a systematic review'. *Arthritis Care Res* 63: 65–78.

Primary analyses showed that the cost per QALY from following a biologic treatment strategy £41 600 for patients with severe RA and £51 100 for patients with only moderate to severe RA. However, additional analyses showed that in patients with poor prognostic markers the cost per QALY fell to £25 300 for those with severe RA and to £28 500 for those with moderate to severe RA. On balance the cost-effectiveness of biologics used to treat RA in England seemed questionable. However, it met current accepted levels in those RA patients with the worst prognoses.

Jansen et al.[47] studied biologics from the US societal perspective for treating patients with moderately to severely active RA who had inadequate responses to conventional disease-modifying drugs. They found that biologic sequences were associated with greater treatment benefit, including more QALYs and greater treatment-related costs than conventional disease-modifying drugs. ICERs for biologics ranged from $126 000 to $140 000 per QALY gained. These cost-effectiveness ratios fell below what is typically claimed to be the US-specific willingness to pay threshold. Alternative scenarios that evaluated the effects of homogeneous patients, dose increases, increased costs of hospitalization for severely physically impaired patients, and a lower baseline HAQ Disability Index score resulted in similar ratios.

Reducing costs of biologics

One factor reducing biologic costs is the introduction of biosimilars. As these cost less than the originator molecules they will reduce acquisition costs of the drugs. However, as Mehr and Brook have indicated[48] the way in which biosimilars will enter clinical practice will be complex and unpredictable. In England the introduction of infliximab and etanercept biosimilars has reduced National Health Service costs. The cumulative cost savings over 2 years is in the region of £40 million.[49]

Another approach to reducing costs and improving cost-effectiveness is to taper or stop biologics when patients have achieved stable low disease activity or remission. The economic analysis of one tapering trial, the Spacing of TNF-blocker injections in RA Study (STRASS) trial showed tapering was associated with less QALYs gain and reduced costs.[50] No conclusion was made about the overall benefit of this approach as there is no overall consensus

on how to assess the economic impact of less effective treatments. Aletaha et al.[51] developed a 5-year economic model to compare withdrawal, tapering, or maintenance of biologics in patients with RA who had achieved remission or low disease activity. They based their approach on meta-analysing 14 different studies. Biologic withdrawal and tapering incurred comparable 5-year total costs. These were lower than those incurred by maintaining biologics. But disease control was better when biologics were maintained. They also found it difficult to conclude whether lower costs or better control should be the primary driver of management in this setting.

Comparing intensive conventional disease-modifying drugs with biologics

In recent years several head-to-head trials have compared intensive treatment strategies using low cost conventional drugs and biologics. Within the trial period these studies usually show both treatments are effective with little to choose between them. Consequently, the lower cost conventional drug treatments are inevitably more cost-effective. An example of this approach is shown in the TACIT trial in established RA,[52] which compared intensive combinations using conventional disease-modifying drugs with starting tumour necrosis inhibitors in active disease.

A comparable trial in established RA, the RACAT trial,[53] assessed the benefits of triple therapy using conventional disease-modifying drugs with starting etanercept. The analysis compared treatments both during the trial and subsequently in a lifetime model which extrapolated costs and outcomes by using a decision analytic cohort model. During the trial using etanercept with methotrexate as first-line therapy provided marginally more QALYs but also had substantially higher drug costs. The lifetime analysis suggested that first-line etanercept with methotrexate would result in 0.15 additional lifetime QALY, but this gain would cost an incremental $77 290. The consequent ICER was $521 520 per QALY per patient. The conclusion was that initiating biologic therapy without trying triple therapy first increases costs while providing minimal incremental benefit.

One further comparative recent trial, the TEAR trial in early RA, has included an economic evaluation.[54] This trial compared immediate or delayed etanercept or triple therapy. The economic analysis

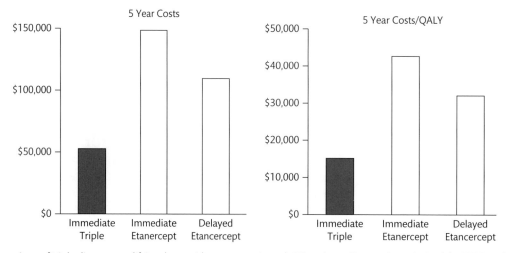

Figure 22.4 Comparison of triple disease-modifying drugs with etanercept in early RA patients. Economic analysis of the TEAR trial.
Source: data from Jalal H, et al (2016) 'Cost-Effectiveness of Triple Therapy Versus Etanercept Plus Methotrexate in Early Aggressive Rheumatoid Arthritis'. *Arthritis Care Res* 68: 1751–7.

involved a cohort model using individual-level data from the trial, published literature, and supplemental clinical data. The immediate strategies were more effective than step-up strategies. When etanercept was part of the treatment strategies they were more costly due to treatment cost differences. Over 1–2 years immediate triple therapy was the least expensive and most effective strategy. Over 5 years immediate etanercept was slightly more effective but was substantially more expensive. The ICER of $12.5 million per QALY. These findings are shown in **Figure 22.4**.

Developing areas

The treatment of RA continues to evolve. There is considerable current interest in treat-to-target strategies using a range of different drug therapies. There is some evidence that this is cost-effective,[55] though more research is needed to be certain. New drugs are also being developed including Janus kinase inhibitors such as tofacitinib and baricitinib. The evidence of their cost-effectiveness is currently incomplete but preliminary studies show they achieve broadly similar benefits at comparable drug costs to existing biologics.[56,57] Further research is needed to define their overall value.

Conclusions

RA remains an expensive disease for patients and healthcare funders. It also has substantial societal costs. Over the last three or four decades the management of RA has changed. Less is spent on hospital care and more is spent on drugs, particularly biologics. However, the total healthcare expenditure is relatively unchanged.

Long established drugs such as methotrexate and combinations of different conventional disease-modifying drugs are effective and cost-effective. Biologics are more expensive and potentially more effective. The economic assessment of when to start high cost biologics and which patients to use them in is complex and controversial. They need to be given to some patients but should not be used in all patients. Biosimilars and biologic tapering may limit costs but could also result in more biologics being used.

Economic considerations should not determine treatment decisions exclusively. But they cannot be ignored in formulating rational management policies. Given the nature of the models there is bound to be some uncertainty in economic assessments and results can vary depending on the assumptions made in modelling and the underlying data. However, as knowledge matures the models are gradually becoming more informative. This is one area where the efforts of the rheumatology community can help to reduce these uncertainties further by collecting the long-term data required for economic analysis. Now that the costs of biologics in England exceed one billion pounds annually, this is going to be an area of ongoing debate and controversy.

REFERENCES

1. Meerding WJ, Bonneux L, Polder JJ, Koopmanschap MA, van der Maas PJ. Demographic and epidemiological determinants of healthcare costs in Netherlands: cost of illness study. *BMJ* 1998;317:111–15.
2. Charlson ME, Charlson RE, Peterson JC, Marinopoulos SS, Briggs WM, Hollenberg JP. The Charlson comorbidity index is adapted to predict costs of chronic disease in primary care patients. *J Clin Epidemiol* 2008;61:1234–40.
3. Meenan RF, Yelin EH, Henke CJ, Curtis DL, Epstein WV. The costs of rheumatoid arthritis. A patient-oriented study of chronic disease costs. *Arthritis Rheum* 1978;21:827–33.
4. Stone CE. The lifetime economic costs of rheumatoid arthritis. *J Rheumatol* 1984;11:819–27.
5. Gabriel SE, Crowson CS, Luthra HS, Wagner JL, O'Fallon WM. Modeling the lifetime costs of rheumatoid arthritis. *J Rheumatol* 1999;26:1269–74.
6. Cooper NJ. Economic burden of rheumatoid arthritis: a systematic review. *Rheumatology* 2000;39:28–33.
7. Pugner KM, Scott D, Holmes JW, Hieke K. The costs of rheumatoid arthritis: an international long-term view. *Semin Arthritis Rheum* 2000;29:305–20.
8. Cooper NJ, Mugford M, Symmons DP, Barrett EM, Scott DG. Total costs and predictors of costs in individuals with early inflammatory polyarthritis: a community-based prospective study. *Rheumatology* 2002;41:767–74.
9. Merkesdal S, Ruof J, Schöffski O, Bernitt K, Zeidler H, Mau W. Indirect medical costs in early rheumatoid arthritis: composition of and changes in indirect costs within the first three years of disease. *Arthritis Rheum* 2001;44:528–34.
10. Hallert E, Husberg M, Jönsson D, Skogh T. Rheumatoid arthritis is already expensive during the first year of the disease (the Swedish TIRA project). *Rheumatology* 2004;43:1374–82.
11. Hallert E, Husberg M, Skogh T. Costs and course of disease and function in early rheumatoid arthritis: a 3-year follow-up (the Swedish TIRA project). *Rheumatology* 2006;45:325–31.
12. Hallert E, Husberg M, Kalkan A, Skogh T, Bernfort L. Early rheumatoid arthritis 6 years after diagnosis is still associated with high direct costs and increasing loss of productivity: the Swedish TIRA project. *Scand J Rheumatol* 2014;43:177–83.
13. Nikiphorou E, Davies C, Mugford M, et al. Direct health costs of inflammatory polyarthritis 10 years after disease onset: results from the Norfolk Arthritis Register. *J Rheumatol* 2015;42:794–8.
14. Kvamme MK, Lie E, Kvien TK, Kristiansen IS. Two-year direct and indirect costs for patients with inflammatory rheumatic joint diseases: data from real-life follow-up of patients in the NOR-DMARD registry. *Rheumatology* 2012;51:1618–27.
15. Kalkan A, Hallert E, Bernfort L, Husberg M, Carlsson P. Costs of rheumatoid arthritis during the period 1990–2010: a register-based cost-of-illness study in Sweden. *Rheumatology* 2014;53:153–60.
16. Eriksson JK, Johansson K, Askling J, Neovius M. Costs for hospital care, drugs and lost work days in incident and prevalent rheumatoid arthritis: how large, and how are they distributed? *Ann Rheum Dis* 2015;74:648–54.
17. Huscher D, Mittendorf T, von Hinüber U, et al. Evolution of cost structures in rheumatoid arthritis over the past decade. *Ann Rheum Dis* 2015;74:738–45.
18. Hresko A, Lin J, Solomon DH. Medical care costs associated with rheumatoid arthritis in the us: a systematic literature review and meta-analysis. *Arthritis Care Res (Hoboken)* 2018;70(10):1431–8.
19. Hu H, Luan L, Yang K, Li SC. Burden of rheumatoid arthritis from a societal perspective: a prevalence-based study on cost of illness for patients with rheumatoid arthritis in China. *Int J Rheum Dis* 2018;21(8):1572–80.
20. Ackerman IN, Pratt C, Gorelik A, Liew D. The projected burden of osteoarthritis and rheumatoid arthritis in Australia: a population-level analysis. *Arthritis Care Res (Hoboken)* 2018;70(6):877–83.

21. Hallert E, Husberg M, Kalkan A, Bernfort L. Rheumatoid arthritis is still ex pensive in the new decade: a comparison between two early RA cohorts, diagnosed 1996–98 and 2006–09. *Scand J Rheumatol* 2016;*45*:371–8.

22. Helewa A, Bombardier C, Goldsmith CH, Menchions B, Smythe HA. Cost-effectiveness of inpatient and intensive outpatient treatment of rheumatoid arthritis. A randomized, controlled trial. *Arthritis Rheum* 1989;*32*:1505–14.

23. Edelson JT, Tosteson AN, Sax P. Cost-effectiveness of misoprostol for prophylaxis against nonsteroidal anti-inflammatory drug-induced gastrointestinal tract bleeding. *JAMA* 1990;*264*:41–7.

24. Thompson MS, Read JL, Hutchings HC, Paterson M, Harris ED Jr. The cost effectiveness of auranofin: results of a randomized clinical trial. *J Rheumatol* 1988;*15*:35–42.

25. Bulpitt CJ, Fletcher AE. Measuring costs and financial benefits in randomized controlled trials. *Am Heart J* 1990;*119*:766–71.

26. Lambert CM, Hurst NP. Health economics as an aspect of health outcome: basic principles and application in rheumatoid arthritis. *Br J Rheumatol* 1995;*34*:774–80.

27. McCabe CJ, Akehurst RL. Health economics in rheumatology. *Baillieres Clin Rheumatol* 1997;*11*:145–56.

28. Bakker CH, Rutten-van Mölken M, van Doorslaer E, Bennett K, van der Linden S. Health related utility measurement in rheumatology: an introduction. *Patient Educ Couns* 1993;*20*:145–52.

29. Verhoeven AC, Bibo JC, Boers M, Engel GL, van der Linden S. Cost-effectiveness and cost-utility of combination therapy in early rheumatoid arthritis: randomized comparison of combined step-down prednisolone, methotrexate and sulphasalazine with sulphasalazine alone. COBRA Trial Group. *Br J Rheumatol* 1998;*37*:1102–9.

30. The EuroQol Group: EuroQol—a new facility for the measurement of health-related quality of life. *Health Policy* 1990;*16*:199–208.

31. Bansback N, Marra C, Tsuchiya A, et al. Using the health assessment questionnaire to estimate preference-based single indices in patients with rheumatoid arthritis. *Arthritis Rheum* 2007;*57*:963–71.

32. Hernández Alava M, Wailoo A, Wolfe F, Michaud K. A comparison of direct and indirect methods for the estimation of health utilities from clinical outcomes. *Med Decis Making* 2014;*34*:919–30.

33. Kobelt G, Jönsson L, Lindgren P, Young A, Eberhardt K. Modeling the progression of rheumatoid arthritis: a two-country model to estimate costs and consequences of rheumatoid arthritis. *Arthritis Rheum* 2002;*46*:2310–19.

34. Kobelt G, Lindgren P, Lindroth Y, Jacobson L, Eberhardt K. Modelling the effect of function and disease activity on costs and quality of life in rheumatoid arthritis. *Rheumatology* 2005;*44*:1169–75.

35. Tosh J, Brennan A, Wailoo A, Bansback N. The Sheffield rheumatoid arthritis health economic model. *Rheumatology* 2011;*50*(Suppl 4):26–31.

36. Kobelt G, Lindgren P, Young A. Modelling the costs and effects of leflunomide in rheumatoid arthritis. *Eur J Health Econ* 2002;*3*:180–7.

37. Schädlich PK, Zeidler H, Zink A, et al. Modelling cost effectiveness and cost utility of sequential DMARD therapy including leflunomide for rheumatoid arthritis in Germany: II. The contribution of leflunomide to efficiency. *Pharmacoeconomics* 2005;*23*:395–420.

38. Tosh JC, Wailoo AJ, Scott DL, Deighton CM. Cost-effectiveness of combination non-biologic disease-modifying antirheumatic drug strategies in patients with early rheumatoid arthritis. *J Rheumatol* 2011;*38*:1593–600.

39. Wailoo A, Hernández Alava M, Scott IC, Ibrahim F, Scott DL. Cost-effectiveness of treatment strategies using combination disease-modifying anti-rheumatic drugs and glucocorticoids in early rheumatoid arthritis. *Rheumatology* 2014;*53*:1773–7

40. Davies LM, Fargher EA, Tricker K, Dawes P, Scott DL, Symmons D. Is shared care with annual hospital review better value for money than predominantly hospital-based care in patients with established stable rheumatoid arthritis? *Ann Rheum Dis* 2007;*66*:658–63.

41. Choi HK, Seeger JD, Kuntz KM. A cost-effectiveness analysis of treatment options for patients with methotrexate-resistant rheumatoid arthritis. *Arthritis Rheum* 2000;*43*:2316–27.

42. Wong JB, Singh G, Kavanaugh A. Estimating the cost-effectiveness of 54 weeks of infliximab for rheumatoid arthritis. *Am J Med* 2002;*113*:400–8.

43. Jobanputra P, Barton P, Bryan S, Burls A. The effectiveness of infliximab and etanercept for the treatment of rheumatoid arthritis: a systematic review and economic evaluation. *Health Technol Assess* 2002;*6*:1–110.

44. van der Velde G, Pham B, Machado M, et al. Cost-effectiveness of biologic response modifiers compared to disease-modifying antirheumatic drugs for rheumatoid arthritis: a systematic review. *Arthritis Care Res* 2011;*63*:65–78.

45. Joensuu JT, Huoponen S, Aaltonen KJ, Konttinen YT, Nordström D, Blom M. The cost-effectiveness of biologics for the treatment of rheumatoid arthritis: a systematic review. *PLoS One* 2015;*10*:e0119683.

46. Stevenson MD, Wailoo AJ, Tosh JC, et al. The cost-effectiveness of sequences of biological disease-modifying antirheumatic drug treatment in England for patients with rheumatoid arthritis who can tolerate methotrexate. *J Rheumatol* 2017;*44*:973–980.

47. Jansen JP, Incerti D, Mutebi A, et al. Cost-effectiveness of sequenced treatment of rheumatoid arthritis with targeted immune modulators. *J Med Econ* 2017;*20*:703–14.

48. Mehr SR, Brook RA. Factors influencing the economics of biosimilars in the US. *J Med Econ* 2017;*20*:1268–71.

49. Aladul MI, Fitzpatrick RW, Chapman SR. Impact of infliximab and etanercept biosimilars on biological disease-modifying antirheumatic drugs utilisation and NHS budget in the UK. *BioDrugs* 2017;*31*(6):533–44.

50. Vanier A, Mariette X, Tubach F, Fautrel B; STRASS Study Group. Cost-effectiveness of TNF-blocker injection spacing for patients with established rheumatoid arthritis in remission: an economic evaluation from the spacing of TNF-blocker injections in rheumatoid arthritis trial. *Value Health* 2017;*20*:577–85.

51. Aletaha D, Snedecor SJ, Ektare V, Xue M, Bao Y, Garg V. Clinical and economic analysis of outcomes of dose tapering or withdrawal of tumor necrosis factor-α inhibitors upon achieving stable disease activity in rheumatoid arthritis patients. *Clinicoecon Outcomes Res* 2017;*9*:451–8.

52. Scott DL, Ibrahim F, Farewell V, et al. Tumour necrosis factor inhibitors versus combination intensive therapy with conventional disease-modifying anti-rheumatic drugs in established rheumatoid arthritis: TACIT non-inferiority randomised controlled trial. *BMJ* 2015;*350*:h1046.

53. Bansback N, Phibbs CS, Sun H, et al. Triple therapy versus biologic therapy for active rheumatoid arthritis: a cost-effectiveness analysis. *Ann Intern Med* 2017;*167*:8–16.

54. Jalal H, O'Dell JR, Bridges SL Jr, et al. Cost-effectiveness of triple therapy versus etanercept plus methotrexate in early aggressive rheumatoid arthritis. *Arthritis Care Res (Hoboken)* 2016;*68*:1751–7.

55. Wailoo A, Hock ES, Stevenson M, et al. The clinical effectiveness and cost-effectiveness of treat-to-target strategies in rheumatoid arthritis: a systematic review and cost-effectiveness analysis. *Health Technol Assess* 2017;*21*:1–258.

56. Claxton L, Jenks M, Taylor M, et al. An economic evaluation of tofacitinib treatment in rheumatoid arthritis: modeling the cost of treatment strategies in the United States. *J Manag Care Spec Pharm* 2016;*22*:1088–102.

57. Ren S, Bermejo I, Simpson E, et al. Baricitinib for previously treated moderate or severe rheumatoid arthritis: an evidence review group perspective of a NICE single technology appraisal. *Pharmacoeconomics* 2018;*36*(7):769–78.

23

Rheumatoid arthritis and work

Suzanne Verstappen, Cheryl Jones, Abdullah Houssien, and James Galloway

Introduction: Why should rheumatoid arthritis impact upon work?

A hallmark of rheumatoid arthritis (RA) is inflammation and subsequent damage to joints of the hands, feet, ankles, knees, and shoulders. Other symptoms include pain and fatigue. Considering most occupations, it is predictable that RA has substantial impact upon ability to work. Throughout history there have been notable examples of people living with RA. The works of Pierre-Auguste Renoir, the impressionist artist, developed RA during his career but was viewed by other young artists as one of the greatest and most important modern artists at the time. While Christiaan Barnard, the first surgeon to successfully perform a human heart transplant, had to retire early due to the disease others continued to have successful careers despite having RA. The actress Kathleen Turner remained active in both theatre and films and Dorothy Hodgkin, a British chemist, won the Nobel prize in Chemistry in 1964 for the development of protein crystallography.

Loss of work due to rheumatic and musculoskeletal diseases (RMDs), including RA, causes a major socioeconomic burden to society. In Europe, RMDs affect more than 4 million people with an estimated societal cost of 0.5–2% of the gross domestic product.[1,2] It is thus not surprising that, in the recent action plan for the prevention and control of non-communicable diseases in the World Health Organization (WHO) European Region, a call for prevention of disability, including work disability, and promotion of bone, joint, and muscle health from school age onwards were key priority areas endorsed by WHO Europe.[3] The peak age of onset for both men and women is before the age of ~65 years, typically the age of retirement in most countries—meaning that most people who develop RA are of working age at diagnosis[4,5] (**Figure 23.1**). For many people work is important, improving self-esteem and self-worth, and contributing to financial independence.[6] As highlighted in other places in this textbook, the treatment of RA has evolved enormously over the last 20 years with the advent of targeted therapies. However, the impact of treatment upon work outcomes has been more challenging to modify. This chapter will review the impact, including economic aspects, of RA on work, personal, and environmental factors associated with work outcomes and management of problems at work or work loss. First, however, we will give a brief description on definitions and measurement of work outcomes.

Definitions of work outcomes

Indicators of work outcomes include a reduction in working performance/ability/productivity while at work due to ill health (presenteeism), absence from work due to ill health (i.e. absenteeism), and work disability (see **Table 23.1**).[7] Environmental factors (e.g. job demands, company size, help colleagues) or personal factors (e.g. age, income) may influence the impact RA has on absenteeism and presenteeism. In addition, RA is a condition that fluctuates over time, where disease flares are followed by periods of low disease activity or remission. **Figure 23.2** shows an example of the impact of such fluctuations on absenteeism and presenteeism over time for a person with RA influenced by an environmental factor such as job demand.[8,9] A person with a more demanding job, but comparable changes in disease activity over time, may be more likely to take a day of sick leave compared to someone who has a less demanding job and will be able to go to work but performs less well due to ill health (**Figure 23.2**). When it becomes difficult to continue working while ill, people with RA may become work disabled or retire early due to ill health.

Measurement of absenteeism and work disability

Absenteeism is relatively simple to measure using simple counts of the amount of time absent from work due to ill health (hours, days sick leave) or rate of people who become work disabled due to ill health. Published literature evaluating absenteeism and work disability have predominantly relied on self-report or using data from social security systems or insurance payed sick days to estimate absenteeism and work disability. Data from social security systems are especially available in Scandinavian countries. When interpreting and comparing results from studies evaluating absenteeism and work disability one has to consider the definitions used in these studies (e.g. work disability due to RA, job loss, early retirement due to ill health, any sick leave, any absence from work, work ability),[10,11] and whether it is RA-specific absenteeism or due to ill health. In this chapter we use absenteeism, including sick leave, and work disability encompassing all the different definitions.

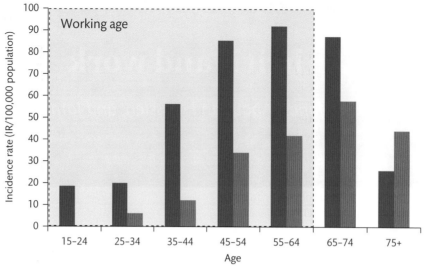

Figure 23.1 Age- and sex-specific rheumatoid arthritis (RA) incidence rates (IR)/100 000 population; female RA patients and male RA patients. Estimates are based on 2010 ACR/EULAR criteria for RA.

Source: data from Humphreys et al. The incidence of rheumatoid arthritis in the UK: comparisons using the 2010 ACR/EULAR classification criteria and the 1987 ACR classification criteria. Results from the Norfolk Arthritis Register (2013) *Ann Rheum Dis*, 72:1315-20.

Table 23.1 Outcome and cost indicators of work outcomes.

Component	Perspective	
	Outcome state	**Cost indicator**
Absenteeism indicators	Number of days/hours of work (e.g. sick leave), work disability, early retirement due to ill health, change in number of hours worked	Cost of time away from work
Presenteeism indicators	Difficulties at work, at-work productivity loss due to ill health	Worker productivity loss expressed in hours translated into costs

Source: data from Beaton et al. (2009) Measuring Worker Productivity: Frameworks and Measures, *J Rheumatol*, 36 (9):2100-2109.

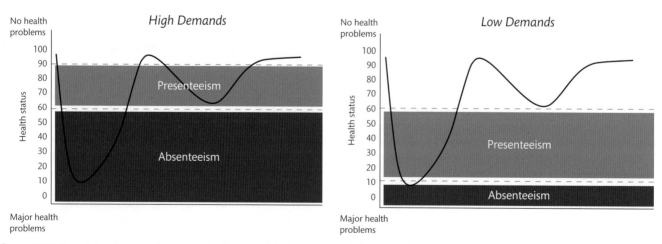

Figure 23.2 Association between fluctuations in disease activity in patients with rheumatoid arthritis on presenteeism and absenteeism in context of job demands.

Source: data from Tang et al (2001) Measuring the Impact of Arthritis on Worker Productivity: Perspectives, Methodologic Issues, and Contextual Factors, *J Rheumatol* 38:1776-80; and Verstappen (2015) Rheumatoid arthritis and work: The impact of rheumatoid arthritis on absenteeism and presenteeism *Best Pract Res Clin Rheumatol* 496-511.

Measurement of presenteeism

Research on the impact of presenteeism has become of greater interest because of evidence that suggests that presenteeism accounts for a greater proportion of the total impact of lost productivity.[12] In a Canadian study,[13] presenteeism, and work disability caused by RA and osteoarthritis (OA) found 49% of participants reported presenteeism, 29% reported absenteeism, 10% reported reduced work hours, and 11% reported they had either ceased working or had changed their job. The authors stated that such evidence indicates that presenteeism is a dominant cause of lost productivity, therefore considering the impact of absenteeism, work disability, and job loss only is not sufficient when estimating the impact of lost productivity caused by RA.[14] However, in contrast to absenteeism, presenteeism is more difficult to identify and measure because the person is at work and may still contribute to output.

There is a lack of available objective measures that can be used to measure presenteeism; this has led to the development of numerous self-report multi-item and single-item measures of presenteeism.[15–17] The Outcome Measures in Rheumatology group (OMERACT) have been identifying and validating self-report measures to identify and measure lost productivity for use in RA. In 2016, OMERACT recommended five self-reported questionnaires as suitable for use in the context of RA.[17] These measures vary in construct (e.g. productivity, ability, employability), recall period (e.g. current, today, 7 days, 1 month), reference (e.g. no reference, compared to colleagues), and attributes (e.g. generic, RA) which can result in variation of levels of presenteeism.[17,18] To illustrate the variation between estimates of presenteeism a study by Zhang et al.[19] compared the estimates of presenteeism caused by OA and RA using four self-report questionnaires including: the Health and Labour Questionnaire (HLQ)[20]; the Work Limitations Questionnaire (WLQ)[21]; Health and Work Performance Questionnaire (HPQ)[22]; and the Work Productivity and Activity Impairment Questionnaire (WPAI).[23] The construct to measure the level of presenteeism included in the questionnaires and the recall period varies; for example, the WPAI uses a 0–10 Likert scale to measure work performance whereas the HLQ asks participants to report the number of extra hours needed to complete their work. For the purpose of the study by Zhang et al., reported presenteeism levels were converted into lost productive hours and extrapolated over a 2-week recall period to allow comparison across studies (Table 23.2). Levels of presenteeism varied substantially

between the four measures. In an international qualitative study (across seven countries), including patients with RA and OA, most patients said that a recall period of 7 days up to a month accurately reflected the impact their disease had while at work.[18] This study also highlighted cross-cultural differences when defining the construct of a questionnaire (e.g. performance, productivity, ability) and when evaluating the impact of presenteeism it is important to consider these differences

Impact of RA on presenteeism, absenteeism, work disability

Until a few years ago, the focus of research in people with RA was mainly on absenteeism and work disability. With the advance of biologic therapy and early and aggressive treatment strategies in people with RA, the focus has shifted to presenteeism as well. Notably, sick leave and work disability are already increased prior to diagnosis of RA and remain higher compared to the general population after diagnosis (Figure 23.3).

A study conducted using data from 32 high- and low-income countries found that the probability of continuing to work was 80% at 2 years and 68% at 5 years, for both men and women.[24] In a review published in 2004, it was estimated that approximately 40–50% of RA study populations became work disabled within the first 5 years[10] (Figure 23.4). Country specific estimates were also reported. The Netherlands reported 37% of the RA population below the age of 65 years were work disabled compared to 9% of the general population. In the United Kingdom, RA patients were 32 times more likely to stop their job due to health reasons compared with healthy controls. In the United States, labour participation was reported to be 20% lower for males with RA and 25% lower for females with RA. Most of the studies included in this review were conducted before the introduction of biologic therapies, and the possible advantages of these drugs and more aggressive treatment strategies were not evaluated. In contrast to work disability, sick leave has been less well investigated. In a review by Lenssinck et al., the average number of sick leave days ranged between 0.1 and 11 per month[11] (Figure 23.5). As previously highlighted, levels of presenteeism vary across studies or even within studies depending on which measure of presenteeism has been used. Comparing four global measures of presenteeism (HLQ, WLQ, HPQ, WPAI), extrapolated 2-week levels of presenteeism ranging from 1.6 to 14.2 (Table 23.2).[19]

Despite the introduction of biologics and more aggressive treatment strategies, rates of sick leave and work disability remain higher in the RA population compared to the general population.[25] This may partly be explained by the fact that in many countries biologics are only prescribed after failure of at least two scDMARDs.[26] Since many people already struggle with their work during the early phases of the disease, some patients stop working before being eligible for biologics. In the British Society of Rheumatology Biologics Register for RA (BSRBR-RA), with patients having a median disease duration of 11 years at start of biologic therapy in 2010, use of biologics did not prevent patients with RA from becoming work disabled compared to the csDMARD group. However, those patients who responded to treatment were more likely to remain in work.[27] In this UK study, only a very few patients who were not working at start of biologic therapy regained paid employment. In

Table 23.2 Average number of lost productive hours and the cost of presenteeism in the past 2 weeks using four self-reported instruments.

Instrument	Recall period	Average lost productive hours (SD)	Cost over 2-week period
HLQ	1 week	1.6 (3.9)	CAN$30.03
WLQ	2 weeks	4.0 (3.9)	CAN$83.05
HPQ	2 weeks	13.5 (12.5)	CAN$284.07
WPAI	1 week	14.2 (16.7)	CAN$258.10

HLQ, Health and Labour Questionnaire; WLQ, Work Limitations Questionnaire; HPQ, WHO Health and Work Performance Questionnaire; WPAI, Work Productivity and Activity Impairment Questionnaire.
Source: data from Zhang et al.(2010), Productivity Loss Due to Presenteeism Among Patients with Arthritis: Estimates from 4 Instruments *J Rheumatol*;37(9):1805–14.

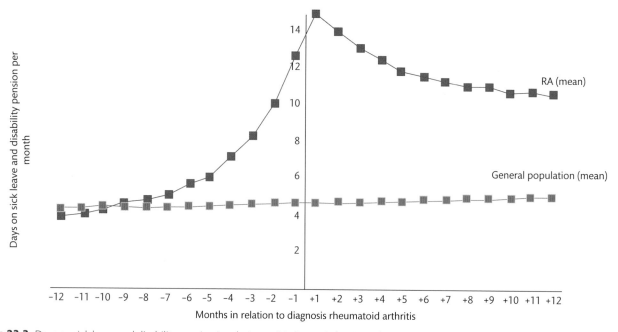

Figure 23.3 Days on sick leave and disability pension in relation to RA diagnosis (patients diagnosed 1999–2007; n = 3029). General population comparators matched 5:1 on age (± 1 year), sex, education level, and county.

Adapted from Neovius et al. (2011) How large are the productivity losses in contemporary patients with RA, and how soon in relation to diagnosis do they develop? *Ann Rheum Dis*;70 (6):1010–15 with permission from the BMJ Publishing Group.

a Dutch cohort of RA patients with a median disease duration of less than 5 years, 11.8% of patients who were not working at the start of the study, 11.8% regained employment again within 2 years after commencing antitumour necrosis factor alpha (anti-TNF) therapy.[28] In a Swedish cohort of patients commencing anti-TNF therapy, the probability of regaining work ability in those work disabled at start of therapy was 35% in those with a disease duration of <5 years compared to 14% in those with a disease duration of ≥5 years.[29] Only a few clinical trials have investigated the association between early biologic therapy use and absenteeism.[9,11] In the study by Bejarano et al.,[30] including patients with RA with <1.0 year disease duration, the percentage of work time lost in patients who

received adalimumab plus methotrexate was significantly lower than in patients who only received methotrexate (18.4% (SD 34.1) vs. 8.6% (SD 22.3), respectively) over a 56-week period, although the primary endpoint of number of patients with all-cause job loss and/or imminent job loss at 16 weeks was not met. In another study investigating response to etanercept plus methotrexate in patients with early RA, after adjustment for baseline characteristics, American College of Rheumatology 70 (ACR70) responders were 72% likely to miss work than ACR20 non-responders. In many, but not all, observational studies and randomized controlled trials (RCTs), a reduction in presenteeism levels has been observed in people with RA treated with a biologic.[9] Unfortunately, follow-up

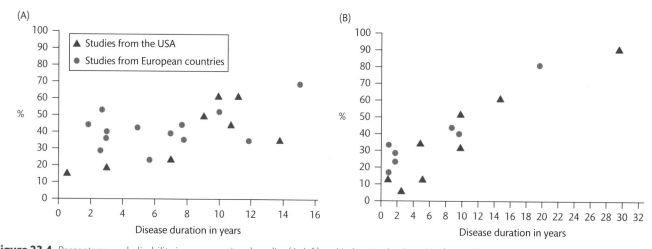

Figure 23.4 Percentage work disability in cross-sectional studies (A, left) and in longitudinal studies (B, right) by increasing disease duration.

Reprinted from Verstappen et al. (2004) Overview of work disability in rheumatoid arthritis patients as observed in cross-sectional and longitudinal surveys *Arthritis Rheum* 51(3):488–97 with permission from Wiley.

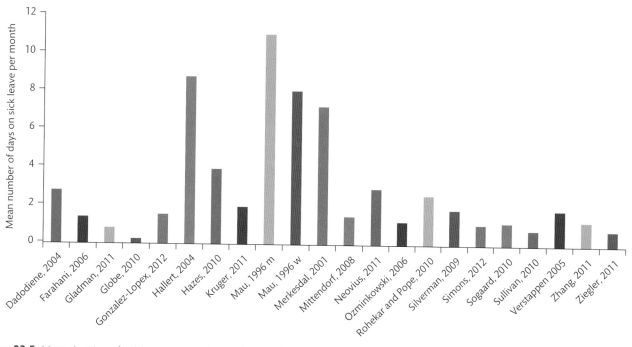

Figure 23.5 Mean duration of sick leave per month in patients with rheumatoid arthritis in paid employment. Data obtained from observational studies.

Source: data from Lenssinck et al (2013) Consequences of inflammatory arthritis for workplace productivity loss and sick leave: a systematic review. *Ann Rheum Dis*, 72:493–505.

duration of these studies was relatively short (<12 months) and it is unknown what the long-term consequences of using biologic therapy on presenteeism is.

In addition to clinically managing the disease, to improve work outcomes in patients with RA we also need to gain a better understanding which personal and environmental factors are associated with absenteeism, work disability, and presenteeism (see Figure 23.6). By understanding these factors, we should be able to provide better interventions or advice to people with RA and thus prevent problems at work and absenteeism. Whereas some of these factors may moderate the effect of an intervention with worker productivity loss, or mediate the association, most of the research to date has focused simply on the associated personal and environmental factors of absenteeism, work disability, and presenteeism.

Factors associated with absenteeism and work disability

There have been many studies exploring factors associated with work outcomes in RA[10,31] with the majority of the studies evaluating possible associations with work disability or job loss and to a lesser extent with sick leave or presenteeism. For the purpose of this chapter, we will separate factors associated with work outcomes into three groups: personal factors, disease-related factors, and environmental factors. For most studies the association between these factors and work outcomes is presented adjusting for other factors. It is essential to consider all studies in the context of the era in which they were undertaken, factors included and adjusted for, and whether they are cross-sectional or longitudinal studies.

Personal factors

Increased age is consistently associated with work disability.[31] It may be financially less burdensome for people to leave the workforce if they are close to retirement age. A German RA cohort demonstrated that the chance of work disability doubles with every 10-year increase of age.[32] Puolakka et al. similarly showed significant associations with age and work outcomes in a Finnish RA cohort.[33] Similar to studies looking at work disability, age has also been found to be associated with absenteeism, especially in large Scandinavian studies. Olofsson et al. reported on a Swedish RA inception cohort and observed that every 10 years increase in age was associated with 66 more days of absenteeism.[29] They also showed that women had on average 61 more days sick-leaved than men. In a Finnish study by Martikainen et al.[34] translating number of days absent and number of days work disabled into productivity costs, increased age was associated with a higher probability of work absence. Gender was not associated with work absence or not, but in those who reported work absence men had higher productivity cost losses than women. Other studies showed conflicting results which may be due to geographical variation.[35,36]

Gender has been extensively studied as a predictor of work disability and absenteeism. The context of gender as a determinant of work disability and sick leave is complex and conflicting.[10,31] Historically, studies typically reported males being disproportionately affected in terms of work disability. More recent studies show inconsistent associations, and vary by year of data collection and geographical region. It is important to consider that older studies typically recruited from populations in which it was social norm for women to often adopt the role of housewife. The traditional concept of work disability inevitably does not capture the impact of RA

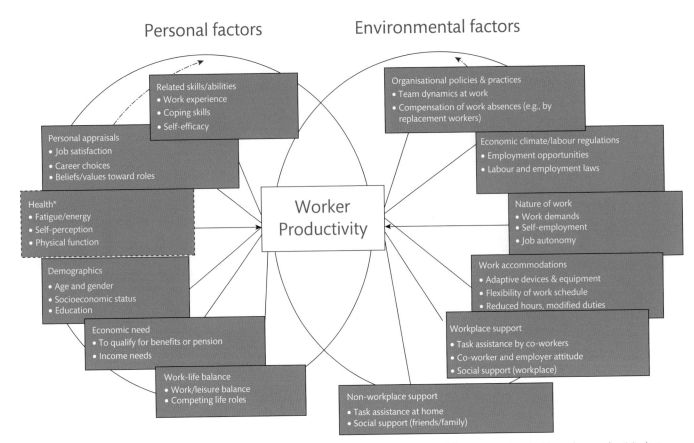

Figure 23.6 Conceptual representation of the interaction between personal and environmental factors associated with worker productivity loss.
Source: data from Sandqvist, Jan L. and Henriksson, Chris M. (2004) Work functioning: A conceptual framework *Work* 23(2):147–57.

upon unpaid housework. Two studies from China and South Korea in 2011 showed an association between female gender and greater loss in work productivity.[37,38] In a Norwegian cohort including patients with RA aged less than 45 years, female patients had a fourfold independent increased risk of becoming work disabled compared to male patients.[39] In another Norwegian study including patients with RA aged <67 years, female gender was also an independent predictor with female patients having a threefold increased risk of new work disability over 7 years.[40]

Lower educational level is significantly associated with worse work outcomes, with people of lower educational status being more likely to leave the workforce[31,41,42] and reporting more days on leave.[29,36] It is likely that patients with lower education and low socioeconomic status are more often employed in physically demanding occupations. There are very consistent data that show individuals with RA working in a manual type of job are more likely to become work disabled.[31,43–47] When evaluating the association between socioeconomic status and work outcomes, one has to consider causality. Many studies are cross-sectional and socioeconomic status could be a cause for work disability. However, it is also possible that socioeconomic status has changed because people had to stop working or change their job and earn less because of their RA. In those patients from lower socioeconomic backgrounds other characteristics affecting health, such as smoking and obesity (which may potentially mediate worse outcomes via a direct impact upon disease severity and other morbidities), could possibly impact on work outcomes. A study from China confirmed smoking to be associated

with poor work outcomes.[47] Extremes of weight (underweight or obese) have also been associated with adverse work outcomes.[31,48] Acknowledging the growing burden of obesity worldwide, this is likely to become a key factor in years to come, although to date relatively little information is published.

Disease related factors

Considering the gap in sick leave and disability pension data between people with RA and the general population, it is to be expected that factors associated with the disease will have an impact on work outcomes, and this is indeed supported by the published literature. Longer disease duration, higher disease activity, higher individual components of disease activity scores all correspond to an increased risk of work disability. Flare in RA is an important concept, and it is accepted that RA, even in the era of biologic therapy, is characterized by fluctuations in disease severity. Very little has been published up on the impact of flare on work outcomes. A study published in 2016 by Bertin compared people who are currently experiencing flares to people without flares and observed a risk ratio for work disability of 1.95 (95%CI 1.16–3.28).[49] Another earlier study from 2007 shows the similar strong relationship between the occurrence of flares and work disability.[50] Few studies investigated the association between a disease activity score such as the 28 joint Disease Activity Score (DAS28). DAS28 was independently associated with work ability in one study, but when investigating the association between individual components of DAS28 objective inflammatory markers (C-reactive protein (CRP)/erythrocyte sedimentation rate (ESR) or number of swollen joints) no association with work ability was found.[29] The latter finding has been confirmed in some, but not all, studies in which there was a lack of association between specific biomarkers of disease (radiographic damage, swollen joint count, ESR, CRP, and rheumatoid factor) and work outcomes.[10,11,31] Markers of physical disability such as the Health Assessment Questionnaire (HAQ) show clear associations with both work disability, absenteeism, and reduced worker productivity.[27,29,31,36,40,43,49,51–53] There is some evidence, but inconsistent, that important patient-reported outcomes such as morning stiffness, fatigue, and pain are associated with increased absenteeism and work disability.[10,31,54] With many patients experiencing morning stiffness, it is surprising that hardly any study has evaluated the association between morning stiffness which might lead to absenteeism or arriving late and more stressful working day. Results from a survey among French RA patients aged <60 years reported that 74.7% of 93 patients who stopped working fatigue (75%), morning stiffness or pain (25%) and difficulty getting around (25%) were the main reasons to stop working.[49] In a German prospective study, severe morning stiffness was associated with early retirement.[41] Older studies exploring the relevance of extra-articular manifestations of RA have shown conflicting results. In a more recent study in the Early RA Network inception cohort, the adjusted Hazard Ratio for claiming benefits was 1.77 (95%CI 1.17–2.70).[43] In the era of modern therapeutics, the prevalence of true extra-articular manifestations (e.g. vasculitis) has vastly declined and this aspect of disease is less relevant in contemporary practice.

Comorbidity

People with RA are at increased risk of a number of comorbidities. Two common comorbidities that accompany RA are cardiovascular disease and fibromyalgia. While it can be argued that such comorbidities could be the result of RA as an extra-articular manifestation, most studies investigating work outcomes have categorized these entities as comorbidities. Most studies looked at the number of comorbidities, rather than individual comorbidities, with each additional comorbid illness increasing the risk of impaired work productivity by 50%.[31] Three studies demonstrate the link between cardiovascular comorbidity and work disability, with a range of two- to fivefold increase in job loss compared to non-affected patients.[28,55,56] Wolfe et al.[57] reported that patients with fibromyalgia have a risk ratio of 4.0 (3.5–4.6) p = 0.0001 for job loss.

Mental health comorbidity was infrequently considered in older studies, but in recent years has started to emerge as a key determinant of work outcomes.[31] RMDs, including RA, and mental health are the two main causes for work loss in Europe. When investigating these two morbidities it is important to acknowledge that they are not individual morbidities, and many people with RA have concomitant mental health problems.[58] To date, few studies looking at work disability have captured mental health comorbidity in a detailed manner. Those studies that have reported on mental health as a predictor in patients with RA have shown consistent and large effect sizes. A German cohort applying the Patient Health Questionnaire depression score (PHQ-9), a threefold increase risk of work disability was observed in those with moderate depression (odds ratio

2.98 (95%CI 1.3–6.88, p<0.0001) and the risk rose further if patient had severe depression.[32] Mental health comorbidity was also investigated by Gonzalez-Lopez in 2013, depression was associated with a relative risk of absenteeism of 3.2 (95%CI 1.1–9.6, p = 0.03).[36] Importantly the association between absenteeism and mental health comorbidity have been demonstrated in very early disease duration cohorts.[59] There is an increasing awareness among healthcare professionals, researchers, and policy-makers that possible interventions to prevent work loss should encompass a more holistic approach and not just focusing on one disease. When discussing problems at work, it is therefore important to gain an understanding of possible other diseases that may impact on problems at work as well.

Environmental factors associated with work disability

When reviewing published literature of work outcomes, it is apparent that the continent and more specifically the country in which people reside has a relationship with work disability.[10,60] There is enormous variation across the globe with respect to societal support for people with long-term health conditions. It was not surprising that in countries where there are more robust support mechanisms, the level of reported work disability seems to be higher. Work by Sokka et al. included data from 32 different countries, and each country was categorized as high or low income.[24] Patients in higher-income countries were more likely to stop work earlier (with less severe markers of disease) compared to those in lower income countries. However, patients in low-income countries had lower overall odds of employment compared to higher-income countries.

The work environment has shown to affect the likelihood of remaining in employment following the diagnosis of RA. The most well investigated work-related factor is job type (manual versus non-manual) and job demands; with the majority of studies showing an increased risk in work disability and sick leave in those having a manual job or physical demanding job.[10,31] Other factors studied that negatively impact upon work outcomes include, negative events at work, low workplace autonomy, workplace adjustments, low control over work tasks or scheduling, low coworker/supervisor support, support at work, physically demanding roles, frequent manual handling of materials, company size, and challenges with commuting.[10,59,61–66] Prevention of sick leave and work disability may often require minor adjustments to the working environment and in many countries legislations are in place and employers are required to make reasonable adjustments or provide training to change job.

Factors associated with presenteeism

Determinants of presenteeism have not been studied to the same extent as those variables that predict work disability. Based on cross-sectional analysis, worse mental health, greater physical role limitations, treatment with biologics, low job satisfaction, and greater work instability were associated with increased levels of presenteeism.[67] A UK study showed that higher levels of pain and fatigue were significant predictors for productivity loss.[35] A Dutch study from 2005 also identified fatigue as a marker of presenteeism, along with having a manual job.[65] In a Chinese study, manual work, smoking, and not having health insurance were the main predictors for reduced productivity at work.[47] With respect to the association between disease activity and presenteeism, a recent study confirmed that low reduced pain and achieving remission protect against work productivity loss compared to low disease activity, although work-related factors were not included in the model.[68]

Economic impact of absenteeism and presenteeism

In addition to impact of RA on work from the healthcare perspective and the patient's perspective, the socioeconomic burden of presenteeism, absenteeism, and work disability is huge. However, to interpret the costs, reported studies, and policy documents, it is important to have some understanding how absenteeism and presenteeism are valued. Transforming absenteeism levels into costs is relatively simple by translating counts of the amount of time (hours, days) into costs spent away from work or receiving work disability benefits or not. However, the majority of self-report presenteeism questionnaires have not been developed using economic theory meaning that the rationale, construct, and development of the questionnaires have not been consistent, potentially leading to variation in design.[69]

The authors acknowledged that extrapolating presenteeism has led to overestimations of the cost of presenteeism. There are two common methods used to value the cost impact of absenteeism and presenteeism caused by RA: the human capital approach (HCA) and the friction cost approach (FCA).

The HCA values the amount of productivity loss by multiplying the amount of time an individual is unproductive during a working week by the hourly wage[70]; many argue that the HCA overestimates the cost of productivity loss.[71-73] In 1992, an alternative method called the FCA was proposed.[71] The FCA calculates the cost of lost productivity by totalling the hours not worked up to the moment the replacement employee is hired. Once the sick employee has been replaced the FCA assumes that initial production levels are restored. In a recent review, the economic burden associated with RA was reported using the HCA and FCA. The cost of RA using the HCA was estimated at €21 900 per patient, per year compared to €14 889 per patient, per year when the FCA was applied.[74]

Evidence suggests that the cost of absenteeism and presenteeism caused by RA is substantial; however, the true value of the impact of RA on absenteeism and presenteeism is unknown.[75] Research is currently focusing on refining methods used to estimate absenteeism and presenteeism to more accurately estimate the impact caused by RA.

Economic burden

RA has a direct and negative impact on productivity. Productivity is an economic concept and is defined as the ratio of inputs (land, labour, capital) used per unit of output.[76] Several reviews have estimated the economic burden associated with RA.[74,77-79] A systematic review by Lundkvist et al.[77] in 2008 reported the economic burden of RA which included direct costs (healthcare), indirect costs (lost productivity), and costs of informal care. The total cost of RA per year in the United States was estimated to be €41.631 billion and €45.263 billion in Europe, translating to a cost per patient, per year of €21 000 in the United States and €13 500 in Europe. In Europe, the largest cost driver was lost productivity, representing 37% of the total cost of RA. In the United States, the biggest cost drivers were drugs (34%), medical care excluding drugs (21%), and costs of lost production (20%).

Prevention and management of worker productivity loss in people with rheumatoid arthritis

For many people with RA, work is an important health outcome. Many rheumatologists may enquire about employment as a matter of course when people are diagnosed, but how frequently does work continue to re-emerge on the agenda during the consultation in rheumatology clinics? Data from the Early Inflammatory Arthritis national audit in the United Kingdom showed that 69% of patients recalled their clinician asking about employment.[80] However, many people with musculoskeletal diseases including RA see their GP as their first port of call to discuss problems at work. In another UK survey, 35% of the respondents mentioned that they expect the GP to provide some support and advice on disease management and work.[81] With a growing area of complex therapeutic decisions and disease management in primary and secondary care, squeezed in to brief healthcare visits, it is vital that healthcare professionals working with RA recognize the enormous importance of work as a part of someone's overall well-being. Although the rheumatologists and GPs may not have the specialist expertise in providing patient tailored advice related to their work problems, they could however be key in directing the patient to the right services such as occupational health services, occupational physicians, or other services. However, according to WHO Europe, less than 10% of the working population has access to these services in many European countries. Especially advice from consultants in occupational medicine or occupational therapists may not always be readable available for those being self-employed or working in small or medium sized companies.

Interestingly, limited RCTs have been conducted investigating non-pharmacological interventions, often with a limited scope (e.g. physical exercise, job accommodation assessment, education), and not all these interventions have been promising.[82,83] In a UK feasibility RCT, including patients with RA, patients received either job retention vocational rehabilitation (VR) or written information only.[84] Participants found VR more acceptable than written information. VR resulted in greater reduction of presenteeism, absenteeism, perceived risk of job loss, and improvement in pain and health status. A Dutch RCT in patients with RA evaluating the effectiveness of an integrated care intervention of the workplace compared to usual care, no significant difference in at-work productivity loss (i.e. presenteeism) was found between the two intervention groups.[85] There is more scope in further evaluating non-pharmacological interventions combined with pharmacological interventions adapting a more holistic approach.

In addition to help from healthcare professionals, employers can play a major role in helping people with RA to prevent presenteeism and absenteeism. There is, however, a lack of awareness among employers and colleagues about chronic fluctuating diseases such as RA. It is therefore not surprising that patients with RA often experience a lack of understanding from their employer, who may struggle to understand the fact that the disease fluctuates over time and that it affects people of all ages and not just old people. Furthermore, due to better treatments people may not always present with 'visible' symptoms such as deformed joints, but still remain to have an active and painful disease. Other challenges people with RA often face to remain in work include: demanding job role; RA-related symptoms (e.g. fatigue); no reasonable adjustments; commute to work; and flexible working (NRAS).[86] Some of these are relatively easy to make and can make a huge difference for those with problems who want to remain in work. To make these adjustments, conversations with employers and colleagues have to be held but patients may be reluctant to have these conversations.[87] Some patients may have concerns about the consequences (e.g. less support, credibility, less career progression opportunities, and even loss of one's job) of openly discussing their disease with their employer or line manager.[87,88]

In conclusion, work productivity is a complex construct and in addition to treating patients with RA to target, and thus reducing the initial impact of RA on work productivity, a more holistic approach regarding preventing problems at work and work loss should be applied also taking into account environmental factors (e.g. job type, company size, flexibility to work), other morbidities (e.g. mental health), and personal factors (e.g. age, family circumstances, education).

Prevention of problems at work and likely work loss is of great importance, because once people with RA are out of the workforce it is very difficult to regain employment again.[51] A first step towards prevention of problems at work and work loss is raise awareness among healthcare professionals, employers, and policy-makers about the impact of RA on work and to gain a better understanding about the challenges people with RA experience to stay in work.

Recommendations:

- Preventing problems at work and work loss needs a holistic approach considering personal, disease-related, and work-related factors.
- Increase awareness about the challenges people with rheumatoid arthritis experience to stay in work.
- Ask about employment and any problems may have at work in clinic—not just at diagnosis but also during later stages of the disease.
- Monitor outcomes and calculate costs using validated tools and instruments underpinned by economic theory.
- Where possible try to direct people with rheumatoid arthritis having problems to the right services. Consider type of work and engage with employers.
- Address other health problems that may affect problems at work, especially mental health.

REFERENCES

1. Bevan S. Economic impact of musculoskeletal disorders (MSDs) on work in Europe. *Best Pract Res Clin Rheumatol* 2015;29(3):356–73.
2. Bevan S QT, McGee R, Mahdon M, Vavrovsky A, Barham L, The Work Foundation. *Fit for Work? Musculoskeletal Disorders in the European Workforce*, 2009. Available at: http://www.bollettinoadapt.it/old/files/document/3704FOUNDATION_19_10.pdf
3. World Health Organization (WHO). *Action Plan for the Prevention and Control of Noncommunicable Diseases in the WHO European Region.* Geneva, Switzerland: World Health Organization (WHO), 2016.
4. Humphreys JH, Verstappen SM, Hyrich KL, et al. The incidence of rheumatoid arthritis in the UK: comparisons using the 2010 ACR/EULAR classification criteria and the 1987 ACR classification criteria. Results from the Norfolk Arthritis Register. *Ann Rheum Dis* 2013;72(8):1315–20.
5. Symmons D, Turner G, Webb R, et al. The prevalence of rheumatoid arthritis in the United Kingdom: new estimates for a new century. *Rheumatology (Oxf)* 2002;41(7):793–800.
6. Black C. *Working for a Healthier Tomorrow. Dame Carol Black's Review of the Health of Britain's Working Age Population*, 2008. Available at: https://www.rnib.org.uk/sites/default/files/Working_for_a_healthier_tomorrow.pdf
7. Beaton D, Bombardier C, Escorpizo R, et al. Measuring worker productivity: frameworks and measures. *J Rheumatol* 2009;36(9):2100–09.
8. Tang K, Escorpizo R, Beaton DE, et al. Measuring the impact of arthritis on worker productivity: perspectives, methodologic issues, and contextual factors. *J Rheumatol* 2011;38(8):1776–90.
9. Verstappen SM. Rheumatoid arthritis and work: the impact of rheumatoid arthritis on absenteeism and presenteeism. *Best Pract Res Clin Rheumatol* 2015;29(3):495–511.
10. Verstappen SM, Bijlsma JW, Verkleij H, et al. Overview of work disability in rheumatoid arthritis patients as observed in cross-sectional and longitudinal surveys. *Arthritis Rheum* 2004;51(3):488–97.
11. Lenssinck ML, Burdorf A, Boonen A, et al. Consequences of inflammatory arthritis for workplace productivity loss and sick leave: a systematic review. *Ann Rheum Dis* 2013;72(4):493–505.
12. Hemp P. *Presenteeism: At Work—But Out of It. Harvard Business Review*, October 2004. Available at: https://hbr.org/2004/10/presenteeism-at-work-but-out-of-it
13. Li X, Gignac MA, Anis AH. The indirect costs of arthritis resulting from unemployment, reduced performance, and occupational changes while at work. *Med Care* 2006;44(4):304–10.
14. Zhang W, Anis AH. The economic burden of rheumatoid arthritis: beyond health care costs. *Clin Rheumatol* 2011;30(Suppl 1):S25–S32.
15. Brooks A, Hagen SE, Sathyanarayanan S, et al. Presenteeism: critical issues. *J Occup Environ Med* 2010;52(11):1055–67.
16. Tang K, Boonen A, Verstappen SM, et al. Worker productivity outcome measures: OMERACT filter evidence and agenda for future research. *J Rheumatol* 2014;41(1):165–76.
17. Beaton DE, Dyer S, Boonen A, et al. OMERACT filter evidence supporting the measurement of at-work productivity loss as an outcome measure in rheumatology research. *J Rheumatol* 2016;43(1):214–22.
18. Leggett S, van de Zee-Neuen, Boonen A, et al. Content validity of global measures for at-work productivity in patients with rheumatic diseases: an international qualitative study. *Rheumatology (Oxf)* 2016;55(8):1364–73.
19. Zhang W, Gignac MA, Beaton D, et al. Productivity loss due to presenteeism among patients with arthritis: estimates from 4 instruments. *J Rheumatol* 2010;37(9):1805–14.
20. van Roijen L, Essink-Bot ML, Koopmanschap MA, et al. Labor and health status in economic evaluation of health care. The

Health and Labor Questionnaire. *Int J Technol Assess Health Care* 1996;*12*(3):405–15.

21. Lerner D, Amick BC, III, Rogers WH, et al. The Work Limitations Questionnaire. *Med Care* 2001;*39*(1):72–85.

22. Kessler RC, Barber C, Beck A, et al. The World Health Organization Health and Work Performance Questionnaire (HPQ). *J Occup Environ Med* 2003;*45*(2):156–74.

23. Reilly MC, Gooch KL, Wong RL, et al. Validity, reliability and responsiveness of the Work Productivity and Activity Impairment Questionnaire in ankylosing spondylitis. *Rheumatology (Oxford)* 2010;*49*(4):812–19.

24. Sokka T, Kautiainen H, Pincus T, et al. Work disability remains a major problem in rheumatoid arthritis in the 2000s: data from 32 countries in the QUEST-RA study. *Arthritis Res Ther* 2010;*12*(2):R42.

25. Neovius M, Simard JF, Klareskog L, et al. Sick leave and disability pension before and after initiation of antirheumatic therapies in clinical practice. *Ann Rheum Dis* 2011;*70*(8):1407–14.

26. Putrik P, Ramiro S, Kvien TK, et al. Variations in criteria regulating treatment with reimbursed biologic DMARDs across European countries. Are differences related to country's wealth? *Ann Rheum Dis* 2014;*73*(11):2010–21.

27. Verstappen SM, Watson KD, Lunt M, et al. Working status in patients with rheumatoid arthritis, ankylosing spondylitis and psoriatic arthritis: results from the British Society for Rheumatology Biologics Register. *Rheumatology (Oxf)* 2010;*49*(8):1570–7.

28. Manders SH, Kievit W, Braakman-Jansen AL, et al. Determinants associated with work participation in patients with established rheumatoid arthritis taking tumor necrosis factor inhibitors. *J Rheumatol* 2014;*41*(7):1263–9.

29. Olofsson T, Petersson IF, Eriksson JK, et al. Predictors of work disability during the first 3 years after diagnosis in a national rheumatoid arthritis inception cohort. *Ann Rheum Dis* 2014;*73*(5):845–53.

30. Bejarano V, Quinn M, Conaghan PG, et al. Effect of the early use of the anti–tumor necrosis factor adalimumab on the prevention of job loss in patients with early rheumatoid arthritis. *Arthritis Care Res* 2008;*59*(10):1467–74.

31. de Croon EM, Sluiter JK, Nijssen TF, et al. Predictive factors of work disability in rheumatoid arthritis: a systematic literature review. *Ann Rheum Dis* 2004;*63*(11):1362–7.

32. Callhoff J, Albrecht K, Schett G, et al. Depression is a stronger predictor of the risk to consider work disability in early arthritis than disease activity or response to therapy. *RMD Open* 2015;*1*(1):e000020.

33. Puolakka K, Kautiainen H, Pekurinen M, et al. Monetary value of lost productivity over a five year follow up in early rheumatoid arthritis estimated on the basis of official register data on patients' sickness absence and gross income: experience from the FIN-RACo trial. *Ann Rheum Dis* 2006;*65*(7):899–904.

34. Martikainen JA, Kautiainen H, Rantalaiho V, et al. Long-term work productivity costs due to absenteeism and permanent work disability in patients with early rheumatoid arthritis: a nationwide register study of 7831 patients: *J Rheumatol* 2016;*43*(12):2101–5.

35. Bansback N, Zhang W, Walsh D, et al. Factors associated with absenteeism, presenteeism and activity impairment in patients in the first years of RA. *Rheumatology (Oxf)* 2012;*51*(2):375–84.

36. Gonzalez-Lopez L, Morales-Romero J, Vazquez-Villegas ML, et al. Factors influencing sick leave episodes in Mexican workers with rheumatoid arthritis and its impact on working days lost. *Rheumatol Int* 2013;*33*(3):561–9.

37. Langley PC, Mu R, Wu M, et al. The impact of rheumatoid arthritis on the burden of disease in urban China. *J Med Econ* 2011;*14*(6):709–19.

38. Kwon JM, Rhee J, Ku H, et al. Socioeconomic and employment status of patients with rheumatoid arthritis in Korea. *Epidemiol Health* 2012;*34*:e2012003.

39. Wallenius M, Skomsvoll JF, Koldingsnes W, et al. Comparison of work disability and health-related quality of life between males and females with rheumatoid arthritis below the age of 45 years. *Scand J Rheumatol* 2009;*38*(3):178–83.

40. Odegard S, Finset A, Kvien TK, et al. Work disability in rheumatoid arthritis is predicted by physical and psychological health status: a 7-year study from the Oslo RA register. *Scand J Rheumatol* 2005;*34*(6):441–7.

41. Westhoff G, Buttgereit F, Gromnica-Ihle E, et al. Morning stiffness and its influence on early retirement in patients with recent onset rheumatoid arthritis. *Rheumatology (Oxf)* 2008;*47*(7):980–4.

42. Eberhardt K, Larsson BM, Nived K, et al. Work disability in rheumatoid arthritis--development over 15 years and evaluation of predictive factors over time. *J Rheumatol* 2007;*34*(3):481–7.

43. McWilliams DF, Varughese S, Young A, et al. Work disability and state benefit claims in early rheumatoid arthritis: the ERAN cohort. *Rheumatology (Oxf)* 2014;*53*(3):473–81.

44. Dadoniene J, Stropuviene S, Venalis A, et al. High work disability rate among rheumatoid arthritis patients in Lithuania. *Arthritis Rheum* 2004;*51*(3):433–9.

45. Young A, Dixey J, Kulinskaya E, et al. Which patients stop working because of rheumatoid arthritis? Results of five years' follow up in 732 patients from the Early RA Study (ERAS). *Ann Rheum Dis* 2002;*61*(4):335–40.

46. Chorus AM, Miedema HS, Wevers CJ, et al. Labour force participation among patients with rheumatoid arthritis. *Ann Rheum Dis* 2000;*59*(7):549–54.

47. Zhang X, Mu R, Wang X, et al. The impact of rheumatoid arthritis on work capacity in Chinese patients: a cross-sectional study. *Rheumatology (Oxf)* 2015;*54*(8):1478–87.

48. Wolfe F, Michaud K. Effect of body mass index on mortality and clinical status in rheumatoid arthritis. *Arthritis Care Res (Hoboken)* 2012;*64*(10):1471–9.

49. Bertin P, Fagnani F, Duburcq A, et al. Impact of rheumatoid arthritis on career progression, productivity, and employability: the PRET Study. *Joint Bone Spine* 2016;*83*(1):47–52.

50. Reisine S, Fifield J, Walsh S, et al. Work disability among two cohorts of women with recent-onset rheumatoid arthritis: a survival analysis. *Arthritis Care Res* 2007;*57*(3):372–80.

51. Verstappen SM, Boonen A, Bijlsma JW, et al. Working status among Dutch patients with rheumatoid arthritis: work disability and working conditions. *Rheumatology (Oxf)* 2005;*44*(2):202–6.

52. Shanahan EM, Smith M, Roberts-Thomson L, et al. Influence of rheumatoid arthritis on work participation in Australia. *Intern Med J* 2008;*38*(3):166–73.

53. Mussen L, Boyd T, Bykerk V, et al. Low prevalence of work disability in early inflammatory arthritis (EIA) and early rheumatoid arthritis at enrollment into a multi-site registry: results from the catch cohort. *Rheumatol Int* 2013;*33*(2):457–65.

54. Lacaille D, White MA, Backman CL, et al. Problems faced at work due to inflammatory arthritis: new insights gained from understanding patients' perspective. *Arthritis Rheum* 2007;*57*(7):1269–79.

55. Kerola AM, Kauppi MJ, Nieminen T, et al. Psychiatric and cardiovascular comorbidities as causes of long-term work disability among individuals with recent-onset rheumatoid arthritis. *Scand J Rheumatol* 2015;*44*(2):87–92.

56. Witney AG, Treharne GJ, Tavakoli M, et al. The relationship of medical, demographic and psychosocial factors to direct and indirect health utility instruments in rheumatoid arthritis. *Rheumatology (Oxf)* 2006;*45*(8):975–81.

57. Wolfe F, Michaud K. Severe rheumatoid arthritis (RA), worse outcomes, comorbid illness, and sociodemographic disadvantage characterize RA patients with fibromyalgia. *J Rheumatol* 2004;*31*(4):695–700.

58. Matcham F, Rayner L, Steer S, et al. The prevalence of depression in rheumatoid arthritis: a systematic review and meta-analysis. *Rheumatology (Oxf)* 2013;*52*(12):2136–48.

59. Geuskens GA, Hazes JM, Barendregt PJ, et al. Predictors of sick leave and reduced productivity at work among persons with early inflammatory joint conditions. *Scand J Work Environ Health* 2008;*34*(6):420–9.

60. van der Zee-Neuen A, Putrik P, Ramiro S, et al. Large country differences in work outcomes in patients with RA—an analysis in the multinational study COMORA. *Arthritis Res Ther* 2017;*19*(1):216.

61. Chorus AM, Miedema HS, Wevers CW, et al. Work factors and behavioural coping in relation to withdrawal from the labour force in patients with rheumatoid arthritis. *Ann Rheum Dis* 2001;*60*(11):1025–32.

62. Hoving JL, van Zwieten MC, Van der MM, et al. Work participation and arthritis: a systematic overview of challenges, adaptations and opportunities for interventions. *Rheumatology (Oxf)* 2013;*52*(7):1254–64.

63. Allaire S, Wolfe F, Jingbo NIU, et al. Current risk factors for work disability associated with rheumatoid arthritis: recent data from a US national cohort. *Arthritis Care Res* 2009;*61*(3):321–8.

64. Lacaille D, Sheps S, Spinelli JJ, et al. Identification of modifiable work-related factors that influence the risk of work disability in rheumatoid arthritis. *Arthritis Care Res* 2004;*51*(5):843–52.

65. de Croon EM, Sluiter JK, Nijssen TF, et al. Work ability of Dutch employees with rheumatoid arthritis. *Scand J Rheumatol* 2005;*34*(4):277–83.

66. Mancuso CA, Rincon M, Sayles W, et al. Longitudinal study of negative workplace events among employed rheumatoid arthritis patients and healthy controls. *Arthritis Rheum* 2005;*53*(6):958–64.

67. van Vilsteren M, Boot CR, Knol DL, et al. Productivity at work and quality of life in patients with rheumatoid arthritis. *BMC Musculoskelet Disord* 2015;*16*:107.

68. Kim D, Kaneko Y, Takeuchi T. Importance of obtaining remission for work productivity and activity of patients with rheumatoid arthritis. *J Rheumatol* 2017;*44*(8):1112–17.

69. Jones C, Payne K, Gannon B, et al. Economic theory and self-reported measures of presenteeism in musculoskeletal disease. *Curr Rheumatol Rep* 2016;*18*(8):53.

70. van den Hout WB. The value of productivity: human-capital versus friction-cost method. *Ann Rheum Dis* 2010;*69* (Suppl 1):i89–i91.

71. Koopmanschap MA, Rutten FF. A practical guide for calculating indirect costs of disease. *Pharmacoeconomics* 1996;*10*(5):460–6.

72. Jacob-Tacken KH, Koopmanschap MA, Meerding WJ, et al. Correcting for compensating mechanisms related to productivity costs in economic evaluations of health care programmes. *Health Econ* 2005;*14*(5):435–43.

73. Pauly MV, Nicholson S, Polsky D, et al. Valuing reductions in on-the-job illness: 'presenteeism' from managerial and economic perspectives. *Health Econ* 2008;*17*(4):469–85.

74. Boonen A, Severens JL. The burden of illness of rheumatoid arthritis. *Clin Rheumatol* 2011;*30* (Suppl 1):S3–8.

75. Filipovic I, Walker D, Forster F, et al. Quantifying the economic burden of productivity loss in rheumatoid arthritis. *Rheumatology (Oxf)* 2011;*50*(6):1083–90.

76. Sloman J, Garratt D, Guest J. *Economics*, 8th edition. Harlow, UK: Pearson, 2012.

77. Lundkvist J, Kastang F, Kobelt G. The burden of rheumatoid arthritis and access to treatment: health burden and costs. *Eur J Health Econ* 2008;*8*(Suppl 2):S49–S60.

78. Kobelt G, Jonsson B. The burden of rheumatoid arthritis and access to treatment: outcome and cost-utility of treatments. *Eur J Health Econ* 2008;*8*(Suppl 2):95–106.

79. Cooper NJ, Mugford M, Scott DG, et al. Secondary health service care and second line drug costs of early inflammatory polyarthritis in Norfolk, UK. *J Rheumatol* 2000;*27*(9):2115–22.

80. Ledingham JM, Snowden N, Rivett A, et al. Patient- and clinician-reported outcomes for patients with new presentation of inflammatory arthritis: observations from the National Clinical Audit for Rheumatoid and Early Inflammatory Arthritis. *Rheumatology (Oxf)* 2017;*56*(2):231–8.

81. Verstappen S. *Working with a Musculoskeletal Condition: What Do Patients Want to Discuss With Healthcare Professionals?* Fit for Work UK Blog, 2018

82. Hoving JL, Lacaille D, Urquhart DM, et al. Non-pharmacological interventions for preventing job loss in workers with inflammatory arthritis. *Cochrane Database Syst Rev* 2014(11): CD010208.

83. Gignac MA, Jetha A, Bowring J, et al. Management of work disability in rheumatic conditions: a review of non-pharmacological interventions. *Best Pract Res Clinical Rheumatol* 2012;*26*(3):369–86.

84. Hammond A, O'Brien R, Woodbridge S, et al. Job retention vocational rehabilitation for employed people with inflammatory arthritis (WORK-IA): a feasibility randomized controlled trial. *BMC Musculoskelet Disord* 2017;*18*(1):315.

85. van Vilsteren M, Boot CR, Twisk JW, et al. One-year effects of a workplace integrated care intervention for workers with rheumatoid arthritis: results of a randomized controlled trial. *J Occup Rehabil* 2017;*27*(1):128–36.

86. National Rheumatoid Arthritis Society (NRAS). *Work Matters: A UK Wide Survey of Adults with Rheumatoid Arthritis and Juvenile Idiopathic Arthritis on the Impact of their Disease on Work*. 2017. Available at: https://www.nras.org.uk/data/files/Publications/Work%20Matters.pdf

87. Gignac MA, Cao X. 'Should I tell my employer and coworkers I have arthritis?' A longitudinal examination of self-disclosure in the work place. *Arthritis Rheum* 2009;*61*(12):1753–61.

88. Gignac MA. Arthritis and employment: an examination of behavioral coping efforts to manage workplace activity limitations. *Arthritis Rheum* 2005;*53*(3):328–36.

SECTION 6
Non-drug treatments

24 **Physical activity and exercise** *285*
   Lindsay M. Bearne and Christina H. Opava

25 **Foot health** *297*
   Heidi J. Siddle and Anthony C. Redmond

26 **Occupational therapy** *311*
   Alison Hammond, Joanne Adams, and Yeliz Prior

27 **Self-management: A patient's perspective** *321*
   Marieke M.J.H. Voshaar

Physical activity and exercise

Lindsay M. Bearne and Christina H. Opava

Disabilities targeted by physical activity and exercise interventions in rheumatoid arthritis

It is widely understood that physical activity and exercise provides many health benefits for the general population as well as for people with long-term conditions. Physical activity and exercise interventions are also recommended in the management of specific disabilities associated with rheumatoid arthritis (RA). These include reduced physical fitness such as aerobic capacity, motor function, flexibility, and neuromuscular function; subjective symptoms such as pain, fatigue, and psychological distress; and limited performance of activities of daily living.

People with RA appear to have considerably reduced physical fitness such as *aerobic capacity*. For example, physical activity energy expenditure, when measured using the gold standard objective measure (doubly labelled water, see section 2), is considerably reduced. Similarly, aerobic capacity is reduced to below the tenth percentile of VO_{2max} compared to normative values[1] although the findings of studies comparing the VO_{2max} of people with RA to healthy controls are conflicting.

Reduced motor function, that is, muscle strength and endurance, is described in subgroups of people with RA. Quadriceps muscle strength is decreased among postmenopausal women with RA compared to age-matched controls[2] and significant reductions in quadriceps, foot and ankle strength compared to healthy controls may also occur.[3] Grip strength and pinch grips are reduced compared to controls, not only in people with active RA, but also among those in remission.[4,5] However, physiological properties of muscle, such as specific force, contractile properties, voluntary activation capacity, and contraction velocity, are not compromised in people with stable RA despite deficits in physical function, which indicates that resistance exercise has the potential to elicit a similar response in people with RA as in healthy populations.[6]

Decreased flexibility and joint range-of-motion is well recognized in people with RA and may be the result of acute inflammation and subsequent excess of joint fluid, but may also follow long-standing inflammation with joint destruction, dislocation, or degradation of the structures surrounding joints.

Neuromuscular function may be impaired in people with RA and poor **balance and proprioception** may be part of the increased risk of falls described for this subpopulation.[7] The strongest risk factors identified in people with RA have some overlap with the risk factors identified in the elderly population (i.e. fall history and multiple medication use) while others are disease-specific, such as swollen/tender lower extremity joints and fatigue. Additional disability-related predictors of falls in people with RA include pain, fear of falling, activity limitation, and impaired lower-limb muscle strength and balance.[8]

Symptoms related to RA, such as **fatigue** (Chapter 21) and **psychological distress** (Chapter 20), are common in RA and are complexly related to each other as well as to disease activity, physical activity, and physical fitness.[9-11] Despite adequately controlled inflammation, **pain** and **activity limitation** are still pronounced among patients with RA, even in early disease.[12] While exercise-related improvements of basic body functions may translate to improved performance of activities, the physiological mechanisms behind non-inflammatory pain in RA are not fully understood. They are, however, commonly considered to be multifactorial and include both peripheral mechanisms (e.g. peripheral joint damage),[13] possibly inducing peripheral sensitization, and central mechanisms amplifying ascending nociceptive signalling due to sensitization in ascending nociceptive pathways, increased descending facilitation, and/or impaired descending inhibitory pathways.[13,14] Central sensitization seems to be present in people with RA (e.g. indicated by lower pain thresholds in joints as well as non-inflamed tissue),[14,15] and hypersensitivity to thermal stimuli at both non-articular and articular sites.[16] Furthermore, a general increase in pain sensitivity in patients with long-standing RA (>5 years) compared to those with more recent onset (<1 year) indicate that the generalized alteration of pain processing is due to sensitization of central nociceptive neurons and/or increased activity in the descending facilitatory pathways since no malfunction of conditioning pain modulation is present.[14]

In addition to the RA-related disabilities generally targeted by physical activity and exercise, increased risk of cardiovascular disease (CVD) (see Chapter 14) or inflammation (disease activity) may also be the focus of physical activity and exercise interventions. Thus, physical activity and exercise are among the most commonly recommended non-pharmacological interventions to reduce these common disabilities and symptoms.

Physical activity and exercise–definitions and recommendations

Definitions

Physical activity is a multifaceted construct defined as 'any bodily movement produced by skeletal muscles that requires energy expenditure beyond resting expenditure'.[17,18] It includes transportation such as walking or cycling, occupational, domestic, and leisure time physical activity such as play, games, or sports. **Health-enhancing physical activity** (HEPA) is any physical activity that produces health benefits and could encompass planned, structured **exercise**, which is purposive, as the objective is improvement or maintenance of one or more component(s) of physical fitness. **Therapeutic exercise** is prescribed, usually by a healthcare or fitness professional, to prevent or reduce impairments of body functions and structures or health-related risk factors, improve, restore, or enhance activities and participation and optimize health, fitness, or sense of well-being[19] (Figure 24.1).

Failure to meet recommended levels of moderate-to-vigorous physical activity is defined as **physical inactivity**.[20] However, **sedentary behaviour** is not just a lack of physical activity. It is specifically described as any waking behaviour characterized by an energy expenditure of 1.5 the metabolic equivalent of task (see section 3) or less while in a sitting or reclining posture.[21] This definition acknowledges the importance of posture but also energy expenditure in defining sedentary activities.

Recommendations

In recognition that the overall volume of physical activity is more important than frequency or duration alone, the World Health Organization physical activity guidelines for the general population recommend that adults aged between 18 and 64 years complete at least 150 minutes of moderate intensity (in bouts of at least 10 minutes) or 75 minutes of vigorous-intensity aerobic physical activity per week or an equivalent combination of moderate-intensity and high-intensity activity. Muscle-strengthening activities involving major muscle groups on two or more days a week are also advised.[18] Guidance for older adults (≥65 years) and adults between 50 and 64 years with long-term conditions is similar, although aerobic activities tailored to baseline fitness and activities to increase or maintain flexibility at least twice a week for a minimum of 10 minutes are advised.[22] Adults with poor mobility, should also perform physical activity to enhance balance and prevent falls on three or more days per week.[18]

As there is a dose-response relationship to physical activity, adults who are inactive, with a high level of sedentary behaviour,[20] should be encouraged to complete small increases in activity and minimize sedentary behaviour, even if it is below the recommendation as this will still produce health benefits.[23,24]

People with RA should thus aim to achieve the HEPA recommendations for the general population, taking into account baseline activity level, disease activity and symptoms[22,25] and incorporate therapeutic exercise prescriptions.[22,26] Therapeutic exercise should include a tailored, progressive programme of moderate- to high-intensity aerobic training and resistance training of all muscle groups and individuals with pain or dysfunction in the wrist and hands are recommended to complete a tailored strengthening and stretching exercise programme.[27]

Measures of physical activity in people with RA

Physical activity is typically expressed as energy expenditure, for example as the metabolic equivalent (MET) of the activity,[28] as kilocalories per kilogram of body mass per minute (kcal·kg−1·min−1)[28] or as the duration, frequency, and intensity of the physical activity performed. Measures of physical activity can be broadly categorized as either direct, objective measures, indirect, subjective measures, or as clinical measures of physical fitness. Comprehensive assessment of physical activity is multifaceted and multipurpose. It may be used to guide prescription of HEPA and therapeutic exercise, to evaluate the effect of interventions or to monitor behaviour and provide feedback on individual performance.

Objective measures of physical activity

Objective measures of physical activity include: direct or indirect calorimetry; doubly labelled water method; direct observation; heart rate and activity monitoring.

Direct or indirect calorimetry or doubly labelled water method[29] determine physical activity-associated energy expenditure through measuring heat production, oxygen consumption, or carbon dioxide production. These measures are accurate but time and resource intensive, burdensome, and difficult to interpret in individuals with RA due to variations in metabolism.[30,31]

Direct observation of physical activity categorizes, codes, and quantifies observed behaviour. It provides contextual information about physical activity behaviour but not energy expenditure. It is useful for recording physical activity in those who have recall difficulties such as children,[32] but is seldom used in people with RA.

Heart rate monitoring is a simple assessment of cardiorespiratory stress during physical activity based on the linear relationship between heart rate and oxygen consumption during moderate-vigorous activity. There are discrepancies at very high and low

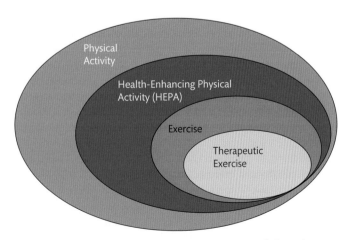

Figure 24.1 Relationship between different concepts of physical activity and exercise.

intensity physical activity[33,34] and heart rate is influenced by factors other than energy expenditure (e.g. disease, caffeine consumption, temperature).[33,34]

Activity monitors capture aspects of bodily movement. **Pedometers** typically measure step counts and estimate distance walked but do not assess intensity, frequency, or duration of activity. While they are reliable in the healthy population who walk at least 0.9 m/s, many underestimate steps taken at slower gait speeds[35] or irregular and unsteady gait patterns,[36] such as in people with RA. **Accelerometers** measure accelerations during movement in either one (usually vertical), two (vertical and mediolateral or vertical and anterior-posterior), or three planes (vertical, mediolateral, and anterior-posterior). The units of acceleration recorded during physical activity are transformed into a count/unit of time and translated into measures of energy expenditure or activity intensity, frequency, and duration.[37] Accelerometers have superior psychometric properties than pedometers[36] although gait disturbances in people with RA alters the validity and reliability of some devices.[38,39] **Multisensory monitors** combine data from biaxial accelerometers, heat flux (heat being dissipated by the body), galvanic signal (onset, peak, and recovery of maximal sweat rates), and skin temperature to quantify physical activity.[40] They have good psychometric properties in the general population[41] and, in people with RA,[40,42] quantify activity at low intensities and are easy to use and acceptable.[40,42,43] While activity and multisensory monitors provide useful estimates of physical activity, they are often costly and, as they are only worn for limited time periods (typically 3–7 days, 7–10 hours/day), it could be questioned if these measures represent habitual activity.

Subjective measures of physical activity

Subjective measures of physical activity include questionnaires, rating scales and activity diaries/logs/short text messages. They are simple and easy to administer, resource efficient and are useful in determining discrete levels of activity (high, moderate, low, inactive) and for repeated measurements, particularly across groups.[44–46] However, the data gathered are variable.[47] All subjective measures are at risk of reporter recall bias, social desirability bias and other external factors (i.e. complexity of the self-report method, age, and seasonal variation).[34,48–50]

Questionnaires aim to identify the dimensions and domains of physical activity using either self-administered responses or interviews. Some questionnaires can be used to estimate energy expenditure although, in the general population, results from validation studies comparing questionnaires to doubly labelled water are inconsistent.[51] Overall, questionnaires correlate and agree with other construct criteria measures for vigorous-intensity physical activity, but they are less accurate for light- to moderate-intensity activity.[52]

Rating scales, such as the Rate of Perceived Exertion (RPE),[53] rate perceived exertion and may be used to guide exercise intensity. The RPE, or derivations of this scale (e.g. Category Ratio scale, the Borg CR10 Scale)[54] are widely used in people with RA.

Activity logs, diaries, or short text messages require individuals to detail their physical activity in real time either in a predetermined time frame or as an activity–by–activity record.[34,48–50] They overcome some of the disadvantages of recall errors but can be burdensome.

Measures of physical fitness

The VO$_{2max}$ test is the criterion measure of **aerobic capacity** which determines the rate of oxygen uptake during an incremental exercise test to maximum exercise intensity (ml/kg/min).[55] It requires individuals to exercise to maximal intensities, is resource intensive and complex, limiting its application to practice. Consequently submaximal tests, such as the Åstrand bicycle ergometer method,[55] treadmill tests,[56] step tests,[57] or five-minute walking test[58] may be used to estimate VO$_{2max}$ and are valid and reliable clinical tests in people with RA.[56,58–60]

Muscle strength is determined by the maximum amount of torque that can be generated in one maximal muscle contraction (one-repetition maximum, 1RM) or predicted using submaximal tests (e.g. 10 RM) in people with arthritis.[61] **Muscular endurance** is assessed by the ability of a muscle group to execute repeated contractions over time or to maintain a maximal voluntary contraction until fatigue, such as timed standing.[62]

Detailed assessment of **body composition** (e.g. dual-energy X-ray absorptiometry or magnetic resonance imaging) is resource intensive so anthropometric assessments are more frequently used in practice. Body mass index assesses whole-body obesity, although caution is required when applying standard thresholds for obesity in people who are at risk of altered body composition, such as those with RA. Waist circumference or waist to hip ratio are alternative measures of central adiposity although the psychometric properties of these measures are uncertain in people with RA. Bioelectrical impedance analysis (measurement of electrical impedance through body tissues) is easy to complete and relatively inexpensive but still lacks in validity and reliability compared with other, more advanced, methods in people with RA.

Flexibility or joint range of movement is commonly assessed using goniometry although the measurement properties of this method tend to be poor.[63,64] The Escola Paulista de Medicina (EPM)-range of motion scale[65] measures ten distinct movements of small and large joints and is valid, reliable, and sensitive to change in people with RA.[63] Wearable devices to assess joint range of movement in people with RA[66] are being developed but the measurement properties are not established.[66]

Neuromuscular activity can be determined by the Berg Balance Scale, a 14-item performance scale,[67] and the figure-of-eight walk.[68] Both are reliable measures of balance in people with RA, although the figure-of-eight walk has greater discriminative ability than the Berg Balance Scale in people with moderate disability.[69] Joint position sense (the ability to reproduce a joint angle) estimates proprioceptive ability in people with arthritis.[4,70] Measures of functional performance provide an estimation of sensorimotor performance and control. Examples include grip ability test[71] or 8 foot get up and go.[72]

HEPA, physical inactivity, and sedentary behaviour in people with RA

People with RA tend to complete predominantly low- to moderate-intensity physical activity and spend more time doing light and moderate activities and less time completing vigorous activities

Table 24.1 Summary of key physical outcomes and measures for HEPA and exercise in people with RA

Type of activity	Proposed outcome	Clinical outcome measurement in people with RA
Aerobic	Improves or maintains cardiorespiratory fitness	Physiological measures (e.g. heart rate), Body movement (e.g. step count, 3-dimensional body accelerations, multisensor devices). Self-reported activity (e.g. questionnaires activity logs) Aerobic fitness—Maximal or submaximal tests (e.g. 5-minute walk test assessment of VO_{2max})
Motor function	Improves or maintains skeletal muscle strength, power, endurance, and mass	Strength—1 repetition maximum or predicted from submaximal strength test (e.g. grip strength tests) Endurance—Repetitions to fatigue Body composition/mass—anthropomentic measures (e.g. BMI, waist circumference or waist to hip ratio), bioelectrical impedance analysis
Flexibility or range-of-motion	Improves or maintains joint range of movement and muscle length	Joint range of movement (e.g. goniometry), Battery tests (e.g. EPM-ROM)[65]
Neuromuscular	Improves or maintains motor control, balance proprioception	Motor control (e.g. grip ability test)[71] Balance (e.g. Berg balance scale)[67] Proprioception (e.g. joint position sense)

EPM-ROM—Escola Paulista de Medicina (EPM)-range of motion scale.

than healthy controls.[1] Consequently, physical activity levels among most people with RA tend to be too low to reach current HEPA recommendations and lower than among healthy controls.[73–75] Huge variations in the percentage of people with RA meeting the current physical activity recommendations are reported; from 29%[74] to 70%[73] (Table 24.1) However, methodological variations hamper comparison between studies which prohibits definitive conclusions. Data from 21 countries suggests that only 13.8% of all individuals with RA perform planned and structured exercise at least three times per week although this ranges from 6% in Argentina to 32% in Finland.[76] The proportion of people that self-report maintained HEPA levels over the past 6 months or more is only 22%, indicating that sustaining HEPA behaviour is more challenging than adopting a new HEPA behaviour.[73]

Physical inactivity and sedentary behaviour are also more frequent in people with RA (~10.3 daily hours) than among the general adult population (~7.5 daily hours), but similar to that in populations with other rheumatic diseases (~9.1 daily hours) and other long-term conditions such as type 2 diabetes, cardiovascular diseases, and obesity (~9.4 daily hours).[77] The prevalence of physical inactivity (defined as no regular weekly exercise) is high in most countries: >80% in seven countries; 60–80% in 12 countries; and 45% and 29%, respectively, in two countries. Physical inactivity is associated with female sex, older age, lower education, obesity, comorbidity, low functional capacity, or higher levels of disease activity, pain, and fatigue.[76]

A range of psychosocial, sociodemographic, and physical factors are associated with HEPA behaviour in people with RA. Correlates of sufficient HEPA (i.e. meeting recommendations) include perception of good health, high motivation, or self-efficacy, positive previous experience of physical activity, high outcome expectations, and good social support.[73] Insufficient HEPA, on the other hand, is more common in older people, females, those with low education level, several comorbidities, fatigue, perceived high activity limitation, coerced regulation style, and certain biochemical markers.[78] Predictors of trajectories to sustained higher HEPA over time include male sex, already established physical activity at baseline, less activity limitation, good social support, and high self-efficacy for

exercise.[79] Identified predictors of not sustaining HEPA over time are, adjusting for disease activity, older age, poor mental health, poor health perception, and overweight/obesity.[74]

Overall, studies indicate that most individuals with RA accumulate insufficient activity to meet HEPA recommendations. Since physical inactivity and sedentary behaviour in adults with autoimmune rheumatic diseases is associated with poor health-related outcomes such as worse disease symptoms and disability, interventions aimed at minimizing physical inactivity and breaking up sedentary time, which are often overlooked modifiable risk factors, should be integrated into the management of people with RA.[25,77]

Benefits of therapeutic exercise on disability

Findings from systematic reviews and meta-analyses based on randomized controlled trials with detailed descriptions of the exercise type, frequency, duration and intensity[80–82] suggest there is moderate-quality evidence that short-term (8–12 weeks) land-based aerobic exercise of moderate to high intensity augments aerobic capacity, but does not improve muscle strength in people with RA. Short-term (8–12 weeks) water-based aerobic exercise of moderate to high intensity also enhances oxygen uptake. Short-term (12–26 weeks) land-based combinations of aerobic and resistance exercise of moderate to high intensity improves both oxygen uptake and muscle strength. These exercise combinations also reduce activity limitation and improves both oxygen uptake and muscle strength if performed on a long-term basis (52–104 weeks). Most interventions evaluate exercise prescribed for three times/week for at least 30 minutes at a time. Aerobic exercise interventions usually consist of cycling on stationary bikes, walking on treadmills, or using rowing ergometers, aerobic walking, swimming, or water aerobics, jogging or running, low-impact aerobics, or sports or games. Resistance training was performed as functional exercises, strength training programmes using gym equipment or rubber exercise bands, or as circuit interval training.[80,82] However, few studies evaluate the effects of resistance training independently and the heterogeneous review and meta-analysis methodologies may influence findings. For example, another meta-analysis suggests that resistance exercise results in statistically significant, and possibly clinically relevant, improvements in muscle strength, walking capacity, and reduced activity limitation without aggravating inflammation.[83] Additionally, aerobic and resistance exercise has the potential to reduce body mass index (BMI) as well as increase muscle mass and reduce fat tissue.[84,85]

While flexibility and range-of-motion exercise is generally recommended to people with RA, evidence is limited except in the hand, where range of motion exercises improves finger extension.[86]

Neuromuscular exercise is often recommended to improve balance and proprioception and thus reduce the risk of falls and fall-related fractures among persons with RA.[8] However, there is limited research examining the efficacy of balance training alone in people with RA,[81,87] although exploratory research appears promising.[88,89]

Fatigue[10,90] and pain[90,91] are reduced, particularly in the short term, following aerobic exercise, although the effects tend to be small. Exercise activates pain inhibitory mechanisms with subsequent increase of pain thresholds during muscle contraction in people with RA that have increased pain sensitivity but, unlike people with conditions associated with central pain sensitization, such as fibromyalgia or chronic fatigue syndrome, individuals with RA have typical exercise-induced hypoalgesia during muscle contractions.[92]

Cardiorespiratory aerobic conditioning in people with stable RA appears to improve quality of life and activity limitation.[91] Exercise may also improve sleep quality and disturbances.[93]

Evidence is growing that supported, home-based, upper extremity exercise improves hand function, pain, and grip strength in the short-term, and upper limb function and pinch strength in the longer term, with no adverse effects on pain or disease activity.[86]

Exercise interventions vary but usually include strength, flexibility, and functional exercise. Longer therapy duration and higher therapy intensity seem to result in better outcomes.[86,94] Interventions are acceptable to people with RA[95,96] and improve performance of on activities of daily living, work, and physical and emotional roles.[96]

The role of therapeutic exercise in reducing risk of comorbidity

Lack of HEPA and excessive sedentary behaviour are predictors of morbidity and mortality among individuals with long-term conditions such as type 2 diabetes, cardiovascular diseases, and obesity. The interrelationships between body composition, physical inactivity, RA, and CVD are complex and physical inactivity increases both BMI and the CVD risk profile.[97] Conversely, low BMI, which is related to rheumatoid cachexia (low muscle mass and high fat accumulation),[98] also represents a CVD risk in people with RA.[99] Empirical evidence indicates that a six-month individualized aerobic and resistance exercise programme confers significant improvements in VO_{2max}, blood pressure, triglycerides, high density lipoprotein, total cholesterol:HDL ratio, BMI, body fat, and 10-year CVD event probability. Notably, change in VO_{2max} was the strongest predictor for the observed improvements in all the assessed CVD risk factors and thus, should be targeted in exercise programmes which aim to reduce CVD risks.[85]

HEPA, therapeutic exercise, and inflammation

RA used to be a contraindication for therapeutic exercise as it was hypothesized to exacerbate systemic and local inflammation and aggravate joint destruction. Thus, bed rest, rather than exercise, was generally recommended.[100,101] However, evidence from contemporary clinical exercise studies suggests that exercise might decrease inflammatory activity.[102,103] Similarly, the fear of exercise aggravating joint destruction is largely unsupported. Only one study suggests that exercise might slightly increase the destruction of large joints that are already severely affected at start of a high-intensity exercise programme.[104] This potential risk may be negated with careful selection of exercises for the affected joints and may be outweighed by beneficial effects of therapeutic exercise.

The physiology underpinning the potential reduction of inflammation following exercise are suggested to be cytokine-driven mechanisms involving IL-6, IL-10 and IL-1 receptor antagonist (IL-1ra), exercise-mediated changes in body composition and improvement in endothelial function after individualized exercise.[105] Six months' combined aerobic and resistance training may thus attenuate C-reactive protein (CRP) expression which is likely to be due to a concomitant reduction in body fat.[85] Furthermore, both micro- and macrovascular function may improve within 3 months of commencing an individualized aerobic and resistance exercise in people with RA and may be accounted for by concomitant reductions in inflammation following exercise.[106] A meta-analysis including participants with inflammatory rheumatic conditions suggests high to moderate-quality evidence for small beneficial effects on disease activity scores and joint damage following cardiorespiratory and strength exercises complying with the American College of Sports Medicine's recommendations. There was also moderate-quality evidence for small beneficial effects on erythrocyte sedimentation rate (ESR) but no exercise effect on CRP.[90]

Economic evaluation of HEPA and therapeutic exercise programmes

The cost-effectiveness or cost-utility of HEPA or therapeutic exercise programmes targeting people with RA are largely unknown. However, it seems that long-term high-intensity supervised exercise provides insufficient health improvement in comparison with conventional physiotherapy to justify the additional cost.[107] In contrast, a physiotherapist-led education, self-management and upper limb exercise training programme is cost-effective from both a healthcare and societal perspective when assessed against the standards set by the National Institute for Clinical Excellence and leads to lower healthcare costs and work absence.[108] A 1-year HEPA coaching programme is cost-effective, but only if targeted towards people with more severe disease[109] while a tailored home-based hand exercise programme is a worthwhile, low-cost intervention.[96]

Overall, HEPA and therapeutic exercise programmes are most cost-effective, at least on a societal level, if directed towards people more affected by RA and are predominantly home-based interventions which support self-management rather than supervised programmes delivered in healthcare facilities. However, economic analysis of the potential, long-term, preventive effects of short-term HEPA or exercise programmes have not been studied in people with RA.

Recommending HEPA for people with RA

While there is strong evidence for beneficial effects of adhering to HEPA recommendations in the general population, evidence is lacking in specific subpopulations, such as RA. However, it is likely that people with RA will have similar benefits and there are detailed recommendations to guide the design of HEPA programmes[22,25] (see section 2.2). Walking also may be a feasible and acceptable form of HEPA.[110–112] Since HEPA is predominantly integrated into an individual's everyday life, away from healthcare facilities, adherence can be challenging. Despite limited evidence for interventions to improve HEPA adherence, health professionals are recommended to consider a range of aspects that may influence adherence when prescribing HEPA.[25,113]

Evidence-based prescription of HEPA and therapeutic exercise

There are three types of physical activity-related interventions to be considered for persons with RA. One is therapeutic exercise, which predominantly aims to improve or retain function and reduce disability, a second option is HEPA and a third possibility is reducing or breaking up prolonged sedentary time. The latter two options aim to reduce symptoms and the risk of comorbidity. It is crucial that an intervention is tailored to each person's physical (e.g. fitness) and psychological capacity, such as their attitudes, beliefs and motivation, as well as their social and physical environment[114] as these all influence an individual's willingness and ability to adopt and sustain a new activity programme.

To optimize the **physical benefits** of HEPA and therapeutic exercise interventions, four aspects need to be specified. These are the (i) type of activity (e.g. aerobic capacity, motor function, flexibility or neuromuscular function); (ii) frequency of activity performance (i.e. number of sessions, episodes, or bouts per specified timeframe); (iii) duration of activity performance (i.e. length of time for each bout); and (iv) intensity (metabolic demand of an activity), such as rate of energy expenditure during aerobic activity or the magnitude of the force exerted during resistance exercise. The requirements for beneficial aerobic and strengthening exercise programmes are specified in Table 24.2. Prescription of intensities for these types of activity should be based on an initial physical fitness testing of aerobic capacity, 1 RM or other physical capacities at target for an actual intervention. The same tests also need to be repeated regularly during an intervention as improvements in physical capacity will form the basis for adjustments to the intervention. It is, however, important to bear in mind that much lower intensities/loads should be applied initially and increased during a 2–3-week period to reach the recommended level. Exercise prescriptions may also need to be adjusted during disease flares.[82]

Pain is often considered, by health professionals and individuals with RA, to represent a barrier to HEPA and therapeutic exercise. While acute pain might represent a barrier to activity, prolonged pain generally does not. Nevertheless, increased activity often confers increased discomfort such as foot pain, hand pain, and general muscle soreness initially that needs to be addressed. Provision of appropriate information (e.g. on footwear, orthotics, or alternative grips), to minimize the impact of initial discomfort should be given. Absolute physical contraindications to HEPA or therapeutic exercise in people with RA are rare, but relative contraindications, such as high inflammatory activity and severe joint destruction should be considered when prescribing HEPA and therapeutic exercise, as should the presence of comorbidities such as pericarditis, heart failure, pleuritis, pulmonary fibrosis, vasculitis, or kidney enlargement. Clearance from an appropriate medical practitioner is recommended and most of the time relative contraindications can be overcome by careful tailoring of interventions and supervision by experienced physiotherapists or suitably qualified fitness professionals in a clinical setting. Such tailoring may include heart rate monitoring, appropriate selection of exercises, and positions to spare affected joints.

Introducing potentially burdensome health behaviour changes, such as adopting and maintaining HEPA or therapeutic exercise, is challenging.[115,116] A person's attitudes, belief, and motivation (psychological capacity) and environment are crucial to successful

Table 24.2 Evidence-based recommendations of type, frequency, duration, and intensity/load of exercise for patients with RA

Type	Frequency	Duration	Intensity/load[1]
Aerobic capacity	3 times/week	30–75 minutes/time	65–80% of VO_{2max}[2] 14–17 Borg RPE[3] scale (6–20)
Muscle strength	2–3 times/week	3 sets × 8–12 repetitions for each of 8–10 large muscle groups	70% of 1 RM[4]
Aerobic capacity+ muscle strength	2–3 times/week	30–90 minutes/time	75–85% of VO_{2max} 70% of 1 RM
Flexibility	2–3 times/week	4 times (10–30 s) for all major muscle groups	

[1] Denotes the intensity/load to be reached during an exercise period through progressive increase from moderate intensity (40–59% of VO_{2max} or 12–13 on Borg RPE scale) and lower load in % of 1 RM

[2] VO_{2max} = Maximum oxygen uptake

[3] RPE = Rating of perceived exertion

[4] 1 RM = the highest load that can be lifted through the entire range of movement one time only

Source: data from Swärdh E and Brodin N (2016) 'Effects of aerobic and muscle strengthening exercise in adults with rheumatoid arthritis: a narrative review summarising a chapter in physical activity in the prevention and treatment of disease (FYSS 2016)' *Br J Sports Med.* 50(6):362-7.

Table 24.3 Characteristics of a traditional didactic approach and a self-management approach to implement HEPA

	Information about HEPA	Goal-setting for HEPA	Patient role	Main components
Traditional didactic approach	Given by the therapist	Set by the therapist, maybe discussed with the patient	Expected to be rationale and adhere to the advice given by the therapist	Information, advice, prescription of HEPA, follow-up
Self-management approach	Need of information explored by motivational interviewing and given after permission from the patient	Set by the patient, developed in interaction with the therapist to ensure realistic, progressive goals	Expected to have the resources to manage behaviour change into HEPA by learning self-regulatory skills	Patient-centred **communication strategy** (e.g. motivational interviewing) to explore motivation and readiness to change. **Behaviour change strategy** using SMART* goal-setting and planning, monitoring, and facilitating own HEPA behaviour, making plans to prevent relapse into sedentary habits, follow-ups

* specific, measurable, achievable, relevant and time bound.
Reprinted from Demmelmaier I, Åsenlöf P., and Opava C (2013) 'Supporting stepwise change: improving health behaviors in rheumatoid arthritis with the example of physical activity' *Int. J. Clin. Rheumatol.* 8(1):89–94 with permission Future Medicine.

adoption and maintenance of new behaviours. Concepts such as readiness to change (willingness to adopt HEPA or a therapeutic exercise regimen), self-efficacy (belief in the ability to perform a certain HEPA or therapeutic exercise programme), fear-avoidance (avoiding activity due to fear of causing damage or increasing pain), and autonomous motivation (belief that a HEPA or therapeutic exercise regimen is goal set by themselves) might be useful to incorporate. Hence, HEPA and exercise prescriptions should, in addition to tests of physical capacity, be based on a person's psychological capacity (e.g. readiness to change and motivation and designed to increase self-efficacy and reduce fear-avoidance beliefs). Expanding use of theory (e.g. Transtheoretical Model, the Social Learning/Cognitive Theory, or the Self-regulation Theory) in the design, evaluation, and interpretation of PA interventions have been suggested.[117] For more information on concepts and behaviour change theories please consult chapters on self-management and psychological approaches in this book (Chapters 26 and 27).

Supporting HEPA and therapeutic exercise

Many health professionals in rheumatology are trained with a strong biomedical bias focusing on physical aspects of functioning and disability in their evaluations and interventions. However, when supporting the adoption and maintenance of new health behaviours, such as HEPA and therapeutic exercise, a wider approach that combines biomedical knowledge with skills to guide behaviour change is required. Such an approach includes, not only the specification of physical activity by type, frequency, duration, and intensity, but also consideration of the psychosocial and environmental determinants of the behaviour.[118,119] Furthermore, skills to support evidence-based behaviour change strategies such as specific goal setting, action planning, and self-monitoring of physical activity may be necessary.[25,120]

For this, a shift away from a traditional, didactic, information provision to person-directed self-management intervention is required[121] (Table 24.3). Motivational interviewing could be part of such self-management support and aims to enhance a person's knowledge and understanding, motivation and readiness to change by discussing and exploring ways to minimize resistance and ambivalence towards HEPA and therapeutic exercise. It aims to encourage ownership of goals, enhance self-efficacy, and assumes competency

(i.e. possessing the resources and knowledge to identify their own needs, goals, and engage in HEPA or therapeutic exercise).[122]

New approaches and work modes are challenging for professionals, but the provision of education and skills training will enhance their use among health professionals in rheumatology so they can best support people with RA to adopt and maintain HEPA and therapeutic exercise.

Key points

1. Therapeutic exercise to target disability and risk of comorbidity is recommended in management of RA.

2. HEPA and disrupting sedentary behaviour are recommended for the general population and, although lacking strong evidence, should also confer health benefits in people with RA.

3. Evidence-based prescription of HEPA and therapeutic exercise requires evaluation of physical and psychological capacity, motivation, and contextual factors.

4. A person-centred, self-management approach, rather than a traditional didactic approach, is optimal to facilitate adoption and maintenance of HEPA and therapeutic exercise.

REFERENCES

1. Munsterman T, Takken T, Wittink H. Are persons with rheumatoid arthritis deconditioned? A review of physical activity and aerobic capacity. *BMC Musculoskelet Disord* 2012;13(1):202.

2. Fridén C, Thoors U, Glenmark B, et al. Higher pain sensitivity and lower muscle strength in postmenopausal women with early rheumatoid arthritis compared with age-matched healthy women–a pilot study. *Disability Rehabil* 2013;35(16):1350–6.

3. Carroll M, Joyce W, Brenton-Rule A, Dalbeth N, Rome K. Assessment of foot and ankle muscle strength using hand held dynamometry in patients with established rheumatoid arthritis. *J Foot Ankle Res* 2013;6(1):10.

4. Bearne LM, Coomer AF, Hurley MV. Upper limb sensorimotor function and functional performance in patients with rheumatoid arthritis. *Disability Rehabil* 2007;29(13):1035–9.

5. Romero-Guzmán AK, Menchaca-Tapia VM, Contreras-Yáñez I, Pascual-Ramos V. Patient and physician perspectives of hand

function in a cohort of rheumatoid arthritis patients: the impact of disease activity. *BMC Musculoskelet Dis* 2016;*17*(1):392.

6. Matschke V, Murphy P, Lemmey AB, Maddison P, Thom JM. Skeletal muscle properties in rheumatoid arthritis patients. *Med Sci Sports Exerc* 2010;*42*(12):2149–55.

7. Stanmore EK, Oldham J, Skelton DA, et al. Fall incidence and outcomes of falls in a prospective study of adults with rheumatoid arthritis. *Arthritis Care Res* 2013;*65*(5):737–44.

8. Stanmore EK, Oldham J, Skelton DA, et al. Risk factors for falls in adults with rheumatoid arthritis: a prospective study. *Arthritis Care Res* 2013;*65*(8):1251–8.

9. Katz P. Causes and consequences of fatigue in rheumatoid arthritis. *Curr Opin Rheumatol* 2017;*29*:269–76.

10. Rongen-van Dartel S, Repping-Wuts H, Flendrie M, et al. Effect of aerobic exercise training on fatigue in rheumatoid arthritis: a meta-analysis. *Arthritis Care Res* 2015;*67*(8):1054–62.

11. Sturgeon JA, Finan PH, Zautra AJ. Affective disturbance in rheumatoid arthritis: psychological and disease-related pathways. *Nat Rev Rheumatol* 2016;*12*(9):532–42.

12. Ahlstrand I, Thyberg I, Falkmer T, Dahlström Ö, Björk M. Pain and activity limitations in women and men with contemporary treated early RA compared to 10 years ago: the Swedish TIRA project. *Scand J Rheumatol* 2015;*44*(4):259–64.

13. Boyden SD, Hossain IN, Wohlfahrt A, Lee YC. Non-inflammatory causes of pain in patients with rheumatoid arthritis. *Curr Rheumatol Rep* 2016;*2016*(18):30.

14. Leffler AS, Kosek E, Lerndal T, Nordmark B, Hansson P. Somatosensory perception and function of diffuse noxious inhibitory controls (DNIC) in patients suffering from rheumatoid arthritis. *Eur J Pain* 2002;*6*:161–76.

15. Meeus M, Vervisch S, De Clerck LS, Moorkens G, Hans G, Nijs J. Central sensitization in patients with rheumatoid arthritis: a systematic literature review. *Semin Arth Rheum* 2012;*41*:556–67.

16. Edwards RR, Wasan AD, Bingham CO, Bathon J, Haythornthwaite JA, Smith MT. Enhanced reactivity to pain in patients with rheumatoid arthritis. *Arthritis Res Ther* 2009;*11*:R61.

17. Caspersen CJ, Powell KE, Christenson GM. Physical activity, exercise, and physical fitness: definitions and distinctions for health-related research. *Public Health Rep* 1985;*100*(2):126–31.

18. World Health Organization (WHO). *Global Recommendations on Physical Activity for Health*. Geneva, Switzerland: WHO, 2010. Available at: https://www.who.int/dietphysicalactivity/global-PA-recs-2010.pdf

19. Kisner C, Colby L. *Therapeutic Exercise: Foundations and Techniques*, 7th edition. Philadelphia, PA: F.A. Davis Company, 2017.

20. Fenton SA, Veldhuijzen van Zanten JJ, Duda JL, Metsios GS, Kitas GD. Sedentary behaviour in rheumatoid arthritis: definition, measurement and implications for health. *Rheumatology (Oxf)* 2018;*57*(2):213–26.

21. Mansoubi M, Pearson N, Clemes SA, et al. Energy expenditure during common sitting and standing tasks: examining the 1.5 MET definition of sedentary behaviour. *BMC Public Health* 2015;*15*(1):516.

22. Nelson ME, Rejeski WJ, Blair SN, et al. Physical activity and public health in older adults: recommendation from the American College of Sports Medicine and the American Heart Association. *Circulation* 2007;*116*(9):1094.

23. Department of Health. *Start Active, Stay Active: Report on Physical Activity in the UK-GOV UK*. London, UK: UK Government, 2016.

24. Garber CE, Blissmer B, Deschenes MR, Franklin BA, Lamonte MJ, Lee I-M, et al. American College of Sports Medicine position stand. Quantity and quality of exercise for developing and maintaining cardiorespiratory, musculoskeletal, and neuromotor fitness in apparently healthy adults: guidance for prescribing exercise. *Med Sci Sports Exerc* 2011;*43*(7):1334–59.

25. Osthoff A-KR, Niedermann K, Braun J, et al. 2018 EULAR recommendations for physical activity in people with inflammatory arthritis and osteoarthritis. *Annals Rheum Dis* 2018;*77*(9):1251–60.

26. Pedersen BK, Saltin B. Exercise as medicine—evidence for prescribing exercise as therapy in 26 different chronic diseases. *Scand J Med Sci Sports* 2015;*25*(Suppl 3):1–72.

27. National Institute for Health and Care Excellence (NICE). *Rheumatoid Arthritis: The Management of Rheumatoid Arthritis in Adults [CG79]*. London, UK: The National Collaborating Centre for Chronic Conditions, 2015. Available at: https://www.nice.org.uk/guidance/cg79

28. McArdle W, Katch F, Katch V. Energy expenditure during rest and physical activity. In: McArdle WD KF, Katch VL (eds). *Essentials of Exercise Physiology*, 4th edition, pp. 237–62. Baltimore, MD: Lippincott Williams & Wilkins, 2011.

29. Ainslie P, Reilly T, Westerterp K. Estimating human energy expenditure: a review of techniques with particular reference to doubly labelled water. *Sports Med* 2003;*33*:683–98.

30. Metsios GS, Stavropoulos-Kalinoglou A, Panoulas VF, et al. New resting energy expenditure prediction equations for patients with rheumatoid arthritis. *Rheumatology* 2008;*47*(4):500–6.

31. Rall L, Roubenoff R. Rheumatoid cachexia: metabolic abnormalities, mechanisms and interventions. *Rheumatology* 2004;*43*(10):1219–23.

32. McKenzie TL. Use of direct observation to assess physical activity. In: Welk G (ed.). *Physical Activity Assessments for Health-Related Research*. Champaign, IL: Human Kinetics, 2002, pp. 179–95.

33. Strath SJ, Swartz AM, Bassett Jr DR, O'Brien WL, King GA, Ainsworth BE. Evaluation of heart rate as a method for assessing moderate intensity physical activity. *Med Sci Sports Exerc* 2000;*32*(9 Suppl):S465–70.

34. Vanhees L, Lefevre J, Philippaerts R, et al. How to assess physical activity? How to assess physical fitness? *Eur J Cardiovasc Prev Rehabil* 2005;*12*(2):102–14.

35. Crouter S, Schneider P, Karabulut M, Bassett DJ. Validity of 10 electronic pedometers for measuring steps, distance, and energy cost. *Med Sci Sports Exerc* 2003;*35*:1455–60.

36. Schneider P, Crouter S, Lukajic O, Bassett D. Accuracy and reliability of 10 pedometers for measuring steps over a 400-m walk. *Med Sci Sports Exerc* 2003; (35):1779–84.

37. Semanik P, Song J, Chang RW, Manheim L, Ainsworth B, Dunlop D. Assessing physical activity in persons with rheumatoid arthritis using accelerometry. *Med Sci Sports Exerc* 2010;*42*(8):1493.

38. Backhouse MR, Hensor EM, White D, Keenan A-M, Helliwell PS, Redmond AC. Concurrent validation of activity monitors in patients with rheumatoid arthritis. *Clin Biomech* 2013;*28*(4):473–9.

39. Yamada M, Aoyama T, Mori S, et al. Objective assessment of abnormal gait in patients with rheumatoid arthritis using a smartphone. *Rheumatol Int* 2012;*32*(12):3869–74.

40. Almeida GJ, Wasko MC, Jeong K, Moore CG, Piva SR. Physical activity measured by the SenseWear Armband in women with rheumatoid arthritis. *Phys Ther* 2011;*91*(9):1367–76.

41. Malavolti M, Pietrobelli A, Dugoni M, et al. A new device for measuring resting energy expenditure (REE) in healthy subjects. *Nutr Metab Cardiovasc Dis* 2007;17(5):338–43.

42. Tierney M, Fraser A, Purtill H, Kennedy N. Study to determine the criterion validity of the SenseWear Armband as a measure of physical activity in people with rheumatoid arthritis. *Arthritis Care Res* 2013;65(6):888–95.

43. Tierney M, Fraser A, Kennedy N. Users' experience of physical activity monitoring technology in rheumatoid arthritis. *Musculoskeletal Care* 2013;11(2):83–92.

44. Corder K, van Sluijs EM, Wright A, Whincup P, Wareham NJ, Ekelund U. Is it possible to assess free-living physical activity and energy expenditure in young people by self-report? *Am J Clin Nutr* 2009;89(3):862–70.

45. Shephard RJ. How much physical activity is needed for good health? *Int J Sports Med* 1999;20(1):23–7.

46. Shephard RJ. Limits to the measurement of habitual physical activity by questionnaires. *Br J Sports Med* 2003;37(3):197–206;

47. van Poppel MNM, Chinapaw MJM, Mokkink LB, van Mechelen W, Terwee CB. Physical activity questionnaires for adults. *Sports Med* 2010;40(7):565–600.

48. Klesges RC, Eck LH, Mellon MW, Fulliton W, Somes GW, Hanson CL. The accuracy of self-reports of physical activity. *Med Sci Sports Exerc* 1990;22(5):690–7.

49. Uitenbroek DG. Seasonal variation in leisure time physical activity. *Med Sci Sports Exerc* 1993;25(6):755–60.

50. Durante R, Ainsworth BE. The recall of physical activity: using a cognitive model of the question-answering process. *Med Sci Sports Exerc* 1996;28(10):1282–91.

51. Westerterp KR. Assessment of physical activity: a critical appraisal. *Eur J Appl Physiol* 2009;105(6):823–8.

52. Jacobs DR, Jr., Ainsworth BE, Hartman TJ, Leon AS. A simultaneous evaluation of 10 commonly used physical activity questionnaires. *Med Sci Sports Exerc* 1993;25(1):81–91.

53. Borg G. Perceived exertion as an indicator of somatic stress. *Scand J Rehabi Med* 1970;2(2):92.

54. Borg G. *Borg's Perceived Exertion and Pain Scales*. Champaign, IL: USA Human Kinetics, 1998.

55. Åstrand I. Aerobic work capacity in men and women with special reference to age. *Acta Physiologica Scandinavica Supplementum* 1960;49(169):1.

56. Minor M, Johnson J. Reliability and validity of a submaximal treadmill test to estimate aerobic capacity in women with rheumatic disease. *J Rheumatol* 1996;23(9):1517–23.

57. Siconolfi SF, Garber CE, Lasater TM, Carleton RA. A simple, valid step test for estimating maximal oxygen uptake in epidemiologic studies. *Am J Epidemiol* 1985;121(3):382–90.

58. Price LG, Hewett JE, Kay DR, Minor MA. Five-minute walking test of aerobic fitness for people with arthritis. *Arthritis Rheumatol* 1988;1(1):33–7.

59. Cooney JK, Moore JP, Ahmad YA, et al. A simple step test to estimate cardio-respiratory fitness levels of rheumatoid arthritis patients in a clinical setting. *Int J Rheumatol* 2013;2013:174541.

60. Nordgren B, Fridén C, Jansson E, et al. Criterion validation of two submaximal aerobic fitness tests, the self-monitoring Foxwalk test and the Åstrand cycle test in people with rheumatoid arthritis. *BMC Musculoskelet Disord* 2014;15(1):305.

61. McNair PJ, Colvin M, Reid D. Predicting maximal strength of quadriceps from submaximal performance in individuals with knee joint osteoarthritis. *Arthritis Care Res* 2011;63(2):216–22.

62. Ekdahl C, Broman G. Muscle strength, endurance, and aerobic capacity in rheumatoid arthritis: a comparative study with healthy subjects. *Ann Rheum Dis* 1992;51(1):35–40.

63. Boström C, Harms-Ringdahl K, Nordemar R. Clinical reliability of shoulder function assessment in patients with rheumatoid arthritis. *Scand J Rheumatol* 1991;20(1):36–48.

64. Jha B, Ross M, Reeves SW, Couzens GB, Peters SE. Measuring thumb range of motion in first carpometacarpal joint arthritis: the inter-rater reliability of the Kapandji Index versus goniometry. *Hand Therapy* 2016;21(2):45–53.

65. Ferraz M, Oliveira LM, Araujo P, Atra E, Walter S. EPM-ROM Scale: an evaluative instrument to be used in rheumatoid arthritis trials. *Clin Exp Rheumatol* 1990;8(5):491–4.

66. Small D, Gardiner P, Connolly J, et al. AB1196-HPR A comparison of patient preference and usability between two electronic goniometric gloves in the measurement of joint movement in patients with rheumatoid arthritis. *Ann Rheum Dis* 2017;76:1530–1.

67. Berg K, Wood-Dauphinee S, Williams J. The Balance Scale: reliability assessment with elderly residents and patients with an acute stroke. *Scand J Rehabil Med* 1995;27(1):27–36.

68. Hess RJ, Brach JS, Piva SR, Van Swearingen JM. Walking skill can be assessed in older adults: validity of the Figure-of-8 Walk Test. *Phys Ther* 2010;90(1):89–99.

69. Norén AM, Bogren U, Bolin J, Stenström C. Balance assessment in patients with peripheral arthritis: applicability and reliability of some clinical assessments. *Physiother Res Int* 2001;6(4):193–204.

70. Hurkmans E, Van Der Esch M, Ostelo R, Knol D, Dekker J, Steultjens M. Reproducibility of the measurement of knee joint proprioception in patients with osteoarthritis of the knee. *Arthritis Care Res* 2007;57(8):1398–403.

71. Dellhag B, Bjelle A. A grip ability test for use in rheumatology practice. *J Rheumatol* 1995;22(8):1559–65.

72. Wilkinson TJ, Lemmey AB, Clayton RJ, Jones JG, O'Brien TD. The 8-foot up and go test is the best way to assess physical function in the rheumatoid arthritis clinic. *Rheumatol Adv Pract* 2018;2(1):rkx017.

73. Demmelmaier I, Bergman P, Nordgren B, Jensen I, Opava CH. Current and maintained health-enhancing physical activity in rheumatoid arthritis: a cross-sectional study. *Arthritis Care Res* 2013;65(7):1166–76.

74. Iversen MD, Frits M, von Heideken J, Cui J, Weinblatt M, Shadick NA. Physical activity and correlates of physical activity participation over three years in adults with rheumatoid arthritis. *Arthritis Care Res* 2017;69(10):1535–45.

75. Manning VL, Hurley MV, Scott DL, Bearne LM. Are patients meeting the updated physical activity guidelines? Physical activity participation, recommendation, and preferences among inner-city adults with rheumatic diseases. *J Clin Rheumatol* 2012;18(8):399–404.

76. Sokka T, Häkkinen A, Kautiainen H, et al. Physical inactivity in patients with rheumatoid arthritis: data from twenty-one countries in a cross-sectional, international study. *Arthritis Care Res* 2008;59(1):42–50.

77. Pinto AJ, Roschel H, de Sá Pinto AL, et al. Physical inactivity and sedentary behavior: overlooked risk factors in autoimmune rheumatic diseases? *Autoimmun Rev* 2017;16(7):667–74.

78. Larkin L, Kennedy N. Correlates of physical activity in adults with rheumatoid arthritis: a systematic review. *J Phys Activity Health* 2014;11(6):1248–61.

79. Demmelmaier I, Dufour AB, Nordgren B, Opava CH. Trajectories of physical activity over two years in persons with rheumatoid arthritis. *Arthritis Care Res* 2016;68(8):1069–77.

80. Hurkmans E, van der Giesen FJ, Vliet Vlieland TP, Schoones J, Van den Ende EC. Dynamic exercise programs (aerobic capacity and/or muscle strength training) in patients with rheumatoid arthritis. *Cochrane Database Syst Rev* 2009;(4):CD006853.

81. Osthoff A-KR, Juhl CB, Knittle K, et al. Effects of exercise and physical activity promotion: meta-analysis informing the 2018 EULAR recommendations for physical activity in people with rheumatoid arthritis, spondyloarthritis and hip/knee osteoarthritis. *RMD Open* 2018;4(2):e000713.

82. Swärdh E, Brodin N. Effects of aerobic and muscle strengthening exercise in adults with rheumatoid arthritis: a narrative review summarising a chapter in Physical activity in the prevention and treatment of disease (FYSS 2016). *Br J Sports Med* 2016;50(6):362–7.

83. Baillet A, Vaillant M, Guinot M, Juvin R, Gaudin P. Efficacy of resistance exercises in rheumatoid arthritis: meta-analysis of randomized controlled trials. *Rheumatology* 2011;51(3):519–27.

84. Lemmey AB, Chester K, Wilson S, Casanova F, Maddison PJ. Effects of high-intensity resistance training in patients with rheumatoid arthritis: a randomized controlled trial. *Arthritis Rheum* 2009;61:1726–34.

85. Stavropoulos-Kalinglou A, Metsios GS, van Zanten JJV, Nightingale P, Kitas GD, Koutedakis Y. Individualised aerobic and resistance exercise training improves cardiorespiratory fitness and reduces cardiovascular risk in patients with rheumatoid arthritis. *Ann Rheum Dis* 2013;72(11):1819–25.

86. Hammond A, Prior Y. The effectiveness of home hand exercise programmes in rheumatoid arthritis: a systematic review. *Br Med Bull* 2016;119(1):49–62.

87. Silva K, Imoto AM, Almeida G, Atallah A, Peccin MS, Trevisani VFM. Balance training (proprioceptive training) for patients with rheumatoid arthritis. *Cochrane Database Syst Rev* 2010;(5):CD007648.

88. da Silva KNG, de Paiva Teixeira LEP, Imoto AM, Atallah ÁN, Peccin MS, Trevisani VFM. Effectiveness of sensorimotor training in patients with rheumatoid arthritis: a randomized controlled trial. *Rheumatol Int* 2013;33(9):2269–75.

89. Williams SB, Brand CA, Hill KD, Hunt SB, Moran H. Feasibility and outcomes of a home-based exercise program on improving balance and gait stability in women with lower-limb osteoarthritis or rheumatoid arthritis: a pilot study. *Arch Phys Med Rehabil* 2010;91(1):106–14.

90. Sveaas S, Berg I, Fongen C, Provan S, Dagfinrud H. High-intensity cardiorespiratory and strength exercises reduced emotional distress and fatigue in patients with axial spondyloarthritis: a randomized controlled pilot study. *Scand J Rheumatol* 2018;47(2):117–21.

91. Baillet A, Zeboulon N, Gossec L, et al. Efficacy of cardiorespiratory aerobic exercise in rheumatoid arthritis: meta-analysis of randomized controlled trials. *Arthritis Care Res* 2010;62(7):984–92.

92. Löfgren M, Opava CH, Demmelmaier I, et al. Pain sensitivity at rest and during muscle contraction in persons with rheumatoid arthritis. A sub study within the Physical Activity in Rheumatoid Arthritis 2010 study. *Arthritis Res Ther* 2018;20(48).

93. McKenna S, Donnelly A, Fraser A, Comber L, Kennedy N. Does exercise impact on sleep for people who have rheumatoid arthritis? A systematic review. *Rheumatol Int* 2017;37(6):963–74.

94. Bergstra S, Murgia A, Te Velde A, Caljouw S. A systematic review into the effectiveness of hand exercise therapy in the treatment of rheumatoid arthritis. *Clin Rheumatol* 2014;33(11):1539–48.

95. Bearne LM, Manning VL, Choy E, Scott DL, Hurley MV. Participants' experiences of an Education, self-management and upper extremity eXercise Training for people with Rheumatoid Arthritis programme (EXTRA). *Physiotherapy* 2017;103(4):430–8.

96. Lamb SE, Williamson EM, Heine PJ, et al. Exercises to improve function of the rheumatoid hand (SARAH): a randomised controlled trial. *Lancet* 2015;385(9966):421–9.

97. Zegkos T, Kitas G, Dimitroulas T. Cardiovascular risk in rheumatoid arthritis: assessment, management and next steps. *Ther Adv Musculoskelet Dis* 2016;8(3):86–101.

98. Summers GD, Metsios GS, Stavropoulos-Kalinoglou A, Kitas GD. Rheumatoid cachexia and cardiovascular disease. *Nat Rev Rheumatol* 2010;6(8):445.

99. Maradit-Kremers H, Crowson CS, Nicola PJ, et al. Increased unrecognized coronary heart disease and sudden deaths in rheumatoid arthritis: a population-based cohort study. *Arthritis Rheumatol* 2005;52(2):402–11.

100. Alexander G, Hortas C, Bacon P. Bed rest, activity and the inflammation of rheumatoid arthritis. *Rheumatology* 1983;22(3):134–40.

101. Smith R, Polley H (eds). *Rest Therapy for Rheumatoid Arthritis*. Mayo Clinic Proceedings, 1978.

102. Bearne L, Scott D, Hurley M. Exercise can reverse quadriceps sensorimotor dysfunction that is associated with rheumatoid arthritis without exacerbating disease activity. *Rheumatology* 2002;41(2):157–66.

103. Stenström CH, Minor MA. Evidence for the benefit of aerobic and strengthening exercise in rheumatoid arthritis. *Arthritis Care Res* 2003;49(3):428–34.

104. Munneke M, De Jong Z, Zwinderman AH, et al. Effect of a high-intensity weight-bearing exercise program on radiologic damage progression of the large joints in subgroups of patients with rheumatoid arthritis. *Arthritis Care Res* 2005;53(3):410–17.

105. Metsios GS, Stavropoulos-Kalinoglou A, Kitas GD. The role of exercise in the management of rheumatoid arthritis. *Expert Rev Clin Immunol* 2015;11:1121–30.

106. Metsios GS, Stavropoulos-Kalinoglou A, van Zanten JJV, et al. Individualised exercise improves endothelial function in patients with rheumatoid arthritis. *Ann Rheum Dis* 2014;73(4):748–51.

107. Van den Hout WB, de Jong Z, Munneke M, Hazes JMW, Breedveld FC, Vliet Vlieland TPM. Cost-utility and cost-effectiveness of a long-term high-intensity exercise program compared to conventional physical therapy in patients with rheumatoid arthritis. *Arthritis Care Res* 2005;53:39–47.

108. Manning VL, Kaambwa B, Ratcliffe J, et al. Economic evaluation of a brief education, self-management and upper limb exercise training in people with rheumatoid arthritis (EXTRA) programme: a trial-based analysis. *Rheumatology* 2015;54:302–9.

109. Brodin N, Lohela-Karlsson M, Swärdh E, Opava CH. Cost-effectiveness of a one-year coaching program for healthy physical activity in early rheumatoid arthritis. *Disability Rehabil* 2015;37:757–62.

110. Baxter SV, Hale LA, Stebbings S, Gray AR, Smith CM, Treharne GJ. Walking is a feasible physical activity for people with

rheumatoid arthritis: a feasibility randomized controlled trial. *Musculoskeletal Care* 2016;*14*:47–56.

111. Elramli AS, Paul L, Gill JM, et al. *Effectiveness of Community-Based Physical Activity on Step Count and Sedentary Behaviour in Patients with Rheumatoid Arthritis Within the First Five Years of Diagnosis.* Dundee, UK: Scottish Society for Rheumatology Autumn Meeting, 2016.

112. Semanik P, Wilbur J, Sinacore J, Chang RW. Physical activity behavior in older women with rheumatoid arthritis. *Arthritis Care Res* 2004;*51*(2):246–52.

113. Ezzat AM, MacPherson K, Leese J, Li LC. The effects of interventions to increase exercise adherence in people with arthritis: a systematic review. *Musculoskeletal Care* 2015;*13*(1):1–18.

114. Michie S, van Stralen MM, West R. The behaviour change wheel: a new method for characterising and designing behaviour change interventions. *Implementation Science* 2011;*6*(1):42.

115. Law RJ, Markland DA, Jones JG, Maddison PJ, Thom JM. Perceptions of issues relating to exercise and joint health in rheumatoid arthritis: a UK-based questionnaire study. *Musculoskeletal Care* 2013;*11*(3):147–58.

116. van Zanten JJV, Rouse PC, Hale ED, et al. Perceived barriers, facilitators and benefits for regular physical activity and exercise in patients with rheumatoid arthritis: a review of the literature. *Sports Med* 2015;*45*(10):1401–12.

117. Demmelmaier I, Iversen MD. How are behavioral theories used in interventions to promote physical activity in rheumatoid arthritis? A systematic review. *Arthritis Care Res (Hoboken)* 2018;*70*(2):185–96.

118. Kibblewhite JR, Hegarty RSM, Stebbings S, Treharne GJ. The role of enjoyment in exercise for people with arthritis: four different viewpoints from a Q-methodology study. *Musculoskeletal Care* 2017;*15*(4):324–32.

119. Bauman AE, Sallis JF, Dzewaltowski DA, Owen N. Toward a better understanding of the influences on physical activity: the role of determinants, correlates, causal variables, mediators, moderators, and confounders. *Am J Prev Med* 2002;*23*:5–14.

120. Michie S, Richardson M, Johnston M, et al. The behavior change technique taxonomy (v1) of 93 hierarchically clustered techniques: building an international consensus for the reporting of behavior change interventions. *Ann Behav Med* 2013;*46*(1):81–95.

121. Demmelmaier I, Åsenlöf P, Opava CH. Supporting stepwise change. Improving health behaviors in rheumatoid arthritis with physical activity as the example. *Int J Clin Rheumatol* 2013;*8*(1):89–94.

122. Miller W, Rollnick S. *Motivational Interviewing: Preparing People for Change* New York, NY: Guilford, 2002.

25

Foot health

Heidi J. Siddle and Anthony C. Redmond

Rheumatoid arthritis and foot disease

The development and severity of foot problems in people with rheumatoid arthritis (RA) increases with the duration of persistent synovitis.[1-6] The mechanical stresses associated with weight-bearing, together with synovitis, are likely to contribute to bone damage and deformity in the foot. In addition, active inflammation weakens the multiple soft tissue structures such as ligaments, joint capsules, and tendons which play an important part in supporting the alignment of the foot. Hence, foot pain and pathomechanical deformities are the result of an ongoing process associated with synovitis, weight-bearing, and ambulation.

Prevalence of foot disease

The initial symptoms of RA are usually reported in the hands, however cross-sectional studies of patient-reported foot involvement have continually demonstrated foot symptoms early in the disease.[7-12] The forefoot, namely across the metatarsophalangeal (MTP) joints has been identified as the most frequent site.[3,7,9,11,13] In two recent UK cohort studies of people with RA, 93.5% of people reported experiencing foot pain during the course of their disease[11] with a similar number experiencing current foot problems.[14]

Despite the introduction of biological disease-modifying antirheumatic drugs (DMARDs), the prevalence of foot pain and foot joint involvement does not appear to be reducing[9,15] although the severity has probably reduced. Furthermore, although treatment strategies such as treat to target are being instigated with the aim of reaching disease remission, there is evidence to suggest that there are still painful and/or swollen MTP joints in a substantial proportion of patients classified as being in disease remission (Disease Activity Score for 28 joints [DAS28] <2.6).[16,17]

Prevalence studies of erosive foot disease in RA have not been undertaken using MR and ultrasound imaging, which are known to detect erosions much earlier in the disease process. Conventional radiographic data, both at onset and during the course of the disease, report destructive changes, specifically erosions most frequently seen at the fifth MTP joint.[7,18] As well as the MTP joints, the talonavicular joint is affected in about a third of people with RA.[3] Radiographic changes in the ankle (tibiotalar joint) and subtalar joint occur in about a quarter of patients, with subtalar joint pathology greatly increasing between 5 and 10 years of disease duration and regularly preceding changes in the ankle joint. Rearfoot and ankle disease is usually seen subsequent to midtarsal and MTP joint radiographic changes.[3,13,19]

Forefoot disease

Forefoot involvement has been identified in up to 45% of the patients at the start of their disease; this is in comparison to only 17% of patients complaining of rearfoot or ankle involvement.[9] 'Walking on pebbles/marbles/stones' is a sensation that people with RA often describe under the MTP joints. These symptoms can be described by those who are newly diagnosed and present with no obvious forefoot deformity; as well as those who have long standing disease and significant forefoot deformity.

Synovitis of the MTP joints in both early and active disease results in localized pain and swelling, leading to the sensation just described. Due to the symmetrical nature of the disease it usually affects all the MTP joints, leading to deformities such as hallux valgus, separation of the toes by synovitis, known as the 'daylight' sign, forefoot widening, hammer and claw toes, subluxation and dislocation of the joints, and plantar bursae[2,10,20] (Figure 25.1A and B). Persistent synovitis results in in stretching and weakening of the joint capsule and loss of integrity of the stabilizing structures, such as the collateral ligaments and plantar plate.[21,22] Subluxation and eventually dislocation of the MTP joints occurs, together with an imbalance between the intrinsic and extrinsic muscles of the foot resulting in sometimes severe forefoot and toe deformity.[13]

Studies during the past ten years suggest that the combination of inflammatory and mechanical factors have a role to play in determining severity of pathology at the MTP joints in people with RA and ultimately symptoms in the forefoot.[23-25] Magnetic resonance imaging (MRI) studies have demonstrated that damage to plantar stabilizing structures such as the capsule and plantar plate of the MTP joints is more common at the fifth MTP joint, the most common site of erosions in the painful forefoot of patients with RA.[26-28]

Midfoot disease

Flattening of the medial longitudinal arch, also known as **pes planovalgus deformity**, is a characteristic change reported in up to half of patients with RA and frequently described as 'my arch has dropped' (**Figure 25.1**C). Arthritis of the talonavicular and subtalar

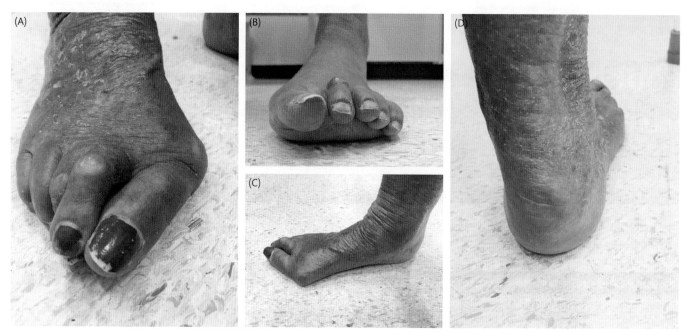

Figure 25.1 (A) Hallux valgus deformity with forefoot widening, hammer, and claw toe deformities. (B) Daylight sign, subluxation, and dislocation of the MTP joints and associated hammer deformity of the lesser toes. (C) Flattening of the medial longitudinal arch. (D) Rear foot valgus deformity.

joints were reported to be much more common in patients with RA and a flattening of the foot, but the pathomechanical process leading to this complex deformity has not been fully described. Arthritis at these joints, typically reported later on in the disease, results from mechanical stresses on weakened and inflamed joints and soft tissue structures, including the tibialis posterior tendon.[3,21] Tibialis posterior tendon pathology such as tenosynovitis and tendinopathy are associated with the pes plano valgus deformity. Recent electromyography studies highlight the combination of inflammation and mechanical dysfunction leading to foot impairment and disability.[29] A study of lateral weight-bearing X-rays proposed two different patterns of flattening of the foot in people with RA; plantar dislocation of the talar head and subluxation of the subtalar joint, and the subtalar joint disease without destruction of the talonavicular joint.[30] Further appropriate imaging of this complex 3D structure would provide a better insight into the mechanism of pathology.

Rearfoot and ankle disease

An everted or valgus deformity of the rearfoot (**Figure 25.1D**) is an identifiable feature of foot disease in people with RA and is typically described with reduced range of motion at the tibiotalar (ankle) and subtalar joints. The severity of rearfoot valgus deformity has been shown to progress with disease duration, especially in the first five years, despite clinical synovitis diminishing after ten years.[2-4,21,31] However, although stiffness and resulting reduced range of motion is described, the rearfoot valgus deformity is initally a mobile deformity which can be functionally improved with the use of foot orthoses (see later section on assessing the foot in RA).

An inverted or varus rearfoot deformity is rarely described and in only a small proportion (16%) of people with RA.[3,13,32] Clinically it is understood that persistent forefoot pain from MTP joint synovitis or mechanical disease as a result of synovitis, results in patients

walking on the outside of their feet in an attempt to avoid loading the metatarsal heads, resulting in a varus rearfoot deformity.[33]

Functional changes in the foot in rheumatoid arthritis

At their most simple the functional changes occurring in RA can be quantified by observing the speed of the patient's walking and overt aspects such as symmetry and length of stride. These are typically known as the temporal and spatial parameters and can be observed qualitatively, or measured directly using a tape measure and stopwatch, or more technologically advanced methods such as the GaitRite walkway (https://www.gaitrite.com). More detailed measurement of functional change such as the pressures underneath the feet or movements in specific joints require more technologically advanced methods.

Spatial and temporal changes

Pain in the forefoot, and sometimes midfoot and hindfoot joints leads to early changes in the gait in people with RA. The walking speed (gait velocity) decreases quite early in the progression of RA as cadence and stride length are reduced. The double support period increases to minimize the forces passing through the foot, and hesitation in loading the forefoot changes the distribution of pressure and delays the onset of loading.[21,34] The dynamic nature of the walking cycle is reduced and this leads to a reduction of the vertical load passing through the feet.

Some specific foot impairments will also change certain gait parameters. Locke and colleagues (1984) showed that in a sample of people with ankle and subtalar joint pain, walking speed was reduced by approximately one-third and single support time by 25%.[35] Rearfoot pain and deformity seem to be more important than forefoot pathology in the effect on function although the forefoot is a commonly reported symptom site.[36] As the disease progresses either chronologically or by severity, the effects become profound, with walking speed falling to half the normal in one study of long standing (25 year), radiologically severe patients.

Foot deformities tend to be mild and reversible or reducible initially, and functional foot orthoses have been shown both to improve function and even slow the progression of further deformity in early disease.[37] In the longer term, untreated synovitis in the rearfoot joints leads to systematic changes in rearfoot structure and function[38] and in time bony adaptation occurs and the changes become irreversible. The altered function, combined with bearing weight on the joint and changes in soft tissue laxity, cause the rearfoot to move into a more pronated position, with the heel becoming more valgus and the tibia becoming more internally rotated.[3,38,39] Functionally, this results in excessive and prolonged rearfoot eversion with the tendency to more extreme eversion increasing as the subtalar joint becomes unstable.

Plantar pressures

It is common to see severe hallux valgus-type deformity in people with RA, with the hallux deviating laterally and the lesser toes subluxed dorsally and hammered at the proximal interphalangeal (PIP) joints.[40] Combined with displacement of the fat pads, bursitis and in more severe cases rupture of the plantar plates and joint restraining soft tissues[26] there can be a significant increase in the pressures under the MTP joints[41] which in turn is associated with greater impairment.[42] Plantar pressure data show the areas of increased pressure to be more localized as shown in **Figure 25.2A** and patients often describe the feeling of 'walking on pebbles'.

Clinically, any sites of forefoot plantar callus indicate localized high pressure and should be checked for during clinical examination. In most instances, the callus has an underlying adventitious bursa and both structures serve to increase the contact area over which the forces are distributed.

Varus deformities of the rearfoot are relatively rare,[10] and usually occur as a direct consequence of functional compensation strategies such as inversion of the forefoot when medial MTP joints are painful.

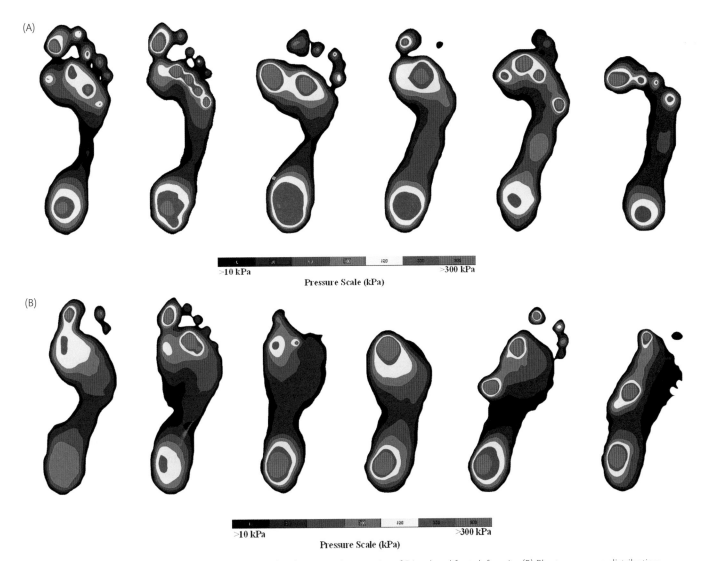

Figure 25.2 (A) Plantar pressure distributions associated with progressing severity of RA-related foot deformity. (B) Plantar pressure distribution associated with valgus deformity, medial loading, and ultimately collapse of the medial arch.

In patients with severe disease, the erosion of the MTP joints can lead to a highly characteristic medialized and localized distribution in the forefoot joints. At the same time the medial drift of the rearfoot and subluxation of the joints of the medial arch lead to patterns of loading across the foot, including the arch area, that are obviously pathological as shown in **Figure 25.2B**.

Such high pressures, particular over areas of tissue that are not intended to be directly weight-bearing can cause significant discomfort. More importantly however, in this group of people who already have increased cardiovascular risk and potential for skin damage due to steroid use, there is an elevated risk of tissue breakdown and significant increases in pressure should be taken seriously in those with longstanding RA.

Kinematics and kinetics

In the past 20 years there have been significant advances in motion analysis and in associated computational modelling techniques. In the research sector these have led to improvements in our understanding of both underlying pathologies in the foot and in the related treatments. The equipment required to study the foot in RA at this level of detail is complex and expensive and so any biomechanical evaluation beyond the simple investigation of temporal and spatial parameters and plantar pressures is beyond the scope of this chapter.

Measurement of impact and outcome

Objective measures

As noted in the previous section, objective measures represent the gold standard for investigating function. Many centres have adopted systems such as GaitRite, although simple approaches using basic instrumentation such as stopwatch and tape measure have been in use for many years. Walking speed, such as measured by the time it takes the patient to walk a set distance or a timed up and go test are useful indicators of a patient's overall function and are useful measures both of baseline disease impact and of treatment effect.[43]

Subjective measures and patient-reported outcomes

Although objective measures of function can provide useful information, they are often inconvenient to collect and do not capture the broader effect of impaired function on the patient's life experience. A range of more subjective patient-reported outcome measures (PROMs) have been developed in rheumatology and are used widely in both clinical and research settings. To anyone working in rheumatology some of the generic PROMs are almost universal and most readers will be familiar with staples such as the Stanford Health Assessment Questionnaire (HAQ). Depending on the requirement for specific aspects of the clinical picture, these rheumatology-specific PROMs can be supplemented with other measures to capture more general health (e.g. the SF-36 or EQ-5D) or specific dimensions of health for example, behavioural change associated with a chronic condition such as captured by the Sickness Impact Profile. Similarly, a number of PROMs have been developed that are aimed specific organ systems or body regions and a number exist for evaluating the foot either specifically in those with RA or more generally.

Foot-specific PROMs

Foot Function Index (FFI)

The FFI was originally developed as an outcome measure for patients with RA although has since been used in a range of chronic conditions.[44] The FFI captures three subscales: pain, disability, and activity limitation. It is self-administered by the patients who respond to anchor questions by marking a 100 mm visual analogue scale in response to multiple questions. Aggregate subscale scores are derived by dividing the actual score by the maximum possible score on the subscale.[44] Test-retest agreement is high overall but varies for the subscales. Moderate concurrent validity has been established but the responsiveness has been criticised.[45] The FFI, as an older measure, was not developed using robust modern psychometric principles and has been criticised for favouring disease related factors at the expense of factors such as footwear, participation restriction, and psychosocial dimensions. The use of visual analogue scales has fallen from favour in recent years, with patients sometimes reporting difficulties with understanding how to complete the form.[46,47]

Foot Impact Scale (FIS)

The FIS was the first foot-specific measure to be developed using the needs-based approach[48] and as such was the first foot-specific PROM to go beyond basic quantification of foot health status.[49] The FIS captures information in eight main themes which are mapped onto two subscales, one encompassing the International Classification of Functioning, Disability and Health (ICF)'s classification of 'Impairments' combined with items relating to footwear or shoes; and one relating to the ICF classifications of activity limitation and participation restriction. The FIS was validated in detail against the Rasch model and has robust psychometric properties. The test-retest reliability is high, with an intraclass correlation coefficient (ICC) of 0.84 and there is good concurrent validity relative to other measures. As with the FFI just discussed, the responsiveness is relatively poor however, which limits its usefulness to baseline evaluations but the FIS represents the current state-of-the-art in foot-specific quality of life measurement for patients with RA.

The Manchester Foot Pain and Disability Questionnaire (MFPDQ)

The MFPDQ measure comprises 19 short statements with trichotomous responses. It has been subjected to a rigorous validation process[50] and several independent studies. It is widely used in rheumatology, in studies of long-term conditions and especially with patients in the community setting. It is self-administered, quick and easy to score, and yields a single index score making it easy to interpret. Because it is not disease specific, the MFPDQ demonstrated a ceiling effect for people with RA[51] so its use is probably limited in acute or severe populations. The MFPDQ is our first choice however, for evaluating foot health status in our non-rheumatoid arthritis patients.

Assessing the foot in rheumatoid arthritis

Clinical assessment of the feet

Our starting point for assessment of the foot in people with RA is simply for the clinician to ask the question, 'Have you had any problems with your feet recently?' Many rheumatologists note that in a busy clinical setting, getting the patient to remove shoes and hosiery is not practical logistically. Nonetheless we know that foot involvement is extremely common in people with RA and contend that asking the opening question takes next to no time and should be a part of every consultation. If then the patient does report having foot problems there is arguably a medical and moral imperative for the assessor to act further. Being pressed for time would not be seen as reason enough to ignore a patient's overtly expressed concern about most other comorbidities. If and when it does become necessary to assess the foot and ankle, an assessor with the requisite skill and training need take no more than 1 minute per foot for an initial assessment. The Regional Examination of the Musculoskeletal System (REMS) is a good starting point for a whole lower limb approach[52] and for a more detailed foot examination, we have described extensively a Leeds foot assessment protocol which is a comprehensive assessment of foot problems based on the widely used approach of History → Observation→ Examination. A detailed description of this assessment protocol can be found elsewhere.[53]

In routine practice, a simple assessment can be made of the patient walking, followed by observation of the legs and feet while standing still, with final observations made with the patient seated or lying supine (i.e. non-weight-bearing). It is also helpful to observe the transition between non-weight-bearing and weight-bearing to observe changes that occur as the limb accepts weight.

When examining specific ankle and foot pathology, it is useful to conduct a systematic observation of the overall foot shape and palpation of the relevant joint margins (ankle, subtalar, midfoot joints, and MTP joints), soft tissue structures, and insertions to isolate inflamed or damaged tissues. Active movement of the ankle is evaluated with the patient moving the joint themselves to a degree that they are comfortable with the assessor estimating direction, range, and quality of motion, and noting any related pain. Finally, the assessment concludes with clinician-assisted passive motions of ankle, subtalar, midfoot, and forefoot joints, noting pain, direction, range, and quality of movement. This 1-minute protocol is enough to differentiate ankle involvement from subtalar disease, identify midfoot disease, and isolate and quantify forefoot joint involvement.

Imaging assessment of the feet

The most commonly used imaging modality is plain X-ray, although plain radiographs are limited to the assessment of existing bony anatomy and joint damage. Foot X-rays are usually taken non-weight-bearing, which is adequate for evaluating erosive change in people with RA but gives a poor representation of the bony relationships as they would align during weight-bearing. Even in non-weight-bearing radiography, because of the complexity of the foot anatomy, it is important to give careful consideration to the orientation of the joint requiring investigation and to order views appropriate to this orientation. Standard antero-posterior and lateral views give limited visualization of the mid and hindfoot joint particularly. Increasingly, weight-bearing X-ray views are available and these provide much better representation of the relative alignment

and likely mechanical function of the foot during activities of daily living. Again, weight-bearing X-ray views should be ordered with consideration of the orientation of the specific joints of interest.

Other useful imaging modalities are MRI, ultrasound, computed tomography (CT), and scintigraphy.[54] Plain X-ray is usually the starting point because of lower cost and good access, but these enhanced modalities can provide useful diagnostic information, particularly about the soft tissues. Scintigraphy has largely been superseded by MRI, although the complex anatomy of the foot again provides challenges in interpreting MRI and CT imaging and many radiologists find subtle findings difficult to assess.

Ultrasound is being used increasingly in rheumatology and is useful around the multitude of small, dynamic structures in the foot, most of which lie close to the surface. Ultrasound can provide imaging at high resolutions and the ability to acquire imaging of structures dynamically is helpful in identifying precisely which tissues might be associated with symptoms. Features such as power Doppler are also of increasing importance in RA, often in the initial diagnosis and subsequently, in both systemic treat-to-target type protocols and also in identifying isolated sites of persisting inflammation.[54]

Other assessments

As noted previously people with RA often have range of comorbidities that place them at risk of poorer tissue viability and it is common practice to evaluate the neurological and vascular systems in at-risk patients. Hand-held Doppler ultrasound or photoplethysmography units represent portable and relatively inexpensive methods for monitoring the peripheral vasculature, and neurological status can be assessed using monofilaments or vibration perception meters.

In summary, much of the reticence relating to assessment of the foot seems to be due to the complexity of the anatomy and the perception of the level of skill required to undertake detailed assessments. The by-product of this is a degree of associated reticence to even open the dialogue with patients about the existence of any foot problems. We advocate an approach which starts with at least having the conversation, to be followed up by a very brief and straightforward assessment that is well within the expertise of almost all clinicians. More detailed assessments are many and varied but there are usually options for onward referral if higher levels of training and skill are required for further follow-up.

Foot health interventions

Disease-specific management

Providers of healthcare

National Institute for Health and Care Excellence (NICE) have acknowledged the knowledge and expertise of podiatrists in assessing and managing foot and ankle conditions specifically by recommending that all people with RA and foot problems should have access to a podiatrist for assessment and periodic review of their foot health needs.[55] Unfortunately not all patients and rheumatology services have direct access to podiatrists[56,57] and therefore it is important to educate and encourage the rheumatology community to ask patients about their feet so that problems are identified early. It is also important to ensure that podiatrists do not consider the foot in isolation of the rest of the person and their systemic disease, particularly in the early stages of the disease and during a flare, and develop links with the rheumatology MDT.

Patient education and self-management

Foot health guidelines recommend that patient education is included in the management of foot problems for all people with RA,[58] regardless of the lack of patient and/or health professional awareness of this need.[59] However, the impact of routine foot health education on foot-specific outcomes has not been determined.

Foot health education for people with RA can be delivered by a clinician on a one-to-one basis or to a group, verbally and/or with supplementary written information, or through signposting to internet resources.[60,61] Unfortunately foot health education is rarely considered within the medical consultation despite patients requiring health professionals to identify their foot education health needs. Tailored foot health education should begin at the initial diagnosis.[59]

The FOOTSTEP self-management programme is the only programme developed to enable elderly adults who would normally seek foot care through podiatry services to undertake their own basic foot care.[62] When this programme was applied in people with RA who had established disease 43% were physically unable to adequately undertake some aspects of the self-management programme.[63] Hence foot health self-management strategies should be considered in the context of the whole disease and not just the foot problems.

Inflammatory and/or mechanical management

As discussed earlier in this chapter, despite the introduction of biological therapies for the management of systemic disease, foot involvement, including synovitis often persists in clinical disease remission.[9,15,17,64] The current 'treat-to-target' paradigm of care for managing RA aims to achieve clinical disease remission and target treatment strategies at individual patients' disease activity.[65] It has been recognized that both inflammatory and mechanical-related foot pathology have a significant impact on mobility and functional capacity in the majority of patients with RA.[66] As such a new paradigm of foot healthcare has been proposed for patients with early disease that promotes the 'tight control' and 'treat-to-target' principles but with a focus on local disease in the foot.[67] The paradigm promotes the early detection of joint disease utilizing the MTP joint squeeze test, a combination of targeted therapy at inflammatory lesions and associated mechanically-based impairments. These include ultrasound-guided corticosteroid injections and custom orthoses, using disease measures (DAS) imaging methods and foot outcome measures to achieve 'tight control' of foot arthritis and monitor disease. These principles also provide an opportunity to optimize treatment in those patients with persistent inflammatory foot and ankle involvement.

Highlighting region-specific management strategies

Directing interventions at specific regions in the foot (i.e. the forefoot, midfoot, rearfoot and ankle) has provided an optimal clinical approach to managing local inflammatory and mechanical disease.[33] Swelling in the forefoot in early disease as well as deformity, such as subluxation of the MTP joints and hallux valgus deformity, in established disease require accommodation in footwear and

off-loading approaches. The midfoot typically requires support as the arch begins to collapse, while treatment of the typical rearfoot valgus deformity involves correcting and stabilizing the rearfoot, particularly in early disease to reduce the progression and development of deformity. Evidence from a large randomized controlled trial (RCT) demonstrates that foot orthoses used in early disease to treat rearfoot valgus deformity reduce pain and disability and slow progression of rearfoot deformity.[68]

Tissue viability, skin, and nail care

Nail care, both of the fingernails as well as toenails, provides challenges for people with RA who have lost strength or movement in their hands to be able to use nail cutting equipment or who are unable to reach their feet due to painful joints. An ingrowing toe nail (onychocryptosis) is a condition in which a spike, shoulder, or serrated edge of the nail has pierced the skin of the sulcus and penetrated the dermal tissues, often as a result of inappropriate or inadequate nail care (**Figure 25.3A**). This poses increased infection risk for those who are immunosuppressed and particularly those taking biological therapies. Suspension of biological therapy following guidelines, along with antibiotics and podiatry treatment, including nail avulsion typically results in a successful outcome for patients.[69]

Neuropathy

Sensorimotor type peripheral neuropathy occurs in the foot and ankle of people with RA.[70–72] However the prevalence varies significantly, with some studies suggesting over half of those with RA may have some neurological deficit in their feet.[73,74] Unlike in the diabetic foot, the clinical implications of neuropathy in RA remain unclear.

Vascular disease

People with RA are at an increased risk of peripheral arterial disease,[75] although the devastating effects seen in people with diabetes are not seen in those with RA. Vasculitis, inflammation of the blood vessels, has previously been associated with ulceration located on the dorsum of the foot and the lower leg.[76] However, in recent studies of patients with RA and ulceration only affecting their feet, vasculitis has not been identified in these cohorts of patients.[77,78] Improved systemic disease control in patients with RA is probably the reason for a reduced prevalence in recent years.

Ulceration/Wound care

Epidemiological studies and case series have reported that ulceration in RA occurs at multiple sites and usually on the pressure-vulnerable bony sites in the forefoot; these include the dorsal aspect of hammer toes (48%) (**Figure 25.3B**), the plantar aspect of metatarsal heads (32%) (**Figure 25.3C**) and the medial aspect of the first MTP joint in patients with hallux valgus (20%).[77,79,80] A recent multicentre, observational study to determine the predictors of foot ulceration in patients with RA showed that risk of ulceration rose with increasing loss of sensation and foot deformity as well as with vascular insufficiency.[80] Although often clinically perceived as the cause, raised plantar pressures did not predict the risk of foot ulceration.

Wound care is multifaceted and should include dressings, managing vascular complications, and addressing the need for off-loading or accommodating deformity when indicated. Wound dressings have several properties that are beneficial, however none

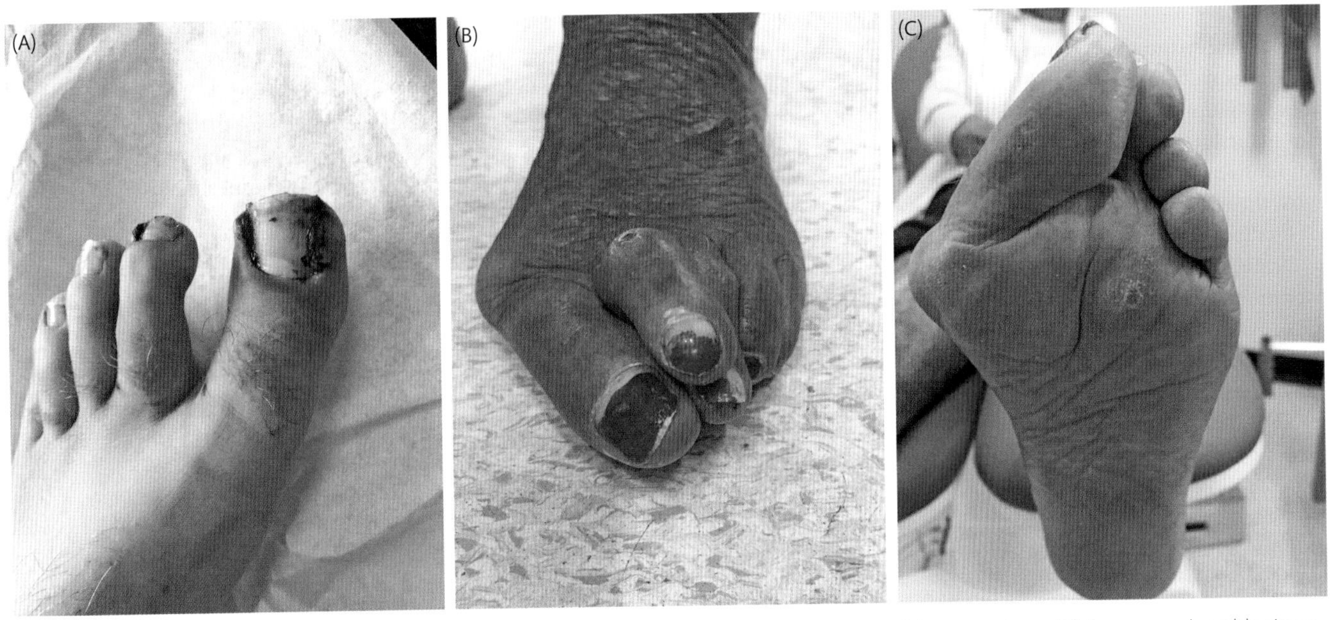

Figure 25.3 (A) Onychocryptosis of the hallux nail. (B) Previous ulceration site to the dorsal aspect of the second toe. (C) Pressure-vulnerable site to the plantar aspect of the third MTP joint.

have been formally evaluated in people with RA who have foot ulceration. A cushioning dressing, usually a foam dressing will help an often painful ulcer site, as well as absorbing exudate. Bulky dressings, particularly for interdigital ulcers, potentially increase pressure in these areas. It is widely recommended by podiatrists that adherent dressings are avoided as they usually cause a deterioration of the both the wound bed and the surrounding fragile tissues.

Off-loading

Accommodation and off-loading are essential to accelerate healing and prevent ulceration. The provision of footwear and foot orthoses will be discussed in further detail next. Traditional methods of off-loading high-pressure sites can be used such as the Aircast Pneumatic Walkers. These are effective but often people with RA find them difficult to use. Hand impairments pose difficulties in getting them on and take off, and where muscle weakness is present in the lower limb, they typically feel heavy and cumbersome to the patient. Alternatively, lightweight forefoot and rearfoot 'off-loader' boots are available which people with RA tolerate much better.

Infection

People with RA are at an increased risk of infection compared to the general population,[81] with the rate of serious skin and soft tissue infections increased in those taking anti-TNF biological therapies.[82] As highlighted earlier, people with RA and foot deformity are at risk of ulceration and therefore their risk of infection at the ulcer site is increased especially if they are taking a biological therapy.

Identifying the presence of infection in wound sites can be difficult in patients with RA; *Staphylococcus aureus* appears to be the most common microorganism.[83] As with any infection, DMARDS and biological therapies should be suspended until the infection has resolved and the course of antibiotics has been completed. Unfortunately, this may cause a flare of the inflammatory disease, which will potentially delay wound healing[78] and therefore it is

recommended that patients are restarted on their systemic medication as soon as the infection has resolved and the wound is improving.

The risk of skin and nail infections highlight the importance of checking the feet as a source of potential infection in patients commencing biological therapies, advocating the need for foot health teams and rheumatology teams to work closely together.

Callus debridement

Subluxation or dislocation of the MTP joints are subject to excessive shear and compressive stresses during gait, frequently resulting in the build-up of painful plantar callosities over the metatarsal heads.[31] Reduction of callus to reduce peak pressures, prevent ulceration, and aid wound healing has been firmly established in patients with diabetes.[84,85] A full RCT has demonstrated that the long-term benefits of sharp scalpel debridement of painful forefoot plantar callosities in RA, when undertaken in conjunction with a combined therapeutic approach (prescription of orthoses and footwear), produced no additional benefit over the combined therapeutic approach alone. As well as questioning the efficacy of callus removal in this group of patients this RCT provides evidence to highlight that the causes of forefoot pain in RA are unlikely to be solely attributed to plantar callosities.[86] However, sharp scalpel debridement is still recommended in cases where an underlying tissue breakdown/ulceration is suspected.

Footwear

Footwear is considered the first line of support when managing musculoskeletal problems associated with the foot and ankle. However, in the presence of pain and deformity inappropriate or ill-fitting footwear can exacerbate impairments or indeed result in new problems such as ulceration. It is recommended that footwear has a fastening (i.e. laces, Velcro, or a buckle) to ensure that it stays firmly fitted to the foot. A wide, deep toe box is essential particularly in the presence of forefoot deformity and a stiff sole to provide support with shock absorption to reduce pressure. As well as avoiding high heels it is equally important to avoid a completely flat shoe, such as the 'ballet pump' style shoe.

In the first instance advice and education regarding the style and fit of footwear should be provided[60,61] but when foot impairments negate the ability to wear 'high street' footwear NICE recommend that therapeutic footwear should be available for all people with RA if indicated.[55] However, the need to change existing footwear styles poses many personal challenges for patients, including cost as well as loss of choice, dignity, and style associated with wearing 'beautiful' shoes. These feelings have been highlighted by females with RA who report feeling, shame, anger, and sadness when wearing such footwear and this is exacerbated during social activities and often seen as a final and symbolic marker of RA on the person's self-perception and their changed lives.[87,88] Despite the challenges highlighted there is growing evidence that specialist accommodative footwear and adaptions such as rocker shoes may be effective in reducing foot pain in RA.[87,89-91]

Foot orthoses

Clinical management guidelines and recommendations for people with RA advocate the use of foot orthoses in managing foot problems.[55,92-95] The most recent evidence from systematic reviews with meta-analyses indicate that foot orthoses may be beneficial in reducing pain and elevated forefoot pressures in RA.[96,97] Previously we have proposed a disease-staged approach to prescribing foot orthoses for people with RA, based on our clinical experience and the minimal evidence available.[33] In early RA there is evidence to support the use of custom designed orthoses[68] (Figure 25.4A), based on the kinematic alterations in foot function which have been detected early in the disease process.[98] However, NHS podiatry departments with restricted budgets and time constraints experience difficulty accessing custom-made devices for patients. Preliminary evidence suggests that people with early RA (less than 2 years disease duration) benefit from using cheaper and more accessible off-the-shelf prefabricated foot orthoses (Figure 25.4B), with the majority of their pain reduction occurring within the first 3 months

of use, but with some small further symptomatic improvement up to 6 months.[99] However, this does need to be confirmed using more robust research methodology. Overall, functional optimization appears to be the most feasible approach for orthoses prescription in early RA and has the potential to provide superior mode-of-action responses when patients present with biomechanical foot problems compared to standard devices.[100]

As mentioned earlier in this chapter there is often persistent foot pain and disability despite the use of biologic therapies and treat-to-target strategies.[15,17,64] Recent evidence predicts more favourable foot pain and disability outcomes when people with RA and foot problems are treated earlier in the course of their disease with foot orthoses.[101] Hence, early and targeted intervention with foot orthoses provides an ideal opportunity to reduce the impact of the disease on the foot and ankle.[67]

Injection techniques

Foot and ankle injections are generally used as therapy (corticosteroid) but can also be used as a diagnostic aid (local anaesthetic) to determine which structure is the most troublesome. The close proximity of multiple joints in the foot often creates difficulty in localizing the exact cause of the pain[102] which can result in the wrong placement of the injection and subsequently leading to poor clinical outcome.

The main indications for giving corticosteroid local injections in the foot and ankle are acute inflammation, tendinopathy, and fasciopathy. Hence, the aim when injecting an inflamed or swollen joint is not to place the needle tip within the joint cavity but to place it within the joint capsule.

The use of ultrasound to guide injections in to the foot and ankle has been shown to have an impact on clinical decision making, leading the physician to change the diagnosis in 32.4% of sites imaged and subsequently alter the planning of corticosteroid injections in to the foot and ankle in 82.5% of patients.[103] Although ultrasound guidance significantly improves the accuracy of joint injections,[73] there is differing evidence surrounding the short-term symptomatic treatment effect.[103,104] Furthermore, access to ultrasound machines and clinicians who are appropriately trained is still limited

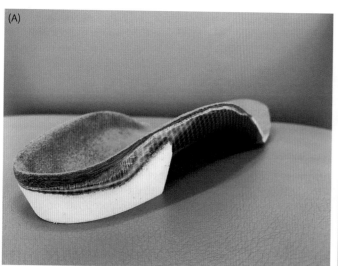
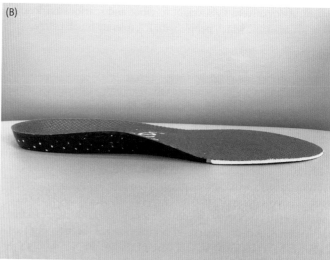

Figure 25.4 (A) Carbon fibre custom designed foot orthoses. (B) Prefabricated foot orthoses.

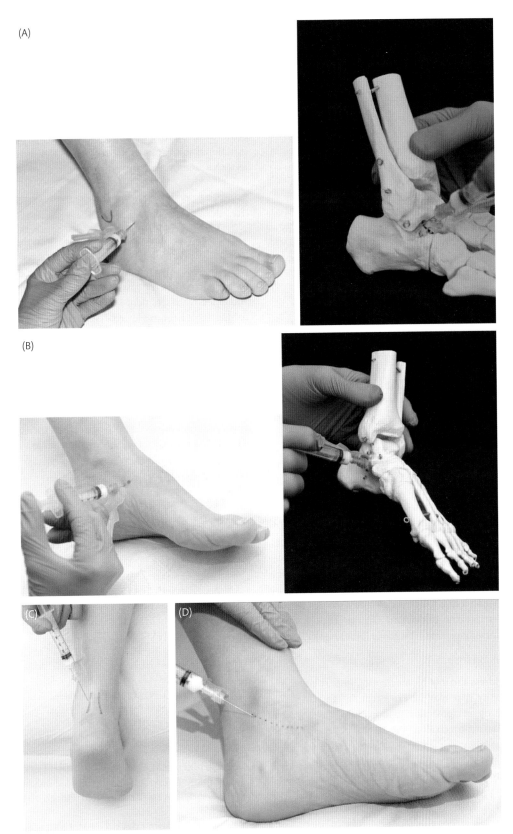

Figure 25.5 (A) Injection of corticosteroid injection into the subtalar joint via the sinus tarsi (lateral malleolus outlined in red). (B) Injection of the talonavicular joint just proximal to the tuberosity of the navicular. (C) Injection in to the retrocalcaneal bursa is approached at an angle to one side of the Achilles tendon (marked in red) close to its insertion into the calcaneum. (D) Injection of the tibialis posterior tendon sheath is made along the axis of the tendon at the level of the medial malleolus, using a proximal approach.

and therefore techniques for giving 'blind' injections in the foot and ankle are provided.

We advocate correcting or improving any biomechanical problems using orthoses and/or footwear prior to injecting foot and ankle, which is likely to reduce the risk of the problem reoccurring. It would be inappropriate to inject multiple sites of disease activity/inflammation in the foot and ankle particularly in the presence of persistent disease; in such cases we would recommend a review of systemic therapy first. When injecting corticosteroid in to a weight-bearing joint it is advisable to rest the joint for 24–48 hours[105] to ensure the steroid preparation stays in the joint and maximum benefit is achieved.

It is beyond the scope of this chapter to detail every foot and ankle injection but we have provided advice on injecting some of the more complex structures relevant to people with RA; the subtalar joint, talonavicular joint, retrocalcaneal bursitis, and tibialis posterior tendon sheath.

Subtalar joint

Injecting through the sinus tarsi provides a simpler approach without imaging (**Figure 25.5A**). Palpating anterior to the lateral malleolus you will be able to locate the sinus tarsi space. The needle (either a 21 or 23 gauge) is directed towards the tip of the medial malleolus, without encountering any bony obstruction, and inserted to a depth of 1–2 cm; inject 40 mg of methylprednisolone.

Talonavicular joint

Identify the tuberosity of the navicular, the superficial joint line of the talonavicular joint just is proximal to the navicular tuberosity. Using a 25 g 'orange' needle inject perpendicular to the skin (**Figure 25.5B**); 20 mg of methylprednisolone or equivalent is recommended.

Retrocalcaneal bursitis

We would recommend that this injection is performed with ultrasound guidance to determine the depth of the bursa. If it is possible, it is ideal if the patient lies prone with their foot hanging over the edge of the treatment couch and held in a dorsiflexed position. The bursa is approached at an angle to one side of the Achilles tendon close to its' insertion into the calcaneum (**Figure 25.5C**); inject 20 mg of methylprednisolone using a 23-gauge (blue) needle.

Tibialis posterior tendon sheath

It is imperative to address the foot biomechanics, in particular any subtalar joint instability that may be exacerbating tenosynovitis/tendinopathy of the tibialis posterior tendon. Insert a 23-gauge needle from a proximal approach along the axis of the tendon at the level of the medial malleolus (**Figure 25.5D**). If resistance is felt it is possible the needle tip is within the substance of the tendon and the needle should be withdrawn slightly, due to risk of rupture, before injecting 20 mg of methylprednisolone; the injected steroid can typically be seen and felt up the tendon sheath.

Exercise

Although current guidelines identify the need to encourage patients to undertake exercise, these are not specific to the foot and ankle.[55] It is important to acknowledge that people with RA may require other foot health management strategies first to ensure they are able to take part in exercise therapy, for example that they are wearing the most supportive and comfortable footwear and provided with orthoses for any additional joint protection needed.

Historically, people with RA have been advised to avoid weight-bearing exercise and concentrate on isometric non-weight-bearing exercises and range of motion exercise in order to avoid aggravating joint inflammation and accelerating joint damage. However, the benefits of high-intensity progressive resistance training have shown significant improvements in increasing the physical capacity and functional ability of people with RA as well as reducing pain and fatigue without exacerbating disease activity or joint pain.[106–109]

Conclusion

This chapter has discussed and emphasized the effects that a complex multisystem disease such as RA has on a weight-bearing structure. The foot is frequently described by people with RA as 'the first to be affected but the last to be treated'. An overview of subjective and objective assessment tools, including clinical and imaging modalities have been reviewed. This chapter encourages the clinician to ask the important question, 'Have you had any problems with your feet recently?' and provides a simple assessment approach and knowledge of further assessment strategies to ensure that the foot is adequately assessed to avoid long-term complications. The relevant non-surgical foot health management strategies have been highlighted for people with RA who frequently present with both inflammatory and mechanical disease in their feet, with the aim of minimizing the impact on the foot and ankle.

REFERENCES

1. Vainio K. The rheumatoid foot; a clinical study with pathological and roentgenological comments. *Ann Chir Gynaecol Fenn Suppl* 1956;45(1):1–107.
2. Spiegel TM, Spiegel JS. Rheumatoid arthritis in the foot and ankle—diagnosis, pathology, and treatment. The relationship between foot and ankle deformity and disease duration in 50 patients. *Foot Ankle* 1982;2(6):318–24.
3. Bouysset M, Bonvoisin B, Lejeune E, Bouvier M. Flattening of the rheumatoid foot in tarsal arthritis on X-ray. *Scand J Rheumatol* 1987;16(2):127–33.
4. Michelson J, Easley M, Wigley FM, Hellmann D. Foot and ankle problems in rheumatoid arthritis. *Foot Ankle Int* 1994;15(11):608–13.
5. Shi K, Tomita T, Hayashida K, Owaki H, Ochi T. Foot deformities in rheumatoid arthritis and relevance of disease severity. *J Rheumatol* 2000;27(1):84–9.
6. Bouysset M, Tebib J, Noel E, et al. Rheumatoid flat foot and deformity of the first ray. *J Rheumatol* 2002;29(5):903–5.
7. van der Leeden M, Steultjens MP, Ursum J, et al. Prevalence and course of forefoot impairments and walking disability in the first eight years of rheumatoid arthritis. *Arthritis Rheum* 2008;59(11):1596–602.
8. Fleming A, Crown JM, Corbett M. Incidence of joint involvement in early rheumatoid arthritis. *Rheumatol Rehabil* 1976;15(2):92–6.
9. Grondal L, Tengstrand B, Nordmark B, Wretenberg P, Stark A. The foot: still the most important reason for walking incapacity in rheumatoid arthritis: distribution of symptomatic joints in 1,000 RA patients. *Acta Orthop* 2008;79(2):257–61.

10. Kerry RM, Holt GM, Stockley I. The foot in chronic rheumatoid arthritis: a continuing problem. *Foot* 1994;4(4):201–3.

11. Otter SJ, Lucas K, Springett K, et al. Foot pain in rheumatoid arthritis prevalence, risk factors and management: an epidemiological study. *Clin Rheumatol* 2010;29(3):255–71.

12. Rydgren L, Fredrikson E. The development of foot deformities in early rheumatoid arthritis. *Br J Rheumatol* 1996;35(abstracts suppl 1):198.

13. Vidigal E, Jacoby RK, Dixon AS, Ratliff AH, Kirkup J. The foot in chronic rheumatoid arthritis. *Ann Rheum Dis* 1975;34(4):292–7.

14. Wilson O, Hewlett S, Woodburn J, Pollock J, Kirwan J. Prevalence, impact and care of foot problems in people with rheumatoid arthritis: results from a United Kingdom based cross-sectional survey. *J Foot Ankle Res* 2017;10(1):46.

15. Otter SJ, Lucas K, Springett K, et al. Comparison of foot pain and foot care among rheumatoid arthritis patients taking and not taking anti-TNFalpha therapy: an epidemiological study. *Rheumatol Int* 2011;31(11):1515–19.

16. Fransen J, Creemers MC, Van Riel PL. Remission in rheumatoid arthritis: agreement of the disease activity score (DAS28) with the ARA preliminary remission criteria. *Rheumatology* 2004;43(10):1252–5.

17. van der Leeden MS, Van Schaardenburg D, Dekker J. Forefoot disease activity in rheumatoid arthritis patients in remission: results of a cohort study. *Arthritis Res Ther* 2010;12(1):R3.

18. Hulsmans HM, Jacobs JWG, van der Heijde DMFM, et al., The course of radiologic damage during the first six years of rheumatoid arthritis. *Arthritis Rheum* 2000;43(9):1927–40.

19. Belt EA, Kaarela K, Mäenpää H, Kauppi MJ, Lehtinen JT, Lehto MU. Relationship of ankle joint involvement with subtalar destruction in patients with rheumatoid arthritis. A 20-year follow-up study. *Joint Bone Spine* 2001;68(2):154–7.

20. Dixon AS. Medical aspects of the rheumatoid foot. *Proc R Soc Med* 1970;63(7):677–9.

21. Keenan MA, Peabody TD, Gronley JK, Perry J. Valgus deformities of the feet and characteristics of gait in patients who have rheumatoid arthritis. *J Bone Joint Surg* 1991;73(2):237–47.

22. Jaakkola JI, Mann RA. A review of rheumatoid arthritis affecting the foot and ankle. *Foot Ankle Int* 2004;25(12):866–74.

23. Davys HJ, Turner DE, Helliwell PS, Conaghan PG, Emery P, Woodburn J. Debridement of plantar callosities in rheumatoid arthritis: a randomized controlled trial. *Rheumatology (Oxf)* 2005;44(2):207–10.

24. Tuna H, Birtane M, Taştekin N, Kokino S. Pedobarography and its relation to radiologic erosion scores in rheumatoid arthritis. *Rheumatol Int* 2005;26(1):42–7.

25. Siddle HJ, Hensor EMA, Hodgeson RJ, et al. Anatomical location of erosions at the metatarsophalangeal joints in patients with rheumatoid arthritis. *Rheumatology (Oxf)* 2014;53(5):932–6.

26. Siddle HJ, Hodgson RJ, Hensor EMA, et al. Plantar plate pathology is associated with erosive disease in the painful forefoot of patients with rheumatoid arthritis. *BMC Musculoskelet Disord* 2017;18(1):308.

27. Siddle HJ, Hodgson RJ, O'Connor P, et al. Magnetic resonance arthrography of lesser metatarsophalangeal joints in patients with rheumatoid arthritis: relationship to clinical, biomechanical, and radiographic variables. *J Rheumatol*, 2012;39(9):1786–91.

28. Siddle HJ, Hodgson RJ, Redmond AC, et al. MRI identifies plantar plate pathology in the forefoot of patients with rheumatoid arthritis. *Clin Rheumatol* 2012;31(4):621–9.

29. Barn R, Turner DE, Rafferty D, Sturrock RD, Woodburn J. Tibialis posterior tenosynovitis and associated pes plano valgus in rheumatoid arthritis: electromyography, multisegment foot kinematics, and ultrasound features. *Arthritis Care Res (Hoboken)* 2013;65(4):495–502.

30. Hattori T, Hashimoto J, Tomita T, Kitamura T. Radiological study of joint destruction patterns in rheumatoid flatfoot. *Clin Rheumatol* 2008;27(6):733–7.

31. Woodburn J, Helliwell PS. Relation between heel position and the distribution of forefoot plantar pressures and skin callosities in rheumatoid arthritis. *Ann Rheum Dis* 1996;55(11):806–10.

32. Bouysset M, Tebib J, Weil G, et al. The rheumatoid heel: its relationship to other disorders in the rheumatoid foot. *Clin Rheumatol* 1989;8(2):208–14.

33. Helliwell P, Woodburn J, Redmond A, Turner D, Davys H. The Foot and Ankle in Rheumatoid Arthritis. A Comprehensive Guide. London, UK: Churchill Livingstone Elsevier, 2007.

34. Turner DW, Helliwell JP. Pes planovalgus in RA: a descriptive and analytical study of foot function determined by gait analysis. *Musculoskeletal Care* 2003;1(1):23–33.

35. Locke M, Perry J, Campbell J, Thomas L. Ankle and subtalar motion during gait in arthritic patients. *Phys Ther* 1984;64(4):504–9.

36. Platto MJ, O'Connell PG, Hicks JE, Gerber LH. The relationship of pain and deformity of the rheumatoid foot to gait and an index of functional ambulation. *J Rheumatol* 1991;18(1):38–43.

37. Woodburn J, Helliwell PS, Barker S. Changes in 3D joint kinematics support the continuous use of orthoses in the management of painful rearfoot deformity in rheumatoid arthritis. *J Rheumatol* 2003;30(11):2356–64.

38. Woodburn J, Udupa JK, Hirsch BE, et al. The geometric architecture of the subtalar and midtarsal joints in rheumatoid arthritis based on magnetic resonance imaging. *Arthritis Rheum* 2002;46(12):3168–77.

39. Bouysset M, Tebib JG, Weil G, Lejeune E, Bouvier M. Deformation of the adult rheumatoid rearfoot. A radiographic study. *Clin Rheumatol* 1987;6(4):539–44.

40. Weinfeld SB, Schon LC. Hallux metatarsophalangeal arthritis. *Clin Orthop Relat Res* 1998;349:9–19.

41. Woodburn J, Stableford Z, Helliwell PS. Preliminary investigation of debridement of plantar callosities in rheumatoid arthritis. *Rheumatology* 2000;39(6):652–4.

42. Schmiegel A, Rosenbaum D, Schorat A, et al. Assessment of foot impairment in rheumatoid arthritis patients by dynamic pedobarography. *Gait Posture* 2008;27(1):110–14.

43. Barkham N, Coates LC, Keen H, et al. Double-blind placebo-controlled trial of etanercept in the prevention of work disability in ankylosing spondylitis. *Ann Rheum Dis* 2010;69(11):1926–8.

44. Budiman-Mak E, Conrad KJ, Roach KE. The Foot Function Index: a measure of foot pain and disability. *J Clin Epidemiol* 1991;44(6):561–70.

45. Kuyvenhoven MM, Gorter KJ, Zuithoff P, Budiman-Mak E, Conrad KJ, Post MW. The foot function index with verbal rating scales (FFI-5pt): a clinimetric evaluation and comparison with the original FFI. *J Rheumatol* 2002;29(5):1023–8.

46. Essink-Bot ML, Krabbe PF, Bonsel GJ, Aaronson NK. An empirical comparison of four generic health status measures. The Nottingham Health Profile, the Medical Outcomes Study 36-item Short-Form Health Survey, the COOP/WONCA charts, and the EuroQol instrument. *Medical Care* 1997;35(5):522–37.

47. Macran S, Kind P, Collingwood J, Hull R, McDonald I, Parkinson L. Evaluating podiatry services: testing a treatment specific measure of health status. *Quality of Life Res* 2003;12(2):177–88.

48. McKenna S, Doward LC. The needs-based approach to quality of life assessment. *Value in Health* 2004;7(Suppl 1):S1–S3.

49. Helliwell P, Reay N, Gilworth G, et al. Development of a foot impact scale for rheumatoid arthritis. *Rheumatology* 2005;53(3):418–22.

50. Garrow AP, Papageorgiou AC, Silman AJ, et al. Development and validation of a questionnaire to assess disabling foot pain. *Pain* 2000;85(1–2):107–13.

51. Helliwell PS. Lessons to be learned: review of a multidisciplinary foot clinic in rheumatology. *Rheumatology* 2003;42(11):1426–7.

52. Coady D, Walker D, Kay L. Regional Examination of the Musculoskeletal System (REMS): a core set of clinical skills for medical students. *Rheumatology* 2004;43(5):633–9.

53. Helliwell P, Woodburn J, Redmond A, Turner D, Davys H. *The Foot and Ankle in Rheumatoid Arthritis: A Comprehensive Guide.* Edinburgh, UK: Churchill Livingstone, 2006.

54. Redmond A, Helliwell PS, Robinson P. Investigating foot and ankle problems. In: Conaghan PG, O'Connor P, Isenberg DA (eds). *Oxford Specialist Handbook in Radiology: Musculoskeletal Imaging.* Oxford, UK: Oxford University Press, 2010.

55. National Institute for Health and Care Excellence (NICE). *Rheumatoid Arthritis: National Clinical Guideline for Management and Treatment in Adults.* London, UK: Royal College of Physicians (UK), 2009.

56. Redmond A, Waxman R, Helliwell P. Provision of foot health services in rheumatology in the UK. *Rheumatology (Oxf)* 2006;45(5):571–6.

57. Ndosi M, Ferguson R, Backhouse MR, et al. National variation in the composition of rheumatology multidisciplinary teams: a cross-sectional study. *Rheumatol Int* 2017;37(9):1453–9.

58. Williams AE, Davies S, Graham A, et al. Guidelines for the management of the foot health problems associated with rheumatoid arthritis. *Musculoskeletal Care* 2011;9(2):86–92.

59. Graham AS, Stephenson J, Williams AE. A survey of people with foot problems related to rheumatoid arthritis and their educational needs. *J Foot Ankle Res* 2017;10:12.

60. Graham AS, Hammond A, Walmsley S, Williams AE. Foot health education for people with rheumatoid arthritis—some patient perspectives. *J Foot Ankle Res* 2012;5(1):23.

61. Graham AS, Hammond A, Williams AE. Foot health education for people with rheumatoid arthritis—the practitioner's perspective. *J Foot Ankle Res* 2012;5(1):2.

62. Waxman R, Woodburn H, Powell M, Woodburn J, Blackburn S, Helliwell P. FOOTSTEP: a randomized controlled trial investigating the clinical and cost effectiveness of a patient self-management program for basic foot care in the elderly. *J Clin Epidemiol* 2003;56(11):1092–9.

63. Semple R, Newcombe LW, Finlayson GL, Hutchison CR, Forlow JH, Woodburn J. The FOOTSTEP self-management foot care programme: are rheumatoid arthritis patients physically able to participate? *Musculoskeletal Care* 2009;7(1):57–65.

64. Wechalekar MD, Lester S, Hill CL. Active foot synovitis in patients with rheumatoid arthritis: unstable remission status, radiographic progression, and worse functional outcomes in patients with foot synovitis in apparent remission. *Arthritis Care Res (Hoboken)* 2016;68:1616–23.

65. Smolen JS, Breedveld FC, Burmester GR, et al. Treating rheumatoid arthritis to target: 2014 update of the recommendations of an international task force. *Ann Rheum Dis* 2016;75(1):3–15.

66. Wickman A, Pinzur MS, Kadanoff R, Juknelis D. Health-related quality of life for patients with rheumatoid arthritis foot involvement. *Foot and Ankle Inter* 2004;25(1):19–26.

67. Woodburn J, Hennessy K, Steultjens MP, McInnes IB, Turner DE. Looking through the 'window of opportunity': is there a new paradigm of podiatry care on the horizon in early rheumatoid arthritis? *J Foot Ankle Res* 2010;3:8.

68. Woodburn J, Barker S, Helliwell PS. A randomized controlled trial of foot orthoses in rheumatoid arthritis. *J Rheumatol* 2002;29(7):1377–83.

69. Davys HJ, Woodburn J, Bingham SJ, Emery P. Onychocryptosis (ingrowing toe nail) in patients with rheumatoid arthritis on biologic therapies. *Rheumatology* 2006;45(Suppl 1):i171.

70. Lanzillo B, Pappone N, Crisci C, di Girolamo C, Massini R, Caruso G. Subclinical peripheral nerve involvement in patients with rheumatoid arthritis. *Arthritis Rheum* 1998;41(7):1196–202.

71. Nadkar MY, Agarwal R, Samant RS, et al. Neuropathy in rheumatoid arthritis. *J Assoc Physicians India* 2001;49:217–20.

72. Agarwal, V., Singh R, Wiclaf, et al. A clinical, electrophysiological, and pathological study of neuropathy in rheumatoid arthritis. *Clin Rheumatol* 2008;27(7):841–4.

73. Wilson O, Kirwan JR. Measuring sensation in the feet of patients with rheumatoid arthritis. *Musculoskeletal Care* 2006;4(1):12–23.

74. Rosenbaum D, Schmiegel A, Meermeier M, Gaubitz M. Plantar sensitivity, foot loading and walking pain in rheumatoid arthritis. *Rheumatology (Oxf)* 2006;45(2):212–14.

75. Alkaabi JK, Ho M, Levison R, Pullar T, Belch JJF. Rheumatoid arthritis and macrovascular disease. *Rheumatology (Oxf)* 2003;42(2):292–7.

76. Cawley MI. Vasculitis and ulceration in rheumatic diseases of the foot. *Baillieres Clin Rheumatol* 1987;1(2):315–33.

77. Siddle HJ, Firth J, Waxman R, Nelson EA, Helliwell PS. A case series to describe the clinical characteristics of foot ulceration in patients with rheumatoid arthritis. *Clin Rheumatol* 2012;31(3):541–5.

78. Shanmugam VK, Demaria DM, Attinger CE. Lower extremity ulcers in rheumatoid arthritis: features and response to immunosuppression. *Clin Rheumatol* 2011;30(6):849–53.

79. Firth J, Hale C, Helliwell P, Hill J, Nelson EA. The prevalence of foot ulceration in patients with rheumatoid arthritis. *Arthritis Rheum* 2008;59(2):200–5.

80. Firth J, Waxman R, Law G, et al. The predictors of foot ulceration in patients with rheumatoid arthritis. *Clin Rheumatol* 2013;33(5):615–21.

81. Doran MF, Crowson CS, Pond GR, O'Fallon WM, Gabriel SE. Frequency of infection in patients with rheumatoid arthritis compared with controls: a population-based study. *Arthritis Rheum* 2002;46(9):2287–93.

82. Dixon WG, Watson K, Lunt M, et al. Rates of serious infection, including site-specific and bacterial intracellular infection, in rheumatoid arthritis patients receiving anti-tumor necrosis factor therapy: results from the British Society for Rheumatology Biologics Register. *Arthritis Rheum* 2006;54(8):2368–76.

83. Fitzgerald P, Siddle HJ, Backhouse MR, Nelson EA. Prevalence and microbiological characteristics of clinically infected foot-ulcers in patients with rheumatoid arthritis: a retrospective exploratory study. *J Foot Ankle Res* 2015;8:38.

84. Murray HJ, Young MJ, Hollis S, Boulton AJ. The association between callus formation, high pressures and neuropathy in diabetic foot ulceration. *Diabet Med* 1996;13(11):979–82.

85. Young MJ, Cavanagh PR, Thomas G, Johnson MM, Murray H, Boulton AJ. The effect of callus removal on dynamic plantar foot pressures in diabetic patients. *Diabet Med* 1992;9(1):55–7.

86. Siddle HJ, Redmond AC, Waxman R. Debridement of painful forefoot plantar callosities in rheumatoid arthritis: the CARROT randomised controlled trial. *Clin Rheumatol* 2013;32(5):567–74.

87. Williams AE, Nester CJ, Ravey MI. Rheumatoid arthritis patients' experiences of wearing therapeutic footwear—a qualitative investigation. *BMC Musculoskelet Disord* 2007;8:104.

88. Williams AE, Nester CJ, Ravey MI, Kottink A, Klapsing MG. Women's experiences of wearing therapeutic footwear in three European countries. *J Foot Ankle Res* 2010;3:23.

89. Dahmen R, Siemonsma PC, Boers M, Lankhorst GJ, Roorda LD. Use and effects of custom-made therapeutic footwear on lower-extremity related pain and activity limitations in patients with rheumatoid arthritis: a prospective observational cohort study. *J Rehabil Med* 2014;46:561–7.

90. Bagherzadeh Cham M, Ghasemi MS, Forogh B, Sanjari MA, Zabihi Yeganeh M, Eshraghi A. Effect of rocker shoes on pain, disability and activity limitation in patients with rheumatoid arthritis. *Prosthet Orthot Int* 2014;38(4):310–5.

91. Cho NS, Hwang JH, Chang HJ, Koh EM, Park HS. Randomized controlled trial for clinical effects of varying types of insoles combined with specialized shoes in patients with rheumatoid arthritis of the foot. *Clin Rehabil* 2009;23(6):512–21.

92. Gossec L, Pavy S, Pham T, et al. Nonpharmacological treatments in early rheumatoid arthritis: clinical practice guidelines based on published evidence and expert opinion. *Joint Bone Spine* 2006;73(4):396–402.

93. Luqmani R, Hennell S, Estrach C, et al. British Society for Rheumatology and british health professionals in Rheumatology guideline for the management of rheumatoid arthritis (the first two years). *Rheumatology (Oxf)* 2006;45(9):1167–9.

94. Forestier R, André-Vert J, Guillez P, et al. Non-drug treatment (excluding surgery) in rheumatoid arthritis: clinical practice guidelines. *Joint Bone Spine* 2009;76(6):691–8.

95. SIGN. *SIGN 123: Management of Early Rheumatoid Arthritis. A National Clinical Guideline.* Edinburgh, UK: Royal College of Physicians, 2011. Available at: https://www.sign.ac.uk/assets/sign123.pdf

96. Hennessy K, Woodburn J, Steultjens M. Custom foot orthoses for rheumatoid arthritis: a systematic review. *Arthritis Care Res (Hoboken)* 2012;64(3):311–20.

97. Conceição CS, Gomes Neto M, Mendes SM, Sá KN, Baptista AF. Systematic review and meta-analysis of effects of foot orthoses on pain and disability in rheumatoid arthritis patients. *Disabil Rehabil* 2015;37(14):1209–13.

98. Turner DE, Helliwell PS, Emery P, Woodburn J. The impact of rheumatoid arthritis on foot function in the early stages of disease: a clinical case series. *BMC Musculoskelet Disord* 2006;7:102.

99. Cameron-Fiddes V, Santos D. The use of 'off-the-shelf' foot orthoses in the reduction of footsymptoms in patients with early rheumatoid arthritis. *Foot* 2013;23:123–9.

100. Gibson KS, Woodburn J, Porter D, Telfer S. Functionally optimized orthoses for early rheumatoid arthritis foot disease: a study of mechanisms and patient experience. *Arthritis Care Res (Hoboken)* 2014;66(10):1456–64.

101. van der Leeden M, Fielder K, Jonkman A, et al. Factors predicting the outcome of customised foot orthoses in patients with rheumatoid arthritis: a prospective cohort study. *J Foot Ankle Res* 2011;4:8.

102. Hay SM, Cooper JR, Getty CJM. Diagnostic injections of the hindfoot joints in patients with rheumatoid arthritis prior to surgical fusion. *Foot* 1999;9(1):40–3.

103. d'Agostino MA, Ayral X, Baron G, Ravaud P, Breban M, Dougados M. Impact of ultrasound imaging on local corticosteroid injections of symptomatic ankle, hind-, and mid-foot in chronic inflammatory diseases. *Arthritis Rheum* 2005;53(2):284–92.

104. Cunnington J, Marshall N, Hide G, et al. A randomized, double-blind, controlled study of ultrasound-guided corticosteroid injection into the joint of patients with inflammatory arthritis. *Arthritis Rheum* 2010;62(7):1862–9.

105. Chakravarty K, Pharoah PD, Scott DG. A randomized controlled study of post-injection rest following intra-articular steroid therapy for knee synovitis. *Br J Rheumatol* 1994;33(5):464–8.

106. Rall LC, Roubenoff R. Body composition, metabolism, and resistance exercise in patients with rheumatoid arthritis. *Arthritis Care Res* 1996;9(2):151–6.

107. de Jong Z, Munneke M, Lems WF, et al. Slowing of bone loss in patients with rheumatoid arthritis by long-term high-intensity exercise: results of a randomized, controlled trial. *Arthritis Rheum* 2004;50(4):1066–76.

108. de Jong Z, Munneke M, Zwinderman AH, et al. Is a long-term high-intensity exercise program effective and safe in patients with rheumatoid arthritis? Results of a randomized controlled trial. *Arthritis Rheum* 2003;48(9):2415–24.

109. Lemmey AB. Rheumatoid cachexia: the undiagnosed, untreated key to restoring physical function in rheumatoid arthritis patients? *Rheumatology (Oxf)* 2016;55(7):1149–50.

26

Occupational therapy

Alison Hammond, Joanne Adams, and Yeliz Prior

Introduction

Rheumatology occupational therapy in the United Kingdom has been a specialist area of practice for nearly 40 years. Therapists most often work in secondary care as part of rheumatology teams. The National Institute for Health and Care Excellence (NICE) Guidelines for management and treatment of adults with rheumatoid arthritis (RA) emphasize the importance of access to specialist occupational therapists.[1] A recent survey identified 75% of rheumatology teams have access to occupational therapy, although funded staffing levels varied considerably across the United Kingdom, impacting on the range of services offered.[2]

Impact of rheumatoid arthritis on lifestyle and how occupational therapy helps

Occupational therapy integrates the provision of self-management, physical, psychological, and social interventions to enable people to maximize their occupational performance, that is to perform their activities and participate in the social roles that are necessary and meaningful to them. Rheumatoid arthritis impacts on lifestyle from an early stage of the disease. Some 60% of people with rheumatoid arthritis have hand and activities of daily living (ADL) problems, 60% with household, leisure, and social activities, 28–40% stop work within five years of diagnosis and 50% by 10 years.[1,3] Once unemployed, people are unlikely to return to work, with potentially serious personal and financial consequences.[4] Accordingly, these figures suggest some two-thirds of people with rheumatoid arthritis could benefit from occupational therapy to help with hand and ADL problems, leisure and social activities, and at least a half with work problems. Adjusting to and living with a progressive and variable chronic disease can lead to a range of emotional reactions, which vary over time (e.g. stress, depression, anxiety, anger) impacting on family, social and work relationships, activity ability, and participation. Loss of valued activities is associated with poorer psychological status, functional and disease outcomes.[5] Occupational therapists have training in both physical and psychological therapies and are well-placed to support people through such transitions.

Occupational therapists use a wide range of interventions: improving upper limb function through hand exercise, ergonomics, assistive devices, and orthoses; fatigue management; pain and mood management (e.g. stress management, relaxation training, mindfulness); activity and environmental modifications; ADL training; transport and mobility advice; benefits and community resources advice. Avocational counselling (i.e. advice and practical assistance with leisure, voluntary work, and adult education opportunities) is highly valued by people with rheumatoid arthritis, as they regularly comment 'there is more to life than just looking after yourself, the family, the house, and working'. As work problems occur early, timely identification of work problems is essential so that therapists can provide stay at work (job retention) work rehabilitation and advice to reduce negative long-term personal, health, social, and financial consequences of unemployment or early retirement.[1] A major focus is self-management education to help people manage pain, fatigue, frustration, and difficulties performing daily roles. Occupational therapists provide interventions to enable people to make changes so they can maintain or adapt their valued activities and roles. Consequently, occupational therapists commonly use motivational interviewing, counselling, and cognitive-behavioural approaches to facilitate people making cognitive and health behavioural changes.

Two case studies help to illustrate the impact of rheumatoid arthritis on people's lifestyles and on what an occupational therapist can offer. The examples are for: early (see **Box 26.1**) and established (see **Box 26.2**) rheumatoid arthritis.

Impact of rheumatoid arthritis on hand function

Good hand function is essential for daily, work, leisure, and social activities and thus a focus of occupational therapy programmes. Frustration performing activities because of limited grip and hand pain is common among people with rheumatoid arthritis. In spite of recent advances in biological treatment for rheumatoid arthritis, persistent active disease remains common and hand impairment and dysfunction continue to be prevalent and progressive for many.[6] Hand impairment and hand function thus remain an important consideration for all the rheumatology team. Hand function can progressively worsen over time.[7] Recent evidence indicates that for some patients, hand function can improve within 3 months

Box 26.1 Early rheumatoid arthritis case study (Eliza Huey)

Eliza is a 41-year-old woman, recently diagnosed with rheumatoid arthritis. She reports pain, swelling, and stiffness in her hands, wrists, and hips, as well fatigue. She has been on disease-modifying antirheumatic drug (DMARD) combination therapy (methotrexate and sulfasalazine) for 5 weeks and experienced multiple side effects, such as nausea, headaches, and dizziness.

The occupational therapist assessed Eliza: she works full-time as a marketing manager in a small firm and is a single mother of two school-age children. She has been on sick leave from work since being diagnosed, as she was unable to cope with the demands of her full-time job. A work assessment identified her main problems in getting back to work: getting up and ready in the morning; negotiating rush hour traffic doing the school run; and then commuting to work. Eliza found early mornings particularly difficult due to morning stiffness, having had no refreshing sleep in weeks and fatigue on wakening.

During goal setting, a return-to-work programme was negotiated with Eliza. Occupational therapy involved: liaising with the rheumatologist for a steroid injection to relieve symptoms while waiting for DMARDs to take effect; supporting Eliza in negotiating a graded return to work with her employer, that is, working flexible hours to avoid the morning rush hour and working from home 1 day a week; fatigue management training, particularly on sleep hygiene and activity pacing; and training in ergonomics (joint protection) at work and home to help reduce pain and fatigue and make activities easier. She was also offered the opportunity to attend the department's self-management education programme in future.

of starting medical treatment, although such improvements plateau over 3 years to leave ongoing hand function limitations.[8] Women report more hand pain than men and hand pain and dysfunction are more closely related to disease activity than articular wrist and hand joint damage, with localized synovitis contributing substantially to hand dysfunction.[9,10] Hand deformities, if present, are an indicator of disease severity. The impact of rheumatoid arthritis on hand function remains significant.

Box 26.2 Established rheumatoid arthritis case study (Alex Nielson)

Alex is a 61-year-old man with rheumatoid arthritis, which was successfully managed with DMARDs (i.e. methotrexate) until recently. Due to problems with kidney function he had to come off his DMARD. This resulted in a flare, which left him with hand, knee, and foot pain and fatigue.

The occupational therapist assessed Alex: he previously led an active lifestyle; enjoyed cycling, dog walking, and playing an instrument. He took early retirement recently, with a view to spending more time with his partner, having outdoor holidays, and playing the French horn in a local brass band. Since the flare he has been unable to walk his dog, as he cannot hold the lead because of pain and swelling in his hand joints. Hand and knee pain also mean he cannot ride his bike or play his French horn. He is depressed, due to loss of his life roles as an engineer, an active partner, dog walker, musician, and cyclist, all of which had provided him with a sense of belonging and self-worth.

Occupational therapy involved: using mindfulness training and motivational interviewing to help Alex identify and modify negative thought patterns and develop problem-solving skills to overcome barriers to participation in his valued life activities; and fatigue management training. A graded approach to physical exercise (through graded walking and cycling programmes, and hand exercises) enabled Alex to start riding his bike and play his horn again. Recommending a waist-band dog lead with Halti collar helped him to walk his dog again.

Muscle cachexia, lower bone density and weakening of ligaments and capsular soft tissue associated with rheumatoid inflammatory processes contribute to loss of hand functional ability.[11] These pathological processes contribute to muscle imbalance between the extrinsic and intrinsic hand muscle groups so that the hand is unable to work smoothly and efficiently. Such muscle imbalances in turn contributes to progressive changes in biomechanical forces when the wrist and hand are used functionally. This chain of events can contribute to further muscle imbalance, reduced range of wrist and hand joint motion, grip strength, and functional ability.[12] The hand unit can become less flexible and the hand arches less able to adapt and accommodate the different grips necessary for daily hand use. Associated rheumatoid hand deformities can include z type collapse of the thumb alongside swan-neck and boutonnière finger deformities and distal radio ulnar joint instability.[13] Such changes cause further reductions in hand function, strength, and dexterity for people ageing with rheumatoid arthritis.

While general activity limitations are multifactorial for people with rheumatoid arthritis, greater hand pain, reduced grip strength, and hand range of motion are most associated with self-reported disability.[12] Thus hand function contributes substantially to an individual's ability to carry out daily activities and work. Although rheumatoid disease processes are now more effectively controlled than in previous years, hand impairment and dysfunction remain significant issues for people living with rheumatoid arthritis. As such, reducing hand pain and improving grip and hand function remain important targets for sustained interdisciplinary team attention.[9]

Assessment

Assessment is the foundation for identifying the impact of rheumatoid arthritis on the client's lifestyle, physical and psychological abilities, and hand and upper limb function. During any assessment, the reason for problems will be explored: is it pain, fatigue, stiffness, physical limitations, environmental factors, psychological factors, lack of confidence (self-efficacy) or lack of information? Following assessment, the therapist and client collaboratively identify treatment priorities and goals and will then re-assess therapy outcomes following treatment.

Assessing activities and participation

Assessments are designed to evaluate occupations. Occupation, in this sense, can be any activity deemed important and meaningful to an individual, ranging from daily personal activities, such as eating, dressing, mobility, engagement in sexual activities, and domestic activities, such as housework, gardening, shopping and caring, through to task specific activities, such as driving and communication. It also includes other key aspects of people's lives such as work, leisure, social activities, education, rest, civic life, and spiritual activities.

Assessments include

The Canadian Occupational Performance Measure (COPM) identifies occupational performance issues and measures individuals' perception of change in occupational performance and satisfaction. It has good clinical utility, is easy to access with a manual and training resources available online.[14] A semi-structured interview, taking about 40 minutes, is used to aid the client identify daily occupations of importance that they want, need, or are expected to do but have difficulty with. Once all relevant issues are identified, the client rates the personal importance of these activities on a 10-point scale (1 poor to 10 good/high), they select five key problems, and these form the basis of treatment goals. The client then rates performance and satisfaction with performance on a 10-point scale. Following treatment, the client re-rates performance and satisfaction. The COPM has good validity, reliability, and responsiveness to change, with a two-point change in performance/satisfaction being clinically significant.

The Evaluation of Daily Activity Questionnaire (EDAQ) is a patient-reported outcome measure (PROM). It includes 138 activities commonly identified as problematic by people with rheumatoid arthritis and musculoskeletal conditions. Activities are grouped into 14 subscales, each of which is reliable and valid, and can be scored and used separately or combined into two components of self-care and mobility.[15] The EDAQ is currently available in English, German, and Dutch. Clients can be given or mailed the EDAQ prior to a therapy appointment and complete it at home in their own time, allowing reflection on abilities and solutions already in use. During the appointment, the therapist can quickly focus on those personal, household, caring, mobility, communication, leisure, and social activities the client reports difficulty with. This speeds up assessment allowing more time to focus on identifying and trying solutions. The EDAQ and manual are freely available online.[16]

The Work Experience Survey Work—Rheumatic Conditions was developed in the United States and is modified for the United Kingdom.[17,18] This semi-structured interview identifies information about work and medical history and includes eight subscales identifying work barriers: getting ready for/travel to work; workplace access; completing job activities: physical demands; mental demands; time, energy, emotional demands; relationships with people at work; environmental factors; and company policies; job satisfaction and life-work balance. Together the client and therapist identify the three main areas to focus on and jointly agree a work rehabilitation plan.

The Work Activities Limitations Scale is a 12-item PROM, which is reliable, valid, and responsive to change. This can be quickly completed to identify key difficulties. It is as a quick method of evaluating outcomes of work interventions.[19]

Activity diaries are also valuable in identifying how a client spends a typical week and weekend day. Each day in the diary is divided into half-hour slots. This helps identify the balance of activities and rest within a person's day and night, and aids the client reflecting on activity difficulties, pain, and fatigue experienced through the day, as well as their work-leisure-personal life balance. Several diary designs are available.

Assessing hand function

Assessment of hand impairment and function starts with clinical hand examination following the three principles of observation, feel, and move.[20,21] Therapists may use the Jamar dynamometer to evaluate grip strength, although the GRIPPIT dynamometer is more sensitive for those with weaker grip and measures both peak and sustained grip strength. Patient-reported outcome measures

(PROMS) are an excellent way to assess the personal impact of hand impairment. General functional outcomes, such as the Arthritis Impact Measurement Scale II, include some hand specific components. However, regional questionnaires, such as the Michigan Hand Outcomes Questionnaire[22] will give more detailed results and are also useful for audit and research. The Disability Arm Shoulder and Hand questionnaire (DASH)[23] is useful in clinical practice, freely available, and easy to administer. Both have sound psychometric properties in rheumatoid arthritis populations.

Assessing educational needs and psychological status

Self-management education needs can be assessed using the Educational Needs Assessment Tool, including 39 items, many of which are relevant to occupational therapy. This can be used to develop educational priorities, and inform goal setting and shared decision-making.[24] Psychological assessments are less commonly used in practice as therapists tend to rely on observation and interview and using their psychological and counselling skills to appraise status. However, useful measures are the Hospital Anxiety and Depression Scale, which has been shown to have high clinical utility and is free of physical symptoms, such as insomnia and weight loss, as well as distinguishing well between anxious and depressive states and examining the impact of cognition on depression or anxiety.[25] Self-efficacy for using self-management methods can also be assessed using the Rheumatoid Arthritis Self-efficacy Scale.[26] This identifies confidence to use health behaviours and is a relevant outcome measure for self-management interventions.

Interventions

Interventions selected are based on the occupational performance limitations identified through assessment, consideration of the client's adjustment to living with their condition, their psychological status, and self-management education needs. Occupational performance can be affected by limited:

- knowledge of rheumatoid arthritis, its management and progress;
- knowledge and skills to adopt ergonomic approaches to reduce pain, fatigue, and joint strain;
- energy to manage a full day of activity and ability to balance rest and activity;
- range of movement, muscle strength and endurance;
- self-efficacy to use self-management approaches and redesign lifestyle.

Comprehensive occupational therapy programmes maintain activity ability, participation, and increase self-management in rheumatoid arthritis.[27–30] A recent systematic review identified there was strong evidence supporting the use of: self-management and patient education provided by occupational therapists using cognitive-behavioural approaches; and ergonomics/joint protection (**Figure 26.1**). Comprehensive occupational therapy, including self-management education and work rehabilitation, has been shown to improve self-reported coping, function, pain, and work productivity.[28,29]

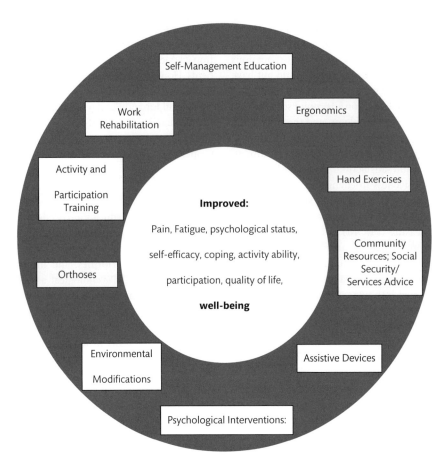

Figure 26.1 Impact of comprehensive occupational therapy in arthritis.

Ergonomics

Ergonomic approaches aim to reduce pain and fatigue during daily activities, work, and leisure. These include:

- Altered movement patterns and use of proper joint and body mechanics.
- Restructuring activities, work simplification, and altering the environment.
- Using ergonomic equipment and assistive technology.
- Activity pacing, planning, prioritizing, and problem-solving to modify activities and routines.

Ergonomic approaches are also termed joint protection and energy conservation techniques. Many people find their own ways through trial and error of reducing pain, fatigue, and consequently frustration, to make activities easier but this often takes time. Ergonomics education applies a systematic approach to enabling people to change habits, find new solutions, and speed up change. Education should be provided when clients are experiencing pain, particularly in the hands, and fatigue, which is not being controlled by medication. If they have little or no pain and fatigue, with few or no activity limitations, they are unlikely to perceive the need to change and education may be of little value. Effective teaching techniques must be used to enable people to make sufficient ergonomic changes to gain benefits. Several randomized controlled trials of group ergonomics education (joint protection) demonstrate using cognitive-behavioural and self-efficacy enhancing approaches are significantly more effective than traditional teaching techniques in improving use of ergonomics, activity ability, and reducing hand pain, general pain, and early morning stiffness.[31] Benefits continued for four years and the behavioural group had fewer hand deformities.[32] However, education must be timed appropriately and provided applicable to clients' needs, as those with less than 6 months disease duration, minimal hand pain, or activity problems did not benefit.[33] An individual programme, based on similar approaches, also demonstrated significant improvements in use of ergonomics, grip strength, and self-efficacy.[34]

Hand ergonomics includes changing movement patterns to limit: using strong, sustained grips, and twisting movements; lifting heavy objects; and tight, prolonged key, tripod, and pinch grips. These help reduce forces on metacarpophalangeal, wrist, and thumb joints and thus reduce hand pain and muscle fatigue. The rapid decline in hand function early in rheumatoid arthritis suggests effective ergonomic education should be provided when increased pain and reduced grip strength are impacting hand function.

Changes recommended include:

- altering movement patterns and use of proper joint and body mechanics. Examples include: using two hands to lift items; holding objects closer to the body when lifting; changing positions regularly; avoiding prolonged sitting and standing; ensuring work surfaces are within the reach envelope; maintaining efficient working postures when working; sitting correctly using ergonomic chairs. Poor posture and positioning have greater energy demands which increase muscle fatigue and pain.

- Restructuring activities, work simplification, and altering the environment. Examples include: filling a kettle with a lightweight jug; shopping via the internet; reordering sequences of activities to increase efficiency; eliminating unnecessary tasks; keeping frequently used equipment within the reach envelope; decluttering and using efficient storage methods.
- Using ergonomic equipment and assistive technology. Examples include: reducing effort required by using ergonomically designed equipment with universal design features, such as non-slip larger handles and lighter weight; avoiding lifting by using wheels.
- Activity pacing, planning, and prioritizing. Pacing examples include: taking microbreaks for 30 seconds every 10 minutes while stretching and bending joints being used in sustained positions; periodic rest breaks or 'moving round' 5 minutes every hour to allow muscle recovery time. Sleep hygiene principles include: using supportive pillows and mattresses; having a regular bedtime and relaxing evening routine; and avoiding stimulants. Planning examples include: balancing activities to alternate between light, medium, and heavy tasks during the day and week; avoiding a 'boom and bust' cycle of doing too much on good days, with consequences of resultant crashes. Fatigue activity diaries can be particularly helpful in enabling people to perceive such patterns.
- Active problem-solving. Teaching people a structured approach to analysing activities, breaking these down into separate tasks and evaluating the movements, psychological demands and equipment used, enable people to apply ergonomic techniques themselves to identify better solutions to making activities easier.

A multimodal group programme delivered by a psychologist and occupational therapist, including cognitive-behavioural approaches to enable improved activity pacing and alter cognitions about fatigue and improve mood, has been shown to be effective in reducing fatigue in those with moderate to severe fatigue.[35]

Hand exercises and orthoses

Hand exercises should be taught alongside ergonomics education. Reducing hand pain and muscle fatigue through ergonomics mean clients are better able to increase and maintain hand exercise frequency and improve grip strength. The provision of effective hand exercise programmes, and wrist and hand orthotics, are supportive and practical ways to reinforce individuals' abilities to contribute to their self-management of any hand pain or dysfunction experienced.

There is strong evidence hand exercise programmes of high intensity (i.e. daily with 30 repetitions of medium resistance exercises for 10–20 minutes, cumulatively) lead to significantly better outcomes in function, pain and grip strength than low-intensity (i.e. range of movement or low resistance exercises at lower frequency).[36] Supervised hand exercise training (once a week for 4–6 weeks) using cognitive-behavioural approaches, is essential to enable people to perform high intensity medium resistance exercises, as many have concerns about whether this is safe initially.[36] This is a cost-effective approach to helping people to manage their hand dysfunction.[36] The SARAH trial is one such high intensity, individually tailored, programme delivered using a health psychology approach with 1 ×/week sessions over 6 weeks, plus a home programme continued during and after, leading to significant and clinically effective results after 12 months and is strongly recommended for clinical practice.[37] It is essential to regularly prompt people to continue hand exercises. Effectiveness decreases over time if exercise is not maintained.[38]

Wrist and hand orthoses remain a popular conservative approach. A review of the effectiveness of hand and wrist orthoses identified just two types had sufficiently robust research evidence to support their effectiveness in reducing pain and increasing hand function. A functional elastic wrist orthosis to provide support to the wrist and hand during daily tasks can provide pain relief and improve function. Swan-neck deformity splints also have strong evidence that they improve hand dexterity.[39]

Recently it has been identified that long-term adherence to self-management strategies, such as ergonomics, hand exercise programmes, and orthotic wear, can be improved by carefully considering the social context within which people live.[40] Occupational therapists are ideally placed to maximize upon this considered approach in their daily collaborative practice with patients.

Activities of daily living

Joint pain impacts on independence, self-esteem, has considerable effects on personal relationships and reduces quality of life. Therapists' skills in ergonomics and theoretical understanding of the impact of the environment and personal factors on individual's performance enable detailed analysis of activity limitations. Occupational therapists work collaboratively with clients to identify solutions, the need for assistive technology and environmental adaptations to prevent or reduce future dependency and maintain independence. ADL training is provided through tailored interventions for individuals as well as via self-management education programmes, such as the Lifestyle Management for Arthritis Programme employed UK wide.[41] Assistive technology (e.g. electric tin openers, bottle openers, adapted knives) helps reduce pain and fatigue and minimizes biomechanical stress and forces placed on joints during activity, as well as minimising risks associated with undertaking the task.

Sexual activities are a central aspect of being human. Rheumatoid arthritis affects the sexual lives of individuals. Many are afraid that they will be in pain, or will cause their partner pain, and sore joints limit initiating sexual relations. Occupational therapists can help by offering a safe environment to discuss such issues, and provide psychological support, reassurance, and practical advice to address sexual issues, within the therapist's boundaries of expertise. For those not wanting to discuss sexual matters, it is helpful to offer written information and the option to seek help in the future.

While there have been considerable improvements in the treatment of inflammatory arthritis using biologic agents and most clients report much improvement, individuals can still have difficulties in performing ADL through previous biomechanical damage causing joint pain, stiffness, fatigue, as well as experiencing anxiety and depression.[42] Additionally, socioeconomic and environmental factors, such as access to help and support, education, and health and social care, can determine health-related quality of life outcomes. While independence in ADL may be the central aim, interdependence may be the best choice for some. Person-centred occupational therapy is used to initiate therapy goals to ensure the individual reaches their optimum function. Occupational therapists can also provide advice on social security and other financial benefits, third-sector support, housing adaptations, and refer on to social services, as applicable.

Work and leisure rehabilitation

Many factors influence work instability and disability including: greater pain, hand pain and fatigue; unadapted work environments and equipment; physically demanding jobs; poor work self-efficacy; increasing stress or low mood related to work difficulties; lack of support, autonomy and participation in decision-making in the workplace; and limited use of self-management strategies.[43] Fatigue can have an additional impact on cognitive ability. Job retention work rehabilitation has the potential to prevent or postpone work disability through modifying such factors. For example, those with workplace ergonomic modifications are 2.5 times less likely to stop work. Work rehabilitation should be provided early, when work instability develops. However, many with arthritis lack access to work rehabilitation and may not even be aware of work information booklets available.

Two trials in the United States demonstrated reduced job loss following work rehabilitation in people with a variety of rheumatic conditions.[44,45] The intervention has been adapted for the United Kingdom and tested in a feasibility study with people with rheumatoid arthritis or early inflammatory arthritis. The intervention was delivered by occupational therapists, who received 3 days' training in work rehabilitation and a work solutions manual. The trial included people on biologics who, though reporting they 'felt the best they had ever been', still experienced work difficulties due to joint pain, fatigue, and lack of confidence. Work rehabilitation included: assessment using the WES-RC; the participant and therapist mutually agreeing priority work problems; and action planning. A tailored, individualized programme was then provided including, as appropriate: applying ergonomic, fatigue, and stress management approaches to the workplace; recommendations for assistive technology/equipment adaptation, workplace/work station modification, transport advice; practical advice and support enabling participants to disclose their condition and negotiate job modifications with employers; explaining rights under the Equality Act 2010 and what are 'reasonable adjustments'; psychological support, through listening to and discussing work problems, encouraging ability and confidence in solving work problems, managing arthritis when working and continuing working in future; advice on other ADL and hand function difficulties affecting work ability; provision of relevant work and self-management advice booklets and other information as appropriate; and referral to relevant rehabilitation and employment services. Participants were offered a work site visit, if needed. The intervention was provided for on average 4 hours in four monthly meetings, including a telephone review about 2 months after the final treatment session, to discuss progress making changes. Although a feasibility study, the results at 9-month follow-up demonstrated a larger effect size in reducing work instability, work limitations, physical ability, pain, and perceived health compared to those receiving work information booklets only.[43] This now is being testing in a randomized controlled trial.

As the disease progresses, people steadily give up leisure and social activities and reduce household activities in order to retain the energy to work. People give up between a third to two-thirds of their leisure and non-work activities meaning life becomes increasingly unbalanced.[46,47] Being prescribed biologics means many are enabled to remain in or return to work and increase or resume participation in leisure and social activities they previously abandoned or were unable to take up. Increasing participation enables people to redefine their sense of self, increase self-confidence, and many perceive themselves as becoming a healthier person. This improvement leads to testing new boundaries but many find they still cannot do all they want to, and continue to have an imbalance between work and other activities: 'I push myself a bit more.'[42] Occupational therapists enable people to effectively develop or take on new activities and social roles. Leisure and social activities are of central importance in people's lives, providing meaning and enjoyment. Limiting these can lead to low mood and increased distress. Therapists therefore identify problems and recommend solutions and strategies to increase participation in non-vocational activities to facilitate occupational balance.

Psychological interventions

'When we are no longer able to change a situation, we are challenged to change ourselves.'

Viktor Frankl 1905–1997

Occupational therapists are well-placed to facilitate a holistic approach addressing the rehabilitation needs of individuals with rheumatoid arthritis, due to their dual training in physical and psychological therapies. The underpinning philosophy of occupational therapy is that therapists must be mindful of individuals' psychosocial needs and the impact of these needs on their health behaviours. Occupational therapists apply psychological theories of learning, motivation, personality, and emotion to understand and facilitate health behaviour change, which underpins rehabilitation interventions for rheumatoid arthritis.

Occupational therapists often come into contact with people with rheumatoid arthritis who are trying to make sense of what is happening to them and coming to terms with the prospect of living with a chronic condition. At this stage, many are dealing with uncertainties around their differential diagnosis, treatment regimen, and impact of these on their family and work commitments, as they try to process information acquired from a variety of sources (e.g. consultations with their GP, rheumatologist, health professionals, and from information leaflets, internet based-sources, and friends) as to how they should manage their condition. This transitional process, more often than not, is accompanied with severe joint pain and fatigue and associated symptoms of sleeplessness, stress, anxiety, and depression. Hence individuals often present to occupational therapy with complex psychological needs, regardless of the nature of the referral.

Rheumatology occupational therapists employ advanced communication skills and therapeutic use of self, which are integral to the outcome of the occupational therapy process. These help maximize the development of a collaborative relationship that underpins engagement of individuals in an effective therapeutic alliance to maintain participation, motivation, involvement, and autonomy. The therapist's warmth and genuineness, listening skills, reading non-verbal cues, and ability to express and manage emotions within interactions are linked to the perceived efficacy of the relationship and to individual satisfaction. People with rheumatic conditions may have limited motivation to make necessary health behaviour changes to improve their health outcomes, due to their symptoms of pain and fatigue. Many are also ambivalent about change and implementing strategies to make the required changes happen.

Rheumatology occupational therapists may employ motivational interviewing techniques to help resolve an individual's ambivalence to change and aid goal setting. Occupational therapists play a key role in facilitating behaviour change, through the use of enabling strategies and being mindful of the individual's roles, values, meanings, attitudes, beliefs, and social context. Psychological interventions used by occupational therapists to support people with rheumatic conditions may include:

- self-esteem and self-efficacy building (e.g. problem-solving, empowerment, assertiveness, self-monitoring and management, shared decision-making);
- developing coping skills and techniques (e.g. relaxation and stress management skills, mood management, pain and fatigue management, mindfulness).

Self-management education

Psychological interventions are integrated into self-management education. Occupational therapists often coordinate and lead arthritis self-management programmes, along with the multidisciplinary team. Key features of effective self-management programmes delivered either in groups, mailed or via the internet are: duration of at least 6 weeks to enable participants to develop skills, with sufficient practice, and instigate changes with support; explicit use of social cognitive theory and cognitive-behavioural approaches; individualized weekly action plans with weekly progress review; a leader manual protocolizing delivery with participant handbooks; and led by the same trained leaders. Exercise and graded home aerobic exercise (e.g. walking, Tai Chi) are key features alongside exercise action-planning with clear details about exercise performance.[48]

Programmes provided by occupational therapists in the United Kingdom include the Looking After Your Joints Programme[31,32] and the modular Lifestyle Management for Arthritis Programme (LMAP), developed from this.[41] The LMAP starts with education about rheumatoid arthritis and its management, enabling participants to evaluate the impact of their condition on their valued activities and daily lives in order to help them reflect on importance, confidence, and readiness for making changes. The programme content includes: ergonomics, hand exercises, fatigue, pain and mood management and exercise (stretch, strength, a walking programme, and an introduction to the Tai Chi for Arthritis Programme). The programme uses individual action planning and weekly reviews of progress, practice, and feedback and home programmes to facilitate change. The LMAP results in significant improvements in pain, fatigue, functional ability, self-efficacy, and use of health behaviours.[41]

Future developments in occupational therapy

Rheumatology occupational therapy services have gone through a considerable change in the last decade. Health and social care initiatives for care in the community and self-management, advancements in early recognition of rheumatoid arthritis in primary care and increased use of biologic agents are helping reduce functional limitations and future disability. Although most rheumatology occupational therapy services in the United Kingdom are still based in outpatient departments in secondary care, there is increasing pressure to relocate to primary care musculoskeletal services. Rheumatology occupational therapists working in primary care can support the management of rheumatoid arthritis in the community and early recognition and referral of people with inflammatory arthritis to secondary care rheumatology teams to ensure optimal treatment outcomes. With better symptom control, more people with rheumatoid arthritis are able to continue working and thus occupational therapists can increasingly focus on provision of work rehabilitation to enable people to remain working and financially independent. Greater recognition of the psychological impact of rheumatoid arthritis will also mean therapists will increasingly use their extensive psychological skills in providing psychological support, psychological therapies, and enabling occupational balance to improve mood.

Likewise, health and social care is moving towards digital/ mobile health technologies (mHealth). In 2017, the Office of National Statistics, identified 90% of households in the UK have internet access, an increase from 57% in 2006. Emerging social media and digital technologies have shifted individuals' roles from consumers of health information to both consumers and coproducers by commenting and sharing health experiences and offering solutions to problems.[48,49] Such platforms enable people with health conditions to engage with one another, providing information on experiences, treatment, and symptoms that satisfy other peoples' information needs, thus increasing self-efficacy and self-worth. Given limited access to specialist occupational therapists, online platforms have the potential to enable therapists to: help people access PROMS online to facilitate personal problem identification and problem-solving; and design and provide online self-management education and rehabilitation interventions to extend access to practical solutions. The use of online platforms and apps, for example, the MSKHUB (a self-management platform at the University of Salford[50]) and the future SARAH trial online hand exercise programme (Oxford University) can help people with rheumatoid arthritis self-manage and be actively involved in their care.

Conclusion

People highly value being independent in performing their daily activities, work, social, and leisure occupations, maintaining a normal life and having a balance between different occupations and rest. They perceive these as central to good health. Occupational therapy promotes health by enabling clients to maintain independence and live a balanced lifestyle pursuing the activities and participating in the social roles meaningful to them.

REFERENCES

1. National Collaborating Centre for Chronic Conditions. *Rheumatoid Arthritis: National Clinical Guideline for Management and Treatment in Adults*. London, UK: Royal College of Physicians, 2009.
2. Ndosi M, Ferguson R, Backhouse M, et al. National variation in the composition of rheumatology multidisciplinary teams: a cross sectional study. *Rheumatol Int* 2017;*37*(9):1453–9.
3. National Rheumatoid Arthritis Society. *The Economic Burden of Rheumatoid Arthritis*. Maidenhead, UK: NRAS, 2010.

4. Verstappen SMM, Boonen A, Bijlsma JWJ, et al. Working status among Dutch patients with rheumatoid arthritis: work disability and working conditions. *Rheumatology* 2004;*44*:202–6.

5. Katz PP, Yelin EH. The development of depressive symptoms among women with rheumatoid arthritis. *Arthr Rheum* 1995;*38*:49–56.

6. Horsten, NCA, Ursum J, Roorda LD, et al. Prevalence of hand symptoms, impairments and activity limitations in rheumatoid arthritis in relation to disease duration. *J Rehab Med* 2010;*42*(10):916–21.

7. Kapetanovic MC, Lindqvist E, Nilsson JÅ, et al. Development of functional impairment and disability in rheumatoid arthritis patients followed for 20 years: relation to disease activity, joint damage, and comorbidity. *Arthritis Care Res (Hoboken)* 2015;*67*(3):340–8.

8. Björk M, Thyberg I, Haglund L, et al. Hand function in women and men with early rheumatoid arthritis. A prospective study over three years (the Swedish TIRA project). *Scand J Rheumatol* 2006;*35*:15–19.

9. Thyberg I, Dahlström Ö, Björk M, et al. Hand pains in women and men in early rheumatoid arthritis, a one-year follow-up after diagnosis. The Swedish TIRA project. *Disabil Rehabil* 2016;*39*:(3):291–300.

10. Erol AM, Ceceli E, Uysal Ramadan S, et al. Effect of rheumatoid arthritis on strength, dexterity, coordination and functional status of the hand: the relationship with magnetic resonance imaging findings. *Acta Rheumatol Port* 2016;*41*(4):328–37.

11. Glinatsi D, Baker JF, Hetland ML, et al. Wrist inflammation as assessed by magnetic resonance imaging is associated with patient-reported physical impairment, global disease activity and pain in early rheumatoid arthritis: long-term results from two randomized controlled trials *Ann Rheum Dis* 2017;*76*:1707–15.

12. Andrade JA, Brandão MB, Raquel C, et al. Factors associated with activity limitations in people with rheumatoid arthritis. *Am J Occup Ther* 2016;*70*:1–7.

13. Adams BD. Management of the distal radioulnar joint in rheumatoid arthritis. In: Chung K (ed.). *Clinical Management of the Rheumatoid Hand, Wrist, and Elbow*, pp. 97–104. Cham, Switzerland: Springer, 2016.

14. The Canadian Occupational Performance Measure. Available at: http://www.thecopm.ca

15. Hammond A, Tennant A, Tyson S, et al. The reliability and validity of the English version of the evaluation of daily activity questionnaire in people with rheumatoid arthritis. *Rheumatology* 2015;*54*(9):1605–15.

16. Hammond A, Tennant A, Tyson S. *The Evaluation of Daily Activity Questionnaire: User Manual v3*. Salford, UK: University of Salford, 2018. Available at: http://usir.salford.ac.uk/30752/

17. Allaire S, Keysor J. Development of a structured interview tool to help patients identify and solve rheumatic condition related work barriers. *Arthritis Care Res* 2009;*61*:988–95.

18. Hammond A, Woodbridge S, O'Brien R et al. *The UK Work Experience Survey for Persons with Rheumatic Conditions (UK WES-RC) Manual Version 3.1*. Salford, UK: University of Salford, 2018. Available at: http://usir.salford.ac.uk/29320

19. Beaton D, Tang K, Gignac MAM, et al. Reliability, validity and responsiveness of five at-work productivity measures in patients with rheumatoid arthritis or osteoarthritis. *Arthr Care Res* 2010;*62*;28–37.

20. Versus Arthritis. Examination of the hand and wrist video. https://www.versusarthritis.org/about-arthritis/healthcare-professionals/useful-resources/regional-examination-of-the-musculoskeletal-system/examination-of-the-hand-and-wrist-video/

21. Whalley K, Bradley S, Adams J. Ch. 37: Hand therapy. In: Curtin M, Egan M, Adams J (eds). *Occupational Therapy for People Experiencing Illness, Injury or Impairment: Promoting Occupation and Participation*, 7th edition, pp. 523–40. New York, NY: Elsevier, 2017.

22. Chung KC, Pillsbury MS, Walters MR, et al. Reliability and validity testing of the Michigan hand outcomes questionnaire. *J Hand Surg Am* 1998;*23*:575–87.

23. Hudak P, Amadio PC, Bombardier C, et al. Development of an upper extremity outcome measure: the DASH (Disabilities of the Arm, Shoulder, and Hand). *Am J Ind Med* 1996;*29*:602–8.

24. Ndosi M, Tennant A, Bergsten U, et al. Cross-cultural validation of the educational needs assessment tool in RA in 7 European countries. *BMC Musculoskelet Disord* 2011;*12*:110.

25. Smarr K, Keefer A. Measures of depression and depressive symptoms: Beck Depression Inventory-II (BDI-II), Center for Epidemiologic Studies Depression Scale (CES-D), Geriatric Depression Scale (GDS), Hospital Anxiety and Depression Scale (HADS), and Patient Health Questionnaire-9 (PHQ-9). *Arth Care Res* 2011;*63*(S11):S454–66.

26. Hewlett S, Cockshott Z, Kirwan J, et al. Development and validation of a self-efficacy scale for use in British patients with rheumatoid arthritis (RASE). *Rheumatology* 2001;*40*:1221–30.

27. Hammond A, Young A, Kidao R. A randomised controlled trial of occupational therapy for people with early rheumatoid arthritis. *Ann Rheum Dis* 2004;*63*:23–30.

28. Siegel P, Tencza M, Apodaca B, et al. Effectiveness of occupational therapy interventions with adults with rheumatoid arthritis: a systematic review. *Am J Occup Ther* 2016;*71*:7101180050.

29. Macedo A, Oakley SP, Panayi GS, et al. Functional and work outcomes improve in patients with rheumatoid arthritis who receive targeted, comprehensive occupational therapy. *Arthr Care Res* 2009;*61*:1522–30.

30. Mathieux R, Marotte H, Battistini L, et al. Early occupational therapy programme increases hand grip strength at 3 months: results from a randomized, blind, controlled study in early rheumatoid arthritis. *Ann Rheum Dis* 2009;*68*:400–3.

31. Hammond A, Freeman K. One-year outcomes of a randomised controlled trial of an educational-behavioural joint protection programme for people with rheumatoid arthritis. *Rheumatology* 2001;*40*:1044–51.

32. Hammond A, Freeman K. The long-term outcomes of a randomised controlled trial of an educational-behavioural joint protection programme for people with rheumatoid arthritis. *Clin Rehabil* 2004;*18*:520–8

33. Freeman K, Hammond A, Lincoln NB. Use of cognitive behavioural arthritis education programmes in newly diagnosed rheumatoid arthritis. *Clin Rehabil* 2002;*16*; 828–36.

34. Niedermann K, Buchi S, Ciurea A, et al. Six and 12 months' effects of individual joint protection education in people with rheumatoid arthritis: a randomized controlled trial. *Scand J Occup Ther* 2012;*19*:360–9.

35. Hewlett S, Ambler N, Almeida C, et al. Self-management of fatigue in rheumatoid arthritis: a randomised controlled trial of group cognitive-behavioural therapy. *Ann Rheum Dis* 2011;*70*:1060–7.

36. Hammond A, Prior Y. The effectiveness of home hand exercise programmes in rheumatoid arthritis: a systematic review. *Br Med Bull* 2016;*119* (1):49–62.

37. Lamb S, Williamson E, Heine P, et al. Exercises to improve function of the rheumatoid hand (SARAH): a randomized controlled trial. *Lancet* 2015;*385*(9966):421–9.

38. Williamson E, McConkey C, Heine P, et al. Hand exercises for patients with rheumatoid arthritis: an extended follow-up of the SARAH randomized controlled trial. *BMJ Open* 2017;*7*:e013121.

39. Royal College of Occupational Therapists. *Hand and Wrist Orthoses for Rheumatological Conditions in Adults*. London, UK: Royal College of Occupational Therapists, 2015.

40. Ong BN, Rogers A, Kennedy A, et al. Behaviour change and social blinkers? The role of sociology in trials of self-management behaviour in chronic conditions. *Sociol Health Illn* 2014;*36*:226–38.

41. Hammond A, Bryan J, Hardy A. Effects of a modular behavioural arthritis education programme: a pragmatic parallel group randomized controlled trial. *Rheumatology* 2008;*47*:1712–18.

42. McArthur MA, Goodacre L. 'Better not best': a qualitative exploration of the experiences of occupational gain for people with inflammatory arthritis receiving anti-TNFα treatment. *Disabil Rehabil* 2015;*37*:854–63.

43. Hammond A, O'Brien R, Woodbridge S, et al. Job retention vocational rehabilitation for employed people with inflammatory arthritis (WORK-IA): a feasibility randomized controlled trial. *BMC Musculoskelet Dis* 2017;*18*:315.

44. Allaire SH, Li W, La Valley MP. Reduction of job loss in persons with rheumatic diseases receiving vocational rehabilitation: a randomized controlled trial. *Arthritis Rheum* 2003;*48*:3212–18.

45. Keysor JJ, LaValley MP, Brown C, et al. Efficacy of a work disability prevention program for people with rheumatic and musculoskeletal conditions: the Work It Study Trial. *Arthritis Care Res (Hoboken)* 2018;*70*(7):1022–9.

46. Prior Y, Amanna AE, Bodell SJ, et al. A qualitative evaluation of occupational therapy-led work rehabilitation for people with inflammatory arthritis: participants' views. *Br J Occup Ther* 2017;*80*:39–48.

47. Reinseth L, Espnes GA. Women with rheumatoid arthritis: non-vocational activities and quality of life. *Scand J Occ Ther* 2007;*14*:108–15.

48. Iversen M, Hammond A, Betteridge N. Self-management of rheumatic diseases: state of the art and future directions. *Ann Rheum Dis* 2010;*69*:955–63.

49. Adams SA. Sourcing the crowd for health services improvement: the reflexive patient and 'share-your-experience' websites. *Social Sci Med* 2011;*72*:1069–76.

50. The Musculoskeletal Hub: online health assessment, community and self-management website. Salford, UK: University of Salford, 2017. Available at: https://mskhub.com

27

Self-management: A patient's perspective

Marieke M.J.H. Voshaar

Introduction

When I received my rheumatoid arthritis (RA) diagnosis at age 19, I had no concept of how my life would change. RA will have an impact on every part of your life. The challenge that I recognize now, 30 years later, is that these changes are not all negative. The way in which you perceive the illness, using skills that are not overly affected by the condition to adjust your life to enjoy it, and applying new abilities that are developed or strengthened by the condition are only a few examples of how your life changes with a lifelong progressive condition.

Several intrinsic and extrinsic factors are of huge importance how you will manage to live with a condition such as RA. Many studies have been conducted to explore which factors are essential to optimize quality of life for RA patients. As we learn that a personalized approach in many fields (e.g. personalized medicine, personalized care) reach optimal results, managing your own condition depends on intrinsic and extrinsic factors that are different for every individual patient. Personality, skills, and beliefs are different in each person, but extrinsic factors that cannot be influenced by the patient also play a role. For example, the local healthcare services, healthcare professionals, and educational programmes available can have a significant effect on the way you deal with your condition.

The combination of extrinsic and intrinsic factors forms a major part of how you can self-manage your condition, as they govern how you perceive your disease activity and can work your life around this. Furthermore, receiving adequate support from those around you is crucial for successful self-management. This includes your social circle, healthcare professionals, and your employer.

Your social environment—your relatives, partners, and friends—are important to help manage the emotional and psychological consequences that are associated with RA. Healthcare professionals are essential in aiming for disease control, and with the improvements in available medication, your employer also has an increased role in your self-management. By making reasonable adjustments in employment and career planning, developing guidelines that facilitate the re-integration of the patient into the workplace, and building daily routines and activities within the full capabilities of their employees with RA, employers can help alleviate patient burdens such as depression, isolation, and lowered self-esteem.

A PERSONAL PERSPECTIVE

My diagnosis of rheumatoid arthritis came out of nowhere. There was very little known family history, and like most members of the general public I was under the assumption that RA was a condition that only affected older people. The information available to the patient at the time of my diagnosis was less accessible to the layperson and offered a less positive prognosis than you would receive now, partially because of progress in medication development and partially owing to a greater focus on the patient-centred approach.

I was told to prepare for a future with fewer opportunities because of my disability, and that I should give up finishing my studies as the expectation of finding a job was negligible. After the first emotional shock—denial, anger, and grief—I came up with a roadmap or business plan on how I wanted to organize my life. My first step was to gain information, so I could work out who could provide each area of support to help me overcome the negative aspects of living with RA.

My primary goal was to control disease activity. I was lucky to be treated by a very wise professor, who already applied a shared decision-making process in his practice, before the concept was in common use. However, I realized that different sorts of support were going to be required in order to manage my new life with RA. Even with my roadmap in place, disease-related setbacks are inevitable, from social problems such as the temporary loss of social engagement or fewer opportunities in your career, or physical issues such as enduring another medical intervention.

However, over time I learnt the best way to manage my condition was by adjusting my goals. Despite the difficulties that living with a chronic condition have caused, valuable experiences have also opened themselves up to me as a direct consequence of RA. Fulfilling positions as a patient research partner, developing this into the role of a researcher, and championing the value of patient views as a key component of research are just some examples. Exploring and recognizing these opportunities can increase your self-confidence, strengthen self-esteem, and decrease prevalent psychological comorbidities.

To me, self-management means the having the decisive role in the management of my own life, with me in the driving seat rather than my condition.

For many RA patients, goal adjustment is a continuous necessity owing to the often unpredictable course of the condition. Therefore, from a patient perspective, it may be helpful to suggest that self-management skills need to be supported by multiple parties throughout the course of RA, via a needs-based strategy. How self-management is defined in the literature and in practice will be described in this chapter.

The requirement for self-management

Patients with a chronic condition are expected to take responsibility for the day-to-day care of their chronic illness. Applying self-management skills in daily life is an essential component to facilitating their care,[1] and although modifications to patient lifestyles can be necessary in rheumatoid arthritis, these techniques can increase quality of life.

It has been shown that teaching and enabling self-management skills can decrease the occurrence of comorbidities such as depression,[2] Furthermore, self-management can also reinforce positive behaviours that affect disease activity, such as medication adherence.[3]

Teaching patients to apply and optimize their self-management skills is therefore important to improve health outcomes. Although self-management of chronic illness is widely recognized as an essential part of rheumatoid arthritis care, many patients have difficulty managing their condition properly.[4] Recognition of these difficulties has led to the development of many self-management support programmes over recent years, with varying

What is self-management?

The holistic and patient-centred view of self-management is presented in the Barlow's definition, 'the individual's ability to manage the symptoms, treatment, physical, and psychosocial consequences and lifestyle changes inherent in living with a chronic condition and to affect the cognitive, behavioural and emotional responses necessary to maintain a satisfactory quality of life'.[5]

Self-management is often linked with patient education, but although education offers information and technical skills, a more nuanced approach to the subject is required.

Lorig et al. (2003) described self-management interventions as problem focused, action oriented, and with an emphasis on patient-generated care plans.[6] Schulman-Green et al. (2012) identified three categories of self-management processes from the perspective of the chronically ill: focusing on illness needs, activating resources, and living with a chronic illness.[7]

- **Focusing on illness needs** refers to tasks associated with medical topics, such as learning about RA, taking medicines, and practical symptom management.
- **Activating resources** refers to various services such as healthcare and social support.
- **Living with a chronic illness** encompasses processes related to daily life (e.g. housekeeping or occupational work), and emotional coping strategies for adjusting to living with RA.

Self-management can therefore be seen as a combination of patient education and medical management (focusing on illness needs) and the process of developing and maintaining new meaningful behaviours to combat mortality and morbidity, improve quality of life, and boost economic productivity (activating resources and living with a chronic illness).[8]

Health professionals often view self-management interventions as the result of structured education to develop patients' illness management skills, whereas Kralik et al. (2003) and Bode et al. (2008) have shown that patients with arthritis view the interventions as a way to bring order into their lives, help recognize boundaries, mobilize resources, cope with change, and plan, pace, and prioritize.[9,10]

These definitions of self-management can be combined, as there is overlap (see **Figure 27.1**). The **Illness needs** circle represents the first step, with the health professional's view of patient self-management techniques. The second step represents the views of the patient about the use of developing self-management skills (**Activating resources** and **Living with a chronic condition**). When the physical needs are cared for, resources must be activated to live with a chronic condition such as RA. This leads to step 3 (**Improving quality of life**)—how can self-management add to improving quality of life.

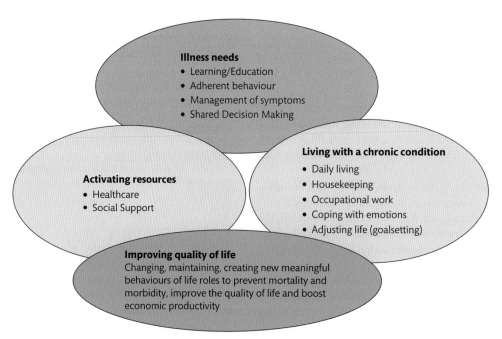

Figure 27.1 Model capturing definitions of self-management.

Definitions of self-management have changed over time, and one explanation may be that healthcare is changing from physician-centred to patient-centred care, in which the health professional and the patient together engage in shared decision-making.[3] It may be expected that the role of the health professional will change: after the first priority of aiming for remission or low disease activity, the more informed patient expects their physician to act as a collaborator in developing treatment plans. However, despite the increasing focus on improving self-management skills, it must be remembered that not all patients have the same chances or capabilities to be involved in their treatments, and therefore self-management should be approached not as a definition, but as a question, 'What does this patient need to self-manage their condition?'

Self-management over the past decade

Chronic disease self-management programmes are developed to introduce and educate participants in the core elements of the practice, including:

- Problem solving
- Decision-making
- Resource utilization
- Taking action
- Forming partnerships with healthcare providers[6,11]

The development of these programmes started in the 1980s, with the Arthritis Self-Management Program (ASMP). Designed to enhance wellbeing and quality of life, Lorig et al. demonstrated that knowledge leads to behaviour change.[12] Participants linked program satisfaction with an increased sense of disease control, and the Social Cognitive Theory of Bandura (SCT) was selected as a framework for change.[11,13] Modern self-management interventions emphasize patient-centred care plans that include educational, behavioural, and cognitive approaches.[6,14,15] Reviews of RA self-management programmes have shown that the explicit use of SCT or cognitive-behavioural therapy (CBT) led to significant short-term improvements in function,[11,16–18] although these effects are rarely sustained. Despite the good results shown by some self-management interventions,[14,15,19–26] barriers to their implementation remain, including difficulties in involving patients, physicians, and organizations; problems with accurate evaluation, and economic constraints.

Results of different self-management programmes

Self-management programmes can differ in both leadership and delivery method, and evaluation of these interventions concludes that different types result in different health outcomes.[27,28] Programmes can be led by peers (people having RA), laypeople (people not having RA), and health professionals, with delivery methods including face-to-face, over the telephone, or online. Most research into the effectiveness of self-management programmes focuses on face-to-face group interventions, with one-on-one health professional approach least evaluated in the literature.[29]

Peer-led telephone support has been shown to be effective for certain health conditions in a review of seven randomized controlled trials[30] although the conclusions did mention that few of the studies were of high quality, and there was a subsequent requirement for well-designed randomized controlled studies to better clarify the cost and clinical effectiveness for this style of programme. Small-group intervention led by peer instructors also showed significant improvements in health behaviours, self-efficacy, and health status, as well as fewer visits to the emergency department.[31] People with arthritis have also reported that becoming a self-management leader showed positive changes both in themselves and in course participants, including a reduction in pain, and an increased willingness to 'get on with life'.[32]

Lay-led self-management programmes are becoming increasingly common as a way to promote self-care for people with chronic conditions, however an analysis of the health outcomes only shows small, short-term improvements.[33]

Health professionals also offer many self-management programmes, often provided to small groups of patients. Most programmes resulted in small to moderate improvements in self-efficacy, exercise, and general health, with a reduction in depression and anxiety.[34–37]

Self-management interventions can successfully improve involvement in exercise and relaxation in housebound older adults, although long-term effects are rarely shown among arthritis patients with regard to these programmes. However, as the increase in exercise participation was maintained for up to eight months following the intervention,[38,39] and in conjunction with a growing older population, the functional gains that can be achieved could be translated into a larger overall beneficial effect.[40]

New delivery methods are currently being developed for these interventions. Online programme development has shown positive results in health status measures (health distress, activity limitation, self-reported global health, and pain) and improvements in self-efficacy for up to 1 year.[41] The Expert Patients Programme, an online peer-led self-management intervention, showed significant improvements for most of the health measures evaluated in a review of the outcomes, and concluded that it appeared to decrease symptoms, improve behaviours and self-efficacy, and reduced healthcare use for up to a year.[42] A mail-delivered arthritis tool-kit also proved effective in improving health status, behaviour, and self-efficacy variables for up to 9 months.[43] Smartphone technology is also a developing delivery system. Applications can be used without special training, and can feature user-friendly graphics and animations, with the potential for multilanguage provision with only minor changes to the intervention. They are also widely available, which could increase programme provision in rural and remote areas, and can be used at any time, helping those patients who work full time to access self-management interventions (such as MyRA). Despite these advantages, the use of smartphone apps can be limited by age, gender, and socioeconomic factors. Continuous utilization may result in several problems. Existing medical apps for people with rheumatic diseases represent a lack of high quality for longitudinal assessment for RA disease activity. According to a review of 2017[44] current apps fall into two categories; simple calculators primarily for rheumatologists and data tracking tools for people with RA. These tracking tools are not uniformly collecting data using validated instruments or composite disease activity measures. Another systematic review of 2018[45] describes that most current RA apps do not provide a comprehensive experience for individuals with RA. Areas for optimization include the implementation of smartphone accessibility features and secure methods of protecting individual health information. Once greater adoption, standardization, and implementation of relevant RA measures are in place within electronic health records, patient care will improve and the ability to learn from aggregate experiences will then increase. More responsive and better treatment results will be provided by incorporating passive and patient-reported outcomes in self-management apps and subsequently integrating these data into the patient's health record.[46]

Self-management support by health professionals

It is clear that supporting self-management skills is an essential component in improving quality of life for RA patients, but increased support of these programmes by health professionals would be beneficial for successful implementation for those people living with chronic illnesses.

Although primary care plays an important role in providing self-management education and support, owing to its reach and increasingly central role in the control of RA,[47,48] general practitioners have been reluctant to refer patients to external self-management programmes. This may because of a fear of fragmenting care, and ambiguity over the benefits to the patient.[49] Support for self-management has been difficult to embed within the primary care community, with a perceived lack of relevance and a view that enacting strategies for self-management was not a professional priority. However, successful management of chronic illnesses such as RA require an integrated approach, with active participation by the patient, their family, and the healthcare professional. Treatment will only reach optimum results when the patient and professional work in a mutual partnership, rather than focusing on the traditional concept of patient compliance and adherence.[4,45,46]

A second barrier to healthcare professionals providing adequate support for self-management is a failure to engage with and identify patients' support needs. In a study of Belgian GPs, Sunaert et al. (2011) found that the professionals were initially reluctant to refer diabetes patients to a self-management programme, and concerns over the value of these resources, difficulties with patient selection, and an increased administrative load were all cited as reasons to refer patients.[49] One possible solution may be to enhance primary care priorities, linking patients' broader systems of implementation networks and resources with pre-existing professional strategies. Furthermore, in a 2014 paper on rheumatology clinicians, it was shown that only brief training was required to implement skills that supported patient self-management.[50] As focus shifts from clinicians' agendas to those of the patient, the professionals reported that by eliciting the patients' self-reported priorities, theoretically-driven strategies such as goal setting could be used. Owing to difficulties with long-term maintenance of self-management,[51] it will be important to research the feasibility of embedding these facilitating techniques within the rheumatology clinical team. If this is possible, within a supportive clinical team with an understanding of self-management, then both patient access to these techniques and ability to maintain the strategies over a longer period

would be achieved.[14,50] Improving clinicians' skills to help patients with managing their conditions has been identified as a priority for service development,[52] but educational programmes should also be adapted for nurses.[53]

Nurses are assigned a major role in self-management support, with the expectation that they understand how living with a chronic disease impacts the daily life of their patients,[54] but also require increased training in facilitating self-management.

Broadly, nurses appear to have four major perceptions of what self-management support entails[53]:

- Coach type: focusing on the patient's daily life activities
- Clinician type: achieving adherence to treatment
- Gatekeeper type: reducing healthcare costs
- Educator type: instructing patients in illness management

While nurses tend to act on a single dominant perspective out of these four types, they should be aware that both their work environment, and the personal preferences of the patient may require a flexible approach and modifying the support they provide to best reflect the needs of the patient.

Despite the increase in patient-centred care as a concept, Wilson et al. (2006) found that within community, primary, and secondary care settings nurses reported anxiety over expert patients, with links to a lack of professional confidence and fears with regard to litigation,[55] however this view was reduced in nurse specialists. The nurse specialists had confidence in their empirical knowledge,[56] which resulted in an openness to encourage the patient perspective, but perceived competence still plays a role.[57] Compared to other health professionals, nurses were the most capable of meeting the emotional needs of the patient. Although this is a major element of self-management[7] many general nurses reported not perceiving this as a key aspect of their role.[55] Further research into the factors that result in the different responses of nurse specialists and generalist nurses may be useful in developing training programmes to ensure a better response to the expert patient, and an increased level of support for self-management techniques.

Patients' need for self-management support

Despite many self-management programmes being developed, positive effects have been modest.[1,4,58,59]

Patients expect healthcare professionals to fulfil a comprehensive role,[60] and patients with a chronic condition need instrumental, psychosocial, and relational support from healthcare professionals, family, friends, and fellow patients to successfully manage their condition.[61,62] For support to be successful, patients and professionals need to work as a collaborative partnership. Patient needs are changing over time,[61] which makes it essential to have regular assessment. Those that offer support to patients can be divided into those with strong ties (family etc.) and weaker ties (less intimate, more distanced contacts). While patients tend to rely on people with strong ties for the most support, those with weaker ties appear more durable and less liable to loss.[63] Weak ties are useful when help from a stronger tie would be inconvenient, impractical, or unwanted, encompassing a tension between the need to be seen as managing adequately without the help of others, but at the same time needing to accept external support. Intimate relationships with strong ties can overstep established boundaries maintaining a level of independence. Weak ties are valuable because they do not implicate burden or stigma about the receipt of help associated with the intense involvement of closer ties pervading more intimate caring relationships.[64] Moreover, weak ties are often based on reciprocating actions (payment, being friends) and therefore rendering the dependence/independence balance, which is experienced as less stressful, more durable, and sustainable than other ties.[63] The nature of the chronic condition is not decisive for the support needs of patients.[65] Inner negotiations to balance self-management practices and life goals were found to be crucial for integrating self-management. This balance could be disturbed by experiencing new or increased symptoms, perceiving new health threats, not experiencing the anticipated effects of self-management, or encountering new information about possible self-management practices.[66,67] In these cases, the patient needs to find a new temporary balance by shifting to another self-management strategy.

The individual context of each patient also affects conditions for self-management integration. Overarching factors include age, ethnicity, gender, and the psychological profile of the patient (including personal feelings about the disease).[61] Patients with comorbidities have also been found to encounter problems with performing self-management, with greater difficulties integrating practices into daily life.[67–73] Some common barriers are depression, weight problems, and difficulty in exercising, fatigue, and pain. Lack of support from family members and poor communication with physicians also cause complications.[74] Problems with accessing self-management resources can also negatively impact the patient's ability to successfully obtain necessary support. Access can be hindered by physical symptoms, difficulties with transportation, and insufficient insurance coverage, as well as a general lack of awareness that the resources are available. In the latter case, poor health literacy can arise when patients are from socially disadvantaged backgrounds. Therefore, healthcare professionals need to facilitate self-management integration tailored to the individual patient's lifestyle and experience,[67] and ensure ongoing communication with both the patient and supper providers to adjust plans if circumstances change.[7]

Suggestions to improve self-management programmes

All chronic illness support, including self-management programmes, require an ongoing relationship between the patient and provider, including considerations of individual barriers as described in the previous section.[75,76] It is essential to both identify and engage with the patient's support requirements; continuous dialogue to improve self-management programmes is an essential part of providing adequate health support as a health professional.[77] However, as the effects of such programmes have been found to be limited, methods of improving integration into patients' lives is vital. Furthermore, although short-term effects are generally observed, long-term changes in health status are not convincingly demonstrated, indicating a requirement for more effective engagement. This may be through facilitating a broader understanding of the aims of the programme into the person's wider support networks, or making participation easier through mobile technology. This could help engage patients

and sustain beneficial changes in behaviour,[78] which in turn may improve the transfer of short-term benefits to long-term improvement in outcomes.[79] It is also necessary to provide sufficient information on the aims of self-management programmes, which should manage the patient's expectations while sustaining intrinsic motivation.[36] Further strategies need to be found to improve the efficacy of these schemes.

REFERENCES

1. van Houtum L, Rijken M, Heijmans M, Groenewegen P. Self-management support needs of patients with chronic illness: do needs for support differ according to the course of illness? *Patient Educ Couns* 2013;93(3):626–32.
2. Vermaak V, Briffa NK, Langlands B, Inderjeeth C, McQuade J. Evaluation of a disease specific rheumatoid arthritis self-management education program, a single group repeated measures study. *BMC Musculoskelet Disord* 2015;16:214.
3. Voshaar MJ, Nota I, van de Laar MA, van den Bemt BJ. Patient-centred care in established rheumatoid arthritis. *Best Pract Res Clin Rheumatol* 2015;29(4–5):643–63.
4. Newman S, Steed K, Mulligan K. Self-management interventions for chronic illness. *Lancet* 2004;364(9444):1523–37.
5. Barlow J, Wright C, Sheasby J, Turner A, Hainsworth J. Self-management approaches for people with chronic conditions: a review. *Patient Educ Counsel* 2002;48(2):177–87.
6. Lorig KR, Holman H. Self-management education: history, definition, outcomes, and mechanisms. *Ann Behav Med* 2003;26(1):1–7.
7. Schulman-Green D, Jaser S, Martin F, et al. Processes of self-management in chronic illness. *J Nurs Scholarsh* 2012;44(2):136–44.
8. Redman BK. The ethics of self-management preparation for chronic illness. *Nurs Ethics* 2005;12(4):360–9.
9. Bode C, Taal E, Emon PAA, et al., Limited results of group self-management education for rheumatoid arthritis patients and their partners: explanations from the patient perspective. *Clin Rheumatol* 2008;27(12):1523–8.
10. Kralik D, Koch T, Price K, Howard N. Chronic illness self-management: taking action to create order. *J Clin Nurs* 2004;13(2):259–67.
11. Iversen MD, Hammond A, Betteridge N. Self-management of rheumatic diseases: state of the art and future perspectives. *Ann Rheum Dis* 2010;69(6):955–63.
12. Lorig KR. Arthritis self-management: a patient education program. *Arthritis Rheum* 1993;36(4):439–46.
13. Bandura A. Self-efficacy: toward a unifying theory of behavioral change. *Psychol Rev* 1977;84(2):191–215.
14. Dures E, Hewlett S. Cognitive-behavioural approaches to self-management in rheumatic disease. *Nat Rev Rheumatol* 2012;8(9):553–9.
15. Garnefski N, Kraaij V, Benoist M, Bout Z, Karels E, Smit A. Effect of a cognitive behavioral self-help intervention on depression, anxiety, and coping self-efficacy in people with rheumatic disease. *Arthritis Care Res (Hoboken)* 2013;65(7):1077–84.
16. Niedermann K, Fransen J, Knols R, Uebelhart D. Gap between short- and long-term effects of patient education in rheumatoid arthritis patients: a systematic review. *Arthritis Rheum* 2004;51(3):388–98.

17. Riemsma RP, Taal E, Kirwan JR, Rasker JJ. Systematic review of rheumatoid arthritis patient education. *Arthritis Rheum* 2004;*51*(6):1045–59.

18. Nunez DE, Keller CD, Fau-Ananian C, Ananian CD. A review of the efficacy of the self-management model on health outcomes in community-residing older adults with arthritis. *Evid Based Nurs* 2009;*6*(3):130–48.

19. Goeppinger J, Lorig KR, Ritter PL, Mutatkar S, Villa F, Gizlice Z. Mail-delivered arthritis self-management tool kit: a randomized trial and longitudinal followup. *Arthritis Rheum* 2009;*61*(7):867–75.

20. Goeppinger J, Armstrong B, Schwartz T, Ensley D, Brady TJ. Self-management education for persons with arthritis: managing comorbidity and eliminating health disparities. *Arthritis Rheum* 2007;*57*(6):1081–8.

21. Lorig KR, Ritter PL, Laurent DD, Plant K. The internet-based arthritis self-management program: a one-year randomized trial for patients with arthritis or fibromyalgia. *Arthritis Rheum* 2008;*59*(7):1009–17.

22. Lorig K, Ritter K, Plant K. A disease-specific self-help program compared with a generalized chronic disease self-help program for arthritis patients. *Arthritis Rheum* 2005;*53*(6):950–7.

23. Lorig KR, Sobel DS, Ritter PL, Laurent D, Hobbs M. Effect of a self-management program on patients with chronic disease. *Eff Clin Pract* 2001;*4*(6):256–62.

24. Nour K, Laforest S, Gauvin L, Gignac M. Long-term maintenance of increased exercise involvement following a self-management intervention for housebound older adults with arthritis. *Int J Behav Nutr Phys Activity* 2007;*4*(22):1–8.

25. Nour K, Laforest S, Gauvin L, Gignac M. Behavior change following a self-management intervention for housebound older adults with arthritis: an experimental study. *Int J Behav Nutr Phys Act* 2006;*3*:12.

26. Foster G, Taylor SJ, Eldridge SE, Ramsay J, Griffiths CJ. Self-management education programmes by lay leaders for people with chronic conditions. *Cochrane Database Syst Rev* 2007;(4):CD005108.

27. Kendall E, Ehrlich C, Sunderland N, Muenchberger H, Rushton C. Self-managing versus self-management: reinvigorating the socio-political dimensions of self-management. *Chronic Illn* 2011;*7*(1):87–98.

28. Glasgow NJ, Jeon YH, Kraus SG, Pearce-Brown CL. Chronic disease self-management support: the way forward for Australia. *Med J Aust* 2008;*189*(S10):S14–16.

29. Cameron KA. Healthy aging: programs that make a difference-part 1. *Consult Pharm* 2012;*27*(4):239–53.

30. Dale J, Caramlau IO, Lindenmeyer A, Williams SM. Peer support telephone calls for improving health. *Cochrane Database Syst Rev* 2008;(4):CD006903.

31. Lorig KR, Sobel DS, Ritter PL, Laurent D, Hobbs M. Effect of a self-management program on patients with chronic disease. *Eff Clin Pract* 2001;*4*(6):256–62.

32. Hainsworth J, Barlow J. Volunteers' experiences of becoming arthritis self-management lay leaders: 'It's almost as if I've stopped aging and started to get younger!'. *Arthritis Rheum* 2001;*45*(4):378–83.

33. Foster G, Taylor SJ, Eldridge SE, Ramsay J, Griffiths CJ. Self-management education programmes by lay leaders for people with chronic conditions. *Cochrane Database Syst Rev* 2007(4):CD005108.

34. Goeppinger J, Armstrong B, Schwartz T, Ensley D, Brady TJ. Self-management education for persons with arthritis: managing comorbidity and eliminating health disparities. *Arthritis Rheum* 2007;*57*(6):1081–8.

35. Warsi A, Wang PS, LaValley MP, Avorn J, Solomon DH. Self-management education programs in chronic disease: a systematic review and methodological critique of the literature. *Arch Intern Med* 2004;*164*(15):1641–9.

36. Bode C, Taal E, Emons PA, et al. Limited results of group self-management education for rheumatoid arthritis patients and their partners: explanations from the patient perspective. *Clin Rheumatol* 2008;*27*(12):1523–8.

37. Garnefski N, Kraaij V, Benoist M, Bout Z, Karels E, Smit A. Effect of a cognitive behavioral self-help intervention on depression, anxiety, and coping self-efficacy in people with rheumatic disease. *Arthritis Care Res (Hoboken)* 2013;*65*(7):1077–84.

38. Nour K, Laforest S, Gauvin L, Gignac M. Behavior change following a self-management intervention for housebound older adults with arthritis: an experimental study. *Int J Behav Nutr Phys Act* 2006;*3*:12.

39. Nour K, Laforest S, Gauvin L, Gignac M. Long-term maintenance of increased exercise involvement following a self-management intervention for housebound older adults with arthritis. *Int J Behav Nutr Phys Act* 2007;*4*:22.

40. Nunez DE, Keller C, Ananian CD. A review of the efficacy of the self-management model on health outcomes in community-residing older adults with arthritis. *Worldviews Evid Based Nurs* 2009;*6*(3):130–48.

41. Lorig KR, Ritter PL, Laurent DD, Plant K. The internet-based arthritis self-management program: a one-year randomized trial for patients with arthritis or fibromyalgia. *Arthritis Rheum* 2008;*59*(7):1009–17.

42. Lorig KR, Ritter PL, Dost A, Plant K, Laurent DD, McNeil I. The Expert Patients Programme online, a 1-year study of an Internet-based self-management programme for people with long-term conditions. *Chronic Illn* 2008;*4*(4):247–56.

43. Goeppinger J, Lorig KR, Ritter PL, Mutatkar S, Villa F, Gizlice Z. Mail-delivered arthritis self-management tool kit: a randomized trial and longitudinal followup. *Arthritis Rheum* 2009;*61*(7):867–75.

44. Grainger R, Townsley H, White B, Langlotz T, Taylor WJ. Apps for people with rheumatoid arthritis to monitor their disease activity: a review of apps for best practice and quality. *JMIR Mhealth Uhealth* 2017;*5*(2):e7.

45. Luo D, Wang P, Lu F, Elias J, Sparks JA, Lee YC. Mobile apps for individuals with rheumatoid arthritis: a systematic review. *J Clin Rheumatol* 2019;*25*(3):133–41.

46. Dixon W, Michaud K. Using technology to support clinical care and research in rheumatoid arthritis. *Curr Opin Rheumatol* 2018;*30*(3):276–81.

47. Holman H, Lorig K. Patient self-management: a key to effectiveness and efficiency in care of chronic disease. *Public Health Rep* 2004;*119*(3):239–43.

48. Carryer J, Budge C, Hansen C, Gibbs K. Providing and receiving self-management support for chronic illness: patients' and health practitioners' assessments. *J Prim Health Care* 2010;*2*(2):124–9.

49. Truglio J, Graziano M, Vedanthan R, et al. Global health and primary care: increasing burden of chronic diseases and need for integrated training. *Mt Sinai J Med* 2012;*79*(4):464–74.

50. Kennedy A, Rogers A, Chew-Graham C, et al. Implementation of a self-management support approach (WISE) across a health system: a process evaluation explaining what did and did not work for organisations, clinicians and patients. *Implement Sci* 2014;*9*:129.

51. Sunaert P, Vandekerckhove M, Bastiaens H, et al. Why do GPs hesitate to refer diabetes patients to a self-management education program: a qualitative study. *BMC Fam Pract* 2011;*12*:94.

52. Dures E, Hewlett S, Ambler N, Jenkins R, Clarke J, Gooberman-Hill R. Rheumatology clinicians' experiences of brief training and implementation of skills to support patient self-management. *BMC Musculoskelet Disord* 2014;*15*:108.

53. Abraham C, Gardner B. What psychological and behaviour changes are initiated by 'expert patient' training and what training techniques are most helpful? *Psychol Health* 2009;*24*(10):1153–65.

54. Newman S, Steed L, Mulligan K. Self-management interventions for chronic illness. *Lancet* 2004;*364*(9444):1523–37.

55. van Hooft SM, Dwarswaard J, Jedeloo S, Bal R, van Staa A. Four perspectives on self-management support by nurses for people with chronic conditions: a Q-methodological study. *Int J Nurs Stud* 2015;*52*(1):157–66.

56. Alleyne G, Hancock C, Hughes P. Chronic and non-communicable diseases: a critical challenge for nurses globally. *Int Nurs Rev* 2011;*58*(3):328–31.

57. Wilson PM, Kendall S, Brooks F. Nurses' responses to expert patients: the rhetoric and reality of self-management in long-term conditions: a grounded theory study. *Int J Nurs Stud* 2006;*43*(7):803–18.

58. Henderson S. Power imbalance between nurses and patients: a potential inhibitor of partnership in care. *J Clin Nurs* 2003;*12*(4):501–8.

59. Williams GC, McGregor HA, King D, Nelson CC, Glasgow RE. Variation in perceived competence, glycemic control, and patient satisfaction: relationship to autonomy support from physicians. *Patient Educ Couns* 2005;*57*(1):39–45.

60. Warsi A, Wang PS, LaValley MP, Avorn J, Solomon DH. Self-management education programs in chronic disease: a systematic review and methodological critique of the literature. *Arch Intern Med* 2004;*164*(15):1641–9.

61. Gardetto NJ. Self-management in heart failure: where have we been and where should we go? *J Multidiscip Healthc* 2011;*4*:39–51.

62. Elissen A, Nolte E, Knai C, et al. Is Europe putting theory into practice? A qualitative study of the level of self-management support in chronic care management approaches. *BMC Health Serv Res* 2013;*13*:117.

63. Dwarswaard J, Bakker EJ, van Staa A, Boeije HR. Self-management support from the perspective of patients with a chronic condition: a thematic synthesis of qualitative studies. *Health Expect* 2016;*19*(2):194–208.

64. Thirsk LM, Clark AM. What is the 'self' in chronic disease self-management? *Int J Nurs Stud* 2014;*51*(5):691–3.

65. Rogers A, Brooks H, Vassilev I, et al. Why less may be more: a mixed methods study of the work and relatedness of 'weak ties'

66. Pickard S. The 'good carer': moral practices in late modernity. *Sociology* 2010;*44*(3):471–87.

67. van Houtum L, Rijken M, Heijmans M, Groenewegen P. Patient-perceived self-management tasks and support needs of people with chronic illness: generic or disease specific? *Ann Behav Med* 2015;*49*(2):221–9.

68. Hibbard JH, Mahoney ER, Stock R, Tusler M. Do increases in patient activation result in improved self-management behaviors? *Health Serv Res* 2007;*42*(4):1443–63.

69. Audulv A, Asplund K, Norbergh KG. The integration of chronic illness self-management. *Qual Health Res* 2012;*22*(3):332–45.

70. Bai YL, Chiou CP, Chang YY. Self-care behaviour and related factors in older people with Type 2 diabetes. *J Clin Nurs* 2009;*18*(23):3308–15.

71. Carbone ET, Rosal MC, Torres MI, Goins KV, Bermudez OI. Diabetes self-management: perspectives of Latino patients and their health care providers. *Patient Educ Couns* 2007;*66*(2):202–10.

72. Clark DO, Frankel RM, Morgan DL, et al. The meaning and significance of self-management among socioeconomically vulnerable older adults. *J Gerontol B Psychol Sci Soc Sci* 2008;*63*(5):S312–19.

73. Egede LE, Ellis C, Grubaugh AL. The effect of depression on self-care behaviors and quality of care in a national sample of adults with diabetes. *Gen Hosp Psychiatry* 2009;*31*(5):422–7.

74. Kerr EA, Heisler M, Krein SL, et al. Beyond comorbidity counts: how do comorbidity type and severity influence diabetes patients' treatment priorities and self-management? *J Gen Intern Med* 2007;*22*(12):1635–40.

75. Schnell-Hoehn KN, Naimark BJ, Tate RB. Determinants of self-care behaviors in community-dwelling patients with heart failure. *J Cardiovasc Nurs* 2009;*24*(1):40–7.

76. Jerant AF, von Friederichs-Fitzwater MM, Moore M. Patients' perceived barriers to active self-management of chronic conditions. *Patient Educ Couns* 2005;*57*(3):300–7.

77. Carryer J, Budge C, Hansen C, Gibbs K. Providing and receiving self-management support for chronic illness: patients' and health practitioners' assessments. *J Prim Health Care* 2010;*2*(2):124–9.

78. Kennedy A, Rogers A, Chew-Graham C, et al. Implementation of a self-management support approach (WISE) across a health system: a process evaluation explaining what did and did not work for organisations, clinicians and patients. *Implement Sci* 2014;*9*:129.

79. Niedermann K, Fransen J, Knols R, Uebelhart D. Gap between short- and long-term effects of patient education in rheumatoid arthritis patients: a systematic review. *Arthritis Rheum* 2004;*51*(3):388–98.

SECTION 7
Drug treatments

28 Analgesics, opioids, and NSAIDs *331*
    Mark D. Russell and Nidhi Sofat

29 Glucocorticoids *339*
    Johannes W.G. Jacobs, Marlies C. van der Goes,
    Johannes W.J. Bijlsma, and José A.P. da Silva

30 Conventional disease-modifying drugs *355*
    David L. Scott

31 Tumour necrosis factor inhibitors *371*
    Peter C. Taylor and Nehal Narayan

32 Interleukin-6 inhibitors *389*
    Neelam Hassan and Ernest Choy

33 B-cell therapies *399*
    Md Yuzaiful Md Yusof, Edward M. Vital, and Maya H. Buch

34 Biosimilars *411*
    Vibeke Strand, Jeffrey Kaine, and John Isaacs

35 Immunogenicity in response to biologic
    agents *425*
    Meghna Jani, John Isaacs, and Vibeke Strand

36 The use of JAK inhibitors in the treatment of
    rheumatoid arthritis *443*
    Katie Bechman, James Galloway, and Peter C. Taylor

37 Combination therapy in rheumatoid arthritis *457*
    Ben G.T. Coumbe, Elena Nikiphorou, and Tuulikki Sokka-Isler

38 Translation of new therapies: From bench to
    bedside *463*
    Jeremy Sokolove

39 Adverse events in clinical studies in rheumatoid
    arthritis *471*
    Mark Yates and James Galloway

28

Analgesics, opioids, and NSAIDs

Mark D. Russell and Nidhi Sofat

Introduction

Rheumatoid arthritis (RA) is a chronic, progressive autoimmune disease characterized by joint pain, stiffness, and systemic inflammation. There have been major advances in our understanding of RA pathophysiology in recent decades, partly driven by therapeutics targeting cytokine pathways including TNF alpha, IL-6, IL-1, and JAK/STATs. Synovitis, a classical feature of rheumatoid arthritis, generates bioactive lipids, kinins, and cytokines. Cytokines released in the arthritic joint, together with other inflammatory mediators including leukotrienes and prostaglandins, contribute to nociceptive pain inputs in RA. In this chapter, we discuss nociceptive treatment targets for pain in RA, including non-steroidal anti-inflammatory drugs (NSAIDs). Sustained nociceptive input, as found in RA, can lead to changes in central pain processing. Nociceptive input is increased following local sensitization of peripheral nerves within the joint. Coupled with inflammation, it is known that major mediators of pain include neuropeptides (e.g. calcitonin gene-related peptide CGRP) and neurotrophins such as nerve growth factor (NGF), each of which can also sensitize peripheral nerves. Immune cells within the CNS directly contribute to developing central sensitization through the generation of cytokines such as IL-1. Interest has therefore grown in analgesics for RA pain that may target the CNS, including opiates and centrally acting analgesics. In this chapter, we discuss the scientific basis of pain in RA, followed by treatments currently widely used in clinical practice, including NSAIDs, opioids, and centrally acting analgesics.

Mechanisms of pain in rheumatoid arthritis

With the advent of new therapies for RA over the last two decades, people with this chronic condition have many more favourable outcomes than they did in the past.[1] Several large randomized controlled trials that underpin the use of disease-modifying antirheumatic drugs (DMARDs) showed statistically significant reductions in pain, stiffness, and swelling with improved health-related quality of life.[2] However, despite often apparent successful inhibition of inflammation by oral DMARDs and/or biologic therapies such as

TNF inhibitors, people with RA often describe pain as being constantly present, and often rate it to be at significant levels.[3] In observational studies of people starting timely DMARD treatment, the mean levels of pain remain significant at follow-up.[4,5] The aetiology of RA pain can be complex, with pain being a major component of flare-ups of RA. Traditionally, RA pain has been described as nociceptive in nature, largely mediated by synovitis, with inflammatory mediator release including prostaglandins, leukotrienes, and cytokines such as TNF alpha, IL-1, and IL-6. Suppression of inflammation often leads to reductions in synovitis and pain, as is well demonstrated after successful treatment with DMARDs. However, people with RA often report changes in pain symptoms during the day, including week to week. Fatigue and mood, in addition to joint swelling, can influence pain and contribute to flare-ups.[6] Interestingly, not all RA flares are associated with noticeable joint swelling or increases in erythrocyte sedimentation rate (ESR) or C-reactive protein (CRP). Painful flares in RA without evidence of inflammation have sometimes been termed 'fibromyalgic rheumatoid' flare-ups in disease activity.[7-9] Non-inflammatory rheumatoid flare-ups may be characterized by high pain reporting when assessing people on Visual Analogue Scale (VAS) for pain, but who have controlled inflammation on evaluation by the Disease Activity Score 28 (DAS28), with low levels of ESR and/or CRP, joint swelling, or synovitis.[10] It may therefore be that by better identifying nociceptive pain features in RA, these are best targeted with agents that suppress inflammation, including DMARDs and NSAIDs. More recently, interest has grown in central sensitization in RA, with the possibility that centrally acting analgesics could be a treatment target. In cases where NSAIDs are contraindicated or lose efficacy, centrally acting analgesics may provide a realistic alternative for pain management in RA (e.g. amitriptyline and gabapentinoids). The evidence for distinct pain-targeting medications, with their pharmacological action in RA, is discussed in subsequent sections. For a summary of analgesics which may be of benefit in RA, please see **Table 28.1**.

Figure 28.1 shows the known mechanisms driving pain in rheumatoid arthritis at the local joint level, dorsal root ganglion, and central neural level. Potential therapeutic options targeted at specific components of pain are also shown.

Table 28.1 Summary of agents currently in use for pain management in rheumatoid arthritis

Non-steroidal anti-inflammatory drugs (NSAIDs)	
Non-COX selective	Diclofenac, ibuprofen, naproxen, piroxicam
COX-2 selective	Celecoxib, etoricoxib, meloxicam
Analgesic (inhibitor of prostaglandin synthesis)	Paracetamol (UK, Europe) Acetaminophen (US)
Opioids	Codeine, dihydrocodeine
Serotonin noradrenaline reuptake inhibitors (SNRIs)	Duloxetine, venlafaxine
Selective serotonin reuptake inhibitors (SSRIs)	Fluoxetine, paroxetine
Gabapentinoids	Gabapentin, pregabalin
Tricyclic antidepressant	Amitriptyline, nortriptyline

Non-steroidal anti-inflammatory drugs

NSAIDs have been important tools in the management of pain and inflammation in RA patients for many decades. The analgesic and anti-inflammatory properties of NSAIDs are mediated through the inhibition of cyclooxygenase (COX)-associated prostaglandin production. In addition to many other physiological actions, prostaglandins form part of the inflammatory cascade associated with RA, and contribute to the sensitization of peripheral and central neurons to painful stimuli.[11] The use of NSAIDs can lead to rapid improvements in symptoms, including pain and stiffness, making them effective analgesics for the management of active RA.

Following their introduction into clinical practice, a large number of studies have been performed to compare the efficacy and safety

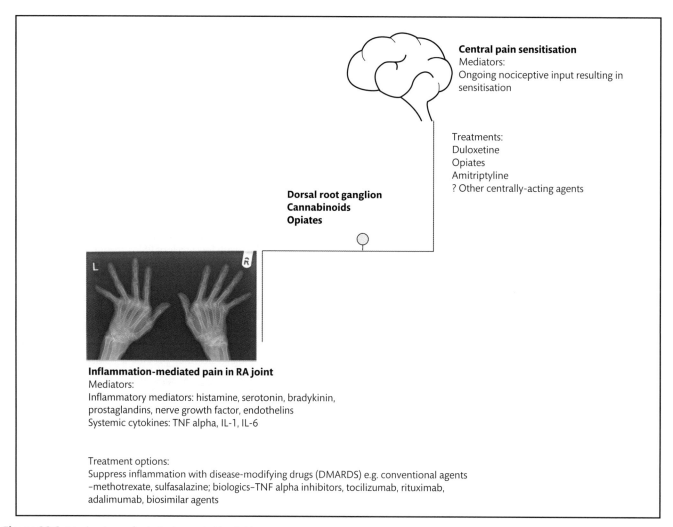

Central pain sensitisation
Mediators:
Ongoing nociceptive input resulting in sensitisation

Treatments:
Duloxetine
Opiates
Amitriptyline
? Other centrally-acting agents

Dorsal root ganglion
Cannabinoids
Opiates

Inflammation-mediated pain in RA joint
Mediators:
Inflammatory mediators: histamine, serotonin, bradykinin, prostaglandins, nerve growth factor, endothelins
Systemic cytokines: TNF alpha, IL-1, IL-6

Treatment options:
Suppress inflammation with disease-modifying drugs (DMARDS) e.g. conventional agents –methotrexate, sulfasalazine; biologics–TNF alpha inhibitors, tocilizumab, rituximab, adalimumab, biosimilar agents

Figure 28.1 Mechanisms of pain in rheumatoid arthritis.

of NSAIDs in the management of RA. Aspirin was the benchmark against which many novel NSAIDs were tested in early clinical studies. In the majority of these studies, the efficacy of newer NSAIDs, including ibuprofen and naproxen, was found to be similar to aspirin but with improved tolerability and safety profiles.[12,13] However, the risk of adverse events even with the newer generation of NSAIDs remains a major concern, reflecting the many physiological roles of prostaglandins. A multitude of studies have reported increases in cardiovascular risk, hypertension, acute and chronic renal dysfunction, hepatotoxicity, and bleeding risk with NSAID use. Perhaps most feared is the potential for NSAID-induced gastrointestinal (GI) bleeding and perforation. This is a particular concern for RA patients, where the risks of chronic NSAID use may be compounded by the presence of comorbidities and other GI-toxic medications, including steroids. Gastrointestinal adverse events are up to 10-times more common in regular users of NSAIDs than non-users, depending on the number of additional risk factors and the age of the patient.[14–16] Importantly, the elevated risk of GI complications is present from the first dose of an NSAID.[17,18] Careful consideration must therefore be given to both short and long-term NSAID prescriptions.

Non-selective NSAIDs, for example ibuprofen and naproxen, inhibit both the COX-1 and COX-2 isoenzymes. Whereas COX-2 is an inducible mediator of inflammation and nociception, COX-1 has important constitutive actions in maintaining the gastrointestinal mucosal barrier through prostanoid production. COX-2 selective inhibitors have been developed with the aim of preserving the analgesic and anti-inflammatory properties of non-selective NSAIDs, while reducing the risk of gastrointestinal toxicity through preservation of the actions of COX-1.[19] Numerous head-to-head trials have confirmed these findings of comparable efficacy and improved gastrointestinal safety with COX-2 selective inhibitors in patients with RA.[19-22] In one study, celecoxib—a COX-2 selective inhibitor—and naproxen both showed superior analgesic and anti-inflammatory effects relative to placebo, with maximal efficacy reached within 2 weeks.[19] Following 12 weeks of therapy, 26% of naproxen-treated patients had developed gastroduodenal ulcers on endoscopic examination, compared to only 4% of placebo-treated patients and 4–6% of celecoxib-treated patients. In the CLASS study, high-dose celecoxib treatment resulted in fewer gastrointestinal ulcers and complications than ibuprofen or diclofenac in RA and osteoarthritis (OA) patients.[21] Reductions in hepatotoxicity and renal toxicity were also noted in the celecoxib cohort. A recent Cochrane Group review of celecoxib use in RA supported these findings, with symptomatic improvements that were at least comparable to non-selective NSAIDs, combined with a 12% absolute reduction in gastroduodenal ulcers larger than 3 mm with celecoxib relative to non-selective NSAIDs.[23] The COX-2 inhibitor, etoricoxib, has also been shown to produce rapid, sustained improvements in efficacy outcomes, comparable to that of naproxen.[24] One study did, however, report a dose-related increase in hypertension-related adverse events with etoricoxib over naproxen.

Studies have also compared the gastrointestinal toxicity of COX-2 inhibitors and non-selective NSAIDs with concomitant gastroprotection. In a study of over 4000 *Helicobacter pylori*-negative OA and RA patients, clinically significant gastrointestinal events were more frequent in patients taking diclofenac and omeprazole, a proton pump inhibitor, than those taking celecoxib; occurring in 3.8% and 0.9% of patients, respectively.[25] It has also been suggested that proton pump inhibitors, when used chronically, may be associated with an increased incidence of gastrointestinal infections and fractures.

The excitement surrounding COX-2 inhibitors was tempered by the cardiovascular risk signals that arose from the Vioxx Gastrointestinal Research (VIGOR) study in 2004. In a study of over 8000 patients with RA, VIGOR compared the gastrointestinal safety profile of the COX-2 inhibitor, rofecoxib, and naproxen.[26] Again, comparable efficacy was demonstrated between the two study treatments, and significantly fewer upper gastrointestinal events occurred in the rofecoxib cohort than the naproxen cohort, with a relative risk of 0.5. However, higher rates of myocardial infarction were noted with rofecoxib (0.4%) relative to naproxen (0.1%). The difference in infarction rates was primarily evident in the subgroup of study participants at high risk for myocardial infarctions but not on low-dose aspirin therapy. This increased risk of vascular events was explained theoretically by the COX-2-mediated inhibition of prostacyclin, in the absence of inhibition of COX-1-derived thromboxane A_2 production—resulting in a prothrombotic state. The authors of the VIGOR study also noted that naproxen has a prominent inhibitory action on thromboxane production and, thus, platelet aggregation, and may therefore be relatively cardioprotective when compared to other non-selective NSAIDs.

The cardiovascular risks associated with COX-2 inhibitors and other NSAIDs have since been assessed in numerous additional studies. The APPROVe study—designed to assess the effects of rofecoxib on the prevention of adenomatous polyps—showed an increased incidence of thrombotic events, particularly myocardial infarctions and ischaemic strokes, with rofecoxib versus placebo (relative risk of 1.92).[27] A dose-related increase in cardiovascular and cerebrovascular events was also noted in a study of high-dose celecoxib for the prevention of polyps.[28] Initial meta-analyses supported earlier hypotheses by demonstrating increased vascular event rates with the COX-2 inhibitor class of drugs, ibuprofen and diclofenac, but not naproxen.[29] This contrasted data obtained from the Alzheimer's Disease Anti-Inflammatory Prevention Trial (ADAPT), suggestive of increased cardiovascular and cerebrovascular event rates with naproxen.[30]

The high COX-2 inhibitor doses employed in many of these studies, combined with the low overall incidence of cardiovascular events, precluded firm conclusions about the relative safety of COX-2 inhibitors and non-selective NSAIDs. The recently published PRECISION study addressed many of these questions. The safety profiles of celecoxib, naproxen and ibuprofen were compared prospectively against placebo in over 24 000 RA and OA patients with increased cardiovascular risk.[31] A lower dose of celecoxib was employed, with mean daily dosages of the three active mediations being 209 mg, 852 mg, and 2045 mg, respectively, for an average treatment duration of 20 months. Gastroprotection was provided for all patients in the form of a proton pump inhibitor, and concomitant low-dose aspirin usage was permitted. No significant differences were noted between the three medications in the primary composite outcome of time to occurrence of cardiovascular death, non-fatal myocardial infarction, or non-fatal stroke. The event rate for serious gastrointestinal events was significantly lower with celecoxib than either naproxen or ibuprofen, despite the use of gastroprotection in all patients. Serious renal adverse events and the rates of hospitalization for hypertension were less frequent with celecoxib than ibuprofen, but not significantly different between celecoxib and naproxen. In a post-hoc analysis of the study data, the risk of major toxicity events was elevated for both naproxen and ibuprofen relative to celecoxib.[32] In terms of analgesic efficacy, naproxen was more effective than either celecoxib or ibuprofen, albeit very modestly—with VAS reductions from baseline of 10.2, 9.3, and 9.5 mm, respectively (on a scale of 0–100 mm). No significant differences in global assessments of arthritis or the Health Assessment Questionnaire disability index were noted between the three treatments.

Ultimately, the decision to commence a COX-2 selective or non-selective NSAID requires a case-by-case assessment of gastrointestinal, cardiovascular, hepatic, and renal risk factors, in consultation with the patient. In patients with acceptable risk profiles, oral NSAIDs should be used at the lowest effective dose for the shortest possible period of time. There should be close monitoring for adverse effects, and coprescription of gastroprotection should be strongly considered when non-selective NSAIDs are used. Particular attention should also be paid to minimizing other cardiovascular risk factors, for example, hypertension and diabetes.

Topical NSAIDs, in the forms of gels and solutions, may be useful for patients with localized areas of pain and inflammation. Plasma concentrations of NSAIDs applied topically are much reduced relative to oral administration[33]—lowering the potential for systemic adverse effects. In a retrospective analysis, no association was found between topical NSAID use and upper GI bleeding and perforations, after adjustment for confounding factors.[34] Unfortunately, only limited data are available for topical NSAID use in RA, with most evidence being derived from studies of OA patients. In a systematic review,[35] topical diclofenac and topical ketoprofen were more effective than placebo at reducing pain in OA patients, with 60% of participants reporting much reduced pain. However, the effects of topical placebo were high: 50% obtained clinical improvement, double that of oral placebo. From the limited available safety data, systemic side effects from topical NSAIDs were not found to be significantly different to placebo.

Paracetamol

The low cost and favourable side effect profile of paracetamol (acetaminophen) makes it an attractive treatment option for a range of painful musculoskeletal conditions. It is frequently chosen as a first-line analgesic for RA patients with risk factors that preclude the safe use of NSAIDs. A trial of paracetamol is also recommended for patients who have had inadequate pain relief with NSAIDs or those with chronic NSAID requirements.[36] In such patients, the concomitant use of paracetamol may reduce the requirement for NSAIDs and, thus, potentially reduce toxicity.

Despite our limited understanding of its mechanism of action, paracetamol is thought generally to have predominantly analgesic, rather than anti-inflammatory, properties. There are some data to suggest that paracetamol does indeed reduce inflammation in arthritis patients. In a small study of participants with knee OA,[37] reductions in knee effusion volumes and synovial tissue volumes were comparable between paracetamol and NSAIDs. As noted by the authors of this study, it is not clear whether these proposed anti-inflammatory actions occur directly or through the inhibition of neurogenic inflammation.

A paucity of available data makes it challenging to draw evidence-based conclusions about paracetamol's efficacy in RA. A Cochrane Group systematic review, published in 2008, identified only four suitable studies comparing paracetamol and NSAIDs in the management of RA.[38] Although limited by the small number of subjects and the potential for bias, a preference for NSAIDs over paracetamol was reported by the majority of patients and investigators. A more recent review of 12 short-term, randomized controlled trials—including the four aforementioned studies—found weak evidence favouring paracetamol over placebo in terms of efficacy[39]; with a suggestion of additive analgesic effects when paracetamol was coadministered with NSAIDs. In a survey study of 1800 rheumatology patients (including 825 patients with RA), three-quarters of RA patients reported at least some efficacy with paracetamol—the majority reporting either slight efficacy (38.5%) or moderate efficacy (31.8%). However, 65% of RA patients found paracetamol to be either much less effective or somewhat less effective than NSAIDs, with 23% reporting similar benefits and 12% reporting a preference for paracetamol.[40]

Recently, paracetamol's efficacy in the management of other painful musculoskeletal conditions, including OA, has been called into question. A systematic review and meta-analysis, published in 2015, noted only modest short-term effects on measures of pain and disability with paracetamol versus placebo in patients with OA of the hip or knee: the largest observed effect size being a 4-point reduction on a 0–100 mm pain scale.[41] The safety of regular paracetamol use has also been challenged. While the dangers of paracetamol at above-therapeutic doses are well known, it has typically been regarded as safe at therapeutic doses—an important factor favouring its use in many painful conditions. However, when taken at the recommended maximum daily dosage of 4 grams, a surprising number of healthy adults show hepatic enzyme elevations: 31–44% of participants were found to have alanine aminotransferase (ALT) levels over three times the upper limit of normal in one study.[42] The clinical significance of these transient hepatic enzyme elevations, particularly in patients with pre-existing liver disease, remains unclear but warrants further investigation. A dose reduction may be required in patients with chronic malnutrition or high alcohol intake, and in patients weighing less than 50 kg. Education about the paracetamol content of combination analgesics will also help to lower the potential for unintentional paracetamol overdoses.

Opioids

Opioids have well-established roles in the management of acute and chronic pain. They act on a range of opioid receptors present in the brain, spinal cord, and peripheral sensory neurons, as well as the gastrointestinal tract. In RA, weak opioids, including codeine and tramadol, are typically used as second-line or adjuvant analgesics in patients who have achieved inadequate pain relief with, or been unable to tolerate, NSAIDs and paracetamol. Strong opioids, such as morphine and buprenorphine, are reserved for patients with severe pain who have failed treatment with paracetamol, NSAIDs, and weak opioids.

Despite a recent US study demonstrating that 60% of RA patients are intermittent or regular opioid users,[43] only a small number of studies have examined their efficacy and safety in patients with RA. The vast majority of these studies are more than 10 years old and involve fewer than 100 subjects, with a significant potential for the introduction of bias. Of the six studies comparing opioids against placebo in a published systematic review, five studies reported improvements in at least one efficacy measure with opioids over placebo.[44] Of the studies with comparable efficacy outcome measures, there was an 18% improvement in patients' global impressions of their RA symptoms with opioids. Despite the short treatment duration in these studies (1–6 weeks), approximately half of the participants experienced adverse events with opioids—with an odds ratio of 3.9 when compared with placebo—resulting in treatment withdrawal for 1 in 6 participants.

Although highly variable from patient to patient, adverse effects are common with both weak and strong opioids. Frequently reported adverse effects include constipation, nausea and vomiting, drowsiness, and mental clouding. These often improve with continued opioid use but can be severe, particularly in elderly patients due to comorbidities, frailty, and the use of other medications. An individual risk-benefit assessment is warranted, with cautious dose titration and close monitoring for adverse effects if the decision is made to commence opioids. Concomitant administration of laxatives and antiemetics can help improve tolerability. Of note, chronic opioid use has also been associated with detrimental effects on bone metabolism and an increased fracture risk.[45] Suggested mechanisms include opioid effects on osteoblast activity and opioid-induced androgen deficiency, coupled with a heightened falls risk due to side effects such as confusion and drowsiness.

Consideration must be given to individual variability in drug metabolism. Codeine is converted into morphine, its active metabolite, by the hepatic CYP2D6 enzyme. Approximately 5–10% of individuals carry two inactive alleles of the *CYP2D6* gene, resulting in poor analgesic efficacy even with higher doses of codeine.[46] In contrast, 1–2% of individuals have more than two functional copies of the *CYP2D6* gene: increasing the potential for opiate toxicity. Similarly, tramadol and oxycodone are substrates of the CYP2D6 enzyme and, thus, may also vary in their metabolism between patients.

A contributing factor to the widespread use of opioids in RA is likely to be their availability in a range of formulations. Tablet burden is important in treatment concordance in patients with RA. This is particularly true of patients with chronic RA pain, who may be on multiple daily analgesic medications, in addition to DMARDs and other treatments. 'Too many pills' was reported by 63% of patients as being a specific barrier to optimal pain management in one study; second only to concerns about adverse effects.[47] Several opioids, including fentanyl and buprenorphine, are available in transdermal, slow-release preparations. These preparations can help to reduce tablet burden in RA patients with severe, chronic pain, by providing consistent background analgesia for up to a week per patch. Tablet burden can also be reduced through the use of combination analgesics. Codeine, in combination with paracetamol, has been shown to be produce effective pain relief in RA patients,[48] with adverse event rates comparable to placebo in one small study. Tramadol, in combination with paracetamol, also reduces pain scores significantly, albeit modestly, relative to placebo.[49] However, high adverse event rates with combination tramadol-paracetamol resulted in discontinuations in 1 in 5 active drug participants in one study of RA patients.[49] Tramadol's ability to lower seizure thresholds is another important consideration—particularly in patients with a history of epilepsy and those on tricyclic antidepressants.

A major concern with the use of opioids for many patients and clinicians is the potential for drug dependency, tolerance, and addiction. Fear of addiction to analgesics has been reported as a barrier to adequate pain relief in a third of RA patients.[47] However, data from a range of oncological and non-oncological conditions, including RA, have shown that opioids can be used effectively in the management of severe pain, with a relatively low risk of dependence.[50] In a retrospective analysis of rheumatology patients treated with codeine and/or oxycodone, evidence of opioid tolerance and abuse was found in 3% of long-term opioid users.[51] In this study, opioids were highly effective at controlling pain; reducing pain scores from 8.2 to 3.6 on a 0–10 scale. Furthermore, 80% of patients reported sustained analgesic efficacy over time. For RA patients with severe pain resistant to other treatments, fear of addiction should not therefore preclude a trial of opioids, provided there is regular clinical review. In cases of increasing opioid requirements, there should be a low threshold for consideration of other contributing factors including fibromyalgia, depression, and anxiety, which were strong, independent predictors of opioid use in a recent, large database study of people with RA.[43]

Centrally acting analgesics

Despite large improvements in our ability to manage RA with DMARDs and analgesic agents, a significant proportion of patients still experience chronic pain. This pain can occur at sites not obviously affected by inflammation and at times when other markers of disease activity appear relatively quiescent. Increasingly, we are recognizing the importance of peripheral and central sensitization in the persistence of rheumatoid pain.[52]

The pro-inflammatory cascade associated with RA can lead to sensitization of peripheral nociceptors and neurons to painful stimuli.[53] Chronic exposure to painful stimuli produces a stream of afferent signals to pain-processing areas of the central nervous system. Over time, these regions also undergo sensitization,[54] amplifying the response to painful stimuli. Sensitization can be demonstrated in RA patients using an array of techniques. These include quantitative sensory testing, with lowered pressure-pain thresholds and high temporal summation correlating with measures of disease activity,[55] and brain MRI, highlighting structural changes in regions associated with pain processing.[56] The use of more discriminatory pain measurement tools, such as painDETECT, highlights a neuropathic component of pain in a significant number of people with RA.[7,57]

Centrally acting analgesic agents are attractive management options for RA patients with evidence of pain sensitization. These agents include antidepressants, such as duloxetine and amitriptyline, and neuromodulators, such as gabapentin and pregabalin. Centrally acting analgesics are effective in the management of a number of chronic pain conditions, including fibromyalgia and neuropathic pain.[58,59] The analgesic effects of tricyclic antidepressants become apparent at relatively low doses, with a quicker onset of action than their antidepressant effects.[60] However, experience with centrally acting analgesics in RA pain is relatively limited. A systematic review of antidepressants for pain management in RA found only eight studies suitable for inclusion, all of which assessed tricyclic antidepressants against a range of control therapies.[60] Unfortunately, a high risk of bias was present in the majority of these studies and conclusions on efficacy were not possible: two studies showed improvements in pain outcomes with tricyclic antidepressants over placebo, whereas five studies showed no difference in pain outcomes. Tricyclic antidepressants were associated with a greater number of minor adverse events (including anticholinergic, central nervous system and GI side effects) but not treatment withdrawals, relative to placebo. In a study of amitriptyline versus paroxetine (a selective serotonin reuptake inhibitor) in RA patients with depression, similar improvements in measures of pain, depression, and disability were seen in both treatment cohorts, although fewer adverse events were noted with paroxetine.[61]

Studies assessing the effects of neuromodulating agents in the management of RA pain are even fewer in number. A systematic review, published in 2012, found only four studies suitable for inclusion, none of which investigated widely used agents such as gabapentin or pregabalin.[62] Two studies assessed the efficacy and safety of nefopam, a centrally acting analgesic thought to act upon monoamine neurotransmitter pathways. Nefopam reduced mean pain levels by 21 mm on a 0–100 mm VAS scale, but was associated with high adverse event and dropout rates when compared with placebo. A study of topical capsaicin—a component of chilies and an inhibitor of the neuropeptide, substance P—reduced mean pain levels by 34 mm after 2 weeks of therapy in patients with OA and RA-related knee pain. As might be expected, a large proportion of participants (44%) reported burning at the site of capsaicin application, however only 2% of participants withdrew because of this.

In view of their efficacy in other chronic pain conditions, a trial of centrally acting analgesics may be appropriate as an adjunct therapy for RA patients with persistent pain, particularly if there is a suspected neuropathic or fibromyalgic component. The use of pain assessment tools such as painDETECT can help support these treatment decisions. Screening for comorbid depression, anxiety and fibromyalgia should also be performed: in one cross-sectional study, a diagnosis of fibromyalgia was made in 15% of RA patients, with dual diagnosis being associated with greater functional impairment.[63] The decision to commence an agent such as amitriptyline or gabapentin must also be weighed against the potential for adverse effects. Whereas a mild sedative effect might benefit a patient with pain and sleep disturbance, it could detriment the safety of a frail, elderly patient.

Conclusion

Pain in RA is complex and multifactorial. Studies demonstrate that cytokines are major contributors to the inflammation-mediated pain in RA. Therapeutic targets aimed at inhibiting inflammatory pain in RA include NSAIDs, which are often used in addition to conventional DMARD therapies. In this chapter, we have discussed the rationale for treatments for RA pain based on trial evidence, which favours NSAIDs as the analgesics of choice. Long-term use of NSAIDs for RA pain is not recommended due to the higher burden of adverse effects associated with chronic use, including gastrointestinal, cardiovascular, and renal complications. There is some evidence for opioids and paracetamol as alternative analgesics in RA.

More recent data suggests that people with RA demonstrate evidence of peripheral and central pain sensitization, and 'fibromyalgic rheumatoid' phenotypes have been described. Further studies are required of agents that target centrally mediated pain in RA, including amitriptyline and the gabapentinoids. Treatment of RA pain requires careful patient evaluation, consideration of other therapies that the patient is taking, and prescription of analgesics based on specific patient needs.

REFERENCES

1. Feldmann M, Maini RN. Anti-TNF alpha therapy of rheumatoid arthritis: what have we learned? *Ann Rev Immunol* 2001;*19*:163–96.
2. Wailoo A, Hock ES, Stevenson M, et al. The clinical effectiveness and cost-effectiveness of treat-to-target strategies in rheumatoid arthritis: a systematic review and cost-effectiveness analysis. *Health Technol Assess* 2017;*21*(17):1–258.
3. Roche PA, Klestov AC, Heim HM. Description of stable pain in rheumatoid arthritis: a 6-year study. *J Rheumatol* 2003;*30*:1733–8.
4. McWilliams DF, Walsh DA. Factors predicting pain and early discontinuation of tumour necrosis factor-alpha inhibitors in people with rheumatoid arthritis: results from the British Society for Rheumatology Biologics Register. *BMC Musculoskel Disord* 2016;*17*:337.
5. McWilliams DF, Zhang W, Mansell JS, et al. Predictors of change in bodily pain in early rheumatoid arthritis: an inception cohort study. *Arthritis Care Res (Hoboken)* 2012;*64*:1505–13.
6. Bingham CO, 3rd, Pohl C, Woodworth TG, et al. Developing a standardised definition for disease 'flare' in rheumatoid arthritis (OMERACT 9 Special Interest Group) *J Rheumatol* 2009;*36*:2335–41.
7. Ahmed S, Magan T, Vargas M, et al. Use of the painDETECT tool in rheumatoid arthritis suggests neuropathic and sensitization components in pain reporting. *J Pain Res* 2014;*7*:579–88.
8. Hewlett S, Sanderson T, May J, et al. 'I'm hurting, I want to kill myself': rheumatoid arthritis flare is more than a high joint count—an international patient perspective on flare where medical help is sought. *Rheumatology (Oxf)* 2012;*51*:69–76.
9. Pollard LC, Kingsley GH, Choy EH, et al. Fibromyalgic rheumatoid arthritis and disease assessment. *Rheumatology (Oxf)* 2010;*49*:924–8.
10. McWilliams DF, Ferguson E, Young A, et al. Discordant inflammation and pain in early and established rheumatoid arthritis: latent class analysis of Early Rheumatoid Arthritis Network and British Society for Rheumatology biologics register data. *Arthritis Res Ther* 2016;*18*:295.
11. Crofford LJ. Use of NSAIDs in treating patients with arthritis. *Arthritis Res Ther* 2013;*15*(Suppl 3):S2.
12. Pinals RS, Frank S. Relative efficacy of indomethacin and acetylsalicylic acid in rheumatoid arthritis. *N Engl J Med* 1967;*276*(9):512–14.
13. Blechman WJ, Schmid FR, April PA, et al. Ibuprofen or aspirin in rheumatoid arthritis therapy. *JAMA* 1975;*233*(4):336–40.
14. Henry D, Dobson A, Turner C. Variability in the risk of major gastrointestinal complications from nonaspirin nonsteroidal anti-inflammatory drugs. *Gastroenterology* 1993;*105*(4):1078–88.
15. MacDonald TM, Morant SV, Robinson GC, et al. Association of upper gastrointestinal toxicity of non-steroidal

anti-inflammatory drugs with continued exposure: cohort study. *BMJ* 1997;*315*(7119):1333–7.

16. Gabriel SE, Jaakkimainen L, Bombardier C. Risk for serious gastrointestinal complications related to use of nonsteroidal anti-inflammatory drugs. A meta-analysis. *Ann Intern Med* 1991;*115*(10):787–96.

17. Hunt RH, Lanas A, Stichtenoth DO, et al. Myths and facts in the use of anti-inflammatory drugs. *Ann Med* 2009;*41*(6):423–37.

18. Matsumoto AK, Melian A, Mandel DR, et al. A randomized, controlled, clinical trial of etoricoxib in the treatment of rheumatoid arthritis. *J Rheumatol* 2002;*29*(8):1623–30.

19. Simon LS, Weaver AL, Graham DY, et al. Anti-inflammatory and upper gastrointestinal effects of celecoxib in rheumatoid arthritis: a randomized controlled trial. *JAMA* 1999;*282*(20):1921–8.

20. Emery P, Zeidler H, Kvien TK, et al. Celecoxib versus diclofenac in long-term management of rheumatoid arthritis: randomised double-blind comparison. *Lancet* 1999;*354*(9196):2106–11.

21. Silverstein FE, Faich G, Goldstein JL, et al. Gastrointestinal toxicity with celecoxib vs nonsteroidal anti-inflammatory drugs for osteoarthritis and rheumatoid arthritis: the CLASS study: a randomized controlled trial. Celecoxib Long-term Arthritis Safety Study. *JAMA* 2000;*284*(10):1247–55.

22. Feng X, Tian M, Zhang W, et al. Gastrointestinal safety of etoricoxib in osteoarthritis and rheumatoid arthritis: A meta-analysis. *PLoS One* 2018;*13*(1):e0190798.

23. Fidahic M, Jelicic Kadic A, Radic M, et al. Celecoxib for rheumatoid arthritis. *Cochrane Database Syst Rev* 2017;*6*:CD012095.

24. Matsumoto A, Melian A, Shah A, et al. Etoricoxib versus naproxen in patients with rheumatoid arthritis: a prospective, randomized, comparator-controlled 121-week trial. *Curr Med Res Opin* 2007;*23*(9):2259–68.

25. Chan FK, Lanas A, Scheiman J, et al. Celecoxib versus omeprazole and diclofenac in patients with osteoarthritis and rheumatoid arthritis (CONDOR): a randomised trial. *Lancet* 2010;*376*(9736):173–9.

26. Bombardier C, Laine L, Reicin A, et al. Comparison of upper gastrointestinal toxicity of rofecoxib and naproxen in patients with rheumatoid arthritis. VIGOR Study Group. *N Engl J Med* 2000;*343*(21):1520–8.

27. Bresalier RS, Sandler RS, Quan H, et al. Cardiovascular events associated with rofecoxib in a colorectal adenoma chemoprevention trial. *N Engl J Med* 2005;*352*(11):1092–102.

28. Solomon SD, McMurray JJ, Pfeffer MA, et al. Cardiovascular risk associated with celecoxib in a clinical trial for colorectal adenoma prevention. *N Engl J Med* 2005;*352*(11):1071–80.

29. Kearney PM, Baigent C, Godwin J, et al. Do selective cyclo-oxygenase-2 inhibitors and traditional non-steroidal anti-inflammatory drugs increase the risk of atherothrombosis: meta-analysis of randomised trials. *BMJ* 2006;*332*:1302.

30. ADAPT Research Group. Cardiovascular and cerebrovascular events in the randomized, controlled Alzheimer's Disease Anti-Inflammatory Prevention Trial (ADAPT). *PLoS Clin Trials* 2006;*1*(7):e33.

31. Nissen SE, Yeomans ND, Solomon DH, et al. Cardiovascular safety of celecoxib, naproxen, or ibuprofen for arthritis. *N Engl J Med* 2016;*375*(26):2519–29.

32. Solomon DH, Husni ME, Libby PA, et al. The risk of major NSAID toxicity with celecoxib, ibuprofen, or naproxen: a secondary analysis of the PRECISION trial. *Am J Med* 2017;*130*(12):1415–22.e4.

33. Kienzler JL, Gold M, Nollevaux F. Systemic bioavailability of topical diclofenac sodium gel 1% versus oral diclofenac sodium in healthy volunteers. *J Clin Pharmacol* 2010;*50*(1):50–61.

34. Evans JM, McMahon AD, McGilchrist MM, et al. Topical non-steroidal anti-inflammatory drugs and admission to hospital for upper gastrointestinal bleeding and perforation: a record linkage case-control study. *BMJ* 1995;*311*(6996):22–6.

35. Derry S, Conaghan P, Da Silva JA, et al. Topical NSAIDs for chronic musculoskeletal pain in adults. *Cochrane Database Syst Rev* 2016;*4*:CD007400.

36. Whittle SL, Colebatch AN, Buchbinder R, et al. Multinational evidence-based recommendations for pain management by pharmacotherapy in inflammatory arthritis: integrating systematic literature research and expert opinion of a broad panel of rheumatologists in the 3e Initiative. *Rheumatology (Oxf)* 2012;*51*(8):1416–25.

37. Brandt KD, Mazzuca SA, Buckwalter KA. Acetaminophen, like conventional NSAIDs, may reduce synovitis in osteoarthritic knees. *Rheumatology (Oxf)* 2006;*45*(11):1389–94.

38. Wienecke T, Gøtzsche PC. Paracetamol versus nonsteroidal anti-inflammatory drugs for rheumatoid arthritis. *Cochrane Database Syst Rev* 2004;(1):CD003789.

39. Hazlewood G, van der Heijde DM, Bombardier C. Paracetamol for the management of pain in inflammatory arthritis: a systematic literature review. *J Rheumatol Suppl* 2012;*90*:11–16.

40. Wolfe F, Zhao S, Lane N. Preference for nonsteroidal antiinflammatory drugs over acetaminophen by rheumatic disease patients: a survey of 1,799 patients with osteoarthritis, rheumatoid arthritis, and fibromyalgia. *Arthritis Rheum* 2000;*43*(2):378–85.

41. Machado GC, Maher CG, Ferreira PH, et al. Efficacy and safety of paracetamol for spinal pain and osteoarthritis: systematic review and meta-analysis of randomised placebo controlled trials. *BMJ* 2015;*350*:h1225.

42. Watkins PB, Kaplowitz N, Slattery JT, et al. Aminotransferase elevations in healthy adults receiving 4 grams of acetaminophen daily: a randomized controlled trial. *JAMA* 2006;*296*(1):87–93.

43. Curtis JR, Xie F, Smith C, et al. Changing trends in opioid use among patients with rheumatoid arthritis in the United States. *Arthritis Rheumatol* 2017;*69*(9):1733–40.

44. Whittle SL, Richards BL, Husni E, et al. Opioid therapy for treating rheumatoid arthritis pain. *Cochrane Database Syst Rev* 2011;(11):CD003113.

45. Coluzzi F, Pergolizzi J, Raffa RB, et al. The unsolved case of 'bone-impairing analgesics': the endocrine effects of opioids on bone metabolism. *Ther Clin Risk Manag* 2015;*11*:515–23

46. Dean L. *Codeine Therapy and CYP2D6 Genotype. Medical Genetics Summaries.* 2012. Available at: http://www.ncbi.nlm.nih.gov/books/NBK100662/

47. Fitzcharles MA, DaCosta D, Ware MA, et al. Patient barriers to pain management may contribute to poor pain control in rheumatoid arthritis. *J Pain* 2009;*10*(3):300–5.

48. Boureau F, Boccard E. Placebo-controlled study of the analgesic efficacy of a combination of paracetamol and codeine in rheumatoid arthritis. *Acta Ther* 1991;*17*:123–36.

49. Lee EY, Lee EB, Park BJ, et al. Tramadol 37.5-mg/acetaminophen 325-mg combination tablets added to regular therapy for rheumatoid arthritis pain: a 1-week, randomized, double-blind, placebo-controlled trial. *Clin Ther* 2006;*28*(12):2052–60.

50. Minozzi S, Amato L, Davoli M. Development of dependence following treatment with opioid analgesics for pain relief: a systematic review. *Addiction* 2013;*108*(4):688–98.

51. Ytterberg SR, Mahowald ML, Woods SR. Codeine and oxy-codone use in patients with chronic rheumatic disease pain. *Arthritis Rheum* 1998;*41*(9):1603–12.

52. Buskila D, Langevitz P, Gladman DD, et al. Patients with rheumatoid arthritis are more tender than those with psoriatic arthritis. *J Rheumatol* 1992;*19*(7):1115–19.

53. Van Laar M, Pergolizzi JV, Mellinghoff H-U, et al. Pain treatment in arthritis-related pain: beyond NSAIDs. *Open Rheumatol J* 2012;*6*:320–330.

54. Magliano M, Morris V. *Use of Analgesics in Rheumatology.* Arthritis Research Campaign, 2002. Available at: https://www.versusarthritis.org/

55. Lee YC, Bingham CO 3rd, Edwards RR, et al. Pain sensitization is associated with disease activity in rheumatoid arthritis patients: a cross-sectional study. *Arthritis Care Res (Hoboken)* 2018;*70*(2):197–204.

56. Wartolowska K, Hough MG, Jenkinson M, et al. Structural changes of the brain in rheumatoid arthritis. *Arthritis Rheum* 2012;*64*(2):371–9.

57. Freynhagen R, Baron R, Gockel U, et al. painDETECT: a new screening questionnaire to identify neuropathic components in patients with back pain. *Curr Med Res Opin* 2006;*22*(10):1911–20.

58. Macfarlane GJ, Kronisch C, Dean LE, et al. EULAR revised recommendations for the management of fibromyalgia. *Ann Rheum Dis* 2017;*76*(2):318–28.

59. Lynch ME. Antidepressants as analgesics: a review of randomized controlled trials. *J Psychiatry Neurosci* 2001;*26*(1):30–6.

60. Richards BL, Whittle SL, Buchbinder R. Antidepressants for pain management in rheumatoid arthritis. *Cochrane Database Syst Rev* 2011;(11):CD008920.

61. Bird H, Broggini M. Paroxetine versus amitriptyline for treatment of depression associated with rheumatoid arthritis: a randomized, double blind, parallel group study. *J Rheumatol* 2000;*27*(12):2791–7.

62. Richards BL, Whittle SL, Buchbinder R. Neuromodulators for pain management in rheumatoid arthritis. *Cochrane Database Syst Rev* 2012;*1*:CD008921.

63. Naranjo A, Ojeda S, Francisco F, et al. Fibromyalgia in patients with rheumatoid arthritis is associated with higher scores of disability. *Ann Rheum Dis* 2002;*61*(7):660–1.

29

Glucocorticoids

Johannes W.G. Jacobs, Marlies C. van der Goes, Johannes W.J. Bijlsma, and José A.P. da Silva

Introduction

Because of their effectiveness, versatility, and low cost, glucocorticoids are used in most vasculitic, allergic, sterile (auto)inflammatory and autoimmune conditions, including rheumatic diseases, such as rheumatoid arthritis (RA). Basic mechanisms and effects, indications, adverse events, and monitoring of glucocorticoid therapy in RA, together with new developments, are discussed here with emphasis on clinically relevant implications.

Pharmacology

Structure and classification

Steroid hormones are characterized by a sterol skeleton, hence their designation 'steroids'. On the basis of their main functions, steroid hormones can be classified into sex hormones, mineralocorticoids (so designated because they affect the electrolyte and fluid balance), and glucocorticoids (which affect the glucose metabolism and immune regulation). Mineralocorticoids and glucocorticoids are synthesized in the adrenal cortex, hence the terms 'corticosteroid' and 'corticoid' for these hormones. It is more precise to use the term glucocorticoid than the term corticosteroid when referring to one of the glucocorticoid drugs.[1] The main natural (i.e. endogenous human) glucocorticoid is cortisol (hydrocortisone). Natural glucocorticoids also have mineralocorticoid effects, but synthetic glucocorticoid drugs have less mineralocorticoid and markedly more glucocorticoid potency.

Absorption and protein binding

Most orally administered glucocorticoids are absorbed readily, probably within about 30 minutes. The bioavailability of prednisone and prednisolone is high. The affinity of the individual glucocorticoids to bind to plasma proteins (transcortin, also called corticosteroid-binding globulin, and albumin) varies. Transcortin binds glucocorticoids more strongly than does albumin; only unbound glucocorticoids are pharmacologically active. In liver disease, hypoalbuminemia, increasing the unbound pharmacologically active fraction of glucocorticoids, and the reduced liver metabolic clearance of glucocorticoids, lead to increased effects and adverse effects of glucocorticoids, implying a need for dose adjustment.

Conversion into active hormones and vice versa, metabolism

Glucocorticoids with an 11-keto instead of an 11-hydroxy group, such as cortisone and prednisone, are inactive (prohormones), because of their very low affinity for the glucocorticoid receptor. To become effective, they must be metabolized by the liver into their biologically active 11-hydroxy configurations, cortisol, and prednisolone, respectively. Prednisone and prednisolone preparations are considered approximately bioequivalent, but severe liver disease should prompt the prescription of prednisolone instead of prednisone.

The intracellular enzyme 11β-hydroxysteroid dehydrogenase (11β-HSD) type 1 predominantly activates glucocorticoid prohormones, although this enzyme can also promote the reverse reaction, leading to inactivation of active glucocorticoids. In contrast, the isoenzyme 11β-HSD type 2 only converts active glucocorticoids into their inactive forms. Tissue levels of active glucocorticoids depend on their serum concentration and on the local availability and activity of these isoenzymes and of the glucocorticoid inactivating enzyme 5alpha-reductase,[2,3] which are influenced by inflammation, leading to higher local glucocorticoid levels in synovial tissue.

Glucocorticoids have carry-on biological effects which last longer than expected from their plasma half-lives. This allows for once daily dosing of prednisone/prednisolone for RA. Maximal effects of glucocorticoids lag behind peak serum concentrations. The serum half-life of prednisolone is increased by decreased rates of metabolism in patients with renal disease or liver cirrhosis, and in elderly patients, which means that a given dose may have a greater effect in such conditions. Several other pharmacological mechanisms may be involved in the variability of glucocorticoid sensitivity in patients.[4] Prednisolone partially is removed by haemodialysis, but, overall, the amount removed does not require dose adjustment.

Nomenclature for glucocorticoid dosages

A standardization of the terminology for glucocorticoid dosages has been proposed, based on the probability of adverse effects, pharmacodynamics, and predominant mechanisms of action. This is expressed in prednisone equivalents: low dose: ≤7.5 mg daily; medium dose: >7.5—≤30 mg daily; high dose: >30—≤100 mg daily; very high dose: >100 mg daily; pulse therapy: ≥250 mg daily for one to a few days.[1]

Drug interactions

Cytochrome P450 (CYP) is a family of isozymes responsible for the biotransformation of several drugs. Drug interactions can be based either on induction (upregulation) or on inhibition (downregulation) of these enzymes. A clinically relevant example of induction of CYP isozymes, particularly CYP3A4, leading to reduced glucocorticoid levels, is rifampicin-induced non-responsiveness to prednisone in inflammatory diseases.[5] Inhibitors of CYP, for example ketoconazole, may cause higher glucocorticoid levels. However, ketoconazole in higher dosages also diminishes endogenous glucocorticoid synthesis justifying its use in the treatment of Cushing syndrome and disease. Grapefruit juice inhibits CYP, but this is likely to be of limited clinical significance.[6]

Molecular mechanisms of action

Glucocorticoids influence about 1% of the entire genome, which accounts for an exceptionally broad spectrum of effects. These genomic effects of glucocorticoids occur predominantly at low and medium dosages, while at high dosages and beyond both genomic and non-genomic mechanisms take place.

Genomic molecular mechanisms

Glucocorticoids exert their main actions through the cytosolic glucocorticoid receptors (GR), which are present in almost all tissues.[7] These genomic actions are described in **Figure 29.1**.

The concept that transactivation is responsible for most adverse effects of glucocorticoid therapy led to the development of selective glucocorticoid receptor agonists, which predominantly induce transrepression. However, reality is not so simple. For example, transactivation also yields anti-inflammatory effects via upregulation of the synthesis of anti-inflammatory proteins.[8] Furthermore, the wanted immunosuppressive effect is dependent on transrepression, but is also associated with increased infection risk, one of the major adverse effects of glucocorticoids.

Glucocorticoids also act in the translational and post-translational phases of protein synthesis.[9] As an example, glucocorticoids may inhibit protein synthesis, e.g. of interleukin (IL)-1, IL-6, granulocyte-macrophage colony-stimulating factor (GM-CSF), and inducible cyclooxygenase (COX)-2, by decreasing the stability of messenger ribonucleic acid (mRNA) via induction of ribonucleases by glucocorticoid-GR complexes.

Non-genomic molecular mechanisms

Compared to genomic effects, non-genomic effects are more rapid, occurring within seconds or minutes. However, clinical effects of non-genomic mechanisms cannot be discriminated from clinical effects of genomic mechanisms. Non-genomic actions may involve membrane-bound GRs. Dexamethasone targets these receptors on T lymphocytes, rapidly impairing T lymphocyte receptor signalling and immune response.[10] Other non-genomic actions, without involvement of GRs, occur via physicochemical interactions with biological membranes, altering cell function. An example is the inhibition by glucocorticoids of calcium and sodium cycling across the plasma membrane of immune cells, which contributes to rapid immunosuppression and reduced inflammation.

Immunosuppressive and immunomodulatory effects

Glucocorticoids downregulate virtually every step of the inflammatory and immune response (see **Figure 29.2**), including the activation, proliferation, differentiation, and survival of a variety of inflammatory cells.[11] The production of pro-inflammatory cytokines, such as IL-1β and tumour necrosis factor (TNF) is decreased and consequently IL-1 and TNF-induced production of metalloproteinases, especially collagenase and stromelysin, which

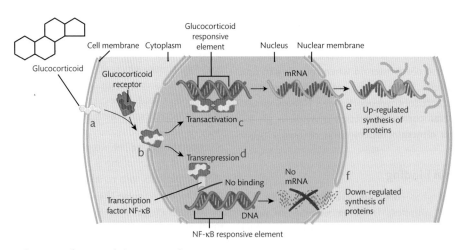

Figure 29.1 Genomic mechanisms of action of glucocorticoids.
Genomic mechanisms require (a) passing of glucocorticoid molecules through the cell membrane, (b) binding to the cytosolic glucocorticoid receptor to form monomer or dimer complexes and migration of these complexes into the nucleus where they finally influence gene expression and protein synthesis via (c) transactivation, or (d) transrepression. Dimers of the complex glucocorticoid-GR bind to glucocorticoid-responsive elements in DNA, and lead to (e) increased synthesis (transactivation) of certain regulatory proteins, mainly those responsible for unwanted metabolic effects of glucocorticoids. Monomers of the glucocorticoid-GR complex inhibit nuclear transcriptional factors, such as NF-κB, resulting in (f) downregulation (transrepression) of (predominantly pro-inflammatory) protein synthesis.

mRNA, messenger RNA; NF-κB, nuclear factor kappa B.

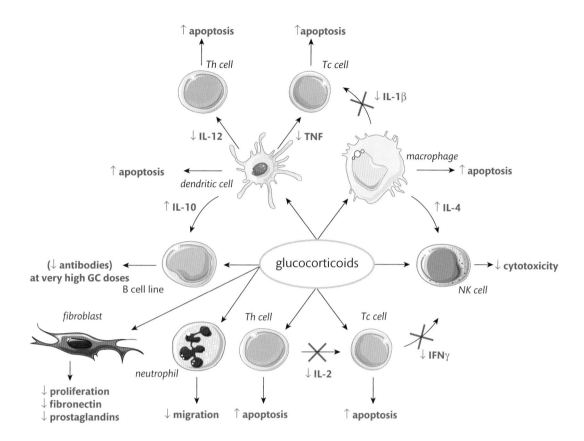

Figure 29.2 Glucocorticoid effects (in red type) on the interplay of inflammatory cells and cytokines. A simplified model.

↓, decreased; ↑, increased; GC, glucocorticoid; IFNγ, interferon-γ; NK cell, natural killer cell; Tc-cell, cytotoxic T lymphocyte; Th-cell, T-helper lymphocyte; red cross, inhibition of cellular (inter)action. Adapted from Sternberg EM. (2006) 'Neural regulation of innate immunity: a coordinated nonspecific host response to pathogens'. *Nat Rev Immunol* 6:318–28 with permission from Springer Nature.

are the main effectors of cartilage degradation in the chronic inflamed joint. The production of anti-inflammatory cytokines, such as IL-4 and IL-10, is stimulated by glucocorticoids. Downregulation of adhesion molecules decreases tissue migration of neutrophils and thus increases their number in the circulation.

Glucocorticoids also inhibit the formation of arachidonic acid metabolites, such as prostaglandins and leukotrienes, several of which are strongly pro-inflammatory. This inhibition is mediated by induction of lipocortin (an inhibitor of phospholipase A2), and inhibition of the cytokine-induced production of COX-2 in monocytes/macrophages, fibroblasts, and endothelial cells, see **Figure 29.3**. Glucocorticoids also inhibit the enzyme-inducible nitric oxide synthase which generates nitric oxide that is involved in vasodilatation at the site of inflammation.

All these effects result in the inhibition of immune and inflammatory responses with rapid and sustained effects on the corresponding symptoms as well on the structural and systemic consequences.

Use of glucocorticoids in RA

Indications

Glucocorticoids are frequently applied in RA: worldwide estimates of the percentages of patients with RA who are on treatment with glucocorticoids at any given time range from 15 to 90%. Aims and indications of this therapy are, first, symptomatic relief: reduction of signs and symptoms, exacerbations, and disease complications and, second, inhibition of development of joint damage in early RA.

Reduction of signs and symptoms

For its symptomatic effect, glucocorticoid therapy is often started and maintained at a low dose in RA, as additional therapy to disease-modifying antirheumatic drugs (DMARDs). Glucocorticoid therapy, even at doses of less than 10 mg prednisolone equivalent/day, are highly effective in relieving symptoms in patients with active RA. Clinical experience is that after some months, the beneficial effects of glucocorticoids often seem to diminish, but if this therapy is tapered off and stopped, patients frequently experience aggravation of symptoms. Although this can be seen especially in the early phases of treatment, it has been demonstrated also after long-term glucocorticoid therapy. The aggravation of disease following termination of treatment may simply be a reflection of the effectiveness of glucocorticoids, but we must also consider the possible contribution of tertiary adrenal insufficiency following the withdrawal of long-term medication.

In case of severe exacerbations or complications of RA, glucocorticoid pulse therapy may be used as a resource, as discussed next.

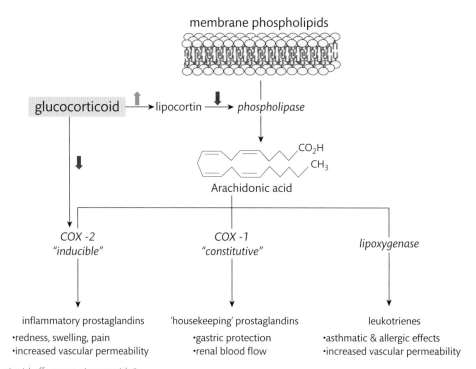

Figure 29.3 Glucocorticoid effects on eicosanoids.*

*Eicosanoids are cell signalling molecules with a molecular structure similar to that of arachidonic acid.
Green up-arrow, stimulation; red down-arrow, inhibition; COX, cyclooxygenase.

Inhibition of progression of joint damage (DMARD effect)

Glucocorticoids used to be considered merely symptomatic interventions. In 1995, joint-preserving effects of 7.5 mg of prednisolone daily were proven for the first time. This study included patients with RA of short and intermediate duration, and glucocorticoids were compared to placebo, in addition to classic DMARDs, for 2 years.[12] Comparable results were obtained in early RA, in two subsequent trials with a similar design, using 5 mg[13] or 7.5 mg[14] of prednisolone daily for 2 years.

In 2002, the results of the Utrecht study on the effects of 10 mg of prednisolone daily, for 2 years, in DMARD-naïve patients with early RA were published.[15] This is the only placebo-controlled trial in which prednisolone was applied as DMARD-monotherapy as first step; other DMARDs were added only as rescue, which would be considered unethical nowadays. The progression of radiologic joint damage was inhibited by prednisolone in these patients. This study reported that the prednisolone group showed a significant decrease in the need for additional interventions: 40% decrease for intra-articular glucocorticoid injections, 49% decrease in acetaminophen use, and 55% decrease in the use of non-steroidal anti-inflammatory drugs (NSAIDs).[16] In an extension of this study, at 3 years after the end of the 2-year initial follow-up, after which prednisolone therapy was tapered off and stopped, yearly radiological progression, albeit substantial, was statistically significantly less in the former prednisolone group.[17]

The concept that glucocorticoids effectively reduce joint damage, both during treatment and for years after its cessation, is also supported by the COBRA trial, published in 1997.[18] In the long-term, beneficial effects continued to be observed regarding radiologic damage, among patients who had received the combination strategy with glucocorticoids during the early phase of the disease.[19,20] Other

studies have been performed with glucocorticoids in early RA, also showing beneficial clinical results and DMARD effects.[21,22] Damage prevention, although at a minor level and at the expense of greater toxicity, was demonstrated with monthly intramuscular injection of 120 mg depot methylprednisolone acetate.[23]

Negative studies on the effect of glucocorticoids upon radiologic damage have also been published.[24-26] Nonetheless, the evidence that glucocorticoids actually are DMARDs, endowed with joint-sparing effects which persist after therapy is stopped, remains very robust. A meta-analysis on radiographic outcome analysed 15 studies on glucocorticoids (two with negative results), including a total 1414 patients; most studies employed a dose of 5–10 mg/day of prednisolone equivalent during 1–2 years. Because different methods had been used in the individual trials, radiographic scores were expressed as percentage of the maximum possible score for the specific radiographic assessment used. The standardized mean difference in progression was 0.40 in favour of strategies using glucocorticoids (95% confidence interval, 0.27–0.54). This was considered a conservative estimate because the most conservative estimate of the difference in each study had been chosen.[27]

The glucocorticoid studies described earlier had no tight control or treat-to-target design. This was the primary research question of the second Computer-Assisted Management in Early RA clinical trial (CAMERA-II): whether prednisone would still have disease-modifying properties in early RA, when added to an effective,[28] tight control, methotrexate-based computer-assisted strategy aimed at remission (treat-to-target).[29] Erosive joint damage after 2 years of therapy was limited in both strategy groups, but it was significantly less in the group also receiving prednisone (n = 117), compared to the group receiving placebo (n = 119). The strategy with prednisone also yielded more clinical improvement: earlier suppression of disease activity parameters, earlier sustained remission (after 6 months of therapy compared to after 11 months), and significantly less need of anti-TNF therapy to achieve remission. The frequency of nausea and elevated serum transaminases was less in the prednisone strategy group, compared to the placebo strategy group, probably because doses of methotrexate were significantly lower in the prednisone strategy group, in which nevertheless RA was suppressed quicker and more effectively. In the prednisone strategy group, mean weight gain after 2 years was 2.9 kg, which was significantly higher than the gain of 1.3 kg in the placebo strategy group. However, in an additional analysis, the extra weight gain in the prednisone strategy group seemed at least partly attributable to improved disease control (active disease induces weight loss) by prednisone.[30] Weight gain, probably also by this mechanism, also has been shown to be an effect of anti-TNF therapy.[31,32] There was no difference in bone mineral density after 2 years between the strategy groups (both received osteoporosis prophylaxis), nor was there a decrease of bone mineral density within each group.[33] At 2 year post-trial follow-up, the median erosion score and need for adding anti-TNF therapy were still significantly lower in the former prednisone strategy group.[34]

The joint-sparing effect of glucocorticoids is predominantly characterised by slowing down of joint erosion formation and much less by inhibition of joint narrowing. The joint-preserving effect is probably based on the inhibition of pro-inflammatory cytokines such as IL-1 and TNFα,[35] which activate osteoclasts leading to bone resorption, periarticular osteopenia, and formation of bone erosions in RA. Furthermore, fibroblast proliferation and IL-1 and TNF-induced metalloproteinase synthesis are inhibited by glucocorticoids, retarding bone and cartilage destruction in inflamed joints of patients with early RA.[27,36,37]

It has not been investigated properly, whether or not glucocorticoids also inhibit progression of joint damage in RA of longer duration than 2 years. A so-called window of opportunity may exist for the treatment of RA in its early phases.[38] If this window is real, effective treatment with glucocorticoids and (other) DMARDs in this early phase results in a positive effect that lasts for a long time, moulding RA into a subsequent disease profile that is less aggressive and easier to control. This opportunity could be lost if treatment starts later or treatment could be less effective.

Prevention of (rheumatoid) arthritis

It has been tried to prevent arthralgia or preclinical arthritis from progressing to arthritis. Two placebo-controlled trials,[39,40] failed to demonstrate that intramuscular glucocorticoid injections might prevent arthritis development in patients with (very) early arthritis or individuals with arthralgia and RA-related autoantibodies. However, in another placebo-controlled double-blind trial, these injections postponed the need for DMARD therapy and prevented 1 in 10 patients from progressing into RA, within a follow-up of 12 months.[41] The latter result needs to be confirmed by further research.

Application and administration

For glucocorticoids as DMARDs in early RA, two dosing strategies are predominantly used: (1) a stable regime of 5–10 mg of prednisone equivalent per day during the first 2 years of the disease; or (2) higher starting doses (e.g. 15–60 mg/day), followed by rapid tapering and continuation of a lower dose or stopping. In later disease, systemic glucocorticoids are also frequently used as adjuvant

therapy in periods of flare or in patients with persistently active disease despite optimal use of other DMARDs. Local joint and soft tissue injections are still a very important resource in daily practice, to be used as needed.

The specific indication and aim of therapy determine route of administration, choice of drug (pharmacological properties), and dose. Clinical efficacy and speed of onset of action are related to the glucocorticoid dose and type and route of administration. The risk of adverse effects of glucocorticoid therapy in RA is dependent on patient factors (age, comorbidity, and comedication), glucocorticoid dose, type and route of administration, and treatment duration.

Oral therapy

Following current practice and recommendations, glucocorticoid therapy in RA should always be given in combination with other DMARDs and tapered when possible.[42,43] The term glucocorticoid-sparing drugs is not used for these other DMARDs in this context, although any effective DMARD added to the therapeutic regime facilitates to taper off and sometimes to stop the glucocorticoid therapy.[44,45]

Pulse therapy; other (very) high dose glucocorticoid bridging therapies

This is used in RA primarily for rapid disease suppression –often to bridge the delay of effect of recently initiated DMARD therapy–, and as treatment of flares and severe complications such as rheumatoid vasculitis. In active RA, the duration of the effects varies, but the beneficial effects generally last for about 6 weeks.[46] Pulse therapy is given typically as ≥250 mg prednisone equivalent daily for one to a few days, intravenously, but schemes with other dosages and routes of administration (oral, intramuscular) are also used frequently as bridging strategy. For instance, methylprednisolone 120 mg or triamcinolone 80 mg as single intramuscular injection.[47]

Local injection therapy

Local injection therapy should, first of all, be based on a proper diagnosis of the problem at hand. One should realize that also in RA, cholesterol deposition, gouty arthritis and (concomitant) bacterial infections may occur, so polarization microscopy and cultures should be considered, especially if the aspect of aspirated fluid is different than expected, or on clinical indication, such as fever. The diagnosis of soft tissue pain must also be accurate, as some causes are not amenable to local treatment (e.g. referred pain). The physician should be experienced with the injection technique, as accuracy of injection also could significantly influence the clinical effect.[48] Ultrasound-guided injection may be applied to improve accuracy and effectiveness of injection therapy.[49,50]

Triamcinolone and methylprednisolone are commonly used glucocorticoids for local soft tissue injection. Triamcinolone is less soluble than methylprednisolone and thus has a longer local effect, but also a less rapid onset of action and a higher risk of local complications, such as subcutaneous tissue (fat) atrophy, especially on atrophic skin and on areas overlying superficial bone. In such cases, one could also choose a more soluble glucocorticoid preparation; another prudent measure is to mix the glucocorticoid preparation with lidocaine to dilute it, and to inject only a small volume. Other reasons to mix the glucocorticoid with a local anaesthetic are diagnostic (relieved pain immediately after injection indicates accurate placement of injection), therapeutic (immediate effect),

Table 29.1 Examples of materials to be used for specific local injections

Disorder/site	Syringe (cc)	Needle (G, length)	Triamcinolone (40 mg/ml)	Lidocaine
Small joint, intra-articular	1	25 G, 1.6 cm (⅝″)	0.25–0.5 cc	0–0.25 cc, 2%
Large joint, intra-articular	2	21 G, 3–5 cm (1¼–2″)	0.5–1 cc	0.5–1 cc, 2%
Tenosynovitis	1	25 G, 1.6 cm (⅝″)	0.25 cc	0.25–0.75 cc, 2%
Subacromial space (bursa)	5	21 G, 3–5 cm (1¼–2″)	1 cc	4 cc, 2%
Biceps tendon Bursitis, in general	2	23 G, 3 cm (1¼″)	1 cc	1 cc, 2%
Epicondylitis	2	25 G, 1.6 cm (⅝″)	0.5 cc	1.5 cc, 2%
Finger flexor tendon	1	25 G, 1.6 cm (⅝″)	0.5 cc	0.5 cc, 2%
Greater trochanter (bursa)	10	21 G, 5 cm (2″) *	1 cc	9 cc, 1%
Carpal tunnel	1	25 G, 1.6 cm (⅝″)	0.5 cc	none
Meralgia paresthetica	5	23 G, 3 cm (1¼″)	1 cc	4 cc, 2%

* longer in obese patients.

Box 29.1 Adverse reactions of local glucocorticoid injections

During injection—within 1 hour
- Vasovagal reaction/collapse
- Pain at the injection site
- Symptoms of nerve damage (injection carpal tunnel)
- Local ecchymosis, bleeding
- Anaphylaxis (lidocaine)

Within hours—1 day
- Pain at the injection site
- Post-injection flare of pain and inflammation (glucocorticoid crystal-induced)
- Facial flushing
- Menstrual irregularity
- Disturbance diabetic control

After some days
- Infection

After some days to weeks
- Tendon rupture

After weeks
- Subcutaneous tissue/fat atrophy
- Skin depigmentation

---

and preventive (diminishing post-injection pain and flare).[51,52] The physician should become acquainted with details of techniques, post-injection care, and risks associated with local injections, described in dedicated reviews and monographies. Examples of materials that can be used for injections at specific sites and for different indications are given in **Table 29.1**.

Rest of the injected area or joint for 24 hours and graded reintroduction of usual use over 2–4 weeks is a common sensible recommendation, but is not backed-up by evidence. Patients should be advised that post-injection pain and even glucocorticoid crystal-induced synovitis may occur in the first 48 hours, which should be treated with local application of cold, and acetaminophen or NSAID. A flare starting more than 48 hours after injection suggests infection and should prompt contact with the physician. This is the most worrisome complication. The reported infection rate of joints following local injections with glucocorticoids is low, ranging from one case in 13 900 to 77 300 injections.[53–55] Adverse effects of local glucocorticoid injections and typical intervals with which they occur are given in the Box 29.1.

Adverse effects and events

Glucocorticoids have a wide range of potential adverse effects—see **Figure 29.4**.

Often, however, both patients and physicians do not fully realize that toxicity is closely dependent on dose and duration: the adverse effect spectrum of the low-dose glucocorticoids used in RA markedly differs from that of high-dose glucocorticoids.[56,57] This likely increases anxiety related to treatment, decreases adherence, and jeopardizes the optimum use of glucocorticoids for the benefit of patients.

Robust data on the incidence of adverse effects of glucocorticoids, especially low dose, are scarce and of limited quality. Most data are derived from observational studies, which tend to overestimate adverse effects of medication, especially due to bias by indication. Furthermore, not all adverse events are adverse effects of glucocorticoids; they could also be manifestations of the disease (i.e. RA, see **Figure 29.5**).

In fact, data obtained from randomized prospective clinical studies such as CAMERA-II,[29] just described, indicate that the adverse effects of low-to-medium dose chronic glucocorticoid therapy, are mild. Indeed, by inhibiting the inflammatory process, glucocorticoids in lower doses may actually counteract several negative effects of the disease, and reduce the need for high dosages of other DMARDs, decreasing the risk of adverse effects of these drugs.

Infections

Clearly the risk of infection associated with glucocorticoid therapy is dose-dependent.[58] Infection risk also increases with higher age and longer duration of treatment.[59–61] With the doses used in the treatment of RA, typically low-dose, randomized prospective studies of up to 2 years duration indicate that there is not increased risk of infection,[62] while observational studies do suggest an increased

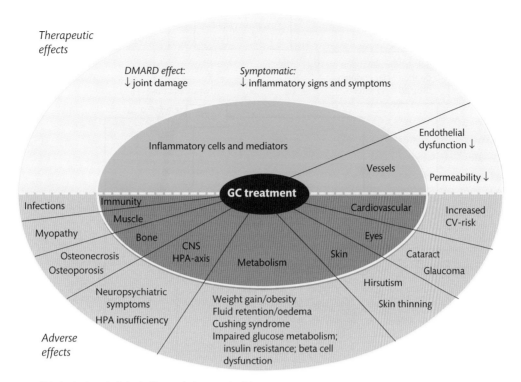

Figure 29.4 Spectrum of biological and clinical effects of glucocorticoids.
Upper, green part: therapeutic effects. Lower, red part: spectrum of adverse effects dependent on dose and duration of the glucocorticoid therapy. DMARD, disease-modifying antirheumatic drug; CNS, central nervous system; HPA, hypothalamic–pituitary–adrenal; CV, cardiovascular.

risk. The actual truth for this application of glucocorticoid therapy is difficult to establish: while randomized clinical trials have several limitations such as patient selection, resulting in inclusion of patients with less (co)morbidity compared to patients in observational studies, and limited patient numbers and duration of exposure, observational studies are unavoidably affected by bias by indication, because they are not randomized.[63] Anyway, in patients on long-term glucocorticoid therapy, especially older people and those with comorbidities and on immunosuppressive comedications,

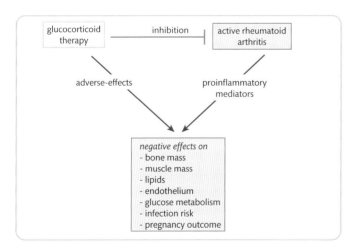

Figure 29.5 Interactions between glucocorticoid therapy, RA disease activity, and negative clinical effects.
Glucocorticoids can have adverse effects, but suppress disease activity and by this mechanism also suppress negative consequences of active RA. Several negative consequences of active RA match adverse effects of glucocorticoids.

physicians should anticipate a dose-dependent increased risk of infections with both typical and atypical microorganisms. Furthermore, clinicians should be aware that glucocorticoids (and biological DMARDs) may blunt classic clinical symptoms and signs of infection and delay the diagnosis.

Before start of chronic glucocorticoid therapy >20 mg prednisone equivalents per day, which would be rather unusual in RA, clinicians should assess the patient's vaccination history and mend vaccination deficiencies.[64,65] However, internationally accepted, glucocorticoid-specific guidelines on vaccination are lacking.

Patients with RA undergoing hand and wrist surgery while on glucocorticoids at low dose appear to have no increased risk of wound infection or disturbed wound healing.[66]

Suppression of hypothalamic–pituitary–adrenal axis

Chronic administration of glucocorticoids suppresses the production of corticotropin-releasing hormone (CRH) and adrenocorticotropic hormone (ACTH) and results in atrophy of adrenal cortex due to lack of stimulation. This atrophy takes time to recover when glucocorticoid therapy is stopped and this may result in transient adrenal insufficiency, which is designed 'tertiary' adrenal insufficiency based on the suppression of CRH.[67] (see Figure 26.6).

The clinical spectrum of tertiary adrenal insufficiency may vary from mild symptoms, such as fatigue and muscle weakness and pain, mimicking disease flare, to more serious signs and symptoms, such as nausea, vomiting, weight loss, and hypotension. If in doubt, it seems prudent to treat patients as having adrenal insufficiency. Laboratory results are, next to a low serum cortisol, low ACTH levels, in contrast to patients with primary adrenal insufficiency, who have elevated ACTH levels.

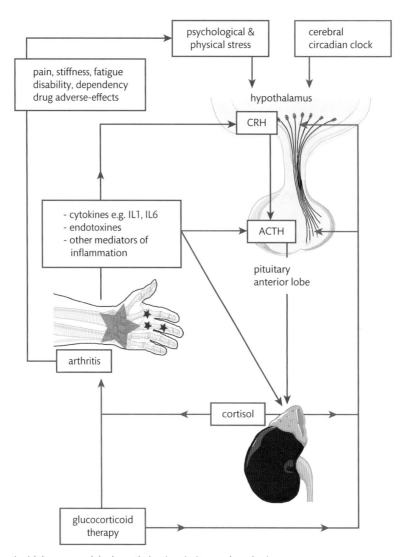

Figure 29.6 Arthritis, glucocorticoid therapy, and the hypothalamic–pituitary–adrenal axis.
Green arrows: suppression of arthritis and of the hypothalamic–pituitary–adrenal axis; red arrows: stimulation of the hypothalamic–pituitary–adrenal axis.

Reliable prediction of glucocorticoid-induced adrenal insufficiency is impossible, but some degree is to be expected if prednisone equivalent doses of more than 5 mg for a few weeks are stopped suddenly or when patients on low-dose glucocorticoid therapy are faced with stressful situations, such as major surgery.

The outer cortical zone involved in mineralocorticoids (aldosterone) biosynthesis is functionally independent of ACTH and stays intact; typically, no major electrolyte abnormalities in the blood occur and mineralocorticoid supplementation is not necessary.

Tapering

It is recommended that glucocorticoids be tapered to their lowest effective dose—and, if possible, discontinued—as soon as the disease or complication being treated is under control.[42,43] The evidence of joint-sparing effects of glucocorticoids, at least for two years of treatment in early disease, may lead some clinicians to prolong this treatment. Tapering must be done carefully to avoid disease flares, and adrenal insufficiency. Gradual tapering permits recovery of adrenal function. There is no standard scheme for tapering; it depends on individual's characteristics, disease activity, indications for the glucocorticoid therapy, doses and duration of therapy, and clinical response. In general, the lower the dose, the smaller the taper steps. To taper high-dose prednisone for severe complications of RA, decrements of 10–5 mg every 1–2 weeks can be used to 30 mg; then 2.5 mg/day decrements every 2–4 weeks until 15 mg/day; thereafter, tapering steps of 1 mg each month or 2.5 mg every 7 weeks. To taper low-dose glucocorticoid therapy in RA, several schemes have been used.[68,69]

Stress regimes

Patients on long-term glucocorticoid medication should be instructed to double their daily glucocorticoid dose, or increase the dose to at least 15 mg prednisolone daily or equivalent, if they develop fever attributed to infection, and to seek medical help. In case of major surgery, given the unreliable prediction of adrenal suppression, many physicians recommend 'stress doses' of glucocorticoids, even for patients considered at low risk of adrenal suppression. A classic stress scheme consists of 100 mg of hydrocortisone intravenously just before surgery, followed by an additional 100 mg every 6 hours for 3 days. However, this is based on anecdotal information and is not always necessary.[70] Although conclusive evidence is scarce, other regimes with lower doses are used. These include a continuous intravenous infusion of 100 mg of hydrocortisone the first day of surgery, followed by 25–50 mg of hydrocortisone every 8 hours for 2 or 3 days. Another option is to administer the usual dose of oral glucocorticoid orally (or the equivalent parenterally) on the day of surgery, followed by 25–50 mg of hydrocortisone every 8 hours for 2 or 3 days. In cases of minor surgery, it is probably sufficient to double the oral daily dose or to increase the dose to 15 mg of prednisolone or equivalent daily for 1–3 days. The clinical utility of testing the functioning of the hypothalamic–pituitary–adrenal axis in patients on glucocorticoids to determine the perioperative glucocorticoid regimen has not been established.

Gastrointestinal adverse effects

Literature data on the risk of peptic ulcer associated with oral glucocorticoids are inconclusive. Glucocorticoids inhibit the production of COX-2 without hampering the production of COX-1 (see **Figure 29.3**), which is in line with studies that found no increased risk of peptic complications. However, glucocorticoids may induce ulcerogenic mechanisms.[71] In other studies, a relative risk of serious upper gastrointestinal peptic complications of about 2 was found.[72] When glucocorticoids are used in combination with non-steroidal anti-inflammatory drugs (NSAIDs), the relative risk of peptic ulcer disease and associated complications is estimated at about 4,[73] although this risk has been questioned.[74] Similar risks were found in a more recent publication.[75] Active RA and higher age are also risk factors for peptic ulcer disease, and should be taken into account when considering gastroprotective measures. Glucocorticoids have also been associated with an increased risk of diverticular perforation of the colon,[76] and with pancreatitis, (odds ratio 1.53, 95% confidence interval 1.27–1.84).[77]

Negative effects on bone

Osteoporosis

Glucocorticoids are associated with increased generalized bone loss and risk for osteoporotic fractures. The same holds true for active inflammatory diseases, such as RA, due to the production of inflammatory mediators that negatively affect bone, such IL-1 and TNF. Glucocorticoids inhibit these effects of disease but this cannot balance the negative generalized effects of glucocorticoids on bone. Glucocorticoids decrease intestinal absorption and increase renal excretion of calcium, decrease the number and function of osteocytes and osteoblasts, while increasing the number and function of osteoclasts. Furthermore, they reduce mechanical load on bones, via loss of muscle mass,[78,79] which contributes to a decrease in bone mineral density (BMD). Vertebral fractures associated with glucocorticoid therapy tend to occur at a higher BMD than fractures related to postmenopausal osteoporosis. This is due to negative effects of glucocorticoids also on bone structure, decreasing bone strength, and an increase in the risk of falls due to glucocorticoid-associated muscle atrophy,[80,81] see **Figure 29.7**. This must be taken into consideration when interpreting BMD, as it underestimates the risk of glucocorticoid-associated fractures.[31]

Osteonecrosis

In RA, osteonecrosis is a rare event, even at high dosages and pulse therapy.[46] It occurs relatively frequently in systemic lupus erythematosus (SLE), which has been attributed to the disease itself and to the higher doses of glucocorticoids applied in this disease.[82]

Glucocorticoid-induced myopathy

Weakness in proximal muscles, especially of the lower extremities, may indicate glucocorticoid-induced myopathy, especially in patients receiving high doses (>30 mg/day prednisone or equivalent). It is often suspected, but infrequently found in low to moderate doses. Glucocorticoid-induced myopathy results from increased protein breakdown and decreased protein synthesis.[83] Diagnosis is clinical and can be confirmed by a muscle biopsy specimen that reveals atrophy of type II fibres and lack of inflammation; there is no elevation of serum muscle enzymes. Treatment consists of withdrawal of the glucocorticoid if possible.

Cardiovascular and metabolic adverse effects and events

The risk of adverse cardiovascular events is increased in patients with RA,[84] and in other inflammatory rheumatic diseases such as psoriatic arthritis, SLE, and ankylosing spondylitis. The European League Against Rheumatism (EULAR) recommendations for cardiovascular disease risk management in patients with RA and other forms of inflammatory joint disorders recommend that a multiplication factor of 1.5 should be applied to cardiovascular risk scores for patients with severe or long-standing RA, irrespective of therapy.[84] This increased risk is probably caused by negative effects of the chronic inflammation itself, via known and unknown disease-related mechanisms.

The negative metabolic effects of glucocorticoids, such as glucose intolerance, obesity, dyslipidaemia and hypertension suggest that they enhance cardiovascular risk.[84] Medium and high doses of glucocorticoids, but also NSAIDs, ciclosporin, and leflunomide may cause or aggravate hypertension, but this is not observed with low doses of synthetic glucocorticoids.[85] Several observational studies have described a dose-dependent increase of the cardiovascular risk in association with glucocorticoid therapy, especially with doses above 8–15 mg/day prednisolone equivalent, and with high cumulative dosages. However, these data incorporate an elevated risk of bias by indication, as both RA and glucocorticoids are associated with such events. Furthermore, glucocorticoids in fact reduce the inflammation-mediated cardiovascular risk. A prospective cohort study concluded that the cardiovascular risk attributed to glucocorticoids in observational studies indeed probably is overestimated.[86] So, the interactions between inflammatory disease, glucocorticoid therapy, and cardiovascular disease are intricate, see **Figure 29.5**.

Glucocorticoids increase hepatic glucose production, induce insulin resistance, and probably also have a direct effect on the β cells of the pancreas, resulting in enhanced insulin secretion. It may take only a few weeks before medium glucocorticoid doses cause hyperglycaemia, but in pulse therapy this effect is present within hours. Active RA is associated with similar negative effects on glucose tolerance,[87,88] which can be abrogated by effective control of inflammation by DMARDs, including low-dose chronic glucocorticoid therapy.[87,89] Worsening of glucose control in patients with established diabetes mellitus is to be expected on medium to high glucocorticoid doses. In previously non-diabetic subjects, an odds ratio of 1.8 for the need to initiate antihyperglycaemic drugs during chronic

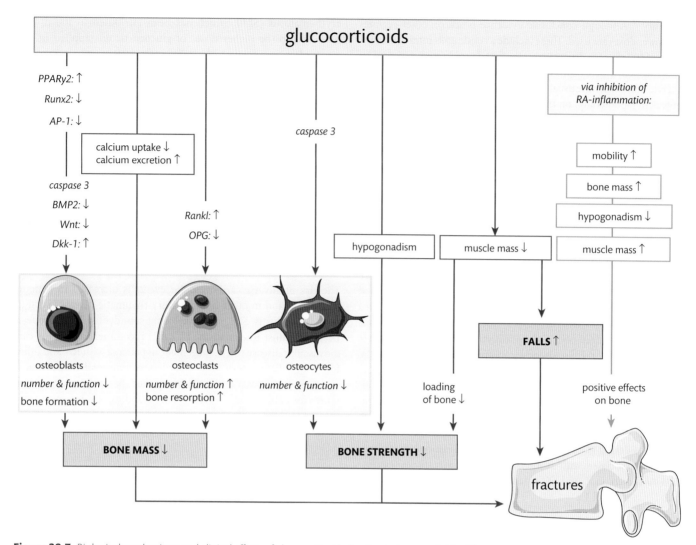

Figure 29.7 Biological mechanisms and clinical effects of glucocorticoids, leading to increased risk of fractures.
Fractures, especially of vertebral bodies, ribs, hips, and wrists, have been described in up to 30–50% of patients on long-term glucocorticoid therapy. Many of the vertebral fractures are asymptomatic. This has been used as an argument to propose that BMD should be combined with morphometric vertebral fracture assessment in patients on glucocorticoid therapy. PPAR γ2, peroxisome proliferator-activated receptor-γ2; Runx2, Runt-related transcription factor 2; AP-1, activator protein-1; BMP2, bone morphogenetic protein 2; Wnt, Wnt signaling pathway; Dkk-1, dickkopf-1; RANKL, nuclear factor-κB ligand; OPG, osteoprotegerin.

glucocorticoid therapy in doses of 10 mg or more of prednisone or equivalent per day was seen; the odds ratio was 3 for 10–20 mg, 5.8 for 20–30 mg, and 10.3 for 30 mg or more daily.[89] The risk is likely higher in patients with other risk factors for diabetes mellitus, such as a family history of the disease, advanced age, obesity, and previous gestational diabetes. Usually, glucocorticoid-induced diabetes is reversible when the drug is discontinued, unless there was pre-existing glucose intolerance.

A Cushingoid phenotype of centripetal fat accumulation with thin extremities with atrophic skin and bruising is a characteristic feature of patients exposed to long-term high-dose glucocorticoids[90,91]; low-dose glucocorticoids for a prolonged period in patients with RA caused only minor effects in fat distribution and body weight.[13,15] Potential mechanisms are manifold and have not been fully elucidated.[92] Patients with active inflammatory diseases tend to lose weight due to catabolic inflammatory mediators, an effect that is counteracted by effective medication, including glucocorticoids.[30–32]

Adverse effects on the eyes

Cataract

Glucocorticoids stimulate the formation of cataract, especially the posterior subcapsular type,[93] but also the cortical type, with an odds ratio of 2.6.[94] The likelihood and severity of this adverse effect depend on dose and duration of treatment. In patients treated with prednisone at a dose of 15 mg or more daily for at least 1 year, cataract is observed frequently, but cataract may also develop with long-term, low-dose therapy.[95] These cataracts are usually bilateral and slowly progressing.

Glaucoma

Glucocorticoids may cause or aggravate glaucoma, especially in patients with high myopia, those with a family history of open-angle glaucoma, and those receiving high doses. Checks of intraocular pressure in these patients are warranted.[96] If intraocular pressure is found to be increased, patients need to be treated with medications to reduce it, often for a prolonged period after stopping the glucocorticoid.[97] Topical application of a glucocorticoid in the eye has a more pronounced effect on intraocular pressure than does systemic therapy.[98]

Adverse effects on skin and hair

Clinically relevant adverse effects of high-dose and long-term glucocorticoids on skin include Cushingoid appearance, easy bruising, ecchymoses, skin atrophy, striae, disturbed wound healing, acne, perioral dermatitis, hyperpigmentation, facial redness, mild hirsutism, and thinning of pubic and scalp hair. The physician may consider these changes to be of minor clinical importance, but they frequently are disturbing to the patient.[90] The spectrum of these adverse effects is dependent on duration of therapy and dose.[95] Usage of 10 mg prednisone equivalent/day by patients with ankylosing spondylitis was associated with 12.6 events per 1000 patient years for non-infectious cutaneous adverse effects, including acne and easy bruising.[99] In RA-patients on low-to-medium glucocorticoid doses, easy bruising/ecchymosis, skin atrophy, and impaired wound healing were associated with current and cumulative glucocorticoid use, whereas there was low occurrence of abnormal stretch marks, acne, perioral dermatitis, alopecia, and hirsutism, which were not statistically significantly associated with glucocorticoid use.[91]

Psychological adverse effects

High-dose glucocorticoid treatment is associated with a variety of cognitive and behavioural symptoms.[100,101] A history of psychiatric illness seems not to predict occurrence of such effects,[101] although there are studies that found the opposite.[102] Previous glucocorticoid-induced psychiatric disturbances or previous treatment(s) free of such disturbances do not clearly predict recurrent or new onset psychological adverse effects in a patient.[103] Although most attention is drawn towards to infrequent overt psychiatric disturbances (e.g. depression and mania), less florid psychological manifestations, which may cause distress to patients, occur more frequently, also at medium doses. These include depressed or elated mood (euphoria), insomnia, irritability, emotional instability, anxiety, memory failure, and other cognition impairments; they may also occur on withdrawal of glucocorticoids. Their exact incidence is unknown, but they are rarely of relevance in the typical low dosages used in RA.

Pregnancy and lactation

The fetus is protected from several exogenous (i.e. maternal) glucocorticoids, such as cortisol and prednisolone, thanks to the placenta. In contrast, dexamethasone freely crosses this barrier, resulting in a maternal-to-fetal blood concentration ratio of about 1:1. So if a pregnant woman has to be treated with glucocorticoids, prednisone, prednisolone, and methylprednisolone would be good choices with low risk for the unborn child. Low to moderate doses of prednisone seem to be safe.[104,105] If the unborn child has to be treated (e.g. to induce lung maturation in a fetus at risk of preterm delivery), fluorinated glucocorticoids, such as betamethasone or dexamethasone, are indicated.

Prednisolone and prednisone are excreted in small quantities in breast milk, but breastfeeding is generally considered safe. The exposure of the infant seems minimized if breastfeeding is avoided during the first 4 hours after (methyl)prednisolone dosing.[104,106] Medium and high dosed glucocorticoids may, even when applied as local injection, suppress lactation.[107]

Prophylactic measures and monitoring

Some prophylactic measures during glucocorticoid therapy are evidence based. If comedication with an NSAID is needed, consider cotreatment with a proton pump inhibitor or misoprostol, and/or prescribe a COX-1 sparing NSAID, dependent on the individual patient's risk of peptic ulcer and cardiovascular disease. Adequate use of calcium, vitamin D, and bisphosphonates according to national or international guidelines minimizes the risk of osteoporosis, as also shown in the CAMERA-II study.[29]

Recommendations have been formulated on the management of systemic glucocorticoid therapy in rheumatic diseases,[108] as well on monitoring of patients receiving low-dose glucocorticoid therapy.[109] For patients receiving medium or high doses of glucocorticoids, good clinical practice monitoring should be intensified; recommendations on the use of these doses have been published.[96] In future clinical trials of glucocorticoid-based therapies for RA, comprehensive monitoring and reporting of treatment-related adverse effects is advised, to obtain more reliable data on the spectrum, incidence, and severity of adverse effects.[109] To assess glucocorticoid-related adverse effects and glucocorticoid-sparing effects of additional drugs, a glucocorticoid toxicity index has been developed.[110]

New developments

Increased knowledge about modes of action of glucocorticoids and pathophysiological backgrounds of rheumatic diseases creates opportunities for new developments to optimize the effects and to decrease adverse effects of these agents.[95,111] For instance, a modified-release prednisone tablet is available. When taken in the evening, the delayed prednisone release mimics the natural circadian rhythm of cortisol and effectively targets the nocturnal release of pro-inflammatory cytokines, especially IL-6. This results in more reduction of morning stiffness in RA compared to taking prednisone early in the morning.[112,113] Combining glucocorticoids with agents that selectively amplify their anti-inflammatory activity (e.g. the platelet-activation blocking agent dipyridamole) could improve the risk:benefit ratio by reducing the effective dose,[114] but this combination has not found its way to the clinic. Another group of such compounds that was under development is that of nitro steroids,[115] but their development seems to have been stopped.[111] Glucocorticoid-containing liposomes, which accumulate at sites of inflammation, enabling less-frequent dosing, are also being studied.[116,117] Selective glucocorticoid receptor agonists causing less DNA-dependent transactivation than conventional glucocorticoids could be associated with fewer metabolic and endocrine adverse effects, but the dogma that transrepression is responsible for immunosuppression and transactivation for adverse effect of glucocorticoids seems too simple,[111] accounting for the delay in the development of these drugs.

REFERENCES

1. Buttgereit F, da Silva JA, Boers M, et al. Standardised nomenclature for glucocorticoid dosages and glucocorticoid treatment regimens: current questions and tentative answers in rheumatology. *Ann Rheum Dis* 2002;61:718–22.

2. Hardy R, Rabbitt EH, Filer A, et al. Local and systemic gluco-corticoid metabolism in inflammatory arthritis. *Ann Rheum Dis* 2008;67:1204–10.

3. Nanus DE, Filer AD, Hughes B, et al. TNFalpha regulates cortisol metabolism *in vivo* in patients with inflammatory arthritis. *Ann Rheum Dis* 2015;74:464–9.

4. Barnes PJ, Adcock IM. Glucocorticoid resistance in inflammatory diseases. *Lancet* 2009;373:1905–17.

5. Carrie F, Roblot P, Bouquet S, Delon A, Roblot F, Becq-Giraudon B. Rifampin-induced nonresponsiveness of giant cell arteritis to prednisone treatment. *Arch Intern Med* 1994;154:1521–4.

6. Varis T, Kivisto KT, Neuvonen PJ. Grapefruit juice can increase the plasma concentrations of oral methylprednisolone. *Eur J Clin Pharmacol* 2000;56:489–93.

7. Cain DW, Cidlowski JA. Immune regulation by glucocorticoids. *Nat Rev Immunol* 2017;17:233–47.

8. Vandevyver S, Dejager L, Tuckermann J, Libert C. New insights into the anti-inflammatory mechanisms of glucocorticoids: an emerging role for glucocorticoid-receptor-mediated transactivation. *Endocrinology* 2013;154:993–1007.

9. Czock D, Keller F, Rasche FM, Haussler U. Pharmacokinetics and pharmacodynamics of systemically administered glucocorticoids. *Clin Pharmacokinet* 2005;44:61–98.

10. Harr MW, Rong Y, Bootman MD, Roderick HL, Distelhorst CW. Glucocorticoid-mediated inhibition of Lck modulates the pattern of T cell receptor-induced calcium signals by down-regulating inositol 1,4,5-trisphosphate receptors. *J Biol Chem* 2009;284:31860–71.

11. Coutinho AE, Chapman KE. The anti-inflammatory and immunosuppressive effects of glucocorticoids, recent developments and mechanistic insights. *Mol Cell Endocrinol* 2011;335:2–13.

12. Kirwan JR. The effect of glucocorticoids on joint destruction in rheumatoid arthritis. The Arthritis and Rheumatism Council Low-Dose Glucocorticoid Study Group. *N Engl J Med* 1995;333:142–6.

13. Wassenberg S, Rau R, Steinfeld P, Zeidler H. Very low-dose prednisolone in early rheumatoid arthritis retards radiographic progression over two years: a multicenter, double-blind, placebo-controlled trial. *Arthritis Rheum* 2005;52:3371–80.

14. Svensson B, Boonen A, Albertsson K, van der HD, Keller C, Hafstrom I. Low-dose prednisolone in addition to the initial disease-modifying antirheumatic drug in patients with early active rheumatoid arthritis reduces joint destruction and increases the remission rate: a two-year randomized trial. *Arthritis Rheum* 2005;52:3360–70.

15. Van Everdingen AA, Jacobs JW, Siewertsz Van Reesema DR, Bijlsma JW. Low-dose prednisone therapy for patients with early active rheumatoid arthritis: clinical efficacy, disease-modifying properties, and side effects: a randomized, double-blind, placebo-controlled clinical trial. *Ann Intern Med* 2002;136:1–12.

16. Van Everdingen AA, Siewertsz Van Reesema DR, Jacobs JW, Bijlsma JW. The clinical effect of glucocorticoids in patients with rheumatoid arthritis may be masked by decreased use of additional therapies. *Arthritis Rheum* 2004;51:233–8.

17. Jacobs JW, Van Everdingen AA, Verstappen SM, Bijlsma JW. Followup radiographic data on patients with rheumatoid arthritis who participated in a two-year trial of prednisone therapy or placebo. *Arthritis Rheum* 2006;54:1422–8.

18. Boers M, Verhoeven AC, Markusse HM, et al. Randomised comparison of combined step-down prednisolone, methotrexate and sulphasalazine with sulphasalazine alone in early rheumatoid arthritis. *Lancet* 1997;350:309–18.

19. Landewé RB, Boers M, Verhoeven AC, et al. COBRA combination therapy in patients with early rheumatoid arthritis: long-term structural benefits of a brief intervention. *Arthritis Rheum* 2002;46:347–56.

20. van Tuyl LH, Boers M, Lems WF, et al. Survival, comorbidities and joint damage 11 years after the COBRA combination therapy trial in early rheumatoid arthritis. *Ann Rheum Dis* 2010;69:807–12.

21. Goekoop-Ruiterman YP, de Vries-Bouwstra JK, Allaart CF, et al. Clinical and radiographic outcomes of four different treatment strategies in patients with early rheumatoid arthritis (the BeSt study): a randomized, controlled trial. *Arthritis Rheum* 2008;58:S126–S135.

22. Ter Wee MM, den Uyl D, Boers M, et al. Intensive combination treatment regimens, including prednisolone, are effective in treating patients with early rheumatoid arthritis regardless of additional etanercept: 1-year results of the COBRA-light open-label, randomised, non-inferiority trial. *Ann Rheum Dis* 2014;74:1233–40.

23. Choy EH, Kingsley GH, Khoshaba B, Pipitone N, Scott DL. A two year randomised controlled trial of intramuscular depot steroids in patients with established rheumatoid arthritis who have shown an incomplete response to disease-modifying antirheumatic drugs. *Ann Rheum Dis* 2005;64:1288–93.

24. Hansen M, Podenphant J, Florescu A, et al. A randomised trial of differentiated prednisolone treatment in active rheumatoid arthritis. Clinical benefits and skeletal side effects. *Ann Rheum Dis* 1999;58:713–18.

25. Paulus HE, Di Primeo D, Sanda M, et al. Progression of radiographic joint erosion during low dose corticosteroid treatment of rheumatoid arthritis. *J Rheumatol* 2000;27:1632–7.

26. Capell HA, Madhok R, Hunter JA, et al. Lack of radiological and clinical benefit over two years of low dose prednisolone for rheumatoid arthritis: results of a randomised controlled trial. *Ann Rheum Dis* 2004;63:797–803.

27. Kirwan JR, Bijlsma JW, Boers M, Shea BJ. Effects of glucocorticoids on radiological progression in rheumatoid arthritis. *Cochrane Database Syst Rev* 2007;(1):CD006356.

28. Verstappen SM, Jacobs JW, van der Veen MJ, et al. Intensive treatment with methotrexate in early rheumatoid arthritis: aiming for remission. Computer-Assisted Management in Early Rheumatoid Arthritis (CAMERA, an open-label strategy trial). *Ann Rheum Dis* 2007;66:1443–9.

29. Bakker MF, Jacobs JW, Welsing PM, et al. Low-dose prednisone inclusion in a methotrexate-based, tight control strategy for early rheumatoid arthritis: a randomized trial. *Ann Intern Med* 2012;156:329–39.

30. Jurgens MS, Jacobs JW, Geenen R, et al. Increase of body mass index in a tight controlled methotrexate-based strategy with prednisone in early rheumatoid arthritis: side effect of the prednisone or better control of disease activity? *Arthritis Care Res (Hoboken)* 2013;65:88–93.

31. Marouen S, Barnetche T, Combe B, Morel J, Daien CI. TNF inhibitors increase fat mass in inflammatory rheumatic disease: a systematic review with meta-analysis. *Clin Exp Rheumatol* 2017;35:337–43.

32. Sfriso P, Caso F, Filardo GS, et al. Impact of 24 months of anti-TNF therapy versus methotrexate on body weight in patients with rheumatoid arthritis: a prospective observational study. *Clin Rheumatol* 2016;35:1615–18.

33. van der Goes MC, Jacobs JW, Jurgens MS, et al. Are changes in bone mineral density different between groups of early

rheumatoid arthritis patients treated according to a tight control strategy with or without prednisone if osteoporosis prophylaxis is applied? *Osteoporos Int* 2013;*24*:1429–36.

34. Safy M, Jacobs J, IJff ND, Bijlsma J, van Laar JM, de Hair M. Long-term outcome is better when a methotrexate-based treatment strategy is combined with 10 mg prednisone daily: follow-up after the second Computer-Assisted Management in Early Rheumatoid Arthritis trial. *Ann Rheum Dis* 2017;*76*:1432–35.

35. Moreland LW, Curtis JR. Systemic nonarticular manifestations of rheumatoid arthritis: focus on inflammatory mechanisms. *Semin Arthritis Rheum* 2009;*39*:132–43.

36. Boumpas DT, Chrousos GP, Wilder RL, Cupps TR, Balow JE. Glucocorticoid therapy for immune-mediated diseases: basic and clinical correlates. *Ann Intern Med* 1993;*119*: 1198–208.

37. DiBattista JA, Martel-Pelletier J, Wosu LO, Sandor T, Antakly T, Pelletier JP. Glucocorticoid receptor mediated inhibition of interleukin-1 stimulated neutral metalloprotease synthesis in normal human chondrocytes. *J Clin Endocrinol Metab* 1991;*72*:316–26.

38. O'Dell JR. Treating rheumatoid arthritis early: a window of opportunity? *Arthritis Rheum* 2002;*46*:283–5.

39. Bos WH, Dijkmans BA, Boers M, van de Stadt RJ, van Schaardenburg D. Effect of dexamethasone on autoantibody levels and arthritis development in patients with arthralgia: a randomised trial. *Ann Rheum Dis* 2010;*69*:571–4.

40. Machold KP, Landewé R, Smolen JS, et al. The Stop Arthritis Very Early (SAVE) trial, an international multicentre, randomised, double-blind, placebo-controlled trial on glucocorticoids in very early arthritis. *Ann Rheum Dis* 2010;*69*:495–502.

41. Verstappen SM, McCoy MJ, Roberts C, Dale NE, Hassell AB, Symmons DP. Beneficial effects of a 3-week course of intramuscular glucocorticoid injections in patients with very early inflammatory polyarthritis: results of the STIVEA trial. *Ann Rheum Dis* 2010;*69*:503–9.

42. Smolen JS, Landewé R, Bijlsma J, et al. EULAR recommendations for the management of rheumatoid arthritis with synthetic and biological disease-modifying antirheumatic drugs: 2016 update. *Ann Rheum Dis* 2017;*76*(6):960–77.

43. Singh JA, Saag KG, Bridges SL, Jr., et al. 2015 American College of Rheumatology guideline for the treatment of rheumatoid arthritis. *Arthritis Rheumatol* 2016;*68*:1–26.

44. Seror R, Dougados M, Gossec L. Glucocorticoid sparing effect of tumour necrosis factor alpha inhibitors in rheumatoid arthritis in real life practice. *Clin Exp Rheumatol* 2009;*27*:807–13.

45. Fortunet C, Pers YM, Lambert J, et al. Tocilizumab induces corticosteroid sparing in rheumatoid arthritis patients in clinical practice. *Rheumatology (Oxf)* 2015;*54*:672–7.

46. Weusten BL, Jacobs JW, Bijlsma JW. Corticosteroid pulse therapy in active rheumatoid arthritis. *Semin Arthritis Rheum* 1993;*23*:183–92.

47. de Jong PH, Hazes JM, Han HK, et al. Randomised comparison of initial triple DMARD therapy with methotrexate monotherapy in combination with low-dose glucocorticoid bridging therapy; 1-year data of the tREACH trial. *Ann Rheum Dis* 2014;*73*:1331–9.

48. Eustace JA, Brophy DP, Gibney RP, Bresnihan B, FitzGerald O. Comparison of the accuracy of steroid placement with clinical outcome in patients with shoulder symptoms. *Ann Rheum Dis* 1997;*56*:59–63.

49. Chen MJ, Lew HL, Hsu TC, et al. Ultrasound-guided shoulder injections in the treatment of subacromial bursitis. *Am J Phys Med Rehabil* 2006;*85*:31–5.

50. Cunnington J, Marshall N, Hide G, et al. A randomized, double-blind, controlled study of ultrasound-guided corticosteroid injection into the joint of patients with inflammatory arthritis. *Arthritis Rheum* 2010;*62*:1862–9.

51. Berger RG, Yount WJ. Immediate 'steroid flare' from intraarticular triamcinolone hexacetonide injection: case report and review of the literature. *Arthritis Rheum* 1990;*33*:1284–6.

52. Goldfarb CA, Gelberman RH, McKeon K, Chia B, Boyer MI. Extra-articular steroid injection: early patient response and the incidence of flare reaction. *J Hand Surg [Am]* 2007;*32*:1513–20.

53. Hollander JL. Intrasynovial corticosteroid therapy in arthritis. *Md State Med J* 1970;*19*:62–6.

54. Gray RG, Tenenbaum J, Gottlieb NL. Local corticosteroid injection treatment in rheumatic disorders. *Semin Arthritis Rheum* 1981;*10*:231–54.

55. Seror P, Pluvinage P, d'Andre FL, Benamou P, Attuil G. Frequency of sepsis after local corticosteroid injection (an inquiry on 1160000 injections in rheumatological private practice in France). *Rheumatology (Oxf)* 1999;*38*:1272–4.

56. da Silva JAP, Jacobs JWG, Kirwan JR, et al. Safety of low dose glucocorticoid treatment in rheumatoid arthritis: published evidence and prospective trial data. *Ann Rheum Dis* 2006;*65*:285–93.

57. Strehl C, Bijlsma JW, de Wit M, et al. Defining conditions where long-term glucocorticoid treatment has an acceptably low level of harm to facilitate implementation of existing recommendations: viewpoints from an EULAR task force. *Ann Rheum Dis* 2016;*75*:952–7.

58. Wilson JC, Sarsour K, Collinson N, et al. Serious adverse effects associated with glucocorticoid therapy in patients with giant cell arteritis (GCA): a nested case-control analysis. *Semin Arthritis Rheum* 2017;*46*(6):819–27.

59. Dixon WG, Kezouh A, Bernatsky S, Suissa S. The influence of systemic glucocorticoid therapy upon the risk of non-serious infection in older patients with rheumatoid arthritis: a nested case-control study. *Ann Rheum Dis* 2011;*70*:956–60.

60. Wolfe F, Caplan L, Michaud K. Treatment for rheumatoid arthritis and the risk of hospitalization for pneumonia: associations with prednisone, disease-modifying antirheumatic drugs, and anti-tumor necrosis factor therapy. *Arthritis Rheum* 2006;*54*:628–34.

61. Migita K, Sasaki Y, Ishizuka N, et al. Glucocorticoid therapy and the risk of infection in patients with newly diagnosed autoimmune disease. *Medicine (Baltimore)* 2013;*92*(5):285–93.

62. Dixon WG, Suissa S, Hudson M. The association between systemic glucocorticoid therapy and the risk of infection in patients with rheumatoid arthritis: systematic review and meta-analyses. *Arthritis Res Ther* 2011;*13*:R139.

63. Santiago T, da Silva JA. Safety of glucocorticoids in rheumatoid arthritis: evidence from recent clinical trials. *Neuroimmunomodulation* 2015;*22*:57–65.

64. van Assen S, Agmon-Levin N, Elkayam O, et al. EULAR recommendations for vaccination in adult patients with autoimmune inflammatory rheumatic diseases. *Ann Rheum Dis* 2011;*70*:414–22.

65. Caplan A, Fett N, Rosenbach M, Werth VP, Micheletti RG. Prevention and management of glucocorticoid-induced side effects: a comprehensive review: infectious complications and vaccination recommendations. *J Am Acad Dermatol* 2017;*76*:191–8.

66. Jain A, Witbreuk M, Ball C, Nanchahal J. Influence of steroids and methotrexate on wound complications after elective rheumatoid hand and wrist surgery. *J Hand Surg Am* 2002;*27*:449–55.

67. Charmandari E, Nicolaides NC, Chrousos GP. Adrenal insufficiency. *Lancet* 2014;*383*:2152–67.

68. Pincus T, Swearingen CJ, Luta G, Sokka T. Efficacy of prednisone 1–4 mg/day in patients with rheumatoid arthritis: a randomised, double-blind, placebo-controlled withdrawal clinical trial. *Ann Rheum Dis* 2009;*68*:1715–20.

69. Hickling P, Jacoby RK, Kirwan JR. Joint destruction after glucocorticoids are withdrawn in early rheumatoid arthritis. Arthritis and Rheumatism Council Low Dose Glucocorticoid Study Group. *Br J Rheumatol* 1998;*37*:930–6.

70. Marik PE, Varon J. Requirement of perioperative stress doses of corticosteroids: a systematic review of the literature. *Arch Surg* 2008;*143*:1222–6.

71. Filaretova L, Podvigina T, Bagaeva T, Morozova O. Dual action of glucocorticoid hormones on the gastric mucosa: how the gastroprotective action can be transformed to the ulcerogenic one. *Inflammopharmacology* 2009;*17*:15–22.

72. Garcia Rodriguez LA, Hernandez-Diaz S. The risk of upper gastrointestinal complications associated with nonsteroidal anti-inflammatory drugs, glucocorticoids, acetaminophen, and combinations of these agents. *Arthritis Res* 2001;*3*:98–101.

73. Piper JM, Ray WA, Daugherty JR, Griffin MR. Corticosteroid use and peptic ulcer disease: role of nonsteroidal anti-inflammatory drugs. *Ann Intern Med* 1991;*114*:735–40.

74. Filaretova L, Podvigina T, Bagaeva T, Bobryshev P, Takeuchi K. Gastroprotective role of glucocorticoid hormones. *J Pharmacol Sci* 2007;*104*:195–201.

75. Tseng CL, Chen YT, Huang CJ, et al. Short-term use of glucocorticoids and risk of peptic ulcer bleeding: a nationwide population-based case-crossover study. *Aliment Pharmacol Ther* 2015;*42*:599–606.

76. Humes DJ, Fleming KM, Spiller RC, West J. Concurrent drug use and the risk of perforated colonic diverticular disease: a population-based case-control study. *Gut* 2011;*60*:219–24.

77. Sadr-Azodi O, Mattsson F, Bexlius TS, Lindblad M, Lagergren J, Ljung R. Association of oral glucocorticoid use with an increased risk of acute pancreatitis: a population-based nested case-control study. *JAMA Intern Med* 2013;*173*:444–9.

78. Weinstein RS. Clinical practice. Glucocorticoid-induced bone disease. *N Engl J Med* 2011;*365*:62–70.

79. Kuchuk NO, Hoes JN, Bijlsma JWJ, Jacobs JWG. Glucocorticoid-induced osteoporosis: an overview. *Int J Clin Rheumatol* 2014;*9*:311–26.

80. Weinstein RS. Glucocorticoids, osteocytes, and skeletal fragility: the role of bone vascularity. *Bone* 2010;*46*:564–70.

81. Diacinti D, Guglielmi G, Pisani D, et al. Vertebral morphometry by dual-energy X-ray absorptiometry (DXA) for osteoporotic vertebral fractures assessment (VFA). *Radiol Med* 2012;*117*:1374–85.

82. Shigemura T, Nakamura J, Kishida S, et al. Incidence of osteonecrosis associated with corticosteroid therapy among different underlying diseases: prospective MRI study. *Rheumatology (Oxf)* 2011;*50*:2023–8.

83. Schakman O, Kalista S, Barbe C, Loumaye A, Thissen JP. Glucocorticoid-induced skeletal muscle atrophy. *Int J Biochem Cell Biol* 2013;*45*:2163–72.

84. Agca R, Heslinga SC, Rollefstad S, et al. EULAR recommendations for cardiovascular disease risk management in patients with rheumatoid arthritis and other forms of inflammatory joint disorders: 2015/2016 update. *Ann Rheum Dis* 2017;*76*:17–28.

85. Panoulas VF, Douglas KM, Stavropoulos-Kalinoglou A, et al. Long-term exposure to medium-dose glucocorticoid therapy associates with hypertension in patients with rheumatoid arthritis. *Rheumatology (Oxf)* 2008;*47*:72–5.

86. van Sijl AM, Boers M, Voskuyl AE, Nurmohamed MT. Confounding by indication probably distorts the relationship between steroid use and cardiovascular disease in rheumatoid arthritis: results from a prospective cohort study. *PLoS One* 2014;*9*:e87965.

87. Wasko MC, Kay J, Hsia EC, Rahman MU. Diabetes mellitus and insulin resistance in patients with rheumatoid arthritis: risk reduction in a chronic inflammatory disease. *Arthritis Care Res (Hoboken)* 2011;*63*:512–21.

88. Hoes JN, van der Goes MC, van Raalte DH, et al. Glucose tolerance, insulin sensitivity and beta-cell function in patients with rheumatoid arthritis treated with or without low-to-medium dose glucocorticoids. *Ann Rheum Dis* 2011;*70*:1887–94.

89. den Uyl D, van Raalte DH, Nurmohamed MT, et al. Metabolic effects of high-dose prednisolone treatment in early rheumatoid arthritis: balance between diabetogenic effects and inflammation reduction. *Arthritis Rheum* 2012;*64*:639–46.

90. van der Goes MC, Jacobs JW, Boers M, et al. Patient and rheumatologist perspectives on glucocorticoids: an exercise to improve the implementation of the European League Against Rheumatism (EULAR) recommendations on the management of systemic glucocorticoid therapy in rheumatic diseases. *Ann Rheum Dis* 2010;*69*:1015–21.

91. Amann J, Wessels AM, Breitenfeldt F, et al. Quantifying cutaneous adverse effects of systemic glucocorticoids in patients with rheumatoid arthritis: a cross-sectional cohort study. *Clin Exp Rheumatol* 2017;*35*(3):471–6.

92. Lee MJ, Pramyothin P, Karastergiou K, Fried SK. Deconstructing the roles of glucocorticoids in adipose tissue biology and the development of central obesity. *Biochim Biophys Acta* 2014;*1842*:473–81.

93. Carnahan MC, Goldstein DA. Ocular complications of topical, peri-ocular, and systemic corticosteroids. *Curr Opin Ophthalmol* 2000;*11*:478–83.

94. Klein BE, Klein R, Lee KE, Danforth LG. Drug use and five-year incidence of age-related cataracts: the Beaver Dam Eye Study. *Ophthalmology* 2001;*108*:1670–4.

95. Huscher D, Thiele K, Gromnica-Ihle E, et al. Dose-related patterns of glucocorticoid-induced side effects. *Ann Rheum Dis* 2009;*68*:1119–24.

96. Duru N, van der Goes MC, Jacobs JW, et al. EULAR evidence-based and consensus-based recommendations on the management of medium to high-dose glucocorticoid therapy in rheumatic diseases. *Ann Rheum Dis* 2013;*72*:1905–13.

97. Garbe E, LeLorier J, Boivin JF, Suissa S. Risk of ocular hypertension or open-angle glaucoma in elderly patients on oral glucocorticoids. *Lancet* 1997;*350*:979–82.

98. Tripathi RC, Parapuram SK, Tripathi BJ, Zhong Y, Chalam KV. Corticosteroids and glaucoma risk. *Drugs Aging* 1999;*15*: 439–50.

99. Zhang YP, Gong Y, Zeng QY, Hou ZD, Xiao ZY. A long-term, observational cohort study on the safety of low-dose glucocorticoids in ankylosing spondylitis: adverse events and effects on bone mineral density, blood lipid and glucose levels and body mass index. *BMJ Open* 2015;*5*:e006957.

100. Wolkowitz OM, Burke H, Epel ES, Reus VI. Glucocorticoids. Mood, memory, and mechanisms. *Ann N Y Acad Sci* 2009;*1179*:19–40.

101. Kenna HA, Poon AW, de los Angeles CP, Koran LM. Psychiatric complications of treatment with corticosteroids: review with case report. *Psychiatry Clin Neurosci* 2011;*65*:549–60.

102. Fardet L, Petersen I, Nazareth I. Suicidal behavior and severe neuropsychiatric disorders following glucocorticoid therapy in primary care. *Am J Psychiatry* 2012;*169*:491–7.

103. Warrington TP, Bostwick JM. Psychiatric adverse effects of corticosteroids. *Mayo Clin Proc* 2006;*81*:1361–7.

104. Temprano KK, Bandlamudi R, Moore TL. Antirheumatic drugs in pregnancy and lactation. *Semin Arthritis Rheum* 2005;*35*:112–21.

105. Ostensen M, Khamashta M, Lockshin M, et al. Anti-inflammatory and immunosuppressive drugs and reproduction. *Arthritis Res Ther* 2006;*8*:209.

106. Cooper SD, Felkins K, Baker TE, Hale TW. Transfer of methylprednisolone into breast milk in a mother with multiple sclerosis. *J Hum Lact* 2015;*31*:237–9.

107. Babwah TJ, Nunes P, Maharaj RG. An unexpected temporary suppression of lactation after a local corticosteroid injection for tenosynovitis. *Eur J Gen Pract* 2013;*19*:248–50.

108. Hoes JN, Jacobs JW, Boers M, et al. EULAR evidence-based recommendations on the management of systemic glucocorticoid therapy in rheumatic diseases. *Ann Rheum Dis* 2007;*66*:1560–7.

109. van der Goes, Jacobs JWG, Boers M, et al. Monitoring adverse events of low-dose glucocorticoids therapy: EULAR recommendations for clinical trials and daily practice. *Ann Rheum Dis* 2010;*69*:1913–19.

110. Miloslavsky EM, Naden RP, Bijlsma JW, et al. Development of a Glucocorticoid Toxicity Index (GTI) using multicriteria decision analysis. *Ann Rheum Dis* 2016;*76*(3):543–6.

111. Strehl C, van der Goes MC, Bijlsma JW, Jacobs JW, Buttgereit F. Glucocorticoid-targeted therapies for the treatment of rheumatoid arthritis. *Expert Opin Investig Drugs* 2017;*26*:187–95.

112. Buttgereit F, Doering G, Schaeffler A, et al. Efficacy of modified-release versus standard prednisone to reduce duration of morning stiffness of the joints in rheumatoid arthritis (CAPRA-1): a double-blind, randomised controlled trial. *Lancet* 2008;*371*:205–14.

113. Bijlsma JW, Jacobs JW. Glucocorticoid chronotherapy in rheumatoid arthritis. *Lancet* 2008;*371*:183–84.

114. Jacobs JW, Bijlsma JW. Innovative combination strategy to enhance effect and diminish adverse effects of glucocorticoids: another promise? *Arthritis Res Ther* 2009;*11*:105.

115. Baraldi PG, Romagnoli R, Del Carmen NM, et al. Synthesis of nitro esters of prednisolone, new compounds combining pharmacological properties of both glucocorticoids and nitric oxide. *J Med Chem* 2004;*47*:711–19.

116. Vanniasinghe AS, Bender V, Manolios N. The potential of liposomal drug delivery for the treatment of inflammatory arthritis. *Semin Arthritis Rheum* 2009;*39*:182–96.

117. van den Hoven JM, Hofkens W, Wauben MH, et al. Optimizing the therapeutic index of liposomal glucocorticoids in experimental arthritis. *Int J Pharm* 2011;*416*:471–77.

30

Conventional disease-modifying drugs

David L. Scott

Introduction

Disease-modifying antirheumatic drugs (DMARDs) are a diverse range of drugs that are used to treat rheumatoid arthritis (RA). They have become a dominant therapeutic group. These drugs are considered together because they are conventional drugs which not only improve the symptoms of RA but also, to greater or lesser extents, modify its course.

Our current perspective about these drugs goes back to the early 1980s.[1,2] Initially several different names were applied for these various drugs. Such terms included 'second-line drugs',[3] 'slow-acting antirheumatic drugs' and 'remission inducing drugs'.[4] These names derive from the order in which they were used, implied by second line; their speed of onset, which is implied by slow-acting; or their impact on remission, which is implied by remission inducing, all had disadvantages. Consequently, the term DMARDs has been generally adopted within rheumatology.

The introduction of biologics and new oral kinase inhibitors has influenced terminology. Many experts now refer to these long-established drugs as conventional DMARDs, in contrast to biologic DMARDs. Some experts have taken the classification further by terming these drugs as conventional synthetic (csDMARDs) as opposed to biologic (bDMARDs) and targeted synthetic (tsDMARDs) such as Janus kinase inhibitors.[5] Whether this more complex terminology will generally prevail is uncertain.

Currently used conventional DMARDs

Many different drugs have been considered to be DMARDs. However, in modern practice there are only four drugs which are used to any great extent. Methotrexate is the dominant DMARD. Other commonly used DMARDs include sulfasalazine, leflunomide, and hydroxychloroquine. There are number of infrequently used or historic DMARDs that are given to occasional patients. The various DMARDs are shown in **Table 30.1**.

DMARDs can be used as monotherapy or in combinations. Their use in combinations can be with other DMARDs, with biologics or with the newer Janus kinase inhibitors. Methotrexate is not only the most widely used DMARD in monotherapy, but is also the main DMARD used in combinations both with other conventional DMARDs and with biologics and Janus kinase inhibitors. Sulfasalazine and leflunomide are also used both as monotherapy and in combinations, but usually with other conventional DMARDs. In contrast hydroxychloroquine is predominantly used in combinations with other conventional DMARDs and has only a limited role as a monotherapy.

Impacts of DMARDs

These drugs reduce joint inflammation. Successful treatment with DMARDs reduces the number of active joints and the severity of joint inflammation. This is shown by reductions in the numbers of tender joints and swollen joints. There are associated reductions in joint pain and stiffness, including early morning stiffness. Patients' and clinicians' overall assessments of their disease are also often measurably reduced by DMARD use.

Improvements in joint inflammation are also associated with reductions in raised acute phase reactants such as the erythrocyte sedimentation rate (ESR) and C-reactive protein levels (CRP). Although many other proteins change as part of the acute phase reactant response to treatment, these are not usually measured in routine clinical practice. There are practical benefits in measuring CRP levels, but the ESR has a strong historic base and remains widely measured.

Improvements in synovitis brought about by DMARDs are mirrored by improvements in physical function and increases in health-related quality of life (HRQOL). These benefits extend across many aspects of health and include reductions in fatigue. Finally, the progression of joint damage is slowed by most DMARDs, and this impact is the main reason they are considered 'disease-modifying' treatments.

There are many different ways of measuring these impacts of DMARDs. However, current practice usually restricts these to a few regularly collected assessments. These usually include:

- Joint counts: numbers of tender and swollen joints—counting either 28 joints or extended 66 and 68 joints
- Patients' and clinicians' overall assessments of disease activity on 100 mm visual analogue scales
- ESR and CRP levels
- Physical Function assessed using the Health Assessment Questionnaire (HAQ)

Table 30.1 Current disease-modifying antirheumatic drugs

Dominant	Methotrexate
Frequently used	Sulfasalazine, hydroxychloroquine, leflunomide
Rarely used	Ciclosporin
Historic	Injectable gold azathioprine, penicillamine, chloroquine

These measures are often combined. In clinical practice the disease activity score for 28 joints (DAS28) is widely used; it incorporates tender joint counts, swollen joint counts, patient global assessments, and ESR. In trials the American College of Rheumatology (ACR) 20, 50, and 70 response criteria are widely used. There are many other measures which can be used. The combined assessments are also used to assess active disease, low disease activity, and remission. These various issues are considered in detail in Chapter 15.

The benefits of DMARDs need to be balanced against the many adverse events they can cause. Some harms are common to most DMARDs. These include changes in blood cells and liver toxicity. Other harms are unique to specific DMARDs. An example is ocular toxicity with hydroxychloroquine. These adverse events are considered in detail with each of the different DMARDs.

General features of DMARDs

Starting DMARDs

DMARDs are known to be effective in RA of high disease activity. Such patients have DAS28 scores greater than 5.1 and usually have 3–6 or more tender and swollen joints. In patients with high disease activity, there is a strong case for treatment with DMARDs.

Historically DMARDs were not started when RA was first diagnosed. However, this approach changed many years ago. International expert opinion now strongly favours starting DMARDs as soon as patients are known to have RA.[5–7] This approach is supported by a large range of clinical guidelines. In the UK national guidance is that patients should start DMARDs within 6 weeks of diagnosis[6]; European and North American guidelines also support similar early use though they were less specific about timelines.

The place of methotrexate as the dominant DMARD means that most guidance recommends preferentially starting patients on methotrexate unless there are reasons to use an alternative DMARD. For example, in younger women with RA who are considering becoming pregnant an alternative DMARD to methotrexate may be preferred.

Some guidance suggests it is sensible to start patients on DMARD monotherapy, which usually means methotrexate. Other guidance recommends considering combination therapy with either DMARDs and short-term steroids or combinations of two or more DMARDs. Intensive treatment can be given to all patients or to those with indicators of severe disease, such strong seropositivity for rheumatoid factor (RF) and/or anticitrullinated protein antibody (ACPA), and having an elevated acute phase response. This is an area of ongoing controversy. To an extent all the guidance implies giving intensive DMARD combinations, or combinations of methotrexate and biologics, to patients with early active RA who fail to respond to methotrexate monotherapy, or other DMARD monotherapy if methotrexate is contraindicated.

In established RA patients may start a new DMARD or combination therapy with DMARDs if their disease has flared, if they have persistently active disease while taking another DMARD or if they have to stop current DMARDs due to toxicity.

Monitoring DMARDs

The risks of haematologic and hepatic toxicity means most DMARDs require regular monitoring with blood and liver function tests. There is considerable uncertainty about the optimal amount and duration of monitoring. Some expert groups have suggested initially monitoring every 1–4 weeks and then gradually extending the duration between tests[8]; other guidance is more flexible about the frequency of monitoring, which can be a minimum of 8–12 weeks in some patients.[5,7]

This practice began because it was possible to predict patients at risk of marrow toxicity with gold injections by prospective monitoring; such an approach substantially improved safety risks. With modern treatment the risks are less clear cut and the benefits of monitoring are more questionable.[9–12] However, in some patients' adverse events involving the blood and liver can be detected on monitoring and such reactions carry substantial risks for patients. Consequently, monitoring has become part of the standard approach to DMARD as well as bDMARD treatment.

Stopping DMARDs

DMARDs are stopped for toxicity and for loss of effect and also for other patient and disease related factors. Often these different reasons overlap. The frequency of stopping DMARD monotherapies because of toxicity or loss of effect is high. More than half of patients initiating DMARDs discontinue treatment over the next 2–3 years. Retention rates differ across DMARDs, with patients remaining on methotrexate longer than other DMARDs. This finding has been confirmed in many different observational studies.[13–15] Two examples of varying retention rates with different DMARDs are shown in **Figure 30.1**. The reasons that patients remain on methotrexate for longer than other DMARDs are uncertain, but they almost certainly underlie the adoption of methotrexate as the key DMARD.

There has been considerable interest in why patients discontinue DMARDs. One observational study from England highlighted the importance of adverse events and found that three-quarters of patients who stopped methotrexate did so for adverse effects, particularly gastrointestinal problems.[16] A detailed evaluation of why RA patients start and stop DMARDs using data from rheumatology practices in Northern California suggested two things. Firstly, there has been a decline in year-to-year stopping of all DMARDs over time. This gradual reduction in the frequency of stopping DMARDs is likely to reflect the increasing treatment options over the last 30 years and rheumatologists being less concerned about marginally abnormal laboratory tests while patients receive DMARDs. Secondly, some factors including Hispanic ethnicity, using oral glucocorticoids, and having more tender joints, predict starting and stopping DMARDs. These latter factors relate to more frequent

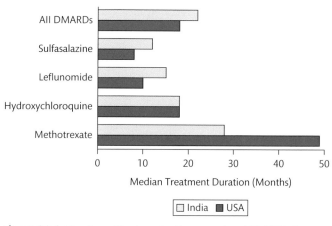

Figure 30.1 Duration of treatment with conventional DMARDs in two observational studies from the United States and India.

Source: Data from Maradit-Kremers H *et al* (2006) 'Patient, disease, and therapy-related factors that influence discontinuation of disease-modifying antirheumatic drugs: a population-based incidence cohort of patients with rheumatoid arthritis'. *J Rheumatol* 33: 248–55 and Agarwal S, Zaman T, and Handa R. (2009) 'Retention rates of disease-modifying anti-rheumatic drugs in patients with rheumatoid arthritis'. *Singapore Med J* 50: 686–92.

switches in treatment.[17] Other detailed studies of why patients stop treatment, using questionnaires and qualitative research methods have highlighted a range of patient level factors.[18,19] Apart from sociodemographic factors, patients' beliefs about their illness and its treatment play crucial roles. Low levels of adherence with treatment, and stopping therapy, may be related in part to negative beliefs about medicines and illness in RA.

Tapering DMARDs

When patients have good responses to treatment and enter a period of stable remission or low disease activity while taking DMARDs the benefit of remaining on treatment is often questioned. The benefits of continuing on treatment while in remission need to be weighed against the risks of potential overtreatment and toxicity together with treatment costs. However, the balance of evidence suggests the rates of flares on stopping treatment is sufficiently high to make a uniform strategy of this nature impractical at the present time. Systematic reviews by O'Mahony et al.[20] and by Schett et al.[21] evaluated trials of stopping DMARDs and some observational studies. Both provided evidence of increased flare rates after stopping DMARDs. The complexity of the challenge of DMARD withdrawal is illustrated in an observational study from Finland.[22] In this 15-year follow-up of 87 patients with early RA treated initially with intensive DMARDs, these drugs were discontinued in 20 patients because of remission or symptom-free periods. However, in almost half of the patients the disease flares, and in some cases the flares occurred several years after DMARD discontinuation.

Temporal changes in DMARD use

Over the last 40 years the types of DMARDs used has changed, mainly due to the adoption of methotrexate as the core drug and decline in use of historic DMARDs like gold and penicillamine. A more interesting and important issue is the overall frequency of DMARD use. An observational study by Edwards et al.[23] used the General Practice Research Database in the United Kingdom to look

at changes from 1995 to 2010 in 35 911 RA patients identified from their general practice records. DMARD prescribing was 19–49% in 1995 and increased to 45–74% by 2010. Most of the increase was due to the greater use of methotrexate. There was substantial regional variation in DMARD prescribing and it was relatively low in some areas of the United Kingdom, suggesting many RA patients remained undertreated.

A similar trend has been found studying patients identified via their specialists, though the overall use of DMARDs is greater in this group. Analysis of an open longitudinal cohort of RA patients managed by rheumatologists in the United States[24] evaluated 1507 RA patients managed between 1983 and 2009. During this period the use of any DMARD increased from 71% to 83% of patients, though this included biologics as well as conventional DMARDs. In 2009 they found the most commonly used conventional DMARDs were methotrexate (49%), hydroxychloroquine (30%), leflunomide (13%), and sulfasalazine (7%). They also noted that since 1999 13% to 18% of RA patients managed by specialists were not taking any DMARDs. Hospital-based specialist practice in England showed a comparable change.[25] In evaluations of 1324 RA patients assessed between 1996 and 2014 in adjacent rheumatology units in London the use of any DMARD increased from 61% to 87% of patients. These increases in DMARD use are an international finding and have been replicated in studies in Germany and Australia.[26,27]

Despite the substantial temporal increase in the use of conventional DMARDs in general and methotrexate in particular for RA, there remains a substantial body of expert opinion suggesting methotrexate remains underused. Rohr et al.[28] used a US database covering 274 million people to identify patients diagnosed with RA naive to methotrexate in 2009 and 2012. Of patients with 5-year follow-up data available, oral methotrexate was started in 35 640 in 2009, and 44% continued this dose during the follow-up. Of the 20 041 patients who changed therapy during the study period, 87% had the addition of or switched to a biologic agent, while only 13% changed to subcutaneous methotrexate. Mean doses of methotrexate and the use of subcutaneous treatment were both considered suboptimal.

Cost-effectiveness

DMARD monotherapy, particularly with methotrexate, is the current minimally acceptable standard of care for RA. Cost-effectiveness studies use this approach as a baseline for comparative studies. Economic modelling has compared early intensive treatment with conventional DMARDs against a more delayed approach.[29] Early intervention reduces the progression of joint erosions and subsequent functional disability and therefore increases quality-adjusted life more than delayed treatment and saves long-term costs. When the cost of very early intervention is factored in, the cost-effectiveness ratio of the early DMARD strategy is about $5000 per quality-adjusted life year. This cost falls well within the acceptable limits for treatment approaches. Economic analysis of individual early treatment strategies suggested intensive early treatment with triple DMARD therapy was more cost-effective than initial methotrexate monotherapy alone.[30]

An alternative approach to evaluating the economic benefits of treatment is to assess the costs of poor adherence to early treatment with DMARDs in a cohort of early RA patients. This approach was taken by Pasma and colleagues.[31] They found that incomplete adherence to early treatment with DMARDs, which was seen in about one-fifth of patients, increased healthcare costs substantially.

The health economic benefits of intensive DMARD treatment in early RA are not necessarily seen in established RA.

Methotrexate

Background

During the last 30 years methotrexate has become the most important drug treatment for RA. The balance of its efficacy, safety, ease of administration, and patient acceptability has made it a key treatment option. It is now considered to be the 'anchor drug' in treating inflammatory arthritis, and that this role may have been enhanced by its positive interaction with biologic treatments. Methotrexate is widely recommended as the initial treatment for active RA and it is used in many different clinical settings.

Although many rheumatologists have played roles in its rise to prominence a key contribution was made by Michael Weinblatt, who provided a detailed outline of the growing role of methotrexate in RA.[32] The precursor of methotrexate, an antifolate drug called aminopterin, was used to treat leukaemia in children in the late 1940s. Subsequently it was successfully given to a small number of patients with RA and also patients with psoriasis and psoriatic arthritis.[33] There was evidence these patients benefitted. However, it was some years before the role of methotrexate was developed in RA with observational studies preceded by randomized trials.

Mechanism of action

Aminopterin and subsequently methotrexate were developed as antifolate agents which inhibit the enzyme dihydrofolate reductase. Its effectiveness at high doses to treat leukaemia almost certainly reflects its impact on folate metabolism. However, this has not been considered a key component of its mechanism of action at the low doses of the drug used in RA. Indeed, folic acid is usually coprescribed with methotrexate in RA to minimize the risks of adverse effects, without compromising efficacy, and so it it seems unlikely inhibiting folate metabolism is a critical mechanism in this setting. A range of other mechanisms have been implicated.[34]

These include effects on adenosine signalling, methyl donors, reactive oxygen species, eicosanoids, and metalloproteinase enzymes, cytokine profiles, and adhesion molecule expression. The concept that methotrexate effects adenosine release has held sway for many years.[35] Adenosine is an important anti-inflammatory mediator and influences immune cells. Methotrexate inhibits adenosine metabolism, and this may be important in its effects in RA. However, adenosine has a short half-life *in vivo* and is consequently difficult to measure directly. The available data about the interactions between methotrexate and adenosine metabolism are variable and, so far, have not led to new insights of direct clinical relevance, though it remains an area of interest. On balance research into how methotrexate might work in RA have been relatively inconclusive and have not yet changed the way it is used in practice.

Clinical trials

The most influential trial of methotrexate by Weinblatt and his colleagues was reported in 1985.[36] It was a randomized, placebo-controlled, 24-week crossover study of 35 patients with refractory RA. Patients initially received 7.5 mg methotrexate weekly which was increased to 15 mg weekly at 6 weeks. Clinical improvements occurred as soon as 3 weeks after methotrexate was started. Over 50% of the patients showed substantial improvements in joint tenderness with methotrexate and 39% had substantial improvements in joint swelling (**Figure 30.2**). At 12 weeks RA disease activity improved significantly in methotrexate-treated patients compared to controls taking a placebo. In the second 12 weeks of the study, flares in disease activity were seen after 3–6 weeks in patients who crossed over from methotrexate to placebo therapy.

Another larger 18-week, placebo-controlled trial by Williams and his colleagues in 189 patients with active RA confirmed the efficacy of methotrexate at the same dosage level.[37] Several other trials corroborated these data. As a consequence, it was approved by regulatory agencies for use in active RA, including the Food and Drug Administration (FDA) in the United States in 1986; it gradually become the key drug to use in active RA.

The most recent Cochrane systematic review of methotrexate in RA, from 2014,[38] evaluated 7 trials which had studied 732 patients over 3 months to 1 year. All the trials included patients who have failed previous DMARDs, which were usually historic treatments like injectable gold. Weekly doses of methotrexate ranged between 5 mg and 25 mg. There were statistically significant improvements in a range of measures of disease activity and physical function. There were also more harms with methotrexate and patients were twice more likely to discontinue treatment with methotrexate due to adverse events than were those taking placebo. However, there was no evidence of significantly more serious adverse effects occurred with methotrexate than placebo.

Although the classic early trials used weekly dosing with oral methotrexate, it has always been available for use as a subcutaneous injection. In 2008 Braun et al.[39] reported a trial comparing 15 mg weekly subcutaneous *versus* oral methotrexate in methotrexate-naive patients with active RA. A total of 188 patients were randomized to receive subcutaneous methotrexate and 187 were randomized to receive oral methotrexate. Significantly more patients treated with subcutaneous methotrexate showed some and good clinical responses. The benefit was larger in patients with established RA. Changing from oral to subcutaneous methotrexate increased responder rates. There was no difference in tolerability between the treatments.

The value of subcutaneous methotrexate has been examined in detail over the last decade. A systematic review by Li et al.[40] identified seven studies involving 1335 patients that examined the potential benefits of subcutaneous methotrexate. They found that subcutaneous methotrexate significantly increases the bioavailability of methotrexate, shortens the time to reach maximum concentration, improves clinical response rates, and reduces some adverse events,

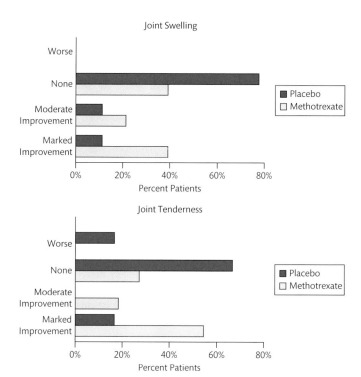

Figure 30.2 Key outcomes in first trial of methotrexate in rheumatoid arthritis.
Source: data from Weinblatt M *et al* (1985) 'Efficacy of low-dose methotrexate in rheumatoid arthritis'. *N Engl J Med* 312: 818–22.

particularly nausea. However, it has no impact on the frequency of treatment failure with methotrexate.

Clinical use

International guidance recommends using methotrexate as part of the first treatment strategy in patients with RA,[41,42] particularly in patients with active disease. The rationale for recommending methotrexate as the first choice DMARD include its efficacy, relative safety, and the possibility of individualizing doses and method of administration. Methotrexate can be used as monotherapy or in combination with other drugs. The value of methotrexate is underlined by the evidence that it seems to reduce comorbidities and mortality in RA.[43,44] Methotrexate dosage should be rapidly increased from an initial dose of 7.5–15.0 mg weekly to maximal levels of 25 mg or even 30 mg weekly. Treatment with methotrexate is usually continued for as long as possible. If the disease flares more drugs are usually added to methotrexate. However, if there are significant adverse events treatment is discontinued.

Most RA patients treated with methotrexate also receive low-dose folic acid, usually given as 5–10 mg weekly on a different day to the methotrexate. There is strong evidence from clinical trials that this reduces adverse effects, particularly gastrointestinal and hepatic adverse effects.[45] Clinicians often give patients higher doses of folic acid to prevent adverse effects. However, one trial by Dhir et al.[46] found no evidence that despite the use of high doses of methotrexate in current practice, there was additional benefit or harm in using a higher dose of folic acid than the usual 5–10 mg/week.

Methotrexate is not suitable for all patients. It is contraindicated in pregnancy and in patients considering pregnancy because it causes embryotoxicity, abortion, and fetal defects.[47] As it affects spermatogenesis and oogenesis it may also decrease fertility. This effect seems reversible after treatment is discontinued. Patients and their partners should be advised to avoid pregnancy until 3 months after cessation of methotrexate therapy. In addition, patients should not breastfeed while taking methotrexate. Finally, the possible risks of effects on reproduction should be discussed with RA patients of childbearing potential before using methotrexate.

Methotrexate needs to be used cautiously in older people and in patients with impaired renal function. This is because its clearance is reduced when creatinine clearance decreases, and such patients require smaller doses.[48] Impaired creatinine clearance is common in elderly patients in whom standard doses may result in more toxicity. An associated issue is that non-steroidal anti-inflammatory drugs also decrease the glomerular filtration rate, particularly in older people. However, the balance of evidence suggests that provided careful monitoring is in place non-steroidal anti-inflammatory drugs can be used with methotrexate.[49]

Adverse reactions

Many different adverse events are seen with methotrexate, though many of these are relatively minor and can often be managed without stopping therapy.[49,50] Common problems include:

a) General non-specific side effects: these include fever, fatigue, and muscle pain.

b) Gastrointestinal problems: these are very common and span anorexia, nausea, vomiting, and diarrhoea. Stomatitis is also common and includes erythema, painful ulcers, and erosions.

c) Skin problems: alopecia is frequent and often concerns women; other skin reactions include urticaria and cutaneous vasculitis.

d) Central nervous system problems: these include headaches, drowsiness, and ataxia.

e) Infections: these involve opportunistic infections with organisms like *Pneumocystis carinii,* fungal infections, and localized or disseminated herpes zoster.

Methotrexate also causes a range of potentially serious adverse events and its use requires regular blood tests, particularly when it is first started. Bone marrow toxicity is one potential major concern: mild to moderate leukopenia, which responds to withdrawal of the drug can occur and occasional patients have pancytopenia, which is potentially fatal.[51] Although it can occur early, within the first few months of starting treatment, which may reflect an idiosyncratic reaction, more often it occurs late, suggesting a cumulative effect, particularly in older people.

Liver toxicity is another clinical challenge. One the one hand mild elevations of transaminase levels and other liver enzymes are common during blood monitoring of methotrexate but serious hepatotoxicity, including fibrosis or cirrhosis is rare, though persistently elevated liver enzyme levels are associated with more serious disease.[52] Conventionally patients taking methotrexate are advised to minimize or completely stop alcohol intake, though some recent evidence suggests such rigorous advice is neither followed nor needed,[53] though controversy remains on how much alcohol is appropriate when taking methotrexate.

Methotrexate also causes a small increase in the risk of lung disease in RA,[54] and particularly pulmonary interstitial disease, which can develop suddenly and may progress to fibrosis. It is sometimes fatal. As interstitial lung disease can occur in RA as an extra-articular feature of the disease unrelated to methotrexate therapy caution is needed in defining cause and effect. However, in patients taking methotrexate the development of a cough is often a warning feature and needs to be fully explored. Patients should usually to have a plain chest X-ray before starting treatment. Some experts also arrange lung function tests.

Vaccinations

Vaccination is a key strategy to reduce infection risk in patients with RA and is advocated in most clinical guidelines. Methotrexate reduces responses to vaccination, particularly pneumococcal vaccination, though its use should not preclude vaccination.[54] A recent trial has shown that temporary discontinuation of methotrexate for 2 weeks after vaccination improves the immunogenicity of seasonal influenza vaccination in RA patients without increasing RA disease activity.[54] This approach is likely to be generally adopted in clinical practice.

Other considerations

Accelerated nodulosis, with small nodules on the fingers or elbows, occurs occasionally during methotrexate therapy.[55] The nodules are histologically indistinguishable from other rheumatoid nodules. Patients are usually seropositive for rheumatoid factor and are aged over 50 years. Although some specialists stop methotrexate others prefer to add an additional drug like hydroxychloroquine.

One unique problem with methotrexate has been the propensity for accidental overdosing, which has often involved clinical staff.[56] One problem is that patients have been prescribed 10 mg tablets weekly instead of 2.5 mg tablets. Patients have also taken methotrexate daily instead of weekly or had their dose increased regularly to toxic levels. For these reasons great caution is needed in ensuring patients receive the correct dose.

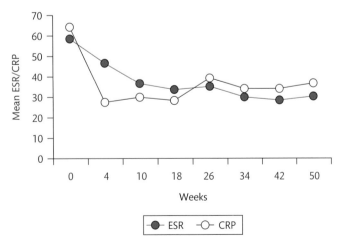

Figure 30.3 Falls in ESR and C-reactive protein during treatment with sulfasalazine.

Source: data from McConkey B et al (1980) 'Sulphasalazine in rheumatoid arthritis'. *Br Med J* 280:442–4.

Sulfasalazine

Background

Sulfasalazine was developed by Nana Svartz in Sweden during the late 1930s as she believed RA had a bacterial origin. Giving sulfonamides and aspirin concomitantly produced no obvious benefits. Consequently, Dr Svartz attempted to combine them chemically. One of the compounds produced was sulfasalazine, which Dr Swartz considered improved RA. It combined sulfapyridine with 5-aminosalicylic acid. However, international research in RA paused in the early 1940s and further development was deferred.[57] Trials in the immediate post-war period were negative in RA.[58] Interest in sulfasalazine was maintained in gastroenterology but not rheumatology.

The use of sulfasalazine was championed by McConkey in Birmingham in the 1970s and 1980s.[59] One key driver was a focus on identifying new treatments that reduced the high ESR and CRP levels that characterize active RA. A small observational study of 74 patients showed that sulfasalazine reduced these acute phase proteins over 12 months.[60] These findings are shown in **Figure 30.3**. This study revitalized interest in the drug and it led to several new clinical trials being undertaken which gave positive results.

Mechanism of action

Although sulfasalazine was developed because of its potential antibacterial effects, the balance of evidence suggests it is effective because it influences a range of immunologic processes.[61] These include effects on inflammatory cells and immunomodulation. There is also some evidence it may influence adenosine metabolism[62] and that it is an inhibitor of nuclear factor kappa B.[63] There is some evidence that sulfapyridine is the active component of sulfasalazine, but as it causes substantial nausea there is no benefit in using it to treat patients.[64]

Clinical trials

The effectiveness of sulfasalazine has been evaluated in two systematic reviews. A Cochrane review[65] evaluated its efficacy in six trials which involved 468 patients. A more extensive systematic review by Weinblatt et al.[66] evaluated 15 trials that included 2 gm/day sulfasalazine as a treatment. The average follow-up time was 36 weeks. Eight of these trials included a placebo group and a further seven trials compared sulfasalazine with hydroxychloroquine (2 trials), penicillamine (3 trials), and gold injections (4 trials). Both systematic reviews concluded sulfasalazine was effective in patients with active RA. The Cochrane review found that compared to placebo the standardized weighted mean difference with sulfasalazine was 0.5 for tender and swollen joint scores and 18 for the ESR.

Clinical use

The conventional target dose of sulfasalazine is 2 gm daily. Patients usually start with 500 mg daily and increase the dose weekly over 1 month. Most patients take two tablets twice daily, and this is usually given in an enteric-coated formulation to minimize gastrointestinal adverse reactions. Some patients receive higher doses, particularly 3 gm daily. There is some evidence that the higher dose level is more effective.[67] When dosage has been stabilized patients usually continue to take the same dose over time.

One particular point of interest about sulfasalazine is that it is one of the few treatments which can be used in patients who are pregnant.[68] It is therefore often recommended for patients who wish to conceive and are pregnant or lactating. Some experts recommend using folic acid supplementation preconception and during pregnancy and suggest that although it is safe to continue during lactation, patients should avoid breastfeeding if their infant is premature or has hyperbilirubinaemia.[69] An associated idiosyncrasy of sulfasalazine is that it can reduce sperm counts in males.[70] This effect has been studied in most detail in patients with inflammatory bowel disease taking sulfasalazine; it is reversed on stopping treatment.

Although sulfasalazine was widely used in the United Kingdom 20 years ago, its role as a monotherapy has declined in recent years and methotrexate has predominated. Elsewhere sulfasalazine was less favoured as a monotherapy. The exception remains its use in female patients who wish to conceive or are pregnant and patients with contraindications to methotrexate. Its use in combinations of disease-modifying drugs remains a major focus on interest. One particular limitation with sulfasalazine is that there is relatively little data about its impact on radiological progression of erosive damage.

Adverse events

In the first few weeks of treatment minor side effects are common, especially upper gastrointestinal problems and nausea. The slow introduction of therapy and the use of enteric coated tablets reduces these problems to an extent. Many other adverse reactions occur within the first few months of starting therapy and these are often relatively trivial and are self-limiting after treatment is stopped. Potentially more serious adverse reactions include leukopenia, rash, abnormal liver function tests, and dyspnoea. About 25% of patients starting treatment stop due to adverse reactions.[70] These reactions also reverse after treatment is stopped. Side effects leading to drug withdrawal after 1 year of therapy are unusual. Treatment is stopped in 20–30% due to adverse reactions.[71] Systematic reviews of toxicity suggest there is no difference in the likelihood of serious adverse events between sulfasalazine and methotrexate, though the chances of withdrawing therapy due to an adverse event is somewhat higher with sulfasalazine.[72] In the initial phases of treatment patients starting sulfasalazine require regular full blood counts and liver function tests; the frequency of these tests can be reduced as treatment becomes sustained.

One unusual adverse event linked to treatment with sulfasalazine is the drug reaction with eosinophilia and systemic symptoms (DRESS) syndrome, which comprises a drug rash with eosinophilia and systemic symptoms. This drug-induced hypersensitivity syndrome, which can mimic a malignant lymphoma, has been reported in occasional patients with RA.[73] Early recognition is essential as the DRESS syndrome has a high mortality rate. It is managed by stopping treatment with sulfasalazine and giving steroids as needed.[74]

Agranulocytosis is also a particular problem with sulfasalazine. One detailed evaluation of 10 000 patients receiving sulfasalazine found it occurred in 6/1000 users who had arthritis, which was substantially higher than in patients with inflammatory bowel disease receiving the drug.[75] It is treated by stopping sulfasalazine and considering the use of broad-spectrum antibiotics and haematopoietic growth factor,[76] which need to be supervised by haematologists.

Leflunomide

Background

Leflunomide was the only conventional DMARD to be specifically developed to treat RA. It was primarily assessed in a series of clinical trials in the 1990s and was found to be both effective and relatively safe. In terms of efficacy, toxicity, and retention on treatment there is relatively little difference between leflunomide and methotrexate. While methotrexate has remained the dominant DMARD for the last two decades or more, leflunomide is less used as a monotherapy in comparison. The reasons for this are not readily discernible. However, it is now unlikely that leflunomide will become a major antirheumatic drug. At the same time, it is used quite often in combination with methotrexate.

Mechanism of action

Leflunomide is a prodrug which is rapidly converted in both the gastrointestinal tract and plasma into an active, open ring malononitrilamide metabolite. It has several potential mechanisms of action.[77] It regulates lymphocyte proliferation through two different mechanisms. Firstly, by inhibiting tyrosine kinases associated with the initial stage of signal transduction. Secondly by inhibiting *de novo* pyrimidine nucleotide biosynthesis, which is generally considered its main impact and may result from non-competitive inhibition of the enzyme dihydroorotate dehydrogenase. There is also evidence that leflunomide modulates inflammation and metalloproteinase induction.

Clinical trials

The most detailed systematic review summarized the results of six trials which enrolled 2044 patients with RA.[78] All the trials were of high quality. The ACR20 response rate with leflunomide is approximately twice that of placebo therapy after both 6 and 12 months of treatment. Other disease activity measures, and assessments of function and radiological progression were also significantly better with leflunomide than with placebo therapy. Its effectiveness was considered comparable with those given by methotrexate at 12 months and sulfasalazine at 6 months. Withdrawal rates and adverse events in patients receiving leflunomide were also not different from those seen with methotrexate and sulfasalazine. Other systematic reviews support the similarity of leflunomide to the dominant DMARDs.[72]

Clinical use

Leflunomide has a long half-life with a slow onset of action and a prolonged effect after stopping treatment. Initially treatment was started by giving patients a loading dose, but this increased adverse events and is not used nowadays. Although the drug could be given intermittently it is conventionally given as 10 mg or 20 mg daily. Many clinicians prefer to start with the lower dose and then increase to 20 mg if there is a clinical need. Leflunomide can be used as a monotherapy in patients who failed to respond or had adverse events with methotrexate.[79] It can also be used in combination with methotrexate, though caution is required about the risks of adverse events.

Preclinical reproductive studies showed leflunomide was found to be embryotoxic and teratogenic. Women treated with leflunomide are advised to avoid pregnancy and it is not recommended for women who wish to conceive. Its long half-life means a considerable wash-out period is required before commencing pregnancy. If women do become pregnant on leflunomide a therapeutic wash-out with cholestyramine is often recommended. However, one study of the actual risks of pregnancy in women who conceived while taking the drug do not suggest the risks are too concerning[80]; a small study of 108 pregnant women found no evidence of a substantial increased risk of adverse pregnancy outcomes due to leflunomide exposure among women who undergo cholestyramine elimination procedure early in pregnancy.

Adverse events

A range of adverse events have been reported with leflunomide, including gastrointestinal upset, hypertension, headache, hepatotoxicity, hair loss, and predisposition to infection and peripheral neuropathy.[81] Some patients have considerable weight loss. Many experts monitor blood pressure during treatment to make certain patients do not have significant problems with hypertension. The frequency of gastrointestinal adverse events is similar to sulfasalazine, but greater than with methotrexate. Serious drug-induced hepatotoxicity is rare. Although leflunomide is often considered to have more risks of adverse events than methotrexate, a retrospective cohort study of a large US insurance claims database, which evaluated 40 594 patients with RA from 1998 to 2000) with 83 143 person-years follow-up, found there were fewer adverse events with leflunomide monotherapy (94 events/1000 patient-years) than methotrexate (145 events/1000 patient-years).[82] There have been concerns about respiratory adverse events with leflunomide but a systematic review, which examined four clinical studies, found no evidence for such an effect.[83] Overall, the adverse event profile with leflunomide is no worse than other conventional DMARDs and may even be better. However, when adverse events occur the long-half-life of leflunomide can be a problem; one option is to use a single day dosing of oral cholestyramine to 'wash-out' the drug and reduce levels by 50%. This approach has been successful in patients with adverse events such as a peripheral neuropathy.[84] Finally as it has limited renal toxicity leflunomide has been used in patients receiving renal dialysis or after renal transplants.[84]

Other conventional DMARDs

Hydroxychloroquine

The antimalarials hydroxychloroquine and chloroquine have both been used to treat RA for several decades. The evidence base for their use is relatively historic. Custom and practice has resulted in hydroxychloroquine becoming the only widely used antimalarial drug in RA and its role is mainly as part of a combination of conventional DMARDs.

The first antimalarial tried with mepacrine, which had been given with some success to patients with systemic lupus erythematosus. As this discoloured the skin, chloroquine was tried as a replacement, with some success.[85] Hydroxychloroquine became the favoured antimalarial because it was considered to have fewer adverse events and was effective.[86] The mechanism of action of hydroxychloroquine is uncertain, but it has a range of immunomodulatory and anti-inflammatory activities.[87]

The Cochrane systematic review of hydroxychloroquine reports on four trials in which 300 patients were randomized to hydrochloroquine and 292 to placebo. There were statistically significant benefits when hydroxychloroquine was compared to placebo. The standardized mean differences for a range of outcome measures ranged from −0.33 to −0.52. There were also significant reductions in the ESR. Although hydroxychloroquine appeared to be effective in treating RA its overall effect was only moderate. However, it also had a low toxicity profile. At the same time there is relatively little evidence that it has any impact in reducing progressive erosive joint damage in RA; it is even less effective than sulfasalazine in reducing damage.[87]

Hydroxychloroquine is given at doses of 200–400 mg daily, in divided doses. As the dose should not exceed 6.5 mg/kg/day calculated from ideal body weight, some patients should only have 200 mg per day. The evidence that higher doses than 200 mg are needed is incomplete.[88] Its favourable toxicity profile means it is sometimes used as a monotherapy in patients with mild disease. However, its predominant current use is as part of a combination therapy.

The main limitation using antimalarials is the potential risk of retinal toxicity, which have been appreciated since these drugs were first used in RA.[89] However, the magnitude of risk, particularly in patients receiving standard doses, has always been difficult to quantify.[90] One recent study assessed hydroxychloroquine retinal toxicity in 123 patients who were using or had used the drug. They found 14% of patients had some evidence of retinal toxicity. Retinal toxicity was associated with duration of hydroxychloroquine use, the daily dose, and the presence of renal disease. Ensuring patients receive less than 5 mg/kg hydroxychloroquine and regular ophthalmic screening were recommended.[91] The precise arrangements for screening vary substantially across different institutions and countries. The most recent national guidelines, from North America.[92] recommend a baseline fundus examination to rule out pre-existing maculopathy with annual screening beginning after 5 years for patients on acceptable doses and without major risk factors. The primary screening tests suggested are automated visual fields plus spectral-domain optical coherence tomography. Modern screening should detect retinopathy before it is visible in the fundus.

A range of other adverse events can occur with hydroxychloroquine. These include rashes, pruritus, and pigmentary changes in the skin; nausea, diarrhoea, and anorexia; dizziness and vertigo; the occasional development of a cardiomyopathy; and occasional blood disorders such as anaemia, agranulocytosis, and thrombocytopenia.

Ciclosporin

There was a strong scientific rationale for using ciclosporin to treat patients with RA based on its specific effects on T-lymphocyte function. Clinical studies showed that ciclosporin is effective in RA at doses of 2.5–5 mg/kg/day. It can be given in a microemulsion-based formulation. Initial low doses are increased depending on the clinical response and monitoring for toxicity.

A systematic review of ciclosporin in RA identified three trials in which 318 patients were enrolled.[93] There were statistically significant decreases in the number of tender and swollen joints compared to placebo. There were also improvements in pain and reductions in disability. However, there are several substantial disadvantages of ciclosporin. Firstly, it has always had only a limited, if any, impact on acute phase measures such as the ESR. This makes it difficult to assess the benefits of treatment.[94] Secondly, and more importantly, there are risks of serious renal toxicity unless the drug is carefully monitored with the dose of ciclosporin adjusted depending on creatinine levels.[95] There are problems with hypertension and interactions with anti-inflammatory drugs like diclofenac. Finally, the benefits of using ciclosporin in combination with methotrexate are uncertain; the extent to which there is a positive interaction is questionable.

As a consequence of these various complexities in assessing the clinical benefits and in monitoring the dose and evaluating toxicity ciclosporin is rarely used to treat RA. There are many effective alternatives that are simpler to use in routine clinical practice.

Azathioprine

The potential of azathioprine to reduce steroid use—its so-called steroid sparing effect—led to its introduction in the 1960s.[96] A small number of clinical trials were undertaken and these provided some indication that azathioprine may benefit patients with RA but the evidence is weak and the effects are small. The Cochrane systematic review analysed three trials involving 81 patients[97]; 40 patients were randomized to azathioprine and 41 to placebo. There was a statistically significant benefit of azathioprine on tender joint scores. However, the trials were small and relatively historic, the clinical benefits were modest and there was no information about the impact on function or other clinically important outcomes. As a consequence, azathioprine has only ever been given to occasional RA patients and has never been a mainstream DMARD.

The toxicity profile of azathioprine is relatively benign and there are no major concerns with it.[98] It has one unique problem with toxicity assessments in that is occasional causes marked bone marrow suppression with leukopenia. The development of severe myelosuppression is often associated with abnormal azathioprine metabolism linked to the thiopurine methyltransferase genetic polymorphism. Pretreatment measures of enzyme activity or genotyping techniques can identify patients homozygous for ineffective enzyme and these patients need to receive low doses of azathioprine or avoid taking the drug completely.[99]

Minor DMARDs

Historically injectable gold, given usually as sodium aurothiomalate and aurothioglucose, was important in developing the concept that there were drugs which could change the course of RA. Identifying injectable gold as a treatment option in active RA and confirming its efficacy in clinical trials took several decades and trials continued into the 1990s. It was conventionally given as weekly intramuscular injections of 50 mg after an initial 10 mg test dose until 1 gm has been received, after which the frequency of injections was reduced, usually to monthly. Treatment was stopped when adverse reactions occurred. Enthusiasts for gold have maintained it is an effective drug without excessive adverse events.[100] However, there are two substantial problems using gold. Firstly, the balance of evidence is that it has more serious toxicity than comparable DMARDs.[101] Secondly, it is a very complex treatment to administer as patients need to be seen weekly and given gold injections by a healthcare professional. Judging the impact of adverse reactions is also relatively challenging. While experts in using gold therapy achieved relatively good outcomes in years gone by it is not a drug that can be used occasionally. The advent of newer treatments with

better efficacy and safety ratios means it is no longer used to any extent at all. Attempts to introduce oral gold in the latter decades of the twentieth century, which ended with the development of auranofin, proved unsuccessful as the drug had insufficient efficacy. Some experts believe its effect is no different from placebo therapy.

Penicillamine was used for several decades to treat active RA. It was an effective oral drug which was evaluated in several trials. Its use was limited by significant toxicity.[102] Some expert reviews of penicillamine consider it was ineffective.[103] The initial dose was 125 mg daily, which was increased after a month to 250 mg daily. Many experts preferred a 'go low go slow' approach and did not increase dosage further; others gave higher long-term doses. In addition to its toxicity penicillamine was subjectively unpleasant to take and many patients only took their doses occasionally.[104] As with gold treatment penicillamine use declined with the advent of new treatments in the twenty-first century.

Finally, when there was a very limited choice of treatments for active RA, particularly in patients with systemic disease, occasional patients were treated with cytotoxic drugs such as cyclophosphamide and chlorambucil.[105] There was some evidence supporting their use when no other alternatives existed. However, with the development of new treatments the rationale for using these toxic treatments has declined and their use is now highly unusual.

Combining conventional DMARDS

Rationale

Patients with RA have always received concomitant treatment with several different drugs. In the twentieth century they often received one DMARD, steroids, and a non-steroidal anti-inflammatory drug. It was therefore only natural that clinicians would want to combine two or more conventional DMARDs. As the DMARDs have different mechanisms of action it was sensible to consider their combination would be more effective than monotherapy without excessive toxicity.

DMARDs can also be combined in two ways. Firstly, they can be started at the same time. Secondly they can be started sequentially, with the first drug followed after a period of delay with the second and, if needed, with a third. Although it is possible to start two or more DMARDs at the same time at the onset of RA, in established disease when patients are already receiving one DMARD, which is often methotrexate, it is easier to add additional DMARDs.

Trials of DMARD combinations started in the 1980s. These early trials showed it was possible to combine drugs, but when their results were analysed in a systematic review, the evidence of efficacy was minimal while their toxicity seems excessive.[106] These early attempts to combine DMARDs aroused interest but were generally unsuccessful.

Triple therapy

The clinical value of DMARD combinations was changed with the introduction of triple therapy using methotrexate, sulfasalazine, and hydroxychloroquine. The first trial of this combination by O'Dell and his colleagues[107] compared triple therapy with methotrexate monotherapy and the combination of sulfasalazine and hydroxychloroquine in 102 RA patients followed for two years. Fifty

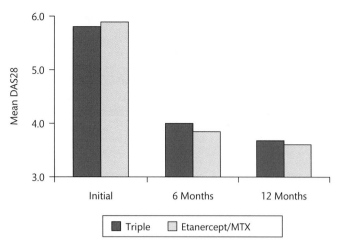

Figure 30.4 Mean disease activity (DAS28 scores) in head-to-head RACAT trial by O'Dell et al. comparing triple therapy (methotrexate, sulfasalazine, and hydroxychloroquine) with etanercept and methotrexate.

Source: data from O'Dell JR et al (2013) 'Therapies for active rheumatoid arthritis after methotrexate failure'. *N Engl J Med* 369:307–18.

of the 102 patients had 50% improvement at 9 months and maintained at least that degree of improvement for 2 years without major drug toxicity. Significantly more patients receiving triple therapy were in this group compared to the control treatments. There were also fewer treatment withdrawals of treatment toxicity with triple therapy than methotrexate monotherapy. This trial changed perceptions of combination DMARDs. A follow-up trials provided supportive evidence that triple therapy is effective and safe[108] and another trial by Saunders et al. showed step-up treatment had similar efficacy to starting all treatments at the same time.[109]

More recent trials have compared triple therapy with the biologic combination of methotrexate and etanercept in both early and established RA.[110,111] In both settings triple therapy has comparable efficacy to biologic treatment. Some of the key outcomes from the Rheumatoid Arthritis Comparison of Active Therapies (RACAT) trial in established rheumatoid arthritis are shown in **Figure 30.4**. The results of this trial suggest that triple therapy achieves similar outcomes to biologics combined with methotrexate. However, there has been substantial controversy about the way non-inferiority is defined in trials of this sort and many experts question the overall comparative benefit of non-biological treatments. As a consequence, they are only used by a minority of rheumatologists in North America. Subsequent follow-up of these patients for just under 1 year showed triple therapy was durable. The likelihood of continuing conventional therapy was 78% for triple therapy versus 63% for the combination of methotrexate with etanercept.[112] Most treatment changes occurred at the start of follow-up. A cost-effectiveness analysis of the RACAT trial showed that etanercept-methotrexate as first-line therapy gave marginally more quality-adjusted life years but had substantially higher treatment costs.[113] Triple therapy was therefore substantially more cost-effective.[114] The conclusion was that initiating biologic therapy without trying triple therapy first increases costs but gives minimal incremental benefit.

Not all experts have such a positive view on triple therapy. A systematic review by Mary et al.[115] of head-to-head trials with biologics identified five trials. American College of Rheumatology and

European League Against Rheumatism (EULAR) response criteria, DAS28, and X-ray progression scores all favoured biologic treatment combined with methotrexate. Functional impairment and rates of adverse events did not differ between treatments. This group recommended using triple therapy in the absence of poor prognostic factors, when there are contraindications to biologic agents, and when treatment strategies are restricted by economic considerations In addition an observational study of treatment retention in over 4000 patients found that in propensity weighted analyses patients were more likely to be persistent and adherent to biologic combination that triple therapy.

Other combinations

Many other DMARD combinations have been evaluated. The evidence supporting their use is variable and they have different risks of benefits. The range of combinations used is summarized in Table 30.2. The most important combination involve methotrexate. A few combinations of non-methotrexate DMARDs have been studied.

The most comprehensive systematic review of different combinations by Hazlewood et al.[116] identified 31 trials of DMARD combinations involving methotrexate. Most evaluated triple therapy (4 trials), or its components—methotrexate with hydroxychloroquine or chloroquine (7 trials) and methotrexate with sulfasalazine (6 trials). All these are effective but triple therapy has some benefits over its components. Three trials combined methotrexate with leflunomide, nine trials combined methotrexate with ciclosporin, and one trial combined it with gold. The comparative efficacy of these combinations is shown in **Figure 30.5**.

Combining leflunomide with methotrexate is effective[117] but there are concerns about the risk of hepatotoxicity[118,119] and also possibly an increased risk of pancytopenia.[120] These potential risks of serious adverse events have restricted the use of this DMARD combination, though it has a role in some patients. Some experts have also produced evidence that the combination of leflunomide with methotrexate is both relatively safe and effective.[120] Combinations of gold and ciclosporin with methotrexate, though effective, involve giving drugs that are difficult to monitor and have potentially high risks of adverse events. These latter combinations are therefore rarely used.

There have been several trials of combinations of DMARDs that do not include methotrexate and there is some evidence these are effective.[121,122] As these mainly involve relatively toxic older DMARDs like injectable gold they are of limited relevance in routine practice settings. An exception is the combination of leflunomide with sulfasalazine, which has been studied in a single small trial[123]; although

Table 30.2 Combinations of conventional disease-modifying drugs

Dominant	Triple therapy (methotrexate, sulfasalazine, hydroxychloroquine)
Sometimes used	Methotrexate/leflunomide, methotrexate/sulfasalazine, methotrexate/hydroxychloroquine
Occasionally used	Sulfasalazine/leflunomide
Rarely used	Methotrexate/injectable gold, methotrexate/ciclosporin, gold/hydroxychloroquine

The use of combinations varies geographically as clinical practice is not uniform. Some countries use more than others of different combinations.

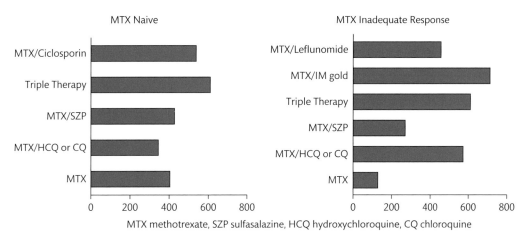

Figure 30.5 Comparison of effects of DMARD combinations on ACR50 responder rates from systematic review.
Source: data from Hazlewood GS et al (2016) 'Methotrexate monotherapy and methotrexate combination therapy with traditional and biologic disease modifying antirheumatic drugs for rheumatoid arthritis: abridged Cochrane systematic review and network meta-analysis'. *Br Med J* 353: i1777.

the results were promising for the combination, the trial was inconclusive and there is no definitive evidence this combination is effective.

Combination DMARDs in early RA

The question of whether or not combination DMARDs should be used in early RA has been studied and reviewed in detail. After carefully evaluating the available evidence some experts believe this approach is valuable. Other experts recommend focusing on initial methotrexate monotherapy. This diversity of opinion reflects three different factors. Firstly, some patients with early active RA improve with relatively simple treatments, including methotrexate monotherapy. Secondly, combinations are more complex to administer and have the potential to increase adverse events. Thirdly, and most critically, it is always possible to step up from methotrexate monotherapy after some months if patients fail to respond. This approach has been used in the Tear trial and similar studies.[110] Consequently the answer to the question hinges on how methotrexate monotherapy is used. The main negative side of using it is failing to increase treatment intensities in non-responders. Provided treatment intensity is increased in the absence of response, the initial DMARD treatment, whether it is methotrexate monotherapy or DMARD combinations, may be of less consequence.

Conclusions

Conventional DMARD therapy has changed substantially over the last 20–30 years. Two key approaches have been identified. Firstly, the dominant role of methotrexate as the anchor drug in rheumatoid arthritis. Secondly, the benefits of combination DMARDs, particularly triple therapy with methotrexate, sulfasalazine, and hydroxychloroquine, or with leflunomide particularly in the United States. The use of these approaches has substantially increased over recent years.[124] As many new effective treatments are being developed for rheumatoid arthritis it seems most likely that use of the conventional DMARDs has now reached its zenith. I anticipate their use will gradually decline in future years and that they will be replaced by more modern treatments.

REFERENCES

1. Hunneyball IM. Recent developments in disease-modifying antirheumatic drugs. *Prog Drug Res* 1980;*24*:101–216.
2. Wright V, Amos R. Do drugs change the course of rheumatoid arthritis? *Br Med J* 1980;*280*:964–6.
3. Steven MM, Hunter JA, Murdoch RM, Capell HA. Does the order of second-line treatment in rheumatoid arthritis matter? *Br Med J* 1982;*284*:79–81.
4. Buer JK. A history of the term 'DMARD'. *Inflammopharmacology* 2015;*23*:163–71.
5. Smolen JS, Landewé R, Bijlsma J, et al. EULAR recommendations for the management of rheumatoid arthritis with synthetic and biological disease-modifying antirheumatic drugs: 2016 update. *Ann Rheum Dis* 2017;*76*:960–77.
6. National Institute for Health and Care Excellence (NICE). *Rheumatoid Arthritis in Adults: Management. Clinical Guideline [CG79]*, 2009 (updated 2015). Available at: https://www.nice.org.uk/Guidance/CG79
7. Singh JA, Saag KG, Bridges SL Jr, et al. 2015 American College of Rheumatology Guideline for the Treatment of Rheumatoid Arthritis. *Arthritis Rheumatol* 2016;*68*:1–26.
8. Chakravarty K, McDonald H, Pullar T, et al.; British Society for Rheumatology, British Health Professionals in Rheumatology Standards, Guidelines and Audit Working Group; British Association of Dermatologists (BAD). BSR/BHPR guideline for disease-modifying anti-rheumatic drug (DMARD) therapy in consultation with the British Association of Dermatologists. *Rheumatology* 2008;*47*:924–5.
9. Comer M, Scott DL, Doyle DV, Huskisson EC, Hopkins A. Are slow-acting anti-rheumatic drugs monitored too often? An audit of current clinical practice. *Br J Rheumatol* 1995;*34*:966–70.
10. Aletaha D, Smolen JS. Laboratory testing in rheumatoid arthritis patients taking disease-modifying antirheumatic drugs: clinical evaluation and cost analysis. *Arthritis Rheum* 2002;*47*:181–8.
11. Kinder AJ, Hassell AB, Brand J, Brownfield A, Grove M, Shadforth MF. The treatment of inflammatory arthritis with methotrexate in clinical practice: treatment duration and incidence of adverse drug reactions. *Rheumatology* 2005;*44*:61–6.
12. Yazici Y. Long-term safety of methotrexate in the treatment of rheumatoid arthritis. *Clin Exp Rheumatol* 2010;*28*(5 Suppl 61):S65–7.

13. Maradit-Kremers H, Nicola PJ, Crowson CS, O'Fallon WM, Gabriel SE. Patient, disease, and therapy-related factors that influence discontinuation of disease-modifying antirheumatic drugs: a population-based incidence cohort of patients with rheumatoid arthritis. *J Rheumatol* 2006;*33*:248–55.

14. Agarwal S, Zaman T, Handa R. Retention rates of disease-modifying anti-rheumatic drugs in patients with rheumatoid arthritis. *Singapore Med J* 2009;*50*:686–92.

15. Curtis JR, Bykerk VP, Aassi M, Schiff M. Adherence and persistence with methotrexate in rheumatoid arthritis: a systematic review. *J Rheumatol* 2016;*43*: 1997–2009.

16. Nikiphorou E, Negoescu A, Fitzpatrick JD, et al. Indispensable or intolerable? Methotrexate in patients with rheumatoid and psoriatic arthritis: a retrospective review of discontinuation rates from a large UK cohort. *Clin Rheumatol* 2014;*33*: 609–14.

17. Solomon DH, Tonner C, Lu B, et al. Predictors of stopping and starting disease-modifying antirheumatic drugs for rheumatoid arthritis. *Arthritis Care Res* 2014;*66*:1152–8.

18. Kumar K, Raza K, Nightingale P, Horne R, Chapman S, Greenfield S, Gill P. Determinants of adherence to disease modifying anti-rheumatic drugs in White British and South Asian patients with rheumatoid arthritis: a cross sectional study. *BMC Musculoskelet Disord* 2015;*16*:396.

19. Pasma A, Schenk C, Timman R, et al. Does non-adherence to DMARDs influence hospital-related healthcare costs for early arthritis in the first year of treatment? *PLoS One* 2017;*12*:e0171070.

20. O'Mahony R, Richards A, Deighton C, Scott D. Withdrawal of disease-modifying antirheumatic drugs in patients with rheumatoid arthritis: a systematic review and meta-analysis. *Ann Rheum Dis* 2010;*69*:1823–6.

21. Schett G, Emery P, Tanaka Y, et al. Tapering biologic and conventional DMARD therapy in rheumatoid arthritis: current evidence and future directions. *Ann Rheum Dis* 2016;*75*:1428–37.

22. Tiippana-Kinnunen T, Paimela L, Kautiainen H, Laasonen L, Leirisalo-Repo M. Can disease-modifying anti-rheumatic drugs be discontinued in long-standing rheumatoid arthritis? A 15-year follow-up. *Scand J Rheumatol* 2010;*39*:12–18.

23. Edwards CJ, Campbell J, van Staa T, Arden NK. Regional and temporal variation in the treatment of rheumatoid arthritis across the UK: a descriptive register-based cohort study. *BMJ Open* 2012;*2*:e001603.

24. Kim SC, Yelin E, Tonner C, Solomon DH. Changes in use of disease-modifying antirheumatic drugs for rheumatoid arthritis in the United States during 1983–2009. *Arthritis Care Res* 2013;*65*:1529–33.

25. Mian AN, Ibrahim F, Scott IC, et al. Changing clinical patterns in rheumatoid arthritis management over two decades: sequential observational studies. *BMC Musculoskelet Disord* 2016;*17*:44.

26. Fassmer AM, Garbe E, Schmedt N. Frequency and trends of disease-modifying antirheumatic drug (DMARD) use in Germany. *Pharmacol Res Perspect* 2016;*4*:e00254.

27. Donges E, Staatz C, Benham H, Kubler P, Hollingworth SA. Patterns in use and costs of conventional and biologic disease-modifying anti-rheumatic drugs in Australia. *Clin Exp Rheumatol* 2017;*35*(6):907–12.

28. Rohr MK, Mikuls TR, Cohen SB, Thorne JC, O'Dell JR. Underuse of methotrexate in the treatment of rheumatoid arthritis: a national analysis of prescribing practices in the US. *Arthritis Care Res* 2017;*69*:794–800.

29. Finckh A, Bansback N, Marra CA, et al. Treatment of very early rheumatoid arthritis with symptomatic therapy, disease-modifying antirheumatic drugs, or biologic agents: a cost-effectiveness analysis. *Ann Intern Med* 2009;*151*:612–21.

30. de Jong PH, Hazes JM, Buisman LR, et al. Best cost-effectiveness and worker productivity with initial triple DMARD therapy compared with methotrexate monotherapy in early rheumatoid arthritis: cost-utility analysis of the tREACH trial. *Rheumatology* 2016;*55*:2138–47.

31. Pasma A, Schenk C, Timman R, et al. Does non-adherence to DMARDs influence hospital-related healthcare costs for early arthritis in the first year of treatment? *PLoS One* 2017;*12*:e0171070.

32. Weinblatt ME. Methotrexate in rheumatoid arthritis: a quarter century of development. *Trans Am Clin Climatol Assoc* 2013;*124*:16–25.

33. Gubner R, August S, Ginsberg V. Therapeutic suppression of tissue reactivity. II. Effect of aminopterin in rheumatoid arthritis and psoriasis. *Am J Med Sci* 1951;*22*:176–82.

34. Brown PM, Pratt AG, Isaacs JD. Mechanism of action of methotrexate in rheumatoid arthritis, and the search for biomarkers. *Nat Rev Rheumatol* 2016;*12*:731–742.

35. Cronstein BN. The mechanism of action of methotrexate. *Rheum Dis Clin North Am* 1997;*23*:739–55.

36. Weinblatt ME, Coblyn JS, Fox DA, et al. Efficacy of low-dose methotrexate in rheumatoid arthritis. *N Engl J Med* 1985;*312*:818–22.

37. Williams HJ, Willkens RF, Samuelson CO Jr, et al. Comparison of low-dose oral pulse methotrexate and placebo in the treatment of rheumatoid arthritis. A controlled clinical trial. *Arthritis Rheum* 1985;*28*:721–30.

38. Lopez-Olivo MA, Siddhanamatha HR, Shea B, Tugwell P, Wells GA, Suarez-Almazor ME. Methotrexate for treating rheumatoid arthritis. *Cochrane Database Syst Rev* 2014;*6*:CD000957.

39. Braun J, Kästner P, Flaxenberg P, et al. Comparison of the clinical efficacy and safety of subcutaneous versus oral administration of methotrexate in patients with active rheumatoid arthritis: results of a six-month, multicenter, randomized, double-blind, controlled, phase IV trial. *Arthritis Rheum* 2008;*58*:73–81.

40. Li D, Yang Z, Kang P, Xie X. Subcutaneous administration of methotrexate at high doses makes a better performance in the treatment of rheumatoid arthritis compared with oral administration of methotrexate: a systematic review and meta-analysis. *Semin Arthritis Rheum* 2016;*45*:656–62.

41. Smolen JS, Landewé R, Bijlsma J, et al. EULAR recommendations for the management of rheumatoid arthritis with synthetic and biological disease-modifying antirheumatic drugs: 2016 update. *Ann Rheum Dis* 2017;*76*:960–77.

42. Singh JA, Saag KG, Bridges SL Jr, et al. 2015 American College of Rheumatology guideline for the treatment of rheumatoid arthritis. *Arthritis Rheumatol* 2016;*68*:1–26.

43. Choi HK, Hernán MA, Seeger JD, Robins JM, Wolfe F. Methotrexate and mortality in patients with rheumatoid arthritis: a prospective study. *Lancet* 2002;*359*:1173–7.

44. Wasko MC, Dasgupta A, Hubert H, Fries JF, Ward MM. Propensity-adjusted association of methotrexate with overall survival in rheumatoid arthritis. *Arthritis Rheum* 2013;*65*:334–42.

45. Shea B, Swinden MV, Ghogomu ET, et al. Folic acid and folinic acid for reducing side effects in patients receiving methotrexate for rheumatoid arthritis. *J Rheumatol* 2014;*41*:1049–60.

46. Dhir V, Sandhu A, Kaur J, et al. Comparison of two different folic acid doses with methotrexate—a randomized controlled trial (FOLVARI Study). *Arthritis Res Ther* 2015;*17*:156.

47. Götestam Skorpen C, Hoeltzenbein M, et al. The EULAR points to consider for use of antirheumatic drugs before pregnancy, and during pregnancy and lactation. *Ann Rheum Dis* 2016;*75*:795–810.

48. Bressolle F, Bologna C, Kinowski JM, Arcos B, Sany J, Combe B. Total and free methotrexate pharmacokinetics in elderly patients with rheumatoid arthritis. A comparison with young patients. *J Rheumatol* 1997;*24*:1903–9.

49. Yazici Y. Long-term safety of methotrexate in the treatment of rheumatoid arthritis. *Clin Exp Rheumatol* 2010;*28*(5 Suppl 61):S65–7; *see also* Colebatch AN, Marks JL, van der Heijde DM, Edwards CJ. Safety of nonsteroidal antiinflammatory drugs and/or paracetamol in people receiving methotrexate for inflammatory arthritis: a Cochrane systematic review. *J Rheumatol Suppl* 2012;*90*:62–73.

50. Albrecht K, Müller-Ladner U. Side effects and management of side effects of methotrexate in rheumatoid arthritis. *Clin Exp Rheumatol* 2010;*28* (5 Suppl 61):S95–101.

51. Lim AY, Gaffney K, Scott DG. Methotrexate-induced pancytopenia: serious and under-reported? Our experience of 25 cases in 5 years. *Rheumatology* 2005;*44*:1051–5.

52. Curtis JR, Beukelman T, Onofrei A, et al. Elevated liver enzyme tests among patients with rheumatoid arthritis or psoriatic arthritis treated with methotrexate and/or leflunomide. *Ann Rheum Dis* 2010;*69*:43–7.

53. Humphreys JH, Warner A, Costello R, Lunt M, Verstappen SMM, Dixon WG. Quantifying the hepatotoxic risk of alcohol consumption in patients with rheumatoid arthritis taking methotrexate. *Ann Rheum Dis* 2017;*76*:1509–1514.

54. Conway R, Low C, Coughlan RJ, O'Donnell MJ, Carey JJ. Methotrexate and lung disease in rheumatoid arthritis: a meta-analysis of randomized controlled trials. *Arthritis Rheumatol* 2014;*66*:803–12; *see also* Subesinghe S, Bechman K, Rutherford AI, Goldblatt D, Galloway JB. A systematic review and metaanalysis of antirheumatic drugs and vaccine immunogenicity in rheumatoid arthritis. *J Rheumatol* 2018;*45*(6):733–44; *see also* Park JK, Lee YJ, Shin K, et al. Impact of temporary methotrexate discontinuation for 2 weeks on immunogenicity of seasonal influenza vaccination in patients with rheumatoid arthritis: a randomised clinical trial. *Ann Rheum Dis* 2018;*77*(6):898–904.

55. Patatanian E, Thompson DF. A review of methotrexate-induced accelerated nodulosis. *Pharmacotherapy* 2002;*22*:1157–62.

56. Sinicina I, Mayr B, Mall G, Keil W. Deaths following methotrexate overdoses by medical staff. *J Rheumatol* 2005;*32*:2009–11.

57. Watkinson G. Sulphasalazine: a review of 40 years' experience. *Drugs* 1986;*32*(Suppl 1):1–11.

58. Svartz N. The treatment of rheumatic polyarthritis with acid azo compounds. *Rheumatism* 1948;*4*:180–5.

59. McConkey B. History of the development of sulphasalazine in rheumatology. *Drugs* 1986;*32* (Suppl 1):12–17.

60. McConkey B, Amos RS, Durham S, Forster PJ, Hubball S, Walsh L. Sulphasalazine in rheumatoid arthritis. *Br Med J* 1980;*280*:442–4.

61. Smedegård G, Björk J. Sulphasalazine: mechanism of action in rheumatoid arthritis. *Br J Rheumatol* 1995;*34*(Suppl 2):7–15.

62. Cronstein BN. The antirheumatic agents sulphasalazine and methotrexate share an anti-inflammatory mechanism. *Br J Rheumatol* 1995;*34* Suppl 2:30–2.

63. Wahl C, Liptay S, Adler G, Schmid RM. Sulfasalazine: a potent and specific inhibitor of nuclear factor kappa B. *J Clin Invest* 1998;*101*:1163–74.

64. Neumann VC, Taggart AJ, Le Gallez P, Astbury C, Hill J, Bird HA. A study to determine the active moiety of sulphasalazine in rheumatoid arthritis. *J Rheumatol* 1986;*13*:285–7.

65. Suarez-Almazor ME, Belseck E, Shea B, Wells G, Tugwell P. Sulfasalazine for rheumatoid arthritis. *Cochrane Database Syst Rev*. 2000;*2*:CD000958.

66. Weinblatt ME, Reda D, Henderson W, et al. Sulfasalazine treatment for rheumatoid arthritis: a metaanalysis of 15 randomized trials. *J Rheumatol* 1999;*26*:2123–30.

67. Pullar T, Hunter JA, Capell HA. Sulphasalazine in the treatment of rheumatoid arthritis: relationship of dose and serum levels to efficacy. *Br J Rheumatol* 1985;*24*:269–76.

68. Götestam Skorpen C, Hoeltzenbein M, Tincani A, et al. The EULAR points to consider for use of antirheumatic drugs before pregnancy, and during pregnancy and lactation. *Ann Rheum Dis* 2016;*75*:795–810.

69. Makol A, Wright K, Amin S. Rheumatoid arthritis and pregnancy: safety considerations in pharmacological management. *Drugs* 2011;*71*:1973–87.

70. Østensen M. Sexual and reproductive health in rheumatic disease. *Nat Rev Rheumatol* 2017;*13*:485–93; *see also* Donovan S, Hawley S, MacCarthy J, Scott DL. Tolerability of enteric-coated sulphasalazine in rheumatoid arthritis: results of a co-operating clinics study. *Br J Rheumatol* 1990;*29*:201–4.

71. Scott DL, Dacre JE. Adverse reactions to sulfasalazine: the British experience. *J Rheumatol Suppl* 1988;*16*:17–21.

72. Donahue KE, Gartlehner G, Jonas DE, et al. Systematic review: comparative effectiveness and harms of disease-modifying medications for rheumatoid arthritis. *Ann Intern Med* 2008;*148*:124–34.

73. Michel F, Navellou JC, Ferraud D, Toussirot E, Wendling D. DRESS syndrome in a patient on sulfasalazine for rheumatoid arthritis. *Joint Bone Spine* 2005;*72*:82–5.

74. Cacoub P, Musette P, Descamps V, et al. The DRESS syndrome: a literature review. *Am J Med* 2011;*124*:588–97.

75. Jick H, Myers MW, Dean AD. The risk of sulfasalazine- and mesalazine-associated blood disorders. *Pharmacotherapy* 1995;*15*:176–81.

76. Andrès E, Maloisel F, Kurtz JE, et al. Modern management of non-chemotherapy drug-induced agranulocytosis: a monocentric cohort study of 90 cases and review of the literature. *Eur J Intern Med* 2002;*13*:324–8.

77. Breedveld FC, Dayer JM. Leflunomide: mode of action in the treatment of rheumatoid arthritis. *Ann Rheum Dis* 2000;*59*:841–9.

78. Osiri M, Shea B, Robinson V, et al. Leflunomide for the treatment of rheumatoid arthritis: a systematic review and metaanalysis. *J Rheumatol* 2003;*30*:1182–90.

79. Maddison P, Kiely P, Kirkham B, et al. Leflunomide in rheumatoid arthritis: recommendations through a process of consensus. *Rheumatology* 2005;*44*:280–6.

80. Chambers CD, Johnson DL, Robinson LK, et al. Birth outcomes in women who have taken leflunomide during pregnancy. *Arthritis Rheum* 2010;*6*:1494–503.

81. Alcorn N, Saunders S, Madhok R. Benefit-risk assessment of leflunomide: an appraisal of leflunomide in rheumatoid arthritis 10 years after licensing. *Drug Saf* 2009;*32*:1123–34.

82. Cannon GW, Holden WL, Juhaeri J, Dai W, Scarazzini L, Stang P. Adverse events with disease modifying antirheumatic drugs (DMARD): a cohort study of leflunomide compared with other DMARD. *J Rheumatol* 2004;*31*:1906–11.

83. Conway R, Low C, Coughlan RJ, O'Donnell MJ, Carey JJ. Leflunomide use and risk of lung disease in rheumatoid arthritis: a systematic literature review and metaanalysis of randomized controlled trials. *J Rheumatol* 2016;43:855–60.

84. Hill CL. Leflunomide-induced peripheral neuropathy: rapid resolution with cholestyramine wash-out. *Rheumatology* 2004;43:809; *see also* Bergner R, Peters L, Schmitt V, Löffler C. Leflunomide in dialysis patients with rheumatoid arthritis--a pharmacokinetic study. *Clin Rheumatol* 2013;32:267–70.

85. Freedman A. Chloroquine and rheumatoid arthritis; a short-term controlled trial. *Ann Rheum Dis* 1956;15:251–7.

86. Hamilton EB, Scott JT. Hydroxychloroquine sulfate ('plaquenil') in treatment of rheumatoid arthritis. *Arthritis Rheum* 1962;5:502–12.

87. Hu C, Lu L, Wan JP, Wen C. The pharmacological mechanisms and therapeutic activities of hydroxychloroquine in rheumatic and related diseases. *Curr Med Chem* 2017;24:2241–9.

88. Tett SE, Cutler DJ, Beck C, Day RO. Concentration-effect relationship of hydroxychloroquine in patients with rheumatoid arthritis--a prospective, dose ranging study. *J Rheumatol* 2000;27:1656–60.

89. Hobbs HE, Sorsby A, Freedman A. Retinopathy following chloroquine therapy. *Lancet* 1959;2:478–80.

90. Scherbel AL, Mackenzie AH, Nousek JE, Atdjian M. Ocular lesions in rheumatoid arthritis and related disorders with particular reference to retinopathy. A study of 741 patients treated with and without chloroquine drugs. *N Engl J Med* 1965;273:360–6.

91. Kim JW, Kim YY, Lee H, Park SH, Kim SK, Choe JY. Risk of retinal toxicity in long-term users of hydroxychloroquine. *J Rheumatol* 2017;44(11):1674–9.

92. Marmor MF, Kellner U, Lai TY, Melles RB, Mieler WF; American Academy of Ophthalmology. Recommendations on screening for chloroquine and hydroxychloroquine retinopathy (2016 revision). *Ophthalmology* 2016;123:1386–94.

93. Wells G, Haguenauer D, Shea B, Suarez-Almazor ME, Welch VA, Tugwell P. Cyclosporine for rheumatoid arthritis. *Cochrane Database Syst Rev* 2000;2:CD001083.

94. Wells G, Tugwell P. Cyclosporin A in rheumatoid arthritis: overview of efficacy. *Br J Rheumatol* 1993;32 Suppl 1:51–6.

95. Dijkmans B, Gerards A. Cyclosporin in Rheumatoid Arthritis. *BioDrugs* 1998;10:437–45.

96. Mason M, Currey HL, Barnes CG, Dunne JF, Hazleman BL, Strickland ID. Azathioprine in rheumatoid arthritis. *Br Med J* 1969;1:420–2.

97. Suarez-Almazor ME, Spooner C, Belseck E. Azathioprine for treating rheumatoid arthritis. *Cochrane Database Syst Rev* 2000;4:CD001461.

98. Singh G, Fries JF, Spitz P, Williams CA. Toxic effects of azathioprine in rheumatoid arthritis. A national post-marketing perspective. *Arthritis Rheum* 1989;32:837–43.

99. Clunie GP, Lennard L. Relevance of thiopurine methyltransferase status in rheumatology patients receiving azathioprine. *Rheumatology* 2004;43:13–18.

100. Rau R. Have traditional DMARDs had their day? Effectiveness of parenteral gold compared to biologic agents. *Clin Rheumatol* 2005;24:189–202.

101. Clark P, Tugwell P, Bennet K, et al. Injectable gold for rheumatoid arthritis. *Cochrane Database Syst Rev* 2000;2:CD000520.

102. Munro R, Capell HA. Penicillamine. *Br J Rheumatol* 1997;36:104–9.

103. Gaujoux-Viala C, Smolen JS, Landewé R, et al. Current evidence for the management of rheumatoid arthritis with synthetic disease-modifying antirheumatic drugs: a systematic literature review informing the EULAR recommendations for the management of rheumatoid arthritis. *Ann Rheum Dis* 2010;69:1004–9.

104. Doyle DV, Perrett D, Foster OJ, Ensor M, Scott DL. The long-term use of D-penicillamine for treating rheumatoid arthritis: is continuous therapy necessary? *Br J Rheumatol* 1993;32:614–17.

105. Luqmani RA, Palmer RG, Bacon PA. Azathioprine, cyclophosphamide and chlorambucil. *Baillieres Clin Rheumatol* 1990;4:595–619.

106. Felson DT, Anderson JJ, Meenan RF. The efficacy and toxicity of combination therapy in rheumatoid arthritis. A meta-analysis. *Arthritis Rheum* 1994;37:1487–91.

107. O'Dell JR, Haire CE, Erikson N, et al. Treatment of rheumatoid arthritis with methotrexate alone, sulfasalazine and hydroxychloroquine, or a combination of all three medications. *N Engl J Med* 1996;334:1287–91.

108. O'Dell JR, Leff R, Paulsen G, et al. Treatment of rheumatoid arthritis with methotrexate and hydroxychloroquine, methotrexate and sulfasalazine, or a combination of the three medications: results of a two-year, randomized, double-blind, placebo-controlled trial. *Arthritis Rheum* 2002;46:1164–70.

109. Saunders SA, Capell HA, Stirling A, et al. Triple therapy in early active rheumatoid arthritis: a randomized, single-blind, controlled trial comparing step-up and parallel treatment strategies. *Arthritis Rheum* 2008;58:1310–17.

110. Moreland LW, O'Dell JR, Paulus HE, et al. A randomized comparative effectiveness study of oral triple therapy versus etanercept plus methotrexate in early aggressive rheumatoid arthritis: the treatment of Early Aggressive Rheumatoid Arthritis Trial. *Arthritis Rheum* 2012;64:2824–35.

111. O'Dell JR, Mikuls TR, Taylor TH, et al. Keystone therapies for active rheumatoid arthritis after methotrexate failure. *N Engl J Med* 2013;369:307–18.

112. Peper SM, Lew R, Mikuls T, et al. Rheumatoid arthritis treatment after methotrexate: the durability of triple therapy versus etanercept. *Arthritis Care Res* 2017;69:1467–72.

113. Bansback N, Phibbs CS, Sun H, et al. Triple therapy versus biologic therapy for active rheumatoid arthritis: a cost-effectiveness analysis. *Ann Intern Med* 2017;167:8–16.

114. Mary J, De Bandt M, Lukas C, Morel J, Combe B. Triple oral therapy versus antitumor necrosis factor plus methotrexate (MTX) in patients with rheumatoid arthritis and inadequate response to MTX: a systematic literature review. *J Rheumatol* 2017;44:773–9.

115. Sauer BC, Teng CC, Tang D, et al. Persistence with conventional triple therapy versus a tumor necrosis factor inhibitor and methotrexate in US veterans with rheumatoid arthritis. *Arthritis Care Res* 2017;69:313–322.

116. Hazlewood GS, Barnabe C, Tomlinson G, Marshall D, Devoe D, Bombardier C. Methotrexate monotherapy and methotrexate combination therapy with traditional and biologic disease modifying antirheumatic drugs for rheumatoid arthritis: abridged Cochrane systematic review and network meta-analysis. *BMJ* 2016;353:i1777.

117. Kremer JM, Genovese MC, Cannon GW, et al. Concomitant leflunomide therapy in patients with active rheumatoid arthritis despite stable doses of methotrexate. A randomized, double-blind, placebo-controlled trial. *Ann Intern Med* 2002;137:726–33.

118. Weinblatt ME, Kremer JM, Coblyn JS, et al. Pharmacokinetics, safety, and efficacy of combination treatment with methotrexate and leflunomide in patients with active rheumatoid arthritis. *Arthritis Rheum* 1999;*42*:1322–8.

119. Weinblatt ME, Dixon JA, Falchuk KR. Serious liver disease in a patient receiving methotrexate and leflunomide. *Arthritis Rheum* 2000;*43*:2609–11.

120. Hill RL, Topliss DJ, Purcell PM. Pancytopenia associated with leflunomide and methotrexate. *Ann Pharmacother* 2003;*37*:149.

121. Choy EH, Smith C, Doré CJ, Scott DL. A meta-analysis of the efficacy and toxicity of combining disease-modifying anti-rheumatic drugs in rheumatoid arthritis based on patient withdrawal. *Rheumatology* 2005;*44*:1414–21.

122. Ma MH, Kingsley GH, Scott DL. A systematic comparison of combination DMARD therapy and tumour necrosis inhibitor therapy with methotrexate in patients with early rheumatoid arthritis. *Rheumatology* 2010;*49*:91–8.

123. Dougados M, Combe B, Cantagrel A, et al. Combination therapy in early rheumatoid arthritis: a randomised, controlled, double blind 52 week clinical trial of sulphasalazine and methotrexate compared with the single components. *Ann Rheum Dis* 1999;*58*:220–5.

124. Mian AN, Ibrahim F, Scott IC, et al. Changing clinical patterns in rheumatoid arthritis management over two decades: sequential observational studies. *BMC Musculoskelet Disord* 2016;*17*:44.

31

Tumour necrosis factor inhibitors

Peter C. Taylor and Nehal Narayan

Introduction

Biological agents inhibiting the actions of tumour necrosis factor (TNF) have significantly altered treatment models for multiple inflammatory disorders. Anti-TNFα is well established as a successful therapy for rheumatoid arthritis (RA), ankylosing spondylitis, and psoriatic arthritis, as well as inflammatory bowel disease. The clinical success of TNFi's has driven the search for other potential molecular targets of disease pathogenesis, and has led to the development of a number of other biologic and small-molecule targeted therapies.

The role of TNFα in rheumatoid arthritis

TNF and TNF receptors belong to a family of molecules (including Fas ligand/Fas) that undertake critical cellular regulatory functions, including apoptosis, and cell activation.[1]

Soluble, biologically active TNFα is generated by the action of the metalloproteinase TNFα converting enzyme, which cleaves off the active form from its 26 kDa transmembrane precursor.[2] Active TNFα binds the TNF receptors TNFR1 (p55, CD120a) and TNFR2 (p75, CD120b), present on many cell types. Whereas TNFR1 is constitutively expressed on all cells (with the exception of erythrocytes), TNFR2 is highly expressed on haematopoietic and endothelial cells.[3]

TNFα is mostly produced by monocytes and macrophages, but other cells found in inflamed RA synovium also produce this cytokine. These include both B and T lymphocytes, as well as synovial fibroblasts.[4] The main contributions of TNFα to inflammation in RA synovium are outlined in **Box 31.1**.

Mechanism of action of TNF inhibitors

The molecular structure of TNFi's differ and currently include mAbs (infliximab, adalimumab and golimumab), either chimeric or human in sequence, a PEGylated Fab fragment (certolizumab), and an IgG1-TNFR2 fusion protein (etanercept). The pharmacological properties of these three anti-TNF subtypes differ with respect to Fc function, binding to membrane bound TNF (tmTNF) and the possible consequences of this, as well as the ability to form complexes. TNFi act on both soluble (sTNF) and tmTNF. The actions of TNFi on tmTNF are well recognized to act via four major mechanisms; reverse signalling, inhibition of ligand activity of tmTNF, antibody dependent cell mediated cytotoxicity, and complement-dependent cytotoxicity. Current evidence demonstrates that not all TNFi are similarly efficacious via these four mechanisms of action.

Reverse signalling

TNF elicited responses (changes induced by TNF receptor activation by its ligand) are regarded as forward signalling. In contrast, when tmTNF producing cells bind to cell surface or soluble receptors, or TNF antibodies, the interaction also induces signalling in tmTNF expressing cells. This is known as reverse signalling.[12]

A crucial component of reverse signalling is thought to be the stimulation of expression of pro-inflammatory genes through the translocation of tmTNF to the nucleus.[13] The critical importance of reverse signalling for the actions of TNFi is evidenced by a study of monocytes derived from the lamina propria and peripheral blood of patients with inflammatory bowel disease (IBD) in which TNFi-dependent induction of apoptosis requires the presence of both tmTNF expressing monocytes and tumour necrosis factor receptor (TNFR) expressing lymphocytes in co-culture.[14] However, not all TNFi are equally effective at inhibition of reverse signalling in this co-culture system in which etanercept was unable to induce T-cell apoptosis, unlike infliximab, adalimumab, and certolizumab.[14] This may explain the lack of efficacy of etanercept for the treatment of IBD.

Inhibition of ligand activity of tmTNF

Ligand activity of tmTNF is inhibited by all TNFi although etanercept reduces tmTNF ligand activity less than other TNFi. For example, infliximab is more potent than etanercept at blocking tmTNF-mediated E-selectin expression on human umbilical vein endothelial cells (HUVEC) endothelial cells (important for leukocyte adhesion in inflammation).[14] In a study of a human lung cancer cell line, etanercept had twofold less activity in inhibition of tmTNF-mediated cell death compared to infliximab, adalimumab, and certolizumab.[15]

Such studies suggest that the observed reduction in efficacy of etanercept at inhibiting ligand activity of tmTNF is due a lower avidity of etanercept with tmTNF and formation of less stable complexes. In support of this possibility, studies of radiolabelled TNFi

> **Box 31.1** Contributory effects of TNFα to inflammation in RA synovium
>
> - Induction of pro-inflammatory cytokines IL-1 and IL-6[5,6]
> - Enhancement of leukocyte migration by increasing permeability of endothelium and expression of adhesion molecules by endothelial cells and leukocytes[7]
> - Activation of neutrophils and eosinophils[8]
> - Induction of synthesis of acute phase reactants[9,10]
> - Induction of matrix metalloproteinase production from synoviocytes and/or chondrocytes, that degrade tissue[11]

indicate that infliximab forms more stable complexes with tmTNF expressed on transfected cells than is the case with etanercept. Furthermore, infliximab binds tmTNF with higher avidity than etanercept.[14]

The influence of an Fc portion of a TNFi on mechanism of action

All three mAbs—adalimumab, infliximab, and golimumab—have human IgG1 Fc, as does etanercept, which has the capability of fixing complement and binding to Fc receptors. In contrast, certolizumab pegol lacks an Fc portion. Several cellular functions, including phagocytosis, antibody dependent cellular cytotoxicity (ADCC), complement-dependent cytotoxicity (CDC), degranulation, cytokine release and regulation of antibody formation might be influenced via the engagement of Fc receptors by TNFi or complexes. Infliximab, adalimumab, and etanercept are all capable of CDC and ADCC, although depending on the assay, the level of ADCC mediated by etanercept is generally reduced compared to infliximab and adalimumab.[16–19] Because of the absence of an Fc region, certolizumab pegol does not mediate cell killing either directly through fixation of complement or via recruitment of effector cells.

The reduced ability of etanercept to induce CDC may be due to the fact that etanercept lacks the CH1 domain that acts to bind complement factor C3.[16]

Although multiple *in vitro* studies have demonstrated TNFi can induce ADCC and CDC, it is uncertain how translatable these findings are to clinical use of TNFi, since such studies used cell lines expressing high levels of tmTNF. This is emphasized by the attempt by Kaymakcalan et al. to confirm *in vitro* findings of a study of tm-TNF transfected cells demonstrating TNFi could activate CDC, using peripheral blood mononuclear cells (PBMCs) from healthy donors, and stimulating with activators of T cells and monocytes. In this setting, CDC could not be induced by any TNFi.[17]

Cellular effects of TNFi

TNFi act in multiple ways to ameliorate inflammation in RA, as demonstrated by a large body of evidence.

Regulation of pro-inflammatory cytokines

Early studies of infliximab demonstrated that TNFi are capable of regulating the production of other cytokines *in vivo*. Following administration of infliximab, a rapid reduction in serum IL-6 concentrations was observed, closely followed by falling serum C-reactive protein (CRP) levels.[18,19] Although IL-1 concentrations are often below the limit of detection in peripheral blood of patients with RA, when it has been detectable, downregulation of IL-1 has been reported in a proportion of patients treated with infliximab.[20] Furthermore, in synovial biopsy specimens taken before and 2 weeks after a single infusion of infliximab 10 mg/kg, computerized image analysis of sections stained for cytokine producing cells demonstrated a reduction in synovial IL-1α in a subgroup.[21]

Modulation of leukocyte cell trafficking

A dose-dependent rise in peripheral blood lymphocyte counts is observed following infliximab infusion with a maximum rise within 24 hours of treatment,[22] implying a reduction in trafficking of lymphocytes into synovial tissues. In keeping with this hypothesis, infliximab therapy is also associated with a reduction in numbers of synovial tissue macrophages and lymphocytes.[23,24] That TNFi modulates inflammatory cell recruitment to inflamed joints was definitively confirmed in a clinical study demonstrating a 40–50% reduction in retention of autologous indium-111-labelled granulocytes in the hands, wrists, and knees 2 weeks after infliximab treatment.[24]

Additionally, in a cohort of 14 patients receiving infliximab therapy, a reduction in histological expression of the synovial cytokine-induced vascular adhesion molecules E-selectin and VCAM-1 was observed 4 weeks after infliximab commencement.[23] Further studies of infliximab demonstrated a significant dose-dependent reduction in soluble serum E-selectin and intercellular adhesion molecule 1 concentrations,[22] and a significantly diminished expression of the chemokines IL-8 and MCP-1 on immunohistochemistry, with a trend toward reduction in a number of other chemokines.[24]

Diminished granulocyte production

The number of peripheral blood granulocytes decreases after infliximab dosing, with maximal reduction within 24 hours.[25] This is thought to be due to reduction in myeloid cell production secondary to downregulation of granulocyte-macrophage colony-stimulating factor (GM-CSF) as a consequence of TNF blockade.

Reduction in tissue oedema, capillary permeability, and synovial angiogenesis

The rapid reduction in joint swelling after TNFi therapy is likely to be secondary to a reduction in tissue oedema and capillary permeability, mediated by vascular endothelial growth factor (VEGF), a cytokine implicated in angiogenesis, known to be elevated in the sera of RA patients.[26] Following infliximab commencement, serum concentrations of VEGF show a dose-dependent reduction. There is also reduction in synovial vascular density and angiogenesis, as assessed by fewer number of vessels expressing the endothelial marker $\alpha_V\beta_3$ integrin.[27]

Clinical imaging evidence of reduction in synovial vascularity following infliximab therapy is provided by power Doppler imaging; several studies demonstrate a reduction in vascularity determined by power Doppler ultrasound in those receiving infliximab compared to those receiving placebo.[28,29]

Reduction in matrix metalloproteinases (MMPs) and receptor activator of nuclear factor κB ligand (RANKL)

Cartilage damage by MMPs is an important contribution to progression of joint damage. Reduction in circulating concentrations of the precursors of MMPs MMP-1 and MMP-3[11] and a significant reduction in synovial tissue expression of matrix metalloproteinases has been observed following TNFi therapy.[30] sRANKL (soluble receptor activator of nuclear factor κB ligand) is recognized to activate bone resorbing osteoclasts in RA, promoting the generation of erosions.[31] Serum levels of sRANKL are known to be elevated in the sera of RA patients. Infliximab therapy normalizes sRANKL,[32] predicting the beneficial effects of anti-TNF therapy on radiographic erosions.

'Originator' biologic TNF inhibitors in clinical practice

Although all biologic TNFi share similar biologic, clinical, and adverse effects, they also differ in their pharmacokinetics and structure.

Five originator TNFi are available for the treatment of RA; infliximab, adalimumab, golimumab, certolizumab and etanercept (see **Figure 31.1**).

Infliximab

Infliximab is a chimeric monoclonal antibody specifically directed against TNFα. The kappa chain variable region, and heavy chain variable region domains of the antigen binding portion of infliximab are murine, and the constant Fc domain is human (see **Figure 31.1**). The drug is produced in a murine myeloma cell line transfected with cloned DNA coding for cA2.[33]

The median terminal half-life is 8–9.5 days, at doses of 3–10 mg/kg. For RA, the recommended dosing of infliximab is 3–10 mg/kg administered via intravenous infusion at 0, 2, and 6 weeks, and then every 8 weeks, along with methotrexate. The Food and Drug Administration (US) (FDA) recommend starting at a dose of 3 mg/kg.[34] Escalation of dose (up to 10 mg/kg) or frequency (every 4–6 weeks) may be necessary in some cases, but are associated with higher risk of infection.[35]

Infliximab key trials

The efficacy and safety of infliximab in RA were initially confirmed in monotherapy trials, in which infliximab was administered after disease-modifying antirheumatic drug (DMARD) washout.

An 8-week open-label trial[36] demonstrated efficacy for two different regimens of infliximab: (1) two infusions of 10 mg/kg 2 weeks apart; and (2) four monthly infusions of 5 mg/kg. Clinical benefits were observed after week 3 and were maximal by week 6 with normalization of CRP levels in almost 90% of patients. Following the last infusion, clinical responses lasted a median of 14 weeks (range, 8–25 weeks).

The ATTRACT trial was a 428-patient randomized controlled trial (RCT) of infliximab (3 mg/kg or 10 mg/kg) compared with placebo given every 4 or 8 weeks in patients with active RA receiving methotrexate (MTX) weekly.[37] Patients who received infliximab (3 or 10 mg/kg) in addition to background MTX therapy showed significantly higher ACR20 responses (50% to 58%) than those taking MTX alone (20%) at 30 weeks. After 54 weeks ACR20 response rates were 42% to 59% in the 3-mg and 10-mg/kg groups.[37] Radiographic damage was progressive in the group receiving MTX plus placebo, increasing by a mean of seven modified total Sharp score (mTSS) units at 1 year. By contrast, both the infliximab-treated groups (3 or 10 mg/kg) showed little change (1.3 and 0.2 units, respectively) after 12 months. At 2 years, 22% of placebo-treated patients showed no evidence of radiographic progression, whereas 43% to 47% of the 3-mg/kg group and 64% of the 10-mg/kg group showed no evidence of radiographic change. In patients without erosions at entry, infliximab plus MTX was revealed to be superior to MTX alone in halting further radiographic progression.[38]

The 12-month ASPIRE trial examined the effects of MTX and infliximab in 1049 patients with early RA with a mean disease duration of 7 months.[39] All patients received MTX weekly (20 mg/wk) and either placebo or infliximab (3 mg/kg or 6 mg/kg). MTX/placebo-treated patients exhibited good ACR20 (54%) and ACR70 (21%) response rates and disease activity score (DAS) remissions (15%); patients treated with MTX/infliximab showed significantly higher ACR20 (62–66%) and ACR70 (33–37%) response rates and DAS remissions (21–33%) at 54 weeks. Radiographic progression was observed primarily in those patients treated only with placebo/MTX. Although 45% of the MTX/placebo-treated patients showed no progression, those receiving infliximab plus MTX demonstrated greater inhibition of structural progression (no progression in 58–59%).

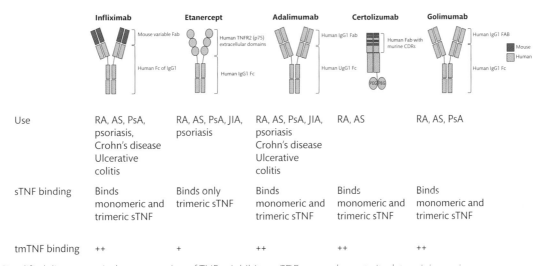

	Infliximab	Etanercept	Adalimumab	Certolizumab	Golimumab
Use	RA, AS, PsA, psoriasis, Crohn's disease Ulcerative colitis	RA, AS, PsA, JIA, psoriasis	RA, AS, PsA, JIA, psoriasis Crohn's disease Ulcerative colitis	RA, AS	RA, AS, PsA
sTNF binding	Binds monomeric and trimeric sTNF	Binds only trimeric sTNF	Binds monomeric and trimeric sTNF	Binds monomeric and trimeric sTNF	Binds monomeric and trimeric sTNF
tmTNF binding	++	+	++	++	++

Figure 31.1 Simplified diagrammatical representation of TNF-α inhibitors. CDR = complementarity determining region.

Etanercept

Etanercept is a soluble p75 TNF receptor fusion protein that consists of 2 p75 TNF receptors bound to the Fc portion of IgG1.[40] Unlike the other TNFi biologics, etanercept binds both lymphotoxin-α and TNFα. The half-life of etanercept is 102 hours, with a range of 4.1–12.5 days. Etanercept is administered once or twice weekly via subcutaneous injection, in doses of 25 mg or 50 mg.

Etanercept key trials

A 6-month RCT compared placebo and etanercept (10 mg or 25 mg) subcutaneously twice weekly[41]; 59% ACR20 and 15% ACR70 response rates were seen in patients taking etanercept 25 mg twice weekly, with lower responses seen with the 10-mg dose. When etanercept was added to long-term MTX, patients receiving etanercept and MTX showed a 71% ACR20 response rate compared with a 27% rate in the placebo plus MTX group.[42] Many of these patients were enrolled in a long-term open-label observational study and exhibited static ACR20, ACR50, and ACR70 response rates over 3 years. Importantly, sustained efficacy allowed for 68% to 85% of patients to decrease their MTX or prednisone doses, and 39% to 59% were able to discontinue MTX and prednisone use after 3 years.[43]

Etanercept was the first biologic therapy to be tested head to head against MTX in an early RA (ERA) trial. This 12-month trial enrolled 632 patients with early RA (mean disease duration, 11 months), who received etanercept (10 or 25 mg twice weekly) or MTX 20 mg/wk.[44] After 12 months, the MTX-treated and 25-mg etanercept-treated groups fared equally well, with ACR20 response rates of 65% and 72%, respectively. The only significant group difference in clinical effects was the more rapid onset of effect in those treated with etanercept in the first 4 months. Serious infectious events were infrequent in both groups (less than 3%). In the second year, a trend toward higher ACR20 responses was seen in the etanercept group compared with the MTX group (72% vs. 59%).[45]

The ERA trial showed that radiographic progression was diminished by both agents when assessed after 6, 12, and 24 months of therapy. In the first year, mTSS showed little change in either the MTX group (1.3 units) or etanercept group (0.8 units) yet results for both were significantly better than their projected rates of radiographic deterioration (estimated to be approximately 9 units/year). In the second year of the trial, significant differences were seen, with etanercept patients showing an increase of only 1.3 mTSS units (no progression in 63%) and MTX patients an increase of 3.2 mTSS units (no progression in 51%). The ERA trial was pivotal in demonstrating the potency of both MTX and etanercept in patients with early, aggressive RA. The additional radiographic advantage of TNF inhibition over MTX in early disease was seen largely in those with erosions at entry into the study.

The TEMPO trial reported the comparative efficacy of MTX, etanercept, and the combination of etanercept plus MTX in 682 patients with active RA with a mean disease duration of 7 years.[46] At both 12 and 24 months the combination of etanercept and MTX was significantly more effective than monotherapy with either MTX or etanercept alone. At 24 months the combination group demonstrated impressive ACR20 (86%) and ACR70 (49%) responses rates and DAS remission (38%). Comparison of MTX-naive and previously treated MTX patients failed to show significant differences in outcomes. The mean mTSS decreased by 0.56 units in patients receiving combination etanercept plus MTX and 78% had no radiographic worsening. By comparison, mTSS increased in those taking etanercept alone (+0.5 units) or MTX alone (+2.8 units), and 60–68% showed no radiographic progression while taking MTX or etanercept, respectively. This study underscores the potential additive clinical and radiographic protection afforded by the combination of MTX and TNFi therapy, especially in patients with aggressive disease.

The COMET trial[47] compared the effects of a combination of etanercept and MTX with MTX alone in 542 MTX-naive patients with early RA (duration of 3 months to 2 years). Half of the patients receiving combined treatment achieved DAS28 remission (less than 2.6) and 80% had no radiographic progression compared with 28% and 59%, respectively, of those taking MTX alone. For a majority of patients with early severe RA, clinical remission and lack of radiographic progression are achievable goals within 1 year of combined treatment with etanercept plus MTX.[47]

Adalimumab

Adalimumab is a recombinant IgG1 monoclonal antibody, fully humanized by phage substitution.[48] The agent binds circulating and cell-bound TNF-α and blocks its interaction with p55 and p75 receptors, inducing lysis of TNF-α expressing cells. Adalimumab is administered subcutaneously rather than by intravenous infusion, and has a terminal half-life of 10–20 days, hence is administered fortnightly.[49]

Adalimumab may be used as monotherapy, or in combination with methotrexate, at recommended dosage of 40 mg fortnightly. Higher dosages (such as 80 mg fortnightly) were used during drug development, but not demonstrated to be more effective in short term studies. A minority of patients may require dose escalation (e.g. 40 mg weekly); in the PREMIER early RA RCT, patients receiving adalimumab monotherapy were more likely to need escalation to weekly adalimumab dosing than those receiving adalimumab with methotrexate (25% compared to 11%, respectively).[50]

Adalimumab key studies

The ARMADA trial studied adalimumab in 271 patients with established RA, and an inadequate response to MTX (MTX-IR).[51] In this 6-month multicentre trial, patients continued to receive stable doses of MTX (mean, 16–17 mg/wk) plus placebo or 20 mg, 40 mg, or 80 mg of adalimumab every 2 weeks. ACR20 response rates were 14%, 48%, 66%, and 66% for those taking placebo, 20 mg adalimumab, 40 mg adalimumab, and 80 mg adalimumab, respectively. In the 4-year open-label extension of this study, responses were sustained in 147 patients who continued with adalimumab therapy.[52]

Another pivotal RCT (DE019) examined efficacy and radiographic outcomes in a 52-week trial in 619 patients in which adalimumab 20 mg or 40 mg every other week or placebo was given to MTX partial responders.[53] ACR20 response rates after 52 weeks were 24% in placebo group, 55% in the 20 mg adalimumab group, and 59% in the 40 mg adalimumab group. Radiographic progression, measured by mTSS, was significantly worse in the placebo group (+2.7 units) compared with the groups receiving adalimumab 20 mg/wk (+0.7 units) and 40 mg every other week (+0.1 units). In the 10-year open-label extension of the study sustained responses were observed, (457 entered, 202 completed) with no change to the expected safety profile.[54]

The PREMIER trial was an important RCT establishing the benefit of administering MTX in combination with adalimumab. This 2-year study evaluated 799 MTX naive patients with RA of duration less than 3 years. Patients were randomized to MTX monotherapy, adalimumab monotherapy, or combination treatment. Adverse event rates were comparable in all three groups. Combination therapy was found to be superior to either monotherapy in ACR20, ACR50, ACR70, and ACR90 response rates at 1 and 2 years. Additionally, there was significantly less radiographic progression (p ≤0.002) in patients receiving combination therapy at both 1 and 2 years of therapy compared to those receiving either MTX or adalimumab monotherapy. A total 49% of patients receiving combination therapy were in disease remission at 2 years (DAS28 <2.6), and 49% had ACR70 response for at least 6 continuous months; rates that are about twofold those found in patients receiving either monotherapy.[50]

Certolizumab pegol

Certolizumab pegol is a human monoclonal antibody to TNFα Fab' fragment that is chemically linked to polyethylene glycol (PEG).[55] The addition of PEG to the Fab' fragment markedly increases the half-life of certolizumab.

Certolizumab pegol is usually administered subcutaneously at doses of 400 mg at weeks 0, 2, and 4 (given as 200 mg twice daily), followed by 200 mg every other week for maintenance, or 400 mg every 4 weeks.

Certolizumab pegol key trials

The RAPID 1[56] and RAPID 2[57] phase 3 RCTs evaluated the efficacy and safety of lyophilized and liquid formulations, respectively, of subcutaneous certolizumab pegol (400 mg at weeks 0, 2, and 4 followed by 200 mg or 400 mg every 2 weeks) plus MTX versus placebo plus MTX for 24 weeks in patients with active RA receiving long-term MTX therapy. Placebo patients went on to receive certolizumab after 24 weeks. Among the 982 patients enrolled in RAPID 1, at week 24 the ACR20 response rates using non-responder imputation for the certolizumab pegol 200-mg and 400-mg groups were 58.8% and 60.8%, respectively, compared with 13.6% for the placebo group. Differences in ACR20 response rates in certolizumab pegol-treated versus placebo-treated patients were significant at week 1 and were sustained to week 52 (p <0.001). The agent also improved physical function as early as week 1 and slowed mean radiographic progression from baseline by week 52, with an increase of 0.4 mTSS units in those receiving 200 mg certolizumab pegol and 0.2 mTSS units in those receiving 400 mg, compared with 2.8 Sharp units in placebo-treated patients (p <0.001). Neither RAPID 1 nor RAPID 2 showed any advantage for 400 mg over 200 mg certolizumab pegol over 52 weeks after induction with 400 mg.

FAST4WARD was a 24-week RCT evaluating certolizumab pegol as monotherapy vs. placebo in 220 DMARD-IR patients.[58] The patients were randomly assigned to receive subcutaneous certolizumab pegol 400 mg (n = 111) or placebo (n = 109) every 4 weeks. The primary endpoint of achievement of ACR20 criteria at week 24 was reached by 45.5% of the certolizumab-treated group and 9.3% of the placebo-treated group (p <0.001). Differences between the certolizumab pegol group and the placebo group in the

ACR20 response rate were statistically significant as early as week 1 through to week 24 (p <0.001). Significant improvements in ACR50, American College of Rheumatology (ACR) components, DAS28(ESR)-3, and all patient-reported outcomes were also observed early in those treated with certolizumab pegol and were sustained throughout the study.

Golimumab

Golimumab is a fully human IgG1 kappa monoclonal antibody, produced by homologous recombination. It is specific for human TNF-α, and binds to both the soluble and transmembrane bioactive forms of human TNF-α.[59] It is administered once every 4 weeks by subcutaneous injection or IV infusion in a dose of 50 mg subcutaneously, or at 2 mg/kg intravenous infusion over 30 minutes at weeks 0 and 4, then every 8 weeks.

Golimumab key trials

In the GO-BEFORE trial, golimumab was administered once every 4 weeks by subcutaneous injection; MTX-naive patients with active RA received golimumab 100 mg alone, golimumab 50 mg or 100 mg in combination with MTX, or MTX alone. When data for three patients who did not receive the study drug but were included in the analysis as non-responders were included, the primary endpoint, achievement of ACR50 criteria by intent-to-treat analysis, was not reached. However, when data for these three patients were excluded, a modified intent-to-treat analysis showed that the proportion of patients achieving ACR50 responses was statistically higher in those receiving golimumab 50 mg every 4 weeks plus MTX than in those receiving MTX alone.[60] ACR20/50/70 response rates were 72.8%, 54.6%, and 38.0% respectively, 84.1% had good to moderate DAS28-CRP response and 72.7% had improvements in physical function.

In the GO-FORWARD RCT, 50-mg and 100-mg doses of golimumab were examined in patients whose disease was active despite ongoing treatment with MTX.[61] At week 14, 55% of patients receiving golimumab 50 mg plus MTX and 56% receiving golimumab 100 mg plus MTX achieved at least 20% improvement in signs and symptoms of RA (ACR20), compared with 33% of patients receiving placebo and MTX (p <0.01 and p <0.001, respectively). Improvements were seen as early as the first clinical assessment, which was 4 weeks after the first golimumab injection, and generally increased over time. At 24 weeks, 68% of patients in the golimumab 50-mg dosing group and 72% of patients receiving golimumab 100 mg experienced clinically relevant improvement in physical function compared with 39% of patients receiving placebo plus MTX (p <0.0001). Data on 313 patients, who received golimumab through to week 256, maintained clinical efficacy with ACR20/50/70 response rates achieved by 63.1%, 40.8% and 24.1%, respectively, of all randomized patients.[62]

GO-AFTER was the first large phase 3 RCT to test the efficacy of TNFi switching in patients in whom the first TNFi failed (TNF-IR).[63] Four hundred and sixty-one (461) TNF-IR patients among whom 25% (n = 115) had received two and 9% (n = 43) three TNFi, were enrolled in this study. Discontinuation of previous TNFi therapy was due to lack of efficacy (58%), intolerance (17%), or other reasons (40%). Patients received subcutaneous placebo, golimumab 50 mg, or golimumab 100 mg every 4 weeks. At baseline, 66% of patients were receiving MTX, 5% were receiving sulfasalazine, and 7% were receiving hydroxychloroquine. Among patients who discontinued a previous TNFi because of lack of efficacy, 35.7% and 42.7% of patients in the golimumab 50-mg and 100-mg groups, respectively, achieved ACR20 responses at week 14 compared with 17.7% in the placebo group. Long-term extension up to 160 weeks, involving 236/459 (51%) patients who continued treatment has been evaluated.[64] Overall at week 160, 63%, 67% and 57% of patients achieved ACR20 response and 59%, 65% and 64% had Health Assessment Questionnaire (HAQ) improvement ≥0.25 unit in Groups 1 (placebo), 2 (golimumab 50 mg), and 3 (golimumab 100 mg), respectively.

The GO-FURTHER phase 3 RCT evaluated the efficacy of intravenous golimumab 2 mg/kg in patients with active RA despite receiving MTX.[65] Patients (n = 592) were randomized (2:1) to receive intravenous golimumab 2 mg/kg, or placebo infusions at weeks 0 and 4 and every 8 weeks; patients continued MTX (15–25 mg/week). At week 14, significantly (p <0.001) larger proportions of golimumab plus MTX than placebo plus MTX patients achieved ACR20 responses (59% vs. 25%, respectively), and greater median improvement in HAQ scores (0.500 vs. 0.125). Serious adverse events were reported by more golimumab plus MTX (4.1%) than placebo plus MTX (2%) patients at week 24. The results up to 1 year follow-up, the patients on intravenous golimumab plus MTX-treated patients demonstrated less radiographic progression than placebo at week 24 (mTSS mean changes 0.03 vs. 1.09; p <0.001) and week 52 (0.13 vs. 1.22; p = 0.001).[66] In addition among patients with ACR20 responses at week 24, approximately 80% maintained these responses up until week 52.

Current guidelines for TNFi therapy commencement

The British Society for Rheumatology (BSR) and National Institute of Healthcare Excellence (NICE) currently recommend positioning of TNFi therapy in patients with active RA who have undergone a trial of 2 synthetic DMARDs, one of which is MTX (unless contraindicated). The BSR recommend the threshold of disease activity for access to a biologic anti-TNF as DAS28 >3.2 with 3 or more swollen and tender joints.[67] However, NICE, the body which determines the disease activity threshold for reimbursement in the United Kingdom recommend a DAS28 of ≥5.[68]

Box 31.2 EULAR 2016 poor prognostic factors for rheumatoid arthritis

- Moderate to high disease activity according to composite measures (after synthetic DMARD therapy)
- High acute phase reactant levels
- High swollen joint counts
- Presence of RF and/or anticitrullinated protein antibody (ACPA), especially at high levels
- Combinations of the above
- Presence of early erosions
- Failure of two or more synthetic DMARDs

Source: data from Smolen J et al (2017) 'EULAR recommendations for the management of rheumatoid arthritis with synthetic and biological disease-modifying antirheumatic drugs: 2016 update'. Ann Rheum Dis 76(6):960–77.

The European League Against Rheumatism (EULAR) 2016 updated recommendations for management of RA suggests that if a first synthetic DMARD (which would usually be methotrexate) fails to achieve the treatment target of at least low disease activity by composite measures (i.e. DAS28 >3.2), and poor prognostic factors are present, addition of a biologic DMARD (such as TNFi therapy), or targeted synthetic DMARD should be considered.[69] Poor prognostic factors are listed in Box 31.2.

The ACR guidance recommends TNFi commencement for those who have moderate or high disease activity despite csDMARD monotherapy or combination csDMARD.[70]

Box 31.3 summarizes major absolute and relative contraindications to anti-TNF-α therapy.

TNFi therapy prescribing in pregnancy

In pregnancy, maternal antibodies are transported across placenta by the neonatal Fc receptor (FcRn) and immunoglobulin concentrations increase in fetal blood from early in the second trimester until delivery. IgG1 is the most efficiently transported immunoglobulin subclass.[71] Other than certolizumab pegol, all the other originator anti-TNFs and currently available biosimilars have an IgG1 Fc portion. In the early days of TNFi therapy, as sporadic reports of pregnancy outcomes in TNFi-treated patients emerged, there was some controversy as to whether there was a causal link to various birth defects and biologic exposure.[72] However, subsequent data was more reassuring, including a report from the BSR registry of 120 pregnancies in 118 women exposed to anti-TNF biologics prior to, or at, conception.[73] Four congenital malformations were noted including congenital hip dislocation and pyloric stenosis.

It is now recognized that it is important for the health of mother and fetus to optimize control of RA disease activity through pregnancy, which may include the use of TNFi, but without concomitant MTX, while remaining mindful of any potential harm to the fetus. EULAR have recently published points to consider for use of antirheumatic drugs in pregnancy and they include the recommendation that among biologics, continuation of TNFi should be considered during the first part of pregnancy. Certolizumab pegol may be considered for use throughout pregnancy due to low rate of transplacental passage.[74] Similarly, the BSR and British Health Professionals in Rheumatology (BHPR) have recently published joint guidelines on prescribing drugs in pregnancy and while breastfeeding.[75] Regarding TNF originator biologics, there is no data for golimumab. But it is recommended that infliximab can be used until week 16 of pregnancy, while etanercept and adalimumab can be used through the first and second trimesters but not the third. The BSR and BHPR recommendations are that certolizumab pegol, lacking an Fc portion and therefore not actively transported to the fetal circulation or into breast milk,[76] can be used throughout. Recent evidence in confirmation of this rationale came from the CRIB study in 14 mother-infant pairs, designed to accurately evaluate the level of placental transfer of certolizumab pegol from mothers to infants, using a highly sensitive CZP-specific assay.[77] Maternal blood levels of certolizumab pegol were all within the expected range at delivery. In contrast, neonatal blood levels were below the lower limit of quantification in 13/14 infant samples at birth and in all infant samples at weeks 4 and 8.[77]

Box 31.3 Summary of contraindications to the use of TNFi therapy

Absolute contraindications
- Presence of serious active infections
- Active mycobacterial tuberculosis infection
- Cardiac failure at New York Heart Association (NYHA) Grade III or IV.

Relative contraindications
- Systemic Lupus Erythematosus, lupus overlap syndrome
- Multiple sclerosis, optic neuritis, demyelinating disorders
- Recurrent or chronic infection
- Hepatitis B infection
- Treated lymphoproliferative disease

Adverse effects of anti-TNF therapy

Multiple adverse effects of TNFi therapy have been identified through both clinical trials and clinical practice (summarized in Box 31.4).

Injection site reactions

During adalimumab and etanercept clinical trials, cutaneous injection site reactions were seen in 20% and 37% of patients respectively.[41,78] However, in clinical practice these are less frequent, and rarely require drug discontinuation. Injection site reactions are usually mild and resolve within 1 week. They are most common during the first 4–8 weeks of drug use, and usually bear no relationship with drug dose, frequency, or presence of antidrug antibodies (ADAbs).

Infusion reactions

Most infliximab infusion reactions occur during or within 2 hours following an infusion, with the majority being mild to moderate in severity and occurring in less than 6% of patients.[79] Common complaints include headache (20%), nausea (15%), urticaria, pruritus, rash, flushing, fever, chills, tachycardia, and dyspnoea. In many, infusion reactions may be the result of a rapid infusion rate, but some may be due to the presence of ADAbs. Infusion reactions are usually transient, are rarely severe, and typically can be controlled by slowing the infusion or treating with paracetamol, non-sedating antihistamines, or short-acting corticosteroids.

More rarely, anaphylactic reactions occur, and for these patients, TNFi should be stopped and supportive or emergency care administered until the patient is stable. Anaphylaxis is likely due to ADAbs which are typically IgG4, but can be IgG1. Immunoglobulin E (IgE) antidrug antibodies have also been occasionally associated with anaphylaxis to infliximab.[80]

Box 31.4 Adverse effects of TNFi therapy

- Injection site reactions
- Infusion reactions
- Cytopenias
- Infections
- Demyelinating disease
- Heart Failure
- Cutaneous reactions
- Malignancy
- Lymphoma
- Induction of antidrug antibodies
- Induction of autoimmunity

Cytopenias

Rare reports of pancytopenia and aplastic anaemia have been described with TNFi therapy, and a small number of these cases have resulted in death. Cytopenias typically developed in the first few weeks after initiation of TNFi therapy. Reasons for this sporadic association are unclear, but cytopenias may be secondary to comorbidities or other myelosuppressive drugs.

The risk of neutropenia in patients taking TNFi is significantly higher in those with a low baseline neutrophil count, and previous history of neutropenia while receiving synthetic DMARDs.[81]

Infections

TNF is a crucial component of the immune response to infection, and use of TNFi therapy has been associated with an increased risk of serious infections. These include typical infections (such as *Streptococcal pneumonia*[82]) and opportunistic infections (OIs). The SAfety Assessment of Biologic ThERapy (SABER) Study assessed the incidence of non-viral OI in a cohort of 33 624 patients with a variety of inflammatory arthritides and IBD. The study demonstrated the rate of non-viral OIs was higher in those patients on TNFi, compared to patients not receiving a bDMARD (2.7 versus 1.7 per 1000 person-years, adjusted hazard ratio (HR) 1.6, 95% CI: 1.0, 2.6).[83] Due to its profound immunosuppressive effects, TNFi are absolutely contraindicated in the presence of active infection.

Current prescribing guidelines caution against the use of TNFi in patients with active serious infection, or in those with chronic, recurrent infections.

To aid clinicians in weighing up the benefits and risks of bDMARD treatment, the Rheumatoid Arthritis Observation of Biologic Therapy (RABBIT) Risk Score was developed. This score estimates the likelihood of a patient developing a serious infection within the next 12 months, based on data from patients with similar risk profiles.[84]

Bacterial infections and TNFi

Streptococcus pneumonia

S. pneumonia is a major cause of mortality and morbidity worldwide[85] and is a common cause of community acquired pneumonia, as well as otitis media. However, in immunocompromised patients, it can cause disseminated infections such as meningitis.[86] It is well established that TNF plays a critical role in host defence against pneumococcal infection. Kirby et al. undertook a study of TNF gene-deficient mice, and mice administered neutralizing monoclonal TNF antibodies, with mice receiving a non-lethal challenge with *S. pneumoniae*. This demonstrated that mice deficient in TNF died more rapidly from infection, and further, were more likely to develop systemic disease.[87] Certainly, disseminated pneumococcal infections have been reported in those receiving TNFi, such as necrotizing fasciitis.[88,89]

Prevention of pneumococcal infection can be achieved through vaccination. TNFi therapy may impair the response to pneumococcal vaccination[90] so the vaccine is usually recommended at 2–3 weeks or longer prior to starting TNFi therapy.[91,92]

Tuberculosis

TNFα has an important role in increasing the ability of activated macrophages to phagocytose and kill mycobacteria. Tuberculosis

(TB) risk incidence on TNFi may be dependent on the background prevalence of TB in various geographic areas.[93,94] Regardless, all studies comparing the risk of TB in patients receiving TNFi therapy to those in a reference population with RA have found increased risk. The BIOBADASER database provides evidence to suggest that TB screening guidelines reduce the risk of TB.[93]

Recommended actions to screen for TB are clinical examination, a chest X-ray within 3 months prior to TNFi initiation. The use of tuberculin skin test is not particularly helpful TB screening test for those on immunosuppressive therapy, where false negative tests may occur. However, interferon gamma release assay is a more sensitive and therefore appropriate screening test for latent TB and in those receiving immunosuppressants.[95]

Legionella pneumophila

Legionella is a well-recognized cause of pneumonia. A 3-year French prospective study of legionella patients receiving TNFi demonstrated an overall annual incidence rate of legionellosis of 4.67 per 100 000 patient-years, using the French population as a reference (95% CI, 0.0–125.7), with highest standardized incidence ratio (SIR) for those receiving infliximab (SIR 15.3, 95% CI 8.5–27.6) or adalimumab (SIR 37.7, 95%CI 21.9–64.9), compared to etanercept (SIR 3.0, 95% CI 1.00–9.2), although it must be recognized that only 27 cases of legionellosis on those receiving TNFi were identified.[96]

Listeria monocytogenes.

Listeriosis is a foodborne illness, and in adults may present with mild gastrointestinal symptoms such as diarrhoea, fever, and muscle aches. In patients receiving TNFi, however, there are multiple reports of more disseminated infection, such as meningitis and endocarditis.[97,98] Dixon et al. reported three cases of listeriosis in 7664 RA patients treated with anti-TNF-α agents.[99] This displays an incidence rate of approximately three cases per 10 000 patient-years, which is much higher than the rate of listeriosis infection in the general population.[100]

A review of the literature in 2013 demonstrated 43 cases of invasive listeria infection in those receiving TNFi, with 22 patients developing neurological involvement (the majority developing meningitis), bacteraemia without infective focus in 11 patients, and bacteraemia with focalization in 9/43 patients (in the form of septic arthritis, cholecystitis, endophthalmitis, splenic abscess, and peritonitis).[100]

Salmonella

Multiple reports suggest that TNFi therapy may increase susceptibility to Salmonella infection.[101–105] One study of patients with inflammatory arthritis demonstrated at least 50% of cases (9/17) of patients with Salmonella on TNFi developed systemic infection, suggesting that TNFi may predispose RA patients to disseminated Salmonella.[104]

Fungal infections and TNFi

Histoplasmosis

Histoplasmosis is the most frequent invasive fungal infection occurring in patients receiving TNFi, with a reported mortality rate of 20%.[106] TNF is well recognized to play a crucial role in host immune response to *Histoplasma capsulatum*.[107] Certainly, in

experimental models of Histoplasma infection, TNF blockade prevented development of a protective immune response[108,109] likely through impairing macrophage activation.[110] A five year study of adverse event reporting of TNFi therapy demonstrated that the incidence of histoplasmosis is higher in patients receiving TNFi monoclonal antibodies, compared to etanercept.[111] Histoplasmosis and blastomycosis infections are particularly common in the US Midwest.

Coccidioidomycosis

This fungus is largely restricted to Western United States (California and Arizona most commonly), Mexico, and parts of central and south America.[112] In most cases in non-immunocompromised individuals not receiving TNFi, there are few symptoms. However, a case series of patients with symptomatic coccidioidomycosis while receiving TNFi demonstrated all patients had pneumonia, with some demonstrating disseminated infection.[113]

Candidiasis

Candida albicans is part of the natural flora of healthy individuals.[114] A recent study demonstrated that TNF inhibits *Candida albicans* biofilm formation, with biofilms being thought to be essential to evading host defence,[115] providing some evidence for a possible contributory mechanism to predisposition to candidiasis for those receiving TNFi therapy. In the United States, there has reportedly been a higher incidence of *Candida* infections among patients treated with infliximab (10.15 cases/100 000 persons) than among patients treated with etanercept (5.31 cases/100 000 persons, p = 0.061).[111]

Aspergillosis

Aspergillus spp are ubiquitous in nature and the spread of infection is usually by inhalation of infectious conidia.[86] A US study of patients receiving TNFi demonstrated a higher incidence of aspergillus infections in those receiving infliximab compared to etanercept (8.63 and 6.19 cases/100 000 persons, p = 0.243, respectively).[111,116] There have been numerous case reports of disseminated aspergillosis in patients receiving TNFi, with predominantly pulmonary involvement.[117–119]

Cryptococcus

This encapsulated fungus is found worldwide, and infection may occur through inhalation after disruption of soil.[86] Although presentation can be varied, lung infection is most common.[86] One retrospective case-control study at a single centre identified 9132 RA patients with a diagnosis of cryptococcal infection between 2001 and 2014. This study demonstrated that adalimumab therapy was associated with a significantly increased risk of cryptococcosis in RA patients (aOR 4.50, 95% CI 1.03–19.66, p = 0.046).[120]

Pneumocystis jirovecii

P. jirovecii causes a non-granulomatous fungal infection, spread via aerosol inhalation. There is a large body of evidence supporting the fact that *P. jirovecii* is an opportunistic infection, with the immunocompromised being at high risk of contracting symptomatic infection.[86] *P. jirovecii* pneumonia (PJP) was described in patients with RA as early as the 1960s, but became more widely recognized after the onset of the AIDS epidemic.[121] In 2007, Kaur and Mahl published a report of 84 cases of PJP in patients on infliximab, reported to the FDA Adverse Event Reporting System between January 1998 and December 2003, with a mortality rate of 27%. Most of these patients had RA, and developed pneumonia after an average of two infusions.[122]

Most studies of patients receiving TNFi have reported incidences of PJP of less than one case per 1000 person-years follow-up[83,99,123-125] supporting the assertion that the risks of PJP chemoprophylaxis likely outweigh the benefits for these patients.[126] Higher prevalence rates of 0.5% have been reported in the context of strict postmarketing surveillance in Japan.[127]

Viral infections

Hepatitis and HIV

Screening for hepatitis B and C is recommended prior to therapy initiation, due to risk of reactivation of latent disease while on TNF inhibitors.[128]

Hepatitis B

Several case reports demonstrate reactivation of hepatitis B during TNFi therapy, with serious consequences, including death.[129-131] Reactivation of viral hepatitis has been more frequently reported for infliximab than for either adalimumab or etanercept. This may be due to the structural differences between these compounds.[132]

Hepatitis C

Aggressive immunosuppression frequently leads to an increase in the levels of hepatitis C virus (HCV) viral load and worsening of liver conditions in transplant patients,[133] possibly through inhibition of TNF-α, which is involved in the apoptotic signalling pathway of hepatocytes infected by HCV. Hence, inhibition of TNF could potentially increase viral replication and worsen the course of chronic hepatitis C.[134]

However, unlike the clinical data for hepatitis B, the risks of continuing TNFi in patients with hepatitis C infection in clinical practice are less clear. In 2011, a systematic review of 37 publications with data on 153 patients who were treated with TNFi in the setting of HCV infection concluded that the safety profile of TNFi to be acceptable in the setting of HCV infection,[135] although the authors did acknowledge a lack of long-term, and large clinical trials data to support this.

This review also demonstrated that etanercept is the TNFi that has been most extensively used in patients with HCV infection, with only one definitely confirmed case of HCV hepatitis worsening.[136] Zein et al. reported a double blinded RCT where etanercept was used as an adjuvant to interferon and ribavirin in patients with chronic hepatitis C infection, and demonstrated significantly greater reduction in HCV viral load at 24 weeks in those receiving etanercept compared to those receiving placebo (63% reduction in ribonucleic acid (RNA) load compared to 24%, p = 0.04).[137]

Indeed, the 2012 Update of the 2008 ACR Recommendations for the use of disease-modifying antirheumatic drugs and biologics in the treatment of RA, recommended that etanercept could potentially be used in patients with hepatitis C.[138] Further, the updated 2015 ACR guidance suggests that RA patients with hepatitis C should be treated the same as RA patients without hepatitis C, although the guidance does state that the strength of evidence to support this is low, with only a small number of RCT done to investigate this.[70] Several direct-acting antivirals have been recently approved for the treatment of hepatitis C and offer cure for the majority of patients.

HIV infection

Patients with HIV are well known to be at risk of opportunistic infection, and it would seem logical therefore to avoid TNFi in this group of patients due to this. Indeed, Aboulafia et al. reported a case of a patient receiving etanercept for psoriatic arthritis. While the etanercept produced an improvement in his arthritis, he developed multiple polymicrobial infections.[139]

There are reports in the literature of successful treatment of RA using TNFi in patients with HIV.[140,141] Cepeda et al. demonstrated that in a cohort of eight HIV-positive patients with inflammatory arthritis (three with RA), TNFi were well tolerated, with no adverse effect on CD4 count or HIV viral load, suggesting that TNFi may be given on a risk benefit basis, if the patient's underlying HIV is controlled, with no evidence of severe immunocompromise (CD4 count of over 200/mm^3 and HIV viral load of less than 60 000/mm^3).[141]

Herpes simplex virus (HSV)

Initial infection with HSV in non-immunocompromised individuals usually causes an asymptomatic or mild self-limiting oral (generally HSV-1) or genital (generally HSV-2) infection, followed by HSV persistence (latency) in nerve ganglia.[86] However, reactivation in immunocompromised patients receiving TNFi can lead to disseminated disease; multiple case reports of HSV encephalitis exist in the literature.[142]

Varicella zoster infection

Patients with RA are recognized to have an increased risk of herpes zoster, the reactivation of varicella zoster infection.[143] In immunocompromised patients, herpes zoster can frequently affect multiple dermatomes, involve the optic nerve, and also become disseminated.[144] McDonald et al. described the occurrence of herpes zoster in 96/3661 RA patients receiving TNFi; of these, 59 were receiving etanercept, 33 infliximab, and 4 receiving adalimumab treatment.[145]

It is also recommended that any patient receiving TNFi, who develops primary varicella zoster, or who has a household contact who develops primary varicella zoster, and the risks of infection are thought to be significant, receive varicella zoster immunoglobulins. Some advocate testing for varicella zoster serology prior to TNFi commencement, to assess immunity.[146] ACR recommends that all patients over 60 should receive herpes zoster vaccine prior to initiation of TNFi.[138] For most patients who meet criteria for herpes zoster vaccination, where reimbursement permits, the recombinant zoster vaccine is preferred over the older live attenuated herpes zoster vaccine (ZVL). For patients who previously received ZVL, revaccination with RSZ is recommended.

Cytomegalovirus (CMV)

It is long established that the majority of individuals will have been exposed to CMV by adulthood.[147] and infection is more frequently asymptomatic, often becoming latent. Multiple reports of disseminated CMV infection in patients receiving TNFi exist in the literature, including retinitis, colitis, hepatitis, and pneumonia.[148-151]

Perioperative TNFi and infection

RA is recognized as an independent risk factor for postoperative infection after orthopaedic surgery, with 2–4 times higher infection rates in RA patients. Some additional work has been undertaken to assess the relationship between peri-operative use of TNFi in RA patients and perioperative infection. For example, one study of 91 RA patients undergoing orthopaedic surgery, demonstrated that 11% of the patients developed a serious postoperative orthopaedic infection.[152] A univariate analysis demonstrated significant association of TNFi with development of serious postoperative infection (OR, 4.4; 95% CI, 1.1–18.41) and remained statistically significant after adjustment for age, sex, disease duration, steroid use, diabetes, and rheumatoid factor seropositivity (OR, 5.3; 95% CI, 1.1–24.9).

To assess whether cessation of TNFi reduces the risk of postoperative infection, a Dutch group conducted a retrospective parallel cohort study of 768 RA patients who underwent elective orthopaedic surgery. One group of patients had stopped TNFi prior to surgery (39 days presurgery for infliximab, 12 days for etanercept, and 56 days for adalimumab), and another continued preoperatively. A control group of patients not receiving TNFi were also included. Infection risk was highest in those who continued TNFi preoperatively (infection risk of 8.7%, compared to 5.8% in those who ceased TNFi, and 4% in those who never received TNFi). Interestingly, wound dehiscence and bleeding occurred more frequently in patients who had continued TNFi therapy.[153]

The British society of Rheumatology recommend that if TNFi are to be stopped prior to surgery, consideration should be given to stopping at a time 3–5 times the half-life for the relevant drug before surgery. Further, TNFi should not be restarted after surgery until there is good wound healing and no evidence of infection.[154] Similarly, the ACR recommend that biologic therapies should be withheld for elective joint replacement surgery, and discontinued for one-dosing cycle before surgery, or surgery should be planned for the end of the bDMARD dosing cycle. ACR further recommends that bDMARDs that were withheld prior to surgery should be restarted with evidence of wound healing and no sign of infection or drainage (approximately 14 days after surgery).[155]

Demyelinating disease

Multiple sclerosis, optic neuritis, and other demyelinating disorders, such as chronic inflammatory demyelinating polyneuropathy, have been described with TNFi use.[156] In 2001, Mohan et al. undertook a review of patients with neurological events suggestive of demyelination during TNFi therapy for inflammatory arthritis, using the FDA adverse events reporting system database. 19 patients with similar neurological events were identified; 17 on etanercept, and 2 receiving infliximab. All neurological events were temporally related to TNFi. All neurologic events improved or resolved on discontinuation of TNFi. One patient exhibited a positive rechallenge phenomenon.[157]

Additionally, TNFi may exacerbate existing demyelinating disease, with one study demonstrating an increase in the number of MS flares in patients receiving TNFi.[158] Therefore, caution should be exercised in commencing TNFi therapy in those with demyelinating disease.

Heart failure

TNF levels are found to be consistently raised in patients with congestive cardiac failure (CCF), and TNF has been shown to negatively affect cardiac contractility.[159] An RCT using high-dose infliximab (at 10 mg/kg) in patients with moderate-to-severe

chronic heart failure demonstrated a significantly higher rate of hospitalization for worsening heart failure, with a HR of 2.84 (1.01–7.97) for patients receiving 10 mg/kg infliximab compared to placebo, and HR of 0.80 (0.22–2.99) for patients receiving 5 mg/kg infliximab compared to placebo.[160] Caution is recommended when using TNFi in patients with CCF, in particular in those with advanced stages of cardiac failure (New York Heart association class III and IV).[161]

Despite the association of TNFi and worsening CCF, there is a long established body of data supporting the idea that TNFi may be beneficial in preventing ischaemic heart disease in RA. Patients with untreated active RA are well recognized to be at risk of atherosclerosis, supported by the fact that cardiovascular disease is a major cause of comorbidity in RA,[162] and other studies that demonstrate carotid artery thickness on ultrasound is increased in patients with RA.[163] In addition, CRP and interleukin (IL) 6 levels are both raised in patients with active RA, and these acute phase reactants are well recognized to be associated with the development of atherosclerosis.[164] However, TNFi have been demonstrated to increase the concentration of high-density lipoprotein (HDL) cholesterol, as well as reduce CRP and IL-6 levels, with consequential likely reduction in cardiovascular risk.[165,166] Indeed, Jacobsson et al. demonstrated in a study of 983 RA patients, that TNFi treatment was associated with a lower incidence of first cardiovascular events than RA patients not receiving TNFi (with age and sex adjusted incidence rate of 14.0/1000 person-years (95% CI 5.7–22.4) in those treated with TNFi, compared with 35.4/1000 person-years (95% CI 16.5–54.4) in those not treated).[167]

Cutaneous reactions

Cutaneous reactions have been ascribed to anti-TNF agents, most usually injection site reactions.

Other skin disorders associated with anti-TNF therapy include lupus-like rashes, psoriasis, leukocytoclastic vasculitis,[168] lichen planus and planus-like eruptions.[169]

Malignancy

RA patients have an increased risk of lymphoma, but not solid malignancies. Much conflicting evidence exists regarding whether TNFi therapy is itself associated with an increased risk of malignancy. In registry studies, no overall increased risk of malignancy was reported in RA patients, regardless of TNFi therapy.[170-172] In patients with prior malignancies, there was a higher risk of a new or recurring malignancy, but this risk was not increased further by exposure to TNFi.[173]

However, another meta-analysis of patients taking TNFi (limited to the monoclonal antibodies) showed more malignancies (0.8%) compared with the placebo-matched population (0.2%), with a pooled OR of 3.3 compared with placebo-treated patients. The risks appear to be dose-dependent, with those receiving high-dose therapy (defined as ≥6 mg/kg infliximab every 8 weeks or ≥40 mg adalimumab every other week) having the greatest risk (odds ratio, 4.3; 95% CI, 1.6–11.8); no important increased risk was seen below these dosages.[174] However, the lower than expected rate of neoplasia in the placebo group has been questioned and may arise from inaccuracies due to short duration of placebo compared with TNFi exposure.

Lymphoma

There were some early reports suggesting that the risk of lymphoma is further increased by TNFi therapy.[170,174,175] However, subsequent studies indicated that the observed increase in risk of lymphoma is secondary to RA disease activity, rather than treatment.[176,177]

Skin cancer

Studies suggest that RA patients treated with TNFi have a significantly increased risk of developing a non-melanoma skin cancer (NMSC); for example, one study of 15 789 patients with RA demonstrated a hazards ratio of 1.24 (p = 0.89), for development of NMSC in those receiving TNFi alone. History of previous malignancy, use of non-steroidal anti-inflammatory drugs (NSAIDs) or glucocorticoids were found to be independent risk factors for developing NMSC.[178] Additionally, RA patients receiving TNFi are at increased risk of developing melanoma, with a recent meta-analysis demonstrating a pooled effect estimate of 1.60 (95% CI 1.16–2.19).[179] Multiple studies recommend vigilance for skin cancers in RA patients receiving TNFi therapy.[178,180]

Current ACR guidelines[70] recommend the use of csDMARDs over biologics in previously treated melanoma and NMSC, and use of rituximab over TNFi in previously treated lymphoproliferative disorders. For previously treated solid organ malignancies, the panel recommends the same RA treatment strategy as for those without malignancy.

Induction of antidrug antibodies

The formation of ADAbs, many of which can be neutralizing, is a concern with TNFi, particularly monoclonal antibodies, such as infliximab and adalimumab. Such antibodies may cause allergic reactions and loss of responsiveness.

The risk of developing ADAbs varies with the type of TNFi therapy, being least common with etanercept, and most common with the mouse/human chimeric monoclonal antibody infliximab.[181] A recent systematic review of 443 studies observed the rate of ADAb formation among bDMARDs across diseases; out of the TNFi studied, the highest overall rates were reported with infliximab (0–83%), adalimumab (0–54%), with lowest rates with etanercept (0–13%) and golimumab (0–19%).[182]

It is well recognized that patients with RA treated with TNFi therapy who develop ADAbs are less likely to achieve a significant clinical response at 6 months (OR 0.03, CI 95%, 0.01–0.22).[183] Discontinuation of the biologic agent has also been shown to be significantly more likely in those with ADAbs compared with those without (for example, in a study of those with adalimumab, hazards ratio 3.0, 95% CI 1.6–5.5 p <0.001).[97] Adjunctive treatment

with a synthetic DMARD, such as methotrexate or leflunomide, has been shown in some studies to reduce the formation of circulating ADAbs, with one systematic review demonstrating a 44% reduction in ADAbs (RR = 0.59, 95% CI 0.50–0.70).[184]

Paradoxical adverse events (PAEs)

PAEs are defined as the occurrence of a pathological condition, during therapy with a bDMARD, that usually responds to this class of drug. Toussirot and Aubin define a true PAE as a condition in which the therapy of concern has proven efficacy for treating. In contrast, a 'borderline' PAE is the an immune-mediate condition observed during bDMARD therapy that does not have proven efficacy in this specific condition, despite a rationale for its use.[185]

Psoriasis is a well-recognized true PAE in those receiving TNFi. A 2010 review identified 207 cases in which psoriatic skin lesions developed in patients treated with TNFi therapy. Partial or complete resolution occurred with treatment for psoriasis, with the majority continuing with TNFi treatment.[186]

A single study of RA patients receiving TNFi demonstrated higher rate of psoriasis in those receiving adalimumab compared to etanercept, and infliximab, with incidence rate ratio (IRR) of 4.6 (1.7–12.1) and 3.5 (1.3–9.3), respectively.[186]

Hidradenitis suppurativa (HS) is a chronic skin disease characterized by recurrent painful inflammatory nodules, abscesses, sinus and fistula formation, involving apocrine gland-bearing areas.[185] One multicentre study, including patients with a variety of different inflammatory diseases, described a large series of cases of new-onset HS on TNFi (mainly adalimumab). Complete resolution of HS was observed after treatment discontinuation or a switch to another biological agent. Rechallenging the drug led to HS relapse in a small number of patients.[187]

Inflammatory bowel disease (IBD)

Toussirot et al. described a series of cases of patients (mostly with ankylosing spondylitis or spondyloarthritis), developing new-onset IBD on TNFi (mostly etanercept). All reported patients had a favourable intestinal outcome after discontinuing the anti-TNF-α agent or after switching to a drug that is a monoclonal antibody.[188]

Numerous 'borderline' PAEs have been reported with TNFi therapy. These are summarized in Box 31.5. Please see Toussirot and Aubin for a full review of borderline PAEs.[185]

Vasculitis and TNFi

A postulated mechanism for the initiation of vasculitis by TNFi is that immune complexes containing the drug may deposit on small vessels and induce local complement activation. The cytokine imbalance that is secondary to TNF inhibition may also play a role, with shift from Th1 to Th2 predominant responses, which can upregulate antibody production.[189]

In general, TNFi are associated most commonly with cutaneous small vessel vasculitis, but systemic involvement with peripheral nerves or kidney has also been observed. The British Society of Rheumatology Biologics Register-RA (BSRBR-RA) cohort study indicates that TNFi associated vasculitis is a rare occurrence, with an incidence of only 15 per 10 000 patients starting a first TNFi.[190]

One retrospective study identified 8 cases of new vasculitis in patients receiving TNFi. The mean time between TNFi initiation and onset of vasculitis was 34.5 months. The skin was most commonly

---

Box 31.5 Borderline PAEs in TNFi therapy

- Uveitis
- Scleritis
- Sarcoidosis
- Granuloma annulare
- Interstitial granulomatous dermatitis
- Vasculitis
- Alopecia areata
- Vitiligo

affected, followed by the peripheral nervous system and kidneys. The most common cutaneous manifestation of TNFi induced vasculitis was purpura, with other manifestations including ulceration, blisters, and erythematous macules. Most patients improved after TNFi discontinuation.[191] In a case series of 39 inflammatory arthritis patients developing vasculitis during TNFi therapy, etanercept was the most frequently incriminated TNFi.[189]

Systemic lupus erythematosus

TNFi therapy is frequently associated with the development of autoantibodies, most commonly antinuclear antibodies (ANA), but also anti-double-stranded deoxyribonucleic acid (anti-dsDNA) antibodies, and antiphospholipid antibodies, frequently without any clinically apparent effects.[99] Seroconversion to ANA positivity has been associated with development of treatment failure to TNFi,[192,193] as well as formation of antidrug antibody (ADAb) or immunogenicity with monoclonal antibody TNFi.[194]

BSRBR-RA found the incidence of TNFi associated systemic lupus erythematosus (SLE) to be a rare occurrence, with an incidence of 10 per 10 000 patients receiving a first TNFi.[190] The most common form of TNFi associated SLE is cutaneous disease. For example, the BSRBR-RA demonstrated that 89% of the cohort receiving TNFi developing lupus-like events had cutaneous disease. The most common cutaneous manifestations include a malar rash, discoid rash, or subacute cutaneous lupus.[190] New arthritis involving large and small joints may also occur, as may fevers/malaise, serositis, and cytopenias. ANA or dsDNA positivity helps confirm the diagnosis, along with the fact that symptoms should resolve on drug discontinuation.

Conclusion

TNFi therapy is well established as a highly effective therapy for RA. TNF blockade in RA consistently decreases disease activity and improves health related quality of life, and lessens or even inhibits radiographic progression of peripheral joint damage.

The success of TNFi has encouraged the development of multiple biologic immunotherapies directed at other therapeutic targets including pro-inflammatory cytokines and key cellular components of inflammation in RA. Better understanding of why some patients and not others respond to TNFi therapy remains the subject of ongoing research. These efforts may yield further clues as to the pathogenesis of RA, and may also provide information to enable future 'precision medicine' tailoring of therapy regimes to the needs of individual patients.

REFERENCES

1. Voss M, Lettau M, Paulsen M, Janssen O. Posttranslational regulation of Fas ligand function. *Cell Commun Signal* 2008;6:11.
2. Idriss HT, Naismith JH. TNF alpha and the TNF receptor superfamily: structure-function relationship(s). *Microsc Res Tech* 2000;50(3):184–95.
3. Parameswaran N, Patial S. Tumor necrosis factor-alpha signaling in macrophages. *Crit Rev Eukaryot Gene Expr* 2010;20(2):87–103.
4. Moelants EA, Mortier A, Van Damme J, Proost P. Regulation of TNF-alpha with a focus on rheumatoid arthritis. *Immunol Cell Biol* 2013;91(6):393–401.
5. McInnes IB, Schett G. Cytokines in the pathogenesis of rheumatoid arthritis. *Nat Rev Immunol* 2007;7(6):429–42.
6. Brennan FM, Maini RN, Feldmann M. TNF alpha--a pivotal role in rheumatoid arthritis? *Br J Rheumatol* 1992;31(5):293–8.
7. Szekanecz Z, Koch AE. Cell-cell interactions in synovitis. Endothelial cells and immune cell migration. *Arthritis Res* 2000;2(5):368–73.
8. Wright HL, Moots RJ, Edwards SW. The multifactorial role of neutrophils in rheumatoid arthritis. *Nat Rev Rheumatol* 2014;10(10):593–601.
9. Badolato R, Oppenheim JJ. Role of cytokines, acute-phase proteins, and chemokines in the progression of rheumatoid arthritis. *Semin Arthritis Rheum* 1996;26(2):526–38.
10. Maini RN, Taylor PC, Paleolog E, et al. Anti-tumour necrosis factor specific antibody (infliximab) treatment provides insights into the pathophysiology of rheumatoid arthritis. *Ann Rheum Dis* 1999;58(Suppl 1I):56–60.
11. Brennan FM, Browne KA, Green PA, Jaspar JM, Maini RN, Feldmann M. Reduction of serum matrix metalloproteinase 1 and matrix metalloproteinase 3 in rheumatoid arthritis patients following anti-tumour necrosis factor-alpha (cA2) therapy. *Br J Rheumatol* 1997;36(6):643–50.
12. Sipos O, Török A, Kalic T, Duda E, Filkor K. Reverse signaling contributes to control of chronic inflammation by anti-TNF therapeutics. *Antibodies* 2015;4(2):123.
13. Domonkos A, Udvardy A, Laszlo L, Nagy T, Duda E. Receptor-like properties of the 26 kDa transmembrane form of TNF. *Eur Cytokine Netw* 2001;12(3):411–19.
14. Scallon B, Cai A, Solowski N, et al. Binding and functional comparisons of two types of tumor necrosis factor antagonists. *J Pharmacol Exp Ther* 2002;301(2):418–26.
15. Nesbitt A, Fossati G, Bergin M, et al. Mechanism of action of certolizumab pegol (CDP870): *in vitro* comparison with other anti-tumor necrosis factor alpha agents. *Inflamm Bowel Dis* 2007;13(11):1323–32.
16. Levin AD, Wildenberg ME, van den Brink GR. Mechanism of action of anti-TNF therapy in inflammatory bowel disease. *J Crohns Colitis* 2016;10(8):989–97.
17. Kaymakcalan Z, Sakorafas P, Bose S, et al. Comparisons of affinities, avidities, and complement activation of adalimumab, infliximab, and etanercept in binding to soluble and membrane tumor necrosis factor. *Clin Immunol* 2009;131(2):308–16.
18. Elliott MJ, Maini RN, Feldmann M, et al. Repeated therapy with monoclonal antibody to tumour necrosis factor alpha (cA2) in patients with rheumatoid arthritis. *Lancet* 1994;344(8930):1125–7.
19. Charles P, Elliott MJ, Davis D, et al. Regulation of cytokines, cytokine inhibitors, and acute-phase proteins following anti-TNF-alpha therapy in rheumatoid arthritis. *J Immunol* 1999;163(3):1521–8.
20. Lorenz HM, Antoni C, Valerius T, et al. *In vivo* blockade of TNF-alpha by intravenous infusion of a chimeric monoclonal TNF-alpha antibody in patients with rheumatoid arthritis. Short term cellular and molecular effects. *J Immunol* 1996;156(4):1646–53.
21. Ulfgren AK, Andersson U, Engstrom M, Klareskog L, Maini RN, Taylor PC. Systemic anti-tumor necrosis factor alpha therapy in rheumatoid arthritis down-regulates synovial tumor necrosis factor alpha synthesis. *Arthritis Rheum* 2000;43(11):2391–6.

22. Paleolog EM, Hunt M, Elliott MJ, Feldmann M, Maini RN, Woody JN. Deactivation of vascular endothelium by monoclonal anti-tumor necrosis factor alpha antibody in rheumatoid arthritis. *Arthritis Rheum* 1996;*39*(7):1082–91.

23. Tak PP, Taylor PC, Breedveld FC, et al. Decrease in cellularity and expression of adhesion molecules by anti-tumor necrosis factor alpha monoclonal antibody treatment in patients with rheumatoid arthritis. *Arthritis Rheum* 1996;*39*(7):1077–81.

24. Taylor PC, Peters AM, Paleolog E, et al. Reduction of chemokine levels and leukocyte traffic to joints by tumor necrosis factor alpha blockade in patients with rheumatoid arthritis. *Arthritis Rheum* 2000;*43*(1):38–47.

25. Taylor PC. Anti-TNFalpha therapy for rheumatoid arthritis: an update. *Intern Med* 2003;*42*(1):15–20.

26. Paleolog EM, Young S, Stark AC, McCloskey RV, Feldmann M, Maini RN. Modulation of angiogenic vascular endothelial growth factor by tumor necrosis factor alpha and interleukin-1 in rheumatoid arthritis. *Arthritis Rheum* 1998;*41*(7):1258–65.

27. Taylor PC. Serum vascular markers and vascular imaging in assessment of rheumatoid arthritis disease activity and response to therapy. *Rheumatology (Oxf)* 2005;*44*(6):721–8.

28. Taylor PC, Steuer A, Gruber J, et al. Comparison of ultrasonographic assessment of synovitis and joint vascularity with radiographic evaluation in a randomized, placebo-controlled study of infliximab therapy in early rheumatoid arthritis. *Arthritis Rheum* 2004;*50*(4):1107–16.

29. Taylor PC, Steuer A, Gruber J, et al. Ultrasonographic and radiographic results from a two-year controlled trial of immediate or one-year-delayed addition of infliximab to ongoing methotrexate therapy in patients with erosive early rheumatoid arthritis. *Arthritis Rheum* 2006;*54*(1):47–53.

30. Catrina AI, Lampa J, Ernestam S, et al. Anti-tumour necrosis factor (TNF)-alpha therapy (etanercept) down-regulates serum matrix metalloproteinase (MMP)-3 and MMP-1 in rheumatoid arthritis. *Rheumatology (Oxf)* 2002;*41*(5):484–9.

31. Geusens P. The role of RANK ligand/osteoprotegerin in rheumatoid arthritis. *Ther Adv Musculoskelet Dis* 2012;*4*(4):225–33.

32. Ziolkowska M, Kurowska M, Radzikowska A, et al. High levels of osteoprotegerin and soluble receptor activator of nuclear factor kappa B ligand in serum of rheumatoid arthritis patients and their normalization after anti-tumor necrosis factor alpha treatment. *Arthritis Rheum* 2002;*46*(7):1744–53.

33. Monaco C, Nanchahal J, Taylor P, Feldmann M. Anti-TNF therapy: past, present and future. *Int Immunol* 2015;*27*(1):55–62.

34. American College of Rheumatology. *Medication Guide: Infliximab*, 2018. Available at: https://www.rheumatology.org/Learning-Center/Medication-Guides/Medication-Guide-Infliximab-Remicade

35. Klotz U, Teml A, Schwab M. Clinical pharmacokinetics and use of infliximab. *Clin Pharmacokinet* 2007;*46*(8):645–60.

36. Elliott MJ, Maini RN, Feldmann M, et al. Treatment of rheumatoid arthritis with chimeric monoclonal antibodies to tumor necrosis factor alpha. *Arthritis Rheum* 1993;*36*(12):1681–90.

37. Lipsky PE, van der Heijde DM, St Clair EW, et al. Infliximab and methotrexate in the treatment of rheumatoid arthritis. Anti-tumor necrosis factor trial in rheumatoid arthritis with concomitant therapy study group. *N Engl J Med* 2000;*343*(22):1594–602.

38. Smolen JS, Han C, Bala M, et al. Evidence of radiographic benefit of treatment with infliximab plus methotrexate in rheumatoid arthritis patients who had no clinical improvement: a detailed subanalysis of data from the anti-tumor necrosis factor trial in rheumatoid arthritis with concomitant therapy study. *Arthritis Rheum* 2005;*52*(4):1020–30.

39. St Clair EW, van der Heijde DM, Smolen JS, et al. Combination of infliximab and methotrexate therapy for early rheumatoid arthritis: a randomized, controlled trial. *Arthritis Rheum.* 2004;*50*(11):3432–43.

40. Haraoui B, Bykerk V. Etanercept in the treatment of rheumatoid arthritis. *Ther Clin Risk Manag* 2007;*3*(1):99–105.

41. Moreland LW, Baumgartner SW, Schiff MH, et al. Treatment of rheumatoid arthritis with a recombinant human tumor necrosis factor receptor (p75)-Fc fusion protein. *N Engl J Med* 1997;*337*(3):141–7.

42. Weinblatt ME, Kremer JM, Bankhurst AD, et al. A trial of etanercept, a recombinant tumor necrosis factor receptor: Fc fusion protein, in patients with rheumatoid arthritis receiving methotrexate. *N Engl J Med* 1999;*340*(4):253–9.

43. Kremer JM, Weinblatt ME, Bankhurst AD, et al. Etanercept added to background methotrexate therapy in patients with rheumatoid arthritis: continued observations. *Arthritis Rheum* 2003;*48*(6):1493–9.

44. Bathon JM, Martin RW, Fleischmann RM, et al. A comparison of etanercept and methotrexate in patients with early rheumatoid arthritis. *N Engl J Med* 2000;*343*(22):1586–93.

45. Genovese MC, Bathon JM, Martin RW, et al. Etanercept versus methotrexate in patients with early rheumatoid arthritis: two-year radiographic and clinical outcomes. *Arthritis Rheum* 2002;*46*(6):1443–50.

46. van der Heijde D, Klareskog L, Rodriguez-Valverde V, et al. Comparison of etanercept and methotrexate, alone and combined, in the treatment of rheumatoid arthritis: two-year clinical and radiographic results from the TEMPO study, a double-blind, randomized trial. *Arthritis Rheum* 2006;*54*(4):1063–74.

47. Emery P, Breedveld FC, Hall S, et al. Comparison of methotrexate monotherapy with a combination of methotrexate and etanercept in active, early, moderate to severe rheumatoid arthritis (COMET): a randomised, double-blind, parallel treatment trial. *Lancet* 2008;*372*(9636):375–82.

48. Mahler SM, Marquis CP, Brown G, Roberts A, Hoogenboom HR. Cloning and expression of human V-genes derived from phage display libraries as fully assembled human anti-TNF alpha monoclonal antibodies. *Immunotechnology* 1997;*3*(1):31–43.

49. Weisman MH, Moreland LW, Furst DE, et al. Efficacy, pharmacokinetic, and safety assessment of adalimumab, a fully human anti-tumor necrosis factor-alpha monoclonal antibody, in adults with rheumatoid arthritis receiving concomitant methotrexate: a pilot study. *Clin Ther* 2003;*25*(6):1700–21.

50. Breedveld FC, Weisman MH, Kavanaugh AF, et al. The PREMIER study: a multicenter, randomized, double-blind clinical trial of combination therapy with adalimumab plus methotrexate versus methotrexate alone or adalimumab alone in patients with early, aggressive rheumatoid arthritis who had not had previous methotrexate treatment. *Arthritis Rheum* 2006;*54*(1):26–37.

51. Weinblatt ME, Keystone EC, Furst DE, et al. Adalimumab, a fully human anti-tumor necrosis factor alpha monoclonal antibody, for the treatment of rheumatoid arthritis in patients taking concomitant methotrexate: the ARMADA trial. *Arthritis Rheum* 2003;*48*(1):35–45.

52. Weinblatt ME, Keystone EC, Furst DE, Kavanaugh AF, Chartash EK, Segurado OG. Long term efficacy and safety of adalimumab plus methotrexate in patients with rheumatoid

arthritis: ARMADA 4 year extended study. *Ann Rheum Dis* 2006;65(6):753–9.

53. Keystone EC, Kavanaugh AF, Sharp JT, et al. Radiographic, clinical, and functional outcomes of treatment with adalimumab (a human anti-tumor necrosis factor monoclonal antibody) in patients with active rheumatoid arthritis receiving concomitant methotrexate therapy: a randomized, placebo-controlled, 52-week trial. *Arthritis Rheum* 2004;50(5):1400–11.

54. Keystone EC, van der Heijde D, Kavanaugh A, et al. Clinical, functional, and radiographic benefits of long-term adalimumab plus methotrexate: final 10-year data in longstanding rheumatoid arthritis. *J Rheumatol* 2013;40(9):1487–97.

55. Goel N, Stephens S. Certolizumab pegol. *MAbs* 2010;2(2):137–47.

56. Keystone E, Heijde D, Mason D, Jr., et al. Certolizumab pegol plus methotrexate is significantly more effective than placebo plus methotrexate in active rheumatoid arthritis: findings of a fifty-two-week, phase III, multicenter, randomized, double-blind, placebo-controlled, parallel-group study. *Arthritis Rheum* 2008;58(11):3319–29.

57. Smolen J, Landewe RB, Mease P, et al. Efficacy and safety of certolizumab pegol plus methotrexate in active rheumatoid arthritis: the RAPID 2 study. A randomised controlled trial. *Ann Rheum Dis* 2009;68(6):797–804.

58. Fleischmann R, Vencovsky J, van Vollenhoven RF, et al. Efficacy and safety of certolizumab pegol monotherapy every 4 weeks in patients with rheumatoid arthritis failing previous disease-modifying antirheumatic therapy: the FAST4WARD study. *Ann Rheum Dis* 2009;68(6):805–11.

59. Kay J, Rahman MU. Golimumab: a novel human anti-TNF-alpha monoclonal antibody for the treatment of rheumatoid arthritis, ankylosing spondylitis, and psoriatic arthritis. *Core Evid* 2010;4159–70.

60. Emery P, Fleischmann RM, Moreland LW, et al. Golimumab, a human anti-tumor necrosis factor alpha monoclonal antibody, injected subcutaneously every four weeks in methotrexate-naive patients with active rheumatoid arthritis: twenty-four-week results of a phase III, multicenter, randomized, double-blind, placebo-controlled study of golimumab before methotrexate as first-line therapy for early-onset rheumatoid arthritis. *Arthritis Rheum* 2009;60(8):2272–83.

61. Keystone EC, Genovese MC, Klareskog L, et al. Golimumab, a human antibody to tumour necrosis factor {alpha} given by monthly subcutaneous injections, in active rheumatoid arthritis despite methotrexate therapy: the GO-FORWARD Study. *Ann Rheum Dis* 2009;68(6):789–96.

62. Keystone EC, Genovese MC, Hall S, et al. Safety and efficacy of subcutaneous golimumab in patients with active rheumatoid arthritis despite methotrexate therapy: final 5-year results of the GO-FORWARD trial. *J Rheumatol* 2016;43(2):298–306.

63. Smolen JS, Kay J, Doyle MK, et al. Golimumab in patients with active rheumatoid arthritis after treatment with tumour necrosis factor alpha inhibitors (GO-AFTER study): a multicentre, randomised, double-blind, placebo-controlled, phase III trial. *Lancet* 2009;374(9685):210–21.

64. Smolen JS, Kay J, Landewe RB, et al. Golimumab in patients with active rheumatoid arthritis who have previous experience with tumour necrosis factor inhibitors: results of a long-term extension of the randomised, double-blind, placebo-controlled GO-AFTER study through week 160. *Ann Rheum Dis* 2012;71(10):1671–9.

65. Weinblatt ME, Bingham CO, 3rd, Mendelsohn AM, et al. Intravenous golimumab is effective in patients with active rheumatoid arthritis despite methotrexate therapy with responses as early as week 2: results of the phase 3, randomised, multicentre, double-blind, placebo-controlled GO-FURTHER trial. *Ann Rheum Dis* 2013;72(3):381–9.

66. Weinblatt ME, Westhovens R, Mendelsohn AM, et al. Radiographic benefit and maintenance of clinical benefit with intravenous golimumab therapy in patients with active rheumatoid arthritis despite methotrexate therapy: results up to 1 year of the phase 3, randomised, multicentre, double blind, placebo controlled GO-FURTHER trial. *Ann Rheum Dis* 2014;73(12):2152–9.

67. Deighton C, Hyrich K, Ding T, et al. BSR and BHPR rheumatoid arthritis guidelines on eligibility criteria for the first biological therapy. *Rheumatology (Oxf)* 2010;49(6):1197–9.

68. Kiely PD, Deighton C, Dixey J, Ostor AJ. Biologic agents for rheumatoid arthritis—negotiating the NICE technology appraisals. *Rheumatology (Oxf)* 2012;51(1):24–31.

69. Smolen JS, Landewe R, Bijlsma J, et al. EULAR recommendations for the management of rheumatoid arthritis with synthetic and biological disease-modifying antirheumatic drugs: 2016 update. *Ann Rheum Dis* 2017;76(6):960–77.

70. Singh JA, Saag KG, Bridges SL, Jr., et al. 2015 American College of Rheumatology Guideline for the treatment of rheumatoid arthritis. *Arthritis Care Res (Hoboken)* 2016;68(1):1–25.

71. Roopenian DC, Akilesh S. FcRn: the neonatal Fc receptor comes of age. *Nat Rev Immunol* 2007;7(9):715–25.

72. Carter JD, Valeriano J, Vasey FB. Tumor necrosis factor-alpha inhibition and VATER association: a causal relationship. *J Rheumatol* 2006;33(5):1014–17.

73. Verstappen SM, King Y, Watson KD, Symmons DP, Hyrich KL. Anti-TNF therapies and pregnancy: outcome of 130 pregnancies in the British Society for Rheumatology Biologics Register. *Ann Rheum Dis* 2011;70(5):823–6.

74. Gotestam Skorpen C, Hoeltzenbein M, et al. The EULAR points to consider for use of antirheumatic drugs before pregnancy, and during pregnancy and lactation. *Ann Rheum Dis* 2016;75(5):795–810.

75. Flint J, Panchal S, Hurrell A, et al. BSR and BHPR guideline on prescribing drugs in pregnancy and breastfeeding-Part II: analgesics and other drugs used in rheumatology practice. *Rheumatology (Oxf)* 2016;55(9):1698–702.

76. Clowse ME, Forger F, Hwang C, et al. Minimal to no transfer of certolizumab pegol into breast milk: results from CRADLE, a prospective, postmarketing, multicentre, pharmacokinetic study. *Ann Rheum Dis* 2017;76(11):1890–6.

77. Mariette X, Forger F, Abraham B, et al. Lack of placental transfer of certolizumab pegol during pregnancy: results from CRIB, a prospective, postmarketing, pharmacokinetic study. *Ann Rheum Dis* 2018;77(2):228–33.

78. Mocci G, Marzo M, Papa A, Armuzzi A, Guidi L. Dermatological adverse reactions during anti-TNF treatments: focus on inflammatory bowel disease. *J Crohns Colitis* 2013;7(10):769–79.

79. Kelsall J, Rogers P, Galindo G, De Vera MA. Safety of infliximab treatment in patients with rheumatoid arthritis in a real-world clinical setting: description and evaluation of infusion reactions. *J Rheumatol* 2012;39(8):1539–45.

80. Vultaggio A, Matucci A, Nencini F, et al. Anti-infliximab IgE and non-IgE antibodies and induction of infusion-related severe anaphylactic reactions. *Allergy* 2010;65(5):657–61.

81. Hastings R, Ding T, Butt S, et al. Neutropenia in patients receiving anti-tumor necrosis factor therapy. *Arthritis Care Res (Hoboken)* 2010;62(6):764–9.

82. Baghai M, Osmon DR, Wolk DM, Wold LE, Haidukewych GJ, Matteson EL. Fatal sepsis in a patient with rheumatoid arthritis treated with etanercept. *Mayo Clin Proc* 2001;76(6):653–6.

83. Baddley JW, Winthrop KL, Chen L, et al. Non-viral opportunistic infections in new users of tumour necrosis factor inhibitor therapy: results of the SAfety Assessment of Biologic ThERapy (SABER) study. *Ann Rheum Dis* 2014;73(11):1942–8.

84. Strangfeld A, Eveslage M, Schneider M, et al. Treatment benefit or survival of the fittest: what drives the time-dependent decrease in serious infection rates under TNF inhibition and what does this imply for the individual patient? *Ann Rheum Dis* 2011;70(11):1914–20.

85. Henriques-Normark B, Tuomanen EI. The pneumococcus: epidemiology, microbiology, and pathogenesis. *Cold Spring Harb Perspect Med* 2013;3(7):pii: a010215.

86. Ali T, Kaitha S, Mahmood S, Ftesi A, Stone J, Bronze MS. Clinical use of anti-TNF therapy and increased risk of infections. *Drug Healthc Patient Saf* 2013;5:579–99.

87. Kirby AC, Raynes JG, Kaye PM. The role played by tumor necrosis factor during localized and systemic infection with Streptococcus pneumoniae. *J Infect Dis* 2005;191(9):1538–47.

88. Chan AT, Cleeve V, Daymond TJ. Necrotising fasciitis in a patient receiving infliximab for rheumatoid arthritis. *Postgrad Med J* 2002;78(915):47–8.

89. Wright SA, Taggart AJ. Pneumococcal vaccination for RA patients on TNF-alpha antagonists. *Rheumatology (Oxf)* 2004;43(4):523.

90. Elkayam O, Caspi D, Reitblatt T, Charboneau D, Rubins JB. The effect of tumor necrosis factor blockade on the response to pneumococcal vaccination in patients with rheumatoid arthritis and ankylosing spondylitis. *Semin Arthritis Rheum* 2004;33(4):283–8.

91. Centers for Disease Control and Prevention (CDC). Use of 13-valent pneumococcal conjugate vaccine and 23-valent pneumococcal polysaccharide vaccine for adults with immunocompromising conditions: recommendations of the Advisory Committee on Immunization Practices (ACIP). *MMWR Morb Mortal Wkly Rep* 2012;61(40):816–19.

92. Fiorino G, Peyrin-Biroulet L, Naccarato P, et al. Effects of immunosuppression on immune response to pneumococcal vaccine in inflammatory bowel disease: a prospective study. *Inflamm Bowel Dis* 2012;18(6):1042–7.

93. Carmona L, Gomez-Reino JJ, Rodriguez-Valverde V, et al. Effectiveness of recommendations to prevent reactivation of latent tuberculosis infection in patients treated with tumor necrosis factor antagonists. *Arthritis Rheum* 2005;52(6):1766–72.

94. Navarra SV, Tang B, Lu L, et al. Risk of tuberculosis with anti-tumor necrosis factor-alpha therapy: substantially higher number of patients at risk in Asia. *Int J Rheum Dis* 2014;17(3):291–8.

95. Hsia EC, Schluger N, Cush JJ, et al. Interferon-gamma release assay versus tuberculin skin test prior to treatment with golimumab, a human anti-tumor necrosis factor antibody, in patients with rheumatoid arthritis, psoriatic arthritis, or ankylosing spondylitis. *Arthritis Rheum* 2012;64(7):2068–77.

96. Lanternier F, Tubach F, Ravaud P, et al. Incidence and risk factors of Legionella pneumophila pneumonia during anti-tumor necrosis factor therapy: a prospective French study. *Chest* 2013;144(3):990–8.

97. Pagliano P, Attanasio V, Fusco U, Mohamed DA, Rossi M, Faella FS. Does etanercept monotherapy enhance the risk of Listeria monocytogenes meningitis? *Ann Rheum Dis* 2004;63(4):462–3.

98. Kelesidis T, Salhotra A, Fleisher J, Uslan DZ. Listeria endocarditis in a patient with psoriatic arthritis on infliximab: are biologic agents as treatment for inflammatory arthritis increasing the incidence of Listeria infections? *J Infect* 2010;60(5):386–96.

99. Dixon WG, Watson K, Lunt M, Hyrich KL, Silman AJ, Symmons DP. Rates of serious infection, including site-specific and bacterial intracellular infection, in rheumatoid arthritis patients receiving anti-tumor necrosis factor therapy: results from the British Society for Rheumatology Biologics Register. *Arthritis Rheum* 2006;54(8):2368–76.

100. Abreu C, Magro F, Vilas-Boas F, Lopes S, Macedo G, Sarmento A. Listeria infection in patients on anti-TNF treatment: report of two cases and review of the literature. *J Crohns Colitis* 2013;7(2):175–82.

101. Netea MG, Radstake T, Joosten LA, van der Meer JW, Barrera P, Kullberg BJ. Salmonella septicemia in rheumatoid arthritis patients receiving anti-tumor necrosis factor therapy: association with decreased interferon-gamma production and Toll-like receptor 4 expression. *Arthritis Rheum* 2003;48(7):1853–7.

102. Rijkeboer A, Voskuyl A, Van Agtmael M. Fatal Salmonella enteritidis septicaemia in a rheumatoid arthritis patient treated with a TNF-alpha antagonist. *Scand J Infect Dis* 2007;39(1):80–3.

103. Bassetti M, Nicco E, Delfino E, Viscoli C. Disseminated *Salmonella paratyphi* infection in a rheumatoid arthritis patient treated with infliximab. *Clin Microbiol Infect* 2010;16(1):84–5.

104. Pena-Sagredo JL, Farinas MC, Perez-Zafrilla B, et al. Non-typhi *Salmonella* infection in patients with rheumatic diseases on TNF-alpha antagonist therapy. *Clin Exp Rheumatol* 2009;27(6):920–5.

105. Keyser FD. Choice of biologic therapy for patients with rheumatoid arthritis: the infection perspective. *Curr Rheumatol Rev* 2011;7(1):77–87.

106. Tsiodras S, Samonis G, Boumpas DT, Kontoyiannis DP. Fungal infections complicating tumor necrosis factor alpha blockade therapy. *Mayo Clin Proc* 2008;83(2):181–94.

107. Cutler JE, Deepe GS, Jr., Klein BS. Advances in combating fungal diseases: vaccines on the threshold. *Nat Rev Microbiol* 2007;5(1):13–28.

108. Deepe GS, Jr., Gibbons RS. T cells require tumor necrosis factor-alpha to provide protective immunity in mice infected with Histoplasma capsulatum. *J Infect Dis* 2006;193(2):322–30.

109. Wallis RS, Broder M, Wong J, Lee A, Hoq L. Reactivation of latent granulomatous infections by infliximab. *Clin Infect Dis* 2005;41(Suppl 3):S194–8.

110. Deepe GS, Jr. Modulation of infection with *Histoplasma capsulatum* by inhibition of tumor necrosis factor-alpha activity. *Clin Infect Dis* 2005;41(Suppl 3):S204–7.

111. Wallis RS, Broder MS, Wong JY, Hanson ME, Beenhouwer DO. Granulomatous infectious diseases associated with tumor necrosis factor antagonists. *Clin Infect Dis* 2004;38(9):1261–5.

112. Saubolle MA, McKellar PP, Sussland D. Epidemiologic, clinical, and diagnostic aspects of coccidioidomycosis. *J Clin Microbiol* 2007;45(1):26–30.

113. Bergstrom L, Yocum DE, Ampel NM, et al. Increased risk of coccidioidomycosis in patients treated with tumor necrosis factor alpha antagonists. *Arthritis Rheum* 2004;50(6):1959–66.

114. Filler SG, Yeaman MR, Sheppard DC. Tumor necrosis factor inhibition and invasive fungal infections. *Clin Infect Dis* 2005;41(Suppl 3):S208–12.

115. Rocha FAC, Alves AMCV, Rocha MFG, et al. Tumor necrosis factor prevents Candida albicans biofilm formation. *Sci Rep* 2017;*7*(1):1206.

116. Wallis RS, Broder M, Wong J, Beenhouwer D. Granulomatous infections due to tumor necrosis factor blockade: correction. *Clin Infect Dis* 2004;*39*(8):1254–5.

117. Manz M, Beglinger C, Vavricka SR. Fatal invasive pulmonary aspergillosis associated with adalimumab therapy. *Gut* 2009;*58*(1):149.

118. Warris A, Bjorneklett A, Gaustad P. Invasive pulmonary aspergillosis associated with infliximab therapy. *N Engl J Med* 2001;*344*(14):1099–100.

119. Lee EJ, Song R, Park JN, et al. Chronic necrotizing pulmonary aspergillosis in a patient treated with a tumor necrosis factor-alpha inhibitor. *Int J Rheum Dis* 2010;*13*(3):e16–19.

120. Liao TL, Chen YM, Chen DY. Risk factors for cryptococcal infection among patients with rheumatoid arthritis receiving different immunosuppressive medications. *Clin Microbiol Infect* 2016;*22*(9):815.e1–3.

121. Wollner A, Mohle-Boetani J, Lambert RE, Perruquet JL, Raffin TA, McGuire JL. Pneumocystis carinii pneumonia complicating low dose methotrexate treatment for rheumatoid arthritis. *Thorax* 1991;*46*(3):205–7.

122. Kaur N, Mahl TC. *Pneumocystis jiroveci* (carinii) pneumonia after infliximab therapy: a review of 84 cases. *Dig Dis Sci* 2007;*52*(6):1481–4.

123. Lichtenstein GR, Feagan BG, Cohen RD, et al. Serious infection and mortality in patients with Crohn's disease: more than 5 years of follow-up in the TREAT registry. *Am J Gastroenterol* 2012;*107*(9):1409–22.

124. Greenberg JD, Reed G, Kremer JM, et al. Association of methotrexate and tumour necrosis factor antagonists with risk of infectious outcomes including opportunistic infections in the CORRONA registry. *Ann Rheum Dis* 2010;*69*(2):380–6.

125. Salmon-Ceron D, Tubach F, Lortholary O, et al. Drug-specific risk of non-tuberculosis opportunistic infections in patients receiving anti-TNF therapy reported to the 3-year prospective French RATIO registry. *Ann Rheum Dis* 2011;*70*(4):616–23.

126. Grubbs JA, Baddley JW. Pneumocystis jirovecii pneumonia in patients receiving tumor-necrosis-factor-inhibitor therapy: implications for chemoprophylaxis. *Curr Rheumatol Rep* 2014;*16*(10):445.

127. Takeuchi T, Taktsuki Y, Nogami Y, et al. Postmarketing surveillance of the safety profile of infliximab in 5000 Japanese patients with rheumatoid arthritis. *Ann Rheum Dis* 2008;67189–94.

128. Karadag O, Kasifoglu T, Ozer B, et al. Viral hepatitis screening guideline before biological drug use in rheumatic patients. *Eur J Rheumatol* 2016;*3*(1):25–8.

129. Ostuni P, Botsios C, Punzi L, Sfriso P, Todesco S. Hepatitis B reactivation in a chronic hepatitis B surface antigen carrier with rheumatoid arthritis treated with infliximab and low dose methotrexate. *Ann Rheum Dis* 2003;*62*(7):686–7.

130. Chung SJ, Kim JK, Park MC, Park YB, Lee SK. Reactivation of hepatitis B viral infection in inactive HBsAg carriers following anti-tumor necrosis factor-alpha therapy. *J Rheumatol* 2009;*36*(11):2416–20.

131. Michel M, Duvoux C, Hezode C, Cherqui D. Fulminant hepatitis after infliximab in a patient with hepatitis B virus treated for an adult onset still's disease. *J Rheumatol* 2003;*30*(7):1624–5.

132. Carroll MB, Bond MI. Use of tumor necrosis factor-alpha inhibitors in patients with chronic hepatitis B infection. *Semin Arthritis Rheum* 2008;*38*(3):208–17.

133. Calabrese LH, Zein N, Vassilopoulos D. Safety of antitumour necrosis factor (anti-TNF) therapy in patients with chronic viral infections: hepatitis C, hepatitis B, and HIV infection. *Ann Rheum Dis* 2004;*63*(Suppl 2):ii18–ii24.

134. Marusawa H, Hijikata M, Chiba T, Shimotohno K. Hepatitis C virus core protein inhibits Fas- and tumor necrosis factor alpha-mediated apoptosis via NF-kappaB activation. *J Virol* 1999;*73*(6):4713–20.

135. Brunasso AM, Puntoni M, Gulia A, Massone C. Safety of anti-tumour necrosis factor agents in patients with chronic hepatitis C infection: a systematic review. *Rheumatology (Oxf)* 2011;*50*(9):1700–11.

136. Pritchard C. Etanercept and hepatitis C. *J Clin Rheumatol* 1999;*5*(3):179.

137. Zein NN. Etanercept as an adjuvant to interferon and ribavirin in treatment-naive patients with chronic hepatitis C virus infection: a phase 2 randomized, double-blind, placebo-controlled study. *J Hepatol* 2005;*42*(3):315–22.

138. Singh JA, Furst DE, Bharat A, et al. 2012 update of the 2008 American College of Rheumatology recommendations for the use of disease-modifying antirheumatic drugs and biologic agents in the treatment of rheumatoid arthritis. *Arthritis Care Res (Hoboken)* 2012;*64*(5):625–39.

139. Aboulafia DM, Bundow D, Wilske K, Ochs UI. Etanercept for the treatment of human immunodeficiency virus-associated psoriatic arthritis. *Mayo Clin Proc* 2000;*75*(10):1093–8.

140. Kaur PP, Chan VC, Berney SN. Successful etanercept use in an HIV-positive patient with rheumatoid arthritis. *J Clin Rheumatol* 2007;*13*(2):79–80.

141. Cepeda EJ, Williams FM, Ishimori ML, Weisman MH, Reveille JD. The use of anti-tumour necrosis factor therapy in HIV-positive individuals with rheumatic disease. *Ann Rheum Dis* 2008;*67*(5):710–12.

142. Bradford RD, Pettit AC, Wright PW, et al. Herpes simplex encephalitis during treatment with tumor necrosis factor-alpha inhibitors. *Clin Infect Dis* 2009;*49*(6):924–7.

143. Smitten AL, Choi HK, Hochberg MC, et al. The risk of herpes zoster in patients with rheumatoid arthritis in the United States and the United Kingdom. *Arthritis Rheum* 2007;*57*(8):1431–8.

144. Mueller NH, Gilden DH, Cohrs RJ, Mahalingam R, Nagel MA. Varicella zoster virus infection: clinical features, molecular pathogenesis of disease, and latency. *Neurol Clin* 2008;*26*(3):675–97, viii.

145. McDonald JR, Zeringue AL, Caplan L, et al. Herpes zoster risk factors in a national cohort of veterans with rheumatoid arthritis. *Clin Infect Dis* 2009;*48*(10):1364–71.

146. Abreu C, Sarmento A, Magro F. Screening, prophylaxis and counselling before the start of biological therapies: a practical approach focused on IBD patients. *Dig Liver Dis* 2017;*49*(12):1289–97.

147. Krech U, Jung M. [Epidemiology, virology and virological diagnosis of cytomegaly]. *Klin Wochenschr* 1973;*51*(11): 529–32.

148. Haerter G, Manfras BJ, de Jong-Hesse Y, et al. Cytomegalovirus retinitis in a patient treated with anti-tumor necrosis factor alpha antibody therapy for rheumatoid arthritis. *Clin Infect Dis* 2004;*39*(9):e88–94.

149. Sari I, Birlik M, Gonen C, et al. Cytomegalovirus colitis in a patient with Behcet's disease receiving tumor necrosis factor alpha inhibitory treatment. *World J Gastroenterol* 2008;*14*(18):2912–14.

150. Mizuta M, Schuster MG. Cytomegalovirus hepatitis associated with use of anti-tumor necrosis factor-alpha antibody. *Clin Infect Dis* 2005;*40*(7):1071–2.

151. Pontikaki I, Gerloni V, Gattinara M, et al. [Side effects of anti-TNFalpha therapy in juvenile idiopathic arthritis]. *Reumatismo* 2006;*58*(1):31–8.

152. Krause ML, Matteson EL. Perioperative management of the patient with rheumatoid arthritis. *World J Orthop* 2014;*5*(3):283–91.

153. den Broeder AA, Creemers MC, Fransen J, et al. Risk factors for surgical site infections and other complications in elective surgery in patients with rheumatoid arthritis with special attention for anti-tumor necrosis factor: a large retrospective study. *J Rheumatol* 2007;*34*(4):689–95.

154. Ding T, Ledingham J, Luqmani R, et al. BSR and BHPR rheumatoid arthritis guidelines on safety of anti-TNF therapies. *Rheumatology* 2010;*49*(11):2217–19.

155. Goodman SM, Springer B, Guyatt G, et al. 2017 American College of Rheumatology/American Association of Hip and Knee Surgeons guideline for the perioperative management of antirheumatic medication in patients with rheumatic diseases undergoing elective total hip or total knee arthroplasty. *Arthritis Care Res (Hoboken)* 2017;*69*(8):1111–24.

156. Kemanetzoglou E, Andreadou E. CNS Demyelination with TNF-alpha Blockers. *Curr Neurol Neurosci Rep* 2017;*17*(4):36.

157. Mohan N, Edwards ET, Cupps TR, et al. Demyelination occurring during anti-tumor necrosis factor alpha therapy for inflammatory arthritides. *Arthritis Rheum* 2001;*44*(12):2862–9.

158. [No authors]. TNF neutralization in MS: results of a randomized, placebo-controlled multicenter study. The Lenercept Multiple Sclerosis Study Group and The University of British Columbia MS/MRI Analysis Group. *Neurology* 1999;*53*(3):457–65.

159. Bozkurt B. Activation of cytokines as a mechanism of disease progression in heart failure. *Ann Rheum Dis* 2000;*59*(Suppl 1):90–3.

160. Chung ES, Packer M, Lo KH, Fasanmade AA, Willerson JT. Randomized, double-blind, placebo-controlled, pilot trial of infliximab, a chimeric monoclonal antibody to tumor necrosis factor-alpha, in patients with moderate-to-severe heart failure: results of the anti-TNF therapy against congestive heart failure (ATTACH) trial. *Circulation* 2003;*107*(25):3133–40.

161. Behnam SM, Behnam SE, Koo JY. TNF-alpha inhibitors and congestive heart failure. *Skinmed* 2005;*4*(6):363–8.

162. Dhawan SS, Quyyumi AA. Rheumatoid arthritis and cardiovascular disease. *Curr Atheroscler Rep* 2008;*10*(2):128–33.

163. Mohan A, Sada S, Kumar BS, et al. Subclinical atherosclerosis in patients with rheumatoid arthritis by utilizing carotid intima-media thickness as a surrogate marker. *Indian J Med Res* 2014;*140*(3):379–86.

164. Held C, White HD, Stewart RAH, et al. Inflammatory biomarkers interleukin-6 and C-reactive protein and outcomes in stable coronary heart disease: experiences from the STABILITY (Stabilization of Atherosclerotic Plaque by Initiation of Darapladib Therapy) trial. *J Am Heart Assoc* 2017;*6*(10):pii: e005077.

165. Irace C, Mancuso G, Fiaschi E, Madia A, Sesti G, Gnasso A. Effect of anti TNFalpha therapy on arterial diameter and wall shear stress and HDL cholesterol. *Atherosclerosis* 2004;*177*(1):113–18.

166. Popa C, Netea MG, Radstake T, et al. Influence of anti-tumour necrosis factor therapy on cardiovascular risk factors in patients with active rheumatoid arthritis. *Ann Rheum Dis* 2005;*64*(2):303–5.

167. Jacobsson LT, Turesson C, Gulfe A, et al. Treatment with tumor necrosis factor blockers is associated with a lower incidence of first cardiovascular events in patients with rheumatoid arthritis. *J Rheumatol* 2005;*32*(7):1213–18.

168. Ramos-Casals M, Roberto Perez A, Diaz-Lagares C, Cuadrado MJ, Khamashta MA. Autoimmune diseases induced by biological agents: a double-edged sword? *Autoimmun Rev* 2010;*9*(3):188–93.

169. Asarch A, Gottlieb AB, Lee J, et al. Lichen planus-like eruptions: an emerging side effect of tumor necrosis factor-alpha antagonists. *J Am Acad Dermatol* 2009;*61*(1):104–11.

170. Geborek P, Bladstrom A, Turesson C, et al. Tumour necrosis factor blockers do nost increase overall tumour risk in patients with rheumatoid arthritis, but may be associated with an increased risk of lymphomas. *Ann Rheum Dis* 2005;*64*(5):699–703.

171. Mercer LK, Lunt M, Low AL, et al. Risk of solid cancer in patients exposed to anti-tumour necrosis factor therapy: results from the British Society for Rheumatology Biologics Register for Rheumatoid Arthritis. *Ann Rheum Dis* 2015;*74*(6):1087–93.

172. Askling J, Fored CM, Geborek P, et al. Swedish registers to examine drug safety and clinical issues in RA. *Ann Rheum Dis* 2006;*65*(6):707–12.

173. Mariette X, Matucci-Cerinic M, Pavelka K, et al. Malignancies associated with tumour necrosis factor inhibitors in registries and prospective observational studies: a systematic review and meta-analysis. *Ann Rheum Dis* 2011;*70*(11):1895–904.

174. Bongartz T, Sutton AJ, Sweeting MJ, Buchan I, Matteson EL, Montori V. Anti-TNF antibody therapy in rheumatoid arthritis and the risk of serious infections and malignancies: systematic review and meta-analysis of rare harmful effects in randomized controlled trials. *JAMA* 2006;*295*(19):2275–85.

175. Setoguchi S, Solomon DH, Weinblatt ME, et al. Tumor necrosis factor alpha antagonist use and cancer in patients with rheumatoid arthritis. *Arthritis Rheum* 2006;*54*(9):2757–64.

176. Askling J, Baecklund E, Granath F, et al. Anti-tumour necrosis factor therapy in rheumatoid arthritis and risk of malignant lymphomas: relative risks and time trends in the Swedish Biologics Register. *Ann Rheum Dis* 2009;*68*(5):648–53.

177. Wolfe F, Michaud K. Biologic treatment of rheumatoid arthritis and the risk of malignancy: analyses from a large US observational study. *Arthritis Rheum* 2007;*56*(9):2886–95.

178. Chakravarty EF, Michaud K, Wolfe F. Skin cancer, rheumatoid arthritis, and tumor necrosis factor inhibitors. *J Rheumatol* 2005;*32*(11):2130–5.

179. Olsen CM, Hyrich KL, Knight LL, Green AC. Melanoma risk in patients with rheumatoid arthritis treated with tumour necrosis factor alpha inhibitors: a systematic review and meta-analysis. *Melanoma Res* 2016;*26*(5):517–23.

180. Mercer LK, Green AC, Galloway JB, et al. The influence of anti-TNF therapy upon incidence of keratinocyte skin cancer in patients with rheumatoid arthritis: longitudinal results from the British Society for Rheumatology Biologics Register. *Ann Rheum Dis* 2012;*71*(6):869–74.

181. van Schouwenburg PA, Rispens T, Wolbink GJ. Immunogenicity of anti-TNF biologic therapies for rheumatoid arthritis. *Nat Rev Rheumat* 2013;*9*(3):164–72.

182. Strand V, Balsa A, Al-Saleh J, et al. Immunogenicity of biologics in chronic inflammatory diseases: a systematic review. *BioDrugs* 2017;*31*(4):299–316.

183. Wu C, Wang S, Xian P, Yang L, Chen Y, Mo X. Effect of anti-TNF antibodies on clinical response in rheumatoid arthritis patients: a meta-analysis. *Biomed Res Int* 2016;*2016*:7185708.

184. Garces S, Demengeot J, Benito-Garcia E. The immunogenicity of anti-TNF therapy in immune-mediated inflammatory diseases: a systematic review of the literature with a meta-analysis. *Ann Rheum Dis* 2013;*72*(12):1947–55.

185. Toussirot E, Aubin F. Paradoxical reactions under TNF-alpha blocking agents and other biological agents given for chronic immune-mediated diseases: an analytical and comprehensive overview. *RMD Open* 2016;*2*(2):e000239.

186. Harrison MJ, Dixon WG, Watson KD, et al. Rates of new-onset psoriasis in patients with rheumatoid arthritis receiving anti-tumour necrosis factor alpha therapy: results from the British Society for Rheumatology Biologics Register. *Ann Rheum Dis* 2009;*68*(2):209–15.

187. Faivre C, Villani AP, Aubin F, et al. Hidradenitis suppurativa (HS): an unrecognized paradoxical effect of biologic agents (BA) used in chronic inflammatory diseases. *J Am Acad Dermatol* 2016;*74*(6):1153–9.

188. Toussirot E, Houvenagel E, Goeb V, et al. Development of inflammatory bowel disease during anti-TNF-alpha therapy for inflammatory rheumatic disease: a nationwide series. *Joint Bone Spine* 2012;*79*(5):457–63.

189. Saint Marcoux B, De Bandt M. Vasculitides induced by TNFalpha antagonists: a study in 39 patients in France. *Joint Bone Spine* 2006;*73*(6):710–13.

190. Jani M, Dixon WG, Kersley-Fleet L, et al. Drug-specific risk and characteristics of lupus and vasculitis-like events in patients with rheumatoid arthritis treated with TNFi: results from BSRBR-RA. *RMD Open* 2017;*3*(1):e000314.

191. Sokumbi O, Wetter DA, Makol A, Warrington KJ. Vasculitis associated with tumor necrosis factor-alpha inhibitors. *Mayo Clin Proc* 2012;*87*(8):739–45.

192. Takase K, Horton SC, Ganesha A, et al. What is the utility of routine ANA testing in predicting development of biological DMARD-induced lupus and vasculitis in patients with rheumatoid arthritis? Data from a single-centre cohort. *Ann Rheum Dis* 2014;*73*(9):1695–9.

193. Pink AE, Fonia A, Allen MH, Smith CH, Barker JN. Antinuclear antibodies associate with loss of response to antitumour necrosis factor-alpha therapy in psoriasis: a retrospective, observational study. *Br J Dermatol* 2010;*162*(4):780–5.

194. Hoffmann JH, Hartmann M, Enk AH, Hadaschik EN. Autoantibodies in psoriasis as predictors for loss of response and anti-infliximab antibody induction. *Br J Dermatol* 2011;*165*(6):1355–8.

32

Interleukin-6 inhibitors

Neelam Hassan and Ernest Choy

Biology of interleukin-6

Interleukin-6 (IL-6) is a 26 kilodalton glycopeptide composed of a four helices joined by disulphide bonds.[1,2] It is a pleiotropic cytokine produced mainly by mononuclear cells, fibroblasts, and endothelial cells.[1] Prior to the identification of the *IL-6* gene on chromosome 7, it has been known as hepatocyte stimulating factor, cytotoxic T-cell differentiation factor, B-cell differentiation factor, B-cell stimulatory factor 2, hybridoma/plasmacytoma growth factor, hepatocyte stimulating factor, monocyte granulocyte inducer type 2, and thrombopoietin based on its diverse biologic effects both on the immune system and homeostasis.[3]

IL-6 signal transduction: Cis- and trans-signalling

IL-6 and the IL-6 family of cytokines, such as interleukin-11 and oncostatin-M, share a unique pathway for cell signalling via the ubiquitously expressed cell surface molecule gp130.[4] Most cytokines, such as tumour necrosis factor alpha (TNFα), cause cellular activation when they bind to membrane-bound cytokine receptors. Membrane IL-6 receptor (IL-6R) is a type-I transmembrane protein. It consists of an immunoglobulin-like domain (D1), the cytokine binding module domains (D2 and D3), and a flexible stalk region followed by the transmembrane and intracellular domains.[2] IL-6R binds to IL-6 through conserved epitopes (known as site I) on the cytokine binding domains. The stalk region of the IL-6R does not take part in signal transduction. Instead, IL-6/IL-6R complex binds to a 130 kilodalton protein, gp130, on cell surface via conserved epitopes (site II and site III) on IL-6. The membrane proximal domains of gp130 are involved in the activation of cytoplasmic Janus-activated tyrosine kinases (JAK1, JAK2, and Tyk2).[5] Dimerization of IL6/IL6R/gp130 complexes lead to phosphorylation of JAKs which drives the subsequent activation of the latent transcription factors signal transducer and activator of transcription-1 and STAT3, and downstream signalling through the ras/mitogen-activated protein kinase cascade and gene transcription.

Cell surface cytokine receptors are often cleaved enzymatically to produce soluble cytokine receptors. In the case of sTNFR, it is a natural antagonist to TNFα as it competes with membrane tumour necrosis factor receptor (TNFR) for TNFα, and downregulates inflammation in RA. In contrast, soluble IL-6R (sIL-6R) is pro-inflammatory rather than anti-inflammatory.[6] Membrane IL-6R

are cleaved by enzymes ADAM-17 and ADAM-10 to form sIL-6R. Circulating IL-6 and sIL-6R form the IL6/IL-6R complex, which binds to cell surface gp130 to trigger cell signalling. This is known as 'trans-signalling' while cell activation via membrane IL-6R is known as 'cis' or 'classical' signalling (**Figure 32.1**). Consequently, through IL-6 trans-signalling, any cell that expresses gp130 can be activated by IL-6 in the presence of sIL-6R. Both membrane-bound and soluble IL-6R are pro-inflammatory. Indeed, sIL-6R protects IL-6 from enzymatic degradation and prolongs the circulating life of IL-6.

A soluble form of gp130 (sgp130) is present in the circulation of healthy individuals.[4] Sgp130 only binds to IL-6 when it is bound to sIL-6R so serves as a natural inhibitor of IL-6 trans-signalling.

Effect of IL-6 on the immune response

IL-6 has a range of effects on both the adaptive and innate immune responses (**Figure 32.2**).

T cells

In autoimmune diseases, Th17 cells have a key role in driving disease development. These CD4+ T cells are so called because they produce IL-17.[7] In collagen-induced arthritis, an animal model of RA, the absence of Th17 cells was associated with resistance to the development of inflammatory arthritis with reduction in bone and joint damage despite activation of Th1 cells and release of Th1-associated cytokines.[8] The development of Th17 cells in these animal models is influenced by the cytokine milieu. In the presence of IL-6 and transforming growth factor β (TGF-β), naïve T cells when stimulated develop into Th17 cells.[9,10] Conversely the production of CD4+CD25+Foxp3+ regulatory T cells that suppress immune responses is reduced.[11] In the absence of IL-6, TGF-β induced the production of CD4+CD25+Foxp3+ regulatory T cells. Hence, IL-6 may have a pivotal role in the development of autoimmune diseases by driving Th17 response.

B cells

The importance of IL-6 in the humoral response was firmly established as IL-6 was identified as a T-cell–derived factor that induced the maturation of B cells into plasma cells. Hence, it was known as B-cell differentiation factor, B-cell stimulatory factor 2,

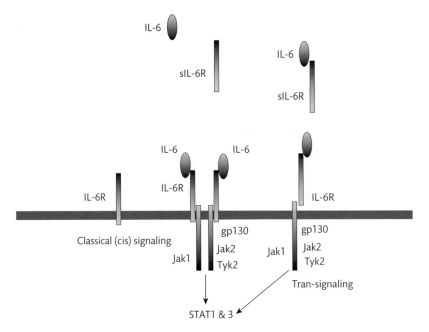

Figure 32.1 IL-6 signalling.

hybridoma/plasmacytoma growth factor prior to the identification of the *IL-6* gene.[12] Indeed, IL-6 deficient mice have diminished antibody response to infection and inflammation.[13] Recently, IL-6 has been shown to induce regulatory B cells, which suppresses B-cell function.[14]

Innate immunity

IL-6 is a key messenger between mesenchymal cells and the innate immune system. During acute inflammation, monocytes, macrophages, and endothelial cells release IL-6, which increases neutrophil adherence to endothelial cells and their transmigration into tissue through release and activation of chemokines and adhesion molecules.[15] IL-6 trans-signalling induces release of chemokine ligand 8 (CXCL8), which leads to increased neutrophil chemotaxis, survival, and activation.[16] Activated neutrophils shed sIL-6R.

Through trans-signalling, stromal cells, which do not express IL-6R, produce monocyte-specific chemoattractants and IL-6. IL-6 released by stromal cells upregulates the expression of M-CSF receptors on monocytes.[17] This allows autocrine feedback of M-CSF to switch monocyte differentiation to macrophages and sustains inflammation.

Recently, activated neutrophils had been shown to release neutrophil extracellular traps (NETs) through autocrine IL-6 signalling.[18] NETs are released during a process known as NETosis, a distinct form of cell death in which the granular and cytosolic contents of the cell are emitted into the extracellular space, together with decondensed chromatin and other nuclear material as NETs.[19] Originally, NETs were considered a strategy employed by neutrophils to immobilize and kill invading pathogens.[20] Recently, NETosis has been associated with autoimmunity as hypercitrullinated proteins have been

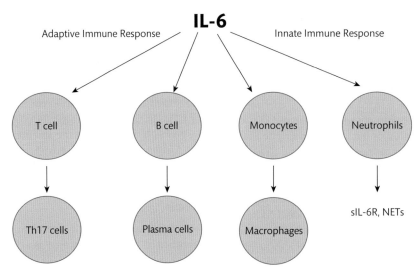

Figure 32.2 Effect of IL-6 on immune responses.

found in NETs.[21] In RA, the percentage of neutrophils undergoing active NETosis correlated positively with anticitrullinated peptide antibody titre.[21]

Role of IL-6 in homeostasis and metabolism

IL-6 has important physiological functions and displays hormone-like properties. These include vascular function, lipid metabolism, insulin resistance, mitochondrial activities, the neuroendocrine system, and maintenance of barrier immunity.[5,18,22,23] IL-6 deficient mice developed obesity, liver inflammation, and insulin resistance but are protected from oestrogen related bone loss and autoimmune diseases.[22,24] Transgenic mice overexpressing IL-6 and sIL-6R, were significantly smaller in size than wild-type mice and did not develop visible fat pads.[25] Classical signalling is important in hepatic control of insulin sensitivity and glucose tolerance,[23] while myocytes from skeletal muscles produce IL-6 during exercise.[26] Furthermore, IL-6 increases fatty acid oxidation, insulin-stimulated glucose uptake, and enhanced expression of the GLUT4 glucose transporter on the plasma membrane of skeletal muscles.

IL-6 stimulates osteoclastogenesis and regulates the expression of RANK ligand (RANKL).[27] It has a major role in bone homeostasis. In a murine model of postmenopausal osteoporosis, IL-6 deficient female mice were protected from osteopenia following ovariectomy.[24] Furthermore, IL-6 levels and IL-6 gene polymorphisms have been associated with bone mineral density alterations in inflammatory diseases.

The role of IL-6 in RA: Articular inflammation and destruction

In RA, both sIL-6R and IL-6 are found in abundance in the synovial joint and sera. Levels of IL-6 and s-IL-6R correlate with disease activity[28] and joint damage.[29] The initial acute inflammatory reaction in the synovial fluid of patients with RA involves an increase in IgM and IgG rheumatoid factors and antibodies to citrullinated peptides in the serum and joints. IL-6 can induce increases in rheumatoid factor by a mechanism thought to involve B-cell differentiation and formation resulting in the production of autoantibodies such as

rheumatoid factor.[30] The articular and systemic effects of IL-6 are summarized in **Figure 32.3**.

Leukocyte trafficking

In the inflamed synovial joint, a large number of activated neutrophils are present. When an irritant was injected into an air pouch underneath the skin of a mouse, leukocytes migrated from the blood and infiltrated the pouch. In IL-6 deficient mice, leukocyte infiltration reduced by 50% primarily due to a reduction in monocyte chemoattractant protein (MCP-1), which recruit monocytes to the site of injury.[15] In *ex-vivo* endothelial cell cultures, IL-6 and sIL-6R in combination induced 6- to 7-fold increase in MCP-1. This was not seen with IL-6 alone highlighting the importance of IL-6 trans-signalling on leukocyte trafficking during acute inflammation. An *ex-vivo* study measured neutrophil adhesion to human umbilical vein endothelial cells co-cultured with synovial fibroblasts or skin from patients with RA on opposite sides of transwells.[31] Neutrophil adherence was enhanced by synovial, but not skin, fibroblasts. IL-6 was present in supernatants and antibody to IL-6, but not TNF or IL-1, abolished neutrophil adhesion to endothelial cells.[31]

Pannus formation

Synovial proliferation and formation of the invasive pannus is a central feature of aggressive and destructive RA. Pannus has been compared to a local tumour in term of its cellular activity, proliferation, and destruction. It is highly vascularized, which is driven by the angiogenic cytokine, vascular endothelial growth factor (VEGF). An *ex-vivo* study found that both TNFα and IL-1 stimulated the release of VEGF by synovial cells. IL-6/sIL-6R complex acts synergistic with TNF and IL-1 resulting in greatly augmented production of VEGF.[32] Inhibiting IL-6 using an anti-IL6R monoclonal antibody significantly reduced the production of VEGF.

Joint damage

Osteoclasts are responsible for bone resorption and erosion in RA.[33] They are derived from mononuclear pluripotential haematopoietic stem cells in the bone marrow. Differentiation of osteoclast precursor cells into osteoclasts and activation are driven by cytokines and growth factors as well as cell surface molecules. One of the key pathways is through the receptor activator of NF-κB (RANK) on the cell surface of the premature osteoclasts. When RANK is engaged

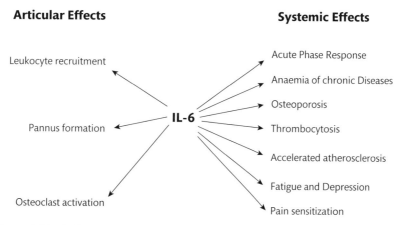

Figure 32.3 Effect of IL-6 in rheumatoid arthritis.

by its cognate ligand RANKL, osteoclast precursors become activated and differentiate into mature osteoclasts.[34] Synovial fluid from patients with RA promotes osteoclastogenesis. Levels of IL-6 and sIL-6R correlated with osteoclast activation which was inhibited by anti-IL-6 monoclonal antibody.[29]

Furthermore, in bovine cartilage, IL-6 and sIL-6R stimulated cartilage catabolism through release of aggrecanases.[35]

The role of IL-6 in RA: Systemic manifestations

In active RA, IL-6 is produced in the synovia, mainly by synovial fibroblasts.[36] Measuring IL-6 in paired samples from patients found higher level in the synovial fluid than the peripheral blood suggesting IL-6 was released into the circulation from the inflamed synovial joint. This accounts for many systemic features of RA (**Figure 32.3**).

Acute phase response

IL-6 is the principal stimulator of the liver to produce acute phase proteins which are used in clinical practice as a measure of systemic inflammation.[37] These include C-reactive protein (CRP), serum amyloid A, haptoglobin, and fibrinogen.[38] Fibrinogen level is the major constituent of the erythrocyte sedimentation rate (ESR).

Anaemia of chronic disease

Anaemia of chronic disease is a feature of severe active RA.[39] Haematological features of anaemia of chronic disease resemble iron deficiency anaemia with a hypochromic, microcytic picture. However, iron replacement therapy is ineffective, ferritin is high, and total iron-binding capacity is low or normal. In healthy animals, infusion of recombinant IL-6 caused decrease in haemoglobin level.[40] In patients with RA who were anaemic, IL-6 levels are significantly elevated in patients when compared with non-anaemic RA patients.[41] The effect of IL-6 on haemoglobin is mediated through the release of hepcidin by hepatocytes as part of the acute phase response. Hepcidin reduces intestinal iron transport and promotes sequestration of iron by macrophages,[42] thereby depriving the bone marrow of iron to manufacture haemoglobin.

Osteoporosis

Systemic osteoporosis, a feature of RA occurs early in the disease.[43] Osteoclast activation by IL-6 is thought to be a key driver as mice deficient of IL-6 are protected from bone loss caused.[24] In contrast, IL-6 transgenic mice showed accelerated bone resorption, reduced bone formation and defective ossification suggesting that IL-6 overexpression lead to osteoporosis due to osteoclast and osteoblast dysregulation.[44]

Thrombocytosis

Patients with active RA often have high platelet count. In mice treated with IL-6, thrombopoietin level is increased.[45] Elevated thrombopoietin level was associated with increased numbers of platelets. Thrombocytosis induced by IL-6 could be abrogated by neutralization of thrombopoietin.

Fatigue and depression

Depression is two to four times more common in patients with RA than in the normal population.[46] Several lines of evidence suggest systemic inflammation may contribute to the high prevalence of depression in RA.[47] Fatigue is a common symptom among patients with RA, which impacts health-related quality of life and physical functioning.[48] The hypothalamic–pituitary–adrenal (HPA) axis has been implicated in the development of fatigue and depression.[49,50] HPA axis dysregulation has been reported in patients with RA and associated with various cytokines, including IL-6.[51]

Nociception

IL-6 signalling has also been implicated in the development of pathological pain. IL-6 deficient mice failed to develop thermal hyperalgesia[52] while transgenic mice overexpressing sgp130Fc in the blood, but not in the central nervous system, showed an increased thermal pain threshold compared to wild-type mice, suggesting that IL-6 trans-signalling impacts on pathological pain.[53]

Cardiovascular disease

Mortality is increased in patients with RA mainly due to higher incidence of cardiovascular events.[54] This increase in cardiovascular risk could not be explained by traditional cardiovascular risk factors. Systemic inflammation as measured by ESR and CRP is a major risk factor. IL-6 released from synovial tissue alters the function of distant tissues, including adipose tissue, skeletal muscle, liver, and the vascular endothelium, and may contribute to the development of accelerated atherosclerosis. IL-6 plasma concentrations are elevated in patients with RA, and the potentially detrimental cardiovascular consequences of these elevations are suggested by research in normal healthy individuals. Circulating IL-6 and CRP levels are predictive of future cardiovascular events in normal healthy individuals.[55,56] In addition, elevated IL-6 level at the time of admission in patients with acute coronary syndromes predicted worse outcomes.[57]

Inhibitors of interleukin-6 in RA

Inhibition of IL-6 signalling can be achieved by monoclonal antibodies targeting IL-6 or IL-6R as they will inhibit both classical and non-classical signalling[58] (**Figure 32.4**). Both tocilizumab and sarilumab are anti-IL-6R monoclonal antibodies which have been licensed for the treatment of RA. Several anti-IL-6 monoclonal antibodies have also been assessed in phase II and III randomized control trials.

a) Anti-IL-6R monoclonal antibodies (tocilizumab, sarilumab, vobarilizumab)

b) Anti-IL-6 monoclonal antibodies (sirukumab, olokizumab, clazakizumab)

Tocilizumab

Tocilizumab (TCZ) was the first humanized anti-IL-6R monoclonal antibody to be developed. It contains a human IgG1 Fc region, which binds to both soluble and membrane-bound IL-6R with high affinity. It prevents the formation of IL-6/IL-6R complex, thereby inhibiting IL-6 signalling. It can be given either subcutaneously or intravenously.

TCZ has been shown to result in significant reduction in disease activity and radiographic joint damage in RA when compared

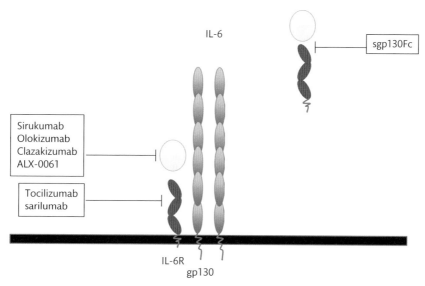

Figure 32.4 Inhibiting IL-6.

to placebo[59,60] and conventional disease-modifying antirheumatic drugs (DMARDs).[61] TCZ also resulted in normalization of CRP levels and reduction in concentration of rheumatoid factor, highlighting the importance of IL-6 in the acute phase and humoral responses.

A large double-blind, double-dummy, parallel-group study in 2010 demonstrated the superiority of TCZ monotherapy over methotrexate (MTX) monotherapy over a 24-week period in patients who had not previously been treated with MTX or biologic agents.[62] A 5-year extension study following up the TCZ monotherapy group was performed, in which almost half of those who transitioned to the extension study required the addition of a DMARD.[63] However of those who continued on TCZ monotherapy, the proportion achieving remission increased at 264 weeks (65.2%) compared to at 24 weeks (40.1%), suggesting TCZ has sustained efficacy over time for some patients.

Other studies evaluated the effect of the addition of TCZ versus placebo in patients who were already on methotrexate[64] and other conventional DMARDs[65] but had failed to respond (DMARD-IR). Rapid improvements were seen in disease activity, but also in physical function, fatigue, and health-related quality of life.

TCZ in combination with MTX (TCZ + MTX) and TCZ monotherapy in MTX-naïve patients with early RA has also been shown to result in significantly greater improvement in radiographic disease progression and physical function than methotrexate alone.[66] This clinical benefit was maintained at 2 years in a follow up study.[67] No statistically significant difference was found in efficacy between the TCZ + MTX and TCZ monotherapy groups.

A more recent 2-year study has demonstrated that TCZ, with or without MTX, was more effective in obtaining sustained remission than MTX in newly diagnosed RA.[68]

A phase III trial of TCZ in combination with MTX in patients who had previously had an inadequate response to at least one TNF inhibitor (TNF-IR) showed that TCZ + MTX was more effective in achieving rapid and sustained improvements in disease activity and patient-reported outcomes compared to placebo with MTX.[69,70] More than 30% of patients in this study had in fact previously failed

treatment with at least two TNFi. This suggests that TCZ is an effective treatment even for those patients who have been previously labelled as having refractory disease.

Only two trials have been performed to date comparing the efficacy of TCZ directly with other biologic agents. A phase 4 superiority study demonstrated that TCZ monotherapy was superior to adalimumab monotherapy (TNFi monoclonal antibody) in reducing the DAS-28-ESR in patients who were intolerant or unable to have methotrexate treatment.[71] A recent global multicentre prospective observational study investigated the effectiveness of TCZ as a first line biologic agent compared to TNFi (etanercept, adalimumab, infliximab, certolizumab or golimumab) in patients who had failed to respond to conventional DMARDs (DMARD-IR).[72] Patients treated with TCZ had a significantly greater improvement in DAS28-ESR and health-related quality of life compared to those on TNFi therapy. Patients on TCZ were also less likely to discontinue the drug compared to those receiving TNFi.

As a consequence of the favourable results from clinical trials, TCZ has been licensed for the treatment of RA, and more recently systemic and polyarticular juvenile idiopathic arthritis. In the United States, TCZ has also been approved for use in giant cell arteritis and as treatment for chimeric antigen receptor (CAR)T cell therapy-induced cytokine release syndrome. The success of tocilizumab has spurred the development of newer biologic agents targeting the IL-6 pathway in RA.

Sarilumab

Sarilumab is a fully human IgG1 monoclonal antibody directed against the IL-6 receptor. Like TCZ, sarilumab binds to both soluble and membrane-bound forms of the receptor with high affinity, thereby inhibiting both cis- and trans- IL-6 mediated signalling. It is administered subcutaneously every fortnight.

Sarilumab in combination with MTX has been demonstrated to improve disease activity, physical function, and radiographic progression at 52 weeks compared to placebo with MTX in MTX-IR RA patients.[73,74] Similar results have also been found when sarilumab is used in combination with other conventional DMARDs in TNF-IR patients.[75]

A recent trial comparing sarilumab with the TNFi, adalimumab, demonstrated that sarilumab monotherapy was superior to adalimumab monotherapy in reducing disease activity and disability in MTX-IR RA patients.[76]

Sarilumab has recently received approval for the treatment of moderate-severe RA in Europe, United States, and Canada.

Vobarilizumab

Vobarilizumab (ALX-0061) is a 26 kilodalton nanobody consisting of an anti-IL6R domain bound to an antihuman serum albumin domain. It has been shown *in vitro* to have a much higher affinity for the soluble IL-6R as opposed to the membrane-bound form.[77] It is thought that preferentially blocking trans-signalling may reduce some of the unwanted consequences of non-specific IL6 blockade and thereby provide an improved safety profile compared to other IL-6R inhibitors.

Vobarilizumab is currently being investigated as a treatment for RA and systemic lupus erythematosus. Preliminary results have recently been presented from two studies in patients with RA. A 12-week phase IIb dose-ranging study for subcutaneous vobarilizumab was conducted in MTX-IR patients with moderate-to-severe RA.[78] Patients were randomized to blinded dose regimens of vobarilizumab monotherapy or open-label TCZ. Vobarilizumab resulted in a reduction in signs and symptoms of RA and improvement in physical function with a similar safety profile to TCZ. A 24-week double-blind phase IIb study of vobarilizumab in combination with MTX also demonstrated an improvement in disease activity compared to placebo in patients with moderate-severe RA.[79] A 2-year open-label extension study in RA patients is currently ongoing.

Sirukumab

Sirukumab is a human monoclonal antibody that selectively binds to the IL-6 cytokine with high affinity, thereby inhibiting both cis- and trans-signalling.

A large phase III multicentre randomized controlled trial in DMARD-IR RA patients demonstrated that sirukumab was superior to placebo in improving disease activity, physical function, and health-related quality of life, as well as inhibiting radiographic disease progression.[80] Improvements occurred as early as 2 weeks and were maintained through to 52 weeks.

Another large multicentre trial examined the effect of sirukumab in more difficult to treat TNF-IR RA patients.[81] Patients were randomly assigned to placebo every 2 weeks, 50 mg sirukumab every 4 weeks, or 100 mg sirukumab every 2 weeks, all given for 52 weeks or less. At week 18, placebo-treated patients meeting early escape criteria (<20% improvement in swollen and tender joint counts) were randomly reassigned to either 50 mg or 100 mg of sirukumab. All remaining placebo-treated patients were subsequently randomly reassigned at week 24 to either sirukumab dose (cross-over). The study demonstrated significant improvement in the signs and symptoms of RA in patients treated with sirukumab compared to placebo. However, five deaths were reported in this study, all of which occurred after week 24 and only in patients treated with sirukumab. These included a cerebrovascular accident (cross-over from placebo to 50 mg sirukumab every 4 weeks), myocardial infarction (early escape from placebo to 100 mg sirukumab every 2 weeks), metastatic breast cancer (randomly assigned to 50 mg sirukumab every 4 weeks), sudden death (randomly assigned to 100 mg sirukumab every 2 weeks), and pneumonia (randomly assigned to 100 mg sirukumab every 2 weeks).

Sirukumab was subsequently refused approval for the treatment of moderate-severe RA by the Food and Drug Administration (FDA) in 2017 due to safety concerns, namely because of an imbalance of deaths between the placebo and active treatment arms through 52 weeks of exposure in pooled placebo-controlled studies.[82] Of a total of 35 deaths in these studies, 34 deaths occurred in sirukumab-treated patients. The major causes of death were cardiovascular events, serious infections, and malignancies.

It is possible that beyond week 18, comparisons of mortality rates were confounded because of transitions from the placebo group to sirukumab treatment due to escape and cross-over, depleting the placebo group of subjects. The adverse events and causes of death noted were also similar in nature to those seen with tocilizumab and sarilumab. However, the increase in overall mortality was seen only with sirukumab. Following the decision by the FDA, the manufacturers of sirukumab have withdrawn applications for global approval for use in RA and further development has been discontinued.

Olokizumab and clazakizumab

Olokizumab and clazakizumab are both humanized monoclonal antibodies which bind to the IL-6 cytokine.

A phase IIb dose-ranging study investigated the efficacy and safety of subcutaneous olokizumab in patients with moderate-severe active RA who had previously failed anti-TNF therapy.[83] Patients were all given background methotrexate and randomized to treatment arms receiving placebo, varying doses/dosage intervals of olokizumab or tocilizumab (TCZ). Olokizumab resulted in significantly greater reductions in disease activity at week 12 compared to placebo at all tested doses and demonstrated a similar efficacy and safety profile to TCZ. A further dose-ranging phase II study evaluating the efficacy of olokizumab compared to placebo in Asian TNF-IR patients showed similar improvements in disease activity.[84]

A phase IIa dose-ranging study demonstrated that intravenous clazakizumab (BMS945429) resulted in significant improvements in disease activity and health-related quality of life at 12 weeks compared to both placebo and MTX in MTX-IR RA patients.[85] A phase IIb dose-ranging study was subsequently performed investigating the efficacy and safety of varying doses/dosage intervals of subcutaneous clazakizumab, with or without MTX, in MTX-IR patients.[86] Patients were randomized to treatment arms receiving placebo with MTX, clazakizumab monotherapy, clazakizumab with MTX, or adalimumab with MTX (which was used as an active comparator). The study was not powered to allow comparisons between clazakizumab doses or between clazakizumab and adalimumab. All doses of clazakizumab resulted in significantly greater reductions in disease activity at 12 and 24 weeks compared to MTX alone, and combination therapy of clazakizumab with MTX generally resulted in higher response rates than clazakizumab monotherapy although only two doses of clazakizumab monotherapy were studied.

However, as of 2017, clazakizumab is no longer under development for RA or any other rheumatologic condition. It is currently being investigated as a therapy to prevent antibody mediated rejection of solid organ transplants.

Adverse effects of IL-6 inhibition

IL-6 inhibitors have been shown to be generally well tolerated although some specific adverse events have been noted in the trials mentioned in section 6. The safety profiles of the IL-6R inhibitors and IL-6 inhibitors appear to be similar suggesting these adverse events are the result of a class effect of IL-6 inhibition.

The most common adverse events seen with IL-6 inhibition are injection site reactions, infections, neutropenia, increases in alanine aminotransferase (ALT) levels and increases in cholesterol levels. More serious adverse events including opportunistic infections and gastrointestinal perforations were rare across all trials. However, it is noted that many of these trials were performed in a selective group of patients, often excluding those with previous history of tuberculosis (TB), concomitant haematological conditions, or diverticular disease, who may be more at risk of these serious adverse events.

Infection will always be a risk with any immunosuppressive treatment and the risk with IL-6R inhibition has been shown to be comparable to TNFi therapy.[71,72] Neutropenia, when it occurred, was often transient and did not lead to serious complications in the majority of cases.[87]

Increases in ALT levels were generally moderate (<3 × upper limit of normal of ALT), dose dependent, and often associated with concomitant DMARD use. No cases of serious liver injury have been reported in trials thus far.

RA is known to be an independent risk factor for cardiovascular disease. However total cholesterol, high density lipoprotein-cholesterol (HDL-C) and low-density lipoprotein-cholesterol (LDL-C) concentrations have been shown to be reduced in active RA and appear to be inversely related to levels of inflammation.[88] The level of these lipids has then been shown to subsequently increase following suppression of inflammation with TNFi treatment and Janus kinase (JAK) inhibitors.[89] Similarly total cholesterol levels have been shown to be increased in a number of trials of both IL-6R and IL-6 inhibitors compared to placebo and DMARDs. The level of LDL cholesterol in particular was shown to have increased even further in the tocilizumab group compared to the adalimumab group in one head-to-head trial.[71]

A phase III multicentre trial examined the effect of IL6-R inhibition with tocilizumab (TCZ) on surrogate markers of cardiovascular risk.[90] Median total cholesterol, LDL-C, and triglyceride levels were increased in those on TCZ compared to those receiving placebo. There were no significant differences in mean small LDL, mean oxidized LDL, or total HDL-C concentrations. However, HDL particles were altered towards an anti-inflammatory composition and reductions were also seen in vascular risk surrogates such as lipoprotein (a).

Interestingly a new study suggests that hypercatabolism of LDL particles may be responsible for the reduced LDL seen in active RA.[91] This hypercatabolism was found to correlate strongly with reduction in serum LDL-C and increase in acute phase reactants, such as CRP. IL-6 inhibition with TCZ normalized this catabolism in a manner associated with the acute phase response, emphasizing the importance of IL-6 as one of the key mediators of inflammation-driven dyslipidaemia.

The net impact on cardiovascular disease (CVD) risk of these changes in lipid concentration secondary to IL-6 inhibition is under investigation. Results of a large phase 4 multicentre clinical trial comparing CVD risk of TCZ versus etanercept (TNFi) have recently been presented.[92] RA patients over the age of 50 with at least one CVD risk factor and inadequate response to at least one conventional DMARD were randomized to receive either TCZ or etanercept and were then followed up for an average period of 3.2 years. A total of 83 major adverse CVD events (MACEs), defined as CVD death, non-fatal myocardial infarction, or non-fatal stroke occurred in the TCZ arm, versus 78 MACEs in the etanercept arm with a hazard ratio of 1.05 (95% confidence interval 0.77–1.43). The study excluded a >43% relative increase in the risk of MACEs with TCZ compared to etanercept.

Future developments

Although IL-6 inhibition has been shown to be an effective and safe treatment for RA, further work is needed to clarify the precise placement of IL-6 inhibitors in the treatment pathway for RA. Few trials have been conducted comparing IL-6 inhibitors with other biologic therapies, and no head-to-head trials have yet been performed comparing the efficacy of different IL-6 inhibitors. It will be important to determine if there are any significant differences between anti-IL6R and anti-IL6 therapies and if there is any benefit to switching between the two if a patient fails to respond to one type of IL-6 inhibitor. Preliminary results from one study have suggested that there may be benefit to switching from one IL-6R inhibitor (TCZ) to another (sarilumab) in non-responders.[93]

The IL-6 pathway remains a major target for drug development for RA and a number of other inflammatory conditions. Newer generation biologics, which aim to selectively inhibit only IL-6 trans-signalling, are currently in development.[94] It is thought that this will reduce the incidence of complications associated with non-specific blockade of IL-6 signalling. Soluble gp130 (sgp130) is a naturally occurring antagonist of trans-IL-6 signalling. Sgp130 binds to the IL-6/sIL-6R complex, preventing it from binding to gp130 on the surface of cells and thereby inhibiting trans-IL-6 signalling. Sgp130 has been shown to reduce disease activity in experimental arthritis mice models, suggesting it may be a potential therapeutic agent for use in the selective blockade of trans-IL6 signalling in RA.[95]

Work is currently underway to identify potential biomarkers, synovial pathotypes, and genes which may help to predict response to the different biologics available. Soluble IL-6R has already been identified as a potential predictor of clinical remission in RA patients treated with TCZ.[96] These biomarkers will be invaluable in directing patients towards specific cytokine-orientated therapies, allowing effective treatment at a much earlier stage in the disease process than is currently possible.

REFERENCES

1. Kishimoto T. Interleukin-6: discovery of a pleiotropic cytokine. *Arthritis Res Ther* 2006;8(Suppl 2):S2.
2. Somers W, Stahl M, Seehra JS. 1.9 A crystal structure of interleukin 6: implications for a novel mode of receptor dimerization and signaling. *EMBO J* 1997;16(5):989–97.
3. Kishimoto T. IL-6: from its discovery to clinical applications. *Int Immunol* 2010;22(5):347–52.

4. Jones SA, Scheller J, Rose-John S. Therapeutic strategies for the clinical blockade of IL-6/gp130 signaling. *J Clin Invest* 2011;*121*(9):3375–83.

5. Liu X, Jones GW, Choy EH, Jones SA. The biology behind interleukin-6 targeted interventions. *Cur Opin Rheumatol* 2016;*28*(2):152–60.

6. Rose-John S, Scheller J, Elson G, Jones SA. Interleukin-6 biology is coordinated by membrane-bound and soluble receptors: role in inflammation and cancer. *J Leukoc Biol* 2006;*80*(2):227–36.

7. Bettelli E, Korn T, Kuchroo VK. Th17: the third member of the effector T cell trilogy. *Curr Opin Immunol* 2007;*19*(6):652–7.

8. Harrington LE, Hatton RD, Mangan PR, et al. Interleukin 17-producing CD4+ effector T cells develop via a lineage distinct from the T helper type 1 and 2 lineages. *Nat Immunol* 2005;*6*(11):1123–32.

9. Kimura A, Naka T, Kishimoto T. IL-6-dependent and -independent pathways in the development of interleukin 17-producing T helper cells. *Proc Natl Acad Sci U S A* 2007;*104*(29):12099–104.

10. Korn T, Mitsdoerffer M, Croxford AL, et al. IL-6 controls Th17 immunity *in vivo* by inhibiting the conversion of conventional T cells into Foxp3+ regulatory T cells. *Proc Natl Acad Sci U S A* 2008;*105*(47):18460–5.

11. Korn T, Anderson AC, Bettelli E, Oukka M. The dynamics of effector T cells and Foxp3+ regulatory T cells in the promotion and regulation of autoimmune encephalomyelitis. *J Neuroimmunol* 2007;*191*(1–2):51–60.

12. Muraguchi A, Hirano T, Tang B, et al. The essential role of B cell stimulatory factor 2 (BSF-2/IL-6) for the terminal differentiation of B cells. *J Exp Med* 1988;*167*(2):332–44.

13. Kopf M, Baumann H, Freer G, et al. Impaired immune and acute-phase responses in interleukin-6-deficient mice. *Nature* 1994;*368*(6469):339–42.

14. Rosser EC, Oleinika K, Tonon S, et al. Regulatory B cells are induced by gut microbiota-driven interleukin-1beta and interleukin-6 production. *Nat Med* 2014;*20*(11):1334–9.

15. Romano M, Sironi M, Toniatti C, et al. Role of IL-6 and its soluble receptor in induction of chemokines and leukocyte recruitment. *Immunity* 1997;*6*(3):315–25.

16. McLoughlin RM, Witowski J, Robson RL, et al. Interplay between IFN-gamma and IL-6 signaling governs neutrophil trafficking and apoptosis during acute inflammation. *J Clin Invest* 2003;*112*(4):598–607.

17. Chomarat P, Banchereau J, Davoust J, Palucka AK. IL-6 switches the differentiation of monocytes from dendritic cells to macrophages. *Nat Immunol* 2000;*1*(6):510–14.

18. Hunter CA, Jones SA. IL-6 as a keystone cytokine in health and disease. *Nat Immunol* 2015;*16*(5):448–57.

19. Fuchs TA, Abed U, Goosmann C, et al. Novel cell death program leads to neutrophil extracellular traps. *J Cell Biol* 2007;*176*(2):231–41.

20. Brinkmann V, Reichard U, Goosmann C, et al. Neutrophil extracellular traps kill bacteria. *Science* 2004;*303*(5663):1532–5.

21. Khandpur R, Carmona-Rivera C, Vivekanandan-Giri A, et al. NETs are a source of citrullinated autoantigens and stimulate inflammatory responses in rheumatoid arthritis. *Sci Transl Med* 2013;*5*(178):178ra40.

22. Matthews VB, Allen TL, Risis S, et al. Interleukin-6-deficient mice develop hepatic inflammation and systemic insulin resistance. *Diabetologia* 2010;*53*(11):2431–41.

23. Wunderlich FT, Strohle P, Konner AC, et al. Interleukin-6 signaling in liver-parenchymal cells suppresses hepatic inflammation and improves systemic insulin action. *Cell Metab* 2010;*12*(3):237–49.

24. Poli V, Balena R, Fattori E, et al. Interleukin-6 deficient mice are protected from bone loss caused by estrogen depletion. *EMBO J* 1994;*13*(5):1189–96.

25. Peters M, Schirmacher P, Goldschmitt J, et al. Extramedullary expansion of hematopoietic progenitor cells in interleukin (IL)-6-sIL-6R double transgenic mice. *J Exp Med* 1997;*185*(4):755–66.

26. Pedersen BK, Febbraio MA. Muscle as an endocrine organ: focus on muscle-derived interleukin-6. *Physiol Rev* 2008;*88*(4):1379–406.

27. Tamura T, Udagawa N, Takahashi N, et al. Soluble interleukin-6 receptor triggers osteoclast formation by interleukin 6. *Proc Natl Acad Sci U S A* 1993;*90*(24):11924–8.

28. Madhok R, Crilly A, Watson J, Capell HA. Serum interleukin 6 levels in rheumatoid arthritis: correlations with clinical and laboratory indices of disease activity. *Ann Rheum Dis* 1993;*52*(3):232–4.

29. Kotake S, Sato K, Kim KJ, et al. Interleukin-6 and soluble interleukin-6 receptors in the synovial fluids from rheumatoid arthritis patients are responsible for osteoclast-like cell formation. *J Bone Miner Res* 1996;*11*(1):88–95.

30. Brozik M, Rosztoczy I, Meretey K, et al. Interleukin 6 levels in synovial fluids of patients with different arthritides: correlation with local IgM rheumatoid factor and systemic acute phase protein production. *J Rheumatol* 1992;*19*(1):63–8.

31. Lally F, Smith E, Filer A, et al. A novel mechanism of neutrophil recruitment in a coculture model of the rheumatoid synovium. *Arthritis Rheum* 2005;*52*(11):3460–9.

32. Hashizume M, Hayakawa N, Suzuki M, Mihara M. IL-6/sIL-6R trans-signalling, but not TNF-alpha induced angiogenesis in a HUVEC and synovial cell co-culture system. *Rheumatol Int* 2009;*29*(12):1449–54.

33. McHugh J. Rheumatoid arthritis: regulating the osteoclast workforce. *Nat Rev Rheumatol* 2017;*13*(9):514.

34. Tanaka S, Tanaka Y, Ishiguro N, Yamanaka H, Takeuchi T. RANKL: a therapeutic target for bone destruction in rheumatoid arthritis. *Mod Rheumatol* 2018;*28*(1):9–16.

35. Flannery CR, Little CB, Hughes CE, Curtis CL, Caterson B, Jones SA. IL-6 and its soluble receptor augment aggrecanase-mediated proteoglycan catabolism in articular cartilage. *Matrix Biol* 2000;*19*(6):549–53.

36. Guerne PA, Zuraw BL, Vaughan JH, Carson DA, Lotz M. Synovium as a source of interleukin 6 *in vitro*. Contribution to local and systemic manifestations of arthritis. *J Clin Invest* 1989;*83*(2):585–92.

37. Dasgupta B, Corkill M, Kirkham B, Gibson T, Panayi G. Serial estimation of interleukin 6 as a measure of systemic disease in rheumatoid arthritis. *J Rheumatol* 1992;*19*(1):22–5.

38. Gabay C, Kushner I. Acute-phase proteins and other systemic responses to inflammation. *N Engl J Med* 1999;*340*(6):448–54.

39. Han C, Rahman MU, Doyle MK, et al. Association of anemia and physical disability among patients with rheumatoid arthritis. *J Rheumatol* 2007;*34*(11):2177–82.

40. Jongen-Lavrencic M, Peeters HR, Rozemuller H, et al. IL-6-induced anaemia in rats: possible pathogenetic implications for anemia observed in chronic inflammations. *Clin Exp Immunol* 1996;*103*(2):328–34.

41. Voulgari PV, Kolios G, Papadopoulos GK, Katsaraki A, Seferiadis K, Drosos AA. Role of cytokines in the pathogenesis of anemia of chronic disease in rheumatoid arthritis. *Clin Immunol* 1999;*92*(2):153–60.

42. Nemeth E, Tuttle MS, Powelson J, et al. Hepcidin regulates cellular iron efflux by binding to ferroportin and inducing its internalization. *Science* 2004;*306*(5704):2090–3.

43. Gough AK, Lilley J, Eyre S, Holder RL, Emery P. Generalised bone loss in patients with early rheumatoid arthritis. *Lancet* 1994;*344*(8914):23–7.

44. De Benedetti F, Rucci N, Del Fattore A, et al. Impaired skeletal development in interleukin-6-transgenic mice: a model for the impact of chronic inflammation on the growing skeletal system. *Arthritis Rheum* 2006;*54*(11):3551–63.

45. Kaser A, Brandacher G, Steurer W, et al. Interleukin-6 stimulates thrombopoiesis through thrombopoietin: role in inflammatory thrombocytosis. *Blood* 2001;*98*(9):2720–5.

46. Sturgeon JA, Finan PH, Zautra AJ. Affective disturbance in rheumatoid arthritis: psychological and disease-related pathways. *Nat Rev Rheumatol* 2016;*12*(9):532–42.

47. Margaretten M, Julian L, Katz P, Yelin E. Depression in patients with rheumatoid arthritis: description, causes and mechanisms. *Int J Clin Rheumtol* 2011;*6*(6):617–23.

48. Pollard LC, Choy EH, Gonzalez J, Khoshaba B, Scott DL. Fatigue in rheumatoid arthritis reflects pain, not disease activity. *Rheumatology (Oxf)* 2006;*45*(7):885–9.

49. Tsigos C, Chrousos GP. Hypothalamic-pituitary-adrenal axis, neuroendocrine factors and stress. *J Psychosom Res* 2002;*53*(4):865–71.

50. Stetler C, Miller GE. Depression and hypothalamic-pituitary-adrenal activation: a quantitative summary of four decades of research. *Psychosom Med* 2011;*73*(2):114–26.

51. Chikanza IC, Petrou P, Kingsley G, Chrousos G, Panayi GS. Defective hypothalamic response to immune and inflammatory stimuli in patients with rheumatoid arthritis. *Arthritis Rheum* 1992;*35*(11):1281–8.

52. Xu XJ, Hao JX, Andell-Jonsson S, Poli V, Bartfai T, Wiesenfeld-Hallin Z. Nociceptive responses in interleukin-6-deficient mice to peripheral inflammation and peripheral nerve section. *Cytokine* 1997;*9*(12):1028–33.

53. Chen Q, Wang WC, Bruce R, et al. Central role of IL-6 receptor signal-transducing chain gp130 in activation of L-selectin adhesion by fever-range thermal stress. *Immunity* 2004;*20*(1):59–70.

54. Choy E, Ganeshalingam K, Semb AG, Szekanecz Z, Nurmohamed M. Cardiovascular risk in rheumatoid arthritis: recent advances in the understanding of the pivotal role of inflammation, risk predictors and the impact of treatment. *Rheumatology (Oxf)* 2014;*53*(12):2143–54.

55. Ridker PM, Rifai N, Stampfer MJ, Hennekens CH. Plasma concentration of interleukin-6 and the risk of future myocardial infarction among apparently healthy men. *Circulation* 2000;*101*(15):1767–72.

56. Ridker PM, Hennekens CH, Buring JE, Rifai N. C-reactive protein and other markers of inflammation in the prediction of cardiovascular disease in women. *N Engl J Med* 2000;*342*(12):836–43.

57. Biasucci LM, Liuzzo G, Fantuzzi G, et al. Increasing levels of interleukin (IL)-1Ra and IL-6 during the first 2 days of hospitalization in unstable angina are associated with increased risk of in-hospital coronary events. *Circulation* 1999;*99*(16):2079–84.

58. Dayer JM, Choy E. Therapeutic targets in rheumatoid arthritis: the interleukin-6 receptor. *Rheumatology (Oxf)* 2010;*49*(1):15–24.

59. Choy EH, Isenberg DA, Garrood T, et al. Therapeutic benefit of blocking interleukin-6 activity with an anti-interleukin-6 receptor monoclonal antibody in rheumatoid arthritis: a randomized, double-blind, placebo-controlled, dose-escalation trial. *Arthritis Rheum* 2002;*46*(12):3143–50.

60. Nishimoto N, Yoshizaki K, Miyasaka N, et al. Treatment of rheumatoid arthritis with humanized anti-interleukin-6 receptor antibody: a multicenter, double-blind, placebo-controlled trial. *Arthritis Rheum* 2004;*50*(6):1761–9.

61. Nishimoto N, Hashimoto J, Miyasaka N, et al. Study of active controlled monotherapy used for rheumatoid arthritis, an IL-6 inhibitor (SAMURAI): evidence of clinical and radiographic benefit from an x ray reader-blinded randomised controlled trial of tocilizumab. *Ann Rheum Dis* 2007;*66*(9):1162–7.

62. Jones G. The AMBITION trial: tocilizumab monotherapy for rheumatoid arthritis. *Expert Rev Clin Immunol* 2010;*6*(2):189–95.

63. Jones G, Wallace T, McIntosh MJ, Brockwell L, Gomez-Reino JJ, Sebba A. Five-year efficacy and safety of tocilizumab monotherapy in patients with rheumatoid arthritis who were methotrexate- and biologic-naive or free of methotrexate for 6 months: the AMBITION study. *J Rheumatol* 2017;*44*(2):142–6.

64. Smolen JS, Beaulieu A, Rubbert-Roth A, et al. Effect of interleukin-6 receptor inhibition with tocilizumab in patients with rheumatoid arthritis (OPTION study): a double-blind, placebo-controlled, randomised trial. *Lancet* 2008;*371*(9617):987–97.

65. Genovese MC, McKay JD, Nasonov EL, et al. Interleukin-6 receptor inhibition with tocilizumab reduces disease activity in rheumatoid arthritis with inadequate response to disease-modifying antirheumatic drugs: the tocilizumab in combination with traditional disease-modifying antirheumatic drug therapy study. *Arthritis Rheum* 2008;*58*(10):2968–80.

66. Burmester GR, Rigby WF, van Vollenhoven RF, et al. Tocilizumab in early progressive rheumatoid arthritis: FUNCTION, a randomised controlled trial. *Ann Rheum Dis* 2016;*75*(6):1081–91.

67. Burmester GR, Rigby WF, van Vollenhoven RF, et al. Tocilizumab combination therapy or monotherapy or methotrexate monotherapy in methotrexate-naive patients with early rheumatoid arthritis: 2-year clinical and radiographic results from the randomised, placebo-controlled FUNCTION trial. *Ann Rheum Dis* 2017;*76*(7):1279–84.

68. Bijlsma JWJ, Welsing PMJ, Woodworth TG, et al. Early rheumatoid arthritis treated with tocilizumab, methotrexate, or their combination (U-Act-Early): a multicentre, randomised, double-blind, double-dummy, strategy trial. *Lancet* 2016;*388*(10042):343–55.

69. Emery P, Keystone E, Tony HP, et al. IL-6 receptor inhibition with tocilizumab improves treatment outcomes in patients with rheumatoid arthritis refractory to anti-tumour necrosis factor biologicals: results from a 24-week multicentre randomised placebo-controlled trial. *Ann Rheum Dis* 2008;*67*(11):1516–23.

70. Strand V, Burmester GR, Ogale S, Devenport J, John A, Emery P. Improvements in health-related quality of life after treatment with tocilizumab in patients with rheumatoid arthritis refractory to tumour necrosis factor inhibitors: results from the 24-week randomized controlled RADIATE study. *Rheumatology* 2012;*51*(10):1860–9.

71. Gabay C, Emery P, van Vollenhoven R, et al. Tocilizumab monotherapy versus adalimumab monotherapy for treatment of rheumatoid arthritis (ADACTA): a randomised, double-blind, controlled phase 4 trial. *Lancet* 2013;*381*(9877):1541–50.

72. Choy EH, Bernasconi C, Aassi M, Molina JF, Epis OM. Treatment of rheumatoid arthritis with anti-tumor necrosis factor or tocilizumab therapy as first biologic agent in a global

comparative observational study. *Arthritis Care Res (Hoboken)* 2017;*69*(10):1484–94.

73. Huizinga TW, Fleischmann RM, Jasson M, et al. Sarilumab, a fully human monoclonal antibody against IL-6Ralpha in patients with rheumatoid arthritis and an inadequate response to methotrexate: efficacy and safety results from the randomised SARIL-RA-MOBILITY Part A trial. *Ann Rheum Dis* 2014;*73*(9):1626–34.

74. Strand V, Kosinski M, Chen CI, et al. Sarilumab plus methotrexate improves patient-reported outcomes in patients with active rheumatoid arthritis and inadequate responses to methotrexate: results of a phase III trial. *Arthritis Res Ther* 2016;*18*:198.

75. Fleischmann R, van Adelsberg J, Lin Y, et al. Sarilumab and nonbiologic disease-modifying antirheumatic drugs in patients with active rheumatoid arthritis and inadequate response or intolerance to tumor necrosis factor inhibitors. *Arthritis Rheum* 2017;*69*(2):277–90.

76. Burmester GR, Lin Y, Patel R, et al. Efficacy and safety of sarilumab monotherapy versus adalimumab monotherapy for the treatment of patients with active rheumatoid arthritis (MONARCH): a randomised, double-blind, parallel-group phase III trial. *Ann Rheum Dis* 2017;*76*(5):840–7.

77. Van Roy M, Van de Sompel A, De Smet K, et al. FRI0021 Alx-0061, an anti-IL-6r nanobody® for therapeutic use in rheumatoid arthritis, demonstrates *in vitro* a differential biological activity profile as compared to tocilizumab [abstract presented at EULAR Congress 2013]. *Ann Rheum Dis* 2013;*72*:A375.

78. Dörner T, Weinblatt M, Beneden KV, et al. FRI0239 Results of a phase 2b study of vobarilizumab, an anti-interleukin-6 receptor nanobody, as monotherapy in patients with moderate to severe rheumatoid arthritis [abstract presented at EULAR Congress 2017]. *Ann Rheum Dis* 2017;*76*:575.

79. Dörner T, Weinblatt M, Durez P, et al. OP0098 Remission and maintenance of efficacy in a phase 2b study of vobarilizumab, an anti-interleukin 6 receptor nanobody, in patients with moderate-to-severe rheumatoid arthritis despite treatment with methotrexate [abstract presented at EULAR Congress 2017]. *Ann Rheum Dis* 2017;*76*:92.

80. Takeuchi T, Thorne C, Karpouzas G, et al. Sirukumab for rheumatoid arthritis: the phase III SIRROUND-D study. *Ann Rheum Dis* 2017;*76*(12):2001–8.

81. Aletaha D, Bingham CO, 3rd, Tanaka Y, et al. Efficacy and safety of sirukumab in patients with active rheumatoid arthritis refractory to anti-TNF therapy (SIRROUND-T): a randomised, double-blind, placebo-controlled, parallel-group, multinational, phase 3 study. *Lancet* 2017;*389*(10075):1206–17.

82. Food and Drug Administration. *Division Summary for the August 2, 2017 AAC Meeting, Biologics License Application (BLA) 761057 for Sirukumab Injection.* Available at: https://www.fda.gov/downloads/AdvisoryCommittees/CommitteesMeetingMaterials/Drugs/ArthritisAdvisoryCommittee/UCM569150.pdf

83. Genovese MC, Fleischmann R, Furst D, et al. Efficacy and safety of olokizumab in patients with rheumatoid arthritis with an inadequate response to TNF inhibitor therapy: outcomes of a randomised Phase IIb study. *Ann Rheum Dis* 2014;*73*(9):1607–15.

84. Takeuchi T, Tanaka Y, Yamanaka H, et al. Efficacy and safety of olokizumab in Asian patients with moderate-to-severe

rheumatoid arthritis, previously exposed to anti-TNF therapy: results from a randomized phase II trial. *Modern Rheumatol* 2016;*26*(1):15–23.

85. Mease P, Strand V, Shalamberidze L, et al. A phase II, double-blind, randomised, placebo-controlled study of BMS945429 (ALD518) in patients with rheumatoid arthritis with an inadequate response to methotrexate. *Ann Rheum Dis* 2012;*71*(7):1183–9.

86. Weinblatt ME, Mease P, Mysler E, et al. The efficacy and safety of subcutaneous clazakizumab in patients with moderate-to-severe rheumatoid arthritis and an inadequate response to methotrexate: results from a multinational, phase IIb, randomized, double-blind, placebo/active-controlled, dose-ranging study. *Arthritis Rheumatol* 2015;*67*(10):2591–600.

87. Moots RJ, Sebba A, Rigby W, et al. Effect of tocilizumab on neutrophils in adult patients with rheumatoid arthritis: pooled analysis of data from phase 3 and 4 clinical trials. *Rheumatology* 2017;*56*(4):541–9.

88. Choy E, Sattar N. Interpreting lipid levels in the context of high-grade inflammatory states with a focus on rheumatoid arthritis: a challenge to conventional cardiovascular risk actions. *Ann Rheum Dis* 2009;*68*(4):460–9.

89. Fleischmann R, Kremer J, Cush J, et al. Placebo-controlled trial of tofacitinib monotherapy in rheumatoid arthritis. *N Engl J Med* 2012;*367*(6):495–507.

90. McInnes IB, Thompson L, Giles JT, et al. Effect of interleukin-6 receptor blockade on surrogates of vascular risk in rheumatoid arthritis: MEASURE, a randomised, placebo-controlled study. *Ann Rheum Dis* 2015;*74*(4):694–702.

91. Robertson J, Porter D, Sattar N, et al. Interleukin-6 blockade raises LDL via reduced catabolism rather than via increased synthesis: a cytokine-specific mechanism for cholesterol changes in rheumatoid arthritis. *Ann Rheum Dis* 2017;*76*(11):1949–52.

92. Giles JT SN, Gabriel SE, Ridker PM, et al. Comparative cardiovascular safety of tocilizumab vs etanercept in rheumatoid arthritis: results of a randomized, parallel-group, multicenter, noninferiority, phase 4 clinical trial [abstract presented at ACR/ARHP Annual Meeting 2016]. *Arthritis Rheum* 2016;*68* (suppl 10).

93. Emery P, van Hoogstraten H, Jayawardena S, Mangan EK, Cejas P, Verschueren P. Efficacy of sarilumab in patients with rheumatoid arthritis who previously received sarilumab or tocilizumab [abstract presented at ACR/ARHP Annual Meeting 2017]. *Arthritis Rheum* 2017;*69*(suppl 10).

94. Lacroix M, Rousseau F, Guilhot F, et al. Novel insights into interleukin 6 (IL-6) cis- and trans-signaling pathways by differentially manipulating the assembly of the IL-6 signaling complex. *J Biol Chem* 2015;*290*(45):26943–53.

95. Nowell MA, Richards PJ, Horiuchi S, et al. Soluble IL-6 receptor governs IL-6 activity in experimental arthritis: blockade of arthritis severity by soluble glycoprotein 130. *J Immunol* 2003;*171*(6):3202–9.

96. Nishina N, Kikuchi J, Hashizume M, Yoshimoto K, Kameda H, Takeuchi T. Baseline levels of soluble interleukin-6 receptor predict clinical remission in patients with rheumatoid arthritis treated with tocilizumab: implications for molecular targeted therapy. *Ann Rheum Dis* 2014;*73*(5):945–7.

33

B-cell therapies

Md Yuzaiful Md Yusof, Edward M. Vital, and Maya H. Buch

Introduction

B-cells have traditionally been considered central to the pathogenesis of rheumatoid arthritis (RA) through antibody-dependent and antibody-independent functions. Owing to the multiple pathogenic roles of B-cells in RA, various strategies for B-cell inhibition have been or are currently being investigated including B-cell depletion, inhibition of B-cell survival factors, inhibition of B-cell receptor signalling, development of B-cell tolerogens, and targeting plasma cells, all with varying degree of success in clinical trials.[1] In this chapter, we will limit our review to the first two strategies, these being the two most evaluated approaches in RA.

A recent advance has focused on blocking B-cell activation and reducing B-cell survival through B-cell activating factor of the tumour necrosis factor (TNF) family (BAFF) and its homologue; a proliferation-inducing ligand (APRIL) inhibition. As with other new therapies, the key clinical questions that need to be addressed include the efficacy and safety of BAFF-inhibitors and a more accurate means of identifying patients likely to respond.

Roles of B cells in rheumatoid arthritis

In healthy individuals, B-lymphocytes are generated in bone marrow with specific antigen reactivity and negative selection against autoreactive B-cells prior to being released into the circulation as transitional cells, ultimately becoming naïve B-cells. Most autoreactive B-cells are removed at two discrete steps in B-cell development; the central B-cell tolerance checkpoint in the bone marrow between early immature and immature B-cells (mostly controlled by intrinsic B-cell factors regulating B-cell receptor and Toll-like receptor) and the peripheral B-cell tolerance checkpoint at transitional stage (involving extrinsic B-cell factors such as regulatory T cells and BAFF). Both checkpoints are defective in RA, resulting in the accumulation of a large number of autoreactive B-cells in the mature naïve B-cell compartment.[2,3]

RA is associated with specific autoantibodies rheumatoid factor (RF) and anticitrullinated protein antibody (ACPA). Autoantibodies can be detected years before clinical symptoms and their presence in individuals with non-specific musculoskeletal pain may predict progression to RA.[4] Far from being mere antibody producers, B-cells may mediate autoimmune disease by acting as efficient antigen presenting cells to T-cells leading to T-cell-mediated inflammation and by being prolific producers of inflammatory cytokines. Recent studies have also shed new light on B-cell regulatory functions in the context of immune-mediated inflammation and reveal their novel roles in bone homeostasis. These multiple pathogenic roles of B-cells are summarized in **Figure 33.1**.

Targeting CD20

CD20 molecule is a 33–37 kDa non-glycosylated phosphoprotein, expressed on the surface of naïve B-cells that have exited the bone marrow to enter blood. CD20 appeared to have no natural ligand and initial studies showed that CD20 knockout mice displayed an almost normal phenotype.[5,6] However, CD20-deficient mice and humans exhibit decreased T-independent immune responses.[7] *In vitro* evidence suggests that it regulates intracellular calcium.[8] CD20 is considered as a general B-cell marker but it is neither expressed on stem cells nor on plasma cells that have returned to the bone marrow. This selective expression on mature B-cells but not on precursors such as stem cells or antibody secreting plasma cells makes it an attractive therapeutic target, particularly from a safety point of view. Depletion via CD20 permits B-cell regeneration and moderate reduction of immunoglobulin levels, at least with initial therapy.

Rituximab

The development of B-cell depletion targeted at the CD20 molecule as a therapeutic modality represented a major advance in RA. Rituximab (RTX) was the first licensed, chimeric anti-CD20 monoclonal antibody (mAb), initially approved in 1997 for the treatment of relapsed or refractory low grade or follicular CD20+ B-cell non-Hodgkin's lymphoma.[9] It has since been licensed for diffuse large B-cell lymphomas, chronic lymphocytic leukaemia (CLL), patients with severe RA who have had an inadequate response or intolerance

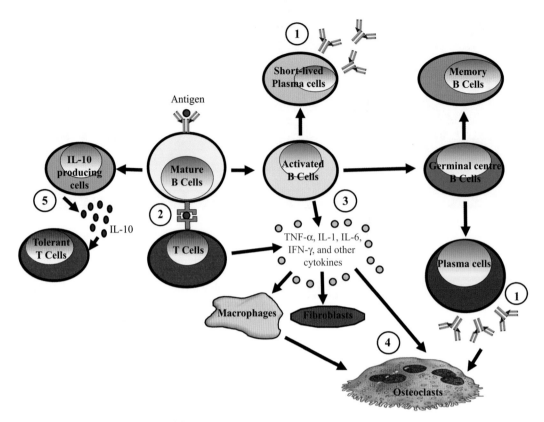

Figure 33.1 Roles of B cells in rheumatoid arthritis. (1) B cells are the source of rheumatoid factor and anticitrullinated protein antibodies, which contribute to immune complex formation and complement activation in the joints. (2) In addition to antibody-dependent function, B cells are highly efficient as antigen presenting cells and in some contexts may have a unique role in activating T cells that cannot be substituted by other types of antigen presenting cells. (3) They may also secrete inflammatory cytokines. (4) Pro-inflammatory cytokines and receptor activator of nuclear factor kappa-B ligand (RANKL) produced by activated B and T cells, macrophages, and synovial fibroblasts promote the differentiation and activation of osteoclasts, leading to bone resorption. (5) There is emerging evidence that specific subsets of B cells can also be immunoregulatory through the provision of interleukin (IL-10) and other mechanisms that have yet to be discovered.

to other disease-modifying antirheumatic drugs (DMARDs) including one or more tumour necrosis factor inhibitors (TNFi-IR) and remission induction of antineutrophil cytoplasmic antibody-associated vasculitis. B-cell killing by rituximab is achieved through a combination of antibody-dependent cell-mediated cytotoxicity (ADCC) in the presence of effector cells, activation of complement resulting in complement-dependent cytotoxicity (CDC) and cross-linking of multiple CD20 molecules, leading to cell death via induction of non-classical apoptosis[10] as depicted in **Figure 33.2**. The first is believed to be the most important mechanism for cell killing.[8] In addition, evidence from haematology patients has shown that targeted epitope expression may decline after infusion of monoclonal antibody (mAb). *In vitro* studies demonstrate that rituximab/CD20 complexes may be removed from B-cells by acceptor cells via Fc-gamma receptor, preventing their killing via an endocytic process called CD20 shaving/trogocytosis.[11]

Rituximab is formulated for intravenous administration and infused over several hours. For RA, clinical pharmacokinetic data are available for two consecutive doses of 500 mg (RTX500) and two doses of 1000 mg (RTX1000) given on days 1 and 15. The mean terminal elimination half-life is approximately 16–16.5 days (after the second infusion) for RTX500 and 18–21 days for RTX1000. There is no difference in pharmacokinetics between first and subsequent cycles of treatment.

Clinical efficacy for rheumatoid arthritis

Initial expectation was that temporary clearance of B-cells (due to sparing of stem cells) might have been sufficient to eliminate pathogenic clones leading to sustained remission after repopulation with a new diverse population of B-cells. However, most patients with RA ultimately relapse after a variable interval following B-cell repopulation, requiring repeat cycles to recapture response.

A series of phase II and III randomized controlled trials (RCTs) have evaluated efficacy of rituximab and their details are summarized in **Table 33.1**.[12–17] In these studies, rituximab was given in two infusions two weeks apart, each preceded by 100 mg of methylprednisolone. However, patient population, rituximab doses, other concomitant therapies, and retreatment intervals varied.

Typically, clinical response to rituximab is captured by approximately 3–4 months. The intravenous glucocorticoid premedication may produce an early, albeit a usually transient, response before 8 weeks. Thus, the latest European consensus recommend that assessment of response should be made at least 16 weeks from the initiation of treatment according to the recommended dosing schedule.[18] Duration of response is variable with the majority of patients experiencing relapse between 6 and 8 months, although some remain well for up to more than 15 months.[19]

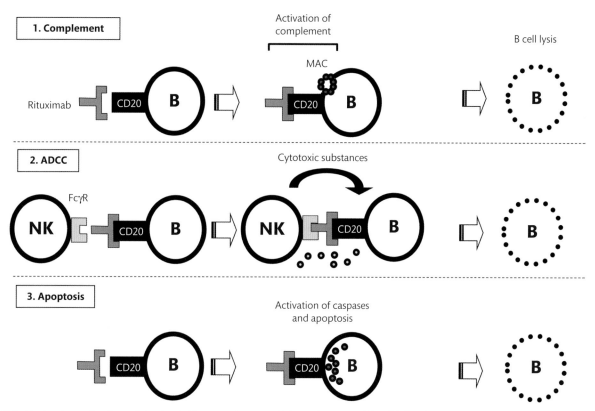

Figure 33.2 Mechanisms of actions of rituximab. There are three possible mechanisms of B-cell killing by rituximab; complement-dependent cytotoxicity (CDC), antibody-dependent cell-mediated cytotoxicity (ADCC), and induction of apoptosis. ADCC is generally believed to be the predominant mechanism. Cell killing depends on Fc-gamma receptor (FcγR) bearing natural killer (NK) cells or monocytes following the binding of rituximab to CD20. However, FcγR-mediated effector mechanisms do not always explain clinical rituximab efficacy in oncological and rheumatological disease, indicating a role for other effector mechanisms.

Radiographic outcomes

The Randomized Evaluation of Long-Term Efficacy of Rituximab in RA (REFLEX)[14] and the International Study in Methotrexate-Naïve Patients Investigating Rituximab's Efficacy (IMAGE)[17] studies reported radiographic data. It is important to highlight that the patient populations in these studies are different. The former enrolled patients who were TNFi-IR and with relatively long disease duration (approximately 12 years) while the IMAGE study recruited methotrexate-naïve patients and with much shorter disease duration (mean disease duration 0.9 months). In the REFLEX study, patients on background methotrexate were randomized to receive either rituximab (2 × RTX1000) or placebo. Following an initial response, retreatment with the same dose was given at time of flare. For those who were initially randomized to placebo, rescue treatment with rituximab could be given. For the purposes of analysis, such patients were still considered part of the 'placebo' group. Radiographs of patients' hands and feet were performed at baseline, week 24 and week 56 and evaluated using the total Genant-modified Sharp score (mTSS) method. The mean change from baseline in the mTSS score at week 56 was significantly lower in the rituximab-treated group (1.00 vs. 2.31, rituximab vs. placebo, p = 0.005); changes in erosion scores (0.59 vs. 1.32, rituximab vs. placebo, p = 0.011) and joint space narrowing (0.41 vs. 0.99, p <0.001); all were significantly in favour of rituximab. Interestingly, patients treated with rituximab

whose clinical outcomes were no better than those receiving placebo still demonstrated less radiographic progression. Sustained inhibition of radiographic progression has been demonstrated at 5 years in the long-term extension (LTE) study and after multiple courses of rituximab.[20]

The IMAGE study of early methotrexate-naïve RA measured similar outcomes in 715 patients randomized equally to three arms of methotrexate alone, methotrexate plus rituximab (2 x RTX500) or methotrexate plus rituximab (2 × RTX1000) doses.[17] At 52 weeks, patients who received higher dose rituximab (2 × RTX1000, either repeated at 6 months in those not in remission or given to those in remission at 6 months if and when disease activity score in 28 joints (DAS28) later worsened) had significantly smaller change in mean mTSS versus methotrexate alone group (0.359 vs. 1.079, p <0.001) and more patients in the former had no progression in mTSS compared to the latter group (63% vs. 53%, p <0.05). Even though statistically significant differences were not observed between patients receiving methotrexate alone and those treated with the lower dose of rituximab (i.e. 2 × RTX500), there was a numerical difference favouring the lower dose of rituximab versus methotrexate alone.

Outcome of repeat cycles

Patients from the three original RCTs were followed up in open-label extension studies. Retreatment with a further 2 × RTX1000 infusion

Table 33.1 Summary of efficacy data from randomized clinical trials of rituximab in rheumatoid arthritis

Study	Population	Group allocation	Endpoints	Main findings	Reference
Edwards et al.	MTX-IR RF positive	1: MTX (n = 40) 2: RTX1000 (n = 40) 3: RTX1000 + CyP (n = 41) 4: RTX1000 + MTX (n = 40) All groups had PO-CS and IV-CS	1: ACR50 at 24 wks 2: DAS28, EULAR, and ACR responses at 24 and 48 wks	All RTX groups were superior to MTX at 6 mo Only groups 3 and 4 were superior to MTX at 12 mo B cells depleted in all RTX groups for 24 wks RF reduced; total Ig remained stable	[12]
DANCER	MTX-IR or TNF-IR RF/CCP positive or negative	1: Placebo 2: Placebo + IV-CS 3: Placebo + IV-CS + PO-CS 4: RTX500 5: RTX500 + IV-CS 6: RTX500 + IV-CS + PO-CS 7: RTX1000 8: RTX1000 + IV-CS 9: RTX1000 + IV-CS + PO-CS All groups had MTX Total N = 465 Retreatment on clinical relapse	1: ACR20 at 24 wks 2: DAS28, EULAR, ACR responses, HAQ, FACIT-F, safety, and HACA at 24 wks	All RTX arms were superior to placebo at 24 wks Time to best response 12 to 24 wks Numerically higher ACR70 and EULAR good responses in RTX 1000 groups vs. RTX 500 CS did not influence efficacy outcomes IV-CS reduced infusion reactions, no added benefit with PO-CS HACA rate: placebo (0.7%), RTX 500 (4.2%) and RTX 1000 (2.7%), but no clinical sequelae in RTX groups	[13]
REFLEX	TNF-IR RF/CCP positive or negative	1: Placebo + MTX (n = 209) 2: RTX1000 + MTX (n = 311) All groups had PO-CS and IV-CS Retreatment on clinical relapse	1: ACR20 at 24 wks 2: DAS28, EULAR, and ACR responses, HAQ, FACIT-F, radiographic, safety at 24 wks	RTX was superior to placebo in all efficacy endpoints at 24 wks Trend to less progression in mTSS score in RTX group Significantly less progression in joint space narrowing score in RTX group Serious infections: placebo = 3.7, RTX = 5.2/100 patient-years	[14]
SERENE	MTX-IR RF/CCP positive or negative	1: Placebo + MTX 2: RTX500 + MTX 3: RTX1000 + MTX Retreatment from 24 wks unless still in remission	1: ACR20 at 24 wks 2: DAS28, EULAR, and ACR responses, HAQ, SF36, FACIT-F at 24 wks	Confirmed similar level of efficacy in RTX group as REFLEX study Further improvement in response rates after retreatment No difference in efficacy between RTX doses Better responses are achieved if RF or CCP positive at RTX baseline	[15]
MIRROR	MTX-IR or TNF-IR RF/CCP positive or negative	1: RTX500 then RTX500 2: RTX500 then RTX1000 3: RTX1000 then RTX1000 Treatment at 0 and 24 wks in all patients All patients received MTX	1: ACR20 at 48 wks 2: DAS28, EULAR, and ACR responses, HAQ, SF36, FACIT-F at 48 wks	Numerically higher ACR response at 48 wks in group 3 vs. other 2 groups Statistically better EULAR response at 48 wks in group 3 46% of ACR20 non-responders at 24 wks responded at 48 wks (group 3) Fewer patients had worse response at 48 wks in group 3	[16]
IMAGE	MTX-naïve, RF-negative patients needed erosions to enter study	1: Placebo + MTX 2: RTX500 + MTX 3: RTX1000 + MTX Retreatment from 24 wks unless still in remission	1: Change in mTSS at 52 wks 2: High-hurdle response (maintenance of ACR70 >6 mo), DAS28, EULAR, and ACR responses, HAQ, SF36, FACIT-F at 52 wks	RTX + MTX was superior to MTX alone in MTX-naïve RA ACR and EULAR responses were not influenced by RTX dose mTSS progression only significantly better vs. placebo with RTX1000 dose	[17]

ACR, American College of Rheumatology; AE, adverse event; CCP, cyclic citrullinated protein; CS, corticosteroid; CyP, cyclophosphamide; DAS28, 28-joint disease activity score; EULAR, European League Against Rheumatism; FACIT-F, Functional Assessment of Chronic Illness Therapy-Fatigue subscale; HACA, human antichimeric antibody; HAQ, Health Assessment Questionnaire; IR, inadequate response; IV-CS, intravenous methylprednisolone 100 mg days 1 and 15; mTSS, total Genant-modified Sharp score; MTX, methotrexate; PO-CS, oral prednisolone 60 mg days 2–7, 30 mg days 8–14; RA, rheumatoid arthritis; RF, rheumatoid factor; RTX500, 2 × 500 mg rituximab; RTX1000, 2 × 1000 mg rituximab; SF-36, 36-item Short Form survey; TNF, tumour necrosis factor.

was administered to those who were deemed responders (by predefined criteria) provided that they had deterioration in disease activity. Data for up to five courses of therapy have been reported.[21] The median treatment interval between the first, second, and third courses in patients with previous TNFi exposure remained stable at approximately 30 weeks. Clinical responses were also sustained during these observations. American College of Rheumatology (ACR) and DAS28 responses were similar after the first and second courses and the proportions of patients achieving 'high-hurdle' end points such as ACR70, DAS28 low disease activity (DAS28 <3.2) and

DAS28 remission (DAS28 <2.6) increased after the second course. Moreover, the change in DAS28 after each course from baseline was consistent, implying cumulative progressive reduction in disease activity with repeat courses of rituximab.

Rituximab retreatment strategies

The optimal retreatment paradigm for rituximab has not been fully determined. The most commonly used paradigm is one of repeated therapy if a patient deteriorates after an initial response as practised in earlier RCTs. Inherent to this is a degree of instability, with potential clinical implications, such as periods of uncontrolled inflammation and more short-term steroid use that can be potentially detrimental to long-term outcomes. Another strategy is fixed retreatment (i.e. every 6 months). Data from the Study of Retreatment With Rituximab in Patients With RA Receiving Background Methotrexate (SUNRISE) trial showed that two courses of 2 × RTX1000 infusions about 6 months apart resulted in improved and sustained ACR20 response at 1 year compared to a single course (54% vs. 45%; p = 0.02), with a similar safety profile.[22] Nevertheless, regular retreatment may risk overtreatment in some patients. Lastly, retreatment can be employed based on treat-to-target approach, in line with the European League Against Rheumatism (EULAR) RA recommendations whereby target of treatment is remission [DAS28 ≥2.6, Simple Disease Activity Index (SDAI) >3.3 or Clinical Disease Activity Index (CDAI) >2.8 or at least low disease activity (LDA)].[23] In a large retrospective pooled analysis of patients from the RCTs, fixed-interval (24 week) treat-to-target strategy was superior in terms of tighter control of disease activity with significantly greater improvements in DAS28 and lower Health Assessment Questionnaire (HAQ)-disability index scores compared to the strategy that retreated patients at the discretion of the physician (as needed, prn).[24] However, there were differences in baseline characteristics in that the 'prn' group had longer RA disease duration and predominantly TNFi-IR compared to the treat-to-target group with shorter disease duration that were mostly biologic-naïve. These factors may have influenced the results of the study.

Rituximab dose

Choosing the right rituximab dose for individual patients remains an unresolved question. A recent systematic review and meta-analysis that included 8 different study populations (6 RCTs and 2 cohort studies) concluded that a lower dose of rituximab (RTX500) than currently licensed (RTX1000) should be the standard regimen for RA. The review reported that RTX500 had similar efficacy and met non-inferiority criteria for most primary outcomes compared to RTX1000.[25] However, careful interpretation of data is needed as these studies recruited different patient populations and were powered for different endpoints.[26] It may not be appropriate to include results and make recommendations for the licensed population (i.e. TNFi-IR from the IMAGE study[17]) where the patients recruited were methotrexate-naïve. Moreover, the results of the non-inferiority analyses were also not consistent for all outcomes particularly the high-hurdle endpoints, such as the ACR70 response, EULAR good response, and LDA at 6 months, which favoured the licensed dose of rituximab. Lastly, in methotrexate-naïve patients, the results from the IMAGE study suggested that the RTX1000 dose was better than RTX500 for inhibition of joint damage during the first 24 months[17] but after this time point and up to 2 years, the radiographic damage was similar between groups. Nevertheless, the 2-year data were insufficiently powered to differentiate radiographic progression statistically between the two rituximab doses.[27] Therefore, the licensed dose of rituximab is still preferable for achievement of LDA and prevention of radiographic progression in patients not responding to methotrexate or TNFi.

With regards to retreatment of patients who respond to an initial course with RTX1000 dose, lower dose of rituximab (RTX500) may be equally effective as RTX1000 at 2 years as evidenced from one RCT.[28] However, longer-term data are needed particularly regarding the outcomes of switching back to the licensed dose following an inadequate response to the lower dose, and whether this can recapture response to therapy.

Managing non-response

It is unclear whether or not all initial non-responders should be retreated with rituximab and the published consensus recommend that alternative agents should be considered in this group of patient.[18] Data from the Methotrexate Inadequate Responders Randomized Study of Rituximab (MIRROR) demonstrated that 46% of patients who failed to achieve an ACR20 response after initial treatment achieved at least an ACR20 response at 48 weeks following their second treatment course.[16] One cohort study showed that such a strategy could be based on B-cell biomarkers using highly sensitive flow cytometry (HSFC). The initial non-responders had higher pre-rituximab plasmablasts compared to responders and only 9% had complete depletion following initial course. Retreatment of the former at 6 months led to complete B-cell depletion. Moreover, 72% of these initial non-responders became EULAR moderate or good responders after retreatment, with the duration of response equivalent to initial responders.[29]

Factors predicting response to rituximab

Antibody status

Studies examining the association between serological status (i.e. RF and/or ACPA) and rituximab treatment outcome in RA were limited by low numbers of seronegative patients. The proportion of seronegative patients recruited in the four major RCTs were: REFLEX (12%),[14] Dose-ranging Assessment International Clinical Evaluation of Rituximab in RA (DANCER) (13%)(13), Study Evaluating Rituximab's Efficacy in Methotrexate Inadequate Responders (SERENE) (17%),[15] and IMAGE (10%).[17] A meta-analysis of these RCTs indicated a modest additional increase in benefit in seropositive over seronegative patients; the reduction in DAS28 was on average 0.35 units greater in the former group (95% confidence interval (CI) 0.12—0.84).[30] The effect of serological status appeared to be greater in patients in the TNFi-IR (REFLEX study) population.

Concomitant disease-modifying antirheumatic drugs

The ACR responses of patients treated with rituximab in combination with methotrexate were numerically superior to those receiving rituximab monotherapy in the phase II trial; ACR20 73% vs. 65%, ACR50 43% vs. 33%, and ACR70 23% vs. 15%, respectively.[12] Moreover, rituximab monotherapy was shown to be more effective than placebo only in achieving ACR20 response but not ACR50 and ACR70 responses. Thus, rituximab is licensed in combination with methotrexate. Data from registry show that use of other concomitant DMARDs such as leflunomide is safe and effective,[31] and reproduces the effect of methotrexate on peripheral B-cell subsets.[32]

Peripheral blood B-cell studies

Treatment with rituximab is followed by peripheral B-cell depletion, evident as early as two weeks after administration of the first infusion. Early studies indicated no relationship between B-cell numbers and clinical response to rituximab when they were measured using conventional cytometry.[33] However, using HSFC, a protocol that was optimized for the detection of plasmablasts, one cohort study reported that persistence of plasmablasts after the first infusion of rituximab was associated with inferior clinical response at 6 months.[34] Moreover, patients with lower numbers of plasmablasts pre-rituximab were associated with plasmablast depletion and good clinical response using RTX500 dose[31] while doses of rituximab even higher than licensed might be employed in those with persistence of plasmablasts after therapy.[32] The application of these biomarkers in a wider practice has not been determined.

Synovial studies

Although treatment with rituximab leads to transient but almost complete depletion of B-cells in the peripheral blood, only partial depletion was reported in the synovial tissue.[35,36] One study performed synovial biopsy before, 4 and 16 weeks post-rituximab and showed that a greater reduction in plasma cells and intimal macrophages in synovial tissue between 4 and 16 weeks were associated with clinical response at 6 months. No baseline tissue biomarkers were predictive of response.[37]

Genetic studies

Pre-rituximab genotyping may be helpful to stratify patients for rituximab therapy and integrate with clinical predictors. Genetic studies have focused on Fc-gamma receptor polymorphisms. The V allele (158VV) polymorphism of the FCGR3A genotype that confers an increased binding affinity for immunoglobulin G (IgG), has been shown to be associated with higher clinical response rates in RA studies.[38,39]

Safety of rituximab

There are no new safety signals including on the risk of infection and malignancies from the long-term data (RCTs + LTE studies up to 11 years) on use of rituximab in RA compared with the extensive data available from haematology and oncology practice.[40,41]

Infusion reactions

Infusion reactions are the most frequent adverse events (AEs) observed during rituximab therapy. Common signs and symptoms include pruritus, urticaria, pyrexia, throat irritation, hypo- and hypertension that are usually mild to moderate in severity. These reactions may be due to cytokine release following B-cell lysis. Up to 30% of patients can be affected but reassuringly the incidence following the second infusion is much lower, possibly because B-cell numbers are already significantly reduced from the first infusion. Only a small number of patients (<1%) experienced a serious infusion reaction (i.e. anaphylaxis and bronchospasm), as reported from RCTs and LTE studies of rituximab in RA.[41] Prophylactic intravenous steroid administration before infusion of rituximab in a phase IIB study reduced infusion reactions from 37% to 29% in patients receiving a first infusion of 1000 mg rituximab.[13] Additionally, in order to minimize the risk of infusion-related reactions, prophylaxis with paracetamol 1 g and diphenhydramine hydrochloride (25–50 mg, or equivalent dose of similar agent) should be given 30–60 minutes before rituximab infusion.[40]

Infections

The rate of rituximab-associated serious infection events (SIE) differed with different treatment-stages in RA.[42] In patients who were TNFi-IR, numerically higher rates of SIEs were recorded in the RTX1000 group compared to placebo; 4.7 versus 3.2/100 patient-years respectively in the DANCER trial[13] and 5.2 versus 3.7/100 patient-years in the REFLEX trial.[14] On the contrary, in patients with early RA who were methotrexate-naïve, the rate of SIE was lower in the two rituximab dosage groups (RTX1000 and RTX500) compared with placebo (3.74, 4.61, and 6.09/100 patient-years, respectively).[17]

With regards to long-term safety from RCTs and LTE studies in RA, the SIE rates in the rituximab-treated group was comparable with the placebo + methotrexate group; 3.76/100 versus 3.79/100 PY, remained stable over time and with multiple courses of rituximab; as depicted in **Figure 33.3**.[41] The commonest infections (>5% patients) reported in rituximab group were upper respiratory tract infections, nasopharyngitis, urinary tract infections, sinusitis, bronchitis diarrhoea, influenza, and gastroenteritis while pneumonia was the commonest SIE (2%).[41] This SIE rate was similar to safety data from long-term follow-up of other biological DMARDs (bDMARDs) in RA (ranging from 3.0 to 5.2/100 patient-years).[43,44]

Opportunistic infections

The immunomodulatory effect of biologic DMARDs has naturally raised concerns with regards to the risk of opportunistic infections. It is worth noting that the risk of individual agents can often be linked to their targets (i.e. cytokine, T-cell modulation, B-cell). With regards to rituximab, serious opportunistic infections from long-term safety data have remained uncommon (rituximab-treated, 0.05 events/100 PY versus placebo, 0.09 events/100 PY).[41]

Tuberculosis (TB)

Only two cases of pulmonary TB, both treated with anti-TB chemoprophylaxis, occurred in the rituximab-treated group in the long-term data from RCTs and LTE studies in RA(41). No cases of extrapulmonary TB or multidrug-resistant TB were observed over a long period of time. Outside the RCTs, reports have included rituximab administered to 7 patients with latent TB and 6 patients with TNFi-associated TB. Over the following year, no patient either developed active TB or had QuantiFERON-TB-Gold In-Tube conversion.[45]

Hepatitis B and C

Data from haematological malignancy have demonstrated hepatitis B virus (HBV) reactivation (sometimes fatal) in rituximab-treated patients.[46,47] In RA, a series of case reports (n = 7) reported HBV reactivation post-rituximab in patients with background chronic hepatitis B infection (only one received antiviral treatment).[48] A small prospective study showed no viral reactivation in any of the vaccinated group (n = 4), resolved HBV infection (n = 12) or chronic HBV infection (n = 2; they received lamivudine and entecavir

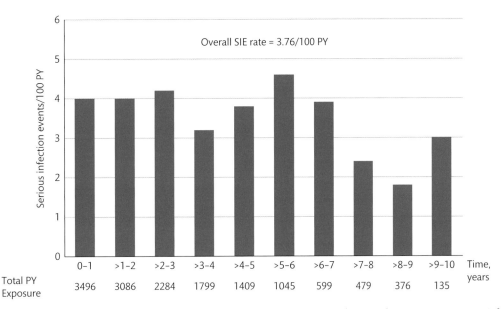

Figure 33.3 Serious infection rates over time during rituximab treatment from RCTs and LTE studies. Bar charts represent serious infection rates over time in 1-year increments in patients who were treated with rituximab.
Reprinted from van Vollenhoven RF et al (2015) 'Long-term Safety of Rituximab: Final Report of the Rheumatoid Arthritis Global Clinical Trial Program over 11 Years'. *J Rheumatol.* 42(10):1761–6 with permission from the *Journal of Rheumatology.*

respectively) and no significant change in protective anti-HBs titres during rituximab treatment.[49]

With regards to hepatitis C virus (HCV) infection, a retrospective study of patients with RA and HCV (without antiviral treatment) compared progression between those were treated either with rituximab or TNFi. No patient developed worsening of clinical HCV after a median follow-up of more than 2 years. However, although the liver transaminases remained stable, viral load was significantly increased in the rituximab group compared to the TNFi; p = 0.003.[50] This might suggest a potential safety concern in patients with HCV infection, without antiviral therapy. To note however, RCTs have demonstrated the efficacy and safety of rituximab in patients with HCV-associated cryoglobulinaemic vasculitis (including in those that failed antiviral therapy).[51]

Herpes zoster

Long-term data from RCTs and LTE studies in RA reported 108 cases of herpes zoster in 100 patients (included two cases of ophthalmic herpes zoster) in the rituximab-treated group compared to 13 cases in the placebo + methotrexate group; rates of 9/1000 PY and 11.7/1000 PY, respectively.[52] This was comparable to the rate of herpes zoster in the general RA population; 11.5/1000 patient-years.[53]

Progressive multifocal leukoencephalopathy

Progressive multifocal leukoencephalopathy (PML) is a rare demyelinating disease of the central nervous system caused by the reactivation of the John Cunningham (JC) virus. Confirmed PML cases from spontaneous reporting and clinical trial sources remain very rare (8 confirmed cases in 271 615 patients treated with rituximab, based on patient market exposure as of November 2013).[41] Therefore, the rate of confirmed PML in patients with RA is 2.95 (95% CI 1.27–5.8) per 100 000 patients, which has remained stable over time (Roche data on file). This incidence is lower compared to patients with Crohn's and multiple sclerosis who were treated with

natalizumab (1/1000)[54] and for psoriasis with efalizumab (1/400).[55] No definite conclusion can be made on the causal link of PML in this series due to small number of cases, background comorbidity (associated with PML) and concomitant DMARDs.

Rituximab-associated neutropenia

Rituximab-associated neutropenia can occur at least 4 weeks following rituximab infusion. It is a recognized complication in B-cell malignancies with an incidence of 3–27%.[56] Data in RA are more limited and the optimal management of these patients has not been defined. Data from a French registry[57] and large cohort studies reported much lower incidences between 1.3 and 3.0% in RA.[58,59] In most cases, neutropenia recovered promptly but counts <0.5 × 10⁹/L were associated with severe non-opportunistic infection requiring treatment with intravenous antibiotic and granulocyte-colony-stimulating factor. Thus, current data suggests retreatment with monitoring is appropriate, with additional caution needed only in severely neutropenic patients.[59]

Hypogammaglobulinaemia

The rituximab consensus update recommend that pre-rituximab immunoglobulin (Ig) levels should be monitored to identify patients who are at greater risk of infection.[18] Data from the French Registry showed that low IgG level (<6 g/L) pre-rituximab was associated with SIE, particularly in the 3 months post-rituximab; 16.2% versus 3.9% without low IgG.[60]

Long-term safety data from RCTs and LTE studies in RA showed cumulative reduction in immunoglobulin levels with repeated courses of therapy. 22.4% (n = 863) of rituximab-treated patients developed low immunoglobulin M (IgM), 3.5% (n = 112) had low IgG and 1.1% (n = 36) had low immunoglobulin A (IgA) levels for ≥4 months and after ≥1 course. Low IgM pre- and post-rituximab was not associated with SIE.[52,60] The rates of SIEs were similar before and during/after low IgG, but both rates were significantly higher than in patients who never developed low IgG.[52]

Immunogenicity

In the pooled analysis of long-term rituximab safety from RCTs and LTE studies, 11% of rituximab-treated patients were found to have human antichimeric antibody (HACA) in at least one visit.[52] However, no relationship between HACA and the dose of rituximab administered, the ability to deplete B-cells, the frequency of infusion reactions, clinical efficacy of the initial dosing or efficacy of retreatment were noted.[21,52]

Malignancy

In earlier RCTs, a history of malignancy was an exclusion criterion for study entry. Data regarding long-term rituximab safety from RCTs and LTE studies reported 109 confirmed non-melanoma skin cancers (NMSC) (0.74 events/100 PY, 95% CI 0.60–0.88) in the rituximab-treated group which was comparable to the placebo plus methotrexate group; (0.81 events/100 PY).[41] There was no evidence of an increased risk of malignancy of any type, over time or rituximab course. The rate of NMSC in the former was also similar to the rates of those in general RA population; 1.17/100 PY[61] and 1.30/100 PY.[62] In patients with a prior history of malignancy, data from the British Society Rheumatology Registry showed that treatment with either rituximab or TNFi did not increase the risk of further malignancy compared to those who were treated with conventional synthetic (csDMARDs); the age- and gender-adjusted hazard ratio of 0.43 (95% CI: 0.10, 1.80) and 0.55 (95% CI: 0.35, 0.86), respectively.[63]

Cardiovascular disease

Long-term rituximab safety data from RCTs and LTE studies reported the rate of myocardial infarction (MI) in the rituximab-treated group was 0.41/100 PY (95% CI 0.31 to 0.54) versus 0.27/100 PY (95% CI 0.09 to 0.84) in the placebo + methotrexate group.[52] Almost all patients affected had ≥1 risk factor for MI. The rate of MI in the former was comparable to the rates in the general RA population (0.48, 95% CI 0.34–0.94 to 0.59 events/100 PY, 95% CI 0.37–0.61).[64] The rate of stroke in the rituximab-treated group was 0.19/100 PY (95% CI 0.13 to 0.29), which was also comparable to the rate in the placebo + methotrexate group; 0.18/100 PY (95% CI 0.05 to 0.72).[52]

Safety in patients with comorbidities

There are limited data from RCTs regarding safety of rituximab in patients with interstitial lung disease (ILD) and bronchiectasis since they are excluded from trial entry due to comorbidity. Indeed, in the only prospective pilot study of ten patients with progressive RA-ILD who were treated with rituximab, the association between significant AE (including two deaths) and either rituximab or underlying disease could not be determined due to the small number of patients.[65] In patients with RA-ILD who received rituximab for arthritis (and stable ILD), one cohort study (albeit non-controlled) reported stable or improved lung disease (assessed by a composite index comprising lung function, high resolution computer tomography score and survival status) over a prolonged follow-up period. Factors that were associated with lung progression included radiographic pattern of usual interstitial pneumonia, previous history of lung progression and pre-rituximab low carbon monoxide diffusing capacity.[66]

Data from the British Rheumatoid Obstructive Airway Disease group that included 68 patients with RA-associated bronchiectasis (RA-BR) bronchiectasis has been reported. In the 12 months pre-rituximab, there was a median (interquartile range) of 3 (1–4)

infective exacerbations per patient. Post-rituximab, 21 patients (31%) had fewer exacerbations compared to baseline; 36 patients (53%) remained stable and 11 patients (16%) had increased exacerbations. When rituximab was compared to a matched TNFi-treated cohort, 8/68 (11.8%) patients discontinued rituximab while 15/46 (32.6%) discontinued TNFi due to respiratory causes including lung-associated deaths. The adjusted 5-year respiratory survival was better in rituximab-treated compared to TNFi-treated RA-BR patients; HR 0.40 (95% CI 0.17–0.96); p = 0.041.[67]

General consideration and strategies to minimize risk of infection

Screening before rituximab

Prior to treatment, an individual therapeutic goal should be established as a shared decision between patients and their treating physicians as well as discussion pertaining to full therapeutic profile of rituximab, including all risks and benefits.[18] Patients should be screened by eliciting a history of concomitant comorbidity, focusing on cardiovascular, pulmonary disease, and infections. The intensity and duration of immunosuppression needs to be considered too. Screening for HBV and HCV infections is recommended as reactivation has been documented in HBsAg-negative as well as HBsAg-positive patients,[68,69] thus stressing the importance of measuring not only HBsAg but also core antibodies against HBc antigen to identify positive carrier status. As long-term data have not shown evidence of an increased frequency of reactivation of tuberculosis in rituximab-treated patients with RA, screening patients systematically for tuberculosis is not necessarily mandated.[42]

Vaccination

Data from RCT and observational studies showed that humoral responses to vaccination to influenza and pneumococcal polysaccharide (T-cell independent antigens) were impaired post-rituximab, but not to tetanus (T-cell dependent antigen).[70,71] This preservation of cellular immunity might explain the low rate of infection among B-cell-depleted patients. Following B-cell repopulation, responses to influenza and pneumococcal polysaccharide were restored. For this reason, any patient considered for rituximab therapy is recommended for any indicated vaccines (hepatitis B for at-risk population, pneumococcus, tetanus toxoid every 10 years, influenza annually) to be completed either 4 weeks before the first (or next planned) course or at least 6 months after the last course.[72]

Monitoring for immunoglobulin levels

Immunoglobulin levels should be measured and monitored prior to initiation and before any retreatment particularly in those who demonstrate low baseline IgG levels[18]. A recent cohort study also advocates that individualized risk-benefit assessment regarding rituximab re-treatment decisions is needed in patients with lower IgG as this is a consistent predictor of SIE, may require treatment with immunoglobulin replacement therapy and may increase infection profiles when rituximab is switched to different bDMARDs.[73]

Cost-effectiveness of rituximab

Rituximab has been shown to be a cost-effective treatment in patients who are TNFi-IR with all four studies (including one RCT although not fully powered) suggesting equivalent/favourable results towards rituximab compared to other TNFi and abatecept.[74-77] In patients with seropositive RA who are biologic-naïve, a recent RCT showed that initial treatment with rituximab was non-inferior to a TNFi and most cost-saving over 12 months.[78]

Rituximab biosimilars

Roche's patent on the reference rituximab MabThera® for RA expired in the European Union in November 2013 and the United States in September 2016. As a result, several manufacturers have developed biosimilars. A biosimilar is defined as a biological product that is highly similar to the reference product notwithstanding minor differences in clinically inactive components, with no clinically meaningful differences between the biological product and the reference product in terms of the safety, purity, and potency of the product. Because of the potential differences in efficacy and immunogenicity from a new manufacturing process, *in vitro* analytical studies and *in vivo* clinical trials are required to confirm clinical equivalence of the biosimilar with the reference rituximab prior to approvals.[79] At the time of writing this chapter, two rituximab biosimilars; Truxima® and Rixathon® have gained marketing approvals in Europe and the United States following RCTs that showed bio- and clinical equivalences to MabThera® in RA.[80,81]

Other type 1 and 2 anti-CD20 molecules

Type I mAbs induce a translocation of CD20 into lipid rafts and efficiently activate the classical pathway of the complement system. Examples of type 1 mAbs include rituximab, ofatumumab, and ocrelizumab. In contrast, type 2 mAb such as obinutuzumab poorly activates complement but directly induces cell death upon binding to CD20 without cross-linking by secondary antibodies. Both types are capable of inducing ADCC in the presence of effector cells.

Ofatumumab is a fully human anti-CD20 mAb that binds to a different epitope than rituximab, is licensed for resistant CLL and has demonstrated efficacy in RA. In a phase III RCT, the primary endpoint was met with a greater proportion of patients on ofatumumab compared with placebo achieving an ACR20 response (50% vs. 27% respectively; p <0.001). Although numerically higher infection rates were reported in ofatumumab versus placebo (32% and 26%), serious infection rates were similar at 2%.[82] Ocrelizumab is a humanized anti-CD20 mAb binding to an overlapping CD20 epitope to rituximab with increased ADCC and reduced CDC properties. It met the primary and secondary endpoints in two parallel phase III RCTs in RA.[83,84] Development in RA however was halted after evidence of increased SIE rates included opportunistic infections, some of which were fatal.[85] These rates were higher in patients who were recruited in Asia versus other countries which might have represented intrinsically increased risk. The drug is still licensed for multiple sclerosis. Obinutuzumab, a type 2, humanized anti-CD20, also binds to a different epitope to rituximab and consists of an Fc region that is glycol-engineered to enhance ADCC. It has been licensed in combination with chlorambucil as a first-line treatment for CLL and is currently being investigated in a phase III trial of lupus nephritis, with a future plan for RA. *In vitro* obinutuzumab demonstrates enhanced depletion compared with rituximab in RA and lupus.[86]

Inhibition of B-cell survival factors

BAFF and APRIL are cytokines that belong to the TNF ligand family. They bind to three receptors and activate their own signalling pathways; BAFF receptor (BAFF-R) binds BAFF strongly, B-cell maturation antigen (BCMA) and TNF receptor superfamily member 13b (TACI) bind both BAFF and APRIL. BAFF and APRIL not only play a crucial role in B-cell homeostasis and the regulation of B-cell maturation but also regulates the function of T-cells by providing costimulatory signals to T-cells in conjunction with T-cell receptor.[87] Elevated BAFF levels have been detected in the serum and synovial fluid of patients with RA.[88]

Progress of BAFF/APRIL inhibition in RA

Belimumab is a fully humanized mAb that specifically binds to and neutralizes the soluble BAFF, thus preventing it from binding to its receptors on the surface of B-cells. In the phase II RCT of patients with moderately active RA who had failed at least one csDMARD, patients were assigned to receive either 1, 4 or 10 mg/kg belimumab infusions or placebo. After 24 weeks, the results showed relatively modest benefit with belimumab, with ACR 20 responses of 35%, 25%, and 28% versus 16%, respectively; the only statistically significant difference was achieved with the lowest dose of belimumab. This was then followed by an optional 24-week extension in which all patients received belimumab. At 48 weeks, ACR20 response increased to 41%.[89] Further studies are evaluating its role in the treatment of RA as monotherapy or in combination with other agents.

Atacicept

Atacicept is a fusion protein containing the extracellular, ligand-binding portion of the receptor TACI and the modified Fc portion of human IgG that blocks BAFF and APRIL. This dual blockade property may provide more potency than blocking BAFF alone with the benefit of also targeting long-lived plasma cells in addition to B-cells. Although pharmacokinetic data from a phase I trial suggested that treatment with atacicept produced significant reduction in immunoglobulin levels as well as a decrease in RF titres in the highest dose group,[90] two phase II RCTs of patients with active RA who were TNFi-IR failed to achieve their primary clinical efficacy endpoints, despite evidence of biologic effects.[91,92]

Conclusion

The introduction of B-cell depletion therapy with rituximab has been a significant addition to the armamentarium of biologics approved for the treatment of RA. It has a unique mechanism of action and mode of administration. In terms of patient selection, rituximab in combination with methotrexate has been shown to be particularly effective in those who are seropositive. Although the licensed population is at least one TNFi-IR, more efficacy data have emerged for use in biologic-naïve including inhibition of radiographic progression. Recent studies have also supported the efficacy of reduced dose and the different retreatment strategies, although long-term data are still needed to establish the optimal approach. Long-term rituximab safety data are reassuring including the risk of infection and malignancies, although Ig monitoring is advised to identify those at higher infection risk. The licensing of rituximab biosimilars will further enhance its cost-effectiveness profile. Future studies will hopefully better characterize the best responder to rituximab and determine its place in the evolving treatment paradigm for RA. BAFF and/or APRIL inhibition are promising alternative strategies for B-cell blockade and several trials are evaluating its efficacy. As with all biologics, long-term safety data will be of paramount importance.

REFERENCES

1. Md Yusof MY, Vital EM, Emery P. B-cell-targeted therapies in systemic lupus erythematosus and ANCA-associated vasculitis: current progress. *Expert Rev Clin Immunol* 2013;9(8):761–72.
2. Samuels J, Ng Y-S, Paget D, Meffre E. Impaired early B-cell tolerance in patients with rheumatoid arthritis. *Arthritis Res Ther* 2005;7(1):P78.
3. Menard L, Samuels J, Ng Y-S, Meffre E. Inflammation-independent defective early B cell tolerance checkpoints in rheumatoid arthritis. *Arthritis Rheum* 2011;63(5):1237–45.
4. Rakieh C, Nam JL, Hunt L, et al. Predicting the development of clinical arthritis in anti-CCP positive individuals with non-specific musculoskeletal symptoms: a prospective observational cohort study. *Ann Rheum Dis* 2015;74(9):1659–66.
5. Uchida J, Lee Y, Hasegawa M, et al. Mouse CD20 expression and function. *Int Immunol* 2004;16(1):119–29.
6. O'Keefe TL, Williams GT, Davies SL, Neuberger MS. Mice carrying a CD20 gene disruption. *Immunogenetics* 1998;48(2):125–32.
7. Kuijpers TW, Bende RJ, Baars PA, et al. CD20 deficiency in humans results in impaired T cell-independent antibody responses. *J Clin Invest* 2010;120(1):214–22.
8. Cragg MS, Walshe CA, Ivanov AO, Glennie MJ. The biology of CD20 and its potential as a target for mAb therapy. *Curr Dir Autoimmun* 2005;8:140–74.
9. McLaughlin P, Grillo-Lopez AJ, Link BK, et al. Rituximab chimeric anti-CD20 monoclonal antibody therapy for relapsed indolent lymphoma: half of patients respond to a four-dose treatment program. *J Clin Oncol* 1998;16(8):2825–33.
10. Boross P, Leusen JH. Mechanisms of action of CD20 antibodies. *Am J Cancer Res* 2012;2(6):676–90.
11. Beum PV, Peek EM, Lindorfer MA, et al. Loss of CD20 and bound CD20 antibody from opsonized B cells occurs more rapidly because of trogocytosis mediated by Fc receptor-expressing effector cells than direct internalization by the B cells. *J Immunol* 2011;187(6):3438–47.
12. Edwards JC, Szczepanski L, Szechinski J, et al. Efficacy of B-cell-targeted therapy with rituximab in patients with rheumatoid arthritis. *N Engl J Med* 2004;350(25):2572–81.
13. Emery P, Fleischmann R, Filipowicz-Sosnowska A, et al. The efficacy and safety of rituximab in patients with active rheumatoid arthritis despite methotrexate treatment: results of a phase IIB randomized, double-blind, placebo-controlled, dose-ranging trial. *Arthritis Rheum* 2006;54(5):1390–400.
14. Cohen SB, Emery P, Greenwald MW, et al. Rituximab for rheumatoid arthritis refractory to anti-tumor necrosis factor therapy: results of a multicenter, randomized, double-blind, placebo-controlled, phase III trial evaluating primary efficacy and safety at twenty-four weeks. *Arthritis Rheum* 2006;54(9):2793–806.
15. Emery P, Deodhar A, Rigby WF, et al. Efficacy and safety of different doses and retreatment of rituximab: a randomised, placebo-controlled trial in patients who are biological naive with active rheumatoid arthritis and an inadequate response to methotrexate (Study Evaluating Rituximab's Efficacy in MTX iNadequate rEsponders (SERENE)). *Ann Rheum Dis* 2010;69(9):1629–35.
16. Rubbert-Roth A, Tak PP, Zerbini C, et al. Efficacy and safety of various repeat treatment dosing regimens of rituximab in patients with active rheumatoid arthritis: results of a Phase III randomized study (MIRROR). *Rheumatology (Oxf)* 2010;49(9):1683–93.
17. Tak PP, Rigby WF, Rubbert-Roth A, et al. Inhibition of joint damage and improved clinical outcomes with rituximab plus methotrexate in early active rheumatoid arthritis: the IMAGE trial. *Ann Rheum Dis* 2011;70(1):39–46.
18. Buch MH, Smolen JS, Betteridge N, et al. Updated consensus statement on the use of rituximab in patients with rheumatoid arthritis. *Ann Rheum Dis* 2011;70(6):909–20.
19. Popa C, Leandro MJ, Cambridge G, Edwards JC. Repeated B lymphocyte depletion with rituximab in rheumatoid arthritis over 7 yrs. *Rheumatology (Oxf)* 2007;46(4):626–30.
20. Keystone EC, Cohen SB, Emery P, et al. Multiple courses of rituximab produce sustained clinical and radiographic efficacy and safety in patients with rheumatoid arthritis and an inadequate response to 1 or more tumor necrosis factor inhibitors: 5-year data from the REFLEX study. *J Rheumatol* 2012;39(12):2238–46.
21. Keystone E, Fleischmann R, Emery P, et al. Safety and efficacy of additional courses of rituximab in patients with active rheumatoid arthritis: an open-label extension analysis. *Arthritis Rheum* 2007;56(12):3896–908.
22. Mease PJ, Cohen S, Gaylis NB, et al. Efficacy and safety of retreatment in patients with rheumatoid arthritis with previous inadequate response to tumor necrosis factor inhibitors: results from the SUNRISE trial. *J Rheumatol* 2010;37(5):917–27.
23. Smolen JS, Breedveld FC, Burmester GR, et al. Treating rheumatoid arthritis to target: 2014 update of the recommendations of an international task force. *Annals Rheum Dis* 2016;75(1):3–15.
24. Emery P, Mease PJ, Rubbert-Roth A, et al. Retreatment with rituximab based on a treatment-to-target approach provides better disease control than treatment as needed in patients with rheumatoid arthritis: a retrospective pooled analysis. *Rheumatology (Oxf)* 2011;50(12):2223–32.
25. Bredemeier M, de Oliveira FK, Rocha CM. Low- versus high-dose rituximab for rheumatoid arthritis: a systematic review and meta-analysis. *Arthritis Care Res (Hoboken)* 2014;66(2):228–35.
26. Vital EM, Md Yusof MY, Emery P. Choosing the right rituximab dose for the right patient: comment on the article by Bredemeier et al. *Arthritis Care Res (Hoboken)* 2014;66(10):1591–3.
27. Tak PP, Rigby W, Rubbert-Roth A, et al. Sustained inhibition of progressive joint damage with rituximab plus methotrexate in early active rheumatoid arthritis: 2-year results from the randomised controlled trial IMAGE. *Ann Rheum Dis* 2012;71(3):351–7.
28. Mariette X, Rouanet S, Sibilia J, et al. Evaluation of low-dose rituximab for the retreatment of patients with active rheumatoid arthritis: a non-inferiority randomised controlled trial. *Ann Rheum Dis* 2014;73(8):1508–14.
29. Vital EM, Dass S, Rawstron AC, et al. Management of nonresponse to rituximab in rheumatoid arthritis: predictors and outcome of re-treatment. *Arthritis Rheum* 2010;62(5):1273–9.
30. Isaacs JD, Cohen SB, Emery P, et al. Effect of baseline rheumatoid factor and anticitrullinated peptide antibody serotype on rituximab clinical response: a meta-analysis. *Ann Rheum Dis* 2013;72(3):329–36.

31. Wendler J, Burmester GR, Sorensen H, et al. Rituximab in patients with rheumatoid arthritis in routine practice (GERINIS): six-year results from a prospective, multicentre, non-interventional study in 2,484 patients. *Arthritis Res Ther* 2014;*16*(2):R80.

32. Vital EM DS, Rawston AC, Emery P. Combination rituximab and leflunomide produces lasting responses in rheumatoid arthritis. *Ann Rheum Dis* 2008;*67*(90).

33. Breedveld F, Agarwal S, Yin M, et al. Rituximab pharmacokinetics in patients with rheumatoid arthritis: B-cell levels do not correlate with clinical response. *J Clin Pharmacol* 2007;*47*(9):1119–28.

34. Dass S, Rawstron AC, Vital EM, Henshaw K, McGonagle D, Emery P. Highly sensitive B cell analysis predicts response to rituximab therapy in rheumatoid arthritis. *Arthritis Rheum* 2008;*58*(10):2993–9.

35. Teng YK, Levarht EW, Toes RE, Huizinga TW, van Laar JM. Residual inflammation after rituximab treatment is associated with sustained synovial plasma cell infiltration and enhanced B cell repopulation. *Ann Rheum Dis* 2009;*68*(6):1011–16.

36. Vos K, Thurlings RM, Wijbrandts CA, van Schaardenburg D, Gerlag DM, Tak PP. Early effects of rituximab on the synovial cell infiltrate in patients with rheumatoid arthritis. *Arthritis Rheum* 2007;*56*(3):772–8.

37. Thurlings RM, Vos K, Wijbrandts CA, Zwinderman AH, Gerlag DM, Tak PP. Synovial tissue response to rituximab: mechanism of action and identification of biomarkers of response. *Ann Rheum Dis* 2008;*67*(7):917–25.

38. Ruyssen-Witrand A, Rouanet S, Combe B, et al. Fcgamma receptor type IIIA polymorphism influences treatment outcomes in patients with rheumatoid arthritis treated with rituximab. *Ann Rheum Dis* 2012;*71*(6):875–7.

39. Quartuccio L, Fabris M, Pontarini E, et al. The 158VV Fcgamma receptor 3A genotype is associated with response to rituximab in rheumatoid arthritis: results of an Italian multicentre study. *Ann Rheum Dis* 2014;*73*(4):716–21.

40. Roche. *Rituximab* [Investigators brochure]. Garden City, UK: Welwyn, 2009.

41. van Vollenhoven RF, Fleischmann RM, Furst DE, Lacey S, Lehane PB. Long-term safety of rituximab: final report of the rheumatoid arthritis global clinical trial program over 11 years. *J Rheumatol* 2015;*42*(10):1761–6.

42. Md Yusof MY, Vital EM, Buch MH. B cell therapies, approved and emerging: a review of infectious risk and prevention during use. *Curr Rheumatol Rep* 2015;*17*(10):65.

43. Westhovens R, Kremer JM, Moreland LW, et al. Safety and efficacy of the selective costimulation modulator abatacept in patients with rheumatoid arthritis receiving background methotrexate: a 5-year extended phase IIB study. *J Rheumatol* 2009;*36*(4):736–42.

44. Klareskog L, Gaubitz M, Rodriguez-Valverde V, et al. Assessment of long-term safety and efficacy of etanercept in a 5-year extension study in patients with rheumatoid arthritis. *Clin Exp Rheumatol* 2011;*29*(2):238–47.

45. Chen YM, Chen HH, Lai KL, Hung WT, Lan JL, Chen DY. The effects of rituximab therapy on released interferon-gamma levels in the QuantiFERON assay among RA patients with different status of Mycobacterium tuberculosis infection. *Rheumatology* 2013;*52*(4):697–704.

46. Tsutsumi Y, Ogasawara R, Kamihara Y, et al. Rituximab administration and reactivation of HBV. *Hepat Res Treat* 2010;*2010*:182067.

47. Singh JA, Wells GA, Christensen R, et al. Adverse effects of biologics: a network meta-analysis and Cochrane overview. *Cochrane Database Syst Rev* 2011(2):CD008794.

48. Nard FD, Todoerti M, Grosso V, et al. Risk of hepatitis B virus reactivation in rheumatoid arthritis patients undergoing biologic treatment: extending perspective from old to newer drugs. *World J Hepatol* 2015;*7*(3):344–61.

49. Mitroulis I, Hatzara C, Kandili A, Hadziyannis E, Vassilopoulos D. Long-term safety of rituximab in patients with rheumatic diseases and chronic or resolved hepatitis B virus infection. *Ann Rheum Dis* 2013;*72*(2):308–10.

50. Lin KM, Lin JC, Tseng WY, Cheng TT. Rituximab-induced hepatitis C virus reactivation in rheumatoid arthritis. *J Microbiol Immunol Infect* 2013;*46*(1):65–7.

51. Sneller MC, Hu Z, Langford CA. A randomized controlled trial of rituximab following failure of antiviral therapy for hepatitis C virus-associated cryoglobulinemic vasculitis. *Arthritis Rheum* 2012;*64*(3):835–42.

52. van Vollenhoven RF, Emery P, Bingham CO, 3rd, et al. Long-term safety of rituximab in rheumatoid arthritis: 9.5-year follow-up of the global clinical trial programme with a focus on adverse events of interest in RA patients. *Ann Rheum Dis* 2013;*72*(9):1496–502.

53. Bongartz T, Orenstein R. Therapy: the risk of herpes zoster: another cost of anti-TNF therapy? *Nat Rev Rheumatol* 2009;*5*(7):361–3.

54. Carson KR, Focosi D, Major EO, et al. Monoclonal antibody-associated progressive multifocal leucoencephalopathy in patients treated with rituximab, natalizumab, and efalizumab: a review from the research on adverse drug events and reports (RADAR) project. *Lancet Oncol* 2009;*10*(8):816–24.

55. Kothary N, Diak IL, Brinker A, Bezabeh S, Avigan M, Dal Pan G. Progressive multifocal leukoencephalopathy associated with efalizumab use in psoriasis patients. *J Am Acad Dermatol* 2011;*65*(3):546–51.

56. Tesfa D, Palmblad J. Late-onset neutropenia following rituximab therapy: incidence, clinical features and possible mechanisms. *Exp Rev Hematol* 2011;*4*(6):619–25.

57. Salmon JH, Cacoub P, Combe B, et al. Late-onset neutropenia after treatment with rituximab for rheumatoid arthritis and other autoimmune diseases: data from the AutoImmunity and Rituximab registry. *RMD Open* 2015;*1*(1):e000034.

58. Tesfa D, Ajeganova S, Hagglund H, et al. Late-onset neutropenia following rituximab therapy in rheumatic diseases: association with B lymphocyte depletion and infections. *Arthritis Rheum* 2011;*63*(8):2209–14.

59. Ferreira JC, Yusof MYM, Das S, Vital EM, Emery P. Rituximab-associated neutropaenia: safety of retreatment rituximab therapy. *Rheumatology* 2015;*54*(suppl 1):i74–i.

60. Gottenberg JE, Ravaud P, Bardin T, et al. Risk factors for severe infections in patients with rheumatoid arthritis treated with rituximab in the autoimmunity and rituximab registry. *Arthritis Rheum* 2010;*62*(9):2625–32.

61. Mellemkjaer L, Linet MS, Gridley G, Frisch M, Moller H, Olsen JH. Rheumatoid arthritis and cancer risk. *Eur J Cancer* 1996;*32A*(10):1753–7.

62. Wolfe F, Michaud K. Biologic treatment of rheumatoid arthritis and the risk of malignancy: analyses from a large US observational study. *Arthritis Rheum* 2007;*56*(9):2886–95.

63. Silva-Fernandez L, Lunt M, Kearsley-Fleet L, et al. The incidence of cancer in patients with rheumatoid arthritis and a prior malignancy who receive TNF inhibitors or rituximab: results from the

British Society for Rheumatology Biologics Register-Rheumatoid Arthritis. *Rheumatology (Oxf)* 2016;*55*(11):2033–9.

64. Dixon WG, Watson KD, Lunt M, et al. Reduction in the incidence of myocardial infarction in patients with rheumatoid arthritis who respond to anti-tumor necrosis factor alpha therapy: results from the British Society for Rheumatology Biologics Register. *Arthritis Rheum* 2007;*56*(9):2905–12.

65. Matteson EL, Bongartz T, Ryu JH, Crowson CS, Hartman TE, Dellaripa PF. Open-label, pilot study of the safety and clinical effects of rituximab in patients with rheumatoid arthritis-associated interstitial pneumonia. *Open J Rheumatol Autoimmune Dis* 2012;*2*(03):53.

66. Md Yusof MY, Kabia A, Darby M, et al. Effect of rituximab on the progression of rheumatoid arthritis-related interstitial lung disease: 10 years' experience at a single centre. *Rheumatology (Oxf)* 2017;*56*(8):1348–57.

67. Md Yusof MY, Iqbal K, Darby M, et al. Effect of rituximab or tumour necrosis factor inhibitors on lung infection and survival in rheumatoid-associated bronchiectasis. *Rheumatology* (Oxf) 2019 kez676 [Epub ahead of print].

68. Pei SN, Chen CH, Lee CM, et al. Reactivation of hepatitis B virus following rituximab-based regimens: a serious complication in both HBsAg-positive and HBsAg-negative patients. *Ann Hematol* 2010;*89*(3):255–62.

69. Koo YX, Tan DS, Tan BH, Quek R, Tao M, Lim ST. Risk of hepatitis B virus reactivation in patients who are hepatitis B surface antigen negative/antibody to hepatitis B core antigen positive and the role of routine antiviral prophylaxis. *J Clin Oncol* 2009;*27*(15):2570–71; author reply 1–2.

70. van Assen S, de Haan A, Holvast A, et al. Cell-mediated immune responses to inactivated trivalent influenza-vaccination are decreased in patients with common variable immunodeficiency. *Clin Immunol* 2011;*141*(2):161–8.

71. Bingham CO, 3rd, Looney RJ, Deodhar A, et al. Immunization responses in rheumatoid arthritis patients treated with rituximab: results from a controlled clinical trial. *Arthritis Rheum* 2010;*62*(1):64–74.

72. van Assen S, Agmon-Levin N, Elkayam O, et al. EULAR recommendations for vaccination in adult patients with autoimmune inflammatory rheumatic diseases. *Ann Rheum Dis* 2011;*70*(3):414–22.

73. Md Yusof MY, Vital EM, McElvenny DM, et al. Predicting severe infection and effects of hypogammaglobulinemia during therapy with rituximab in rheumatic and musculoskeletal diseases. *Arthritis Rheumatol*. 2019 Nov;*71*(11):1812–1823..

74. Manders SH, Kievit W, Adang E, et al. Cost-effectiveness of abatacept, rituximab, and TNFi treatment after previous failure with TNFi treatment in rheumatoid arthritis: a pragmatic multicentre randomised trial. *Arthritis Res Ther* 2015;*17*(1):134.

75. Kielhorn A, Porter D, Diamantopoulos A, Lewis G. UK cost-utility analysis of rituximab in patients with rheumatoid arthritis that failed to respond adequately to a biologic disease-modifying antirheumatic drug. *Curr Med Res Opin* 2008;*24*(9):2639–50.

76. Lindgren P, Geborek P, Kobelt G. Modeling the cost-effectiveness of treatment of rheumatoid arthritis with rituximab using registry data from Southern Sweden. *Int J Technol Assess Health Care* 2009;*25*(2):181–9.

77. Launois R, Payet S, Saidenberg-Kermanac'h N, Francesconi C, Franca LR, Boissier MC. Budget impact model of rituximab after failure of one or more TNFalpha inhibitor therapies in the treatment of rheumatoid arthritis. *Joint Bone Spine* 2008;*75*(6):688–95.

78. Porter D, van Melckebeke J, Dale J, et al. Tumour necrosis factor inhibition versus rituximab for patients with rheumatoid arthritis who require biological treatment (ORBIT): an open-label, randomised controlled, non-inferiority, trial. *Lancet* 2016;*388*(10041):239–47.

79. Vital EM, Kay J, Emery P. Rituximab biosimilars. *Expert Opin Biol Ther* 2013;*13*(7):1049–62.

80. Yoo DH, Suh C-H, Shim SC, et al. A multicentre randomised controlled trial to compare the pharmacokinetics, efficacy and safety of CT-P10 and innovator rituximab in patients with rheumatoid arthritis. *Ann Rheum Dis* 2017;*76*(3):566–70.

81. Smolen JS, Cohen SB, Tony HP, et al. A randomised, double-blind trial to demonstrate bioequivalence of GP2013 and reference rituximab combined with methotrexate in patients with active rheumatoid arthritis. *Ann Rheum Dis* 2017;*76*(9):1598–602.

82. Taylor PC, Quattrocchi E, Mallett S, Kurrasch R, Petersen J, Chang DJ. Ofatumumab, a fully human anti-CD20 monoclonal antibody, in biological-naive, rheumatoid arthritis patients with an inadequate response to methotrexate: a randomised, double-blind, placebo-controlled clinical trial. *Ann Rheum Dis* 2011;*70*(12):2119–25.

83. Rigby W, Tony HP, Oelke K, et al. Safety and efficacy of ocrelizumab in patients with rheumatoid arthritis and an inadequate response to methotrexate: results of a forty-eight-week randomized, double-blind, placebo-controlled, parallel-group phase III trial. *Arthritis Rheum* 2012;*64*(2):350–9.

84. Tak PP, Mease PJ, Genovese MC, et al. Safety and efficacy of ocrelizumab in patients with rheumatoid arthritis and an inadequate response to at least one tumor necrosis factor inhibitor: results of a forty-eight-week randomized, double-blind, placebo-controlled, parallel-group phase III trial. *Arthritis Rheum* 2012;*64*(2):360–70.

85. Emery P, Rigby W, Tak PP, et al. Safety with ocrelizumab in rheumatoid arthritis: results from the ocrelizumab phase III program. *PLoS One* 2014;*9*(2):e87379.

86. Reddy V, Klein C, Isenberg DA, et al. Obinutuzumab induces superior B-cell cytotoxicity to rituximab in rheumatoid arthritis and systemic lupus erythematosus patient samples. *Rheumatology (Oxf)* 2017;*56*(7):1227–37.

87. Vincent FB, Morand EF, Mackay F. BAFF and innate immunity: new therapeutic targets for systemic lupus erythematosus. *Immunol Cell Biol* 2012;*90*(3):293–303.

88. Bosello S, Youinou P, Daridon C, et al. Concentrations of BAFF correlate with autoantibody levels, clinical disease activity, and response to treatment in early rheumatoid arthritis. *J Rheumatol* 2008;*35*(7):1256–64.

89. Stohl W, Merrill JT, McKay JD, et al. Efficacy and safety of belimumab in patients with rheumatoid arthritis: a phase II, randomized, double-blind, placebo-controlled, dose-ranging study. *J Rheumatol* 2013;*40*(5):579–89.

90. Tak PP, Thurlings RM, Rossier C, et al. Atacicept in patients with rheumatoid arthritis: results of a multicenter, phase IB, double-blind, placebo-controlled, dose-escalating, single- and repeated-dose study. *Arthritis Rheum* 2008;*58*(1):61–72.

91. van Vollenhoven RF, Kinnman N, Vincent E, Wax S, Bathon J. Atacicept in patients with rheumatoid arthritis and an inadequate response to methotrexate: results of a phase II, randomized, placebo-controlled trial. *Arthritis Rheum* 2011; *63*(7):1782–92.

90. Genovese MC, Kinnman N, de La Bourdonnaye G, Pena Rossi C, Tak PP. Atacicept in patients with rheumatoid arthritis and an inadequate response to tumor necrosis factor antagonist therapy: results of a phase II, randomized, placebo-controlled, dose-finding trial. *Arthritis Rheum* 2011;*63*(7):1793–803.

34

Biosimilars

Vibeke Strand, Jeffrey Kaine, and John Isaacs

Introduction

Unlike synthetic small molecule drugs, biologic agents, by definition, are produced from living cells. For this reason, it is impossible to manufacture an identical copy of a biologic agent. In fact, a batch of monoclonal antibody or soluble receptor is not a pure drug substance but contains multiple subtly different but highly related products, so-called microheterogeneity. Reference, or innovator, biologics in use today are not identical to the originally licensed products, due to changes in manufacturing or downstream processes that have occurred over the lifetime of the reference products. Nonetheless, as patents expire, it has become possible for copies of reference products to be legally manufactured. To ensure these agents are as close as possible to the reference product (in terms of quality attributes, efficacy, safety, and immunogenicity), stringent regulations have been developed for the manufacture and testing of 'biosimilar' products.[1,2]

Biosimilars have been regulated by EMA since 2005 and more recently by FDA starting in 2010, with passage of the Affordable Care Act as of 2016.[3,4] To date, 35 biosimilars have come to market in the EU. In the United States where only products with >100 amino acid residues are considered biosimilars, six have been approved, but only two have reached the market as the others remain embroiled in patent litigation.[5] Recently an agreement between Abbvie and Amgen would suggest that pathways for distribution and marketing of biosimilar products in the United States will be well established by 2023.[6] Health Canada has approved four biosimilars; Australia eight; and New Zealand five. It is important to distinguish products formally approved by regulatory agencies as biosimilars from those designed as copies or 'biomimics'.[7] Agents in this latter group have not been compared in equivalence trials with the originator biologic agent. Over the past 20 years, following approval of the first biologic agent for treatment of rheumatoid arthritis (RA), a number of manufacturing process changes have been introduced with each product.[8,9] These types of changes range from relatively minor alterations in filtration apparatus or equipment replacement upgrades to major changes in cell culture media or construction of new manufacturing sites (**Figure 34.1A**). According to the potential risk associated with each change, the required characterization of new product lots by regulatory agencies have ranged from analytical data and process studies including stability, to additional

clinical data ensuring comparability between the new and previous lots (**Figure 34.1 B**).[10–13] Failure to adequately regulate these aspects might have significant safety implications, for example opening the door to post-translational modifications that substantially impact a biologic agent's molecular function (**Figure 34.1C**). Largely due to such manufacturing changes (which have resulted in improved efficiency and yield), detailed characterizations of biologic agent lots have led to the ability to fully 'reverse engineer' a biosimilar from the reference product based only on the public knowledge of its primary structure, contained in the patent (**Figure 34.1D**).

Biosimilars: Regulatory definitions

The European Medicines Agency (EMA) requires biosimilars to have **comparable** quality, biologic activity, safety, and efficacy to the reference product based on a comprehensive comparability exercise. The US Food and Drug Administration requires biosimilars to be **highly similar or interchangeable**, with no clinically meaningful differences in terms of safety, purity, and potency. The biosimilar must utilize the same mechanism of action and be expected to produce the same clinical result in any given patient. Both agencies require an entirely independent chemistry, manufacturing, and controls (CMC) section in the regulatory dossier as the biosimilar will have more analytical data than the innovator product. Based on reverse engineering against multiple available lots of the reference product, there will be extensive comparative data between reference product and biosimilar, as well as analyses of both products based on newer techniques and characterizations beyond those previously available. These techniques may identify batch-to-batch variability over and above that already identified with the reference product. It follows that, with increasingly sensitive analytical techniques, the parameters for characterization of the biosimilar will be more stringent than those for the reference product.[14,15]

Characterization of biosimilars

EMA approach

Original EMA guidelines regulating biosimilars were issued in 2005–2006; revisions were finalized and adopted between 2012 and 2014.[16]

(A)

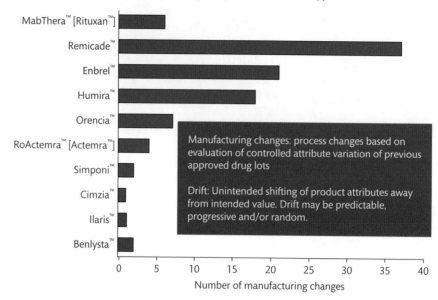

Biologic Drugs May Evolve Over Time:
Manufacturing Changes Vs. Drift

Reported manufacturing changes from time of EU approval

Manufacturing changes: process changes based on evaluation of controlled attribute variation of previous approved drug lots

Drift: Unintended shifting of product attributes away from intended value. Drift may be predictable, progressive and/or random.

Number of manufacturing changes

(B)   Biologic Manufacturers Work with Regulatory Authorities to
Assess Level of Risk Associated with Process Change

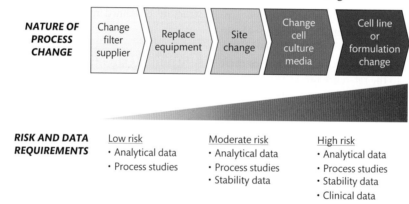

Figure 34.1 (A) Numerous changes in biologic drug manufacturing processes occur routinely during the post-approval life cycle of a biologic agent. The nature of the manufacturing modifications remains proprietary and confidential. However, EMA issues notifications of changes. In contrast, the impact of drift over the life cycle of a biologic is unpredictable. (B) The nature of a manufacturing change determines the quantity and type of supporting data required to evaluate comparability. The theoretical risk of clinical consequence related to production modification determines the need for clinical supporting data. (C) Changes in manufacturing processes may drive changes in naturally occurring post-translational modifications (PTMs). This in turn, may have clinically meaningful effects on both drug activity and metabolism. Post-translational enzymatic modification may potentially increase or decrease drug binding to its epitope as well as change drug clearance mechanisms, affect complement activation or immunoglobulin (Fc) receptor binding, or alter immunogenicity by changes in quaternary structure. (D) To reverse engineer a reference product, a biosimilar developer must create a manufacturing process for that biologic *de novo*.

(A) Adapted from: Schneider CK: Ann Rheum Ds 2013:72: 315–8. (B) Figure adapted from Lee JF, *et al. Curr Med Res Opin* 2012;28:1053-1058. With permission from Informa UK Ltd. (C) Adapted from: Kuhlmann M, Covic A. Nephrol Dial Transplant 2006;21(Suppl 5):4-8. (D) Adapted from: **1.** Roger SD. *Nephrology (Carlton)* 2006;11:341–346. 2. Mellstedt H, et al. *Ann Oncol* 2008;19:411–419.

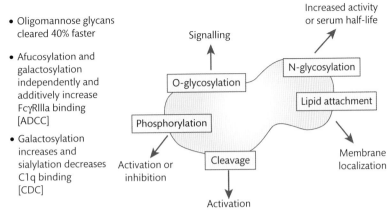

(C) What is the Impact of Post Translational Modifications [PTMs]?

- Oligomannose glycans cleared 40% faster
- Afucosylation and galactosylation independently and additively increase FcγRIIIa binding [ADCC]
- Galactosylation increases and sialylation decreases C1q binding [CDC]

Choice of expression system and manufacturing process can impact many aspects of mAb structure and function – not to mention "drift" over time

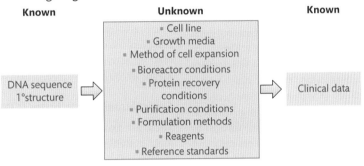

(D) It is Impossible to Precisely Duplicate Another Manufacturer's Biologic Agent

Figure 34.1 (Continued)

These include guidelines on 'Similar biological medicinal products' (October 2014), '. . . Containing biotechnology-derived proteins as active substances . . .' (May 2014) '. . . Non-clinical and clinical issues . . .' (December 2014), as well as 'Procedural advice for users of the centralized procedure for similar biological medicinal products applications (March 2013). Two product class specific guidelines are relevant to monoclonal antibodies (mAbs) and soluble receptors: 'On similar biological medicinal products containing mAbs—non-clinical and clinical issues' and 'Immunogenicity assessment of mAbs intended for *in vivo* clinical use' both adopted May 2012. Recent guidelines, issued in 2016, 'Good pharmacovigilance practices: Product- or population-specific considerations II: Biological medicinal products' applies equally to reference products and biosimilars.[17]

FDA approach

US FDA has issued 11 guidance documents between 2012 and 2017, including draft revisions and final documents.[18] These include: 'Scientific Considerations' (February 2012; final: April 2015), outlining a tiered stepwise approach using the 'totality of the evidence' including an abbreviated development programme

with evaluation of residual uncertainty at each step; 'Quality Considerations' (February 2012; final: April 2015) summarizing extensive structural and functional characterization and identification of critical quality attributes (CQAs). A draft guidance discussing 'Clinical Pharmacology Data' (May 2014) describes a required bridging study to compare pharmacokinetics (PK) and immunogenicity of the biosimilar to both US and ex-US manufactured reference products in healthy volunteers.

Of particular interest are several new types of guidances, designed to facilitate interactions between biosimilar sponsors and the FDA: 'Questions and Answers' (February 2012, final: April 2015); 'Additional Questions and Answers' (draft: May 2015) updated as appropriate; and 'Formal Meetings between FDA and Biosimilar Sponsors' (draft: March 2013), a new paradigm based on the Biosimilar User Fees Act (BSUFA) published in 2012. An additional guidance includes 'Reference product exclusivity', preventing biosimilar application submission until 12 years after the first licensure of the reference product. A draft labelling guidance indicates that only clinical data supporting use of the reference product will be included in the label unless specific differences exist with the biosimilar in terms of administration, preparation, storage, or safety. A final guidance on non-proprietary naming indicates the biosimilar will share the same proper name, not necessarily the generic name (or International Nonproprietary Name (INN)), as the reference product, with a randomly generated four letter suffix to facilitate pharmacovigilance. A recent guidance: 'Determination of Biosimilar Interchangeability' was issued in 2017 outlining the type of trial required to allow an interchangeable biosimilar to be substituted for the reference product 'without intervention of the healthcare provider who prescribed the product'.[19] Such a trial would require at least three switches between a US-produced reference product and the biosimilar with the primary endpoint being equivalent pharmacokinetics; secondary endpoints including efficacy and safety. Additional guidances include 'Statistical Considerations for Analytic Similarity' (30 September 2017) and an 'Processes and further considerations related to post-approval manufacturing changes for biosimilars' (31 March 2019).

Health Canada approach

Health Canada released a Guidance Document in November 2016 summarizing submission requirements for biosimilars compared to a reference product marketed in Canada or bridging from Canadian to a reference product sourced from an International Conference on Harmonization (ICH) country with a history of safe use.[20] The biosimilar submission must provide satisfactory chemistry and manufacturing information; efficacy must be assessed in comparative clinical trials as well as immunogenicity, all using a tiered approach; a postmarketing risk management plan should be part of the submission. Specifically, in contrast to US FDA, their guidance states that healthy volunteers may not be appropriate for PK/PD studies and that labelling will include comparative data between the biosimilar and reference product in tabular form.

Demonstration of biosimilarity

To reverse engineer a biosimilar, the developer must create de novo a manufacturing process for that biologic product (i.e. only the DNA sequence of the reference product and its clinical data are known)—all other data remain proprietary between the sponsor and regulatory agencies. The cell line, growth media, method of cell expansion, bioreactor conditions, protein recovery conditions, purification and formulation methods, reagents and reference standards remain proprietary (**Figure 34.1D**).[21,22] Post-translational modifications may occur during the manufacturing process that can affect the structure and function of a mAb. Glycosylation may increase activity or serum half-life; phosphorylation may affect activation or inhibition of function (**Figure 34.1C**).[23] Thus a detailed series of assays are required to characterize the biosimilar in comparison to the reference product(s).

Physicochemical and functional (biologic) characterization are major initial steps in establishing biosimilarity. Non-clinical studies may include limited toxicology studies, as were performed for the reference product. Each step is designed to decrease residual uncertainty in matching the biosimilar to its reference product using a tiered approach (**Figure 34.2A**).

Structural assays

Structural assays are designed to ascertain the attributes of the biosimilar related to its primary amino acid sequence, any post-translational modifications and the integrity of its secondary, tertiary, and quaternary structure.[16,18] Product related and process related substances, and impurities from the host cells and downstream process must be quantified and fully characterized. Final characterization of the finished drug product including its strength, formulation, and stability must be assessed including its degradation profiles. So-called 'fingerprint' analyses of proposed biosimilar products inform a necessarily detailed structural evaluation as part of the 'totality-of-the-evidence' approach (**Figure 34.2B**).

Functional assays

Biologic and functional activities, including receptor binding and immunochemical properties must be characterized.[16,18] The kinetics and thermodynamics of binding must be ascertained in relationship to the functional activity of the mAb. These include potency assays such as antigen binding, as well as ascertainment of effector functions (antibody dependent cellular cytotoxicity (ADCC)/complement-dependent cytotoxicity (CDC)), Fc receptor family binding activities, neonatal Fc receptor (FcRn) binding and other means to confirm the mechanism of action.

Critical quality attributes (CQAs)

These are features that are important to the identity, purity, biologic activity, and stability of a biologic product and must be characterized within appropriate limits, ranges, or distribution to ensure product quality. They are classified into three tiers depending on their potential impact on clinical activity. Examples of potentially **highly** impactful Tier 1 CQAs for TNF inhibitors (TNFi) include amino acid identity, binding to soluble and transmembrane TNFα and *in vitro* neutralization of TNFα (see **Figure 34.2C**). Examples of Tier 1 CQAs for a cell depleting mAb such as rituximab include: binding to the CD20 antigen, ADCC and CDC (**Figure 34.2C**).

Clinical trials to confirm biosimilarity

Bridging 3-way comparison of PK/Immunogenicity in healthy volunteers

A trial in healthy volunteers is required by FDA to demonstrate PK equivalency between a biosimilar and both US manufactured and ex-US manufactured reference products following a single dose.[18] Clinical PK similarity is required for all three prospectively defined PK endpoints:

- Maximum serum concentration (C_{max})
- Area under the time-concentration curve from first to last time point measured (AUC_{0-t}), and
- Area under the time-concentration curve from first time point extrapolated to infinity ($AUC_{0-\gamma}$).

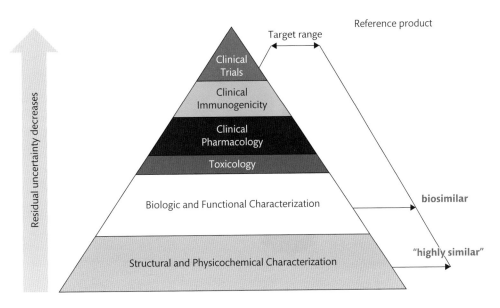

(A) Biosimilars must be Systematically Engineered to Match Reference Product

(B) Fingerprint Analysis of mAbs/Fusion Proteins

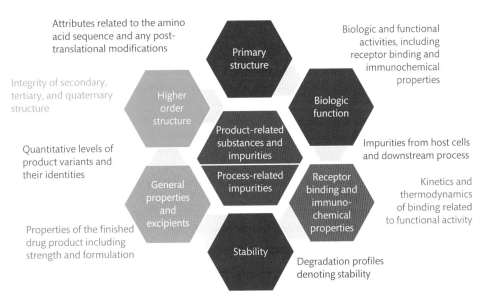

Figure 34.2 Characterization of a biosimilar. (A) Similar to traditional drug development processes, biosimilar development requires what FDA describes as a 'totality-of-the-evidence' approach whereby the majority of data leading to a claim of biosimilarity is generated via extensive analytical evaluation (including PK bioequivalence studies, immunogenicity, and toxicology studies). The financial savings in biosimilar development are due primarily to the extrapolation across indications and the limited clinical trial programme mandated for drug approval. (B) Examples of 'totality-of-the-evidence'. (C) A critical quality attribute (CQA) is a physical, chemical, biological, or microbiological property or characteristic that should be within an appropriate limit, range, or distribution to ensure desired product quality. CQAs may also be important in evaluation of product stability, overall biologic activity, and determination of overall purity. Ongoing evaluation of CQA's is an important aspect of quality risk management with biosimilar production.

www.fda.gov/downloads/AdvisoryCommittees/CommitteesMeetingMaterials/Drugs/AdvisoryCommitteeforPharmaceuticalScienceandClinicalPharmacology/UCM315764

(C) Example of a Biosimilar Monoclonal Antibody and Its CQAs

CQA 2
*Cell Line and
Process Dependent
TNFα neutralization*

Disulfide
integrity

Antigen
binding

Non-CQA

*Cell Line–
Independent
CQA: Primary
Structure*

CQA 1
*Cell Line Dependent
Higher order structure*

Fc-mediated
binding

CQA 4
*Cell Line and
Process Dependent
Content and Product
related impurities*

CQA 3
*Cell Line Dependent
FcRn binding*

Non-CQA

Figure 34.2 Continued

Approximately 90% confidence intervals (CI) of the geometric means of the aforementioned parameters must fall fully between 80% and 125%, a broadly accepted ICH definition of PK equivalency. PK and pharmacodynamic measures (if available) must be assessed, as well as immunogenicity and safety, following the single dose of each product.

Single or multiple active comparator trials for equivalency

Finally, a head-to-head clinical trial of biosimilar and reference product should be performed in at least one of the clinical indications for use of the reference product.[24] The design is based on previous randomized controlled trials (RCTs) of the reference product in an approved clinical indication, and should more stringently demonstrate equivalence, not non-inferiority. The equivalence margin is selected to preserve >70–75% of the effect size seen in a meta-analysis of RCTs of the reference product. The lower limit of the 95% CI for a difference between biosimilar and reference product must not cross the equivalence margin to ensure non-inferiority of the biosimilar. Biosimilar equivalence trials tend to have subtly different designs (**Figure 34.3**), therefore it cannot be stated categorically that they are equivalent to one another (although they are all equivalent to the reference product).[25]

Study populations, treatment regimen, and trial endpoints

A variety of trial designs have been utilized to demonstrate clinical equivalence of a biosimilar to its US/EMA or ex-US/EMA manufactured reference product, with the understanding that this will provide the data for extrapolation of use of the biosimilar to the other clinical indications for which the reference product is approved.[26] It is expected that the population, primary endpoint, sample size, and study duration will be adequately sensitive to detect relevant differences between biosimilar and reference product, should they exist. Typically, only one indication is selected although several TNFi and rituximab biosimilars have been studied in two indications, one with and one without background methotrexate (MTX) therapy, for example, RA and psoriasis (Ps) (TNF inhibitor), or RA and follicular lymphoma (rituximab), as a means to better understand immunogenicity.

Of importance is to select a sensitive endpoint to detect potential clinical differences, as well as the choice of the margin to define equivalence.[25] For TNFi biosimilars, RCTs in RA or Ps have been most frequently selected, based on the sensitivity of the American College of Rheumatology (ACR) response criteria and the Psoriasis Area and Severity Index (PASI) score. For example, these endpoints best distinguished the reference product adalimumab from placebo treatment in four RCTs in RA and two in Ps. Across eight sponsors with adalimumab biosimilars, four have performed trials in RA with endpoints at 12 and/or 24 weeks. Three trials in Ps populations have used PASI75 at 12 or 16 weeks as efficacy endpoints and 1 RCT in both indications was designed specifically to assess different rates of immunogenicity.

The choice of treatment regimen and study population will also be based on prior RCTs utilizing the reference product. Psoriasis (Ps) has been selected as an indication where background MTX therapy is not used, and so potentially more likely to highlight differences in immunogenicity. RA has been selected specifically to study MTX inadequate responders where background therapy should decrease

Biosimilar Clinical Trials: Key Considerations and Decision Points

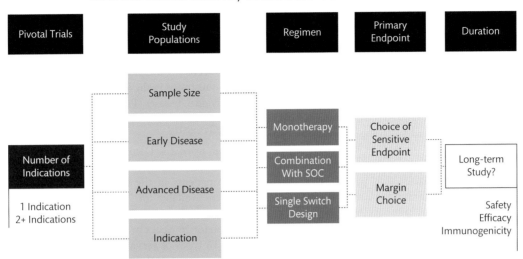

Figure 34.3 Variables to be considered in developing a clinical trial programme for biosimilars. Note that FDA/EMA definitions of biosimilarity allow for extrapolation of data among various patient populations. Trial endpoints may be clinical and/or based on pharmacokinetic and immunogenicity analysis. Some sponsors have chosen to study more than one patient population in multiple trial designs and indications. Implicit in the trial design is that populations studied as well as endpoints, sample sizes, and study duration should be adequately sensitive to detect potential differences between reference product and biosimilar, should they exist.
www.fda.gov/Downloads/Drugs/GuidanceComplianceRegulatoryInformation/Guidances/UCM291128

immunogenicity. Of interest, a single trial in spondyloarthropathy (SpA) without background MTX demonstrated lower levels of immunogenicity than in RA for both reference product and biosimilar, without an obvious explanation other than the difference in underlying disease.[27]

Other decisions include the patient population, whether it be early or advanced disease, and specifically chosen according to prior RCTs with the reference product as well as the ability to accrue patients into an active comparator trial. Some sponsors have allowed previous exposure to biologic agents (<2 agents or non-TNFi's) and others required that they be biologic naïve. Initial concerns about a lack of comparability of results in Crohn's disease populations compared with RA populations have not been confirmed in subsequent investigations, including observational

studies and one RCT.[28,29] Design elements among the numerous adalimumab biosimilars in RA trials exemplifies this variability (Table 34.1).

Single or multiple switch studies

Despite stringent regulatory guidances that define biosimilars to be highly similar or comparable to their reference products, questions remain about switching from originator to biosimilar, particularly mandated 'non-medical' switches.[30] Most of the recent RCTs comparing TNFi or rituximab biosimilars have included a single switch from reference product to biosimilar in an extension phase after the primary endpoint has been reached. Some have transitioned all patients receiving reference product to biosimilar; others have re-randomized patients to continue reference product or switch to

Table 34.1 Key trial design elements for adalimumab biosimilars in RA

Company	Amgen	Boehringer Ingelheim	Fuji Film Kyowa Kirin	Pfizer	Samsung Bioepis
Drug	ABP-501	BI 695501	FKB327	PF-06410293	SB5
Disease activity *	≥6 S, ≥6 T	≥6 S, ≥6 T ESR>28 or CRP>1.0	≥6 S, ≥6 T CRP≥1.0	≥6 S, ≥6 T hsCRP≥0.8	≥6 S, ≥6 T ESR>28 or CRP>1.0
Prior biological Rx	<2	<2	<2	Not permitted	Not permitted
Stable MTX required	7.5–25 mg/wk	15–25 mg/wk	10–25 mg/wk	?dose	10–25 mg/wk
Transition ** design	26 wk OLE	24 wk exten; Humira® vs. ADAbs	OLE 2 arms transition 1 OLE at wk 52	Humira® arm randomized wk s26, wk 52 OLE	Blinded transition wk 24
1° end point	ACR20, 24 wk	ACR20, 12 & 24 wk	ACR 20, 24 wk	ACR 20, 12 wk	ACR 20, 24 wk

*T, tender joints, S, swollen joints **OLE, open-label extension, ADAbs, adalimumab biosimilar

Adapted from Lai Z. and La Noce A. Key design considerations on comparative clinical efficacy studies for biosimilars: adalimumab as an example. *RMD Open* 2016;2:e000154. doi: 10.1136/rmdopen-2015-000154 with permission from the BMJ Publishing Group biosimilar. In general, long-term data after week 52 have included only open-label treatment with the biosimilar.

Now that a guidance defining interchangeability has been released by FDA, requirements for a multiple switch trial are established.[19] To date, two sponsors have initiated RCTs in plaque psoriasis with multiple switches. GP2015 is the only FDA-approved biosimilar of etanercept. The EGALITY trial is a phase III RCT in patients with Ps incorporating two multiple switching arms between GP2015 and etanercept.[31] Patients were randomized to remain on GP2015 or etanercept, or to undergo repeated switching between the two treatments (three switches at 6-week intervals to week 30) and then maintain treatment to week 52. Repeated switching had no impact on efficacy, safety, or immunogenicity.

Recently a multiswitch trial was initiated with BI695501, a biosimilar of adalimumab, in plaque psoriasis, with the intent of securing an interchangeability label when and if ultimately approved.[32]

Longitudinal observational switching studies: NOR-SWITCH and DANBIO registry

NOR-SWITCH

The biosimilar infliximab Remsima® was approved for marketing in Norway in 2013, and in 2015 Celltrion further reduced the price by 69% of the reference product price, thereby making it the preferred product. The Norwegian government assigned 20 million NOK in the national budget for 2014 to perform a switch study. This was an RCT conducted over 12 months which included 498 eligible patients with RA, SpA, psoriatic arthritis (PsA), Ps, CD, or ulcerative colitis (UC) who were on stable treatment with Remicade® for ≥6 months and were randomized blindly to continue it or switch to the biosimilar infliximab.[33] The primary endpoint for non-inferiority was disease worsening across all indications with a margin of +/−15%. In the full analysis set of 481 individuals across all indications non-inferiority was demonstrated in the aggregate, as the trial was not powered for the individual diseases (**Figure 34.4**).

DANBIO registry

Based on price, the Danish government mandated a switch from reference product Remicade® to biosimilar Remsima® in 2015. Of 802 patients in the DANBIO registry receiving infliximab, data were available for 769: RA: 403, SpA: 279 and PsA: 120.[34] Healthcare utilization following this 'non-medical switch' was collected for 26 weeks prior to and 26 weeks following the switch. Use of 16 types of services relevant to the specialty of rheumatology was identified and included outpatient visits, infliximab infusions, nurse counselling, phone consultations, and musculoskeletal ultrasound. No negative impact on disease activity was seen after 12 months although adjusted 1-year CT-P13 retention rate was slightly lower than for INX in a historic cohort.

Prospective open-label observational studies

Numerous pharmaceutical company sponsored trials, have compared a biosimilar product to a reference agent with uniform

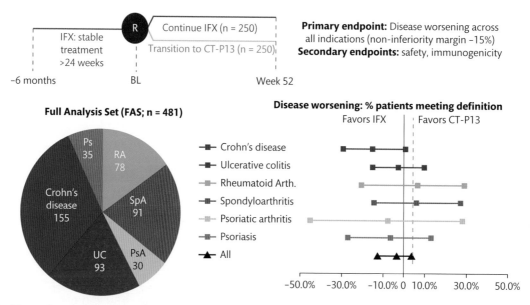

Figure 34.4 The Norwegian government mandated this switch study in 2014. This non-inferiority RCT was conducted over 12 months. 498 eligible patients with RA, SpA, PsA, Ps, CD, or UC on stable Remicade® therapy for ≥6 months were randomized to continue Remicade® or switch to biosimilar infliximab. The primary endpoint for non-inferiority was disease worsening across all indications with a margin of +/−15%. The data analysis was not powered to test non-inferiority for individual disease categories.

Data sourced from Jorgensen KK, Olsen IC, Goll GL et al. Switching from originator infliximab to biosimilar CT-P13 compared with maintained treatment with originator infliximab (NOR-SWITCH): a 52-week, randomised, double-blind, non-inferiority trial. *Lancet* 2017;389:2304–16.

equivalent efficacy, safety, and discontinuation rates (as would be predicted based on biosimilarity).[35,36] However, real-world switching studies may not always reveal similar outcomes. In these studies, 'non-medical switching' from a reference product to a biosimilar has typically been mandated by the government.[33,37] In several studies, a greater reporting of adverse events (AEs) and patient discontinuation occurred consistent with the 'nocebo' response, whereby the patient and/or physician feels that they may have been prescribed an inferior product.[35,38,39] Overall the additional discontinuation rate is approximately 10%. Most investigators consider this due to psychological factors, including expectation bias on the part of patients and/or physicians.

Immunogenicity

Several systematic literature reviews have summarized the immunogenicity of approved biosimilars versus their reference products.[40] The PK variables in the initial bridging studies have supported comparability between the products, as well as by immunogenicity and safety.

Observational studies have shown cross-reactivity (e.g. similar immunodominant epitopes), between reference product and biosimilars, and that assays designed to detect immunogenicity with one will also detect it with the other.

Assays

Current assays for immunogenicity are more sensitive than the enzyme-linked immunosorbent assays (ELISA) or radioimmunoassays (RAI) utilized for reference products at the time of their approval, in which biologic serum levels would interfere with the assay. The newer assays include electrochemiluminescence (ECLIA) or flow-through microfluidic immunoassays, typically performed after acid dissociation to disrupt antidrug antibody (ADAb)-mAb complexes.[41]

Three procedures are performed:

- Screening, for overall ADAb status
- If positive, confirmation using a 'competitive' or 'inhibition' assay, and
- Characterization for neutralizing ADAbs (NAbs)

Data comparing biosimilars to reference products

Overall, immunogenicity has been shown to be comparable between biosimilars and their reference products, but at a higher rate than cited in the original Summary of Product Characteristics or labels of the originators.[39] Newer assays have greater sensitivity, and less interference from circulating drug than the older ELISA and radioimmunoassays. Thus, reported values for ADAb levels of 38% with biosimilar (Amgevita® / Amjevita™ or Amgevita®/Solymbic®) are similar to reference adalimumab in RA with background MTX therapy (38%).[42] Neutralizing antibody (Nab) levels of 9–11% (biosimilar) compare with NAbs of 9–13% (reference adalimumab) in Ps with monotherapy, yet overall immunogenicity was detected in 52% receiving the biosimilar vs. 64% with the reference product.[43] Significantly lower levels were reported with biosimilar (Brenzys™ or Benepali®) vs. reference etanercept: 1% vs. 13.1%, although ADAbs were largely transient without significant differences in safety or circulating

drug levels (which are lower with clinically significant immunogenicity). More patients withdrew due to injection site reactions with the reference product (2 vs. 7) although this did not clearly relate to ADAbs.[44]

Interchangeability and substitution: Unique to United States

As previously noted, interchangeability is a regulatory designation only in the United States. Currently 23 states have legislation that will prevent automatic substitution of the interchangeable biosimilar for the reference product without the approval of the prescribing healthcare provider.[45] It is anticipated that availability of biosimilars will most likely rely more upon the pharmacy benefit managers, based on cost considerations. At this time, it is unclear what advantages a designation of interchangeability will offer.

Extrapolation to other clinical indications

Central to the concept of biosimilarity is the extrapolation of data from a single RCT in one clinical indication to all other indications for which the reference product is approved—thus the significant cost savings in development. While initially met with scepticism, now that multiple biosimilars have been approved and are in use in the EU and ex-US, it has become clear both with registry data and now at least one post-approval RCT that both safety and efficacy data do indeed extrapolate across indications.[46] Initially Health Canada did not approve extrapolation of biosimilar infliximab to Crohn's disease, due to concerns around a possible difference in ADCC potency between biosimilar and reference product. Subsequently, this decision was reversed.[47] Cost savings attributed to biosimilars have markedly increased the availability of biologic therapies across Eastern EU countries with lower gross domestic product (GDP), as well as across the western EU.

Pharmacoeconomic ramifications

Multiple investigations have established varying degrees of bDMARD accessibility among countries, complicating financial projections. Factors include group attributes (country welfare [measured as GDP]) and individual attributes (overall disease activity [measured by DAS], socioeconomic status) as well as acceptability and affordability. Real-world use of bDMARDS varies significantly among less affluent central and eastern European countries with criteria for accessibility being stricter in less affluent countries. Assuming a willingness to replace reference products, the financial ramifications of less expensive biosimilars in these countries is obvious. However, cost savings will benefit the healthcare system as a whole and will not necessarily increase biologic accessibility. This will vary from country to country, and possibly from one healthcare provider to another.

Several recent pharmacoeconomic analyses of the potential for biosimilars to reduce costs and increase patient access to bDMARDs have been published.[48,49] The budgetary impact of switching patients to CT-P13 (biosimilar infliximab) for RA in the United Kingdom, Germany, Italy, the Netherlands, and Belgium on an annual basis ranged from a potential saving of €2.89 million in Belgium (10% discount) to €33.8 million in Germany (30% discount).[50] Similar reports of financial savings following introduction of CT-P13 in other countries including Ireland, Bulgaria, the Czech Republic, Hungary, Poland, Romania, and Slovakia have all been published.[51,52] Real-world data confirm these projections: in both Japan and Norway CT-P13 (renamed infliximab-BS-NK in Japan), is 67% and 69% cheaper, respectively, compared to reference infliximab.[53] To date, over 34 000 patients in >40 countries have been treated with this agent.[54] Fifteen months after introduction of CT-P13 in South Korea about 20% of infliximab claims were for the biosimilar. In the United Kingdom, the National Institute for Health and Care Excellence (NICE) has provided guidance to rheumatologists stating 'treatment should be initiated with the least expensive drug'. At the time of writing most UK rheumatologists will prescribe a biosimilar, when available, for patients initiating a biologic therapy. Switching remains more variable although some payers are starting to mandate non-medical switching for patients with stable, low disease activity on a reference product. Belgium and Germany have developed a quota system, which drives physicians to prescribe biosimilars in up to 40% of their patients. Denmark required non-medical switches to the respective biosimilar as soon as it was available, and data have been collected and published in the DANBIO registry confirming comparability after switching.[33] Despite modest uptake of biosimilars in the United States to date, one recent review predicts potential savings of 54 billion US$ over the next ten years based on 2016 data.[55] A lower to upper saving estimate range from 25 to 150 billion US$ was projected based on rapidly changing aspects of the healthcare and insurance landscape. Several issues unique to the United States are likely to impact biosimilar acceptance. US FDA guidance on differences between biosimilarity and interchangeability are incomplete at this time. This lack of precision in product labelling discourages price competition. Secondly, the complex naming system for each biosimilar agent encourages perceptions of differences and discourages price competition. Automatic dispensing of a biosimilar product by a pharmacy benefit manager programme is likely to be poorly accepted by treating rheumatologists. The lack of a single insurance payer system in the United States precluding significant reductions in price through discounting by pharmaceutical companies is another problem compared with single payer EU countries. Ultimately cost savings will be divided among multiple groups in the United States: pharmaceutical industry, insurance companies, government, and patients, with biosimilar uptake being dependent on all of these aspects contributing to a changing landscape.[56]

Naming and labelling

In the EU biosimilars are referred to by their trade names, which differ from the brand-name reference product, although the INNs

Table 34.2 TNFi and rituximab biosimilars marketed in the EU*

Biosimilar	Company	Name
Infliximab	Celltrion	Remsima Inflectra Flammegis
	Samsung Bioepis	Flixabi
Adalimumab	Amgen	Amgevita Solymbic
	Samsung Bioepis	Imraldi
Etanercept	Sandoz	Erelzi
	Samsung Bioepis	Benepali
Rituximab	Celltrion	Truxima Blitzima Tuxella Ritemvia
	Sandoz	Rixathon Riximuo

* (2016 data)

are the same.[16] In the United States, a randomly generated four-letter suffix is added to the proper US name, not necessarily the INN, and each product has a different brand name.[18]

Postmarketing surveillance

Assuming all postmarketing surveillance of the reference product has been completed, FDA does not mandate further surveillance after biosimilar approval. In contrast, both Health Canada and EMA request postmarketing surveillance plans in conjunction with the biosimilar submission package.[17] The summary of safety concerns should be the same as for the reference product. EMA requires any post authorization risk management plan for a reference product to be similarly applied to the relevant biosimilar.

Real-world use of biosimilars applicable to rheumatoid arthritis

The following tables show the TNFi biosimilars marketed in the EU, United States, and Canada at time of authorship (2017) (Tables 34.2–34.4).

Table 34.3 TNFi biosimilars marketed in the US

Biosimilar	Company	Name
Infliximab	Pfizer	Infliximab-dyyb: Inflectra™
	Merck	Infliximab-abda: Renflexis™
Etanercept	Sandoz	Etanercept-szzs: Erelzi™
Adalimumab	Amgen	Adalimumab-atto: Amjevita™

Table 34.4 TNFi biosimilars marketed in Canada

Biosimilar	Company	Name
Infliximab	Pfizer	Inflectra®
Etanercept	Samsung Bioepis	Benepali®

International consensus and conclusions

For biosimilars to become widely used in clinical rheumatology, both the rheumatologist and their patients' confidence in the regulatory process is mandatory. An international group of experts recently reported their guidance.[57] The ACR has similarly published a 'white paper' outlining its position.[58]

Overarching principles and recommendations are summarized in Box 34.1.

Several unanswered questions still remain. Multiple switch studies between biosimilar and reference products have only recently been initiated. Switching studies using multiple different biosimilars have never been performed. Optimal postmarketing pharmacovigilance of biosimilars, and the design of registries, have not been defined by consensus. These will obviously vary from country to country but attempts at standardization may become important. Legal disputes in the United States among pharmaceutical manufacturers continue to delay accessibility to these agents. Future challenges will continue to make this a rapidly evolving and exciting chapter in rheumatic disease therapeutics.

Box 34.1 Summary of principles and recommendations

1 Treatment of rheumatic diseases is based on a shared decision-making process between patients and their physicians. Patients and healthcare providers should be informed about the nature of biosimilars, their approval process, and their safety and efficacy.

2 A biosimilar is neither better nor worse in efficacy and not inferior in safety to its reference product. Approved biosimilars can be used to treat appropriate patients in the same way as their reference products. The availability of biosimilars must significantly lower the cost of treating an individual patient as well as increase access to optimal therapy for most patients.

3 Relevant preclinical and pivotal clinical trial data should be published. Since a biosimilar is equivalent to the reference product in its physicochemical, functional, and pharmacokinetic properties, confirmation of efficacy and safety in a single indication is sufficient for extrapolation to other diseases for which the reference product has been approved.

4 As no clinically significant differences in immunogenicity between biosimilars and their products have been detected, ADAbs to biosimilars need not be measured in clinical practice.

5 Currently available evidence indicates that a single switch from a reference product to one of its biosimilars is safe and effective; there is no scientific rationale to expect that switching among biosimilars of the same reference product would result in a different clinical outcome. Multiple switching between biosimilars and their reference products or other biosimilars should be assessed in registries.

6 Harmonized methods should be established to obtain reliable pharmacovigilance data, including traceability, about both biosimilars and reference products.

REFERENCES

1. Declerck P, Danesi R, Petersel D, Jacobs I. The language of biosimilars: clarification, definitions, and regulatory aspects. *Drugs* 2017;77:671–7.
2. Doerner T, Strand V, Castanedo-Hernandez G, et al. The role of biosimilars in the treatment of rheumatic diseases. *Ann Rheum Dis* 2013;72(3):322–8.
3. US FDA. *How Drugs Are Developed and Approved*, 2014. Available at: http://www.fda.gov/Drugs/DevelopmentApprovalProcess/HowDrugsareDevelopedandApproved/ApprovalApplications/TherapeuticBiologicApplications/Biosimilars/default.htm
4. European Medicines Agency and the European Commission. *Biosimilars in the EU—Information Guide for Healthcare Professionals.* Available at: http://www.ema.europa.eu/docs/en_GB/document_library/Leaflet/2017/05/WC500226648.pdf
5. Regulatory Affairs Professional Society. *FDA approves 6th Biosimilar in US—Second for Humira*, 2017. Available at: http://www.raps.org/Regulatory-Focus/News/2017/08/28/28340/FDA-Approves-6th-Biosimilar-in-US-Second-for-Humira/
6. Bioworld. *Amgen-Abbvie Agreement Erases Uncertainty for Humira Biosimilar.* Available at: http://www.bioworld.com/content/amgen-abbvie-agreement-erases-uncertainty-humira-biosimilar-0
7. Hassett B, Sheinberg M, Casteneda-Hernandez G, et al. Variability of intended copies for etanercept (Enbrel®): data on multiple batches of seven products. *MAbs* 2018;10(1):166–76.
8. Schiestl M, Stangler T, Torella C, et al. Acceptable changes in quality attributes of glycosylated biopharmaceuticals. *Nat Biotechnol* 2011;29(4):310–12.
9. McCamish M, Woollett G. The state of the art in the development of biosimilars. *Clinical Pharm Ther* 2012;91:405–17.
10. Schneider CK. Biosimilars in rheumatology: the wind of change. *Ann Rheum Dis* 2013;72:315–18.
11. Lee JF Litten JB Grampp G. Comparability and biosimilarity: considerations for the healthcare provider. *Curr Med Res Opin* 2012;28:1053–8.
12. U.S. Food and Drug Administration (FDA). *CMC Postapproval Manufacturing Changes for Specified Biological Products to be Documented in Annual Reports*, 2017. Available at: https://www.fda.gov/downloads/drugs/guidancecomplianceregulatoryinformation/guidances/ucm570441.pdf
13. Ramanan SI, Grampp G. Drift, evolution, and divergence in biologics and biosimilars manufacturing. *BioDrugs* 2014;28:363–72.
14. Kozlowski S, Woodcock J, Midthun K, et al. Developing the nation's biosimilars program. *N Engl J Med* 2011;365:385–8.
15. Reichert JM, Beck A, Iyer H. European Medicines Agency workshop on biosimilar monoclonal antibodies July 2, 2009, London, UK. *MAbs* 2009;1:394–416.
16. European Medicines Agency. *Multidisciplinary: Biosimilar.* Available at: http://www.ema.europa.eu/ema/index.jsp?curl=pages/regulation/general/general_content_000408.jsp&mid=WC0b01ac058002958c
17. European Medicines Agency. *Guidelines on Good Pharmacovigilance Practices (GVP)*, 2017. Available at: http://www.ema.europa.eu/docs/en_GB/document_library/Regulatory_and_procedural_guideline/2017/10/WC500236404.pdf
18. U.S. Food and Drug Administration (FDA). *Compliance Program Guidance Manual (CPGM)*, 2015. Available at: https://www.

fda.gov/Drugs/GuidanceComplianceRegulatoryInformation/Guidances/ucm290967.htm

19. U.S. Food and Drug Administration (FDA). *Considerations in Demonstrating Interchangeability with a Reference Product Guidance for Industry*, 2019. Available at: https://www.fda.gov/downloads/Drugs/GuidanceComplianceRegulatoryInformation/Guidances/UCM537135.pdf

20. Government of Canada. *Biosimilar Biologic Drugs in Canada: Fact Sheet*. Available at: https://www.canada.ca/en/health-canada/services/drugs-health-products/biologics-radiopharmaceuticals-genetic-therapies/applications-submissions/guidance-documents/fact-sheet-biosimilars.html

21. Roger SD. Biosimilars: how similar or dissimilar are they? *Nephrology (Carlton)* 2006;*11*:341–6.

22. Mellstedt H, Niederwieser D, Ludwig H. The challenge of biosimilars. *Ann Oncol* 2008;*19*:411–19.

23. Kuhlmann M, Covic A. The protein science of biosimilars. *Nephrol Dial Transplant* 2006;*21*(Suppl 5):4–8.

24. Doerner T, Strand V, Cornes P, et al. The changing landscape of biosimilars in rheumatology. *Ann Rheum Dis* 2016;*0*:1–9.

25. Kay J, Isaacs JD. Clinical trials of biosimilars should become more similar. *Ann Rheum Dis* 2017;*76*:4–6.

26. Lai Z, La Noce A. Key design considerations on comparative clinical efficacy studies for biosimilars: adalimumab as an example. *RMD Open* 2016;*2*:e000154.

27. Braun J. Letter: response to: 'Infliximab and CT-P13 immuno-genicity assessment in PLANETAS and PLANETRA main and extension studies: utility of laboratory methods description' by Francesca Meacci et al. *Ann Rheum Dis* 2016;*75*:e63.

28. Deiana S, Gabbani T, Annese V. Biosimilars in Inflammatory bowel disease: a review of post-marketing experience. *World J Gastroenterol* 2017;*23*:197–203.

29. The Center for Biosimilars. *New Data Support Switching to Biosimilar CT-P13 in Patients with Crohn's Disease*, 2017. Available at: http://www.centerforbiosimilars.com/news/new-data-support-switching-to-biosimilar-ctp13-in-patients-with-crohns-disease

30. Toussirot E, Marotte H. Switching from originator biological agents to biosimilars: what is the evidence and what are the issues? *RMD Open* 2017;*3*:e000492.

31. Griffiths CE, Thaci D, Gerdes S, et al. The EGALITY study: a confirmatory, randomised, double blind study comparing the efficacy, safety and immunogenicity of GP2015, a proposed etanercept biosimilar, versus the originator product in patients with moderate to severe chronic plaque-type Ps. *Br J Dermatol* 2017;*176*:928–38.

32. U.S. Library of Medicine. *The VOLTAIRE-X Trial Looks at the Effect of Switching Between Humira® and BI 695501 in Patients with Plaque Psoriasis*, 2019. Available at: https://clinicaltrials.gov/ct2/show/NCT03210259

33. Jorgensen KK, Olsen IC, Goll GL, et al. Switching from originator infliximab to biosimilar CT-P13 compared with maintained treatment with originator infliximab (NOR-SWITCH): a 52-week, randomised, double-blind, non-inferiority trial. *Lancet* 2017;*389*:2304–16.

34. Glintborg B, Sørensen IJ, Loft AG, et al. A nationwide non-medical switch from originator infliximab to biosimilar CT-P13 in 802 patients with inflammatory arthritis: 1-year clinical outcomes from the DANBIO registry. *Ann Rheum Dis* 2017;*76*:1426–31.

35. Moots R, Azevedo A Coindreau, JL, et al. Switching between reference biologics and biosimilars for the treatment of rheumatology,

gastroenterology, and dermatology inflammatory conditions: considerations for the clinician. *Curr Rheumatol Rep* 2017;*19*:37.

36. Tweehuysen L, van den Bemt B, van Ingen I. Subjective complaints as main reason for biosimilar discontinuation after open label transitioning from originator to biosimilar infliximab. *Arth Rheum* 2018;*70*(1):60–8.

37. De Cock D, Kearsley-Fleet L, Watson K, Hyrich KL. Switching from RA originator to biosimilar in routine clinical care: early data from the British Society for Rheumatology biologics register for rheumatoid arthritis [abstract]. *Arth Rheum* 2017;*69* (Suppl 10).

38. Tweehuysen L, Huiskes VJB, Van den Bemt BJF, et al. Open label transitioning from originator etanercept to biosimilar SB4 compared to continuing treatment with originator etanercept in a historical cohort in rheumatic diseases in daily practice [abstract]. *Arth Rheum* 2017;*69* (Suppl 10).

39. Rezk M, Pieper B. Treatment outcomes with biosimilars: be aware of the nocebo effect. *Rheumatol Ther* 2017;*4*:209–18.

40. Chingcuaco F, Segal JB, Kim SC, Alexander GC. Bioequivalence of biosimilar tumor necrosis factor-α inhibitors compared with their reference biologics: a systematic review. *Ann Int Med* 2016;*165*(8):565–74.

41. Park W, Hrycaj P, Jeka S, et al. A randomised, double-blind, multicentre, parallel-group, prospective study comparing the pharmacokinetics, safety, and efficacy of CT-P13 and innovator infliximab in patients with ankylosing spondylitis: the PLANETAS study. *Ann Rheum Dis* 2013;*72*:1605–12.

42. Cohen S, Genovese MC, Choy E, et al. Efficacy and safety of the biosimilar ABP 501 compared with adalimumab in patients with moderate to severe rheumatoid arthritis: a randomised, double-blind, phase III equivalence study. *Ann Rheum Dis* 2017;*76*:1679–87.

43. Papp K, Bachelez H, Costanzo A, et al. Clinical similarity of the biosimilar ABP 501 compared with adalimumab after single transition: long-term results from a randomized controlled, double-blind, 52-week, phase III trial in patients with moderate-to-severe plaque psoriasis. *Br J Dermatol* 2017;*177*(6):1562–74.

44. Emery P, Vencovský J, Sylwestrzak A, et al. A phase III randomised, double-blind, parallel-group study comparing SB4 with etanercept reference product in patients with active rheumatoid arthritis despite methotrexate therapy. *Ann Rheum Dis* 2017;*76*:51–7.

45. National Conference of State Legislatures (NCSL). *State Laws and Legislation Related to Biologic Medications and Substitution of Biosimilars*, 2018. Available at: http://www.ncsl.org/research/health/state-laws-and-legislation-related-to-biologic-medications-and-substitution-of-biosimilars.aspx

46. Toussirot E, Marotte H. Switching from originator biological agents to biosimilars: what is the evidence and what are the issues? *RMD Open* 2017;*3*:e000492.

47. Danese S, Fiorino G, Raine T, et al. ECCO position statement on the use of biosimilars for inflammatory bowel disease—an update. *J Crohn's Colitis* 2017;*11*(1):26–34.

48. Lulacsi L, Brodszky V, Baji P, et al. Biosimilars for management of rheumatoid arthritis: economic considerations. *Expert Rev Clin Immunol* 2015;*11*(Suppl 1):S43–S52.

49. Inotai A, Csanadi M, Vitezic D, et al. Policy practices to maximise social benefit from biosimilars. *J Bioequiv Availab* 2017;*9*(4):467–72.

50. Jha A, Upton A, Dunlop WC, et al. The budget impact of biosimilar infliximab (remsima) for the treatment of autoimmune diseases in five European countries. *Adv Ther* 2015;*32*:742–56.

51. McCarthy G, Guy H. Introduction of an infliximab biosimilar (CT-P13): a five-year budget impact analysis for the treatment of rheumatoid arthritis in Ireland. *Value in Health* 2013; PMS22.

52. Brodszky V, Baji P, Balogh O, et al. Budget impact analysis of biosimilar infliximab (CT-P13) for the treatment of rheumatoid arthritis in six Central and Eastern European countries. *Eur J Health Econ* 2014;*15*(Suppl 1):S65–71.

53. Dorner T, Strand V, Cornes P, et al. The changing landscape of biosimilars in rheumatology. *Ann Rheum Dis* 2016;*75*(6):974–82.

54. Jahnsen J. Clinical experience with infliximab biosimilar Remsima (CT-P13) in inflammatory bowel disease patients. *Therap Adv Gastroenterol* 2016;*9*:322–9.

55. Mulcahy AW, Jakub P, Hlavka, Case SR. *Biosimilar Cost Savings in the United States: Initial Experience and Future Potential.* Santa Monica, CA: RAND Corporation, 2017. Available at: https://www.rand.org/pubs/perspectives/PE264.html

56. Frank RG. Friction in the path to use of biosimilar. *Drugs NEJM* 2018;*378*:791–793.

57. Kay J, Schoels MM, Doerner T, et al. Consensus-based recommendations for the use of biosimilars to treat rheumatological diseases. *Ann Rheum Dis* 2017;*77*(2):165–74.

58. Bridges Jr. SL, White DW, Worthing AB, et al. The science behind biosimilars-entering a new era of biologic therapy. *Arth Rheumatol* 2018;*70*:334–44.

35

Immunogenicity in response to biologic agents

Meghna Jani, John Isaacs, and Vibeke Strand

Introduction

Biologic agents such as tumour necrosis factor alpha (TNFα) inhibitors (TNFis) have transformed outcomes in rheumatological conditions such as rheumatoid arthritis (RA). However, up to 40% of patients do not respond to TNFis from the outset or lose response over time. Biologics and biosimilars are biotechnology-derived proteins and have the potential to be highly immunogenic. In a proportion of patients, the immune response provoked by a biologic agent leads to the production of antidrug antibodies (ADAb), or immunogenicity. This is because the immune system can detect minor alterations in the three-dimensional structure between an introduced molecule and a native protein.[1] Antibody formation is a potential hazard of all protein drugs, and has been well described ever since protein therapeutics were introduced.[2] Examples include porcine/bovine insulin, growth hormone, other monoclonal antibodies such as natalizumab (a therapeutic antibody against α4 integrin), therapeutic proteins such as type I interferons in the treatment of multiple sclerosis, and recombinant erythropoietin. Immunogenicity can lead to serious safety concerns, such as pure red cell aplasia leading to profound anaemia in chronic kidney disease treated with erythropoietin.[1,3]

Development of immunogenicity can influence the treatment response to TNFi drugs with the formation of ADAb against monoclonal antibodies, while fusion proteins such as etanercept appear much less immunogenic. The majority of evidence has been described in infliximab and adalimumab-treated patients, in whom development of immunogenicity has been linked with both clinical response and adverse events. The reported prevalence of ADAbs can vary considerably between studies on the same agent. This is because a number of factors can affect immunogenicity. The subject of immunogenicity has also received much recent attention due to the introduction of biosimilars and new therapeutics within the rheumatology armamentarium. In this chapter we review the pharmacological implications of the ADAb response, interpretation of levels based on the techniques used for measurement, the clinical significance in terms of efficacy/safety for each of the available biologics, the issues around biosimilars and immunogenicity, the potential to tolerize to ADAbs, and future directions.

Pharmacological implications of the antidrug antibody response

On-going immunogenic stimulation by a protein therapeutic can have variable consequences depending on the type of antibodies induced: neutralizing or non-neutralizing, the key difference being the effect they have on efficacy. ADAbs are said to be either binding antibodies (non-neutralizing)[4] or neutralizing and can alter pharmacokinetics of the drug, decrease efficacy, and in some cases induce immune complex mediated adverse events. Binding antibodies can either expedite the clearance of the biologic, termed clearing bodies, or can prolong bioavailability, called sustaining bodies.[5] The difference in effects between binding and neutralizing antibodies is attributable to the epitopes they bind to: binding antibodies bind to sites within the biologic drug molecule that do not participate in the interaction with its receptor target, whereas neutralizing antibodies interact with the epitope on the biologic molecule that is functionally relevant for ligand-receptor interaction, thereby compromising therapeutic efficacy.[4] The latter are sometimes referred to as anti-idiotype antibodies. Neutralizing antibodies are primarily composed of IgG isotypes and it is reported that the neutralizing properties of IgG4 subtype is higher than IgG1 and IgG2,[4] both measured by different types of assays covered in Section 4. The presence of ADAbs therefore affects treatment response through limiting both the pharmacokinetics and pharmacodynamics of the drug.[6]

The factors that predispose to immunogenicity

Drug structure and sequence variation

All biologics, due to their protein structure not being identical to endogenous immunoglobulins, are capable of stimulating an immune response and production of ADAbs, which is a typical

T-cell-dependent immune response.[7] Proteins with non-human chimeric sources such as infliximab, have demonstrated considerable immunogenicity in patients,[8] resulting in human antichimeric antibodies. Humanized antibodies contain foreign complementarity determining regions (CDRs) within a human V-region framework, thereby providing immunogenic epitopes. In terms of fully human antibodies, such as adalimumab and golimumab, the gene rearrangements that underpin antibody diversity mean that human CDRs are not germline-encoded and therefore escape central tolerance induction rendering them potentially immunogenic. In addition, allotypes exist in antibody constant and variable regions, providing further potentially immunogenic epitopes. Furthermore, glycosylation, contaminants arising during the formulation process as well as aspects of the drug production process such as presence of aggregates, impurities, and excipients may also contribute.

Individual and treatment related factors

The individual ADAb response is dependent on the immunocompetence of the patient, type of disease, and unknown factors such as genetic predisposition. From a clinician's perspective, modifiable treatment related factors may include the dose/frequency of the biologic, the route of administration, interruption in drug therapy and, importantly, concomitant non-biologics disease-modifying antirheumatic drugs (nbDMARDs).[1] Current evidence suggests concomitant methotrexate (MTX) in particular is associated with lower immunogenicity of TNFi agents, especially in RA,[9] confirmed initially in one of the earliest infliximab trials.[5] ADAbs were inversely associated with infliximab dose (53%, 21%, and 7% in patients receiving 1, 3, and 10 mg/kg monotherapy, respectively), and the use of concomitant MTX at a dose of 7.5 mg/week greatly diminished the appearance of ADAbs, with incidence rates of 15%, 7%, and 0% at the three dose levels. A more recent meta-analysis revealed that the use of immunomodulatory, primarily MTX, reduced the proportion of patients on infliximab and adalimumab with detectable ADAbs by 41% (risk ratio (RR) = 0.59, 95% CI 0.50, 0.70).[10,11] Current evidence indicates that MTX, leflunomide, azathioprine, and mycophenolate mofetil are best at abrogating immunogenicity, perhaps because they are antiproliferative, as long as they are administered before or with the first dose of the protein drug. Other nbDMARDs such as sulfasalazine and hydroxychloroquine may have a more attenuated effect on drug ADAbs and consequently drug levels.[12]

Detection of antidrug antibodies

The detection of ADAbs can often be underestimated due to interference with assays by circulating free drug. Therefore, the timing of the sample is important, preferably before the patient is due their next dose (i.e. trough levels: when the lowest amount of drug is in the bloodstream). ADAbs may be measured in non-trough samples but, due to the presence of free drug, the use of enzyme-linked immunosorbent assays (ELISA) in this setting is less sensitive compared to more drug-tolerant techniques such as radioimmunoassay (RIA).[13,14] Therefore, the type and timing of assays can often explain differences in ADAb rates observed in randomized controlled trials (RCTs) and observational studies.

Measuring immunogenicity

The European Medicines Agency (EMA) and the US Food and Drug Administration (FDA) have developed guidelines for the assessment of the immunogenicity of monoclonal antibodies for *in vivo* clinical use, which outline the mandatory requirements for the approval of biopharmaceuticals.[15,16] However clinical trials have previously underestimated the true prevalence of immunogenicity due to less sensitive tests, with the reported frequency of ADAbs in the Summary of Product Characteristics for monoclonal antibodies being typically low (3–18%). A number of methods have been used in observational studies to detect the presence of ADAbs, including a bridging or double-antigen/sandwich ELISA and the radioimmunoassay (RIA) antigen-binding test (ABT), discussed in more detail next.[17] However, the EMA and FDA insist on more modern assays for new products and biosimilars.

Bridging ELISA test

ELISA tests have been most frequently used to measure immunogenicity in clinical trials due to their simplicity, convenient assay format, low cost, high throughput, and elimination of the need for a special laboratory with radioactivity facilities. Improved assays for detection of ADAbs include the two-site or bridging ELISA test.[16] The drug of interest is bound to a solid matrix, to which patient sera are added and ADAb to the drug are detected using a biotinylated form of the drug of interest (Figure 35.1).

Both Fab arms of the ADAb need to be available for binding (Figure 35.1), which increases susceptibility to drug interference. This was demonstrated in a cohort of 216 RA patients treated with adalimumab for 28 weeks, where 15 trough level serum samples (7%) were positive for ADAb using the bridging ELISA assay only when drug levels were undetectable, compared to 29 (13%) using the RIA.[18] The bridging ELISA also failed to detect the IgG4 ADAb, which plays a prominent role in situations of repeated antigenic stimulation, interferes with efficient binding of the drug and has greater potential for neutralization.[4,19] A previous study in RA found that ADAbs detected against infliximab were predominantly IgG, 36% being IgG4.[20] Human antiglobulins such as rheumatoid factors can also theoretically interfere with ADAb measurement, although the bridging ELISA cannot detect low affinity species due to the need for each arm of the ADAb to bind either the solid surface or the capture reagent. Kappa light chains of infliximab also interfere in measurement, therefore increasing the likelihood of false negative results.

Radioimmunoassay

The RIA ABT uses protein A Sepharose to capture ADAbs from the patient's serum, followed by addition of radio-labelled drug, which will bind to drug-specific antibodies, if present (Figure 35.1). Fluid-phase RIA is not influenced by artefacts induced by solid-phase adsorption of proteins, which constitutes an advantage over solid-phase ELISAs, and better reflecting the situation *in vivo*. The RIA is therefore more specific than the bridging ELISA, less prone to drug interference in the context of trough serum levels,[13,18] can also detect the IgG4 subclass that is functionally monovalent and is less susceptible to artefacts from neo-epitope formation that occur when proteins are fixed to plastic surfaces.[21]

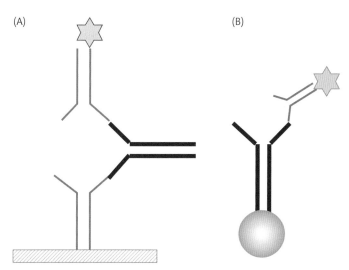

Figure 35.1 Schematic representation of the previous assays to detect ADAbs. (A) Bridging ELISA: anti-TNF drug (blue) is coated on the plate, antidrug antibody (purple) is detected using biotinylated drug. Antidrug antibodies in complex with drug will not be detected using this method, as both Fab arms need to be available. (B) Radioimmunoassay: antibodies to anti-TNF (purple) are captured by protein A-immobilized Sepharose (blue sphere) and detected using radio-labelled drug-F(ab')2.
Source: data from Hart et al. 'Differential effect of drug interference in immunogenicity assays'. *Journal of Immunological Methods* 372 (2011) 196–203.

The need to use radioisotopes, however, makes RIA more complex and expensive than ELISA and, while the RIA only detects IgG1, IgG2, and IgG4 ADAbs, the bridging ELISA will theoretically also detect IgG3, IgA, and possibly IgE antibody classes (but not IgG4). However, when compared directly, the results obtained using a bridging ELISA do not differ substantially from those obtained with the RIA ABT using protein A Sepharose.[18] Furthermore, studies using RIA have shown a significant correlation between ADAb and loss of response to monoclonal antibody therapies in RA as described next. Thus, a major advantage of RIA over bridging ELISAs is the lack of interference from free drug, which means that RIA need not be restricted to testing trough serum samples. However, both techniques have some limitations, hence the need for newer techniques.

Newer techniques

In clinical practice it may not be possible to obtain a trough serum sample in patients on biologic drugs to measure immunogenicity. Therefore, a drug-tolerant assay may be ideal in terms of clinical feasibility. Newer assays have been designed to detect both free and unbound ADAb, even in the presence of high drug levels.[22] Van Schouwenburg and colleagues[13] used a pH-shift-anti-idiotype ABT (PIA) method, in which complexes of TNFi and ADAb are first dissociated by lowering the pH by acid dissociation. Re-association of complexes is prevented by the addition of excess fluid-phase F(ab) fragments of rabbit anti-idiotype antibodies that compete with patient ADAbs for binding to the drug. In a sample of 30 RA patients on adalimumab, the PIA method revealed ADAb in 21 patients while the unmodified ABT detected ADAb in only five.

More recently, three further drug-tolerant assays were developed and, along with the PIA, were compared with the RIA ABT in adalimumab-treated RA patients. These included an

acid-dissociation RIA (similar to PIA, without the addition F(ab) fragments), a temperature-shift RIA (included incubation at 37oC for 16 hours to dissociate drug-antibody complexes) and an electrochemiluminescence-based assay.[23] The percentage of ADAb-positive patients ranged from 51% to 66% between the four assays, with the acid-dissociation RIA identifying the highest number of patients as positive. The clinical significance of these results with respect to treatment response and the role of artefact, however, remain unclear. While possible to perform in a research setting, these tests would be cumbersome to use in clinical practice and would not be utilized without thorough investigation of additional benefit over existing assays.

As per FDA guidance for industry,[13] newer drugs such as biosimilars undergo more robust testing using the more sensitive assays described in this section, in comparison with the reference product RCTs a number of years ago. This in part explains the differences in immunogenicity rates observed in recent trials (discussed more in Section 7). A multitiered evaluation is usually performed with (i) screening, (ii) confirmation, and (iii) characterization stages.[24] The screening assay is conducted for overall presence or absence of ADAbs, and therefore needs to be highly sensitive to detect both low and high affinity species. Techniques such as acid dissociation may be deployed for this stage (Figure 35. 2) within electrochemiluminescence assays or flow-through microfluidic immunoassays. Samples testing positive are subjected to the confirmation assay that determines the specificity of any ADAbs detected to a given product. In this step, unlabelled drug may be added to florescence-labelled samples and the magnitude of inhibition of the signal is then measured. Samples that test positive in the confirmatory assay, should then undergo further characterization assays to detect the neutralizing potential of the ADAbs, or a titering assay.[16]

Table 35.1 outlines the advantages and disadvantages of the different assays for the detection of immunogenicity. ELISA and RIA remain the most commonly used techniques in trials and observational studies. New and emerging assays that circumvent the main shortcoming of drug interference may hold promise in the future, however none are routinely available and accepted yet.

The clinical consequences of immunogenicity

Immunogenicity has the potential to affect the therapeutic potential of a biological drug by affecting drug levels as stated earlier, but also has been associated with safety concerns. This section will review the effect of ADAbs (and TNFi drug levels) on efficacy. The majority of studies have focussed on infliximab and adalimumab-treated patients. The association between drug safety and ADAbs is summarized in 'Effects on drug safety', p. 436 and highlighted in Tables 35.2–35.4.

Infliximab

Infliximab is one of the most studied TNFis in terms of immunogenicity. The 25% chimeric structure of infliximab with its murine V-region theoretically elicits a more pronounced immunogenic response than humanized or fully human monoclonal antibodies. Several observational studies assessing the effect of infliximab on efficacy and safety are summarized in Table 35.2. The bridging ELISA and RIA were utilized most commonly to detect immunogenicity, with rates

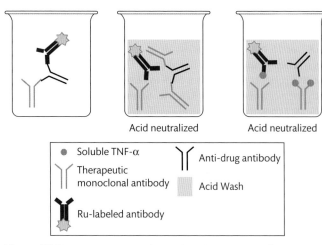

Acid neutralized   Acid neutralized

● Soluble TNF-α

Y Therapeutic
monoclonal antibody

Y Anti-drug antibody

░ Acid Wash

Y Ru-labeled antibody

Figure 35.2 Screening assays: electrochemiluminescence (the current industry standard). The electrochemiluminescence (ECL) platform utilizes a ruthenium-conjugated protein instead of an enzyme conjugate or radio-labelled moiety. An ECL reaction under the appropriate voltage stimulation is caused by reduction of ruthenium ions. As these are recycled, the electrochemical signal is amplified to yield sensitivity. The diagram illustrates how an acid wash is utilized to remove interfering drug to allow detection of antidrug antibodies.

Source: data from Wadhwa M, Knezevic I, Kang HN, et al. (2015) 'Immunogenicity assessment of biotherapeutic products: An overview of assays and their utility'. *Biologicals* 43:298–306.

of ADAbs being reported in 17–54% of RA patients[25,26] (Table 35.2), but now considerably higher in biosimilar studies utilizing more sensitive assays.

Antibodies to infliximab often appear between the third and sixth month of treatment in RA[27]; however, as long as there is still a detectable serum trough level of infliximab, there can continue to be clinical benefit.[24] On the other hand, low trough serum drug levels can herald development of ADAbs to infliximab, which in turn is associated with subsequent treatment failure.[25] Most early observational studies focussed on detection of ADAbs and association with treatment response up to 6–12 months and were of modest size (<100 patients/drug). Despite this, the association of ADAbs to infliximab with reduced serum trough drug levels was clearly demonstrated in the majority of studies. Trough drug levels are practical to obtain in a clinical setting with infliximab, as patients usually require hospital admission for their infusion and a predose sample can be obtained as required.

Few factors have been identified in infliximab studies that directly influence ADAbs and drug levels. The effect of concomitant MTX use has been evaluated in many studies and although there is widespread acceptance that concurrent MTX use is associated with reduced immunogenicity, some observational studies failed to achieve statistical significance.[25,28–31] In cohorts with longer follow-up, the use of MTX was associated with lower levels of ADAb and improved drug survival.[30] Infliximab infusions are normally commenced at 3 mg/kg for RA at 0, 2, 6, and every 8 weeks thereafter. Pascual-Salcedo et al. describes two kinds of response on dose escalation to 5 mg/kg in RA patients who had not responded to infliximab after 14 weeks in association with ADAbs. In a type I response ADAbs disappeared after the dose increase, coinciding with measurable infliximab serum trough levels and an improvement in treatment response. In these cases, ADAbs could be detected again if the dose

Table 35.1 Types of assays used to measure ADAbs in monoclonal antibodies

Assay	Advantages	Disadvantages
1) Bridging/Double antigen/Sandwich ELISA	● Convenient assay format ● Low cost ● High throughput ● Obviates the need for radioactivity	● Does not detect IgG4 antibodies ● High level of drug interference ● Presence of rheumatoid factor can interfere with the assay
2) Radioimmunoassay	● High specificity ● Less prone to drug and rheumatoid factor interference compared to ELISAs ● Detects IgG1, IgG2, and IgG4	● Use of radioisotopes ● Still prone to some drug interference ● More expensive than bridging ELISAs
3) pH-shift anti-idiotype antigen-binding test/ acid-dissociation tests	● Complexes of ADAb bound to drug in serum dissociated by lowering pH ● Can accurately measure ADAb in presence of circulating drug levels and used in many biosimilar studies	● Not tested in many observational studies to date ● Likely to be cumbersome for use in clinical practice ● Expensive
4) Electrochemiluminescence	● Good sensitivity, comparable to RIA and ELISAs ● No radioisotopes used ● Measurement simple and rapid	● Antigen labelling required ● Susceptible to interference by therapeutic, serum components, e.g. multivalent targets ● May not detect IgG4 ● Vendor-specific equipment & reagents
5) Surface plasmon resonance/BIACORE™	● Can detect low affinity antibodies ● Automated	● Expensive ● Needs specific equipment ● Less sensitive than ELISA/ RIA
6) Fluid-phase mobility shift assay	● Can simultaneously measure TNFi level ● Less prone to drug interference ● Detects IgG4	● Not validated in larger studies or rheumatological disorders ● Feasibility in clinical practice undetermined
7) Bioassays	● Functional assay that assesses neutralization potential of antibodies often used for regulatory approval	● Expensive ● Relatively time consuming ● Not readily commercially available for monoclonal antibodies

Table 35.2 Published studies on the impact of anti-infliximab antibodies on safety and efficacy

Authors	Disease	Detection method	(n)	Follow-up	ADAb	Infliximab serum levels (association/timing)	Impact of ADAb on safety (n)	Impact of ADAb on efficacy	Reduction of ADAb on methotrexate	Comments
Haraoui 2006[32]	RA	Double-antigen ELISA	51	Not recorded	27% group 1*, 47% in group 2* (*comments)	Trough levels, inversely correlated	Not recorded	Associated with loss of response	Not recorded	* Group 1 patients achieved and maintained clinical responses with infliximab 3 mg/kg; Group 2 patients required higher doses
Wolbink 2006[33]	RA	RIA	51	1 year	43%	Trough levels, inversely correlated	Positive ADAbs in all 3 patients that had infusion reactions	Inversely correlated (DAS28 scores)	Not reported	29 (57%) patients without detectable ADAbs were significantly more often classified as responders (20/29; 59%) compared with patients with detectable ADAbs (8/22; 36%, p = 0.04)
Bendtzen 2006[29]	RA	RIA	106	6 months	44%	Trough levels, inversely correlated	22 patients had infusion reactions strongly correlated with ADAbs	Inversely correlated (DAS28 scores)	Concomitant MTX associated with lower ADAb	ADAbs developed in 13%, 30%, 44% at time intervals of 1.5, 3, and 6 months
van den Bemt 2008[34]	RA	RIA	18	Up to 16 weeks	22%	Trough levels, inversely correlated	1 lupus-like reaction (in a patient whose infliximab dose was reduced)	Not formally assessed	Not reported	- The aim was to assess if RA patients whose dose had been increased to 5 mg/kg could be reduced safely to standard dose of 3 mg/kg - Majority of patients could dose reduce, with the exception of 2 patients
Radstake 2009[27]	RA	RIA	35	6 months	50%	Trough levels, inversely correlated	Not reported	Inversely correlated (DAS28 and EULAR response criteria)	Not reported	35 infliximab patients, 34 on adalimumab At 6 months, 15 (43%) were good responders, 6 (17%) were moderate and 14 (40%) poor responders with close correlation with the levels of infliximab/adalimumab and ADAb formation
Finckh 2010[25]	RA	Sandwich (indirect) ELISA	64	1 year	17% secondary non-responders, 10% responders	Inversely correlated	Positive ADAbs in all infusion-related reactions (2)	Inversely correlated (DAS28 and EULAR response criteria)	Low patient numbers, not significant	Inclusion criteria included patients who had been on infliximab for 1 year: Secondary non-responders (n = 24) were compared to responders (n = 40)
Pascual-Salcedo 2011[30]	RA	Bridging ELISA	85	4 years + Assessed at 3 time points (6/ 12 months/ 4years+)	32.9%	Trough levels, inversely correlated	Positive ADAbs in all infusion-related reactions (9)	Inversely correlated (DAS28 and EULAR response criteria)	No, but increased survival time on treatment	Patients with ADAbs more often required increased infliximab doses (51.7%) (p = 0.032) and median survival time on treatment was shorter (4.15 vs. 8.89 years) (p = 0.0006)
Ducourau 2011[35]	RA (17), SpA (91)	Double-antigen ELISA	108	Up to 4 years or until treatment discontinued	19%	Trough levels, inversely correlated	52% (n = 11) ADAb +ve patients developed infusion-related reactions (rashes, hyperthermia, Quincke's oedema); Guillain–Barré syndrome (n = 1)	Inversely correlated to BASDAI and DAS28 scores	Yes: SpA patients on monotherapy had a higher rate of ADAbs (32% vs. 0% p = 0.03)	- Only sera with infliximab concentrations of <2 mg/L were tested for ADAbs - Median time to ADAbs detection after initiation was 3.7 months (1.7–26.0 months)

(continued)

Table 35.2 *Continued*

Authors	Disease	Detection method	(n)	Follow-up	ADAb	Infliximab serum levels (association/timing)	Impact of ADAb on safety (n)	Impact of ADAb on efficacy	Reduction of ADAb on methotrexate	Comments
Hoshino 2012[36]	RA	RIA	40	54 weeks (2, 6, 8 weekly thereafter)	35% (The majority of patients (64.3%) had ADAbs at 14 weeks)	Trough levels, inversely correlated	Infliximab-related allergic dyspnoea (n = 1), urticaria (n = 2) in ADAb +ve patients	Inversely correlated (DAS28 higher in ADAb +ve group)	Not significant	Compared with 40 patients on etanercept; none of which had ADAbs detected; etanercept serum trough levels unrelated to disease activity
Krintel 2013[26]	RA	Surface plasmon resonance assay	218	52 weeks	54%	Trough levels—inversely correlated	Increased adverse events in ADAb +ve patients n = 17 with infusion reactions; urticarial: 1 infection: 1 exanthema: 1	Inversely correlated—(DAS28 score)	No association	- Patients evaluated at 2, 6, 14, and 52 weeks - Patients with detectable ADAbs after 6 weeks had an increased risk of adverse drug reactions HR = 5.06 [95% CI 2.36, 10.84; p <0.0001]
Mok 2013[31]	RA (35), PsA (10), AS (12)	RIA	24	Up to 18 months	50%	Trough levels—not systematically evaluated	Not assessed	Inversely correlated	Concomitant MTX associated with lower ADAb but not statistically significant	- Conducted in a Chinese population - Pharmacological assessment at only 1 time point. - ADAb +ve patients had poorer drug survival over 18 months
Eng 2015[37]	RA	RIA	44	Varied—only remission patients included	18%	Trough levels—inversely correlated	Not assessed	Not assessed—all patients in remission as defined with a DAS28 <2.6	Not assessed	Cross-sectional study to assess incidence of ADAb in patients whose disease was classified as in remission
Arstikyte 2015[38]	RA (62), PsA (32), AS (49)	Bridging ELISA	62	Median 28 months	24.6%	Trough levels—inversely correlated	5.3% (n = 3) with ADAbs developed infusion reactions with higher OR (OR 5.88 [95%CI: 1.04–33.28])	Higher OR to change to another biologic or stop treatment	No correlation found in infliximab patients	- ADAbs and drug levels measured only once in patients at different time points - Association of ADAbs with treatment failure, however very wide CI (OR 11.43 [95% CI 1.08–120.93])
Min Jung 2015[39]	RA	Sandwich ELISA	29 (39 AS)	Varied (cross-sectional)	28.8%	Not specified	Not assessed	Inversely correlated	No association	Korean RA and AS patients tested cross-sectionally to assess prevalence of ADAbs - With adalimumab as the referent, infliximab patients had higher OR 9.2 (95% CI: 2.0–41.8)
Moots 2017[40]	RA	RIA	196	Varied (cross-sectional)—mean duration 13.1 months	17.4%	Trough levels inversely correlated	Low numbers but no significant difference between ADAb +ve /-ve patients	Inversely correlated (DAS28 scores)	Concomitant MTX associated with lower ADAbs—but not significant	Multinational cross-sectional study - Trough levels not associated with patient reported outcomes

Studies are listed in chronological order. Where the same study includes multiple disease groups, numbers for each are listed. In studies where multiple biologics are evaluated, n = number of patients on infliximab. Abbreviations: ADAbs, antidrug antibodies; AS, ankylosing spondylitis; BASDAI, Bath Ankylosing Spondylitis Disease Activity Index; DAS28, disease activity score of 28 joints; ELISA, enzyme-linked immunosorbent assay; EULAR, European League Against Rheumatism; MTX, methotrexate; OR, odds ratio; PsA, psoriatic arthritis; RA, rheumatoid arthritis; RIA, radioimmunoassay; SpA, spondyloarthropathy of infliximab was subsequently reduced, with a simultaneous clinical deterioration. In the type II response, ADAbs did not disappear after drug escalation, but instead reached high levels. In some patients this was associated with development of infusion-related reactions (n = 3), which often are associated with ADAbs (sometimes IgE but usually IgG).[30] Currently dose escalation in infliximab-treated RA patients with ADAbs is not recommended as standard due to its unknown effect on safety and possible temporary effect on efficacy.

Adalimumab

Despite adalimumab being a so-called fully human monoclonal antibody against TNF, the antigen-binding site still induces an immune response (see 'Drug structure and sequence variation', p. 425). The reported frequency of ADAbs to adalimumab ranges from 10% to 87% depending on the study (summarized in Table 35.3) and 48–56% with biosimilar adalimumab. The inverse association between trough serum drug levels and ADAbs to adalimumab has been observed in multiple studies,[27,41–46] similar to infliximab.

A landmark study in 2011 was published by Bartelds et al., which systematically followed up a cohort of RA patients on adalimumab.[43] Immunogenicity was detecting using robust methodology, an RIA developed by Sanquin Laboratories[22] with corresponding drug levels tested using an ELISA. An ADAb frequency of 28% was reported after 3 years, about half of which developed within the first 3 months and the majority within 6 months of initiation of therapy. Compared to patients without ADAbs, those with moderate/high antibody titres had significantly lower serum drug concentrations, had poorer drug survival over the course of the study and were less likely to achieve improvement in disease activity, especially if concomitant MTX was not prescribed.

Several studies have assessed the effect of concomitant prescription of MTX on ADAbs in adalimumab-treated patients (Table 35.3). Use and particularly dose of methotrexate at baseline appears to be important at attenuating ADAb levels, with patients on doses between 20 and 25 mg/week less likely to develop immunogenicity compared to those on lower doses.[42,47] In contrast the CONCERTO study, in which MTX-naïve early RA patients were commenced on open-label adalimumab with a blinded variable dose of MTX, suggested that both efficacy and serum adalimumab levels were similar with MTX 10 mg or 20 mg per week.[48]

Patients with more severe disease at baseline, may be more likely to develop ADAbs. In the Netherlands' cohort,[40] RA patients who developed immunogenicity were more likely to have higher DAS28 scores (5.5 vs. 5.1), more erosive disease (83% vs. 70%), longer disease duration (12 vs. 8 years) and higher levels of inflammatory markers. In the national UK cohort[45] patients who developed ADAbs had a significantly longer disease duration compared to those who did not (14 vs. 7 years).

Pharmacological biomarkers such as ADAbs and TNFi drug levels need to be practical to measure in clinical practice, and provide additional clinical value to the clinician and patient over current clinical assessment. At 3 months, ADAb formation and low adalimumab levels have been demonstrated to be significant predictors of European League Against Rheumatism (EULAR) non-response at 12-months (area under receiver operating characteristic (ROC) curve 0.71, 95% confidence intervals [CI] 0.57–0.85).[47] A previous study from the Netherlands' cohort reported that formation of ADAbs to one monoclonal antibody may predict antibody

formation and reduced efficacy to subsequent monoclonal-based treatments.[49] However, in one study patients who developed ADAbs to adalimumab appeared just as likely to respond to etanercept as patients who were previously biologic naïve, thereby providing an alternative treatment strategy if ADAbs are present.[50] Various algorithms have been proposed for adalimumab-treated patients suggesting that, in the presence of ADAbs and low adalimumab levels, switching to another agent may be beneficial.[6,51]

Predictors of adalimumab drug level

The majority of studies described in Table 35.3 focus on detection of immunogenicity and its effect on drug levels and treatment response. The drug level itself reflects the amount of unbound drug available in the serum, available for TNF binding. Subtherapeutic drug levels may result in partial suppression of inflammation leading to flares of the disease. Fewer studies have characterized the direct effect of drug level on treatment response, and its associated predictors, however emerging evidence suggests that drug levels are a more useful biomarker in prediction of response than ADAbs. While this is valid on a population level, more studies are needed to test whether this is true on an individual patient basis, and its specific role in personalized medicine.

One such study was by Pouw et al.,[52] which established the concept of a concentration–effect curve following re-analysis of the data from previously reported Dutch studies.[40,46] Clinical efficacy improved with increasing serum adalimumab concentration and reached a maximum with levels between 5 and 8 µg/ml. Adalimumab concentrations were also significantly different if patients were on concomitant MTX; patients on combination therapy of MTX and adalimumab had higher median drug concentrations compared to patients on monotherapy, with the pharmacokinetic benefit of MTX plateauing at 10 mg per week. This may be due to the direct effect of MTX on ADAb formation, or other unmeasured factors which may influence drug levels such as adherence. A concentration–effect curve in the national UK cohort (Biologics in Rheumatoid Arthritis Genetics and Genomics Study Syndicate [BRAGGSS]) identified a drug level threshold of <5 µg/ml was associated with a lesser improvement in disease activity.[47] The adalimumab level was the best predictor of improvement in DAS28 at 12 months, after adjustment for confounders (regression coefficient 0.060 [95% CI 0.015, 0.10], p = 0.009), compared to measuring ADAbs alone. Additional factors associated with low adalimumab drug levels included a body mass index of ≥30 kg/m² and poor self-reported patient adherence.[44] Use of other nbDMARDS (leflunomide, sulfasalazine, hydroxychloroquine) were also associated with higher adalimumab drug levels compared with adalimumab monotherapy in some studies.[12] However the associations appeared less robust than when MTX was used as the concurrent nbDMARD.

Certolizumab pegol

For newer TNFis for RA such as certolizumab pegol, there are less data on immunogenicity in an observational setting. Certolizumab pegol is a PEGylated Fab' fragment of a humanized TNF inhibitor monoclonal antibody. PEGylation refers to the covalent binding of polyethylene glycol (PEG) molecules to proteins, performed to enhance the molecule's half-life.[55] It has been shown to reduce immunogenicity of some proteins,[57] while increasing it in others by producing antibodies to the PEG residue, in certain cases leading to

Table 35.3 Published studies in rheumatoid arthritis on the impact of antiadalimumab antibodies on safety and efficacy

Authors	Disease	Detection method	(n)	Follow-up	ADAb	Adalimumab serum levels (association and timing)	Impact of ADAb on safety (n)	Impact of ADAb on efficacy	Reduction of ADAb on Methotrexate	Comments
Bender 2007[53]	RA	Sandwich ELISA	15	Up to 18 months	87%	Timing not specified, drug levels not evaluated	ADAb +ve patients also developed exanthema (2) herpes zoster (1)	Inverse correlation (DAS28)	Low numbers but all patients on monotherapy developed ADAbs and dropped out	- One of the first observational studies evaluating ADAb formation and clinical consequences - Patient selection not clear, however, especially high rate of ADAbs reported
Bartelds 2007[41]	RA	RIA	121	6 months	17%	Trough levels—inversely correlated	Not reported	Inversely correlated (DAS28 and EULAR response criteria)	Negatively associated (p <0.0001)	- EULAR non-responders had ADAbs significantly more often than good responders (34% vs. 5%; p = 0.032) - Patients with ADAbs showed reduced improvement in DAS scores
Radstake 2009[27]	RA	RIA	34	6 months	30%	Trough levels—inversely correlated	Not reported	Inversely correlated (DAS28 and EULAR response criteria)	Not reported	35 patients received infliximab; 34 received adalimumab. At 6 months, 15 (43%) were good responders, 6 (17%) were moderate and 14 (40%) poor responders with close correlation between serum levels of infliximab/adalimumab and ADAb formation
Bartelds 2010[49]	RA	RIA	235	28 weeks	20%	Trough levels—inversely correlated	Not reported	Inversely correlated (DAS28 and EULAR response criteria)	Negatively associated	- Patients with anti-infliximab ADAbs were more likely to develop antiadalimumab antibodies than anti-TNF naïve patients (11 (33%) vs. 32 (18%); p = 0.039) - ΔDAS28 was greater for anti-TNF naïve patients (1.7 ± 1.5) than for switchers without anti- infliximab antibodies (ΔDAS28 = 0.9 ± 1.4) (p = 0.009)
Bartelds 2011[43]	RA	RIA	272	3 years	28%	Trough levels—inversely correlated	Not reported	Inversely correlated (DAS28CRP higher in ADAb +ve group)	Negatively associated with use and dose	Majority (67%) developed ADAbs in the first 6 months of treatment, despite 3-year follow-up
Krieckhart 2012[54]	RA	RIA	204	3 years	26%	Not reassessed	Not reported	Patients were more likely to achieve low/ minimal disease activity if they were ADAb -ve	Not reassessed	- Same cohort as the Bartelds study above,[42] but excluded anti-TNF switchers - Comparison of low/minimal disease activity in etanercept and adalimumab-treated patients made after stratification of ADAbs
Mok 2013[31]	RA, PsA (& AS)	RIA	17	Up to 18 months	31%	Trough levels— not systematically evaluated	Not assessed	Inversely correlated	MTX appeared protective but not statistically significant	- Conducted in a Chinese population - Pharmacological assessment at only 1 time point - ADAb +ve patients had poorer drug survival over 18 months
Chen 2015[45]	RA	ELISA & RIA	36	12 months	27.8–36.1%	Trough levels—inversely correlated	Not assessed	Inversely correlated (EULAR response)	Not assessed	Used both RIA and ELISAs to quantify ADAbs in adalimumab patients (27.8% and 36.1% respectively). - Trough serum levels used, but limited conclusions as only 36 patients tested

Eng 2015[37]	RA	RIA	49	Varied—only remission patients included	2%	Trough levels—low drug level in 1 patient	Not assessed	Not assessed—all patients in remission as defined with a DAS28 <2.6	Not assessed	Cross-sectional study to assess incidence of ADAb in patients classified as being in remission
Min Jung 2015[39]	RA	Sandwich ELISA	163 (82 AS)	Varied (cross-sectional)	10% (n = 17)	Unspecified	Not assessed	Inversely correlated	No association	Korean RA and AS patients tested cross-sectionally to assess prevalence of ADAbs
Jani 2015[47]	RA	RIA	160	12 months	24.8%	Random (non-trough) drug levels inversely correlated with ADAbs	Not assessed	Inversely correlated	MTX dose significantly different in ADAb +ve and ADAb –ve patients	- Multicentre national prospective UK study - Combination of detecting ADAbs and low drug level at 3 months post treatment gave an area under the ROC curve of 0.71 for EULAR non-response at 12 months
Moots 2017[40]	RA	RIA	199	Varied (cross-sectional)—mean duration 13.5 months	31.2%	Trough levels inversely correlated	Low numbers but no significant difference between ADAb +ve /–ve patients	Inversely correlated (DAS28 scores)	Concomitant MTX associated with lower ADAbs- but not significant	Multinational cross-sectional study - Trough adalimumab levels additionally associated with HAQ-DI

Studies are listed in chronological order. Where the same study includes multiple disease groups, numbers for each are listed. In studies where multiple biologics are evaluated, n = number of patients on adalimumab. Abbreviations: ADAbs, antidrug antibodies; AS, ankylosing spondylitis; DAS28, disease activity score of 28 joints; ELISA, enzyme-linked immunosorbent assay; EULAR, European League Against Rheumatism; HAQ-DI: Health assessment questionnaire disability index; MTX, methotrexate; PsA, psoriatic arthritis; RA, rheumatoid arthritis; RIA, radioimmunoassay.

loss of efficacy.[57] Golimumab is a fully human monoclonal antibody that inhibits TNF.

Immunogenicity to certolizumab has been assessed mainly in the context of RCTs in which ELISAs were used for detection of ADAbs. With a typical detection rate between 5% and 6%,[58] the proportion of ADAb-positive patients in such trials was too low to assess their effect on treatment response or safety, however neutralizing antibodies have been reported using cell-based assays in one RCT.[59] A recent observational study, that used RIA for measurement of ADAbs, detected that a high proportion of patients on certolizumab (37%) developed ADAbs.[60] ADAbs were significantly associated with low drug levels, which in turn correlated with 12 months EULAR response (β = 0.032 (95% CI 0.0011 to 0.063), p = 0.042). This study demonstrated that even smaller, non-glycosylated fragments might induce immunogenicity. However, due to the nature of the molecule, it may be that the antibody-drug complexes dissociate more readily and are more likely to be detected. Regardless, therapeutic drug monitoring may be useful in certolizumab-treated RA patients in combination with clinical assessment of response.

Golimumab

Prevalence of antigolimumab ADAbs in RCTs typically ranges from 2% to 10%.[61-63] Small observational studies of <50 patients have been performed using the drug in RA.[64,65] Both studies showed that ADAbs were associated with low drug levels which, in turn, were associated with poor treatment response. Patients with golimumab drug levels of >1.4 mg/L appeared more likely sustain a response at 12 months (disease activity score (DAS)<3.2),[64] and drug levels were positively correlated with MTX dosage,[65] as seen in adalimumab and infliximab-treated patients.

Etanercept ADAbs and drug levels

Etanercept is a soluble dimeric fusion protein and has been found to be less immunogenic according to reported data. Most studies to date have either failed to detect ADAbs or have detected them at lower levels compared to monoclonal antibodies (summarized in **Table 35.4**). This is likely because the only foreign part of etanercept is the short linker that connects the soluble receptor domain to the human IgG1 Fc.[66] ADAbs to etanercept were not detected even when more sensitive assay techniques such as RIA were employed.[31,36,67] Therefore, associations with safety outcomes have not been evaluated fully in relation to etanercept immunogenicity.

Where ADAbs were detectable, no correlation was reported with drug levels, adverse reactions, or clinical response in RA.[36,38,39,67,68] This suggests the possibility of binding antibodies (that do not neutralize the effect of the drug) or false positive results, as in the majority of the studies ELISAs of low specificity were used. One early study in RA which assessed immunogenicity to etanercept as its primary endpoint, described ADAbs in 5.6% at any time point in 222 patients using ELISAs.[68] Although most ADAbs were transient over 28 weeks and no effect on efficacy was concluded, the authors reported only 50% of ADAb+ve patients attained ACR20 responses at 6 months (compared to 63% overall in 222 patients). Furthermore, none of the ADAb+ve patients attained ACR70 response, compared to 14% in all patients in the study. Despite being found to be non-neutralizing, ADAbs to etanercept may in some cases affect drug pharmacokinetics.

Patients with RA who do not respond to etanercept may have lower serum trough drug concentrations at 6 months, even without detection of antibodies using RIA,[50] however this has not been shown consistently.[38] Jamnitski et al. also reported that RA patients with the lowest etanercept levels were more likely to be female, have a higher glomerular filtration rate and higher BMI (27.5 kg/m^2 vs. 24.9 kg/m^2) at baseline. Interestingly, the study also reported significantly lower mean MTX doses (but not use) in patients with low vs. high etanercept levels (12.6 vs. 16.9 mg/week). The mechanism of this is unclear in the absence of detectable ADAbs, but along with the studies just described, suggests evaluation of secondary non-response in these patients requires further study and validation in well-characterized cohorts with longer follow-up.

Non-TNFi biologics

Therapeutic drug monitoring and measurement of ADAbs appears to be less useful in the assessment of non-TNFi biologics, primarily due to few data suggesting utility in a real-world setting. Rituximab is a chimeric protein and associated with a high incidence of infusion reactions,[70] although the majority are the consequence of cytokine release in association with B-cell lysis, particularly early in treatment. In rituximab-treated RA patients, one study evaluated 58 patients undergoing treatment, with drug levels and ADAbs measured at 4, 12–16 weeks, or 24 weeks.[71] Only 8.6% of patients had ADAbs detected using a RIA assay and these were associated with low drug levels. A wide variability of serum rituximab levels was observed and were not associated with B-cell depletion or clinical response. Although with the first course of treatment, B-cell depletion abrogates the ADAb response, it returns in some patients with re-administration. In a recent study investigating rituximab-treated lupus patients, ADAbs were measured in a small subset of patients and were discovered in both responders and secondary non-responders[72] suggesting limited clinical utility. Previous pharmacokinetic models have revealed that the mean rituximab elimination was not affected by MTX comedication, gender, or body surface area.[73,74] Therefore, measurement of rituximab drug levels and ADAbs is not currently recommended to guide clinical care.

The few studies that have evaluated immunogenicity to tocilizumab, have found ADAbs were detected in a small proportion of recipients,[75-78] however this may be assay dependent. The ACT-RAY study that utilized a screening assay, followed by a neutralizing assay if positive detected neutralizing antibodies in up to 1.8% (n = 5) of tocilizumab-treated patients.[79] However the risk of hypersensitivity/anaphylactic reactions to tocilizumab is not negligible and has been well described, both in RA and in systemic autoimmune diseases.[70,80] Anaphylactic reactions have been reported in several patients receiving IV tocilizumab, one of which was reported fatal and was the subject of an FDA letter to prescribers. Hypersensitivity reactions often occur during the first or second infusion, and within the initial 20 minutes, suggesting an IgE-mediated mechanism and previous sensitization to the drug.[80] While some subjects demonstrate ADAbs this is not the case in all subjects with hypersensitivity to tocilizumab, and IgE antibodies have not been reported. However, intradermal testing revealed a positive response in 3 of 4 patients with systemic autoimmunity and acute hypersensitivity.[80] Tocilizumab trough levels, either via the subcutaneous or intravenous route (like rituximab), demonstrate a wide variability. Some studies suggest an association of drug levels with treatment response

Table 35.4 Published studies in rheumatoid arthritis on the impact of etanercept drug levels and antidrug antibodies on efficacy and safety

Authors	Disease	Detection method	(n)	Follow-up	ADAb	Etanercept serum levels (association & timing)	Impact of ADAb on safety (n)	Impact of ADAb on efficacy	Reduction of ADAb on Methotrexate	Comments
Dore 2007[68]	RA	ELISA	222	28 weeks (ADAbs assessed at baseline, 24, 28 weeks)	5.6%	Not evaluated	Non-serious infectious events (n = 7), septic arthritis (n = 1) observed in ADAb +ve patients but not felt to be immunogenicity related	Concluded not associated with ADAbs (however, 50% of ADAb +ve patients achieved ACR20 vs. 63% in total group)	Not assessed	- Transient ADAbs observed in 9/12 patients - None of the ADAbs were found to be neutralizing (using a neutralizing ADAb assay) - Injection site reactions reported in 29.3% of all patients
Jamnitski 2011[69]	RA	ELISA	292	24 weeks	None	Trough levels associated with EULAR response	Not assessed	Not assessed	Not assessed	Patients with etanercept levels <2.1 mg/L comprised 40% of all non-responders. - Etanercept drug levels significantly higher in good EULAR responders (compared to moderate and no EULAR responders)
Hoshino 2012[36]	RA	RIA	40	32 weeks (2, 6, 8 weekly thereafter)	None detected	No ADAbs detected, serum trough levels not associated with treatment response	Not assessed	Not assessed	Not assessed	Compared with 40 patients on infliximab (Japanese patients), no etanercept patients had ADAbs detected; etanercept serum trough levels unrelated to disease activity
Mok 2013[31]	RA (35), PsA (10) & AS (12)	RIA	18	Up to 18 months	None detected	Trough levels—not systematically evaluated	Not assessed	Not assessed	Not assessed	- Conducted in a Chinese population - Pharmacological assessment at only 1 time point
Min Jung 2015[39]	RA	Sandwich ELISA	85	Varied (cross-sectional)	1.4% (2)	Unspecified	Not assessed	Not assessed	No association	Korean RA and AS patients tested cross-sectionally to assess prevalence of ADAbs - With adalimumab as the referent, etanercept patients had lower OR of developing ADAbs 0.3 (95% CI: 0.1–0.6)
Arstikyte 2015[38]	RA (62), PsA (32) AS (39)	Bridging ELISA	61	Median 28 months	None detected	Trough levels measured, n = 4 with undetectable levels. No association with response	Not assessed	Not assessed	Not assessed	- ADAbs and drug levels measured only once in patients at different time points - Only 4 patients had undetectable etanercept levels in the study, lack power to determine any effect on efficacy
Jani 2015[47]	RA	RIA	171	12 months	None detected	Association between random drug levels and treatment response not significant after adjustment	Not evaluated	None detected	None detected	Multinational cross-sectional study - Etanercept levels associated with 12-month EULAR response in the age and gender univariate ordinal logistic regression model
Moots 2017[40]	RA	RIA	199	Varied (cross-sectional)—mean duration 14.6 months	None detected	No association with DAS scores, but significantly correlated with CRP	Not evaluated	None detected	None detected	Multinational cross-sectional study - Trough adalimumab levels additionally associated with HAQ-DI

Studies are listed in chronological order. Where the same study includes multiple disease groups, numbers for each are listed. In studies where multiple biologics are evaluated, n = number of patients on etanercept. Abbreviations: ADAbs, antidrug antibodies; AS, ankylosing spondylitis; ELISA, enzyme-linked immunosorbent assay; EULAR, European League Against Rheumatism; MTX, methotrexate; OR, odds ratio; PsA, psoriatic arthritis; RA, rheumatoid arthritis; RIA, radioimmunoassay.

and inflammatory markers such as C-reactive protein (CRP) and ESR,[75,76] however drug levels as low as 1 mg/L were found to be sufficient to normalize CRP. Further work is needed to fully explore the utility of therapeutic drug monitoring in this setting, as well as any clinical consequences of 'overexposure' in terms of drug levels.

The role of immunogenicity on abatacept pharmacokinetics is unclear. Low levels and transient antibodies have been observed in response to intravenous or subcutaneous abatacept in clinical trials (<5%) with no impact on clinical efficacy or safety.[81–83] As with etanercept, the immunogenic portion of abatacept is the linker region and there are no suitable assays designed to detect anti-linker ADAbs. Pharmacokinetic modelling in early abatacept studies assessing the effect of weight-tiered dosing regimens on serum IL-6 concentrations, have demonstrated that doses of >10 mg/kg do not result in additional IL-6 suppression. To date, there have been no concentration–effect models for abatacept to determine the optimal threshold for drug monitoring.

Effect on drug safety

A higher rate of immune-mediated adverse drug reactions has been reported in patients who develop immunogenicity, compared to patients who do not.[26,29,33] Infusion reactions have been associated with ADAbs to infliximab in a number of studies.[26,29,30,33,35,36,38,84] Among all biologics, infliximab and rituximab were associated with the highest relative risk of hypersensitivity reactions compared to any injectable TNFi agent (RR: 26.9 [17.4–41.5]) and 22.2 [11.6–42.4], respectively), followed by tocilizumab and abatacept.[70] Immunogenicity has also been linked to serious adverse events such as thrombotic events, autoimmune reactions such as lupus-like reactions and paradoxical events (e.g. vasculitis-like like reactions), the evidence for which has been reviewed recently.[85] Other allergic adverse events have also been observed in ADAb-positive patients in fewer numbers and include urticaria,[26,36] rashes including exanthema,[26] Quincke's oedema (angioedema), and infliximab-related allergic dyspnoea.[35] Immunogenic reactions in tocilizumab-treated patients such as psoriasiform eruptions and drug reaction with eosinophilia and systemic symptoms syndrome (DRESS)[86] have also been reported but the link with immunogenicity is perhaps less clear.

Due to the rarity of such events and lack of homogeneity in the small observational studies, a robust association between safety and ADAbs to adalimumab has not been clearly established, as in the majority of studies adverse events were not recorded (Table 35.3). Of concern, however, was a study by Korswagen et al.[87] which reported a higher incidence of serious arterial and venous thromboembolic events with ADAbs in the same cohort of RA patients treated with adalimumab reported in the Bartelds et al. study.[42] Three severe thromboembolic events were observed in high titre ADAb-positive patients, including necrosis of the toes, portal/mesenteric vein thrombus and left atrial thrombi, which prompted a retrospective review of all phenotyped patients. Antiadalimumab antibodies were detected in 76 out of 272 (28%) patients. Eight thromboembolic events occurred in the cohort as a whole, four of which had occurred in patients with ADAbs.[87] Although potentially highlighting a signal for concern, the conclusions were limited due to a number of issues with this study.[85] Furthermore, two large prospective observational studies to date evaluating increased thromboembolic risk

in TNFi-treated patients compared to nbDMARD patients did not find an association,[88,89] however ADAb status was not characterized in these patients.

Immune events associated with TNFi agents range from a spectrum of asymptomatic immunological variations to autoimmune clinical manifestations.[82] Antinuclear antibody (ANA) development with TNFi has been described in a large proportion of patients, with seroconversion rates of 31–63% with infliximab, 16–51% with adalimumab and 12–48% with etanercept in prospectively observed RA patients.[90,91] It has been proposed a proportion of patients on monoclonal antibody-based TNFi agents in observational studies may develop ANA and antidouble stranded DNA (dsDNA) antibodies due to immunogenicity that could act as a surrogate marker of impending treatment failure.[92,93] Seroconversion of ANA and dsDNA have also been observed at higher rates in RA[91,94] and psoriasis[92] patients in association with secondary non-response to TNFi, with a direct association with ADAbs seen in infliximab-treated patients.[93] Similarly, in inflammatory bowel disease patients, perinuclear antineutrophil cytoplasmic antibodies (pANCA) positivity has been associated with lower clinical response in monoclonal antibody treated patients.[95] Patients predisposed to developing immunogenicity may also therefore be prone to developing other (auto)antibodies such as ANA, dsDNA, and antineutrophil cytoplasm antibodies (ANCA). Development of lupus and vasculitis-like events occurs much less frequently with an absolute risk of 1/ 1000 patient-years (95% CI: 8, 13) and 15/10 000 patient-years (95% CI: 12, 19) respectively.[96] Factors associated with higher rates of such events are high disease burden, while use of concomant MTX and sulfasalazine appear to be associated with lower rates,[96] similar to features associated with immunogenicity.

Immunogenicity and biosimilars

One of the main concerns of switching from a reference biologic to biosimilars is potential immunogenicity with an associated effect on safety and efficacy profile, as even minor modifications in the molecule can alter immunogenicity.[97] Therefore assessment of biosimilar immunogenicity is conducted in equivalence trials to ensure that the immunogenic potential of the biosimilar is similar to that of the reference product. Clinical trials of infliximab and its biosimilars have been reassuring with comparable rates of ADAbs to biosimilar and reference infliximab (e.g. 48.4% vs. 48.2%).[98] Additionally in conditions in which MTX is not routinely prescribed such as ankylosing spondylitis, ADAbs rates have been within equivalence margins.[99]

Interestingly one phase III etanercept biosimilar trial reported a rate of 13.1% ADAbs with originator etanercept compared to 0.7% with SB4 (biosimilar) at 28 weeks.[100] Immunogenicity testing was performed using a tiered approach: initially using an meso scale discovery (MSD) electrochemiluminescence bridging ELISA (with acid dissociation), followed by neutralizing antibodies measured using a competitive ligand bind assay. Only one sample in the etanercept originator group was found to have neutralizing potential. In the majority of cases, detected ADAbs in both groups appeared transient, being detectable at 4 weeks and disappearing completely by week 8. More sensitive assays were used in this study (requiring an acid-dissociation step, for instance) and ADAbs were measured more frequently and earlier than in previously reported trials and studies. Although in the majority these were non-neutralizing, it does raise the possibility of ADAbs being formed to etanercept,[101] albeit to a lesser extent than to monoclonal antibodies, and highlights the requirement for further exploration in a clinical setting using sensitive assays.

The NOR-SWITCH RCT and DANBIO registry have recently published data from Norway and Denmark as part of their national switch initiatives in infliximab-treated patients.[102,103] Immunogenicity rates within the NOR-SWITCH trial were similar between the biosimilar and the originator (8% vs. 7%), as were infusion reactions (2% vs. 4%). While it recruited a heterogeneous range of diseases, the trial demonstrated non-inferiority in terms of efficacy and safety during a 12-month follow-up, with slightly higher flares in the biosimilar group (29.6% vs. 26.2%). The DANBIO registry observed switched patients to the infliximab biosimilar had retention rates slightly lower than the reference product, with an adjusted absolute difference of 3.4%. This may suggest a 'nocebo effect', unmeasured confounding, or possibly issues of immunogenicity leading to loss of response. While the majority of patients appear to tolerate switching well during the limited follow-up, there may be subgroups of patients who may benefit from remaining on the originator drug (further information in Chapter 34 on biosimilars).

Tolerizing to antidrug antibodies

ADAbs are clearly a significant limitation to therapy with most biologic agents but can they be avoided? A number of observations are potentially relevant to this question:

- The administration of high amounts of soluble protein leads to tolerance induction,[104] potentially explaining data with infliximab whereby higher doses were associated with a lower incidence of ADAb formation.[10]
- Aggregated IgG is highly immunogenic in mice but soluble monomeric IgG can tolerize to aggregated IgG.[105,106]
- Cell-binding monoclonal antibodies are more immunogenic than those that do not bind cells.[103] While the reasons underpinning this observation remain unclear, it may explain why cell-binding TNFi such as infliximab (which can signal via cell surface TNF),[107] and rituximab, appear more immunogenic than, for example, etanercept or tocilizumab.
- The ADAb response is a classical, T-cell dependent immune response.[7]

Taking these factors into account, ADAb to a highly immunogenic cell-binding monoclonal anti-CD8 antibody were prevented in mice by creating non-cell-binding variants. These contained either the anti-CD8 heavy chain combined with an irrelevant light chain, or the anti-CD8 light chain combined with an irrelevant heavy chain.[106] These two variants contained the same T-cell epitopes as the native anti-CD8 antibody but did not bind cells. By pretreating mice with deaggregated preparations of the variants, multiple subsequent administrations of the parent anti-CD8 monoclonal antibody did not provoke an immune response. Subsequently, in a proof of concept clinical study, a non-cell-binding version of alemtuzumab was manufactured which differed by just one amino acid from the

'wild-type' alemtuzumab. Administration of the variant to multiple sclerosis patients prior to therapy with alemtuzumab itself appeared to reduce the incidence of ADAbs.[105]

In practice, it would not be economical to manufacture tolerogenic variants for pretreatment of patients prior to biologic therapy. However, for non-cell-binding therapeutic antibodies there may be the potential to utilize the concept of high zone tolerance although, in this context, aggregates and impurities within biologic preparations could act as potent adjuvants. For cell-binding antibodies one could imagine a biphasic therapeutic that initially tolerizes. For example, the idiotype could be masked by a cleavable peptide, providing a therapeutic antibody that is initially non-binding until it is cleaved either in the circulation or at the site of action, by an endogenous enzyme.[108,109]

Summary

In conclusion, immunogenicity and its effects on drug pharmacokinetics have been described for all monoclonal TNFis. Furthermore, ADAbs have been associated with certain adverse events. Factors affecting immunogenicity are multifactorial, but use of concomitant MTX appears to provide consistent benefit in reducing ADAbs and also certain immune-mediated adverse events. Immunogenicity is also an important consideration when comparing biosimilar biologic agents with their reference product, although data thus far are reassuring in this regard, with no evidence of heightened immunogenicity with biosimilars. Unlike the situation with inflammatory bowel disease, where there are fewer treatment options at present, routine therapeutic drug monitoring, including immunogenicity testing, is not currently widely practised in rheumatology. Evidence on how best to utilize such tests, including well-designed RCTs with assessment of cost-effectiveness, are necessary before wide-scale implementation is contemplated.

REFERENCES

1. Schellekens H. Bioequivalence and the immunogenicity of biopharmaceuticals. *Nat Rev Drug Discov* 2002;1:457–62.
2. Isaacs JD. The antiglobulin response to therapeutic antibodies. *Semin Immunol* 1990;2:449–56.
3. Bendtzen K. Is there a need for immunopharmacologic guidance of anti-tumor necrosis factor therapies? *Arthritis Rheum* 2011;63:867–70.
4. Sethu S, Govindappa K, Alhaidari M, et al. Immunogenicity to biologics: mechanisms, prediction and reduction. *Arch Immunol Ther Exp (Warsz)* 2012;60:331–44.
5. Ponce R, Abad L, Amaravadi L, et al. Immunogenicity of biologically-derived therapeutics: assessment and interpretation of nonclinical safety studies. *Regul Toxicol Pharmacol* 2009;54:164–82.
6. Vincent FB, Morand EF, Murphy K, et al. Antidrug antibodies (ADAb) to tumour necrosis factor (TNF)-specific neutralising agents in chronic inflammatory diseases: a real issue, a clinical perspective. *Ann Rheum Dis* 2013;72:165–78.
7. Isaacs JD, Waldmann H. Helplessness as a strategy for avoiding antiglobulin responses to therapeutic monoclonal antibodies. *Ther Immunol* 1994;1:303–12.

8. Strand V, Balsa A, Al-Saleh J, et al. Immunogenicity of biologics in chronic inflammatory diseases: a systematic review. *BioDrugs* 2017;31:299–316.

9. Jani M, Barton A, Warren RB, et al. The role of DMARDs in reducing the immunogenicity of TNF inhibitors in chronic inflammatory diseases. *Rheumatology (Oxf)* 2014;53:213–22.

10. Maini RN, Breedveld FC, Kalden JR, et al. Therapeutic efficacy of multiple intravenous infusions of anti-tumor necrosis factor alpha monoclonal antibody combined with low-dose weekly methotrexate in rheumatoid arthritis. *Arthritis Rheum* 1998;41:1552–63.

11. Garcês S, Demengeot J, Benito-Garcia E. The immunogenicity of anti-TNF therapy in immune-mediated inflammatory diseases: a systematic review of the literature with a meta-analysis. *Ann Rheum Dis* 2013;72:1947–55.

12. Vogelzang EH, Pouw MF, Nurmohamed M, et al. Adalimumab trough concentrations in patients with rheumatoid arthritis and psoriatic arthritis treated with concomitant disease-modifying antirheumatic drugs. *Ann Rheum Dis* 2015;74:474–5.

13. Jani M, Isaacs JD, Morgan AW, et al. Detection of anti-drug antibodies using a bridging ELISA compared with radio-immunoassay in adalimumab-treated rheumatoid arthritis patients with random drug levels. *Rheumatology (Oxf)* 2016;55:2050–5.

14. Chaparro M, Guerra I, Muñoz-Linares P, et al. Systematic review: antibodies and anti-TNF-α levels in inflammatory bowel disease. *Aliment Pharmacol Ther* 2012;35:971–86.

15. European Medicine Agency. *Guideline on Immunogenicity Assessment of Monoclonal Antibodies Intended for In Vivo Clinical Use*. London, UK: EMA/CHMP/BMWP/86289/2010 Committee for Medicinal Products for Human Use (CHMP), 2012. Available at: https://www.ema.europa.eu/en/documents/scientific-guideline/guideline-immunogenicity-assessment-monoclonal-antibodies-intended-vivo-clinical-use_en.pdf

16. FDA/CDER/CBER. *Assay Development and Validation for Immunogenicity Testing of Therapeutic Protein Products— Guidance for Industry*. US Dep Heal Hum Serv Food Drug Adm, 2016. Available at: https://www.fda.gov/downloads/Drugs/Guidances/UCM192750.pdf

17. Cobbold S, Rebello P, Davies H, et al. A simple method for measuring patient anti-globulin responses against isotypic or idiotypic determinants. *J Immunol Methods* 1990;127:19–24.

18. Hart MH, de Vrieze H, Wouters D, et al. Differential effect of drug interference in immunogenicity assays. *J Immunol Methods* 2011;372:196–203.

19. Aalberse RC, Stapel SO, Schuurman J, et al. Immunoglobulin G4: an odd antibody. *Clin Exp Allergy* 2009;39:469–77.

20. Svenson M, Geborek P, Saxne T, et al. Monitoring patients treated with anti-TNF-alpha biopharmaceuticals: assessing serum infliximab and anti-infliximab antibodies. *Rheumatology (Oxf)* 2007;46:1828–34.

21. Cassinotti A, Travis S. Incidence and clinical significance of immunogenicity to infliximab in Crohn's disease: a critical systematic review. *Inflamm Bowel Dis* 2009;15:1264–75.

22. van Schouwenburg P a, Bartelds GM, Hart MH, et al. A novel method for the detection of antibodies to adalimumab in the presence of drug reveals 'hidden' immunogenicity in rheumatoid arthritis patients. *J Immunol Methods* 2010;362:82–8.

23. Bloem K, van Leeuwen A, Verbeek G, et al. Systematic comparison of drug-tolerant assays for anti-drug antibodies in a cohort of adalimumab-treated rheumatoid arthritis patients. *J Immunol Methods* 2015;418:29–38.

24. Wadhwa M, Knezevic I, Kang HN, et al. Immunogenicity assessment of biotherapeutic products: an overview of assays and their utility. *Biologicals* 2015;43:298–306.

25. Finckh A, Dudler J, Wermelinger F, et al. Influence of anti-infliximab antibodies and residual infliximab concentrations on the occurrence of acquired drug resistance to infliximab in rheumatoid arthritis patients. *Joint Bone Spine* 2010;77:313–18.

26. Krintel SB, Grunert VP, Hetland ML, et al. The frequency of anti-infliximab antibodies in patients with rheumatoid arthritis treated in routine care and the associations with adverse drug reactions and treatment failure. *Rheumatology (Oxf)* 2013;52:1245–53.

27. Radstake TRDJ, Svenson M, Eijsbouts AM, et al. Formation of antibodies against infliximab and adalimumab strongly correlates with functional drug levels and clinical responses in rheumatoid arthritis. *Ann Rheum Dis* 2009;68:1739–45.

28. Wolbink GJ, Aarden LA, Dijkmans B. Dealing with immunogenicity of biologicals: assessment and clinical relevance. *Curr Opin Rheumatol* 2009;21:211–15.

29. Bendtzen K, Geborek P, Svenson M, et al. Individualized monitoring of drug bioavailability and immunogenicity in rheumatoid arthritis patients treated with the tumor necrosis factor alpha inhibitor infliximab. *Arthritis Rheum* 2006;54:3782–9.

30. Pascual-Salcedo D, Plasencia C, Ramiro S, et al. Influence of immunogenicity on the efficacy of long-term treatment with infliximab in rheumatoid arthritis. *Rheumatology (Oxf)* 2011;50:1445–52.

31. Mok CC, van der Kleij D, Wolbink GJ. Drug levels, anti-drug antibodies, and clinical efficacy of the anti-TNFα biologics in rheumatic diseases. *Clin Rheumatol* 2013;32:1429–35.

32. Haraoui B, Cameron L, Ouellet M, et al. Anti-infliximab antibodies in patients with rheumatoid arthritis who require higher doses of infliximab to achieve or maintain a clinical response. *J Rheumatol* 2006;33:31–6.

33. Wolbink GJ, Vis M, Lems W, et al. Development of antiinfliximab antibodies and relationship to clinical response in patients with rheumatoid arthritis. *Arthritis Rheum* 2006;54:711–15.

34. van den Bemt BJF, den Broeder AA, Snijders GF, et al. Sustained effect after lowering high-dose infliximab in patients with rheumatoid arthritis: a prospective dose titration study. *Ann Rheum Dis* 2008;67:1697–701.

35. Ducourau E, Mulleman D, Paintaud G, et al. Antibodies toward infliximab are associated with low infliximab concentration at treatment initiation and poor infliximab maintenance in rheumatic diseases. *Arthritis Res Ther* 2011;13:R105.

36. Hoshino M, Yoshio T, Onishi S, et al. Influence of antibodies against infliximab and etanercept on the treatment effectiveness of these agents in Japanese patients with rheumatoid arthritis. *Mod Rheumatol* 2012;22:532–40.

37. Eng GP, Bendtzen K, Bliddal H, et al. Antibodies to infliximab and adalimumab in patients with rheumatoid arthritis in clinical remission: a cross-sectional study. *Arthritis* 2015;2015:784825.

38. Arstikyte I, Kapleryte G, Butrimiene I, et al. Influence of immunogenicity on the efficacy of long-term treatment with TNF α blockers in rheumatoid arthritis and spondyloarthritis patients. *Biomed Res Int* 2015;2015:604872.

39. Jung SM, Kim H-S, Kim H-R, et al. Immunogenicity of anti-tumour necrosis factor therapy in Korean patients with rheumatoid arthritis and ankylosing spondylitis. *Int Immunopharmacol* 2014;21:20–5.

40. Moots RJ, Xavier RM, Mok CC, et al. The impact of anti-drug antibodies on drug concentrations and clinical outcomes

in rheumatoid arthritis patients treated with adalimumab, etanercept, or infliximab: results from a multinational, real-world clinical practice, non-interventional study. *PLoS One* 2017;12:e0175207.

41. Bartelds GM, Wijbrandts CA, Nurmohamed MT, et al. Clinical response to adalimumab: relationship to anti-adalimumab antibodies and serum adalimumab concentrations in rheumatoid arthritis. *Ann Rheum Dis* 2007;66:921–6.

42. Bartelds G, Krieckaert C. Development of antidrug antibodies against adalimumab and association with disease activity and treatment failure during long-term follow-up. *JAMA* 2011;305:1460–8.

43. Plasencia C, Pascual-Salcedo D, García-Carazo S, et al. The immunogenicity to the first anti-TNF therapy determines the outcome of switching to a second anti-TNF therapy in spondyloarthritis patients. *Arthritis Res Ther* 2013;15:R79.

44. Vogelzang EH, Kneepkens EL, Nurmohamed MT, et al. Anti-adalimumab antibodies and adalimumab concentrations in psoriatic arthritis; an association with disease activity at 28 and 52 weeks of follow-up. *Ann Rheum Dis* 2014;73:2178–82.

45. Chen D-Y, Chen Y-M, Tsai W-C, et al. Significant associations of antidrug antibody levels with serum drug trough levels and therapeutic response of adalimumab and etanercept treatment in rheumatoid arthritis. *Ann Rheum Dis* 2015;74:e16.

46. Zisapel M, Zisman D, Madar-Balakirski N, et al. Prevalence of TNF-α blocker immunogenicity in psoriatic arthritis. *J Rheumatol* 2015;42:73–8.

47. Jani M, Chinoy H, Warren RB, et al. Clinical utility of random anti-TNF drug level testing and measurement of anti-drug antibodies on long-term treatment response in rheumatoid arthritis. *Arthritis Rheumatol* 2015;67:2011–19.

48. Burmester G-R, Kivitz AJ, Kupper H, et al. Efficacy and safety of ascending methotrexate dose in combination with adalimumab: the randomised CONCERTO trial. *Ann Rheum Dis* 2015;74:1037–44.

49. Bartelds GM, Wijbrandts CA, Nurmohamed MT, et al. Anti-infliximab and anti-adalimumab antibodies in relation to response to adalimumab in infliximab switchers and anti-tumour necrosis factor naive patients: a cohort study. *Ann Rheum Dis* 2010;69:817–21.

50. Jamnitski A, Bartelds GM, Nurmohamed MT, et al. The presence or absence of antibodies to infliximab or adalimumab determines the outcome of switching to etanercept. *Ann Rheum Dis* 2011;70:284–8.

51. Garcês S, Antunes M, Benito-Garcia E, et al. A preliminary algorithm introducing immunogenicity assessment in the management of patients with RA receiving tumour necrosis factor inhibitor therapies. *Ann Rheum Dis* 2014;73:1138–43.

52. Pouw MF, Krieckaert CL, Nurmohamed MT, et al. Key findings towards optimising adalimumab treatment: the concentration-effect curve. *Ann Rheum Dis* 2015;74:513–18.

53. Bender NK, Heilig CE, Dröll B, et al. Immunogenicity, efficacy and adverse events of adalimumab in RA patients. *Rheumatol Int* 2007;27:269–74.

54. Krieckaert CL, Jamnitski A, Nurmohamed MT, et al. Comparison of long-term clinical outcome with etanercept treatment and adalimumab treatment of rheumatoid arthritis with respect to immunogenicity. *Arthritis Rheum* 2012;64:3850–5.

55. McDonnell T, Ioannou Y, Rahman A. PEGylated drugs in rheumatology--why develop them and do they work? *Rheumatology (Oxf)* 2014;53:391–6.

56. He XH, Shaw PC, Tam SC. Reducing the immunogenicity and improving the *in vivo* activity of trichosanthin by site-directed pegylation. *Life Sci* 1999;65:355–68.

57. Ganson NJ, Kelly SJ, Scarlett E, et al. Control of hyperuricemia in subjects with refractory gout, and induction of antibody against poly(ethylene glycol) (PEG), in a phase I trial of subcutaneous PEGylated urate oxidase. *Arthritis Res Ther* 2006;8:R12.

58. Choy EHS, Hazleman B, Smith M, et al. Efficacy of a novel PEGylated humanized anti-TNF fragment (CDP870) in patients with rheumatoid arthritis : a phase II double-blinded, randomized, dose-escalating trial. *Rheumatology (Oxf)* 2002;1:1133–7.

59. Fleischmann R, Vencovský J, van Vollenhoven RF, et al. Efficacy and safety of certolizumab pegol monotherapy every 4 weeks in patients with rheumatoid arthritis failing previous disease-modifying antirheumatic therapy: the FAST4WARD study. *Ann Rheum Dis* 2009;68:805–11.

60. Jani M, Isaacs JD, Morgan AW, et al. High frequency of antidrug antibodies and association of random drug levels with efficacy in certolizumab pegol-treated patients with rheumatoid arthritis: results from the BRAGGSS cohort. *Ann Rheum Dis* 2017;76:208–13.

61. Keystone EC, Genovese MC, Klareskog L, et al. Golimumab, a human antibody to tumour necrosis factor {alpha} given by monthly subcutaneous injections, in active rheumatoid arthritis despite methotrexate therapy: the GO-FORWARD Study. *Ann Rheum Dis* 2009;68:789–96.

62. Kay J, Matteson EL, Dasgupta B, et al. Golimumab in patients with active rheumatoid arthritis despite treatment with methotrexate: a randomized, double-blind, placebo-controlled, dose-ranging study. *Arthritis Rheum* 2008;58:964–75.

63. Emery P, Fleischmann RM, Moreland LW, et al. Golimumab, a human anti-tumor necrosis factor alpha monoclonal antibody, injected subcutaneously every four weeks in methotrexate-naive patients with active rheumatoid arthritis. *Arthritis Rheum* 2009;60:2272–83.

64. Kneepkens EL, Plasencia C, Krieckaert CL, et al. Golimumab trough levels, antidrug antibodies and clinical response in patients with rheumatoid arthritis treated in daily clinical practice. *Ann Rheum Dis* 2014;73:2217–19.

65. Chen DY, Chen YM, Hung WT, et al. Immunogenicity, drug trough levels and therapeutic response in patients with rheumatoid arthritis or ankylosing spondylitis after 24-week golimumab treatment. *Ann Rheum Dis* 2015;74:2261–4.

66. Christen U, Thuerkauf R, Stevens R, et al. Immune response to a recombinant human TNFR55-IgG1 fusion protein: auto-antibodies in rheumatoid arthritis (RA) and multiple sclerosis (MS) patients have neither neutralizing nor agonist activities. *Hum Immunol* 1999;60:774–90.

67. Jamnitski A, Krieckaert CL, Nurmohamed MT, et al. Patients non-responding to etanercept obtain lower etanercept concentrations compared with responding patients. *Ann Rheum Dis* 2012;71:88–91.

68. Dore RK, Mathews S, Schechtman J, et al. The immunogenicity, safety, and efficacy of etanercept liquid administered once weekly in patients with rheumatoid arthritis. *Clin Exp Rheumatol* 2007;25:40–6.

69. de Vries MK, Brouwer E, van der Horst-Bruinsma IE, et al. Decreased clinical response to adalimumab in ankylosing spondylitis is associated with antibody formation. *Ann Rheum Dis* 2009;68:1787–8.

70. Yun H, Xie F, Beyl RN, et al. Risk of hypersensitivity to biologic agents among medicare patients with rheumatoid arthritis. *Arthritis Care Res* 2017;69:1526–34.

71. Thurlings RM, Teng O, Vos K, et al. Clinical response, pharmaco-kinetics, development of human anti-chimaeric antibodies, and synovial tissue response to rituximab treatment in patients with rheumatoid arthritis. *Ann Rheum Dis* 2010;69:409–12.

72. Md Yusof MY, Shaw D, El-Sherbiny YM, et al. Predicting and managing primary and secondary non-response to rituximab using B-cell biomarkers in systemic lupus erythematosus. *Ann Rheum Dis* 2017;76(11):1829–36.

73. Ng CM, Bruno R, Combs D, et al. Population pharmacokinetics of rituximab (anti-CD20 monoclonal antibody) in rheumatoid arthritis patients during a phase II clinical trial. *J Clin Pharmacol* 2005;45:792–801.

74. Breedveld F, Agarwal S, Yin M, et al. Rituximab pharmaco-kinetics in patients with rheumatoid arthritis: B-cell levels do not correlate with clinical response. *J Clin Pharmacol* 2007;47:1119–28.

75. Kneepkens EL, van den Oever I, Plasencia CH, et al. Serum tocilizumab trough concentration can be used to monitor systemic IL-6 receptor blockade in patients with rheumatoid arthritis: a prospective observational cohort study. *Scand J Rheumatol* 2017;46(2):87–94.

76. Benucci M, Meacci F, Grossi V, et al. Correlations between immunogenicity, drug levels, and disease activity in an Italian cohort of rheumatoid arthritis patients treated with tocilizumab. *Biol Targets Ther* 2016;10:53–8.

77. Burmester GR, Rubbert-Roth A, Cantagrel A, et al. Efficacy and safety of subcutaneous tocilizumab versus intravenous tocilizumab in combination with traditional DMARDs in patients with RA at week 97 (SUMMACTA). *Ann Rheum Dis* 2016;75:68–74.

78. Burmester GR, Choy E, Kivitz A, et al. Low immunogenicity of tocilizumab in patients with rheumatoid arthritis. *Ann Rheum Dis* 2017;76:1078–85.

79. Dougados M, Kissel K, Sheeran T, et al. Adding tocilizumab or switching to tocilizumab monotherapy in methotrexate inadequate responders: 24-week symptomatic and structural results of a 2-year randomised controlled strategy trial in rheumatoid arthritis (ACT-RAY). *Ann Rheum Dis* 2013;72:43–50.

80. Rocchi V, Puxeddu I, Cataldo G, et al. Hypersensitivity reactions to tocilizumab: role of skin tests in diagnosis. *Rheumatol* 2014;53:1527–9.

81. Genovese MC, Covarrubias A, Leon G, et al. Subcutaneous abatacept versus intravenous abatacept: a phase IIIb noninferiority study in patients with an inadequate response to methotrexate. *Arthritis Rheum* 2011;63:2854–64.

82. Nash P, Nayiager S, Genovese MC, et al. Immunogenicity, safety, and efficacy of abatacept administered subcutaneously with or without background methotrexate in patients with rheumatoid arthritis: results from a phase III, international, multicenter, parallel-arm, open-label study. *Arthritis Care Res (Hoboken)* 2013;65:718–28.

83. Weinblatt ME, Moreland LW, Westhovens R, et al. Safety of abatacept administered intravenously in treatment of rheumatoid arthritis: integrated analyses of up to 8 years of treatment from the abatacept clinical trial program. *J Rheumatol* 2013;40:787–97.

84. Plasencia C, Pascual-Salcedo D, Alcocer P, et al. The timing of serum infliximab loss, or the appearance of antibodies to infliximab (ATI), is related with the clinical activity in ATI-positive patients with rheumatoid arthritis treated with infliximab. *Ann Rheum Dis* 2013;72:1888–90.

85. Jani M, Dixon WG, Chinoy H. Drug safety and immunogenicity of tumour necrosis factor inhibitors: the story so far (in press). *Rheumatology (Oxf)* 2017;57(11):1896–907.

86. Zuelgaray E, Domont F, Peiffer-Smadja N, et al. Tocilizumab-induced drug reaction with eosinophilia and systemic symptoms syndrome in adult-onset still disease. *Ann Intern Med* 2017;167:141–2.

87. Korswagen L a, Bartelds GM, Krieckaert CLM, et al. Venous and arterial thromboembolic events in adalimumab-treated patients with antiadalimumab antibodies: a case series and cohort study. *Arthritis Rheum* 2011;63:877–83.

88. Davies R, Dixon WG, Watson KD, et al. Influence of anti-TNF patient warning regarding avoidance of high risk foods on rates of listeria and salmonella infections in the UK. *Ann Rheum Dis* 2013;72:461–2.

89. Kim SC, Solomon DH, Liu J, et al. Risk of venous thromboembolism in patients with rheumatoid arthritis: initiating disease-modifying antirheumatic drugs. *Am J Med* 2015;128:539.e7–17.

90. Benucci M, Saviola G, Baiardi P, et al. Anti-nucleosome antibodies as prediction factor of development of autoantibodies during therapy with three different TNFalpha blocking agents in rheumatoid arthritis. *Clin Rheumatol* 2008;27:91–5.

91. Takase K, Horton SC, Ganesha A, et al. What is the utility of routine ANA testing in predicting development of biological DMARD-induced lupus and vasculitis in patients with rheumatoid arthritis? Data from a single-centre cohort. *Ann Rheum Dis* 2014;73:1695–9.

92. Pink AE, Fonia A, Allen MH, et al. Antinuclear antibodies associate with loss of response to antitumour necrosis factor-alpha therapy in psoriasis: a retrospective, observational study. *Br J Dermatol* 2010;162:780–5.

93. Hoffmann JHO, Hartmann M, Enk AH, et al. Autoantibodies in psoriasis as predictors for loss of response and anti-infliximab antibody induction. *Br J Dermatol* 2011;165:1355–8.

94. Yukawa N, Fujii T, Kondo-Ishikawa S, et al. Correlation of antinuclear antibody and anti-double-stranded DNA antibody with clinical response to infliximab in patients with rheumatoid arthritis: a retrospective clinical study. *Arthritis Res Ther* 2011;13:R213.

95. Nguyen DL, Nguyen ET, Bechtold ML. pANCA positivity predicts lower clinical response to infliximab therapy among patients with IBD. *South Med J* 2015;108:139–43.

96. Jani M, Dixon WG, Kearsley-Fleet L, et al. Drug-specific risk and characteristics of lupus and vasculitis-like events in patients with rheumatoid arthritis treated with TNFi: results from BSRBR-RA. *RMD Open* 2017;3:e000314.

97. Dörner T, Strand V, Castañeda-Hernández G, et al. The role of biosimilars in the treatment of rheumatic diseases. *Ann Rheum Dis* 2013;72:322–8.

98. Park W, Hrycaj P, Jeka S, et al. A randomised, double-blind, multicentre, parallel-group, prospective study comparing the pharmacokinetics, safety, and efficacy of CT-P13 and innovator infliximab in patients with ankylosing spondylitis: the PLANETAS study. *Ann Rheum Dis* 2013;72:1605–12.

99. Park W, Yoo DH, Miranda P, et al. Efficacy and safety of switching from reference infliximab to CT-P13 compared with maintenance of CT-P13 in ankylosing spondylitis: 102-week data from the PLANETAS extension study. *Ann Rheum Dis* 2017;76(2):346–54.

100. Emery P, Vencovský J, Sylwestrzak A, et al. A phase III randomised, double-blind, parallel-group study comparing SB4 with etanercept reference product in patients with active rheumatoid arthritis despite methotrexate therapy. *Ann Rheum Dis* 2015;76(1):51–7.

101. Meacci F, Manfredi M, Infantino M, et al. Anti-etanercept and anti SB4 antibodies detection: impact of the assay method. *Ann Rheum Dis* 2016;75:e39–e39.

102. Jørgensen KK, Olsen IC, Goll GL, et al. Switching from originator infliximab to biosimilar CT-P13 compared with maintained treatment with originator infliximab (NOR-SWITCH): a 52-week, randomised, double-blind, non-inferiority trial. *Lancet* 2017; 389:2304–16.

103. Glintborg B, Sørensen IJ, Loft AG, et al. A nationwide non-medical switch from originator infliximab to biosimilar CT-P13 in 802 patients with inflammatory arthritis: 1-year clinical outcomes from the DANBIO registry. *Ann Rheum Dis* 2017;0:1426–31.

104. Mitchison N. Induction of immunological paralysis in two zones of dosage. *Proc R Soc L B Biol Sci* 1964;15:272–92.

105. Weigle W. Different types of immunological unresponsiveness. *Adv Exp Med Biol* 1973;29:357–62.

106. Benjamin R, Cobbold S, Clark M, et al. Tolerance to rat monoclonal antibodies. Implications for serotherapy. *J Exp Med* 1986;163:1539–52.

107. Thalayasingam N, Isaacs JD. Anti-TNF therapy. *Best Pract Res Clin Rheumatol* 2011;25:549–67.

108. Somerfield J, Hill-Cawthorne GA, Lin A, et al. A novel strategy to reduce the immunogenicity of biological therapies. *J Immunol* 2010;185:765–8.

109. Waldmann H. Human monoclonal antibodies: the residual challenge of antibody immunogenicity. *Methods Mol Biol* 2014;1060:1–8.

36

The use of JAK inhibitors in the treatment of rheumatoid arthritis

Katie Bechman, James Galloway, and Peter C. Taylor

JAK-STAT biology

Discovery of the JAK-STAT pathway was a landmark breakthrough in cell biology that has advanced our understanding of communication between cells central to host defence. This pathway involves families of proteins, denoted as JAKs (Janus family tyrosine kinases) and STATs (signal transducers and activators of transcription).

The discovery of JAKs and STATs arose from efforts to understand the action of interferons produced in the immune response against viruses. The pathway provided a mechanism to explain how extracellular signals, such as interferons, trigger intracellular responses that alter the expression of genes within the cells.[1] It is now recognized that a wide variety of cytokines, colony-stimulating factors, and hormones use this pathway.

In rheumatoid arthritis (RA), activated B cells, T cells, macrophages, and other leukocytes infiltrate the synovium in response to pro-inflammatory cytokines and chemokines. These activated immune cells produce further pro-inflammatory cytokines, perpetuating the cycle of inflammation and leading to joint damage. Monoclonal antibody technology has enabled the generation of biologics against cytokines or their receptors and immune cell associated molecules.[2] However, despite the success of biologics, targeting a single cytokine does not completely abrogate the pathology of RA for all patients. Furthermore, being large proteins, biologic drugs have the relative disadvantage of requiring parenteral administration. With the advances in understanding of cytokine signalling and small molecular engineering, a question emerged whether targeting intracellular signalling might provide an orally deliverable, safe, and efficacious strategy.[3]

JAK-STAT pathway in inflammation

The JAK-STAT pathway operates downstream of more than 50 cytokines and growth factors, and it is regarded as a central communication node for the immune system.[4] Signalling through the JAK-STAT pathway is initiated when a cytokine binds to its corresponding receptor. This instigates a conformational change in the cytoplasmic portion of the receptor, leading to activation of receptor associated members of the JAK family of kinases.[5] Activated JAKs can phosphorylate tyrosines on their associated receptors. The phosphorylated tyrosines serve as docking sites for STATs and other signalling molecules. Once engaged to the receptor on a tyrosine residue, STATs also become phosphorylated. Activated STATs then dissociate from the receptor, dimerize, and are rapidly transported from the cytoplasm to the nucleus.[5] STATs then bind to members of the GAS (gamma activated site) family of target gene promoters (**Figure 36.1**). This process is fast; newly induced STAT DNA binding activity can be detected in the nucleus within minutes of cytokine binding to its corresponding receptor.[6] This JAK-STAT signalling pathway is regulated by a vast array of intrinsic and environmental stimuli.[7]

Cytokine signalling in the JAK-STAT pathway

Cytokines are crucial in the pathogenesis of RA, promoting autoimmunity and propagating synovial inflammation and joint destruction.[8] Key cytokines include: interferon (IFNα and IFNβ), interleukins (IL-1, IL-6, IL-7, IL-10, IL-12, IL-15, IL-17, IL-18, IL-21, IL-23), transforming growth factor (TGF-β); and tumour necrosis factor (TNF).[8] A subset of these cytokines, important in RA utilize the JAK-STAT pathways to transmit signals (**Figure 36.2**).[9]

In general, cytokines are grouped into super families based on the receptors they bind, which signal through different pathways. Two major classes are type I and type II cytokines. The cytoplasmic domain of type 1 and type 11 receptors signal via the JAK-STAT pathway.

Type I cytokines include cytokines that share the common gamma-chain (γc) cytokine receptor subunit (IL-2, IL-4, IL-7, IL-9, IL-15, and IL-21) the common β-chain (IL-3, IL-5, GM-CSF), signal through the gp130 receptor subunit (IL-6, IL-11, IL-27), and the dimeric cytokine family (IL-12, IL-23, and IL-35). Included in this group is also type 1 hormone-like cytokines (erythropoietin (EPO), thrombopoietin (TPO), G-CSF, growth hormone, and leptin).[3,10,11]

Type II cytokines include type I, II, and III IFNs (IFN-α, IFN-β, IFN-γ, IL-28, and IL-29) and IL-10-related cytokines (IL-10, IL-19, IL-20, IL-22, IL-24, and IL-26).[3,10–12]

Despite their importance in immune-mediated disease, cytokines such as TNF, IL-1, and IL-17 do not signal via the JAK-STAT

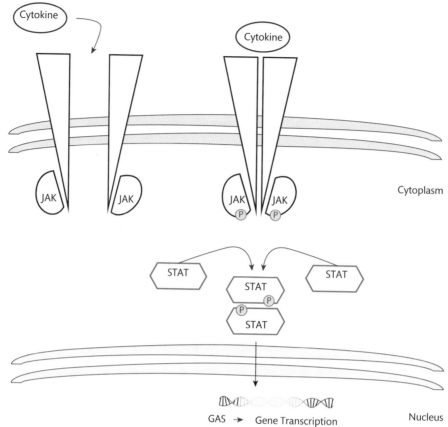

Figure 36.1 The JAK-STAT signalling pathway.

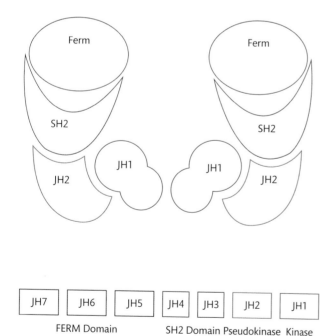

Figure 36.2 Structure of Janus kinase (JAK) and signal transduction and activation of transcription (STAT) molecules.

pathway. However, these cytokines can be induced by cytokines that do signal via this pathway. For example, IL-6 drives the production of TNF and IL-1, and induces the differentiation of type 17 helper T cells, which produce IL-17.[11]

Structure of JAK

JAKs belong to the family of tyrosine kinases enzymes. Kinases are recognized by their ability to catalyse the phosphorylation of tyrosine residues, causing a change in the function of the protein that the kinase is contained in.

All JAKs consist of four structural domains. An alternative nomenclature for the four domains is based on their amino acid sequence, classified as the seven Janus homology (JH) domains (**Figure 36.3A**). The kinase domain (JH1) is the site of catalytic activity and the site which is targeted by JAK inhibitors. The pseudokinase domain (JH2) has a regulatory function, although may have low levels of catalytic activity. The SH2 domain (JH3 and JH4) stabilizes the structural conformation of the enzyme, while the FERM domain (JH5, JH6, and JH7) mediates receptors interaction.[6,13] The name Janus is in reference to the presence of the two faced kinase domains, alluding to the double-faced Roman god of gates and doors.

JAK family

There are four members of the JAK family: JAK1, JAK2, JAK3, and TYK2. An important element of JAK function is the pairing of the JAK kinases; each cytokine receptor requires at least two associated JAKs in order to signal. This may involve identical JAK homodimers (e.g. JAK2/JAK2) or as heterodimers (e.g. JAK1/JAK3).[14] The combination of cytokine signally through JAK-STAT pairing is demonstrated in **Figure 36.3**.

JAK3 only couples to the γc chain of the cytokine receptor and does not associate with any other cytokine receptor. JAK3 is always paired

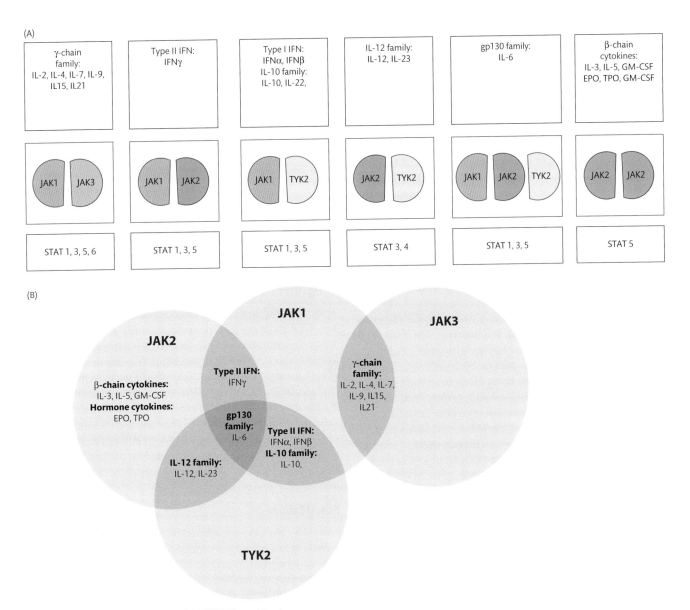

Figure 36.3 Cytokine signally through JAK/STAT combination.

with JAK1 and in this arrangement controls signalling for the γc cytokines (IL-2, IL-4, IL-7, IL-9, IL-15, and IL-21). JAK3 mutations results in severe combined immunodeficiency (SCID) characterized by the lack of T and natural killer (NK) cells, but not B cells.[12,15]

In contrast to JAK3, JAK1 is widely expressed and associates with type I cytokines that use γc chain and gp130 receptor subunit (IL-6) and type II cytokine receptors (IFNs and IL10). In addition to pairing with JAK3, JAK1 also pairs with JAK2 and TYK2.[12]

JAK2 is also widely expressed and associates with type I cytokines that use common β chain (IL-3, IL-5, GM-CSF), gp130 (IL-6) and dimeric receptor (IL-12, IL-23) as well as type 1 hormone-like cytokines (EPO, TPO). JAK2 also associated with IL-10 type II cytokines receptors.[11] JAK2 is the only member of the JAK family that pairs with itself. JAK knockout mice die in early embryogenesis from failure of erythropoiesis.

TYK2 is associated with type I cytokines that use gp130 (IL-6) and dimeric receptor (IL-12, IL-23) as well as type II cytokines receptors (IFNs and IL-10).[5,11]

Structure of STATs

STATs have six essential functional requirements: (a) to bind phosphorylated tyrosines; (b) to themselves become tyrosine phosphorylated; (c) to dimerize; (d) to translocate into the nucleus; (e) to bind DNA; and (f) to modulate gene expression.[6]

Inactive cytoplasmic STATs exist as either monomers or preformed dimers. The conserved SH2 domain on STAT proteins recognizes specific phosphotyrosine motifs. This allows recruitment to the cytokine receptor, association with the activating JAK and homo- or heterodimerization.[5]

There are seven known STATs proteins: STAT1, STAT2, STAT3, STAT4, STAT5a and STAT5b, STAT6. Various cytokines specifically activate certain STAT proteins. This has been demonstrated in knockout mice. For example, STAT1-deficient mice are highly susceptible to microbial and viral infections and tumour formation due to severely impaired IFN responses, with the induction of many well-known IFN-inducible genes being abrogated.[12]

Targeting JAK-STAT pathway with small molecule JAK inhibitors

The human kinome comprises more than 500 kinase enzymes. Over the last 20 years, various kinases have been among the most intensively pursued drug targets. The therapeutic potential of blocking the JAK-STAT pathway was first recognized in the 1990s. A patient with autosomal SCID was identified with a naturally occurring JAK3 mutation, in which a single amino acid substitution prevented JAK3–receptor interaction.[16] Since then, huge efforts have been made to develop small molecules that target this cytokine signalling pathway. JAK inhibitors (also known as Janus kinase inhibitors or 'jakinibs') are small molecules that block the activity of one or more of the Janus kinase family of enzymes (JAK1, JAK2, JAK3, TYK2) thereby interfering with the JAK-STAT signalling pathway.[17]

Therapeutic window

Current JAK inhibitors act by competitively blocking the adenosine triphosphate-binding (ATP) site in the JH1 domain.[15] The binding site has structural similarities with other tyrosine kinases and therefore a potential challenge was to develop small molecules with selectivity for JAK enzymes without unwanted off-target effects. In view of homology between enzymes and the near identical ATP binding sites, a further challenge for medicinal chemists was to develop drug candidates with selectivity for particular members of the JAK family. However, these challenges have been overcome and several drug candidates have progressed to clinical studies. Tofacitinib, for example, selectively inhibits JAKs 1, 3 and 2 at the approved dose but becomes a 'pan JAK' inhibitor at higher doses.[3] Similarly, the inhibition profiles of different JAK inhibitors have been investigated in vitro. In these experiments, the half maximal inhibitory concentration (IC_{50}) required to inhibit JAK activity is measured for each agent. However, these in vitro experiments can produce conflicting results due to differences in the methodology used for in vitro kinase assays and may be difficult to interpret. In general, the JAK inhibitors that have been tested in trials all block more than one JAK enzyme and inhibit the signalling of multiple cytokines. See Table 36.1 for pharmacodynamics for current drugs.[18–20]

Oral availability of JAK inhibitors

In contrast to contemporary biologic disease-modifying antirheumatic drugs (DMARDs), small molecular chemical entities with low molecular weight have the advantage of oral administration.

Table 36.1 Pharmacodynamics of JAK inhibitors; comparison of enzyme and whole cell activity for selective JAK inhibitors (IC_{50} the concentration of an inhibitor where the response is reduced by half)

Drug	IC_{50} (nM)			
	JAK1	JAK2	JAK3	TYK2
Tofacitinib	112	20	1	-
Baricitinib	5.9	5.7	>400	53
Filgotinib	10	28	810	116
Upadacitinib	43	200	2300	4700
Peficitinib	3.9	5.0	0.7	4.8

Furthermore, they can easily penetrate the cell membrane to access the cytoplasm and interfere with intracellular signalling.

Pharmacokinetics

The currently licenced JAK inhibitors demonstrate a non-linear (dose-proportional) pharmacokinetic profile. Tofacitinib and baricitinib are rapidly absorbed (reaching peak concentration by 0.5–1 hour) and eliminated (half-life ~3 hours). The short half-life of JAK inhibitors is a potential advantage over biologics; in the case of an adverse event such as infection, the immunosuppressive effects of the drug can be rapidly reversed.[21] Tofacitinib is metabolized and cleared by the liver (70%) and kidneys (30%). Metabolism is primarily facilitated by CYP3A4 with minor contribution from CYP2C19. Baricitinib undergoes renal excretion through glomerular filtration and active secretion. Less than 10% is metabolized, mediated by CYP3A4.[22,23]

Drug interaction

Tofacitinib exposure is decreased when co-administered with potent CYP inducers (e.g. rifampicin), while exposure is increased when co-administered with potent inhibitors of CYP3A4 (e.g. ketoconazole) or CYP2C19 inhibitors (e.g. fluconazole). The dose of tofacitinib dose should be reduced to 5 mg once daily in patients coprescribed CYP3A4 or CYP2C19 inhibitors. Tofacitinib does not significantly inhibit or induce the pharmacokinetics of other medications.[23] Baricitinib exposure is not affected by co-administration of CYP3A4 or inducers or CYP3A4/CYP2C19 inhibitors but a reduced dose of 2 mg qd is recommended for patients with creatinine clearance of between 30 and 60 ml/minute or those taking OAT3 inhibitors such as probenecid.[23]

Renal failure

Both JAK inhibitors are affected by renal function. Baricitinib dose reduction to 2 mg qd is recommended in patients with a creatinine clearance between 30 and 60 ml/min, or in patients taking OAT3 inhibitors such as probenecid, while use is not recommended in patients with creatinine clearance <30 ml/min. Tofacitinib dose should be reduced to 5 mg once daily in patients with severe renal impairment (creatinine clearance <30 ml/min).[22]

Immunogenicity

Another difficulty seen with protein-based biological therapies compared to small molecules is their immunogenicity. The development of antidrug antibodies has been identified as an important contributor to treatment failure with biologics.[24] This is not seen with small molecules.

Comparison of biologic and small molecule targeting therapy in RA is summarized in Table 36.2.

Currently licenced JAK inhibitors

Tofacitinib

Tofacitinib (formerly designated CP 690 550) was developed by Pfizer and became the first JAK inhibitor to be approved for the treatment of RA by the Food and Drug Administration (FDA) in 2012. The European Medicines Agency (EMA) did not approve tofacitinib until 2017 due to safety concerns.

Table 36.2 Comparison of biologics and small molecules in RA

	Biologics	Small molecules
Target	Extracellular	Intracellular
Mechanism of action	Blocking/depletion	Enzyme inhibition
Specificity	high	Variable
Composition	Protein	Small molecule chemical entity
Molecular weight	>1kDA	<700 Da
Stability	Sensitive to proteases and heat	Mostly stable
Administration	Parenteral	Oral
In vivo half-life	Long	Short
Degradation	Catabolism	Metabolism
Immunogenicity	Immunogenic	No
Cost to manufacture	High	Low/variable

Source: data from Mócsai A, Kovács L, and Gergely P. (2014) 'What is the future of targeted therapy in rheumatology: biologics or small molecules?' *BMC Med* 13(12):43.

Tofacitinib is a potent, selective JAK inhibitor, with minimal effects on other kinases.[25] The drug inhibits JAK3 and JAK1, with some affinity for JAK2 and limited affinity for TYK2. Tofacitinib was originally described as a selective JAK3 inhibitor, with 20-fold selectivity relative to JAK2. However, the observed selectivity varies according to the nature of the assay employed *in vitro*.[26]

In vitro studies have demonstrated tofacitinib to inhibit γc chain cytokines (IL-2, IL-4, IL-7, IL-15, and IL-21) signalling via JAK3; non-γc chain cytokine signalling, including IL-6 induced phosphorylation of STAT3 and STAT1 mediated by JAK1-JAK2; IFN-γ phosphorylation of STAT1 mediated by JAK1-JAK2; and IL-12 and IL-23 mediated phosphorylation of STAT-1 via JAK2-Tyk2.[25] In RA animal models, tofacitinib therapy was associated with a dose-dependent reduction in inflammatory swelling, cell influx, and cartilage damage.[27]

Efficacy studies

Tofacitinib has demonstrated significant efficacy in phase II and III randomized controlled trials (RCTs) in adult RA patients both in combination with csDMARDs, including methotrexate, and as monotherapy. Pivotal RCTs are shown in Table 36.3.

Table 36.3 Tofacitinib pivotal RCT(s)

ORAL Solo	Tofacitinib 5 mg, 10 mg bd, or placebo	DMARD/biologic-IR
ORAL Sync	Tofacitinib 5 mg, 10 mg bd, or placebo with csDMARDs	DMARD-IR
ORAL Scan	Tofacitinib 5 mg, 10 mg bd, or placebo with MTX	MTX-IR
ORAL Standard	Tofacitinib 5 mg, 10 mg bd, or ADA 40 mg or placebo with MTX	MTX-IR
ORAL Step	Tofacitinib 5 mg, 10 mg bd, or placebo with MTX	TNF inhibitors-IR
ORAL Start	Tofacitinib 5 mg, 10 mg bd, or MTX	MTX-naïve RA
ORAL Strategy	Tofacitinib 5 mg, 5 mg with MTX, or ADA 40 mg with MTX	MTX-IR

MTX, methotrexate; ADA, adalimumab; IR, inadequate response.

ORAL Solo was a 6-month RCT of 611 patients with who had failed therapy with a DMARD (DMARD-IR). Patients were randomized to tofacitinib 5 mg bd, 10 mg bd, or placebo bd. Tofacitinib treatment was associated with statistically significant improvement in ACR20, ACR50, and ACR70 response criteria and HAQ-DI scores at month 3. The percentage of patients with a DAS28 of less than 2.6 was not significantly higher with tofacitinib than with placebo.[28] There were statistically significant and clinically meaningful improvements in multiple patient-reported outcomes including; Patient Global Assessment of Disease Activity (PtGA); Patient Assessment of Pain (Pain); Health Assessment Questionnaire-Disability Index (HAQ-DI); Short Form 36 (SF-36) summary and domain scores; Functional Assessment of Chronic Illness Therapy-Fatigue (FACIT-F) at 3 months. Benefits were rapid in onset and significant improvements were reported at week 2 for PtGA, Pain, and HAQ-DI, and differentiation from baseline was seen as early as 3 days after treatment initiation for PtGA and Pain.[29]

ORAL Standard was a 12-month trial randomizing 717 methotrexate (MTX)-IR patients to tofacitinib 5 mg bd, 10 mg bd, adalimumab 40 mg, or placebo (to both tofacitinib and to adalimumab), with MTX. At month 6, ACR 20 response rates were significantly higher among tofacitinib 5 mg or 10 mg arm (51.5% and 52.6%, respectively) and adalimumab arm (47.2%) than placebo arm (28.3%). The authors concluded superior efficacy to placebo and numerically similar to adalimumab, although a formal non-inferiority comparison was not performed.[30] There were clinically meaningful improvements across a broad range of patient-reported outcomes (PROs) at 3 months and sustained to month 12. The greatest improvements were observed with tofacitinib 10 mg twice a day (BID).[31]

ORAL Sync was a 12-month RCT randomizing 792 DMARD-IR patients, to tofacitinib 5 mg bd, 10 mg bd, or placebo bd, with MTX. Tofacitinib treatment was associated with statistically significant improvement in ACR20 response rates. DAS28 less than 2.6 response rates at month 6 were superior in the tofacitinib groups versus placebo. Significant responses were observed by week 2 for ACR20 and ACR50, and by week 4 for ACR70.[32] A significantly greater proportions of patients in both tofacitinib treatment groups versus placebo reported improvements greater than the minimum clinically important differences (MCID) at month 3 across all PROs, except the SF-36 role-emotional domain (significant for tofacitinib 10 mg BID).[33]

ORAL Scan was a 24-month trial designed to assess radiographic preservation with tofacitinib. The study randomized 797 patients who had failed therapy with MTX, to tofacitinib 5 mg bd, 10 mg bd, or placebo bd, with MTX. Both tofacitinib doses demonstrated clinical efficacy. However, the rate of structural damage progression in the placebo treated arm was low and it was not possible to demonstrate structural damage inhibition by changes from baseline in modified Total Sharp score (mTSS) for tofacitinib 5 mg bd although there statistically significant inhibition of radiographic progression (p <0.05), with tofacitinib 10 mg bd.[34]

ORAL Step was a 6-month, trial randomizing 399 patients with an inadequate response to TNF inhibitors (TNF-IR), to tofacitinib 5 mg bd, 10 mg bd, or placebo bd with MTX. Tofacitinib treatment was associated with statistically significant improvement in ACR20, ACR50, and ACR70 response criteria[35] and statistically significant and clinically meaningful improvements in HAQ-DI, PtGA, pain, physical function, HRQOL, and fatigue compared to placebo.[36] The percentage of patients with a DAS28 of less than 2.6 were significant in tofacitinib 10 mg twice-daily group compared to placebo.[35]

ORAL Start was a 24-month RCT randomizing 958 MTX naïve patients to tofacitinib 5 mg bd, 10 mg bd, or MTX. Mean changes in mTSS from baseline to month 6 were significantly smaller in the tofacitinib groups than in the MTX group, but changes were modest in all three groups. ACR70 response at 6 months were significantly higher with 5 mg and 10 mg tofacitinib (26% and 38%, respectively) compared with MTX (12%).[37] There were statistically significant differences in multiple PROs between both tofacitinib doses and MTX. This was first evident at month 1 (PtGA, pain, HAQ-DI, and FACIT-F) and months 3 and 6 in other outcomes. The benefits persisted over the length of the trial.[38]

ORAL Strategy was a 12-month head-to-head, non-inferiority trial randomizing 1146 MTX-IR patients to tofacitinib 5 mg monotherapy, tofacitinib 5 mg plus MTX, or adalimumab 40 mg plus MTX. At 6 months, ACR50 responses were seen in 38%, 46%, and 44%, respectively. Non-inferiority was declared for tofacitinib + MTX versus adalimumab + MTX but not for tofacitinib monotherapy.[39]

Baricitinib

Baricitinib was developed by Eli Lily and approved by the EMA in 2017. Baricitinib was approved by the FDA in 2018 at the lower 2mg once daily dose for the treatment of adults with moderately-to-severely active RA who have had an inadequate response to one or more anti-TNF therapies.

Baricitinib is also regarded as a selective inhibitor of the JAK family without any effect on other kinases.[40] It inhibits JAK1 and JAK2, and to a much lesser extent TYK2. Baricitinib is considered a JAK3 sparing agent with 100-fold selectivity for JAK1 and JAK2.[15]

In vitro studies have demonstrated baricitinib to inhibit interferons (IFNα, IFNγ), common γ-chain cytokines (IL-15, IL-21), IL-6, and IL-27 with dose- and time-dependent inhibition of phosphorylation of STAT3.[40] In RA animal models, baricitinib therapy was associated with a dose-dependent reduction in inflammatory swelling and joint damage, at doses low enough to be devoid of any inhibitory effect on JAK3.[41]

Efficacy studies

Baricitinib has also demonstrated significant efficacy in phase II and III RCTs. The development programme includes one phase 1, three phase II, and four phase III trials. Patients completing phase III RCTs were eligible to enter long-term extension studies including RA-BEYOND and RA-BALANCE specifically for patients in Argentina, Brazil, and China. Pivotal RCTs are shown in Table 36.4.

Table 36.4 Baricitinib pivotal RCT(s)

RA-Begin	Baricitinib 4 mg od, 4 mg od with MTX, or MTX	DMARD-naïve RA
RA-Build	Baricitinib 2 mg, 4 mg od, or placebo with csDMARDs	DMARD-IR
RA-Beam	Baricitinib 4 mg od, ADA 40 mg, or placebo with MTX	DMARD-IR
RA-Beacon	Baricitinib 2 mg, 4 mg, or placebo, with csDMARDs	Biologic-IR

MTX, methotrexate; ADA, adalimumab; IR, inadequately response.

RA-Begin was a 52-week trial randomizing 588 DMARD-naïve patients to once-daily baricitinib 4 mg monotherapy, MTX monotherapy or combination once-daily baricitinib 4 mg and MTX. At 24 week, ACR20 response was significantly higher with baricitinib monotherapy and combination compared to MTX monotherapy. Improvements were observed as early as week 1. Baricitinib was associated with reduction in radiographic progression compared with MTX monotherapy; however, the difference was only statistically significant for baricitinib combination arm.[42] Patients receiving baricitinib had greater levels of pain improvement compared to MTX monotherapy. The time when 50% of patients achieved 70% pain improvement was 20 weeks for MTX, 12 weeks for baricitinib and 8 weeks for baricitinib + MTX.[43]

RA-Build was a 24-week RCT randomizing 684 DMARD-IR patients to receive once-daily baricitinib 2 mg, 4 mg, or placebo with background csDMARDs therapy. ACR20 responses were significantly higher with baricitinib 2 mg and 4 mg compared to placebo as both 12 and 24 weeks. Statistically significant improvements were observed in DAS28, SDAI remission, and HAQ-DI. Radiographic progression was also reduced at 24 weeks in both 2 mg and 4 mg arm compared to placebo.[44]

RA-Beam was a 52-week trial randomizing 1307 MTX-IR patients to once-daily baricitinib 4 mg, adalimumab 40 mg, or placebo, with background MTX therapy. ACR 20 responses were significantly higher with baricitinib compared to placebo at weeks 12 and 24. Baricitinib was also found to be non-inferior to adalimumab for the ACR20 response, with a margin of 12% (70% vs. 61% for adalimumab), and was therefore considered to be significantly superior to adalimumab (p = 0.01). Significantly greater inhibition of radiographic progression was also seen with baricitinib compared to placebo at 24 and 52 weeks.[45] There were significant improvements in HAQ-DI, PtGA, pain, FACIT-F, SF-36 physical component summary score, EQ-5 D, and Work Productivity and Activity Impairment Questionnaire with baricitinib compared with placebo and adalimumab at week 12. Improvement occurred within the first weeks of treatment and were maintained throughout the 52-week trial.[46]

RA-Beacon was a 24-week RCT randomizing 527 bDMARD-IR patients to once-daily baricitinib 2 mg, 4 mg, or placebo, with background DMARD therapy. At week 12, ACR 20 responses were 55% in the baricitinib 4 mg arm compared with 27% in the placebo group (p <0.001). Statistically significant improvements were also observed in DAS28, but not SDAI remission.[47] Patients receiving baricitinib had significantly higher degrees of improvements in most PROs compared with placebo. Improvements were maintained to week 24 and generally more rapid and of greater magnitude with baricitinib 4 mg than 2 mg.[48]

Safety concerns

The Introduction of JAK inhibitors was initially overshadowed by safety concerns, particularly with respect to opportunistic infections observed with higher doses. However, as the phase III trials have emerged and long-term extension data has been evaluated, the absolute risk of serious adverse events appears comparable to biologics. The most important difference appears to be an increased risk of herpes zoster infections. The safety concerns will now be discussed in detail.

Infection

JAK inhibition results in the suppression of multiple integral elements of the immune response. Infection secondary to immunosuppression represents a major concern.[21] Infections, especially nasopharyngitis, upper respiratory tract, urinary tract and herpes zoster are the most frequent adverse events in tofacitinib trial and long-term extension (LTE) studies. The most common serious adverse events were also infections. Glucocorticoids, baseline lymphopenia, line of therapy (third line vs. second), and geographical region (Asia, Europe, and Latin America, versus the United States and Canada) were associated with increased risk of serious infection.[49] The rates of infection do not seem to increase with longer duration of therapy,[49] however, the number were numerically higher in patients receiving 10 mg compared to 5 mg dose or patients also receiving (background DMARDs).[50]

Pooled data from clinical trial and LTE studies reported a serious infection incidence rate of 2.7 per 100 patient-years.[49] Similar findings are noted in baricitinib studies. A pooled analysis of phase I to III clinical trials reported a serious infection incidence rate of 3.2 per 100 patient-years.[51] In interventional studies, the observed risk of serious infections with tofacitinib is comparable to published rates for biologics.[52]

Herpes zoster

The most recognized infectious complication with JAK inhibitors has been the reactivation of varicella zoster virus. The crude incident rate of herpes zoster with tofacitinib is reported at 4.4 per 100 patient-years of treatment.[53] Similar rates are reported with baricitinib (4.3 per 100 patient-years within 24 weeks).[51,54] Overall, when patients from Japan and Korea are included, this is 1.5–2-fold higher than observed in patients on DMARDs or biologics.[55] With tofacitinib, the highest rates are in older patients, with coprescription of glucocorticoids or MTX, and in Asians from Japan and Korea.[53] There are very few cases of multidermatomal or disseminated herpes, and no cases of visceral disease or death.[53]

Opportunistic infections

Tuberculosis is reported with both tofacitinib and baricitinib. Tuberculosis (TB) was the most common opportunistic infections reported but was rare in regions of low and medium TB incidence.[56] With tofacitinib, there were 26 cases of active TB all within the treatment arm, of which 20 occurred in patient receiving the 10 mg dose. All patients were screened. If positive, patients were excluded from phase II trials and only allowed to enter into phase III trials if they started 9-months of isoniazid therapy. Rifampicin was not used as this interacts with tofacitinib.[56] With baricitinib, there were seven cases of TB, two of which had incomplete TB screening. All cases occurred in endemic areas.[51]

Malignancy

Immunomodulatory therapies have been associated with an increased risk of malignancy. This may relate to disturbances in immunosurveillance; the process by which the immune system reduces tumour development, growth, and survival.[57] Complicating this picture, it the known association of lymphoproliferative cancers in patients with autoimmune diseases including RA.[58]

Extensive analysis of biologics, especially TNFi, suggests these agents do not increase the risk of solid organ or lymphoproliferative cancers.[59-61] Theoretical concerns exist regarding the risk of malignancy with JAK inhibitors, as these agents affect both interferons; a central coordinator in tumour immune surveillance and NK cells; lymphocytes known for their ability to kill tumour cells.[57]

An integrated analysis of data from two phase I, nine phase II, six phase III and two LTE studies involving 6194 tofacitinib-treated patients (8.5 years follow-up and 19 406 patient-years' exposure) recorded 173 patients with malignancies and 118 patients with non-melanoma skin cancer (NMSC). The incident rate for malignancies excluding NMSC was 0.9 (95% CI 0.8 to 1.0) per 100 patient-years. The most common cancers were lung (n = 32) followed by breast (n = 25) and lymphoproliferative/lymphoma (n = 19).[49] The standardized incidence ratios for all malignancies and for NMSC were within the expected range seen in patients with moderate-to-severe RA. Additionally, the rate of malignancies remained stable over time.[62]

Less long-term data are available for baricitinib. A safety analysis of eight completed trials and one ongoing LTE study included 3464 baricitinib-treated patients (only 13.5% had exposure data for more than two years). The malignancy rate, excluding NMSC, was reported at 0.7 per 100 patients-years.[51]

Although reassuring, long-term experience with these agents are limited in comparison to the biologic such as TNF inhibitors. Postmarketing surveillance (e.g. drug registries) is essential data to fully evaluate of cancer risk.[21]

Venous thromboembolism (VTE)

The baricitinib RCTs identified an imbalance in the number of VTE events. An analysis of pooled data of 3492 baricitinib-treated patients recorded five episodes of deep vein thrombosis (DVT) or pulmonary embolism (PE) in patients receiving 4 mg, compared to no episode with placebo. All patients with VTE had multiple risk factors. Two VTE events were considered serious. The event rates remained stable over time. The overall incidence rate for DVT/PE was 0.46 per 100 patient-years.[63] The published incidence rate for DVT/PE in the RA population is 0.29 to 0.79 per 100 patient-years.[64] In the European Union, where baricitinib use is approved, the EMA have updated the label with a precaution for patients who have risk factors for DVT and PE, although whether a causal link between baricitinib and VTE exists remains unclear. Analysis of VTE across tofacitinib RCTs showed no evidence of an increased risk of thromboembolic events (IRs 0.1 per 100 patient year (95% CI: 0.0, 0.3) for both 5 mg and 10 mg tofacitinib doses in RA).[65]

Gastrointestinal perforation

There is an elevated incidence of lower intestinal perforations in RA patients receiving IL-6 receptor blocker tocilizumab, with an increased risk in patients within diverticular disease. This has been demonstrated in RCTs and real-world data.[66]

The risk of gastrointestinal (GI) perforation with tofacitinib was evaluated using in a cohort of 4755 with 2329 person-years exposure. Three cases of lower GI perforation were recorded, with an incidence rate of 1.26 per 1000 patient-years. However, the number of cases and exposure time was limited. In comparison to other biologics, there was a greater than twofold risk among tofacitinib users compared to patients receiving TNFi, although this was not statistically significant.[67] Baricitinib safety analysis with 6637 patient-years reported three GI perforations, with an incidence rate of 0.5 per 1000 patient-years.[68]

Laboratory parameters

JAK inhibitors can cause anaemia, neutropenia, and thrombocytopenia but this is rarely of clinical significance. Erythropoietin (EPO), thrombopoietin (TPO), and colony-stimulating factors (CSF) signal via JAK2, and inhibition of this pathway is the likely culprit.

An analysis of tofacitinib from six phase 3 trial and two LTE studies (n = 4858) reported a decreased mean neutrophil counts, a gradual reduction in mean lymphocyte and an increase in mean haemoglobin levels. Changes in haemoglobin levels were paralleled by changes in the opposite direction in markers of RA disease activity. The changes in haematological parameters stabilized over time in the LTE studies.[69] An analysis of data from baricitinib phase II, III, and LTE studies demonstrated one-third of 2451 patients developed treatment-emergent shifts in haemoglobin. A fall in haemoglobin below the lower limit of normal (LLN) was seen in patients taking 2 mg, 4 mg, or placebo, without significant differences between treatment arms. Following an initial decline attributed to phlebotomy, dose-dependent increases in EPO, iron, and total iron binding capacity were observed, with a return to baseline haemoglobin. Adverse events (defined as a shift in haemoglobin from <grade 3 to ≥grade 3) were uncommon and generally not associated with adverse outcomes.[70]

NK development and activation are dependent on cytokines mediated via the JAK-STAT pathway. Both tofacitinib and baricitinib therapy are associated with a fall in NK cell counts; a dose-dependent fall by week 2 of therapy with tofacitinib, while a transient increased is seen in the first 4 weeks of therapy with baricitinib before counts fall below baseline levels.[71,72] No association between baseline or nadir NK cell count and the incidence of serious infection, herpes zoster, or malignancy has been reported so far.[71]

Hypercholesterolemia is also observed with both JAK inhibitors. In four phase II tofacitinib studies, a dose-dependent increase in total, high-density lipoprotein (HDL) and low-density lipoprotein (LDL) cholesterol of 16–30% were observed.[73] In a phase II baricitinib study, a dose-dependent increase in LDL, HDL, and triglycerides were also observed, with an increase in HDL by week 12 that correlated with improvement in DAS28.[74]

Elevations in lipid profile have been observed with biologics, especially the IL-6 receptor blockers tocilizumab, suggesting the mechanism may lie in blockade of the IL-6 pathway. It is not known whether a 5-hydroxy-3-methylglutaryl-coenzyme A reductase inhibitor is responsible for these changes.[73] A study evaluating cholesterol and lipoprotein in patients with active RA and matched healthy volunteers, reported that a fall in cholesterol levels in active RA patients may be driven by increases in cholesterol ester catabolism. In this study, tofacitinib treatment reduced cholesterol ester catabolism, increasing cholesterol levels towards those seen in healthy volunteers.[75]

JAK inhibitors in development

Second generation JAK inhibitors

Next-generation JAK inhibitors have been designed with a view to improved selective affinity for one or more of the four JAK enzymes. The principle aim of these agents is to reduce non-selective pan JAK inhibition, in the hope that this will reduce unwanted adverse effects without a decline in clinical efficacy. Several agents have been developed and are currently being elevated in phase II clinical trials. These include filgotinib and upadacitinib (ABT-494), selective JAK1 inhibitors; peficitinib, a pan JAK inhibitor with only mild inhibition of JAK2 and decernotinib, a selective JAK3 inhibitor. Safety concerns were raised with decernotinib and the manufacturer decided not to proceed with development of this drug for RA.[76]

Upadacitinib

Upadacitinib (code name ABT-494) is developed by AbbVie. It is also a selective JAK1 inhibitor, with 74-fold selectivity for JAK1 over JAK2. This is due to its ability to bind JAK1 at both the ATP binding site of JH1 and at another JAK1 binding site with a less conserved domain[13] (Table 36.1).

Upadacitinib is being evaluated in six global phase III RCTs in RA, but also in psoriatic arthritis, Crohn's disease, ulcerative colitis, and atopic dermatitis.[77] Upadacitinib exposure is weakly decreased with strong inhibition of CYP3A and moderately increased in with broad CYP induction.[78] Approximately 20% is eliminated by the kidneys.[77]

Efficacy

Upadacitinib has been evaluated in two phase IIb trials in subjects with RA who were inadequate responders to methotrexate or antitumour necrosis factor (TNF) therapy. The first, BALANCE I, was a 12-week dose ranging study of 276 patients on stable MTX who had failed TNF. Patients were randomized to upadacitinib 3, 6, 12, or 18 mg twice daily or placebo. At week 12, significantly more patients receiving upadacitinib (53–71%) than those receiving placebo (34%) achieved an ACR20 response, with a dose-response relationship among all doses (p <0.001).[79] The second phase II study, BALANCE II, randomized 300 patients with an inadequate response to MTX to upadacitinib 3, 6, 12, or 18 mg twice daily, 24 mg once daily or placebo with background MTX. Similar findings were noted, with a significant dose response for ACR20 responses compared to placebo. The proportions of patients achieving ACR50 and ACR70 responses were also significantly higher for all upadacitinib doses (except the 12 mg dose for the ACR70 response) than for placebo.[80] For both studies, the onset of action was rapid, with significant differences seen by week 2.

A recent phase III study in DMARD-IR patients randomized 661 to receive once-daily extended-release formulation of urokinase-type plasminogen activator (uPA) at 15 mg or 30 mg, or placebo. Preliminary results demonstrate significantly more patients achieving an ACR20 response (UPA 15 mg 64%, UPA 30 mg 66% vs. placebo 36%) and DAS28-CRP low disease activity (UPA 15 mg 48%, UPA 30 mg 48% vs. placebo 17%) at 12 weeks. Onset of action was rapid and there were significantly greater improvements in PROs (HAQ-DI, morning stiffness and FACIT-F) for both doses versus placebo.[81] A second phase III study in bDMARD-IR population randomized 498 patients to UPA at 15 mg or 30 mg, or placebo, switching up to either UPA 15 mg or UPA 30 mg at week 12. Significantly more patients achieved ACR20 (UPA 15 mg 65%, UPA 30 mg 56% vs. placebo 28%) and DAS28-CRP ≤3.2 (UPA 15 mg 43%, UPA 30 mg 42% vs. placebo 14%) by week 12. At week 24, responses were similar or greater for patients originally on UPA and comparable for patients who switched to UPA after 12 weeks of placebo.[82]

Safety

The mean changes in laboratory parameters (serum transaminase levels and total white blood cells, neutrophils, or lymphocytes) were not influenced by increasing doses of upadacitinib. There was a dose-dependent reduction in haemoglobin levels. There were more cases of haemoglobin reduction at higher doses suggesting that the selectivity for JAK-1 over JAK-2 may reduce with increased exposure. Similarly, there was a greater decrease in NK cell counts at higher doses. Like other JAK inhibitors, a dose-dependent elevation of LDL cholesterol and HDL cholesterol levels was observed; however, the ratio of LDL: HDL remained unchanged.[79]

From both phase two studies, the incidences of adverse events were higher in the upadacitinib treatment groups with a trend towards dose dependency. Patients who completed BALANCE I or II were enrolled into BALANCE-EXTEND, an ongoing, combined open-label extension. Out of 516 pts who completed the 2 RCTs, 494 entered into the extensions study. The adverse event rate was lower than seen in both phase II studies. The incidence rate by 100 patient-years was 3.7 for herpes zoster, 0.8 for malignancy (excl. NMSC), 0.1 for cardiovascular events.[83]

In the phase III studies, the frequency of adverse events was comparable for placebo and UPA 15 mg, but higher for UPA 30 mg. Infection events were similar in all arms, but there were more serious infections and herpes zoster cases in UPA 30.[82] Malignancies were observed in 5 patients through to week 24,[82] and in 2 patients through to 12 weeks.[81] VTE was reported in 2 patients (UPA 15 and 30) during first 12 weeks, and in 4 patients (3 with UPA 15, 1 with UPA 30) from week 12 to 24. All had risk factors for DVT/PE.[82]

Filgotinib

Filgotinib (GLPG0634), is codeveloped by Galapagos and Gilead Sciences. It is a selective JAK1 inhibitor. Although filgotinib inhibits JAK1/JAK2, in whole blood assays it shows 30-fold selectivity for JAK1- over JAK2-dependent signalling (Table 36.1).[76]

Preclinical studies demonstrated that filgotinib forms an active metabolite, that exhibits a similar JAK1 selectivity profile as the filgotinib albeit less potent. This metabolite contributes to the relatively long duration of JAK1 inhibition following filgotinib dosing.[84] Neither filgotinib nor its active metabolite inhibits or induces CYP activity at clinically relevant concentrations.

Efficacy

Filgotinib has been investigated in two phase IIb studies. DARWIN1 was a 24-week trial randomizing 594 patients with an inadequate response to MTX to 50, 100, or 200 mg once or twice-daily filgotinib or placebo, with background MTX therapy. At week 12, ACR 20 responses were significantly higher with filgotinib 100 and 200 mg, with no difference between once-daily and twice-daily regimens. Rapid onset of action and dose-dependent responses were observed for most efficacy endpoints.[85] The DARWIN2 study was a 24-week trial randomizing 283 patients with an inadequate response to MTX to 50, 100 or 200 mg once-daily filgotinib or placebo, as monotherapy. At week 12, significant differences in ACR20 were seen with filgotinib 100 and 200 mg versus placebo, with statistical significance differences in composite measures of remission or response to treatment.[86]

Safety

Dose-dependent changes in laboratory parameters were observed in both DARWIN studies without clinical consequence including; decreases in neutrophil count and platelet counts (the platelet count stabilized at week 4) and mild elevation in creatinine. There were no reductions in absolute lymphocytes or NK cells. The haemoglobin level increased correlates with filgotinib's anti-inflammatory effect and the absence of JAK2 inhibition. There was a dose-dependent elevation in HDL and LDL cholesterol; although the LDL: HDL ratio was reduced.[76]

Patients who completed DARWIN 1 or 2 were enrolled in the DARWIN 3 study, a phase 2 open-label extension study. Preliminary data of 1314 patientyears of exposure confirmed similar rates of serious infections compared to the core studies, however infections decreased over time from 15% (week 0–12) to 5% (week 5–96). There was no active case of tuberculosis. A total of 16 cases of herpes zoster were reported (1.2 per 100 patient-years) and 6 cases of malignancy (excl. NMSC) (0.5 per 100 patient-years).[87]

Filgotinib clinical trial data has been encouraging and within the efficacy range observed in tofacitinib and baricitinib. JAK1 selectivity may have theoretical advantages over these first generation JAK inhibitors, although this is difficult to judge without greater patient exposure data or a head-to-head trial.[76]

Peficitinib

Peficitinib (ASP015K) is JAK inhibitor that inhibits JAK1, JAK2, JAK3, and TYK2 enzyme activities with moderate selectivity for JAK3 inhibition and only mild inhibition of JAK2[18] (Table 36.1).

Efficacy

The efficacy for peficitinib for the treatment of RA has been investigated in three phase II trials. The first, a 12-week study randomizing 281 Japanese patients who has previously received DMARDs or TNF to monotherapy peficitinib 25, 50, 100, or 150 mg once daily or placebo. At week 12, peficitinib 50, 100, and 150 mg showed a significantly greater ACR20 response, with a statistically significant dose response.[18] In the second phase II trial, 289 patients with limited DMARD exposure were randomized peficitinib 25 mg, 50 mg, 100 mg, or 150 mg monotherapy or placebo once daily for 12 weeks. Patients in the peficitinib 100 mg and 150 mg groups achieved a rapid and statistically significant ACR20 response compared with those in the placebo group (p <0.05), reaching statistical significance by week 2.[88] The third phase II study evaluated peficitinib combination therapy with MTX. This 12-week study randomized 378 patients with an inadequate response to MTX to peficitinib 25 mg, 50 mg, 100 mg, or 150 mg or placebo once daily in combination with MTX. At 12 weeks, the ACR20 response rate in only the 50 mg peficitinib group was significantly different compared with placebo. There were no apparent dose-dependent responses and the placebo response rate was high.[89]

Safety

The common changes in laboratory parameters from these three trials included dose-dependent decreases in the absolute neutrophil count, increase in creatinine kinase levels and increases in HDL and LDL. Three serious infections were reported and seven cases of herpes zoster.

Conclusions

Low molecular weight, orally available, 'small molecules' which target and inhibit components of the JAK enzyme inflammatory signalling cascade have been lately considered as an important alternative to biologic therapies for RA. JAK signalling is used by a number of pro-inflammatory cytokines known to be involved in RA pathogenesis, notably IL-6. Therefore, several JAK inhibitors with variable degrees of selectivity and specificity for the JAK enzymes have been investigated in treatment of RA.

To date, two JAK inhibitors, tofacitinib and baricitinib, have been approved for treatment of RA in certain regions. Tofacitinib, a selective oral JAK1/3 inhibitor, has undergone extensive clinical trials of twice daily dosing in RA and is approved for clinical use in over 80 countries. Baricitinib is a novel, potent and selective oral JAK1/2 inhibitor approved by EMA that has been tested in a large phase III programme of once-daily dosing. Both tofacitinib and baricitinib have demonstrated significant clinical improvements, limitation of structural damage, and preservation of function in active RA patients. Both drugs are well tolerated, and only the increased risk of viral infections such as herpes zoster seems to distinguish the safety profile of these targeted synthetic DMARDs from that of bDMARDS.

A number of other investigational oral JAK inhibitors with varying selectivity for the four JAK enzymes are in clinical development including filgotinib and upadacitinib, both of which have greatest affinity for JAK1, and peficitinib, a pan JAK inhibitor with only mild inhibition of JAK2.

It is likely that we will see an expanding choice of approved JAK inhibitors in the clinic but it may not be straightforward to distinguish safety and efficacy differences. There will be close scrutiny of emerging real-world data for safety and sustained efficacy for currently approved and future drugs. Perceived convenience of dosing schedule and cost effectiveness are likely to influence the uptake of these orally available drugs as compared to the longer established and parenterally administered bDMARDs.[90]

REFERENCES

1. Darnell JE, Jr., Kerr IM, Stark GR. JAK-STAT pathways and transcriptional activation in response to IFNs and other extracellular signaling proteins. *Science* 1994;*264*(5164):1415–21.
2. Brennan FM, McInnes IB. Evidence that cytokines play a role in rheumatoid arthritis. *J Clin Invest* 2008;*118*(11):3537–45.
3. O'Shea JJ, Kontzias A, Yamaoka K, Tanaka Y, Laurence A. Janus kinase inhibitors in autoimmune diseases. *Ann Rheum Dis* 2013; *72*(Suppl 2):ii111–15.
4. Villarino AV, Kanno Y, O'Shea JJ. Mechanisms and consequences of JAK-STAT signaling in the immune system. *Nat Immunol* 2017;*18*(4):374–84.
5. Kisseleva T, Bhattacharya S, Braunstein J, Schindler CW. Signaling through the JAK/STAT pathway, recent advances and future challenges. *Gene* 2002;*285*(1–2):1–24.
6. Leonard WJ, O'Shea JJ. JAKs and STATs: biological implications. *Ann Rev Immunol* 1998;*16*:293–322.
7. Aaronson DS, Horvath CM. A road map for those who don't know JAK-STAT. *Science* 2002;*296*(5573):1653–55.
8. McInnes IB, Schett G. Cytokines in the pathogenesis of rheumatoid arthritis. *Nat Rev Immunol* 2007;*7*(6):429–42.

9. Hodge JA, Kawabata TT, Krishnaswami S, et al. The mechanism of action of tofacitinib—an oral Janus kinase inhibitor for the treatment of rheumatoid arthritis. *Clin Exp Rheumatol* 2016; *34*(2):318–28.
10. Ihle JN. Cytokine receptor signalling. *Nature* 1995;*377*(6550):591–9=4.
11. Schwartz DM, Bonelli M, Gadina M, O'Shea JJ. Type I/II cytokines, JAKs, and new strategies for treating autoimmune diseases. *Nat Rev Rheumatol* 2016;*12*(1):25–36
12. O'Shea JJ, Gadina M, Schreiber RD. Cytokine signaling in 2002: new surprises in the JAK/STAT pathway. *Cell* 2002;*109* Suppl:S121–31.
13. Banerjee S, Biehl A, Gadina M, Hasni S, Schwartz DM. JAK-STAT signaling as a target for inflammatory and autoimmune diseases: current and future prospects. *Drugs* 2017;*77*(5):521–46.
14. Murray PJ. The JAK-STAT signaling pathway: input and output integration. *J Immunol* 2007;*178*(5):2623–9.
15. Clark JD, Flanagan ME, Telliez JB. Discovery and development of Janus kinase (JAK) inhibitors for inflammatory diseases. *J Med Chem* 2014;*57*(12):5023–38.
16. Cacalano NA, Migone TS, Bazan F, et al. Autosomal SCID caused by a point mutation in the N-terminus of Jak3: mapping of the Jak3-receptor interaction domain. *EMBO J* 1999;*18*(6):1549–58.
17. Kontzias A, Kotlyar A, Laurence A, Changelian P, O'Shea JJ. Jakinibs: a new class of kinase inhibitors in cancer and autoimmune disease. *Curr Opin Pharmacol* 2012;*12*(4):464–70.
18. Takeuchi T, Tanaka Y, Iwasaki M, Ishikura H, Saeki S, Kaneko Y. Efficacy and safety of the oral Janus kinase inhibitor peficitinib (ASP015K) monotherapy in patients with moderate to severe rheumatoid arthritis in Japan: a 12-week, randomised, double-blind, placebo-controlled phase IIb study. *Ann Rheum Dis* 2016;*75*(6):1057–64.
19. Mócsai A, Kovács L, Gergely P. What is the future of targeted therapy in rheumatology: biologics or small molecules? *BMC Med* 2014;*12*(1):43.
20. Nakayamada S, Kubo S, Iwata S, Tanaka Y. Recent progress in JAK inhibitors for the treatment of rheumatoid arthritis. *BioDrugs* 2016;*30*(5):407–19.
21. Winthrop KL. The emerging safety profile of JAK inhibitors in rheumatic disease. *Nat Rev Rheumatol* 2017;*13*(4):234–43.
22. European Medicines Agency (EMA). *Olumiant*, 2018. Available at: https://www.ema.europa.eu/en/medicines/human/EPAR/olumiant
23. European Medicines Agency (EMA). *Xeljanz*, 2018. Available at: https://www.ema.europa.eu/en/medicines/human/EPAR/xeljanz
24. van Schouwenburg PA, Rispens T, Wolbink GJ. Immunogenicity of anti-TNF biologic therapies for rheumatoid arthritis. *Nat Rev Rheumatol* 2013;*9*(3):164–72.
25. Scott LJ. Tofacitinib: a review of its use in adult patients with rheumatoid arthritis. *Drugs* 2013;*73*(8):857–74.
26. Norman P. Selective JAK inhibitors in development for rheumatoid arthritis. *Expert Opin Investig Drugs* 2014;*23*(8):1067–77.
27. Milici AJ, Kudlacz EM, Audoly L, Zwillich S, Changelian P. Cartilage preservation by inhibition of Janus kinase 3 in two rodent models of rheumatoid arthritis. *Arthriti Res Ther* 2008;*10*(1):R14.
28. Fleischmann R, Kremer J, Cush J, et al. Placebo-controlled trial of tofacitinib monotherapy in rheumatoid arthritis. *N Engl J Med* 2012;*367*(6):495–507.
29. Strand V, Kremer J, Wallenstein G, et al. Effects of tofacitinib monotherapy on patient-reported outcomes in a randomized

phase 3 study of patients with active rheumatoid arthritis and inadequate responses to DMARDs. *Arthritis Res Ther* 2015;17(1):307.

30. van Vollenhoven RF, Fleischmann R, Cohen S, et al. Tofacitinib or adalimumab versus placebo in rheumatoid arthritis. *N Engl J Med* 2012;367(6):508–19.

31. Strand V, van Vollenhoven RF, Lee EB, et al. Tofacitinib or adalimumab versus placebo: patient-reported outcomes from a phase 3 study of active rheumatoid arthritis. *Rheumatology* 2016;55(6):1031–41.

32. Kremer J, Li ZG, Hall S, Fleischmann R, et al. Tofacitinib in combination with nonbiologic disease-modifying antirheumatic drugs in patients with active rheumatoid arthritis: a randomized trial. *Ann Intern Med* 2013;159(4):253–61.

33. Strand V, Kremer JM, Gruben D, Krishnaswami S, Zwillich SH, Wallenstein GV. Tofacitinib in combination with conventional disease-modifying antirheumatic drugs in patients with active rheumatoid arthritis: patient-reported outcomes from a phase III randomized controlled trial. *Arthritis Care Res* 2017;69(4):592–8.

34. van der Heijde D, Tanaka Y, Fleischmann R, et al. Tofacitinib (CP-690,550) in patients with rheumatoid arthritis receiving methotrexate: twelve-month data from a twenty-four-month phase III randomized radiographic study. *Arthritis Rheum* 2013;65(3):559–70.

35. Burmester GR, Blanco R, Charles-Schoeman C, et al. Tofacitinib (CP-690,550) in combination with methotrexate in patients with active rheumatoid arthritis with an inadequate response to tumour necrosis factor inhibitors: a randomised phase 3 trial. *Lancet* 2013;381(9865):451–60.

36. Strand V, Burmester GR, Zerbini CA, et al. Tofacitinib with methotrexate in third-line treatment of patients with active rheumatoid arthritis: patient-reported outcomes from a phase III trial. *Arthritis Care Res* 2015;67(4):475–83.

37. Lee EB, Fleischmann R, Hall S, et al. Tofacitinib versus methotrexate in rheumatoid arthritis. *N Engl J Med* 2014;370(25):2377–86.

38. Strand V, Lee EB, Fleischmann R, et al. Tofacitinib versus methotrexate in rheumatoid arthritis: patient-reported outcomes from the randomised phase III ORAL Start trial. *RMD Open* 2016;2(2):e000308.

39. Fleischmann R, Mysler E, Hall S, et al. Efficacy and safety of tofacitinib monotherapy, tofacitinib with methotrexate, and adalimumab with methotrexate in patients with rheumatoid arthritis (ORAL Strategy): a phase 3b/4, double-blind, head-to-head, randomised controlled trial. *Lancet* 2017;390(10093):457–68.

40. Richez C, Truchetet ME, Kostine M, Schaeverbeke T, Bannwarth B. Efficacy of baricitinib in the treatment of rheumatoid arthritis. *Expert Opin Pharmacother* 2017;18(13):1399–407.

41. Fridman JS, Scherle PA, Collins R, et al. Selective inhibition of JAK1 and JAK2 is efficacious in rodent models of arthritis: preclinical characterization of INCB028050. *J Immunol* 2010;184(9):5298–307.

42. Fleischmann R, Schiff M, van der Heijde D, et al. Baricitinib, methotrexate, or combination in patients with rheumatoid arthritis and no or limited prior disease-modifying antirheumatic drug treatment. *Arthritis Rheumatol* 2017;69(3):506–17.

43. Lee YC, Emery P, Bradley JD, et al. *Remaining Pain in DMARD-Naive Rheumatoid Arthritis Patients Treated with Baricitinib and Methotrexate* [abstract]. *Arthritis Rheumatol* 2017;69(Suppl 10). Available at: http://acrabstracts.org/abstract/remaining-pain-in-dmard-naive-rheumatoid-arthritis-patients-treated-with-baricitinib-and-methotrexate/

44. Dougados M, van der Heijde D. Baricitinib in patients with inadequate response or intolerance to conventional synthetic DMARDs: results from the RA-BUILD study. *Ann Rheum Dis* 2017;76(1):88–95.

45. Taylor PC, Keystone EC, van der Heijde D, et al. Baricitinib versus placebo or adalimumab in rheumatoid arthritis. *N Engl J Med* 2017;376(7):652–62.

46. Keystone EC, Taylor PC, Tanaka Y, et al. Patient-reported outcomes from a phase 3 study of baricitinib versus placebo or adalimumab in rheumatoid arthritis: secondary analyses from the RA-BEAM study. *Ann Rheum Dis* 2017;76(11):1853–61.

47. Genovese MC, Kremer J, Zamani O, et al. Baricitinib in patients with refractory rheumatoid arthritis. *N Engl J Med* 2016;374(13):1243–52.

48. Smolen JS, Kremer JM, Gaich CL, et al. Patient-reported outcomes from a randomised phase III study of baricitinib in patients with rheumatoid arthritis and an inadequate response to biological agents (RA-BEACON). *Ann Rheum Dis* 2017;76(4):694–700.

49. Cohen SB, Tanaka Y, Mariette X, et al. Long-term safety of tofacitinib for the treatment of rheumatoid arthritis up to 8.5 years: integrated analysis of data from the global clinical trials. *Ann Rheum Dis* 2017;76(7):1253–62.

50. Cohen S, Radominski SC, Gomez-Reino JJ, et al. Analysis of infections and all-cause mortality in phase II, phase III, and long-term extension studies of tofacitinib in patients with rheumatoid arthritis. *Arthritis Rheumatol* 2014;66(11):2924–37.

51. Smolen J, Genovese M, Takeuchi T, et al. THU0166 safety profile of baricitinib in patients with active RA: an integrated analysis. *Ann Rheum Dis* 2016;75:243–4.

52. Strand V, Ahadieh S, French J, et al. Systematic review and meta-analysis of serious infections with tofacitinib and biologic disease-modifying antirheumatic drug treatment in rheumatoid arthritis clinical trials. *Arthritis Res Ther* 2015;17:362.

53. Winthrop KL, Yamanaka H, Valdez H, et al. Herpes zoster and tofacitinib therapy in patients with rheumatoid arthritis. *Arthritis Rheumatol* 2014;66(10):2675–84.

54. Fleischmann R, Alam J, Arora V, et al. Safety and efficacy of baricitinib in elderly patients with rheumatoid arthritis. *RMD Open* 2017;3(2):e000546.

55. Curtis JR, Xie F, Yun H, Bernatsky S, Winthrop KL. Real-world comparative risks of herpes virus infections in tofacitinib and biologic-treated patients with rheumatoid arthritis. *Ann Rheum Dis* 2016;75(10):1843–7.

56. Winthrop KL, Park SH, Gul A, Cardiel MH. Tuberculosis and other opportunistic infections in tofacitinib-treated patients with rheumatoid arthritis. *Ann Rheum Dis* 2016;75(6):1133–8.

57. Dunn GP, Koebel CM, Schreiber RD. Interferons, immunity and cancer immunoediting. *Nat Rev Immunol* 2006;6(11):836–48.

58. Thomas E, Brewster DH, Black RJ, Macfarlane GJ. Risk of malignancy among patients with rheumatic conditions. *Intl J Cancer* 2000;88(3):497–502.

59. Mercer LK, Galloway JB, Lunt M, et al. Risk of lymphoma in patients exposed to antitumour necrosis factor therapy: results from the British Society for Rheumatology Biologics Register for Rheumatoid Arthritis. *Ann Rheum Dis* 2017;76(3):497–503.

60. Mercer LK, Lunt M, Low ALS, et al. Risk of solid cancer in patients exposed to anti-tumour necrosis factor therapy: results from the British Society for Rheumatology Biologics Register for Rheumatoid Arthritis. *Ann Rheum Dis* 2015;74(6):1087–93.

61. Askling J, Fahrbach K, Nordstrom B, Ross S, Schmid CH, Symmons D. Cancer risk with tumor necrosis factor alpha (TNF) inhibitors: meta-analysis of randomized controlled trials of adalimumab, etanercept, and infliximab using patient level data. *Pharmacoepidemiol Drug Saf* 2011;20(2):119–30.

62. Curtis JR, Lee EB, Kaplan IV, et al. Tofacitinib, an oral Janus kinase inhibitor: analysis of malignancies across the rheumatoid arthritis clinical development programme. *Ann Rheum Dis* 2016;75(5):831–41.

63. Weinblatt M TP, Burmester GR, Witt S, et al. *Cardiovascular Safety during Treatment with Baricitinib in Rheumatoid Arthritis* [abstract]. *Arthritis Rheumatol* 2017;69(Suppl 10). Available at: http://acrabstracts.org/abstract/cardiovascular-safety-during-treatment-with-baricitinib-in-rheumatoid-arthritis/

64. Ogdie A, Kay McGill N, Shin DB, et al. Risk of venous thromboembolism in patients with psoriatic arthritis, psoriasis and rheumatoid arthritis: a general population-based cohort study. *European Heart J* 2018;39(39):3608–14.

65. Mease PJ, Kremer J, Cohen S, et al. *Incidence of Thromboembolic Events in the Tofacitinib Rheumatoid Arthritis, Psoriasis, Psoriatic Arthritis and Ulcerative Colitis Development Programs* [abstract]. *Arthritis Rheumatol* 2017;69(Suppl 10). Available at: http://acrabstracts.org/abstract/incidence-of-thromboembolic-events-in-the-tofacitinib-rheumatoid-arthritis-psoriasis-psoriatic-arthritis-and-ulcerative-colitis-development-programs/

66. Strangfeld A, Richter A, Siegmund B, et al. Risk for lower intestinal perforations in patients with rheumatoid arthritis treated with tocilizumab in comparison to treatment with other biologic or conventional synthetic DMARDs. *Ann Rheum Dis* 2017;76(3):504–10.

67. Xie F, Yun H, Bernatsky S, Curtis JR. Brief report: risk of gastrointestinal perforation among rheumatoid arthritis patients receiving tofacitinib, tocilizumab, or other biologic treatments. *Arthritis Rheumatol* 2016;68(11):2612–17.

68. Genovese MC, Smolen JS, Takeuchi T, et al. *Safety Profile of Baricitinib for the Treatment of Rheumatoid Arthritis up to 5.5 Years: An Updated Integrated Safety Analysis* [abstract]. *Arthritis Rheumatol* 2017;69 (Suppl 10). Available at: http://acrabstracts.org/abstract/safety-profile-of-baricitinib-for-the-treatment-of-rheumatoid-arthritis-up-to-5-5-years-an-updated-integrated-safety-analysis/

69. Schulze-Koops H, Strand V, Nduaka C, et al. Analysis of haematological changes in tofacitinib-treated patients with rheumatoid arthritis across phase 3 and long-term extension studies. *Rheumatology* 2017;56(1):46–57.

70. Kay J, Harigai M, Rancourt J, et al. FRI0092 Effects of baricitinib on haemoglobin and related laboratory parameters in rheumatoid arthritis patients. *Ann Rheum Dis* 2017;76:513–14.

71. van Vollenhoven RF, Tanaka Y, Lamba M, et al. THU0178 relationship between NK cell count and important safety events in rheumatoid arthritis patients treated with tofacitinib. *Ann Rheum Dis* 2015;74:258–59.

72. Emery P, McInnes I, Genovese M, et al. *Characterisation of Changes in Lymphocyte Subsets in Baricitinib-Treated Patients with Rheumatoid Arthritis in Two Phase 3 Studies* [abstract]. *Arthritis Rheumatol* 2015;67(Suppl 10). Available at: http://acrabstracts.org/abstract/characterization-of-changes-in-lymphocyte-subsets-in-baricitinib-treated-patients-with-rheumatoid-arthritis-in-two-phase-3-studies/

73. McInnes IB, Kim HY, Lee SH, et al. Open-label tofacitinib and double-blind atorvastatin in rheumatoid arthritis patients: a randomised study. *Ann Rheum Dis* 2014;73(1):124–31.

74. Kremer JM, Genovese MC, Keystone E, et al. Effects of baricitinib on lipid, apolipoprotein, and lipoprotein particle profiles in a phase IIb study of patients with active rheumatoid arthritis. *Arthritis Rheumatol* 2017;69(5):943–52.

75. Charles-Schoeman C, Fleischmann R, Davignon J, et al. Potential mechanisms leading to the abnormal lipid profile in patients with rheumatoid arthritis versus healthy volunteers and reversal by tofacitinib. *Arthritis Rheumatol* 2015;67(3):616–25.

76. Taylor PC, Abdul Azeez M, Kiriakidis S. Filgotinib for the treatment of rheumatoid arthritis. *Expert Opin Investig Drugs* 2017;26(10):1181–7.

77. Klünder B, Mohamed M-EF, Othman AA. Population pharmacokinetics of upadacitinib in healthy subjects and subjects with rheumatoid arthritis: analyses of phase I and II clinical trials. *Clin Pharmacokinet* 2018;57(8):977–88.

78. Mohamed MF, Jungerwirth S, Asatryan A, Jiang P, Othman AA. Assessment of effect of CYP3A inhibition, CYP induction, OATP1B inhibition, and high-fat meal on pharmacokinetics of the JAK1 inhibitor upadacitinib. *Br J Clin Pharmacol* 2017;83(10):2242–8.

79. Kremer JM, Emery P, Camp HS, et al. A phase IIb study of ABT-494, a selective JAK-1 inhibitor, in patients with rheumatoid arthritis and an inadequate response to anti-tumor necrosis factor therapy. *Arthritis Rheumatol* 2016;68(12):2867–77.

80. Genovese MC, Smolen JS, Weinblatt ME, et al. Efficacy and safety of ABT-494, a selective JAK-1 inhibitor, in a phase IIb study in patients with rheumatoid arthritis and an inadequate response to methotrexate. *Arthritis Rheumatol* 2016;68(12):2857–66.

81. Burmester GR, Kremer J, van Den Bosch F, et al. *A Phase 3 Randomized, Placebo-Controlled, Double-Blind Study of Upadacitinib (ABT-494), a Selective JAK-1 Inhibitor, in Patients with Active Rheumatoid Arthritis with Inadequate Response to Conventional Synthetic DMARDS* [abstract]. *Arthritis Rheumatol* 2017;69(Suppl 10). Available at: http://acrabstracts.org/abstract/a-phase-3-randomized-placebo-controlled-double-blind-study-of-upadacitinib-abt-494-a-selective-jak-1-inhibitor-in-patients-with-active-rheumatoid-arthritis-with-inadequate-response-to-convention/

82. Genovese MC, Fleischmann R, Combe B, et al. *Upadacitinib (ABT-494) in Patients with Active Rheumatoid Arthritis and Inadequate Response or Intolerance to Biological DMARDS: A Phase 3 Randomized, Placebo-Controlled, Double-Blind Study of a Selective JAK-1 Inhibitor* [abstract]. *Arthritis Rheumatol.* 2017;69(Suppl 10). Available at: http://acrabstracts.org/abstract/upadacitinib-abt-494-in-patients-with-active-rheumatoid-arthritis-and-inadequate-response-or-intolerance-to-biological-dmards-a-phase-3-randomized-placebo-controlled-double-blind-study-of-a-selec/

83. Genovese MC, Kremer J, Zhong S, Friedman A. *Long-Term Safety and Efficacy of Upadacitinib (ABT-494), an Oral JAK-1 Inhibitor in Patients with Rheumatoid Arthritis in an Open Label Extension Study* [abstract]. *Arthritis Rheumatol* 2017;69(Suppl 10). Available at: http://acrabstracts.org/abstract/long-term-safety-and-efficacy-of-upadacitinib-abt-494-an-oral-jak-1-inhibitor-in-patients-with-rheumatoid-arthritis-in-an-open-label-extension-study/

84. Namour F, Diderichsen PM, Cox E, et al. Pharmacokinetics and pharmacokinetic/pharmacodynamic modeling of filgotinib (GLPG0634), a selective JAK1 inhibitor, in support of phase IIB dose selection. *Clin Pharmacokinet* 2015;54(8):859–74.

85. Westhovens R, Taylor PC, Alten R, et al. Filgotinib (GLPG0634/GS-6034), an oral JAK1 selective inhibitor, is effective in combination with methotrexate (MTX) in patients with active

rheumatoid arthritis and insufficient response to MTX: results from a randomised, dose-finding study (DARWIN 1). *Ann Rheum Dis* 2017;76(6):998–1008

86. Kavanaugh A, Kremer J, Ponce L, et al. Filgotinib (GLPG0634/GS-6034), an oral selective JAK1 inhibitor, is effective as monotherapy in patients with active rheumatoid arthritis: results from a randomised, dose-finding study (DARWIN 2). *Ann Rheum Dis* 2017;76(6):1009–19.

87. Alten R, Westhovens R, Kavanaugh A, et al. THU0173 Long term safety and efficacy of filgotinib in a phase 2B open label extension study in patients with rheumatoid arthritis: results up to 144 weeks. *Ann Rheum Dis* 2017;76:267.

88. Genovese MC, Greenwald M, Codding C, et al. Peficitinib, a JAK inhibitor, in combination with limited conventional synthetic disease-modifying antirheumatic drugs in the treatment of moderate-to-severe rheumatoid arthritis. *Arthritis Rheumatol* 2017;69(5):932–42.

89. Kivitz AJ, Gutierrez-Urena SR, Poiley J, et al. Peficitinib, a JAK inhibitor, in the treatment of moderate-to-severe rheumatoid arthritis in patients with an inadequate response to methotrexate. *Arthritis Rheumatol* 2017;69(4):709–19.

90. O'Shea JJ, Laurence A, McInnes IB. Back to the future: oral targeted therapy for RA and other autoimmune diseases. *Nat Rev Rheumatol* 2013;9(3):173–82.

37

Combination therapy in rheumatoid arthritis

Ben G.T. Coumbe, Elena Nikiphorou, and Tuulikki Sokka-Isler

Introduction

The understanding of the pathogenesis and iatrogenic management of rheumatoid arthritis (RA) has come a long way, with multiple therapeutic options currently available.[1-4]

Combination therapies refer to the use of two or more drugs that interact with multiple targets, and their effects may be antagonistic, additive, or synergistic depending on their interactions. Methotrexate has become the 'anchor' drug in treating RA, used in both monotherapy and combination therapy.

The current therapeutic repertoire for RA consists of DMARDs, including conventional synthetic DMARDs (csDMARDs), biologic DMARDs (bDMARDs) and targeted synthetic DMARDs (tsDMARDs). The pathophysiology of RA is complex, involving an interplay between genetic risk factors and environment triggers, and both innate and adaptive immune responses.[1] It is increasingly recognized that multiple complex molecular networks are implicated in disease development and progression in RA.[2] The complexity and plasticity of these molecular networks limits the efficacy of commonly used single molecular drug therapeutics.[3] Increasingly it has been recognized that not only the *combination* of drugs is important but the *timing* of intervention is critical to develop treatment effects adding a temporal dimension.[4] With rising standards of care and outcomes, a greater appreciation of these aspects of treatment is necessary. This reinforces the need to develop clear and effective treatment strategies to achieve expected targets. This chapter addresses the evidence related to the utilization of combination strategies for the management of RA as compared to monotherapy.

Combination therapy with csDMARDs

Evidence from clinical practice shows that DMARD therapy should be introduced in the early stages of managing RA in order to achieve rapid attainment of clinical remission according to treat-to-target principles. Furthermore, combination csDMARD therapy has been shown to control RA more successfully than csDMARD monotherapy. The FIN-RACo (Finnish Rheumatoid Arthritis Combination Therapy) a two year multicentre, randomized trial in early RA, the efficacy and tolerability of combination therapy (sulfasalazine (SSZ), methotrexate (MTX), hydroxychloroquine (HCQ), and prednisolone) compared with DMARD monotherapy, with or without prednisolone had been demonstrated.[5] The study also showed that the frequency of adverse events between combination therapy and monotherapy, was not dissimilar. Longer term follow-up of the FIN-RACo studies have demonstrated that the achievement of tight control at an early stage in RA can lead to lower radiologic progression (Larsen scores) in most RA patients.[6] In support of this study, the TICORA (tight control for rheumatoid arthritis) study, a single-blinded study, demonstrated the value of triple combination therapy (MTX, SSZ, and HCQ) versus DMARD monotherapy, also reducing radiographic damage.[7] This can be considered a landmark study in the new era of targeted biological therapies, as it showed that tight control could be achieved with standard csDMARDs without use of bDMARDs. The BeSt study (Dutch acronym for Behandel-Strategieën, 'treatment strategies'), a multicentre randomized controlled trial (RCT) to assess the clinical and radiographic efficacies of four different treatment strategies in early RA patients demonstrated that initial combination csDMARD therapy was preferable to step-up combination csDMARD therapy and methotrexate (MTX) monotherapy, with earlier functional improvement, less progression of radiographic damage, and fewer adverse effects.[8]

The FIN-RACo trial outlined that the utilization of csDMARD combinations was more effective inducing clinical remission in early RA patients when compared to monotherapy.[9] This study supported previous research which demonstrated the utility and superiority of combination csDMARD therapy, both dual and triple therapy versus monotherapy.[10] The majority of studies related to combination therapy have examined MTX as the anchor drug.[11] The COmbinatietherapie Bij Reumatoide Artritis (COBRA) RCT, demonstrated the advantage of a step-down regimen of prednisolone and combination therapy of MTX and SSZ compared with SSZ monotherapy in DMARD-naïve, early RA patients in terms of disease activity and radiographic progression. The trial also demonstrated that patients had lower total medical costs, fewer adverse effects from therapy, and increased ability to remain in employment.[12] Long-term follow-up from the COBRA RCT demonstrated that the rate of progression of joint damage remained lower in the combination therapy group for up to 4 years after the initial 56-week intervention period. The presence of these durable and lasting effects following initiation of combination therapy on a 'treat-to-target' basis was an important finding.[8,13]

As a result of this evidence, significant interest in evaluating the efficacy of early interventions with combination csDMARDs was created. A recent indirect comparison meta-analysis has shown statistically significant superiority of such combination therapy (triple therapy of MTX, SSZ and HCQ) over both MTX monotherapy and MTX and bDMARD therapy for ACR50 responses in both MTX-naïve and MTX incomplete responders (MTX-IR).[14]

Combinations of csDMARDs and bDMARDs

The body of literature that supports the utilization of csDMARD and bDMARD combination therapy is substantial.[16] Despite this, there remains significant international variability in the access and use of these agents, most notably with regard to patient eligibility, with restrictions on their use being imposed by national bodies, driven by cost. In terms of American and European guidelines, there is no hierarchical positioning for the utilization of different bDMARDs when used in combination with csDMARDs in patients with early RA with low disease activity.[16,17] Within the last decade European Medicines Agency (EMA) or FDA-approved biosimilars have similar efficacy and safety as their respective reference bDMARDs and should be preferred if they cost less.[16] MTX remains the anchor within these combinations, as it is the most widely studied with extensive understanding of its safety and efficacy profile. The OPTIMA (Optimal Protocol for Treatment Initiation With Methotrexate and Adalimumab) trial demonstrated that combination therapy of MTX and adalimumab was superior to monotherapy with MTX and resulted in stable low disease activity and improved structural, clinical, and functional outcomes.[18] This was further supported in the BeSt trial which demonstrated that combination therapy of MTX and infliximab was superior to monotherapy and step-up combination therapy leading to earlier functional improvement, reduced progression of radiographic damage, and fewer adverse effects.[8]

The sustained treatment responses seen with concomittant csDMARD use is underlined by reduced immunogenicity towards bDMARDs, an important cause of therapeutic faiklure, leading to prolonged treatment responses.[19] This rationale was reinforced by a study in the British Society of Rheumatology Biologics Registry (BSRBR) which demonstrated that continuation of background csDMARD use leads to better long-term persistence of remission.[20]

Optimising the use of Methotrexate

The increased concern related to poor treatment-adherence of many patients currently receiving combination therapy is a recognized confounding factor in many RCTs.[4,19] The adverse effects of medications are the major driving factors for discontinuation of combination therapy particularly MTX.[20,21] Some studies suggest that titration to higher oral doses of MTX to initiate faster remission and the utilization of subcutaneous (SC) methotrexate to mitigate adverse effects are underutilized options.[20] It is known that discomfort is associated with oral MTX, in particular nausea and vomiting, can lead to poor adherence and older literature identifies this side effect to be dose dependent.[22] Gastrointestinal absorption limitations have been shown to limit the bioavailability of MTX at higher oral doses and this picture is further complicated by patient heterogeneity.[23] This has led to significant interest in optimizing treatment regimens

to maximize efficacy and minimize adverse effects. Previous studies comparing the efficacy of low dose MTX monotherapy have found that they may be equally effective as high dose monotherapy.[24,25] More recent studies have explored the utilization of alternative routes of administration of MTX in order to reduce systemic exposure to MTX and reported improved tolerance to MTX and higher remission rates as defined by ACR20 and ACR70.[26] Analysis of the bioavailability of MTX given through the SC and oral routes has been compared and has been demonstrated that when the oral MTX dose is increased >15 mg/week the systemic exposure to MTX plateaus. Preferential use of SC MTX, particularly at higher doses, provides a paradigm for overcoming poor adherence and tolerance associated with oral MTX leading to optimization of MTX.

csDMARD and tsDMARD combinations

Novel emerging agents include a new class of DMARDs named targeted synthetic DMARDs (tsDMARDs), which interfere with pathways critical in cytokine signalling in RA pathogenesis, downstream to the site where bDMARDs act, with a high degree of potency.[27,28] One example of this class includes the Janus kinase (JAK) inhibitors, tofacitinib and baricitinib, which have been approved by US FDA and EMA.[29,30] Baricitinib and tofacitinib monotherapy or in combination with MTX were shown to provide early and sustained clinical improvements in patients with various stages of RA, including bDMARD-IR patients, especially TNFi.[31-33] In patients with RA and an inadequate response to csDMARD therapy baricitinib was associated with significant reductions in DAS28 and inhibition of radiographic joint damage.[32] In comparison to tumour necrosis factor (TNF) inhibitors it has been demonstrated that in MTX-IR patients baricitinib in combination with background MTX was associated with significant clinical improvements as compared to MTX and adalimumab.[34] Tofacitinib has been demonstrated to be superior to csDMARDs in the treatment of early MTX-naïve RA as monotherapy when compared to the use of MTX monotherapy in both early (START) and established DMARD-IR RA (SOLO).[35] Tofacitinib has been shown in combination with MTX to be superior to MTX alone in driving significant clinical improvement including physical function over 6 months and with a safety profile not dissimilar to csDMARDs.[36] The effectiveness of combinations of MTX and tofacitinib has been demonstrated in the Oral Rheumatoid Arthritis (ORAL) trials which showed that tofacitinib and MTX had rapid and clinically meaningful improvements in relation to physical function and DAS28 scores over a 6 month period in those who are TNF-IR (STEP).[36] Furthermore the ORAL investigators have demonstrated that in DMARD-IR patients tofacitinib was shown to have similar effectiveness and safety profile when used in monotherapy compared to MTX monotherapy (SOLO), is superior in combination therapy with MTX than monotherapy and non-inferior to TNF inhibitor, adalimumab when in combination with MTX (STANDARD).[28,37-40]

Health economic considerations

Significant challenges related to the financial sustainability of many health systems exist due to the rise of chronic diseases, combined with demographic challenges, progression of medical technologies, and the cost of the b-and tsDMARDs. However, the cost of these new therapies is significant and must be balanced against the economic and societal benefits that medication offers individual patients. The difference in efficacy between DMARD combination treatments, including or excluding bDMARDs, is small. Due to the enormous cost differences.[40] The first results of the NORDSTAR study indicated that during the first 24 weeks in early active RA, there was no major difference between the best conventional active therapy (including triple combination) and the three other arms that included bDMARDs.[40] Therefore, RA guidelines should recommend combination csDMARD treatment before initiation of a bDMARD.[41] It is the principle of early aggressive intervention which is the juncture point where cost considerations become appreciable.

This was demonstrated in the SweFOT trial where combination csDMARD therapy was not substantially worse than a control treatment of csDMARD and bDMARD combination therapy in terms of clinical outcomes at 12 and 24 months follow-up.[42] The TACIT trial further supports that a combination of MTX, SSZ, and HCQ resulted in non-inferior outcomes when compared to the combination of MTX and TNF inhibitor (TNFi) etanercept,[43] in support of previous trials.[44,45] These RCTs have provided considerable evidence to the scientific community and policy makers for the role of combination csDMARD therapy, which costs significantly less than bDMARD combinations.[45] In some countries, including developed countries such as the United Kingdom, the high cost of treatment considerably limits use of this combination and is a major driver of inequity worldwide.[46,47,48] The CARDERA (Combination of Anti-Rheumatic Drugs in Early RA) trial in the United Kingdom has demonstrated a reduction in both primary care and hospital costs as well as clinical effectiveness, with intensive use of two csDMARDs and short-term glucocorticoids (GCs) in RA of <24-months duration.[49] Evidence is growing that csDMARD therapy is as effective as bDMARD + MTX in early and late RA.[40] There is a significant cost reduction in using triple therapy when compared to the use of bDMARDs. Recent analyses have concluded that initiating bDMARDs before trying triple therapy first increases costs while providing minimal incremental benefit.[51]

Consequences of expiration of patents to reduce the medication costs in rheumatology are worth noticing. First was when the patent of bMDARDs expired and the introduction of biosimilars resulted in reduction of prices of the bio originals. The second may have even more profound consequences, namely when the patents of JAK inhibitors expire.[52,53]

Current RA management recommendations

Current recommendations advocate rapid escalation of MTX therapy, maintained according to treat-to-target principles.[52,54,55] Although 30% of patients achieve full clinical remission with MTX monotherapy (oral), 70% require additional step-up treatment, either csDMARDs or bDMARDs. The starting dose of methotrexate should be the full maintenance dose; Canadian and Finnish recommendations state that MTX should be administered subcutaneously right from the start. Canadian and Finnish recommendations state that maintenance MTX should be started subcutaneously. Historically there was significant interest in the use of combination csDMARD therapy compared to monotherapy, however, with

bDMARDs on the market and more recently targeted synthetic DMARDs too, the utilitzation of combination csDMARD therapy appears to have fallen out of favour in some parts of the world. This is reflected in the 2016 RA EULAR guidelines, where use of bDMARDs is advocated when patients do not respond to two csDMARD monotherapies or where failure has occurred with one csDMARD monotherapy and the patient has poor prognostic factors.[16] Within the 2015 ACR guidelines physicians are given the option of using bDMARDs in combination with csDMARD (particularly MTX) in incomplete responders to csDMARD monotherapy before the use of combination csDMARDs.[17] It has been suggested that the health benefits of bDMARDs warrant the additional costs, however, the cost-effectiveness studies supporting this are based on comparison of bDMARD monotherapy with csDMARD monotherapy rather than combination csDMARD therapy in MTX incomplete responders.[51,56] In those who fail to achieve remission, evidence from three trials supports utilization of combination csDMARDs before the utilization of bDMARDs.[8,44,57] Many rheumatologists are reluctant to use this approach and prefer to add a TNFi to MTX.[58] The preferential use of bDMARDs compared to csDMARDs has significant economic consequences resulting from the 10–20 fold differences in cost between them. Thus, the adherence to current guidelines supporting use of bDMARDs may not be possible in all settings.[46,47]

The 2016 EULAR and ACR recommendations have generated debate and controversy in the use of evidence used to support the recommendations.[16,17] There is no question regarding many aspects of the two sets of guidelines including their emphasis on 'treat-to-target' aims, earlier intervention, and efficacy of bDMARDs in MTX-IR patients. However, there are concerns related to the generalisability of the recommendations in low resource settings where access to these agents is limited.[46,47]

The failure to utilize intra-articular GC injections (IAGCIs) into inflamed joints has also been associated with reduced remission rates, higher disease activity, and lower health related quality of life. Hence, IAGCIs should be used as an integral part of the targeted treatment of early RA.[59] Of course, steroids should be used with caution, but their central role in the management of RA cannot be denied.

Uncertainties with combination therapy

Systematic reviews show combining conventional DMARDs, biologics with methotrexate and JAK inhibitors with methotrexate are effective in both early and established RA with head-to-head trials finding no significant difference between strategies. But the trials look at somewhat different patient groups and use variable methods; consequently the results may not be entirely comparable.[60] Persistence with treatment may vary between different therapies, with observational data suggesting it is much lower with triple therapy (methotrexate, sulfasalazine, and hydroxychloroquine) than with TNF inhibitors with methotrexate. This difference has been attributed to greater adverse event rates with sulfasalazine.[61–63] But observational studies of persistence are complex and may reflect differences in specialists' experience using conventional DMARDs. The studies showing poor persistence with triple therapy are from North America, and the historical use of sulfasalazine has been found to be much lower in North America than Europe, particularly

Scandinavian countries, in earlier observational studies. So it is possible specialists vary in how they perceive some combination therapies that based on their prior experience with different drugs.[64]

Overall there is strong evidence favouring the use of combination therapy in many RA patients, but no definitive evidence to prefer one approach over another. The choice of approach should reflect local and national custom and practice, the experience of the clinicians involved and the perspectives of individual patients. What is certainly clear, based on the available evidence, is that csDMARD combination therapy is both clinically effective and cost effective.

Conclusions

The therapeutic armamentarium available for treatment of RA has changed significantly over the past 30 years, transforming the therapeutic landscape and prognosis for a substantial proportion of patients with RA.[67] Combination therapies represent an important therapeutic paradigm for the management of RA. The rationale for combination therapies is clear and demonstrated to bring treatment benefit to patients achieving lower disease activity scores and reduced radiographic progression according to 'treat-to-target' principles. However, it is increasingly viewed that the newer agents, bDMARDs and tsDMARDs, are often viewed as superior to older agents, csDMARDs, where this may not necessarily be. A rigorous evidence-based debate is required involving not only parameters related to disease activity scores and radiographic progression, but related to the cost-effectiveness analysis of using many of these newer agents compared to older csDMARDs.

REFERENCES

1. McInnes IB, Schett G. The pathogenesis of rheumatoid arthritis. *N Engl J Med* 2011;365(23):2205–19.
2. McInnes IB, O'Dell JR. State-of-the-art: rheumatoid arthritis. *Ann Rheum Dis* 2010;69(11):1898–906.
3. He B, Lu C, Zheng G, et al. Combination therapeutics in complex diseases. *J Cell Mol Med* 2016;20(12):2231–40.
4. Miossec P. Drug treatments for rheumatoid arthritis: looking backwards to move forwards. *BMJ* 2015;350:h1192.
5. Möttönen T, Hannonen P, Leirisalo-Repo M, et al. Comparison of combination therapy with single-drug therapy in early rheumatoid arthritis: a randomised trial. FIN-RACo trial group. *Lancet* 1999;353(9164):1568–73.
6. Rantalaiho V, Korpela M, Laasonen L, et al. Early combination disease-modifying antirheumatic drug therapy and tight disease control improve long-term radiologic outcome in patients with early rheumatoid arthritis: the 11-year results of the Finnish Rheumatoid Arthritis Combination Therapy trial. *Arthritis Res Ther* 2010;12(3):R122.
7. Grigor C, Capell H, Stirling A, et al. Effect of a treatment strategy of tight control for rheumatoid arthritis (the TICORA study): a single-blind randomised controlled trial. *Lancet* 2004;364(9430):263–9.
8. Goekoop-Ruiterman YPM, de Vries-Bouwstra JK, Allaart CF, et al. Clinical and radiographic outcomes of four different treatment strategies in patients with early rheumatoid arthritis (the BeSt study): a randomized, controlled trial. *Arthritis Rheum* 2005;52(11):3381–90.
9. Sokka T, Mäkinen H, Puolakka K, Möttönen T, Hannonen P. Remission as the treatment goal--the FIN-RACo trial. *Clin Exp Rheumatol* 2006;24(6 Suppl 43):S74–6.
10. O'Dell JR, Haire CE, Erikson N, et al. Treatment of rheumatoid arthritis with methotrexate alone, sulfasalazine and hydroxychloroquine, or a combination of all three medications. *N Engl J Med* 1996;334(20):1287–91.
11. Tugwell P, Pincus T, Yocum D, et al. Combination therapy with cyclosporine and methotrexate in severe rheumatoid arthritis. The Methotrexate-Cyclosporine Combination Study Group. *N Engl J Med* 1995;333(3):137–41.
12. Boers M, Verhoeven AC, Markusse HM, et al. Randomised comparison of combined step-down prednisolone, methotrexate and sulphasalazine with sulphasalazine alone in early rheumatoid arthritis. *Lancet* 1997;350(9074):309–18.
13. Landewé RBM, Boers M, Verhoeven AC, et al. COBRA combination therapy in patients with early rheumatoid arthritis: long-term structural benefits of a brief intervention. *Arthritis Rheum* 2002;46(2):347–56.
14. Hazlewood GS, Barnabe C, Tomlinson G, Marshall D, Devoe D, Bombardier C. Methotrexate monotherapy and methotrexate combination therapy with traditional and biologic disease modifying antirheumatic drugs for rheumatoid arthritis: abridged Cochrane systematic review and network meta-analysis. *BMJ* 2016;353:i1777.
15. Rein P, Mueller RB. Treatment with biologicals in rheumatoid arthritis: an overview. *Rheumatol Ther* 2017;4(2):247–61.
16. Smolen JS, Landewé R, Bijlsma J, et al. EULAR recommendations for the management of rheumatoid arthritis with synthetic and biological disease-modifying antirheumatic drugs: 2016 update. *Ann Rheum Dis* 2017;76(6):960–77.
17. Singh JA, Saag KG, Bridges SL, et al. 2015 American College of Rheumatology guideline for the treatment of rheumatoid arthritis. *Arthritis Rheumatol* 2016;68(1):1–26.
18. Kavanaugh A, van Vollenhoven RF, Fleischmann R, et al. Testing treat-to-target outcomes with initial methotrexate monotherapy compared with initial tumour necrosis factor inhibitor (adalimumab) plus methotrexate in early rheumatoid arthritis. *Ann Rheum Dis* 2018;77(2):289–92.
19. Rheumatology (Oxford). 2014 Feb;53(2):213–22. doi: 10.1093/rheumatology/ket260. Epub 2013 Aug 14. The role of DMARDs in reducing the immunogenicity of TNF inhibitors in chronic inflammatory diseases. Jani M1, Barton A, Warren RB, Griffiths CE, Chinoy H.
20. Jani M1, Barton A, Warren RB, Griffiths CE, Chinoy H. The role of DMARDs in reducing the immunogenicity of TNF inhibitors in chronic inflammatory diseases. *Rheumatology* (Oxford). 2014 Feb;53(2):213–22. doi: 10.1093/rheumatology/ket260. Epub 2013 Aug 14.
21. Soliman MM, Ashcroft DM, Watson KD, et al. Impact of concomitant use of DMARDs on the persistence with anti-TNF therapies in patients with rheumatoid arthritis: results from the British Society for Rheumatology Biologics Register. *Ann Rheum Dis* 2011;70(4):583–9.
22. Curtis JR, Zhang J, Xie F, et al. Use of oral and subcutaneous methotrexate in rheumatoid arthritis patients in the United States. *Arthritis Care Res* 2014;66(11):1604–11.
23. Nikiphorou E, Negoescu A, Fitzpatrick JD, et al. Indispensable or intolerable? Methotrexate in patients with rheumatoid and

psoriatic arthritis: a retrospective review of discontinuation rates from a large UK cohort. *Clin Rheumatol* 2014;33(5):609–14.

24. Bello AE, Perkins EL, Jay R, Efthimiou P. Recommendations for optimizing methotrexate treatment for patients with rheumatoid arthritis. *Open Access Rheumatol* 2017;9:67–79.

25. Schiff MH, Jaffe JS, Freundlich B. Head-to-head, randomised, crossover study of oral versus subcutaneous methotrexate in patients with rheumatoid arthritis: drug-exposure limitations of oral methotrexate at doses ≥15 mg may be overcome with subcutaneous administration. *Ann Rheum Dis* 2014;73(8):1549–51.

26. Yamanaka H, Inoue E, Tanaka E, et al. Influence of methotrexate dose on its efficacy and safety in rheumatoid arthritis patients: evidence based on the variety of prescribing approaches among practicing Japanese rheumatologists in a single institute-based large observational cohort (IORRA). *Mod Rheumatol* 2007;17(2):98–105.

27. Furst DE, Koehnke R, Burmeister LF, Kohler J, Cargill I. Increasing methotrexate effect with increasing dose in the treatment of resistant rheumatoid arthritis. *J Rheumatol* 1989;16(3):313–20.

28. Braun J, Kästner P, Flaxenberg P, et al. Comparison of the clinical efficacy and safety of subcutaneous versus oral administration of methotrexate in patients with active rheumatoid arthritis: results of a six-month, multicenter, randomized, double-blind, controlled, phase IV trial. *Arthritis Rheum* 2008;58(1):73–81.

29. Pesu M, Candotti F, Husa M, Hofmann SR, Notarangelo LD, O'Shea JJ. Jak3, severe combined immunodeficiency, and a new class of immunosuppressive drugs. *Immunol Rev* 2005;203:127–42.

30. Strand V, Kremer JM, Gruben D, Krishnaswami S, Zwillich SH, Wallenstein G V. Tofacitinib in combination with conventional disease-modifying antirheumatic drugs in patients with active rheumatoid arthritis: patient-reported outcomes from a phase III randomized controlled trial. *Arthritis Care Res* 2017;69(4):592–8.

31. Richez C, Truchetet M-E, Kostine M, Schaeverbeke T, Bannwarth B. Efficacy of baricitinib in the treatment of rheumatoid arthritis. *Expert Opin Pharmacother* 2017;18(13):1399–407.

32. Shi JG, Chen X, Lee F, et al. The pharmacokinetics, pharmacodynamics, and safety of baricitinib, an oral JAK 1/2 inhibitor, in healthy volunteers. *J Clin Pharmacol* 2014;54(12):1354–61.

33. Genovese MC, Kremer J, Zamani O, et al. Baricitinib in patients with refractory rheumatoid arthritis. *N Engl J Med* 2016;374(13):1243–52.

34. Dougados M, van der Heijde D, Chen Y-C, et al. Baricitinib in patients with inadequate response or intolerance to conventional synthetic DMARDs: results from the RA-BUILD study. *Ann Rheum Dis* 2017;76(1):88–95.

35. Fleischmann R, Schiff M, van der Heijde D, et al. Baricitinib, methotrexate, or combination in patients with rheumatoid arthritis and no or limited prior disease-modifying antirheumatic drug treatment. *Arthritis Rheumatol* 2017;69(3):506–17.

36. Taylor PC, Keystone EC, van der Heijde D, et al. Baricitinib versus Placebo or Adalimumab in Rheumatoid Arthritis. *N Engl J Med* 2017;376(7):652–62.

37. Fleischmann RM, Huizinga TWJ, Kavanaugh AF, et al. Efficacy of tofacitinib monotherapy in methotrexate-naive patients with early or established rheumatoid arthritis. *RMD Open* 2016;2(2):e000262.

38. Burmester GR, Blanco R, Charles-Schoeman C, et al. Tofacitinib (CP-690,550) in combination with methotrexate in patients with active rheumatoid arthritis with an inadequate response to

tumour necrosis factor inhibitors: a randomised phase 3 trial. *Lancet* 2013;381(9865):451–60.

39. van Vollenhoven RF, Fleischmann R, Cohen S, et al. Tofacitinib or adalimumab versus placebo in rheumatoid arthritis. *N Engl J Med* 2012;367(6):508–19.

40. van der Heijde D, Tanaka Y, Fleischmann R, et al. Tofacitinib (CP-690,550) in patients with rheumatoid arthritis receiving methotrexate: twelve-month data from a twenty-four-month phase III randomized radiographic study. *Arthritis Rheum* 2013;65(3):559–70.

41. Fleischmann R, Mysler E, Hall S, et al. Efficacy and safety of tofacitinib monotherapy, tofacitinib with methotrexate, and adalimumab with methotrexate in patients with rheumatoid arthritis (ORAL Strategy): a phase 3b/4, double-blind, head-to-head, randomised controlled trial. *Lancet* 2017;390(10093):457–68.

42. Lund Hetland M, Haavardsholm E, Rudin A, et al. A Multicenter Randomized Study in Early Rheumatoid Arthritis to Compare Active Conventional Therapy versus Three Biological Treatments: 24 Week Efficacy and Safety Results of the NORD-STAR Trial [abstract]. *Arthritis Rheumatol.* 2019; 71 (suppl 10). https://acrabstracts.org/abstract/a-multicenter-randomized-study-in-early-rheumatoid-arthritis-to-compare-active-conventional-therapy-versus-three-biological-treatments-2-4-week-efficacy-and-safety-results-of-the-nord-star-trial/.

43. Singh JA, Hossain A, Mudano AS, et al. Biologics or tofacitinib for people with rheumatoid arthritis naive to methotrexate: a systematic review and network meta-analysis. *Cochrane Database Syst Rev* 2017;5:CD012657.

44. Graudal N, Hubeck-Graudal T, Faurschou M, Baslund B, Jürgens G. Combination therapy with and without tumor necrosis factor inhibitors in rheumatoid arthritis: a meta-analysis of randomized trials. *Arthritis Care Res* 2015;67(11):1487–95.

45. van Vollenhoven RF, Geborek P, Forslind K, et al. Conventional combination treatment versus biological treatment in methotrexate-refractory early rheumatoid arthritis: 2 year follow-up of the randomised, non-blinded, parallel-group SweFOT trial. *Lancet* 2012;379(9827):1712–20.

46. Scott DL, Ibrahim F, Farewell V, et al. Randomised controlled trial of tumour necrosis factor inhibitors against combination intensive therapy with conventional disease-modifying antirheumatic drugs in established rheumatoid arthritis: the TACIT trial and associated systematic reviews. *Heal Technol Assess* 2014;18(66):i–xxiv, 1.

47. Moreland LW, O'Dell JR, Paulus HE, et al. A randomized comparative effectiveness study of oral triple therapy versus etanercept plus methotrexate in early aggressive rheumatoid arthritis: the treatment of Early Aggressive Rheumatoid Arthritis Trial. *Arthritis Rheum* 2012;64(9):2824–35.

48. O'Dell JR, Mikuls TR, Taylor TH, et al. Therapies for active rheumatoid arthritis after methotrexate failure. *N Engl J Med* 2013;369(4):307–18.

49. Misra DP, Agarwal V, Sharma A, Wakhlu A, Negi VS. 2016 update of the EULAR recommendations for the management of rheumatoid arthritis: a utopia beyond patients in low/middle income countries? *Ann Rheum Dis* 2017;76(11):e47.

50. Smolen JS, Landewé RBM, van der Heijde D. Response to: '2016 update of the EULAR recommendations for the management of rheumatoid arthritis: no utopia for patients in low/middle-income countries?' by Misra et al. *Ann Rheum Dis* 2017;76(11):e48.

51. Dörner T, Strand V, Cornes P, et al. The changing landscape of biosimilars in rheumatology. *Ann Rheum Dis* 2016;*75*(6):974–82.

52. Wailoo A, Hernández Alava M, Scott IC, Ibrahim F, Scott DL. Cost-effectiveness of treatment strategies using combination disease-modifying anti-rheumatic drugs and glucocorticoids in early rheumatoid arthritis. *Rheumatol* 2014;*53*(10):1773–7.

53. Jalal H, O'Dell JR, Bridges SL, et al. Cost-effectiveness of triple therapy versus etanercept plus methotrexate in early aggressive rheumatoid arthritis. *Arthritis Care Res* 2016;*68*(12):1751–57.

54. Bansback N, Phibbs CS, Sun H, et al. Triple therapy versus biologic therapy for active rheumatoid arthritis: a cost-effectiveness analysis. *Ann Intern Med* 2017;*167*(1):8–16.

55. Müller S, Wilke T, Fuchs A, et al. Non-persistence and non-adherence to MTX therapy in patients with rheumatoid arthritis: a retrospective cohort study based on German RA patients. *Patient Prefer Adherence* 2017;*11*:1253–64.

56. Sauer BC, Teng C-C, Tang D, et al. Persistence with conventional triple therapy versus a tumor necrosis factor inhibitor and methotrexate in US veterans with rheumatoid arthritis. *Arthritis Care Res* 2017;*69*(3):313–22.

57. Visser K, van der Heijde D. Optimal dosage and route of administration of methotrexate in rheumatoid arthritis: a systematic review of the literature. *Ann Rheum Dis* 2009;*68*(7):1094–9.

58. Smolen JS, Landewé R, Breedveld FC, et al. EULAR recommendations for the management of rheumatoid arthritis with synthetic and biological disease-modifying antirheumatic drugs. *Ann Rheum Dis* 2010;*69*(6):964–75.

59. Wailoo AJ, Bansback N, Brennan A, Michaud K, Nixon RM, Wolfe F. Biologic drugs for rheumatoid arthritis in the Medicare program: a cost-effectiveness analysis. *Arthritis Rheum* 2008;*58*(4):939–46.

60. van Vollenhoven RF, Ernestam S, Geborek P, et al. Addition of infliximab compared with addition of sulfasalazine and hydroxychloroquine to methotrexate in patients with early rheumatoid arthritis (SweFOT trial): 1-year results of a randomised trial. *Lancet* 2009;*374*(9688):459–66.

61. Peper SM, Lew R, Mikuls T, et al. Rheumatoid arthritis treatment after methotrexate: the durability of triple therapy versus etanercept. *Arthritis Care Res* 2017;*69*(10):1467–72.

62. Kuusalo LA, Puolakka KT, Kautiainen H, et al. Intra-articular glucocorticoid injections should not be neglected in the remission targeted treatment of early rheumatoid arthritis: a post hoc analysis from the NEO-RACo trial. *Clin Exp Rheumatol* 2016;*34*(6):1038–44.

63. Hughes CD, Scott DL, Ibrahim F; TITRATE Programme Investigators. Intensive therapy and remissions in rheumatoid arthritis: a systematic review. *BMC Musculoskelet Disord* 2018;*19*:389.

64. Erhardt DP, Cannon GW, Teng CC, Mikuls TR, Curtis JR, Sauer BC. Low persistence rates in rheumatoid arthritis patients treated with triple therapy are attributed to adverse drug events associated with sulfasalazine. *Arthritis Care Res* 2019;*71*(10):1326–35.

65. Sauer BC, Teng CC, Tang D, et al. Persistence with conventional triple therapy versus a tumor necrosis factor inhibitor and methotrexate in US veterans with rheumatoid arthritis. *Arthritis Care Res* 2017;*69*:313–22.

66. Bonafede M, Johnson BH, Tang DH, Shah N, Harrison DJ, Collier DH. Etanercept-methotrexate combination therapy initiators have greater adherence and persistence than triple therapy initiators with rheumatoid arthritis. *Arthritis Care Res* 2015;*67*:1656–63.

67. Sokka T, Envalds M, Pincus T. Treatment of rheumatoid arthritis: a global perspective on the use of antirheumatic drugs. *Mod Rheumatol* 2008;*18*(3):228–39.

68. Verschueren P, De Cock D, Corluy L, et al. Effectiveness of methotrexate with step-down glucocorticoid remission induction (COBRA Slim) versus other intensive treatment strategies for early rheumatoid arthritis in a treat-to-target approach: 1-year results of CareRA, a randomised pragmatic open-label superiority trial. *Ann Rheum Dis* 2017;*76*(3):511–20.

69. Meyfroidt S, Van der Elst K, Westhovens R. Methotrexate in combination with other DMARDs is not superior to methotrexate alone for remission induction with moderate-to-high-dose glucocorticoid bridging in early rheumatoid arthritis after 16 weeks of treatment: the CareRA trial. *Ann Rheum Dis* 2015;*74*:27–34.

70. Burmester GR, Pope JE. Novel treatment strategies in rheumatoid arthritis. *Lancet* 2017;*389*(10086):2338–48.

Translation of new therapies: From bench to bedside

Jeremy Sokolove

Introduction

The process of drug development is often long and complex. The vast majority of compounds developed and tested die in the preclinical phase of drug development. A molecule targeting a pathway entering the clinic often has well over a decade of study behind it including work in academic and industry laboratories and even those which survive to enter Phase 1 human trials have a failure rate of over 90%.[1] See **Figure 38.1**.

Initial studies, in academic or industry labs, provide signals from animal studies which help identify pathways which, upon modulation, might ultimately lead to drug efficacy (target identification). Subsequent work, usually in industry laboratories, further validate target pathways identified (target validation) and deliver early hit molecules for testing (lead identification) followed by a series of iteratively improving compounds for further evaluation until a final clinical candidate is achieved (lead optimization). Toxicology studies provide confidence in safety of compounds in early development and, in combination with animal pharmacology, enable the translation of preclinical animal data to project efficacious exposures for first-in-human studies.

However, the process of translating drugs from the bench to the bedside is not a one-way street. In fact, the process of drug development often begins at the bedside. This is related to the fact that the strongest evidence supporting the existence of a drug target in the human, is the ability to demonstrate alteration of the target in the setting of disease relative to the healthy condition.

The current process of drug development in rheumatology and immunology is challenging, in large part due an incomplete understanding of disease pathophysiology. In a disease such as rheumatoid arthritis (RA) there are many overlapping and in some cases redundant pathways activated (or suppressed) as a manifestation of clinical disease. These pathways are also heterogeneous across patients; even among those with what appears to be the same clinical phenotype.[2] RA as described be the current classification criteria,[3] still likely represents a wide variety of molecular subtypes. Thus, the effectiveness of a drug targeting a single pathway will be proportional to the relative dominance of that pathway in each individual RA patient's underlying pathology. This proportionality is evidenced across clinical trials in which success for any given RA therapy is defined by a $\geq 20\%$ improvement in the composite American College of Rheumatology (ACR) score (ACR20).[4] Similarly, with any single therapy to date, less than 30% of patients manifest robust disease control as defined by a $\geq 70\%$ improvement in ACR score (ACR70) or the achievement of 'remission' according to the disease activity score (DAS28 remission).[5] The most logical explanation for the lack of response, or only incomplete abrogation of disease activity, is that there exist collateral pathways which remain unchecked by any single therapy (and in many cases by combinations of currently available therapies).[6] Thus there remains a significant need to develop better therapies for RA patients. These needs can be viewed in many ways, but the following are potential approaches for advancing drug development to better serve patients with RA and related immunologic diseases.

Identification of targets that are more broadly represented across all RA patients

A critical overlying pathway which could influence a broader population of RA patients could help bring a higher percentage of patients responding a therapy. Notably, there is no guarantee that any single therapy would address the issue of 'shallow' responses currently observed in the majority of RA patients.

One potential area that could benefit a wide population of RA patients is the potential to identify mechanisms driving disease initiation. The identification and targeting of a common mechanism driving disease initiation or early propagation of RA could potentially abrogate disease before the development of multiple redundant and collateral pathways of pathologic activation. However, though there has been great progress in this area, studies to date suggest that even in the earliest phases of RA, there are potentially multiple initiating processes.[7] Whether these multitudes of initiating processes might convene on a common and potentially targetable mechanistic pathways remains to be defined.

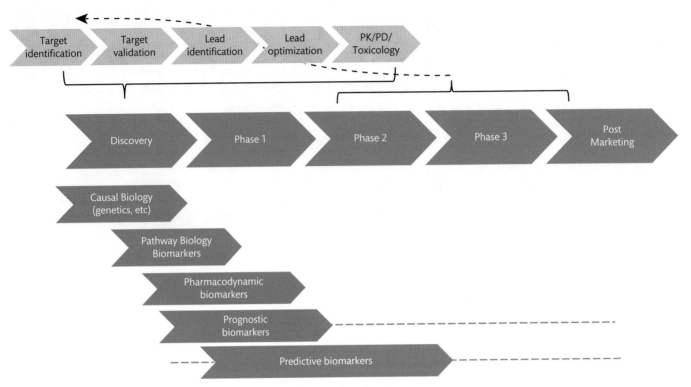

Figure 38.1 Bench to bedside drug development: forward translation and back again.
The process of drug development progresses from discovery efforts focused on target identification to initial and confirmatory clinical trials. At each stage there is requirement and/or opportunity to leverage existing and novel scientific tools to identify markers with the ability to identify causal biology and downstream pathways, as well as markers predictive of natural history or response to therapy. Notably, even with the most potent therapies on the horizon, there is continued need to better define disease subtypes and/or identify novel therapeutic targets. Thus, well curated patient data obtained from clinical trials provides the opportunity to undertake 'reverse translation' in an effort to further the iterative cycle of advancing drug development.

Identification of new targets which are represented in subgroups of RA patients

The concept of personalized medicine suggests that treatments be targeted so as to deliver the **right drug** to the **right patient** at the **right time** and at the **right dose**.[8] If in fact since there are differential pathways at play in each patient, it will be important to identify the relevant pathways for each individual and to tailor therapy to the underlying pathologic pathways. Thus, a major focus of research in RA is aimed at identifying the breadth of pathways potentially activated across the spectrum of RA patients, identifying new targets, and developing new molecules for targeting these newly identified pathways.

Identification of collateral pathways which can be targeted for additive efficacy

Though each of the first two approaches are likely to improve the treatment of RA, it is perhaps naïve to think that a process as molecularly diverse as RA, will, in any given patient, be simplistic enough to rely on any single activation pathway. By the time RA is clinically manifest, it is likely that there are a variety of aberrant pathways at play systemically and at end organ (i.e. the joint and synovium). Notably, rheumatology has already entered into the common practice of utilizing multiple therapeutic drug combinations. Over the prior four to five decades, rheumatologists have likely experimented with every potential combination of available therapy. These combinations have met with some success; the most well studied being the so-called triple therapy of methotrexate, hydroxychloroquine, and sulfasalazine.[9] However, these therapies were chosen from the limited few which were available and combined empirically and with limited understanding of how their individual and combined molecular impact might ultimately deliver therapeutically. More recently, with the advent of biologic therapies, primarily but not limited to tumour necrosis factor (TNF) inhibitors (TNFi), there has again been empiric demonstration that the combination of biologic agents with conventional immunosuppressive therapies provides additive and, in some cases, synergistic benefits.[10] The combination of methotrexate, and ultimately several other conventional synthetic disease-modifying antirheumatic drugs (csDMARDs), is clear and at least one molecular mechanism for this observation has been demonstrated. In addition to the antirheumatic effect of methotrexate or other DMARDs, the prolongation of half-life as well as the ability to abrogate development of an immune response against the biologic therapy (antidrug antibodies) has provided a molecular explanation for the benefits of combination RA therapy.[11] Notably, even with the advent of targeted synthetic disease-modifying antirheumatic drugs (DMARDs) such as Janus kinase (JAK) inhibitors, there still appears to be an additive benefit of methotrexate when added to JAK inhibitor therapy.[12] This implies that even as our armamentarium of highly effective DMARDs grows, each therapy still has gaps in efficacy for which new targets must be identified.

Target identification

Target identification is the process of identifying a direct molecular target with the potential to be modulated for the purpose of therapeutic effect. There are many ways to get to this target, whether it is extrapolation from basic scientific observations, or directed studies within a previously implicated disease process or pathway. The objective is to translate novel and potentially related basic studies to a clinical disease or pathologic condition. The American Physiological Society (APS) has defined translational research as 'the transfer of knowledge gained from basic research to new and improved methods of preventing, diagnosing, or treating disease, as well as the transfer of clinical insights into hypotheses that can be tested and validated in the basic research laboratory'.[13] Though many have implied that the transfer of knowledge is primarily from the basic science lab to the patient in the clinic, the process is in fact a two-way street in which much of the basis for study in the lab is derived from observations of the human clinical condition.

One such example is the identification of so-called 'experiments of nature'. Genetic polymorphisms in laboratory animals or in human populations can result in an identifiable phenotype; sometimes as a disease, sometimes as a protective benefit, sometimes as both. In any case, such observations can generate hypotheses so as to suggest potential targets for drug development.

Conventional and now rapidly advancing tools for generating mutant animals[14] have yielded many models of aberrant inflammation similar to that observed in human arthritis and these models can be interrogated or experimentally manipulated for target identification. Additionally, loss of function mutations ('knock outs') which protect an animal from the development or reduce the severity of an induced immunologic process suggest potentially viable drug targets. However, mutations present from embryogenesis may not represent the impact of modifying the same target in adulthood. As well, animal models of disease often do not fully recapitulate the human disease condition. Perhaps the most crucial limitation is that studies are conducted in genetically homogenous animals, using identical timing and mechanisms of initiation to generate model disease pathology. Thus, the pathways associated with animal models of inflammatory disease are unlikely to represent the much broader spectrum of pathways activated though a variety of mechanisms and across the genetic and environmental diversity of patients with inflammatory arthritis. Thus, it is perhaps not surprising that there are numerous examples of animal models where laboratory observations failed to predict the outcome of clinical studies. The following quote is in reference to mathematical models, but likely is the most succinct and accurate way to describe the use of animal models in when studying disease mechanism and target identification.

'Essentially, all models are wrong, but some are useful'

Perhaps even more rapid in their development than animal models, are technologies which enable rapid and efficient characterization of human genetics.[15] Studying the genetics underlying the predisposition to disease can potentially inform on relevant pathways for therapeutic interventions. Though not always disease-specific, the identification of genetic anomalies which predispose to excess inflammation can identify potential targets for anti-inflammatory therapy. As an example, there are multiple genetic polymorphisms within the type 1 interferon pathway, many of which predispose to either immunodeficiency or pathologic inflammation.[16] Each of the identified mutated proteins provides a possible target for suppression of interferon-mediated inflammation. One example is the association of primary immunodeficiency with mutations within JAK and signal transducers and activators of transcription (STAT) pathway members and the resultant identification of now proven targets for treatment of RA.[17] Similarly, a variety of mutations in the gene coding for Bruton's tyrosine kinase (BTK) are associated with an X-linked agammaglobulinemia as a result of impaired B-cell maturation and differentiation.[18] This observation identified BTK as a potential target for immunosuppression, especially in autoimmunity associated with a state of excessive B-cell activation.

Is it possible that the pathologic pathways underlying RA could be as simple as the genetic polymorphisms which an individual inherits? Given only a 15% concordance for RA among monozygotic twins,[19] this is clearly not the whole story. Even with the most robust of genetic associations, it is still the minority of individuals with RA for whom any of these mutations are present. However, it is still possible that these correlated mutations may point to pathways which are more relevant to disease pathology, at least in a significant subset of RA patients. In fact, it has been suggested that, across multiple well-studied diseases, those drug mechanisms with 'direct genetic support' increases probability of drug success from 2.0% at the preclinical stage to 8.2% for approved compounds.[20]

An example from RA is CTLA4, a component of the T-cell costimulatory pathway within which it exerts a net inhibitory effect on T-cell activation. A non-coding polymorphism, but one which has been suggested to alter the expression ratio of soluble to full length CTLA4, has been associated with development of RA[21] and the drug CTLA4-Ig (abatacept) has proven highly effective for the treatment of RA[22]. Another interesting polymorphism is in the IL-12B gene (the target of the drug ustekinumab) which has been observed to increase risk for Crohn's disease.[23] Though the absence of genetic association certainly does not directly imply lack of causality, it is interesting to note that although both RA and Crohn's are effectively treated with TNFi therapy, targeting IL-12 with ustekinumab has proven effective in Crohn's[24] but with negligible benefit in RA.[25]

Alternatively, since genetics is likely only one piece of many contributing to the end phenotype of RA, translational medicine has been taking an increasing focus on studies starting with human disease tissue and utilizing traditional and rapidly evolving scientific tools to 'back-translate' to identify potential disease targets. This approach has yielded great insight in the field of oncology in which the characterization of directly pathologic mutations, as well as closely associated genetic and epigenetic anomalies, have begun to make personalized medicine a reality for the treatment of a variety of cancers.[26]

Among the translational success stories in RA is the identification of TNF as a pathologic mediator and therapeutic target. Dr Marc Feldman and his team demonstrated the robust expression of TNF in the RA synovium[6] and with Dr Ravinder Maini, demonstrated the profound therapeutic effect of TNF inhibition in RA patients.[27] More recently work at the United States National Institutes of Health by Dr John O'Shea identified experiments of nature involving mutation in the JAK-STAT pathway and subsequently demonstrated pathologic activation of the JAK-STAT pathways in RA and related immunologic diseases.[28] This work helped enable the clinical introduction of small molecule JAK inhibitors including tofacitinib as well as the plethora of JAK inhibitors currently in clinical trials.[29]

However, all is not so straightforward in translational medicine. Based on the aforementioned translational methods, there is at least equally convincing evidence supporting a critical role for the cytokines IL-1 and IL-17 in RA. IL-1 and IL-17 have both been identified at robust levels in the RA synovium and in circulating RA blood.[30,31] And both IL-1 and IL-17 were proven critical in animal models of arthritis in which deficiency or neutralization of IL-1[32] or IL-17[33] was highly efficacious. However, the efficacy of IL-1 blockade in human RA was only marginal[34] (at least relative to that observed with TNF, IL-6, or JAK inhibition), and even less efficacy was observed in clinical studies of IL-17 blockade in RA.[35]

Thus, target identification is a critical step in the course of drug development and there are many existing and evolving tools that can be used to identify such targets. However, it is important to remember that even the best of targets will still face a long and challenging path before it can ever be exploited as a successful therapy in the clinic.

Target validation

Upon identification of a potential target, the process of target validation ensues. This important work provides both additional supportive evidence for a target and begins process of ensuring mechanistic understanding of the means by which a pathway may mediate pathology. The process usually overlaps with the process of target identification and includes *in vitro* and *in vivo* studies of drug targets including use of so-called tool compounds with the ability to affect the implicated pathway. These molecules are rarely those which will be advanced to the clinic but provide the opportunity for pathway interrogation prior to embarking on the long and complex process of identifying and optimization a lead therapeutic compound.

In vitro and *ex-vivo* cellular assays are often used to mimic the pathways implicated *in vivo*. These cell culture systems can be induced via a variety of molecular activators and manipulated by use of tool compounds (usually inhibitors) as well as such techniques as ribonucleic acid (RNA) interference (RNAi), or more recently, with use of CRISPR-mediated genetic manipulation.[36]

Though *in vitro* and cell-based assays are usually cheaper and faster to run than animal studies, the artificial stimuli used for pathway activation are rarely as complex as the processes activated *in vivo*. Thus, pathway manipulation *in vivo* provides significant support for advancing a target toward selection of an ultimate drug candidate.

As with other stages of development in the march from bench to bedside, there are numerous caveats during target validation. Manipulation of potential target pathways in cell culture should be a result of so-called on target effects. However, many tool compounds lack pathway specificity or simply exert their effect through off-target cellular toxicity. Due to similar lack of specificity or due to lack of access of the drug to the target, *in vivo* behaviour of tool compounds may not be always be predictive of the ultimate effects which can be achieved with a more advanced therapeutic compound.

Notably, the process of target validation is critical for the purpose of scientific confirmation of initially promising results. Initial studies identifying potential targets are often performed and published out of academic laboratories. Although most academic labs are scientifically rigorous, clinical experience and several recent comprehensive reports have noted inconsistent ability to replicate academic studies. One report suggested only 11% of published preclinical cancer studies from academic labs could be reproduced by Amgen scientists and another report by scientists at Bayer found that approximately 75% of published academic studies brought in-house could not be reproduced.[37] There are multiple reasons why two labs might generate conflicting data including subtle methodologic, environmental, and reagent differences. But it also highlights the need for vigorous target validation using multiple methodologies before advancing on a campaign to identify lead compounds as well as the extensive follow on preclinical and clinical validation required for drug success.

Lead generation

Once a target is validated, the next step is identification of potential compounds to modulate the implicated pathway. Finding 'hit' compounds can be done in several ways. Humoral mediators such as cytokines and extracellular targets such as receptors can be targeted with antibodies or related large molecular weight proteins. These are generated using immunologic methods coupled with follow on refinement using molecular biology and biochemistry to optimize such molecules. For intracellular targets or other molecular machinery, small molecules are usually required to modulate these pathways. In some cases, pre-existing tool compounds or molecules found in nature may provide a starting point for generating a lead compound. However, most often, leads are identified by high-throughput screening (HTS) of large and relatively diverse chemical libraries.

Notably, the process of HTS typically identifies a significant number of false positives results. Thus, there is often a need to revert back to the cellular assays used for target validation or development of other additional and more specific cellular or chemical screens to confirm specific activity and characterize mechanism of action.

Lead optimization

Chemical screens often identify molecules which, *in vitro*, can perform the desired modulation of a physiochemical pathway. Although a good starting point, the lead compounds identified must undergo an extensive process of lead optimization. This optimization process involves tools from medicinal chemistry as well as increasingly utilizes tools from biochemistry, biophysics, and molecular informatics. The initial hit must be optimized in terms of both physical function as well as chemical properties to function optimally as a drug.

The function of any drug is defined by basic pharmacology—How well does the drug affect its desired function? How tightly does it bind to the target (affinity) and what is its potency (how much drug does it take to get the job done)?

Once the affinity and potency has been determined, there is an iterative process of chemical manipulation based on an extensive wealth of science and use of orthogonal tools which provide additional information to make additional improvements. Medicinal chemists synthesize many closely related compounds designed to improve binding and function. In some cases, a hit compound can be crystalized, including in complex with the target, to define structure-activity relationships (SAR). And more recently, informatics tools have facilitated computer modelling to predict more optimal structural properties. The goal is to achieve improved affinity, avidity, selectivity, and ultimately, improved pharmacologic properties.

But drugs do not function in isolated wells or test tubes. It is critical that a drug has sufficient 'drug-like properties'. Drugs must function in living systems and to do so, they must again maintain biologic potency *in vivo*. There must be ways to administer the drug, assure it reaches the target site of action, and is appropriately cleared by the body. The next round of lead optimization requires consideration of the physiochemical properties of the drug with respect to absorption (solubility), distribution, metabolism, and elimination (ADME).

Pharmacokinetics, pharmacodynamics, and toxicology

Pharmacokinetics (PK) is the characterization of the ADME of a drug when it enters the body, either human or model animal. Sometimes characterized as 'what the body does to a drug', the characterization of PK is critical to begin the process of identifying safe and efficacious drug doses leading up to and upon entering the clinic. However, the level and fate of drug observed in the body is not particularly useful without some metric of correlation with drug effect on the body. Thus pharmacodynamics (PD) has been characterized as 'what a drug does to the body'. The interplay between PK and PD help determine the goal level of drug to be achieved in the body (usually first in an animal model) and thus provide and estimation of dose(s) needed to evaluate effect in the human.

However, there is an additional critical step in drug development which must be considered, and that is drug safety. Most clinicians are aware of the close scrutiny drug safety gets in clinical studies but there are extensive requirements for evaluation before a molecule ever enters a 'first-in-human' study. This process is usually referred to as toxicology or non-clinical safety evaluation.

At least a minimum number of non-clinical safety studies are required for first entering the clinic and then multiple additional studies are conducted before approval and marketing. These include toxicology studies of increasing duration to permit chronic dosing (chronic toxicology studies) and a range of other studies which address other potential risks (i.e. reproduction toxicity studies, genotoxicity studies, carcinogenicity studies, as well a variety of molecule specific studies including but not limited to phototoxicity and immunotoxicity.)

Standard toxicology requires study of a new molecule in two animal species, at least one of which must have similar metabolism to human such that there is adequate evaluation of all relevant human metabolites (usually any metabolite amounting to >10% of the parent compound in humans must be present or separately characterized in the animal).[38] Evaluation is conducted at multiple doses starting at approximately the anticipated efficacious dose and usually two higher doses. Upon completion of the intended dosing duration, a complete pathologic evaluation of multiple organ systems is conducted on all animals. The goal is to identify a level of drug exposure without demonstrable pathology, usually called the 'no-adverse-event level' (NOAEL), and then establish a safety margin between the NOAEL and the intended level to begin testing in humans. In most cases, the US FDA recommends a 10-fold safety margin as a starting dose for non-oncology drug studies. Thus, in combination with preclinical pharmacology, the toxicology margin is used to determine first-in-human dosing.

Translational biomarkers

A biomarker is a characteristic that can be objectively measured as an indicator of normal or pathologic biological processes, or as an indicator of response to therapy.[39] As part of the progression from the lab to the clinic, there is need to develop biomarkers which can be used to define pharmacodynamics effects in preclinical animal models and which can optimally be translated for use in first-in-human studies. Although commonly used to describe a biochemical variable, such as the concentration of a circulating protein or other biomolecule, the broad definition of biomarker can apply to any type of biological data. Some biomarkers focus on anatomical and structural features visualized by radiography, ultrasonography, computed tomography (CT) scanning (for example, positron emission tomography) or MRI (including functional MRI scans that can provide information about the neuronal activity in certain regions of the brain).[40] Other variables considered biomarkers are cellular immune responses, genetic traits, histologic characteristics of diseased tissue and proteins or RNA expressed in tissues.

Notably, most non-oncology indications conduct first-in-human studies in healthy volunteers for the purpose of assessing safety and PK. Since disease abrogation cannot be ascertained in healthy subjects, the ability to assess the effect of a drug and identify the level of drug exposure required to exert a physiologic effect is critical for selection of doses to advance into clinical trials in actual patients. In early stage studies (i.e. preclinical models and human Phase 1), biomarkers of target engagement are needed to confirm and quantify binding of a drug to its intended target and correlate with concurrent drug exposure. The ability to measure the effect of target engagement in terms of a downstream pharmacodynamics effect is also helpful to estimate what level of target binding correlates with what degree of physiologic effect. It could be that only 50% target engagement maximally suppresses pathway activation or alternatively that, even with 100% of the targets occupied, there is still residual downstream pathway activation, perhaps through alternative pathways of activation. Though not confirming that the observed effect will directly correlate with improvement in patients with active disease, the movement of relevant biomarkers provides what is considered 'proof of mechanism'.

Once a drug candidate enters the clinic and for testing in patients, the first study is considered 'proof of concept'. Usually in a small study, there is an attempt to show movement in the level of disease activity. However, the movement of biomarkers closely related to disease activity, especially those which are based in disease mechanism, can provide evidence to support follow on studies in larger populations of patients. When successful, such 'mechanistic biomarkers'[40] could also potentially be translated from the trial setting into clinical use.

The use of 'dynamic' biomarkers measures a change induced by drug treatment. When the change is one that can be observed much earlier than the intended clinical outcome, it can allow shorter and often smaller early phase studies by demonstrating early changes in disease-associated biological processes. Results of dynamic biomarker testing could also provide an early signal for the clinician to initiate or intensify therapy in the setting of highly active disease or, conversely, to withdraw a specific treatment in the setting of a clearly insufficient therapeutic response. Finally, it can also potentially possible to identify patients who have underlying active, if subclinical, disease activity for whom therapy should be escalated in terms of dose or therapeutic regimen.

Another type of biomarker is the prognostic biomarker. This should be differentiated from the predictive biomarker in that it helps identify the trajectory of a disease (rather than response to a specific therapy). An example would be a biomarker such as anti-CCP and/ or rheumatoid factor which have been associated with development of more severe and more rapidly erosive RA. In such a setting, a more aggressive approach to therapy might be chosen in an attempt to more completely control disease activity and to prevent or delay the onset of joint damage and physical disability. One example in RA is the well-described association of anti-CCP and rheumatoid factor antibodies with increased disease severity and erosive potential.[41]

Perhaps the most useful, and to date most elusive, type of biomarker is the predictive biomarker. An initial use of such predictive biomarker is for stratification of patients entering clinical trials. Identifying those most likely to respond to a novel mechanism can result in a larger experimental effect size and thus enable smaller, more efficient clinical trials.

In oncology, the assessment for biomarkers which can predict drug response has become standard in most modern studies for the purpose not only of the study, but ultimately for treatment of patients upon drug approval.[26] This approach, as introduced earlier, is an example of personalized medicine; the ability to deliver the **right drug** to the **right patient** at the **right time** and at the **right dose**. The ability to discern those patients who will respond to a drug and those who will not has potentially huge value in terms of patient care, patient safety, and healthcare costs.[40]

Though there is still much work to be done to help stratify rheumatology patients, there have been multiple promising avenues made toward enriching for responders to specific lines of therapy. An example is use of the well-established RA-associated autoantibodies rheumatoid factor and anti-CCP. In addition to the association with more severe disease activity (as just discussed), the presence of these autoantibodies has been associated with preferential response to some biologic therapies, particularly rituximab[42] and abatacept[43,44]; while no such association has been noted for TNFi treatments. This brings up the mechanistic potential that RA patients driven by a more dominant adaptive immune pathology may preferentially respond to therapies targeting the B cell, T cell, or perhaps the process of T-cell/B-cell interaction. Another such example is the measurement of proteins ICAM1 and CLCL13, both of which were found to be elevated in RA serum. However, in a head-to-head trial of TNFi (adalimumab) versus anti-IL-6R (tocilizumab), elevated serum sICAM1 was associated with better TNFi outcome, while elevated serum CXCL13 was associated with better anti-IL6R outcome. Notably, combining these biomarkers showed that sICAM1^{high}/CXCL13^{low} patients had better treatment outcomes with TNFi therapy and less robust outcomes with anti-IL-6Rα therapy, while sICAM^{low}/CXCL13^{high} patients had better treatment outcomes from anti-IL6Rα therapy and less response from TNFi.[45] Notably, *CXCL13* was identified as highly expressed in RA synovium with a B-cell aggregate-rich synovial lymphoid phenotype again suggesting that these biomarkers may relate to underlying synovial pathotype of RA. However, despite these and many other biomarkers potentially associated with response to certain therapies, the absolute predictive ability of any single biomarker remains relatively small and thus there are growing efforts to bring forward better biomarkers as well efforts to develop multiplex biomarkers[46–48] capable of leveraging measurement of multiple analytes to improve predictive performance, all with the goal of developing an actionable predictive biomarkers.

Finally, in addition to classic protein or cellular biomarkers, network science utilizing systems biology-based and machine learning has the potential to integrate multiple data sources to can uncover complex changes in a biological system.[49] There is growing interest in leveraging large amounts of collected data from which novel machine learning algorithms might be able to piece out a reproducible group of datapoints that predict a clinical outcome.[50] It is possible that in near future, the field will be able to utilize a broad range of clinical datapoints including prospectively clinical characteristics, measured biomarkers, imaging data, as well as other biologic measures such as the status of the autonomic nervous system[51] to predict and define therapeutic response.

Conclusions

Not unlike other fields of medicine, the process of drug discovery in RA is long and complex. If across a single disease such as RA, there are in fact differential biochemical pathways at play in each patient, then there is the opportunity that the same studies which are undertaken to identify novel drug targets could simultaneous leverage the same populations to concurrently identify mechanistic biomarkers which predict therapeutic response. Additionally, biologic and clinical data obtained during the interrogation of any investigated therapy should be fed back into the drug discovery pipeline to help identify new and potentially synergistic therapeutic targets. Such a process could provide a seamless link from drug discovery, to drug development, to clinical care, and back again.

REFERENCES

1. Waring MJ, Arrowsmith J, Leach AR, et al. An analysis of the attrition of drug candidates from four major pharmaceutical companies. *Nat Rev Drug Discov* 2015;14(7):475–86.
2. Firestein GS. Inhibiting inflammation in rheumatoid arthritis. *N Engl J Med* 2006;354(1):80–2.
3. Aletaha D, Neogi T, Silman AJ, et al. 2010 rheumatoid arthritis classification criteria: an American College of Rheumatology/ European League Against Rheumatism collaborative initiative. *Ann Rheum Dis* 2010;69(9):1580–8.
4. Felson DT, Anderson JJ, Boers M, et al. The American College of Rheumatology preliminary core set of disease activity measures for rheumatoid arthritis clinical trials. The Committee on Outcome Measures in rheumatoid arthritis clinical trials. *Arthritis Rheum* 1993;36(6):729–40.
5. Elliot MJ, Maini RN, Feldmann M, et al. Treatment of rheumatoid arthritis with chimeric monoclonal antibodies to tumor necrosis factor alpha. *Arthritis Rheum* 2008;58(2 Suppl):S92–S101.
6. Feldmann M, Maini RN. Perspectives from masters in rheumatology and autoimmunity: can we get closer to a cure for rheumatoid arthritis? *Arthritis Rheum* 2015;67(9):2283–91.
7. McInnes IB, Schett G. The pathogenesis of rheumatoid arthritis. *N Engl J Med* 2011;365(23):2205–19.
8. Camilleri M, Shin A. Lessons from pharmacogenetics and metoclopramide: toward the right dose of the right drug for the right patient. *J Clin Gastroenterol* 2012;46(6):437–9.
9. O'Dell JR, Haire CE, Erikson N, et al. Treatment of rheumatoid arthritis with methotrexate alone, sulfasalazine and hydroxychloroquine, or a combination of all three medications. *N Engl J Med* 1996;334(20):1287–91.
10. Kavanaugh A, Fleischmann RM, Emery P, et al. Clinical, functional and radiographic consequences of achieving stable low

disease activity and remission with adalimumab plus methotrexate or methotrexate alone in early rheumatoid arthritis: 26-
week results from the randomised, controlled OPTIMA study.
Ann Rheum Dis 2013;*72*(1):64–71.

11. Hindryckx P, Novak G, Vande Casteele N, et al. Incidence, prevention and management of anti-drug antibodies against therapeutic antibodies in inflammatory bowel disease: a practical
overview. *Drugs* 2017;*77*(4):363–77.

12. Fleischmann R, Mysler E, Hall S, et al. Efficacy and safety of
tofacitinib monotherapy, tofacitinib with methotrexate, and
adalimumab with methotrexate in patients with rheumatoid arthritis (ORAL Strategy): a phase 3b/4, double-
blind, head-to-head, randomised controlled trial. *Lancet*
2017;*390*(10093):457–68.

13. Hall JE. The promise of translational physiology. *Am J Phys Lung
Cell Mol Physiol* 2002;*283*(2):L235–6.

14. Qin W, Kutny PM, Maser RS, et al. Generating mouse models
using CRISPR-Cas9-mediated genome editing. *Curr Protoc
Mouse Biol* 2016;*6*(1):39–66.

15. Levy SE, Myers RM. Advancements in next-generation
sequencing. *Ann Rev Genomics Hum Genet* 2016;*17*:95–115.

16. Rodero MP, Crow YJ. Type I interferon-mediated monogenic
autoinflammation: the type I interferonopathies, a conceptual
overview. *J Exp Med* 2016;*213*(12):2527–38.

17. O'Shea JJ, Holland SM, Staudt LM. JAKs and STATs in immunity, immunodeficiency, and cancer. *N Engl J Med*
2013;*368*(2):161–70.

18. Vihinen M, Kwan SP, Lester T, et al. Mutations of the human
BTK gene coding for bruton tyrosine kinase in X-linked
agammaglobulinemia. *Hum Mutat* 1999;*13*(4):280–5.

19. Silman AJ, MacGregor AJ, Thomson W, et al. Twin concordance
rates for rheumatoid arthritis: results from a nationwide study. *Br
J Rheumatol* 1993;*32*(10):903–7.

20. Nelson MR, Tipney H, Painter JL, et al. The support of human
genetic evidence for approved drug indications. *Nat Genet*
2015;*47*(8):856–60.

21. Plenge RM, Padyukov L, Remmers EF, et al. Replication of putative candidate-gene associations with rheumatoid arthritis in
>4,000 samples from North America and Sweden: association of
susceptibility with PTPN22, CTLA4, and PADI4. *Am J Human
Genet* 2005;*77*(6):1044–60.

22. Genovese MC, Becker JC, Schiff M, et al. Abatacept for rheumatoid arthritis refractory to tumor necrosis factor alpha inhibition.
N Engl J Med 2005;*353*(11):1114–23.

23. Duerr RH, Taylor KD, Brant SR, et al. A genome-wide association study identifies IL23R as an inflammatory bowel disease
gene. *Science* 2006;*314*(5804):1461–3.

24. Feagan BG, Sandborn WJ, Gasink C, et al. Ustekinumab as induction and maintenance therapy for Crohn's disease. *N Engl J
Med* 2016;*375*(20):1946–60.

25. Smolen JS, Agarwal SK, Ilivanova E, et al. A randomised phase
II study evaluating the efficacy and safety of subcutaneously administered ustekinumab and guselkumab in patients with active
rheumatoid arthritis despite treatment with methotrexate. *Ann
Rheum Dis* 2017;*76*(5):831–9.

26. Li T, Kung HJ, Mack PC, Gandara DR. Genotyping and genomic
profiling of non-small-cell lung cancer: implications for current
and future therapies. *J Clin Oncol* 2013;*31*(8):1039–49.

27. Maini R, St Clair EW, Breedveld F, et al. Infliximab (chimeric
anti-tumour necrosis factor alpha monoclonal antibody) versus
placebo in rheumatoid arthritis patients receiving concomitant

methotrexate: a randomised phase III trial. ATTRACT Study
Group. *Lancet* 1999;*354*(9194):1932–9.

28. O'Shea JJ, Gadina M, Schreiber RD. Cytokine signaling in
2002: new surprises in the JAK/STAT pathway. *Cell* 2002;*109*
Suppl:S121–31.

29. Schwartz DM, Kanno Y, Villarino A, Ward M, Gadina M, O'Shea
JJ. JAK inhibition as a therapeutic strategy for immune and inflammatory diseases. *Nat Rev Drug Discov* 2017;*16*(12):843–62.

30. Eastgate JA, Symons JA, Wood NC, Grinlinton FM, di Giovine
FS, Duff GW. Correlation of plasma interleukin 1 levels with disease activity in rheumatoid arthritis. *Lancet* 1988;*2*(8613):706–9.

31. McInnes IB, Schett G. Cytokines in the pathogenesis of rheumatoid arthritis. *Nat Rev Immunol* 2007;*7*(6):429–42.

32. Geiger T, Towbin H, Cosenti-Vargas A, et al. Neutralization of
interleukin-1 beta activity *in vivo* with a monoclonal antibody
alleviates collagen-induced arthritis in DBA/1 mice and prevents the associated acute-phase response. *Clin Exp Rheumatol*
1993;*11*(5):515–22.

33. Lubberts E, Koenders MI, Oppers-Walgreen B, et al. Treatment
with a neutralizing anti-murine interleukin-17 antibody after
the onset of collagen-induced arthritis reduces joint inflammation, cartilage destruction, and bone erosion. *Arthritis Rheum*
2004;*50*(2):650–9.

34. Cohen SB, Moreland LW, Cush JJ, et al. A multicentre, double
blind, randomised, placebo controlled trial of anakinra (Kineret),
a recombinant interleukin 1 receptor antagonist, in patients with
rheumatoid arthritis treated with background methotrexate. *Ann
Rheum Dis* 2004;*63*(9):1062–8.

35. Blanco FJ, Moricke R, Dokoupilova E, et al. Secukinumab in
active rheumatoid arthritis: a phase III randomized, double-
blind, active comparator- and placebo-controlled study. *Arthritis
Rheumatol* 2017;*69*(6):1144–53.

36. La Russa MF, Qi LS. The new state of the art: Cas9 for gene activation and repression. *Mol Cell Biol* 2015;*35*(22):3800–9.

37. Frye SV, Arkin MR, Arrowsmith CH, et al. Tackling reproducibility in academic preclinical drug discovery. *Nat Rev Drug
Discov* 2015;*14*(11):733–4.

38. Claude JR, Claude N. Safety pharmacology: an essential interface
of pharmacology and toxicology in the non-clinical assessment
of new pharmaceuticals. *Toxicology Letters* 2004;*151*(1):25–8.

39. O'Connell D, Roblin D. Translational research in the pharmaceutical industry: from bench to bedside. *Drug Discovery Today*
2006;*11*(17–18):833–8.

40. Robinson WH, Lindstrom TM, Cheung RK, Sokolove J.
Mechanistic biomarkers for clinical decision making in rheumatic diseases. *Nat Rev Rheumatol* 2013;*9*(5):267–76.

41. Vencovsky J, Machacek S, Sedova L, et al. Autoantibodies can
be prognostic markers of an erosive disease in early rheumatoid
arthritis. *Ann Rheum Dis* 2003;*62*(5):427–30.

42. Isaacs JD, Cohen SB, Emery P, et al. Effect of baseline rheumatoid factor and anticitrullinated peptide antibody serotype on
rituximab clinical response: a meta-analysis. *Ann Rheum Dis*
2013;*72*(3):329–36.

43. Sokolove J, Schiff M, Fleischmann R, et al. Impact of baseline anti-cyclic citrullinated peptide-2 antibody concentration
on efficacy outcomes following treatment with subcutaneous
abatacept or adalimumab: 2-year results from the AMPLE trial.
Ann Rheum Dis 2016;*75*(4):709–14.

44. Gottenberg JE, Courvoisier DS, Hernandez MV, et al. Brief report: association of rheumatoid factor and anti-citrullinated
protein antibody positivity with better effectiveness of

abatacept: results from the pan-European registry analysis. *Arthritis Rheumatol* 2016;*68*(6):1346–52.

45. Dennis G, Jr., Holweg CT, Kummerfeld SK, et al. Synovial phenotypes in rheumatoid arthritis correlate with response to biologic therapeutics. *Arthritis Res Ther* 2014;*16*(2):R90.

46. Yazici Y, Swearingen CJ. MBDA: what is it good for? *Ann Rheum Dis* 2014;*73*(11):e72.

47. Chandra PE, Sokolove J, Hipp BG, et al. Novel multiplex technology for diagnostic characterization of rheumatoid arthritis. *Arthritis Res Ther* 2011;*13*(3):R102.

48. Hueber W, Tomooka BH, Batliwalla F, et al. Blood autoantibody and cytokine profiles predict response to anti-tumor necrosis factor therapy in rheumatoid arthritis. *Arthritis Res Ther* 2009;*11*(3):R76.

49. Manem VSK, Salgado R, Aftimos P, Sotiriou C, Haibe-Kains B. Network science in clinical trials: a patient-centered approach. *Semin Cancer Biol* 2018;*52*(Pt 2):135–50.

50. Wei Z, Wang W, Bradfield J, et al. Large sample size, wide variant spectrum, and advanced machine-learning technique boost risk prediction for inflammatory bowel disease. *Am J Human Genet* 2013;*92*(6):1008–12.

51. Holman AJ, Ng E. Heart rate variability predicts anti-tumor necrosis factor therapy response for inflammatory arthritis. *Auton Neurosci* 2008;*143*(1–2):58–67.

Adverse events in clinical studies in rheumatoid arthritis

Mark Yates and James Galloway

Introduction

When prescribing any therapy, potential benefits must be balanced against risk. This is particularly relevant in rheumatoid arthritis (RA), where many treatments available have important associated adverse events. Awareness of adverse event profiles is crucial in supporting patient-centred care, particularly in situations where comparative efficacy data are sparse. Across the biologic class of therapy, head-to-head trials are infrequent, and it is often easier to make choices based on adverse event profile, rather than efficacy. This chapter will review patterns of adverse events seen with RA treatments, including by organ class. Firstly, it is important that we define what we mean by an adverse event, and how these terms are utilized in clinical studies.

Terminology

The terminology surrounding adverse events and adverse reactions can be confusing and is often used in a contradictory fashion. It is helpful to clarify two definitions before going further. The European Medicines Agency (EMA) in conjunction with the World Health Organization (WHO) defines an **adverse event** as 'any untoward medical occurrence that may present during treatment with a pharmaceutical product, but which does not necessarily have a causal relationship with this treatment'. An **adverse drug reaction** is defined as 'a response to a drug which is noxious and unintended and which occurs at doses normally used in man for prophylaxis, diagnosis, or therapy of disease, or for the modification of physiologic function'.[1] Adverse drug reactions can be further subcategorized.[2]

Dose-related

Typically, a predictable reaction with low mortality, related to the pharmacological action of the medication.

Non-dose-related

Unpredictable with a high mortality. The reaction is not related to the pharmacological action of the medication. An example is drug reaction with eosinophilia and systemic symptoms (DRESS) following sulfasalazine.

Dose-related and time-related

A reaction related to cumulative dose. An example is retinopathy following long-term hydroxychloroquine use.

Time-related

A reaction that develops a period of time after the treatment was commenced. An example is hypogammaglobulinaemia following long-term treatment with rituximab.

Withdrawal

Following discontinuation of a medication. For example, erythrodermatous psoriasis following steroid withdrawal in patients with psoriatic arthritis.

Unexpected therapy failure

Dose-related reaction, often due to drug interactions. For example, inefficacy of steroids when combined with rifampicin, due to liver enzyme upregulation.

A **serious adverse event** or **reaction** can be defined as 'any untoward medical occurrence that at any dose:

- results in death;
- is life-threatening;
- requires inpatient hospitalization or prolongation of existing hospitalization;
- results in persistent or significant disability/incapacity; or
- is a congenital anomaly/birth defect'.

Identifying and attributing adverse events

Attributing an adverse event to a therapy can be challenging, particularly outside of the research setting. This is rarely possible with absolute certainty. We must rely on the probability that a given therapy leads to a particular reaction. This is a crucial distinction, as it prompts those working in pharmacovigilance to consider alternative attribution hypotheses, even when the likelihood of causality is high. Disproving a causal hypothesis can prove very challenging as there may be multiple possible explanations for an event.[3]

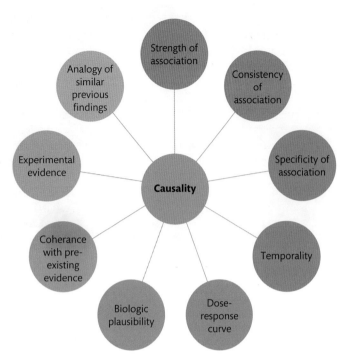

Figure 39.1 Schematic displaying considerations when determining causality.

In 1965 Sir Austin Bradford Hill presented the nine aspects of an association to consider when determining if causality is likely.[4] They are presented in **Figure 39.1**.

Evidence can be pooled from multiple sources to determine the probability of causality.

Clinical trials

This may be the first signal that a therapy is associated with an adverse reaction. Trials are usually relatively short in duration (6–12 months) and primarily designed to test efficacy. Most serious adverse events are relatively rare and may only occur after prolonged exposure. These aspects limit the value of trial data in determining adverse reactions. Clinical trial design follows three phases before licensing takes place:

- Phase I. Healthy volunteer studies designed to evaluate pharmacokinetics and pharmacodynamics;
- Phase II. Studies in patients to identify optimal dosing and test biomarkers or clinical response;
- Phase III. Large double-blind randomized controlled trials (RCTs) in patients to evaluate drug efficacy and safety.

Postmarketing surveillance (PMS)

PMS is a phase IV study after a therapy is licensed where it is assessed in the 'real-world' outside the controlled setting of an RCT for the first time and is a compulsory regulatory requirement. These studies are designed to look at effectiveness, evaluating how well the drug works, outside of a highly selected trial population. In addition, larger sample sizes with longer follow up can provide more robust evidence of adverse reactions than RCTs.[5]

Spontaneous pharmacovigilance

This relies on prescribers and dispensers reporting suspected adverse reactions to a regulatory body on an ad-hoc basis. In the United Kingdom this is carried out via the yellow card system, reporting to the Medicines and Healthcare products Regulatory Agency (MHRA). This allows the MHRA to monitor the safety of therapies and identify any potential adverse drug reactions that have not previously been recognized.

Registries

Registries are a specific example of a phase IV pharmacovigilance study. They typically collect data on patients with a particular diagnosis, therapy choice, or risk factor. An example is the Rheumatoide Arthritis: Beobachtung der Biologika-Therapie (RABBIT) registry, which collects data on patients in Germany with RA prescribed biologic therapy. This has been utilized to characterize associated risks with tumour necrosis factor alpha inhibiting (TNFi) therapy (see Chapter 44 and 45 on registries).

Scope

A multitude of therapies have been utilized for the treatment of RA. Some of which, such as penicillamine, have all but disappeared from use while others, such as non-steroidal anti-inflammatory drugs are no longer prescribed on a long-term basis due to adverse event concerns and the advent of disease-modifying treatments with improved side effect profiles. For this chapter to be as clinically relevant as possible the focus will be on therapies recommended for RA management by the national institute for health and care excellence (NICE):

- Glucocorticoids;
- Conventional synthetic disease-modifying antirheumatic drugs (csDMARDs) including methotrexate, leflunomide, sulfasalazine, and hydroxychloroquine, and;
- Biological disease-modifying antirheumatic drugs (bDMARDs) including tumour necrosis factor alpha (TNFα) inhibitors, tocilizumab, rituximab, abatacept, and Janus kinase (JAK) inhibitors.

Adverse events

Infection

Infections are a major subtype of adverse events associated with RA therapies, which is not surprising given their immuno-suppressive properties. There are data that suggest active RA in itself is a risk factor for infection, so the relative impact of therapies on this risk requires careful consideration.

Glucocorticoids

Oral glucocorticoids (GC) are commonly prescribed in RA to manage disease flares. They suppress cell-mediated immunity via impairment of phagocyte function, a plausible mechanistic pathway for an increased risk of infection. A meta-analysis investigating the association with infection in patients with RA reported that oral GC use had a higher relative risk of lower respiratory tract infections, tuberculosis, postoperative infections, and all site serious infections. These effects were still observed with doses of less than 5 mg a day. Interestingly this was only present in pooled observational data. No significant effect at lower doses was detectable in the meta-analysed RCT data.[6] Uncertainty remains on the safety of low dose oral steroids, although most guidelines now recommend avoidance of long-term steroids where targeted alternatives exist.

Conventional synthetic disease-modifying antirheumatic drugs (csDMARDS)

Methotrexate

Methotrexate (MTX) remains a key therapy 60 years after it was first used in RA. As a monotherapy it is a cost-effective route to remission in a subset of patients with RA and is a key treatment in combination with other csDMARDS and biological disease-modifying therapies. MTX and infection risk in RA is much debated. Research from the early 1990s suggested that patients treated with MTX had a higher frequency of respiratory tract and skin infections.[7] Confounding by indication may have explained this, as those treated with MTX in the study had worse baseline functional scores and were more likely to have severe or uncontrolled RA, potentially explaining the findings. More recent large-scale retrospective studies have reported a slight increased risk of respiratory tract infection but no statistically significant increased risk of infection overall.[8,9] There are case reports proposing a link between MTX and opportunistic infections such as pulmonary aspergillosis,[10] but this is not borne out in larger scale studies.

Sulfasalazine

The mechanism of action in sulfasalazine (SSZ) in RA is not clear but may be related to inhibition of nuclear factor kappa B.[11] SSZ is not associated with increased risk of infection *per se* but may lead to agranulocytosis which predisposes to infections. This is discussed in more detail later.

Leflunomide

Leflunomide (LEF) inhibits ribonucleotide uridine monophosphate pyrimidine, halting the cell cycle in memory T cells and dendritic cells.[12] As with SSZ, LEF does not have a direct link to increased infection risk, but does rarely cause leukopenia, predisposing to viral infections.[13] One challenge when studying leflunomide is that this agent is less frequently used in comparison to other agents and as such safety data are sparser.

Hydroxychloroquine

Hydroxychloroquine (HCQ) has a range of immunomodulatory actions, of which several relate to inhibition of toll-like receptors.[14] It is not immune suppressive, and infections are not considered part of the side effect profile.

Biologic disease-modifying antirheumatic drugs (bDMARDS)

TNF-alpha inhibiting therapies (infliximab, etanercept, adalimumab, golimumab, certolizumabpegol)

TNFi therapies have profoundly advanced the management of RA. Three TNF-alpha molecules combine to form a transmembrane trimer and then binds to their receptors. This leads to proinflammatory cytokine release, upregulation of adhesion molecules, and leukocyte migration.[15] The cytokine TNF is particularly relevant to host defence against intracellular pathogens.

There are currently five TNFi therapies available for prescription in the United Kingdom.

There is a large body of research focussed on serious infection risk (defined as any infection requiring hospitalization and/or parental antimicrobial therapy) with TNFi. Pooled data from RCTs indicate that all five preparations are associated with an increased risk of infection.[16,17] These findings are supported by most analyses from registry data. Dichotomising infection into 'serious' and 'non-serious' of course does not adequately explain the nature of infection risk with TNF-alpha inhibiting therapy. Background population risk of infection will impact on the findings in a given study, impacting on the likelihood that any reported infection does have a true association with TNFi therapy. Table 39.1 details specific infections and their associations with TNF-alpha inhibiting therapy.

Tuberculosis was one of the earliest signals identified for TNF inhibitors[29] and all patients are now routinely screened for latent tuberculosis prior to starting therapy. The careful screening programme has resulted in a dramatic decline in tuberculosis incidence (see Figure 39.2).

Key message: Watch for intracellular pathogens (e.g. tuberculosis and invasive fungal disease)

Interleukin-6 (IL-6) receptor antagonists (tocilizumab)

Tocilizumab is an IL-6 receptor antibody, licensed for use in RA, usually as a second line agent if TNFi fails or is not appropriate. It carries an increased risk of serious infection, broadly in line with the other biologic therapies.[30] IL-6 is a key cytokine in mucosal immunity, which may explain its association with diverticular perforation. As tocilizumab suppresses C-reactive protein (CRP), gastrointestinal (GI) perforation in this setting can present subacutely with a normal CRP. Higher mortality has also been observed follow GI perforation, thought to be due to delayed intervention.[31]

Key message: Beware intestinal perforations and infections presenting with a normal CRP

CD-20 antagonists (rituximab)

Rituximab is a monoclonal anti-CD20 antibody licensed for use in RA. It is typically employed as a second line agent if TNFi is not effective or inappropriate. Repeated doses of rituximab are associated with an increased risk of hypogammaglobinaemia.[32] This predisposes to infection (particularly sinopulmonary), though the majority of patients with depleted immunoglobulins will not sustain serious infection. Immunoglobulin levels should be monitored in patients receiving rituximab, particularly in those with repeated or serious infection. Repeat dosing should be approached with care in patients with declining immunoglobulins, and consideration to alternative agents should be given before immunoglobulins fall below the normal range.

There are case reports of patients developing progressive multifocal leukoencephalopathy (PML) secondary to John Cunningham virus while taking rituximab for RA. The majority of these patients had concurrent malignancy or had taken other immunosuppressant therapies.[33] It is therefore not appropriate to assign causality to rituximab, but given the severity of PML, and the association of rituximab and PML in other diseases, it is good practice to counsel patients on this potential but rare association prior to commencement.

Table 39.1 Infections associated with TNFi therapy

Infection	Detail	Evidence source
Tuberculosis	Increased risk, mainly reactivation of latent disease. Screening for latent disease recommended prior to starting therapy.	Multiple registry data[18]
Septic arthritis	Risk of septic arthritis twice as high in those taking adalimumab, etanercept, or infliximab, compared to those on csDMARDs. Most common organism *Staphylococcus aureus*.	BSRBR registry data[19]
Listeria Monocytogenes	Reported cases, the majority with infliximab treatment.	National adverse event reporting system (USA)[20]
Hepatitis B	Risk of reactivation. HBsAg positive (chronic infection) patients require antiviral prophylaxis. Those that are HBsAg negative but HBcAb positive (resolved infection) require regular monitoring for reactivation. Screening recommended prior to commencement of therapy.	Case reports, small prospective and retrospective studies[21]
Hepatitis C	TNFi therapy should be avoided in acute infection or in those with chronic infection and Child-Pugh class B or C liver disease. Screening recommended prior to commencement of therapy.	National guidelines[22]
Herpes zoster	Most studies report an increased risk, although published data are inconsistent.	Registry data and cohort studies[23,24]
Histoplasmosis	Reactivation of latent disease and de novo infections have been reported with TNF-alpha inhibitors in areas endemic for the fungus.	Retrospective case analysis[25]
Coccidioidomycosis	Fungus spread by spore inhalation. Endemic in regions across the Americas. Increased incidence of acute cases with TNFi.	Retrospective cohort study[26]
Aspergillosis	Invasive disease reported but rare.	Registry data[27]
Cryptococcus	Reported but rare.	Registry data[27]
Pneumocystis pneumonia	Increased risk. Rare but high mortality.	Observational data[28]

There is an association with reactivation of hepatitis B in those with chronic or previously resolved infection.[34] A specific at-risk population are those patients with latent hepatitis B virus, who have prior exposure to the virus, but no circulating antigenaemia. Screening must therefore look for both current hepatitis B infection but also prior exposure by testing hepatitis B core antibody status (see **Figure 39.3**). Patients with prior hepatitis B exposure should be offered viral prophylaxis to prevent this adverse event.

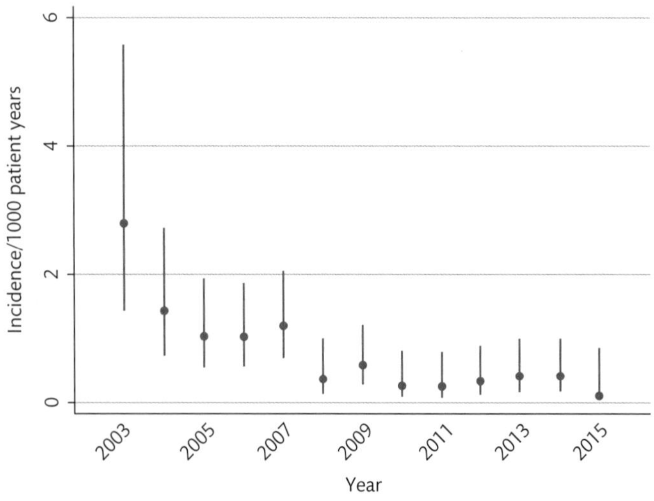

Pneumocystis pneumonia has been reported with rituximab therapy. In the UK registry of biologic therapies, rates of pneumocystis were low in absolute terms, but the greatest excess risk was observed for rituximab.[35]

Key message: Hypogammaglobulinaemia can developed with long-term use. Be vigilant for pneumocystis pneumonia

CTLA4-Immunoglobulin (abatacept)

Abatacept is a fusion protein that binds to CD80 and CD86 on antigen presenting cells. In doing so it inhibits T cells activation. There is an association with infection in pooled trial data, but a head-to-head study suggests there may be a lower risk than that with TNFi.[36,37]

Key message: Considered to have the safest adverse event profile for a biologic with respect to infection

Janus kinase (JAK) inhibitors (tofacitinib and baricitinib)

The introduction of tofacitinib and baricitinib offers a non-injectable therapeutic option for patients with RA who have failed established therapies. Postmarketing data are much less mature for the JAK inhibitor class and so the evidence base for estimating infection risk is smaller. Considering the mechanism of JAK inhibitors, which are canonical interferon signally pathways, as well as the signalling pathway for a number of cytokines, infection risk is an important theoretical concern. The impact on interferon pathways would be anticipated to lower the threshold for viral infections. The existing data for JAK inhibition is reassuring with respect to overall

Figure 39.2 The declining incidence of tuberculosis in RA patients commencing biologic therapy in the United Kingdom.

Source: data from Rutherford AI, Patarata E, Subesinghe S, et al. Opportunistic infections in rheumatoid arthritis patients exposed to biologic therapy: results from the British Society for Rheumatology Biologics Register for Rheumatoid Arthritis. *Rheumatology*. 2018;57(6):997–1001.

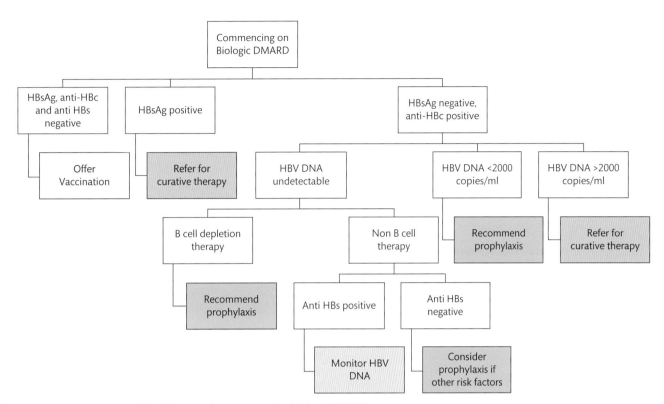

Figure 39.3 Hepatitis B status flow diagram when commencing biologic DMARD.
Source: data from Hepatitis B (chronic): diagnosis and management: NICE; 2017. Available from: https://www.nice.org.uk/guidance/cg165.

infection rates, with trial data suggesting the risks are comparable to TNFi.[38,39] In contrast, reactivation of Zoster is increased to almost 4%, compared to a background rate of just below 1% in the general RA population.[40]

Key message: Increased risk of shingles reactivation

Malignancy

Given the role of the immune system in cancer surveillance, it is a long-held concern that immunosuppressive therapies may predispose to malignancy. RA itself is associated with an increased risk of lymphoma, which makes the task of identifying therapies that increase the risk of cancer all the more challenging. There are few data supporting a link between GCs or the four commonly used csDMARDs and solid organ malignancy. The impact of csDMARD use on skin cancer risk remains uncertain, particularly as basal cell carcinomas are poorly reported in many studies. Also, of note is the occurrence of lymphoproliferative disease in patients on MTX therapy, which regresses on drug withdrawal, and may well be driven by Epstein–Barr virus.[41]

bDMARDs

TNF-alpha inhibiting therapies

When TNFi first launched, perhaps given the name, there was substantial concern regarding cancer risk. Trials due to their small sample size and short follow up were thought unable to provide reassurance. The registers were born out of a desire to specifically look for cancers (the power calculation for the BSRBR was to detect a

doubling in lymphoma risk).[42] The hard work across registers has paid off, as there is now a strong evidence base that shows no link with cancers. Cancer association has been studied in numerous manners:

1. Incident cancers are no more common in TNFi users versus RA patients on csDMARD alone[43–45];
2. In patients who develop cancer, mortality is no different in patients who were on TNFi at the time of diagnosis[46];
3. In patients who commence TNFi after a previous cancer, recurrence rates are no different[47,48];
4. Specific cancer subtypes (including lymphoma) are no different.[49,50]

The question may not be entirely concluded for melanoma, which is a very rare tumour, but for which there is a more specific plausible biologic link.[51]

Other bDMARDs

There is much less information concerning malignancy risk and the other bDMARDs, so it is not possible to draw as strong conclusions as we can with TNFi therapy. The available data suggest we can be reassured that they are broadly in line with what has been seen with TNFi (see **Table 39.2**).

Cardiovascular manifestations

Accelerated atheromatous disease with cardiovascular morbidity and mortality in patients with RA is well documented. There is also a rare association between RA and pericarditis and myocarditis, particularly with active disease. Cardiovascular adverse reactions are

Table 39.2 Malignancy risk for bDMARDs

Therapy	Malignancy risk	Evidence
Tocilizumab	No long-term increased risk seen	Long-term extension of RCT[52]
Rituximab	No long-term increased risk seen	Pooled trial data[32]
Abatacept	No long-term increased risk seen	Pooled trial data[53]
JAK inhibitors	No long-term increased risk seen	Long-term extension of RCT[54]

rarely seen with RA therapies, so the benefit of well controlled RA almost certainly outweighs the additional risk of the adverse events. An exception to this may be GCs.

Glucocorticoids

The dose-dependent adverse cardiovascular effects of GC are well documented but in short, prolonged use predisposes to:

- Hypertension likely related to nitric oxide suppression as well as sodium and fluid retention[55];
- Accelerated atherosclerosis;
- Arrhythmias, most commonly atrial fibrillation or flutter;
- Hyperlipidaemia.

Mineralocorticoid activation may promote myocardial fibrotic re-modelling, predisposing to heart failure.[56] There appears to be a dose-dependent effect, where those on higher doses are at an increased risk of cardiovascular events.[57]

csDMARDs

Cardiovascular complications are rare. Table 39.3 summarizes each of the commonly used csDMARDs and their cardiovascular risk.

bDMARDs

Cardiovascular adverse reactions are very rare, with little evidence supporting significant risk with rituximab, abatacept, or JAK inhibitors.

TNF-alpha inhibitors

TNF levels are elevated in cardiac failure, leading to trials of TNFi as a therapy.[59,60] One of these trials was concluded prematurely because of toxicity concerns, and a subsequent meta-analysis[61] suggested a possible detrimental effect of TNFi in people with moderate-to-severe heart failure. No data have linked TNFi use to incident heart failure.[62] Given this uncertainty, it is recommended that an alternative treatment option is taken in patients with moderate or severe heart failure. If significant heart failure (New York Heart Association (NYHA) Class III or IV) develops while a patient is on TNFi, discontinuation is recommended.

Table 39.3 Commonly used csDMARDs and cardiovascular risk

Drug	Risk
Methotrexate	Appears to reduce risk of cardiovascular events in RA[58]
Sulfasalazine	No known cardiovascular adverse reactions
Leflunomide	Hypertension in subset of patients, particularly if combined with NSAIDs
Hydroxychloroquine	No known cardiovascular adverse reactions

Tocilizumab

Tocilizumab use is associated with an elevation of the low-density lipoprotein to high density lipoprotein ratio, although this has not been followed up with elevated incidence of cardiac events.[63] Lipid derangement rarely prompts a therapy switch, but requires monitoring and intervention with cholesterol lowering agents as appropriate. To date, the rise in lipids has not correlated with an excess cardiovascular risk, although long-term data continue to accumulate to fully answer this question.

Cutaneous reactions

Rashes are commonly reported adverse reactions with RA therapies. They are generally mild and resolve upon therapy discontinuation, but are often distressing for patients, and can progress into more significant reactions.

Glucocorticoids

Thinning of the skin and an associated increased propensity to bruising is common, with increasing risk with higher dosages.

csDMARDs

Methotrexate

MTX therapy is associated with the following cutaneous adverse reactions:

- **Stomatitis**. This can be managed with up-titration of a patient's folic acid dose. In the event of severe ulcers, a temporary reduction in the MTX dose as well as increasing folic acid can be effective. A deterioration in renal function can be a trigger for new onset or worsening stomatitis.
- **Macular punctate rash.** This typically occurs on the knees and elbows, with sparing of the trunk. The rash will usually resolve with MTX dose reduction. If the rash persists after the dose is reduced, MTX should be stopped.
- **Alopecia.** Hair thinning is relatively common and can be very distressing. It does not tend to be extensive and can be mitigated by an increase in folic acid dosage. It usually reverses upon discontinuation.

Sulfasalazine

A pruritic maculopapular rash is reported in around 5% of patients taking SSZ.[64] DRESS syndrome is a rare (1:1000—1:10 000), idiosyncratic reaction that can occur after SSZ exposure. It typically develops 1–8 weeks following initiation of treatment. It is characterized by a cutaneous eruption, haematological abnormalities (eosinophilia and lymphocytosis) and systemic symptoms (including fever, lymphadenopathy, hepatitis, pneumonitis, and carditis). The cutaneous manifestations are variable, but usually begin with widespread erythematous and maculopapular lesions which may evolve into blisters or purpura. Although rare, DRESS caries a mortality of up to 10%.

Leflunomide

A pruritic rash and mild alopecia are common adverse reactions with LEF treatment. They are rarely severe enough to warrant a change in therapy.

Hydroxychloroquine

A pruritic maculopapular rash is common with HCQ therapy. It tends to be allergic in nature, so discontinuation of therapy is appropriate. Long-standing HCQ therapy is associated with cutaneous pigmentation abnormalities, typically with hyperpigmentation of the shins, hyper- or hypopigmentation of oral mucosa, and a lightening of hair colour.

bDMARDs

TNF-alpha inhibiting therapy

A number of cutaneous adverse reactions are associated with TNFi. They are a significant cause of drug discontinuation. Table 39.4 provides a summary.

Tocilizumab

Cutaneous reactions are rare with tocilizumab therapy. Hypersensitivity reactions with a resultant pruritic erythematous rash can occur.

Rituximab

Aside from a pruritic rash associated with a postinfusion reaction (discussed in more detail in this chapter), there is little evidence of cutaneous adverse reactions with rituximab therapy.

Abatacept

A psoriasiform rash is associated with abatacept therapy, with a similar incidence to that of TNFi. Erythema nodosum has also been reported.

JAK inhibition

The evidence to date suggests the JAK inhibitors have no associated adverse skin reactions.

Table 39.4 Summary of cutaneous adverse reactions associated with TNFi

Reaction	Details
Psoriatic skin lesions	Often pustular psoriasis on palms or soles of feet. Most cases respond well to withdrawal of TNFi treatment
Eczematous lesions	Does not usually require discontinuation of therapy
Cutaneous features of systemic lupus erythematosus (SLE)	TNFi-induced SLE is discussed in more detail later
Lichen Planus	Rare, usually requires discontinuation of therapy[65]
Alopecia	Rare, complete, or partial reversal is typical on discontinuation of therapy[66]

Pulmonary manifestations

RA is associated with a range of pulmonary manifestations including pleural effusion, interstitial pneumonitis, pulmonary nodules, and organizing pneumonia. There are some similarities between the RA-related pulmonary manifestations and drug reactions that have historically led to the belief that some of our drugs (particularly MTX) has a causal role to play in the development of lung fibrosis. The risk of pulmonary events associated with any therapy option must be balanced against the risk of active uncontrolled RA.

csDMARDs

There are case reports suggesting an association between both SSZ and LEF to pneumonitis. The authors assert that the data are not convincing for a link with chronic pulmonary toxicity. There is also no evidence to suggest HCQ has an association.[67]

Methotrexate

An association between low dose MTX therapy and pulmonary fibrosis has long been debated. A review of the studies supporting this association reveals a degree of channelling bias whereby patients in historic studies tended to be prescribed MTX if they had active and severe RA while those in comparator groups had less severe disease. This is supported by pooled data from RCTs with subjects who have non-RA diagnoses, which did not show any increased risk of adverse respiratory events with MTX therapy.[68] A meta-analysis of RCTs assessing MTX use in RA reported a small but significant increase in the risk of lung disease, which was driven by increased pneumonitis in the MTX-treated patients.[69] By contrast observational data have shown a beneficial effect of MTX therapy in RA-related interstitial lung disease, with improved survival.[70] Given the available evidence, it is recommended that MTX for RA is used with caution in those with established interstitial lung disease.

bMDARDs

There is insufficient evidence to confirm a link between any of the bDMARDs and pulmonary toxicity. There is a paradox whereby TNFi therapy has been utilized for RA-related pulmonary disease, while there also being reports of granulomatous disease and pulmonary fibrosis in RCTs. Registry data however suggest that TNFi does not increase mortality in patients with RA-related interstitial lung disease.[71]

Neurological and psychiatric reactions

Low mood often coincides with chronic disease, particularly one such as RA that significantly impacts on a patient's functional status. It is important to consider where therapy choices may exacerbate pre-existing mental health problems.

Glucocorticoids

Many patients receiving GC therapy report neurological or psychiatric adverse reactions. They usually present in a dose-dependent manner, so dosage and duration should be carefully considered in patients with symptoms or additional risk factors. Described reactions include:

- **Mood changes.** Elation or hypomania upon commencement of therapy. Depressed mood is more commonly reported with prolonged treatment.

- **Psychosis.** This is rarely seen with high doses.
- **Memory loss.** Commonly reported, particularly in older patients.
- **Suicidal Ideation.** Small increase in absolute risk of suicide with GC therapy, particularly in younger patients.[72]

csDMARDs

Neurological and psychiatric side effects associated with csDMARDs are common but tend to be mild and resolve with a reduction in dose or after stopping therapy. **Table 39.5** summarizes this.

bDMARDs

Headache and dizziness are commonly reported with all of the bDMARDs. These symptoms are typically mild and do not require therapy discontinuation.

TNF-alpha inhibitors

Adverse events reporting data suggest a rare association between TNFi and demyelination, presenting with a range of neurological symptoms including confusion, ataxia, and nerve palsies.[74] The pattern of demyelination typically seen with anti-TNF therapy is monophasic in nature. It is not recommended that patients with established demyelinating disease are commenced on TNFi. This is in part driven by the trial of the anti-TNF agent lenercept for multiple sclerosis (MS), which was halted early after those randomized to anti-TNF experienced a worsening of their MS symptoms.[75]

Hepatic

Many RA therapies have an impact on hepatic function. Often asymptomatic at first, unrecognized impairment can lead to irreversible liver damage as well as impeding or enhancing the metabolism of concomitant medications.

Glucocorticoids

GC therapy does not have any direct adverse impact on hepatocytes, but prolonged use can lead to hyperlipidaemia as described previously in this chapter. This predisposes to fatty liver disease.

csDMARDs

MTX, LEF, and SSZ can all induce a dose-dependent hepatic impairment, ranging from a mild transient transaminase elevation, to (very rarely) severe impairment and irreversible cirrhosis. Regular blood tests, particularly at the onset of therapy, usually allow any impairment to be detected and addressed before significant damage has occurred. For patients with pre-existing hepatic impairment, SSZ is often favoured over LEF and MTX.

Table 39.5 Neurological and psychiatric effects associated with csDMARDs

Drug	Reaction(s)
Methotrexate	Headache, low energy, reduced concentration. Usually improved with up-titration of folic acid
Sulphasalazine	Headache
Leflunomide	Reports of peripheral neuropathy. Resolution tends to be slow but is more likely with prompt discontinuation[73]
Hydroxychloroquine	Headache, tinnitus, insomnia, dizziness

bDMARDs

There is a small risk of hepatic enzyme elevation with TNFi. Pretreatment liver function blood tests are recommended to identify individuals with pre-existing liver disease. Tocilizumab is associated with elevated alanine aminotransferase, which settles upon discontinuation.[76]

Gastrointestinal

Gastrointestinal adverse drug reactions are common and have a significant impact on patients' quality of life. They are a common cause of therapy discontinuation.

Glucocorticoids

Gastric ulcers and gastrointestinal bleeding are associated with GC therapy, particularly when combined with non-steroidal anti-inflammatory drugs (NSAIDs). It is recommended that a proton pump inhibitor is prescribed in prolonged GC use.

csDMARDs

All of the four major csDMARDs can lead to gastrointestinal upset with nausea, abdominal pain, and altered bowel habit. This is more common with LEF therapy, which can cause a profound diarrhoea and substantial weight loss, particularly when a loading dose of 100 mg was routine practice. Up-titration of folic acid with MTX therapy can help alleviate symptoms.

bDMARDs

TNFi, abatacept, and rituximab all have a rare association with mild gastrointestinal upset. As previously discussed, tocilizumab has been associated with gastrointestinal perforation in patients with diverticular disease. An alternative therapy choice is therefore recommended in those with active diverticular disease. Preliminary data suggest that JAK inhibition may also be associated with perforation in those with diverticular disease, although more investigation is required before this can be confirmed.[77]

Administration reactions and hypersensitivity

Many RA therapies have reported hypersensitivity and administration reactions, particularly upon commencement of therapy. It is important clinicians and patients are aware of these reactions prior to starting treatment, in order to enable preventative measures to be taken, and to reduce the risk of therapy discontinuation should a reaction occur.

csDMARDs

Methotrexate

Subcutaneous (SC) administration is usually well tolerated. Erythematous scaly plaques at injection sites have been rarely reported.[78] Anaphylactic reactions have been described, but this is typically with intrathecal therapy for malignancy, rather than with the low oral or SC doses utilized in RA.

Sulfasalazine

DRESS syndrome is a severe hypersensitivity reaction rarely associated with SSZ. Patients present with high fever, a maculopapular or erythrodermic rash, and multiorgan failure secondary to eosinophil infiltration. Typically presenting around 4 weeks after exposure, SSZ discontinuation usually leads to resolution of symptoms. DRESS syndrome carries a mortality rate of around 10%. Despite its rarity, it is recommended that DRESS is discussed during patient pretherapy counselling.

Leflunomide

DRESS syndrome, angioedema, and Stevens Johnson syndrome have all been reported in patients taking LEF therapy. More data are required before it can be concluded there is a significant association between LEF and these severe hypersensitivity reactions.

Hydroxychloroquine

Stevens Johnson syndrome has been reported in patients taking HCQ, but similar to LEF more data are required to investigate if this is significantly associated with HCQ therapy.

bDMARDs

TNF-alpha inhibiting therapy

Mild skin reactions at injection sites are commonly reported with the four SC administered TNFi therapies (etanercept, golimumab, certolizumabpegol, and adalimumab). These typically occur upon commencement of treatment and rarely require intervention. Injection site rotation and topical steroids can be utilized if required. Intravenous (IV) infliximab use is linked to infusion reactions and can be anaphylactic in nature. Pre-administration of an antihistamine and a test dose of infliximab reduces the risk of a severe reaction. A delayed reaction with rash, arthralgia, myalgia, pyrexia, and fatigue can also occur up to 2 weeks postinfusion.

Tocilizumab

Injection site reactions similar to those seen with TNFi are relatively common. Anaphylactic and anaphylactoid reactions have been reported with IV administration but are very rare.

Rituximab

An infusion reaction occurring within 2 hours of exposure is commonly reported in up to 45% of patients upon primary therapy.[79] This is likely due to rituximab binding of CD20 on lymphocytes, leading to B cell cytokine release. The patient will typically report fever, headache, rash, shortness of breath, and facial swelling. Rarely this progress to anaphylactic reaction, but in most patients the symptoms are mild with resolution on discontinuation of the rituximab infusion.

The risk of an infusion reaction can be reduced by slow uptitration of the infusion rate, and premedicating with antihistamines and GCs.

Abatacept

Injection site reactions with SC administration occur in under 5% of patients. Infusion reactions with IV administration have been reported, with anaphylactic reactions at its most severe.

JAK inhibition

There is insufficient evidence to data to confirm any associated hypersensitivity reaction with JAK inhibiting therapy.

Haematological reactions

Various haematological abnormalities occur in RA, including normocytic anaemia, neutropenia, and thrombocytopenia or thrombocytosis.

Table 39.6 Haematological adverse effects associated with csDMARDs

Therapy	Reaction
Methotrexate	Pancytopenia, particularly with renal impairment
Sulfasalazine	Leukopenia, usually mild, but severe agranulocytosis can occur. Haemolytic anaemia, more common in those with glucose-6-phosphate dehydrogenase deficiency
Leflunomide	Very rarely causes leukopenia on its own, but likely increases myelosuppressive effects of MTX when coprescribed
Hydroxychloroquine	No haematological adverse reactions recorded

Glucocorticoids

Neutrophilia is commonly seen with GC therapy, due to reduced endothelial adherence of neutrophils. The resulting leucocytosis can be mistaken as an indicator of bacterial infection.

csDMARDS

csDMARDs commonly lead to haematological abnormalities. Regular blood monitoring is recommended for MTX, SSZ, and LEF. The nature of these adverse reactions is detailed in **Table 39.6**.

bDMARDs

Haematological adverse reactions are not as common with bDMARDs, so recommended monitoring is not as stringent as with csDMARDs. See **Table 39.7** for therapy specific haematological reactions. Thromboembolic events with JAK inhibitors have been a considerable source of controversy. The Federal drug agency (FDA) have only approved the 2 mg dose of baricitinib, due to concerns regarding the risk of thromboembolism and no increase in efficacy in trial data with the 4 mg dose.[80] The EMA has licensed the 4 mg dose. We await results from pharmacovigilance studies and drug registries to further characterize the risk of thromboembolism with JAK inhibitors.

Ophthalmic

Ocular involvement in RA is rare but can result in a significant impact on quality of life. Episcleritis and scleritis are uncommon but

Table 39.7 Haematological adverse effects associated with bDMARDs

Therapy	Reaction
TNF-alpha inhibiting therapy	Mild neutropenia is common. Pancytopenia and aplastic anaemia rarely seen
Tocilizumab	Transient neutropenia is common
Rituximab	Late-onset (months after administration) neutropenia is common. Repeated dosing associated with hypogammaglobulinaemia[32]
Abatacept	No associated haematologic adverse reactions
JAK inhibitors	Mild anaemia, neutropenia, and thrombocytopenia. Increased frequency of venous thromboembolic events

can have significant ophthalmic sequelae. Sicca symptoms are more common, occurring in up to 20% of patients with RA, but can usually be managed successfully with regular artificial tear eye drops.

Glucocorticoids

Oral GC therapy is associated the following ocular adverse reactions:

- Early cataract formation, particularly with doses of more than 10 mg a day;
- Glaucoma, particularly in those with a family history, diabetes, or myopia;
- Exophthalmos;
- Central serous chorioretinopathy. Oedematous separation of the retina from the choroid.

csDMARDs

MTX therapy has been rarely reported to lead to periorbital oedema and blurred vision. HCQ associated retinopathy is well described. Melles and Marmor performed a retrospective case-control study that included over 2000 patients who had been on HCQ for more than five years. They found an overall prevalence of retinopathy of 7.5%, with higher doses, duration of use, and concurrent renal impairment associating with an increased risk of retinopathy.[81] US and UK guidelines recommend that patients have formal retinal screening with ocular coherence tomography when HCQ is commenced, and on an annual basis after 5 years of therapy[82,83] (see Figures 39.4 and 39.5).

bDMARDs

Despite being rarely reported, registry data suggest etanercept may be associated with an increased risk of uveitis.[84] The authors recommend an alternative TNFi is used in patients with a history of uveitis

Bone

RA increases the risk of osteoporosis, predisposing to fragility fractures. It is recommended that patients with RA are assessed for risk factors of osteoporosis and the need for treatment on an annual basis. The impact of therapies on bone turnover is important to consider when making treatment choices in a group already at an increased risk.

Glucocorticoids

The negative impact of prolonged GC therapy on bone turnover leading to osteoporosis is well established. Patients on long-term GCs should undergo regular done mineral density measurement and subsequent treatment for osteoporosis if appropriate. In addition, prolonged high-dose GC treatment has been associated with osteonecrosis.

csDMARDs

MTX when prescribed at high doses for leukaemia has been associated with increased bone resorption. This doesn't appear to be the case with doses used in the treatment of RA. SSZ, LEF, and HCQ are not associated with osteoporosis.

bDMARDs

There is no known association between any of the RA biological therapy options and osteoporosis.

Metabolic and endocrine

Glucocorticoids

Glucose intolerance is common with oral GC therapy, with difficulty in maintaining blood sugar control in those with pre-existing diabetes mellitus. Progression to a novel diagnosis of diabetes is rare in patients who do not have preceding glucose intolerance. Long-term GC therapy suppresses endogenous production of cortisol via the hypothalamic-pituitary-adrenal axis. Sudden cessation of GCs can therefore lead to adrenal insufficiency and a potentially severe Addisonian crisis.

csDMARDs and bDMARDs

Hypothyroidism is a rare adverse reaction of tocilizumab, which has been utilized as a steroid sparing agent in autoimmune thyroid eye disease.[85] Evidence associating TNFi, abatacept, rituximab, JAK

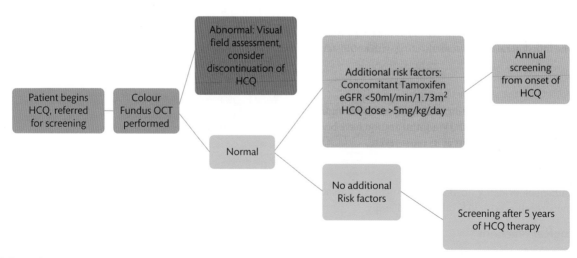

Figure 39.4 Baseline assessment algorithm for HCQ induced retinopathy. OCT = optical coherence tomography.

Source: data from RCOphth. Hydroxychloroquine and Chloroquine Retinopathy: Recommendations on Screening 2018. Available from: https://www.rcophth.ac.uk/standards-publications-research/clinical-guidelines/.

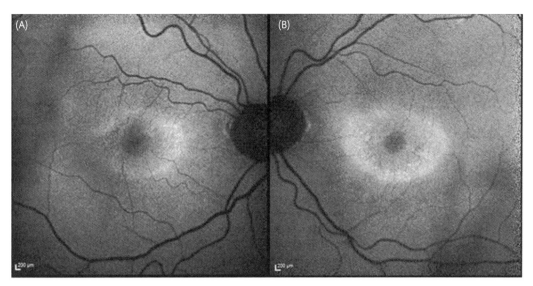

Figure 39.5 Bilateral increased parafoveal autofluorescence signal, seen with HCQ-retinopathy.
Reproduced from Latasiewicz M. et al (2017) Hydroxychloroquine retinopathy: an emerging problem *Eye* 31:972–6 with permission from Springer Nature.

inhibitors, MTX, SSZ, LEF, and HCQ with endocrine or metabolic adverse reactions are rare and inconsistent.

Autoimmune

Development of symptoms consistent with distinct autoimmune disorders is not uncommon in RA, owing to the overlap between these conditions. Rarely, these new symptoms may be attributable to the therapy a patient is receiving.

Glucocorticoids and csDMARDs

GC, MTX, and LEF therapy in RA have no associated autoimmune adverse reactions.

There are case reports suggesting a link between SSZ therapy and granulomatosis with polyangiitis in a small number of cases.[86] More evidence is necessary before this potential association can be confirmed or refuted.

bDMARDs

TNF-alpha inhibiting therapy

Autoantibody development, most commonly antinuclear antibodies (ANA), with TNFi therapy is well described.[87] This can rarely lead to the manifestation of distinct autoimmune diagnoses including:

* Vasculitis. Typically with cutaneous features, and rarely systemic[88];
* Systemic lupus erythematosus. Usually ANA positive, cutaneous features again predominate;
* Uveitis with etanercept (see ophthalmic section). Consider alternative TNFi in patients with a history of uveitis;
* Demyelinating disease (see neurology section). Avoid TNFi in patients with new symptoms of, or established demyelinating disease;
* Psoriasis (see cutaneous section). Does not usually require discontinuation of therapy.[89]

Of the remaining bDMARDs, there are reports describing the development of vasculitis with abatacept therapy.[90]

Conclusion

This chapter provides an overview of drug related adverse events that a rheumatologist should be familiar with. It is by no means exhaustive but highlights the most common and most important issues. The reality is that prescribing medicine for any disease is always a balance between risk and benefit. Unless there is a robust appreciation of risk, such judgements will never be fully informed.

Key messages

* Serious and opportunistic infections are more common with bDMARD therapy.
* There is a potential link between rituximab therapy and PML.
* Solid organ cancer risk is no higher in patients treated with TNFi.
* GCs are associated with significant cardiovascular comorbidity.
* Pustular psoriasis can lead to discontinuation of TNFi.
* MTX, LEF, and SSZ are all associated with hepatic impairment, rarely leading to cirrhosis.
* Tocilizumab is associated with gastrointestinal perforation in those with active diverticular disease.
* SSZ rarely leads to a severe hypersensitivity reaction, DRESS syndrome.
* HCQ, particularly in higher doses and renal impairment, is associated with retinopathy.

REFERENCES

1. European Medicines Agency. *Clinical Safety Data Management: Definitions and Standards for Expedited Reporting*, 1995. Available at: https://www.ema.europa.eu/en/ich-e2a-clinical-safety-data-management-definitions-standards-expedited-reporting

2. Edwards IR, Aronson JK. Adverse drug reactions: definitions, diagnosis, and management. *Lancet* 2000;*356*(9237):1255–9.

3. Caster O, Edwards IR. Reflections on attribution and decisions in pharmacovigilance. *Drug Safety* 2010;*33*(10):805–9.

4. Hill AB. The environment and disease: association or causation? *Proc R Soc Med* 1965;*58*(5):295–300.

5. Suvarna V. Phase IV of drug development. *Perspect Clin Res* 2010;*1*(2):57–60.

6. Dixon WG, Suissa S, Hudson M. The association between systemic glucocorticoid therapy and the risk of infection in patients with rheumatoid arthritis: systematic review and meta-analyses. *Arthritis Res Ther* 2011;*13*(4):R139–R.

7. van der Veen MJ, van der Heide A, Kruize AA, Bijlsma JW. Infection rate and use of antibiotics in patients with rheumatoid arthritis treated with methotrexate. *Ann Rheum Dis* 1994;*53*(4):224–8.

8. Bernatsky S, Hudson M, Suissa S. Anti-rheumatic drug use and risk of serious infections in rheumatoid arthritis. *Rheumatology (Oxf)* 2007;*46*(7):1157–60.

9. Lacaille D, Guh DP, Abrahamowicz M, Anis AH, Esdaile JM. Use of nonbiologic disease-modifying antirheumatic drugs and risk of infection in patients with rheumatoid arthritis. *Arthritis Rheum* 2008;*59*(8):1074–81.

10. O'Reilly S, Hartley P, Jeffers M, Casey E, Clancy L. Invasive pulmonary aspergillosis associated with low dose methotrexate therapy for rheumatoid arthritis: a case report of treatment with itraconazole. *Tuber Lung Dis* 1994;*75*(2):153–5.

11. Wahl C, Liptay S, Adler G, Schmid RM. Sulfasalazine: a potent and specific inhibitor of nuclear factor kappa B. *J Clin Invest* 1998;*101*(5):1163–74.

12. Zhang X, Brunner T, Carter L, et al. Unequal death in T helper cell (Th)1 and Th2 effectors: Th1, but not Th2, effectors undergo rapid Fas/FasL-mediated apoptosis. *J Exp Med* 1997;*185*(10):1837–49.

13. Rozman B. Clinical pharmacokinetics of leflunomide. *Clin Pharmacokinet* 2002;*41*(6):421–30.

14. Kyburz D, Brentano F, Gay S. Mode of action of hydroxychloroquine in RA-evidence of an inhibitory effect on toll-like receptor signaling. *Nat Clin Pract Rheumatol* 2006;*2*(9):458–9.

15. Roach DR, Bean AG, Demangel C, France MP, Briscoe H, Britton WJ. TNF regulates chemokine induction essential for cell recruitment, granuloma formation, and clearance of mycobacterial infection. *J Immunol* 2002;*168*(9):4620–7.

16. Singh JA, Wells GA, Christensen R, et al. Adverse effects of biologics: a network meta-analysis and Cochrane overview. *Cochrane Database Syst Rev* 2011(2):CD008794.

17. Singh JA, Cameron C, Noorbaloochi S, et al. Risk of serious infection in biological treatment of patients with rheumatoid arthritis: a systematic review and meta-analysis. *Lancet* 2015;*386*(9990):258–65.

18. Tubach F, Salmon D, Ravaud P, et al. Risk of tuberculosis is higher with anti-tumor necrosis factor monoclonal antibody therapy than with soluble tumor necrosis factor receptor therapy: the three-year prospective French Research Axed on Tolerance of Biotherapies registry. *Arthritis Rheum* 2009;*60*(7):1884–94.

19. Galloway JB, Hyrich KL, Mercer LK, et al. Risk of septic arthritis in patients with rheumatoid arthritis and the effect of anti-TNF therapy: results from the British Society for Rheumatology Biologics Register. *Ann Rheum Dis* 2011;*70*(10):1810–4.

20. Slifman NR, Gershon SK, Lee JH, Edwards ET, Braun MM. Listeria monocytogenes infection as a complication of treatment with tumor necrosis factor alpha-neutralizing agents. *Arthritis Rheum* 2003;*48*(2):319–24.

21. Vassilopoulos D, Calabrese LH. Management of rheumatic disease with comorbid HBV or HCV infection. *Nat Rev Rheumatol* 2012;*8*(6):348–57.

22. Singh JA, Furst DE, Bharat A, et al. 2012 update of the 2008 American College of Rheumatology recommendations for the use of disease-modifying antirheumatic drugs and biologic agents in the treatment of rheumatoid arthritis. *Arthritis Care Res* 2012;*64*(5):625–39.

23. Galloway JB, Mercer LK, Moseley A, et al. Risk of skin and soft tissue infections (including shingles) in patients exposed to anti-tumour necrosis factor therapy: results from the British Society for Rheumatology Biologics Register. *Ann Rheum Dis* 2013;*72*(2):229–34.

24. Winthrop KL, Baddley JW, Chen L, et al. Association between the initiation of anti-tumor necrosis factor therapy and the risk of herpes zoster. *JAMA* 2013;*309*(9):887–95.

25. Vergidis P, Avery RK, Wheat LJ, et al. Histoplasmosis complicating tumor necrosis factor-alpha blocker therapy: a retrospective analysis of 98 cases. *Clin Infect Dis* 2015;*61*(3):409–17.

26. Bergstrom L, Yocum DE, Ampel NM, et al. Increased risk of coccidioidomycosis in patients treated with tumor necrosis factor alpha antagonists. *Arthritis Rheum* 2004;*50*(6):1959–66.

27. Salmon-Ceron D, Tubach F, Lortholary O, et al. Drug-specific risk of non-tuberculosis opportunistic infections in patients receiving anti-TNF therapy reported to the 3-year prospective French RATIO registry. *Ann Rheum Dis* 2011;*70*(4):616–23.

28. Baddley JW, Winthrop KL, Chen L, et al. Non-viral opportunistic infections in new users of tumour necrosis factor inhibitor therapy: results of the SAfety Assessment of Biologic ThERapy (SABER) study. *Ann Rheum Dis* 2014;*73*(11):1942–8.

29. Keane J, Gershon S, Wise RP, et al. Tuberculosis associated with infliximab, a tumor necrosis factor alpha-neutralizing agent. *N Engl J Med* 2001;*345*(15):1098–104.

30. Smolen JS, Beaulieu A, Rubbert-Roth A, et al. Effect of interleukin-6 receptor inhibition with tocilizumab in patients with rheumatoid arthritis (OPTION study): a double-blind, placebo-controlled, randomised trial. *Lancet* 2008;*371*(9617):987–97.

31. Strangfeld A, Richter A, Siegmund B, et al. Risk for lower intestinal perforations in patients with rheumatoid arthritis treated with tocilizumab in comparison to treatment with other biologic or conventional synthetic DMARDs. *Ann Rheum Dis* 2017;*76*(3):504–10.

32. van Vollenhoven RF, Emery P, Bingham CO, 3rd, et al. Long-term safety of patients receiving rituximab in rheumatoid arthritis clinical trials. *J Rheumatol* 2010;*37*(3):558–67.

33. Clifford DB, Ances B, Costello C, et al. Rituximab-associated progressive multifocal leukoencephalopathy in rheumatoid arthritis. *Arch Neurol* 2011;*68*(9):1156–64.

34. Mitka M. FDA: increased HBV reactivation risk with ofatumumab or rituximab. *JAMA* 2013;*310*(16):1664.

35. Rutherford AI, Patarata E, Subesinghe S, Hyrich KL, Galloway JB. Opportunistic infections in rheumatoid arthritis patients exposed to biologic therapy: results from the British Society for Rheumatology Biologics Register for Rheumatoid Arthritis. *Rheumatology* 2018;*57*(6):997–1001.

36. Maxwell LJ, Singh JA. Abatacept for rheumatoid arthritis: a Cochrane systematic review. *J Rheumatol* 2010;*37*(2):234–45.

37. Schiff M, Weinblatt ME, Valente R, et al. Head-to-head comparison of subcutaneous abatacept versus adalimumab for

rheumatoid arthritis: two-year efficacy and safety findings from AMPLE trial. *Ann Rheum Dis* 2014;73(1):86–94.

38. Strand V, Ahadieh S, French J, et al. Systematic review and meta-analysis of serious infections with tofacitinib and biologic disease-modifying antirheumatic drug treatment in rheumatoid arthritis clinical trials. *Arthritis Res Ther* 2015;17:362.

39. Smolen J, Genovese M, Takeuchi T, et al. THU0166 Safety profile of baricitinib in patients with active RA: an integrated analysis. *Ann Rheum Dis* 2016;75:243–4.

40. Winthrop KL, Curtis JR, Lindsey S, et al. Herpes zoster and tofacitinib: clinical outcomes and the risk of concomitant therapy. *Arthritis Rheumatol (Hoboken)* 2017;69(10):1960–8.

41. Rizzi R, Curci P, Delia M, et al. Spontaneous remission of 'methotrexate-associated lymphoproliferative disorders' after discontinuation of immunosuppressive treatment for autoimmune disease. Review of the literature. *Med Oncol* 2009;26(1):1–9.

42. Watson K, Symmons D, Griffiths I, Silman A. The British Society for Rheumatology biologics register. *Ann Rheum Dis* 2005;64(Suppl 4):iv42–3.

43. Mercer LK, Lunt M, Low AL, et al. Risk of solid cancer in patients exposed to anti-tumour necrosis factor therapy: results from the British Society for Rheumatology Biologics Register for Rheumatoid Arthritis. *Ann Rheum Dis* 2015;74(6):1087–93.

44. Wadstrom H, Frisell T, Askling J. Malignant neoplasms in patients with rheumatoid arthritis treated with tumor necrosis factor inhibitors, tocilizumab, abatacept, or rituximab in clinical practice: a nationwide cohort study from Sweden. *JAMA Intern Med* 2017;177(11):1605–12.

45. Leombruno JP, Einarson TR, Keystone EC. The safety of anti-tumour necrosis factor treatments in rheumatoid arthritis: meta and exposure-adjusted pooled analyses of serious adverse events. *Ann Rheum Dis* 2009;68(7):1136–45.

46. Lunt M, Watson KD, Dixon WG, Symmons DP, Hyrich KL. No evidence of association between anti-tumor necrosis factor treatment and mortality in patients with rheumatoid arthritis: results from the British Society for Rheumatology Biologics Register. *Arthritis Rheum* 2010;62(11):3145–53.

47. Silva-Fernandez L, Lunt M, Kearsley-Fleet L, et al. The incidence of cancer in patients with rheumatoid arthritis and a prior malignancy who receive TNF inhibitors or rituximab: results from the British Society for Rheumatology Biologics Register-Rheumatoid Arthritis. *Rheumatology (Oxf)* 2016;55(11):2033–9.

48. Raaschou P, Soderling J, Turesson C, Askling J. Tumor necrosis factor inhibitors and cancer recurrence in Swedish patients with rheumatoid arthritis: a nationwide population-based cohort study. *Ann Int Med* 2018;169(5):291–9.

49. Askling J, Fored CM, Baecklund E, et al. Haematopoietic malignancies in rheumatoid arthritis: lymphoma risk and characteristics after exposure to tumour necrosis factor antagonists. *Ann Rheum Dis* 2005;64(10):1414–20.

50. Mercer LK, Davies R, Galloway JB, et al. Risk of cancer in patients receiving non-biologic disease-modifying therapy for rheumatoid arthritis compared with the UK general population. *Rheumatology (Oxf)* 2013;52(1):91–8.

51. Raaschou P, Simard JF, Holmqvist M, Askling J. Rheumatoid arthritis, anti-tumour necrosis factor therapy, and risk of malignant melanoma: nationwide population based prospective cohort study from Sweden. *BMJ* 2013;346:f1939.

52. Rubbert-Roth A, Sebba A, Brockwell L, et al. Malignancy rates in patients with rheumatoid arthritis treated with tocilizumab. *RMD Open* 2016;2(1):e000213.

53. Simon TA, Smitten AL, Franklin J, et al. Malignancies in the rheumatoid arthritis abatacept clinical development programme: an epidemiological assessment. *Annals Rheumatic Dis* 2009;68(12):1819–26.

54. Cohen SB, Tanaka Y, Mariette X, et al. Long-term safety of tofacitinib for the treatment of rheumatoid arthritis up to 8.5 years: integrated analysis of data from the global clinical trials. *Ann Rheum Dis* 2017;76(7):1253–62.

55. Kelly JJ, Mangos G, Williamson PM, Whitworth JA. Cortisol and hypertension. *Clin Exp Pharmacol Physiol Suppl* 1998;25:S51–6.

56. Weber KT. Aldosterone in congestive heart failure. *N Engl J Med* 2001;345(23):1689–97.

57. Wei L, MacDonald TM, Walker BR. Taking glucocorticoids by prescription is associated with subsequent cardiovascular disease. *Ann Int Med* 2004;141(10):764–70.

58. De Vecchis R, Baldi C, Palmisani L. Protective effects of methotrexate against ischemic cardiovascular disorders in patients treated for rheumatoid arthritis or psoriasis: novel therapeutic insights coming from a meta-analysis of the literature data. *Anatol J Cardiol* 2016;16(1):2–9.

59. Mann DL, McMurray JJ, Packer M, et al. Targeted anticytokine therapy in patients with chronic heart failure: results of the Randomized Etanercept Worldwide Evaluation (RENEWAL). *Circulation* 2004;109(13):1594–602.

60. Chung ES, Packer M, Lo KH, Fasanmade AA, Willerson JT. Randomized, double-blind, placebo-controlled, pilot trial of infliximab, a chimeric monoclonal antibody to tumor necrosis factor-alpha, in patients with moderate-to-severe heart failure: results of the anti-TNF Therapy Against Congestive Heart Failure (ATTACH) trial. *Circulation* 2003;107(25):3133–40.

61. Gartlehner G, Hansen RA, Jonas BL, Thieda P, Lohr KN. The comparative efficacy and safety of biologics for the treatment of rheumatoid arthritis: a systematic review and meta-analysis. *J Rheumatol* 2006;33(12):2398–408.

62. Joachim L, Anja S, Jörn K, et al. Does tumor necrosis factor α inhibition promote or prevent heart failure in patients with rheumatoid arthritis? *Arthritis Rheum* 2008;58(3):667–77.

63. Kim SC, Solomon DH, Rogers JR, et al. Cardiovascular safety of tocilizumab versus tumor necrosis factor inhibitors in patients with rheumatoid arthritis: a multi-database cohort study. *Arthritis Rheumatol* 2017;69(6):1154–64.

64. Box SA, Pullar T. Sulphasalazine in the treatment of rheumatoid arthritis. *Br J Rheumatol* 1997;36(3):382–6.

65. Asarch A, Gottlieb AB, Lee J, et al. Lichen planus-like eruptions: an emerging side effect of tumor necrosis factor-alpha antagonists. *J Am Acad Dermatol* 2009;61(1):104–11.

66. Bene J, Moulis G, Auffret M, et al. Alopecia induced by tumour necrosis factor-alpha antagonists: description of 52 cases and disproportionality analysis in a nationwide pharmacovigilance database. *Rheumatology (Oxf)* 2014;53(8):1465–9.

67. Roubille C, Haraoui B. Interstitial lung diseases induced or exacerbated by DMARDS and biologic agents in rheumatoid arthritis: a systematic literature review. *Semin Arthritis Rheum* 2014;43(5):613–26.

68. Conway R, Low C, Coughlan RJ, O'Donnell MJ, Carey JJ. Methotrexate use and risk of lung disease in psoriasis, psoriatic arthritis, and inflammatory bowel disease: systematic literature review and meta-analysis of randomised controlled trials. *BMJ* 2015;350:h1269.

69. Conway R, Low C, Coughlan RJ, O'Donnell MJ, Carey JJ. Methotrexate and lung disease in rheumatoid arthritis: a

meta-analysis of randomized controlled trials. *Arthritis Rheumatol (Hoboken)* 2014;*66*(4):803–12.

70. Rojas-Serrano J, Herrera-Bringas D, Pérez-Román DI, Pérez-Dorame R, Mateos-Toledo H, Mejía M. Rheumatoid arthritis-related interstitial lung disease (RA-ILD): methotrexate and the severity of lung disease are associated to prognosis. *Clin Rheumatol* 2017;*36*(7):1493–500.

71. Dixon WG, Hyrich KL, Watson KD, Lunt M, Symmons DP. Influence of anti-TNF therapy on mortality in patients with rheumatoid arthritis-associated interstitial lung disease: results from the British Society for Rheumatology Biologics Register. *Ann Rheum Dis* 2010;*69*(6):1086–91.

72. Fardet L, Petersen I, Nazareth I. Suicidal behavior and severe neuropsychiatric disorders following glucocorticoid therapy in primary care. *Am J Psychiatry* 2012;*169*(5):491–7.

73. Weimer LH, Sachdev N. Update on medication-induced peripheral neuropathy. *Curr Neurol Neurosci Rep* 2008;*9*(1):69.

74. Mohan N, Edwards ET, Cupps TR, et al. Demyelination occurring during anti-tumor necrosis factor alpha therapy for inflammatory arthritides. *Arthritis Rheum* 2001;*44*(12):2862–9.

75. [No authors]. TNF neutralization in MS: results of a randomized, placebo-controlled multicenter study. The Lenercept Multiple Sclerosis Study Group and The University of British Columbia MS/MRI Analysis Group. *Neurology* 1999;*53*(3):457–65.

76. Maini RN, Taylor PC, Szechiński J, et al. Double-blind randomized controlled clinical trial of the interleukin-6 receptor antagonist, tocilizumab, in European patients with rheumatoid arthritis who had an incomplete response to methotrexate. *Arthritis Rheum* 2006;*54*(9):2817–29.

77. Xie F, Yun H, Bernatsky S, Curtis JR. Brief report: risk of gastrointestinal perforation among rheumatoid arthritis patients receiving tofacitinib, tocilizumab, or other biologic treatments. *Arthritis Rheumatol (Hoboken)* 2016;*68*(11):2612–17.

78. Yadlapati S, Efthimiou P. Inadequate response or intolerability to oral methotrexate: is it optimal to switch to subcutaneous methotrexate prior to considering therapy with biologics? *Rheumatol Int* 2016;*36*(5):627–33.

79. Edwards JCW, Szczepański L, Szechiński J, et al. Efficacy of B-cell–targeted therapy with rituximab in patients with rheumatoid arthritis. *N Engl J Med* 2004;*350*(25):2572–81.

80. Nair RN, Nikolov NP, Seymour S, Thanh Hai MT. *Summary of Resubmission and NDA 207924 DPARP/OND Recommendations Baricitinib, a JAK inhibitor for RA: FDA*, 2018. Available at: https://www.accessdata.fda.gov/drugsatfda_docs/nda/2018/207924Orig1s000SumR.pdf

81. Melles RB, Marmor MF. The risk of toxic retinopathy in patients on long-term hydroxychloroquine therapy. *JAMA Ophthalmol* 2014;*132*(12):1453–60.

82. Ledingham J, Gullick N, Irving K, et al. BSR and BHPR guideline for the prescription and monitoring of non-biologic disease-modifying anti-rheumatic drugs. *Rheumatology* 2017;*56*(6):865–8.

83. RCOphth. *Hydroxychloroquine and Chloroquine Retinopathy: Recommendations on Screening*, 2018. Available at: https://www.rcophth.ac.uk/standards-publications-research/clinical-guidelines/

84. Lim LL, Fraunfelder FW, Rosenbaum JT. Do tumor necrosis factor inhibitors cause uveitis? A registry-based study. *Arthritis Rheum* 2007;*56*(10):3248–52.

85. Russell DJ, Wagner LH, Seiff SR. Tocilizumab as a steroid sparing agent for the treatment of Graves' orbitopathy. *Am J Ophthalmol Case Rep* 2017;*7*:146–8.

86. Denissen NH, Peters JG, Masereeuw R, Barrera P. Can sulfasalazine therapy induce or exacerbate Wegener's granulomatosis? *Scand J Rheumatol* 2008;*37*(1):72–4.

87. Atzeni F, Talotta R, Salaffi F, et al. Immunogenicity and autoimmunity during anti-TNF therapy. *Autoimmun Rev* 2013;*12*(7):703–8.

88. Ramos-Casals M, Roberto Perez A, Diaz-Lagares C, Cuadrado MJ, Khamashta MA. Autoimmune diseases induced by biological agents: a double-edged sword? *Autoimmun Rev* 2010;*9*(3):188–93.

89. Collamer AN, Battafarano DF. Psoriatic skin lesions induced by tumor necrosis factor antagonist therapy: clinical features and possible immunopathogenesis. *Semin Arthritis Rheum* 2010;*40*(3):233–40.

90. Carvajal Alegria G, Uguen A, Genestet S, Marcorelles P, Saraux A, Cornec D. New onset of rheumatoid vasculitis during abatacept therapy and subsequent improvement after rituximab. *Joint Bone Spine* 2016;*83*(5):605–6.

SECTION 8
Management and outcomes

40 **Prevention of rheumatoid arthritis** 487
Tom W.J. Huizinga, Annette van der Helm-van Mil,
and Andrew Cope

41 **Treatment targets and remission** 495
Kenneth F. Baker and Arthur G. Pratt

42 **Clinical outcomes** 507
David L. Scott

43 **Clinical recommendations** 519
Anna-Birgitte Aga, Espen A. Haavardsholm, Till Uhlig,
and Tore K. Kvien

44 **European biologics registers** 535
Angela Zink and Anja Strangfeld

45 **Voluntary patient registries** 545
Jeff Greenberg and Sheetal Patel

40

Prevention of rheumatoid arthritis

Tom W.J. Huizinga, Annette van der Helm-van Mil, and Andrew Cope

Introduction

Early initiation of effective disease-modifying antirheumatic drugs (DMARDs) and treat to target therapy adjustments are the keystones of current treatment in rheumatoid arthritis (RA).[1,2] Underlying the relevance of early treatment initiation is the concept of the window of opportunity, which presumes that there is a confined period in which the disease is most susceptible to the disease-modifying effects of treatment.[3,4] Although the precise timelines are not established, it is assumed that the autoimmune process is susceptible to targeting before arthritis becomes clinically evident. At present, treatment of established RA is effective in suppressing inflammation, but its ability to modify the persistent course of the disease is limited.[5] Retrospective nested case-control studies have revealed that RA-related autoantibodies and markers of systemic or local subclinical inflammation can be present years or months before the diagnosis,[6-12] demonstrating that the disease process is evolving long before the disease becomes clinically detectable. Such observations have encouraged a call for 'preventive trials'—treatment initiation in the pre-arthritic phase of the disease process with the ultimate aim of preventing the onset of RA (**Figure 40.1**). This challenge raises questions such as 'how can we accurately identify individuals in the pre-arthritis phases?', 'how can we avoid overtreatment?' and 'how should we currently manage patients that are presumed to be at risk for RA?'. This chapter reviews the current state of knowledge on the identification of patients at risk for RA in different pre-arthritis phases as well as their management.

Management in the pre-arthritis phase: What is the evidence?

Data from clinical trials reporting the impact of treatment initiated in pre-arthritic phase of RA are limited. The first placebo-controlled trial in the pre-arthritis phase in humans was published in 2009 and showed that two intramuscular injections of dexamethasone in seropositive patients with arthralgia decreased the levels of serum autoantibodies, but did not prevent the development of arthritis.[13] More recently, results from the PRAIRI trial demonstrated that a single infusion of rituximab in seropositive patients with arthralgia, together

with signs of systemic and/or local inflammation, delayed but did not prevent the development of clinical arthritis.[14]

The Personalized Risk Estimator of Rheumatoid Arthritis (PRE-RA) Family Study is a prospective, open label, randomized clinical trial targeting first-degree relatives (FDR) of RA patients who do not have RA themselves. While not a clinical trial of an investigational medicinal product (CT-IMP), the goal is to better understand the willingness of at-risk individuals to change lifestyle behaviours, focusing on four behavioural factors linked to RA risk: cigarette smoking, excess body weight, poor oral health, and low fish intake. Such a feasibility study is immensely important for providing a framework for future studies of this type. Consenting individuals are randomized to one of three interventions delivered by online tool:

1. Comparison arm: subjects will receive standard education about RA;
2. PRE-RA Arm: subjects will receive RA education and the PRE-RA tool, adapted from Your Disease Risk, which provides risk estimates for a range of diseases including cancer, heart disease, and type 2 diabetes, to include an absolute lifetime risk estimate;
3. PRE-RA Plus Arm: subjects will receive the same as those randomized to the PRE-RA Arm plus intensive health education, including input from a trained health counsellor. These subjects will also be given advice on how to change and sustain these behaviours. This information will be available to take home.

The primary outcome of the PRE-RA Family Study, measured using a variant of a visual analogue scale—a contemplation ladder, will evaluate the willingness to change any of these four behaviours from baseline to 6 weeks, 6 months, and 12 months. The study started in January 2014. Primary completion was in September 2016 and the study is scheduled to complete in June 2018. According to the publicly available data (clinicaltrials.gov), 238 subjects have been enrolled. This intriguing study, whose design was published in 2014,[15] will provide important insights into the challenges associated with making lifestyle changes for subjects informed about their risk of developing RA. The design will also provide important clues as to the optimal approach for changing and sustaining behaviours over time, although whether the same approaches applied to FDR will have similar impact in the general population will require further study. Regardless of these nuances, one anticipates that a very

To be used in patients with arthralgiaw without clinical arthritis and without other explanation for the arthralgia

AUC 0.93
≥3 items: sens 90%
spec 74%

History taking:
Joint symptoms of recent-onset (duration <1 year)
Symptoms located in MCP-joints
Duration of morning stiffness ≥60 min
Most severe symptoms present in the early morning
Presence of a first-degree relative with RA

Physical examination:
Difficulty with making a fist
Positive squeeze test of MCP-joints

Figure 40.1 The items of the EULAR definition for clinical suspect arthralgia.

large longitudinal clinical trial would follow, requiring an extensive period of follow-up.

For as long as there are no positive results from any of these proof-of-concept studies, there remains no evidence to support the use of DMARDs in patients without clinical arthritis, a notion in line with published recommendations.[1,2] However, as patients may experience pain and functional limitations, pain reduction with non-steroidal anti-inflammatory drugs or other pain killers seems logical, together with close monitoring for the development of clinical arthritis.

The relevance of adequate risk stratification

Risk stratification is an essential requirement to the advancement of research in the prevention of RA. First, adequate risk stratification is crucial when designing and interpreting the results of preventive studies, because the risk of individual persons of developing the disease outcome determines the power of the study. The greater the percentage of persons without a high risk of developing RA in the next 1 or 2 years that are enrolled in prevention studies, the lower the power to detect a significantly protective effect. These persons can be considered as 'non-informative' inclusions. This becomes especially important in the face of the relatively low sample sizes of most preventive trials reported to date.[13,15] This phenomenon was illustrated following application of risk stratification in a post-hoc analysis of the PROMPT trial.[16,17] In this trial, patients with undifferentiated arthritis (UA) were randomized to treatment with methotrexate or placebo in order to prevent RA (primary outcome) or to achieve drug-free remission (secondary outcome). Analysis of the whole group showed that methotrexate neither prevented the development of RA nor induced a state of drug-free remission. Initial post-hoc analysis suggested however that methotrexate had an effect in anticitrullinated protein antibody (ACPA)-positive patients but not in ACPA-negative patients. Although the ACPA-positive patients were at higher risk of RA than ACPA-negative patients, risk stratification based solely on ACPA was rather simplistic.[16] Previous studies on the natural course of UA have shown that only one-third of the UA patients will progress to RA, whereas others will evolve into different diagnoses or their inflammatory arthritis may spontaneously resolve.[18,19] A prediction model of the individual risk of a UA-patient to progress to RA, including data on clinical factors, and

acute phase reactants in addition to autoantibodies, has been derived and validated.[20,21] Repeating the analyses of the PROMPT trial considering only those patients with a high predicted risk of developing RA (>80% in the next year), revealed that methotrexate prevented RA development (number needed to treat of 2) and resulted in more frequent drug-free remission after 5 years of follow-up (0% in the placebo treated group and up to 40% in the group randomized to receive methotrexate).[17] Further stratification for ACPA was also done, showing a preventive effect in ACPA-positive patients with a high predicted risk on RA as well as in ACPA-negative patients with a high predicted risk, whereas no effect was observed in the ACPA-positive or ACPA-negative patients without a high risk on RA (i.e. both these groups contained predominantly 'non-informative inclusions'). In other words, the previous conclusion that methotrexate might only work in ACPA-positive UA was due to the fact that this group included a higher proportion of high-risk patients than ACPA-negative UA in general. Altogether, these data revealed that an important preventive effect was observed only when patients with a high risk on RA were studied (**Figure 40.2**).

Adequate risk stratification also facilitates shared decision-making, as this requires that patients are adequately informed about their risk of RA. Some recent qualitative studies have revealed that persons at risk for RA have difficulties evaluating the risk of developing RA when this risk is expressed as a percentage, and that these patients prefer to receive a yes/no answer on whether or not they will progress to RA.[22–24] This implies that risk prediction tools with high positive and negative predictive values are the most appropriate to facilitate shared decision-making regarding treatment initiation during the symptomatic pre-arthritis phase of the disease.

Finally, successfully translating research results to clinical practice also depends on risk stratification. If the ongoing proof-of-concept studies are positive and provide evidence supporting the treatment of arthralgia in order to prevent clinically apparent persisting arthritis, the next question will be 'whom to treat?'. Insufficient risk stratification at the time that positive proof-of-concept trial results emerge may result in overtreatment of patients that are considered to be only at modest risk of RA. This is highly undesirable, both from the perspective of individual patients and from the socio-economic point of view. Thus, adequate risk stratification is crucial.

What constitutes high risk for a person at risk?

Persons prefer a yes/no answer on the question of whether they will develop RA.[22–24] But, what levels of risk of RA would justify initiation of treatment in the perspective of those at risk, and which factors influence their decision? A recent Swiss study evaluated this question in 32 asymptomatic FDR of RA patients.[25] Hypothetical scenarios consisting of attributes with different levels (risk reduction, risk of mild and serious adverse events and mode of administration) were presented and persons were asked whether they would accept preventive treatment. Overall, the willingness to take preventive medication increased in parallel with the risk of developing RA; 38% of the relatives studied would be willing to take medication if the risk of RA was 40%. Interestingly, several factors were **not** associated with willingness to take preventive medication, including a delay in the

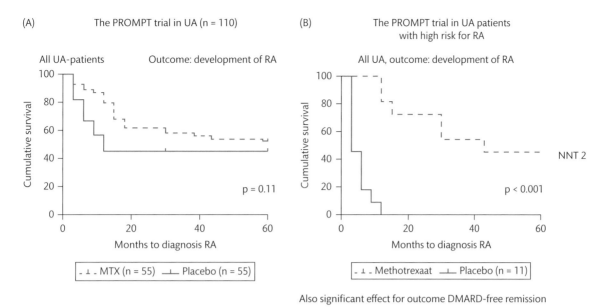

Figure 40.2 (A) the PROMPT study in all patients with UA, and (B) the PROMPT study in only the high-risk patients.
Reprinted from Burgers LE et al (2017) 'Brief Report: Clinical Trials Aiming to Prevent Rheumatoid Arthritis Cannot Detect Prevention Without Adequate Risk Stratification: A Trial of Methotrexate Versus Placebo in Undifferentiated Arthritis as an Example'. *Arthritis Rheumatol* 69(5):926–31 with permission from Wiley and Sons.

onset of RA (instead of its prevention), risk of mild adverse events, and the mode of administration of the medication (oral, injection, infusion).[25] These data clearly illustrate the importance of patient perceptions of the willingness to take preventive medication and the contributing factors that should be taken into account to successfully design preventive trials and implement their results in practice. Patient willingness is of utmost importance as studies in the field of oncology and cardiovascular diseases have shown that adherence to preventive medications is rather poor.[26,27]

Prevention can be initiated at different phases of the disease

The EULAR study group for risk factors for RA has defined several phases of RA development and the definition of these phases is based on our current understanding of the etiopathogenesis of RA. The phases are: genetic and environmental risk factors for RA, autoimmunity associated with RA, symptoms without clinical arthritis and then clinical arthritis (this can be either unclassified arthritis or rheumatoid arthritis).[28] Not all patients will pass every stage and some stages can be present at the same time (e.g. smoking, autoimmunity, and arthritis).

Primary prevention seeks to avoid a disease from developing in the first place. For individuals targeted for primary prevention strategies features of the disease are absent. Good examples include vaccination to protect against foreign pathogens, or smoking cessation. Secondary prevention applies methods to detect and address an existing disease before the onset of symptoms and signs, and before the disease has fully manifest. Treatment of hypertension and hyperlipidaemia are good examples. Tertiary prevention aims to restore the patients with established disease to full health—physical, mental, and social—reducing the harm of active, symptomatic disease, through treatment, lifestyle changes and, where appropriate, a

programme of rehabilitation. This strategy is central to our approach to managing patients with established RA. Rheumatologists also practice quaternary prevention. Here, strategies are actively applied to mitigate against the effects of unnecessary or excessive therapeutic intervention.

With these definitions in mind, what are the options for RA prevention? Primary prevention would necessitate intervention (lifestyle modifications, drug therapy or otherwise) during the asymptomatic phase prior to the detection of RA-associated blood signatures, such as the presence of disease specific autoantibodies. Here, risk would be attributable to genetic, demographic, and lifestyle factors, as well as family history.[29–31] Defining an optimal duration for intervention, which might address lifestyle behaviours, can be challenging, and the risks of therapeutic intervention must be weighed against the relatively modest risk of developing disease over an extended period of time. Secondary prevention strategies seek to target the higher risk individual who has joint symptoms in combination with autoantibodies associated with RA; higher risk is associated with rheumatoid factor and ACPA positivity, in addition to subclinical evidence of synovitis or osteitis, as defined by high resolution imaging. While tertiary prevention is not relevant to the current discussion, concepts of quaternary prevention that address issues around risk and benefit of intervention become highly relevant. Thus, based on our current knowledge and understanding of RA risk, a realistic goal for treating individuals during the preclinical phase of RA most closely aligns with concepts of secondary prevention. With this in mind, the remaining discussion focuses on emerging therapies that aim to prevent (or delay) the onset of established disease in symptomatic individuals deemed to be at high risk.[32–35]

Data suggest that clinical arthritis or evident RA is present in a surprisingly small proportion of the patients referred to secondary care.[36] Furthermore, of all patients with arthralgia without clinical arthritis, rheumatologists consider only a small proportion as being at risk for RA, based on the clinical presentation: clinically suspect arthralgia (CSA). Thus, a Dutch observational study showed that this comprised only 7% of all patients that presented to rheumatologic care without clinical arthritis and with arthralgia that was not otherwise explained.[37] Also in secondary care, pattern recognition, and clinical expertise are important for differentiating arthralgia at risk of RA from other types of arthralgia. It has been reported that the clinical expertise had a high sensitivity (80%), thus few patients presenting with arthralgia who would subsequently progress to RA were missed by their rheumatologists.[36]

Although clinical expertise is regularly used in daily care, its subjectivity is an obvious drawback for research studies. A EULAR taskforce set-out to explicate this particular clinical expertise in defined items that are measurable and reached a definition of arthralgia that is suspicious for progression to RA.[38] This definition is to be used in secondary care in patients with arthralgia in whom the rheumatologist considers that RA is imminent, and more likely than other diagnoses. The clinical definition consists of 7 items; 5 obtained by history taking and 2 by physical examination (**Figure 40.1**). Healthcare systems around the world operate differently with respect to primary care and organ specialists in secondary care (such as internists, gynaecologists, orthopaedists, or surgeons).[39–41] This results in different populations of arthralgia patients. However, all these healthcare systems have rheumatologists who see patients suspected to have RA and therefore the EULAR definition of arthralgia suspicious for progression to RA is applicable in almost all healthcare systems in the world.[42] The aim of this definition is to harmonize the group of patients that rheumatologists consider at risk of RA. Indeed, data have revealed that this definition serves well to exclude some patients that (despite a rheumatologist's suspicion of imminent RA) turn out to be at low risk of RA.[43] The application of this definition in CSA-patients identified a subgroup of patients with a slightly higher risk of subsequent RA.

In conclusion, selecting arthralgia patients with a higher risk for RA, such as patients fulfilling the EULAR definition of arthralgia at risk for RA, seems to offer an optimal starting position to investigate the mechanisms underlying this phase of RA development and for designing preventive trial protocols.

The accuracy of risk prediction depends on the disease stage/the setting

Risk stratification is of utmost importance, as post-test chances highly depend on this risk. This general principle is exemplified for the presence of ACPA (IgG). Two nested case-control studies have estimated that the risk of ACPA-positive individuals in the general population to develop RA is ~5% for the next 5 years, with a lifetime risk of 16%.[6,7] The prevalence of ACPA in the general population is 1–2%,[44–46] and results from the first longitudinal study in this setting suggest that the presence of ACPA in symptom-free persons is associated with a risk of developing RA of 8% after a median of 3 years of follow-up.[44] This means that 92% of the subjects with a positive ACPA-test in the general population has a false-positive result as they will not develop RA in the forthcoming years. Based on the prevalence and positive predictive value (PPV) the number needed to test to identify one RA-patient can be estimated at ~1200. Several

important studies on ACPA-positive arthralgia have been performed in different settings (health fairs, primary care, secondary care, and/ or a combination of these).[47–49] The PPV of ACPA for RA development during the next year ranged, in these studies, between 20 and 34%.[47,48,50] As the number of persons that underwent ACPA testing was not reported, the number needed to test cannot be estimated. A longitudinal observational study in CSA, among patients that were selected by rheumatologists based on the clinical presentation, revealed a prevalence of ACPA of 16%.[11] In CSA, a positive ACPA-test was associated with a risk of 63% to develop clinical arthritis within 1 year, and thus the risk of false-positivity for arthritis development within 1 year was 37%. Based on these data, the number of CSA-patients to test for ACPA in order to have once case of ACPA-positive RA within one year is 10. Hence, the higher the *a priori* risk of RA, the higher is the predictive value of ACPA testing for subsequent RA (higher PPV, lower risk on false-positivity) and thus the lower the number of persons that need to be tested to identify one RA-patient. In the future, it is anticipated that more refined tests that incorporate other structural features of ACPA, such as the presence of specific glycans in the Fab or Fc-part of the ACPA-molecule, will lead to better test performance of ACPA testing.[51,52]

How accurately can we currently identify imminent RA?

The single presence of ACPA in arthralgia that is clinically at risk for RA is insufficient to achieve accurate risk stratification, because the PPV is at its most 63% (implying ≥37% false-positives), and up to half of the newly diagnosed RA patients are ACPA-negative and are missed by this approach (false-negatives). Furthermore, patients have indicated that they prefer a test for which there is a very high likelihood the test that can confirm or exclude imminent RA. Importantly, other biomarkers have been identified. Subclinical joint inflammation, either detected by magnetic resonance imaging (MRI) or by ultrasound, has been proven predictive.[9–11,53] Although further studies are required to evaluate head-to-head the predictive accuracy of subclinical inflammation detected by either imaging modalities, and also to evaluate the minimal region that needs to be imaged for maximal results, current data have already revealed that subclinical inflammation is a predictor that is independent of that of autoantibodies and clinical features.[10,11] Also C-reactive protein has been shown to independently predict RA development.[11] Cellular characteristics of B cells or T cells, and gene expression profiles of whole blood have also been studied; such markers are of interest as they may signify important etiopathogenetic mechanisms.[54–58]

Three studies combined different types of predictors. Unfortunately, they were undertaken in different patient populations (ACPA-positive non-specific musculoskeletal (MSK) symptoms in primary care, autoantibody-positive 'non-further-specified' arthralgia, and CSA in secondary care).[11,47,48] Although the results were promising, none of these models is yet validated in independent patient populations. So, although information on different types of biomarkers is available, current research results were obtained in a variety of patient populations, with significant differences in background risk for RA, which hampers validation.

Examples of current intervention studies

Enrolling in the United States since March 2016 is the Strategy to Prevent the Onset of Clinically Apparent Rheumatoid Arthritis (Stop-RA) study. This multicentre, randomized, double-blind, placebo-controlled clinical trial seeks to test whether hydroxychloroquine, taken at the 200–400 mg dose for 12 months, is both safe and effective for the prevention of RA in 200 subjects who are positive for ACPA (> 2 times the upper limit of normal, equivalent to ≥40 units in the anti-CCP3 assay), with or without arthralgia. This approach is based on the observation that up to 50% of such individuals will develop RA over a period of 3 years, regardless of the presence of other risk factors. The primary outcome is the development of RA at 36 months, as defined by the 2010 ACR/EULAR criteria (≥ 6 points), or by a joint examination consistent with inflammatory arthritis with ≥ 1 erosion confirmed by X-ray imaging of the hands, wrists, and feet. The study is actively recruiting, and the results are expected in the Spring of 2020.

Three RA prevention clinical trials are currently recruiting in Europe as of December 2017. The Arthritis Prevention in the Preclinical Phase of RA with Abatacept (APIPPRA) study recruited its first study subject in December 2014. This multicentre, randomized, double-blind clinical trial is comparing the effects of 12 months treatment with weekly subcutaneous injections of abatacept (125 mg) or placebo on preventing or delaying the onset of clinically apparent arthritis. The primary endpoint is the time to development of three or more swollen joints or fulfilment of the 2010 ACR/EULAR criteria for RA, confirmed by ultrasonography. The study is powered to detect a 50% reduction in arthritis development (from 40% to 20%) in the active treatment arm. Study subjects will receive treatment for 12 months and follow-up for a further 12 months. The APIPPRA study protocol includes a parallel ultrasound study for all participants, overseen by trained ultrasonographers who are blinded to clinical assessments. Extensive biological sampling every 3 months will permit analysis of immunological signatures associated with the at-risk state, progression to arthritis, and with response to intervention. The study is recruiting in the United Kingdom and Netherlands, with outcome data expected in Spring 2020.

A similarly designed RA prevention study is currently enrolling in the Netherlands—the TREAT EARLIER study, in which enrolled subjects who are ACPA positive or negative will be randomized to receive intramuscular steroids and methotrexate or placebo. A combination of clinical and MRI imaging are being used to identify high-risk subjects. The primary outcome will be the frequency of clinically detectable arthritis with a swollen joint count (SJC) of more than two joints, both persisting for at least 4 weeks, obtained after 2 years. Subjects will be treated for 1 year, and followed up for a further year.

Statins attenuate inflammation in individuals with atherosclerosis, as shown in observational studies and in a large randomized controlled trial in which cardiovascular protection was accompanied by a reduction in C-reactive protein levels.[59] Inspired by these observations a nested case-control study from the United Kingdom was performed in a large population-based cohort.[60] The study showed that high-intensity statin treatment was associated with a 23% reduction in the risk of incident RA in comparison to low-intensity statin treatment.[60] Subsequently. the Statins to Prevent RA (STAPRA) study was designed. This is a double-blind, placebo-controlled study that will evaluate whether atorvastatin 40 mg or placebo, taken for up to 3 years, can prevent or delay the development of clinically apparent arthritis. The trial seeks to recruit 220 study subjects, deemed to be at risk by virtue of carrying immunoglobulin M (IgM) rheumatoid factor and ACPA, or high titre ACPA (≥ 3 × upper limit of normal), in the absence of clinically apparent arthritis. The primary outcome is the development of clinical arthritis confirmed by a rheumatologist. It is anticipated that the study will be closed to recruitment by July 2020.

These novel interventional studies share a number of key features. Firstly, stratification has been prioritized with the 'at-risk' individual being defined by the presence of RA-specific autoantibodies in serum, with or without the presence of symptoms, or stratification by imaging. A successful trial outcome will depend on the number of primary outcome events in the placebo arm, permitting meaningful comparison with the active arm. This in turn will be determined by an accurate estimate of the progression to disease of the sample population, which in turn will determine sample size. Secondly, to date these prevention studies include placebo arms, which will have distinct advantages in terms of determining the impact of the targeted approach. Thirdly, rates of progression to disease across populations, is also reflected in the similar sample sizes across studies—being around 200.

Conclusion

The current state-of-the-art highlights several areas for prioritization, in terms of the future research agenda. These include the refinement of risk stratification—adopting algorithms that incorporate both clinical, laboratory, and imaging parameters. The choice and evaluation of molecular or cellular biomarkers that can be incorporated into such algorithms will necessarily be determined by a deeper understanding of the immunobiology that underpins the preclinical phase of RA. This requires dedicated effort and resources to study in depth large cohorts of subjects at risk of RA across the time spectrum. These studies will ultimately determine how best to stratify the at-risk state, and inform therapy decisions, be they lifestyle modifications or targeted therapy.

Acknowledgement

This chapter is based on two other publications:

Cope AP. Emerging therapies for pre-RA, In: *Best Prac Res Clin Rheumatol* 2017;31(1):99–111; and

van Steenbergen HW, da Silva JAP, Huizinga TWJ, van der Helm-van Mil AHM. Preventing progression from arthralgia to arthritis: targeting the right patients. *Nat Rev Rheumatol* 2018;14(1):32–41.

REFERENCES

1. Smolen JS, Landewé R, Breedveld FC, et al. EULAR recommendations for the management of rheumatoid arthritis with synthetic and biological disease-modifying antirheumatic drugs: 2013 update. *Ann Rheum Dis* 2014;73(3):492–509.

2. Combe B, Landewé R, Daien CI, et al. 2016 update of the EULAR recommendations for the management of early arthritis. *Ann Rheum Dis* 2017;76(6):948–59.

3. Boers M. Understanding the window of opportunity concept in early rheumatoid arthritis. *Arthritis Rheum* 2003;48(7):1771–4s.

4. van Nies JA, Tsonaka R, Gaujoux-Viala C, Fautrel B, van der Helm-van Mil AHM. Evaluating relationships between symptom duration and persistence of rheumatoid arthritis: does a window of opportunity exist? Results on the Leiden Early Arthritis Clinic and ESPOIR cohorts. *Ann Rheum Dis* 2015;74(5):806–12.

5. Ajeganova S, van Steenbergen HW, van Nies JAB, Burgers LE, Huizinga TWJ, van der Helm-van Mil AHM. Disease-modifying antirheumatic drug-free sustained remission in rheumatoid arthritis: an increasingly achievable outcome with subsidence of disease symptoms. *Ann Rheum Dis* 2016;75(5):867–73.

6. Nielen MM, van Schaardenburg D, Reesink HW, et al. Specific autoantibodies precede the symptoms of rheumatoid arthritis: a study of serial measurements in blood donors. *Arthritis Rheum* 2004;50(2):380–6.

7. Rantapää-Dahlqvist S, de Jong BA, Berglin E, et al. Antibodies against cyclic citrullinated peptide and IgA rheumatoid factor predict the development of rheumatoid arthritis. *Arthritis Rheum* 2003;48(10):2741–9.

8. Sokolove J, Bromberg R, Deane KD, et al. Autoantibody Epitope Spreading in the Pre-Clinical Phase Predicts Progression to Rheumatoid Arthritis. *PLoS One* 2012;7(5):e35296.

9. van de Stadt LA, Bos WH, Meursinge Reynders M, et al. The value of ultrasonography in predicting arthritis in auto-antibody positive arthralgia patients: a prospective cohort study. *Arthritis Res Ther* 2010;12(3):R98.

10. Nam JL, Hensor EMA, Hunt L, Conaghan PG, Wakefield RJ, Emery P. Ultrasound findings predict progression to inflammatory arthritis in anti-CCP antibody-positive patients without clinical synovitis. *Ann Rheum Dis* 2016;75(12):2060–7.

11. van Steenbergen HW, Mangnus L, Reijnierse M, Huizinga TWJ, van der Helm-van Mil AHM. Clinical factors, anticitrullinated peptide antibodies and MRI-detected subclinical inflammation in relation to progression from clinically suspect arthralgia to arthritis. *Ann Rheum Dis* 2016;75(10):1824–30.

12. van Steenbergen HW, Huizinga TW, van der Helm-van Mil AH. Review: the preclinical phase of rheumatoid arthritis: what is acknowledged and what needs to be assessed? *Arthritis Rheum* 2013;65(9):2219–32.

13. Bos WH, Dijkmans BA, Boers M, van de Stadt RJ, Schaardenburg D. Effect of dexamethasone on autoantibody levels and arthritis development in patients with arthralgia: a randomised trial. *Ann Rheum Dis* 2010;69(3):571–4.

14. Gerlag DM, Safy M, Maijer KL, et al. *A Single Infusion of Rituximab Delays the Onset of Arthritis in Subjects at High Risk of Developing RA* [abstract]. *Arthritis Rheumatol* 2016;68(Suppl 10). Available at: http://acrabstracts.org/abstract/a-single-infusion-of-rituximab-delays-the-onset-of-arthritis-in-subjects-at-high-risk-of-developing-ra/s

15. Sparks JA, Iversen MD, Miller Kroouze R, et al. Personalized risk estimator for rheumatoid arthritis (PRE-RA) family study: rationale and design for a randomized controlled trial evaluating rheumatoid arthritis risk education to first-degree relatives. *Contemp Clin Trials* 2014;39:145–57.

16. van Dongen H, van Aken J, Lard LR, et al. Efficacy of methotrexate treatment in patients with probable rheumatoid arthritis: a double-blind, randomized, placebo-controlled trial. *Arthritis Rheum* 2007;56(5):1424–32.

17. Burgers LE, Allaart CF, Huizinga TWJ, van der Helm-van Mil AHM. Brief report: clinical trials aiming to prevent rheumatoid arthritis cannot detect prevention without adequate risk stratification: a trial of methotrexate versus placebo in undifferentiated arthritis as an example. *Arthritis Rheumatol* 2017;69(5):926–31.

18. Harrison BJ, Symmons DP, Brennan P, Barrett EM, Silman AJ. Natural remission in inflammatory polyarthritis: issues of definition and prediction. *Rheumatology* 1996;35(11):1096–100.

19. van Aken J, van Dongen H, Cessie S le, Allaart CF, Breedveld FC, Huizinga TWJ. Comparison of long-term outcome of patients with rheumatoid arthritis presenting with undifferentiated arthritis or with rheumatoid arthritis: an observational cohort study. *Ann Rheum Dis* 2006;65(1):20–5.

20. van der Helm-van Mil AHM, le Cessie S, van Dongen H, Breedveld FC, Toes REM, Huizinga TWJ. A prediction rule for disease outcome in patients with Recent-onset undifferentiated arthritis: how to guide individual treatment decisions. *Arthritis Rheum* 2007;56(2):433–40.

21. van der Helm-van Mil AHM, Detert J, Cessie SL, et al. Validation of a prediction rule for disease outcome in patients with recent-onset undifferentiated arthritis: moving toward individualized treatment decision-making. *Arthritis Rheum* 2008;58(8):2241–7.

22. Newsum EC, van der Helm-van Mil AH, Kaptein AA. Views on clinically suspect arthralgia: a focus group study. *Clin Rheumatol* 2016;35(5):1347–52.

23. Stack RJ, Stoffer M, Englbrecht M, et al. Perceptions of risk and predictive testing held by the first-degree relatives of patients with rheumatoid arthritis in England, Austria and Germany: a qualitative study. *BMJ Open* 2016;6(6):e010555.

24. Falahee M, Simons G, Buckley CD, Hansson M, Stack RJ, Raza K. Patients' perceptions of their relatives' risk of developing rheumatoid arthritis and of the potential for risk communication, prediction and modulation. *Arthritis Care Res (Hoboken)* 2017;69(10):1558–65.

25. Finckh A, Escher M, Liang MH, Bansback N. Preventive treatments for rheumatoid arthritis: issues regarding patient preferences. *Curr Rheumatol Rep* 2016;18(8):51.

26. Smith SG, Sestak I, Forster A, et al. Factors affecting uptake and adherence to breast cancer chemoprevention: a systematic review and meta-analysis. *Ann Oncol* 2016;27(4):575–90.

27. Naderi SH, Bestwick JP, Wald DS. Adherence to drugs that prevent cardiovascular disease: meta-analysis on 376,162 patients. *Am J Med* 2012;125(9):882–7.e1.

28. Gerlag DM, Raza K, van Baarsen LG, et al. EULAR recommendations for terminology and research in individuals at risk of rheumatoid arthritis: report from the Study Group for Risk Factors for Rheumatoid Arthritis. *Ann Rheum Dis* 2012;71(5):638–41.

29. Bonita R, Beaglehole R, Kjellström T. *Basic Epidemiology*, 2nd edition. Geneva, Switzerland: World Health Organization, 2006, p. 212

30. Frisell T, Holmqvist M, Källberg H, Klareskog L, Alfredsson L, Askling J. Familial risks and heritability of rheumatoid arthritis: role of rheumatoid factor/anti-citrullinated protein antibody status, number and type of affected relatives, sex, and age. *Arthritis Rheum* 2013;65(11):2773–82.

31. Hemminki K, Li X, Sundquist J, Sundquist K. Familial associations of rheumatoid arthritis with autoimmune diseases and related conditions. *Arthritis Rheum* 2009;60(3):661–8.

32. Scott DL, Wolfe F, Huizinga TW. Rheumatoid arthritis. *Lancet* 2010;376(9746):1094–108.

33. van den Dungen C, Hoeymans N, Gijsen R, et al. What factors explain the differences in morbidity estimations among general practice registration networks in the Netherlands? A first analysis. *Eur J Gen Pract* 2008;14(s1):53–62.

34. National Audit Office. *Services for People with Rheumatoid Arthritis*, 2009. Available at: http://www.nao.org.uk/report/services-for-people-with-rheumatoid-arthritis/

35. Emery P, Breedveld FC, Dougados M, Kalden JR, Schiff MH, Smolen JS. Early referral recommendation for newly diagnosed rheumatoid arthritis: evidence-based development of a clinical guide. *Ann Rheum Dis* 2002;61(4):290–7.

36. van Steenbergen HW, van der Helm-van Mil AH. Clinical expertise and its accuracy in differentiating arthralgia patients at risk for rheumatoid arthritis from other patients presenting with joint symptoms. *Rheumatol Oxf Engl* 2016;55(6):1140–1.

37. Steenbergen HW van, Nies JAB van, Huizinga TWJ, Bloem JL, Reijnierse M, Mil AHM van der H. Characterising arthralgia in the preclinical phase of rheumatoid arthritis using MRI. *Ann Rheum Dis* 2015;74(6):1225–32.

38. van Steenbergen HW, Aletaha D, Voorde LJJB de, et al. EULAR definition of arthralgia suspicious for progression to rheumatoid arthritis. *Ann Rheum Dis* 2017;76(3):491–6.

39. Nifelen MM, Spronk I, Davids R. *Incidentie en Prevalentie van Gezondheidsproblemen in de Nederlandse Huisartsenpraktijk in 2014. Uit: NIVEL Zorgregistratie Eerste Lijn*, 2017. Available at: https://www.nivel.nl/nl/NZR/incidenties-en-prevalenties

40. Lamberts H, Wood M. *International Classification of Primary Care*. Oxford, UK: Oxford University Press, 1987.

41. de Rooy DP, van der Linden MP, Knevel R, Huizinga TWJ, van der Helm-van Mil AHM. Predicting arthritis outcomes—what can be learned from the Leiden early arthritis clinic? *Rheumatology* 2011;50(1):93–100.

42. Burgers LE, Siljehult F, ten Brinck RM, van Steenbergen HW. Performance of the EULAR definition of arthralgia suspicious for progression to rheumatoid arthritis [abstract]. *Ann Rheum Dis* 2016; annrheumdis-2016–209846. doi:10.1136/annrheumdis-2016–209846.

43. Newsum EC, de Waal MW, van Steenbergen HW. How do general practitioners identify inflammatory arthritis? A cohort analysis of Dutch general practitioner electronic medical records. *Rheumatology (Oxf)* 2016;55(5):848–53.

44. Hensvold AH, Frisell T, Magnusson PKE, Holmdahl R, Askling J, Catrina AI. How well do ACPA discriminate and predict RA in the general population: a study based on 12 590 population-representative Swedish twins. *Ann Rheum Dis* 2017;76(1):119–25.

45. van Zanten A, Arends S, Roozendaal C, et al. Presence of anticitrullinated protein antibodies in a large population-based cohort from the Netherlands. *Ann Rheum Dis* 2017;76(7):1184–90.

46. Haji Y, Rokutanda R, Kishimoto M, Okada M. *Anti-cyclic Citrullinated Protein Antibody (ACPA) Positivity in General Population and Follow-Up Results for ACPA Positive Persons* [abstract]. *Arthritis Rheumatol* 2016;68 (Suppl 10). Available at: http://acrabstracts.org/abstract/anti-cyclic-citrullinated-protein-antibody-acpa-positivity-in-general-population-and-follow-up-results-for-acpa-positive-persons/

47. van de Stadt LA, Witte BI, Bos WH, van Schaardenburg D. A prediction rule for the development of arthritis in seropositive arthralgia patients. *Ann Rheum Dis* 2013;72(12):1920–6.

48. Rakieh C, Nam JL, Hunt L, et al. Predicting the development of clinical arthritis in anti-CCP positive individuals with non-specific musculoskeletal symptoms: a prospective observational cohort study. *Ann Rheum Dis* 2015;74(9):1659–66.

49. de Hair MJ, Landewé RB, van de Sande MG, et al. Smoking and overweight determine the likelihood of developing rheumatoid arthritis. *Ann Rheum Dis* 2013;72(10):1654–8.

50. van de Stadt LA, de Koning MH, van de Stadt RJ, et al. Development of the anti-citrullinated protein antibody repertoire prior to the onset of rheumatoid arthritis. *Arthritis Rheum* 2011;63(11):3226–33.

51. Rombouts Y, Ewing E, van de Stadt LA, et al. Anti-citrullinated protein antibodies acquire a pro-inflammatory Fc glycosylation phenotype prior to the onset of rheumatoid arthritis. *Ann Rheum Dis* 2015;74(1):234–41.

52. Rombouts Y, Willemze A, van Beers JJBC, et al. Extensive glycosylation of ACPA-IgG variable domains modulates binding to citrullinated antigens in rheumatoid arthritis. *Ann Rheum Dis* 2016;75(3):578–85.

53. Kleyer A, Krieter M, Oliveira I, et al. High prevalence of tenosynovial inflammation before onset of rheumatoid arthritis and its link to progression to RA—a combined MRI/CT study. *Semin Arthritis Rheum* 2016;46(2):143–50.

54. Janssen KMJ, Westra J, Chalan P, et al. Regulatory CD4+ T-cell subsets and anti-citrullinated protein antibody repertoire: potential biomarkers for arthritis development in seropositive arthralgia patients? *PLoS One* 2016;11(9):e0162101.

55. van Beers-Tas MH, Marotta A, Boers M, Maksymowych WP, van Schaardenburg D. A prospective cohort study of 14-3-3η in ACPA and/or RF-positive patients with arthralgia. *Arthritis Res Ther* 2016;18(1):76.

56. Lübbers J, Beers-Tas MH van, Vosslamber S, et al. Changes in peripheral blood lymphocyte subsets during arthritis development in arthralgia patients. *Arthritis Res Ther* 2016;18(1):205.

57. Chalan P, Kroesen B-J, van der Geest KSM, Huitema MG, et al. Circulating CD4+CD161+ T lymphocytes are increased in seropositive arthralgia patients but decreased in patients with newly diagnosed rheumatoid arthritis. *PLoS One* 2013;8(11):e79370.

58. van Baarsen LG, Bos WH, Rustenburg F, et al. Gene expression profiling in autoantibody-positive patients with arthralgia predicts development of arthritis. *Arthritis Rheum* 2010;62(3):694–704.

59. Ridker PM, Danielson E, Fonseca FA, et al. Rosuvastatin to prevent vascular events in men and women with elevated C-reactive protein. *N Engl J Med* 2008;359:2195–207

60. Tascilar K, Dell'Aniello S, Hudson M, Suissa S. Statins and risk of rheumatoid arthritis: a nested case-control study. *Arthritis Rheumatol* 2016;68:2603–11.

41

Treatment targets and remission

Kenneth F. Baker and Arthur G. Pratt

Treating to target

Any modern consideration of the management of rheumatoid arthritis (RA) is underpinned by an appreciation that optimal outcomes for patients are achieved through timely and sustained suppression of immune-mediated inflammation. Faced with a relapsing and remitting systemic disease, clinicians recognize a spectrum of RA 'activity' that not only varies between patients but is dynamic within individuals. By attempting to quantify this disease activity, and so define 'targets' against which treatment intensity may be actively titrated over time, remarkable strides in the condition's prognosis have been achieved. To fully appreciate these concepts and the broadly accepted management strategies that have arisen from them, it is instructive to consider how they have evolved over the past 30 years.

Historical perspective

In the 1980s patients with newly diagnosed RA were typically treated with non-steroidal anti-inflammatory drugs (NSAIDS), rest, and splinting. Conventional synthetic disease-modifying antirheumatic drugs (csDMARDs) including sulfasalazine or methotrexate were reserved for those with established joint damage and disability, who had 'earned' their treatment and the perceived risk of toxicity. Although the Ritchie articular index (RAI) for measuring the extent and intensity of peripheral joint tenderness had been developed 20 years earlier,[1] attempts to incorporate a consideration of inflammatory burden when quantifying RA activity only culminated in the then widely adopted **disease activity score** (DAS) at the end of that decade.[2] Comprising a composite of RAI, a 44-swollen joint count, erythrocyte sedimentation rate (ESR) and patient-reported global assessment of disease activity (recorded on a visual analogue scale; patient VAS), scores could be translated to indicate high, moderate or low disease activity, and even the state of clinical remission—defined as the absence of clinical signs and symptoms of inflammatory disease activity.

A number of landmark studies that followed in the 1990s galvanized support for the notion that a 'window of opportunity' exists in early RA, during which prompt, csDMARD-induced DAS suppression is associated with reduced cumulative radiographic joint damage.[3–5] The emphasis of such studies was the empirical choice and combination of initiator csDMARD(s) for incipient disease control, rather than use of any predetermined DAS target to guide treatment decisions. By contrast, in the TIght COntrol for Rheumatoid Arthritis (TICORA) study of 2004, Grigor et al. drew upon the paradigm of tight glycaemic control as a means of preventing complications in type 1 diabetes mellitus,[6] applying it to RA.[7] They employed an intensive 'step-up' treatment approach, in which a DAS of >2.4 ('moderate' disease activity or greater) recorded at any monthly assessment prompted incremental escalation of csDMARD dose and combination; this approach led to significantly improved outcomes over an 18-month period compared with a less intensive comparator approach in which treatment decisions were not informed by DAS.[7] Since publication of this seminal paper numerous studies (reviewed in [8] and [9]) have reinforced the validity of the so-called **treat-to-target** (T2T) strategy in improving outcomes for newly diagnosed RA. Despite some variation in treatment targets used (discussed in the following sections), T2T has become embedded in clinical practice and is the subject of consensus management recommendations.[10]

Beyond the early arthritis clinic, the value of the T2T approach among patients with established but active RA is generally accepted, though with a more limited evidence base. In a cluster-randomized trial of 384 established RA patients receiving conventional synthetic disease-modifying antirheumatic drugs (DMARD),[11] treatment escalation according to regular DAS28 measurement resulted in twice as many achieving low disease activity (DAS28 ≤3.2) after 24 weeks compared to standard care alone. In contrast, a cluster-randomized trial of 308 established RA patients initiating adalimumab found no significant difference in the primary outcome (change in DAS28 after 12 months) in patients randomized to routine care *versus* T2T strategies based on either DAS28 or swollen joint count.[12] However, time to achieve good/moderate European League Against Rheumatism (EULAR) response was significantly shorter in the T2T groups *versus* routine care, indicating at least some benefit of T2T in this trial.

Questions regarding optimal first-line drug and dose selection, or the virtues of a 'step-down' combination drug approach within the overarching T2T framework, have been the subject of intervening investigations, during which time widespread use of biologic DMARDs (bDMARDs) has also become a reality. In particular, no overt advantage to the first-line use of anti-TNF over csDMARD has been convincingly demonstrated in respect of long-term radiographic damage, disability, or disease activity, assuming T2T adherence.[13]

Tapering oral, intra-articular, and/or intramuscular steroid use is currently an important adjunct to csDMARD initiation in this setting, but the added value of combination csDMARD initiation first line, as opposed to methotrexate alone, is more doubtful and may be associated with a higher rate of adverse events.[14,15]

In summary, the management of RA has changed beyond recognition over the past 30 years, culminating in refinement of a T2T strategy that has revolutionized RA management in the past decade.[16] That the strategy of tailoring treatment escalation decisions against regular disease activity assessments in this way is, almost certainly, more important than the precise escalation sequence, emphasizes the impact of T2T for rheumatology practice. Some caution in attributing all recent improvements in RA outcomes to T2T adoption is prudent, however. A recent systematic review of the clinical- and cost-effectiveness of T2T in RA management highlights several limitations in the current available evidence, including a risk of bias in the published literature and heterogeneity in treatment targets and protocols.[17] These practical considerations of T2T implementation in the clinic are considered in the next section.

Current T2T recommendations

T2T principles and recommendations currently endorsed by the EULAR for the management of RA are summarized in **Table 41.1** and **Figure 41.1**.[10] The aim of the T2T approach is to effect rapid and sustained suppression of inflammatory disease activity in a manner that is both acceptable to the patient and cost-effective for the healthcare provider. To achieve this optimally, national and international treatment recommendations currently converge on the use of low-dose methotrexate as an 'anchor drug' for use in combination with adjunctive glucocorticoids at the time of diagnosis.[15,18,19] Up

to 60% of early RA patients can achieve clinical remission within 4 months using this approach, although significant treatment adjustments are needed in the majority to maintain this state in the longer term[14,20]; treatment intensification involving csDMARD and/or bDMARD permutations will invariably be indicated among the remainder whose disease is not so swiftly suppressed. The ideal frequency of regular disease activity assessments required to such treatment escalation decisions, while not definitive, is suggested to range between monthly and 3-monthly as long as inadequate disease control persists, reducing to every 6 months or longer once achieved (**Table 41.1** and [10]). In practice this will be further influenced by local resource and patient preferences, but the advantages of monthly reviews as implemented by T2T interventional studies in early RA.[7,21] provide compelling justification for the attendant reconfiguration of services required.

Aside from the increased frequency of clinic visits, further potential barriers to the implementation of T2T in clinical practice have been identified, including medication lag time, comorbidities, and patient preference not to escalate treatment.[22] Interventions at the level of the healthcare provider may help address these; in a US study of 23 rheumatology provider sites, a learning collaborative intervention delivered to healthcare professionals resulted in a 5-fold increase in rates of T2T adherence.[23]

Clinical treatment targets

Defining an appropriate treatment target is critical to T2T implementation in daily clinical practice for optimizing RA patient outcomes. This is not as facile as it may first appear, however. In this

Table 41.1 Principles and recommendations for the treatment-to-target of rheumatoid arthritis, as endorsed by the European League Against Rheumatism (EULAR)

Overarching principles	
A	The treatment of rheumatoid arthritis must be based on a shared decision between patient and rheumatologist
B	The primary goal of treating patients with rheumatoid arthritis is to maximize long-term health-related quality of life through control of symptoms, prevention of structural damage, normalization of function, and participation in social and work-related activities
C	Abrogation of inflammation is the most important way to achieve these goals
D	Treatment-to-target by measuring disease activity and adjusting therapy accordingly optimizes outcomes in rheumatoid arthritis
Treat-to-target recommendations	
1	The primary target for treatment of rheumatoid arthritis should be a state of clinical remission
2	Clinical remission is defined as the absence of signs and symptoms of significant inflammatory disease activity
3	While remission should be a clear target, low disease activity may be an acceptable alternative therapeutic goal, particularly in long-standing disease
4	The use of validated composite measures of disease activity, which include joint assessments, is needed in routine clinical practice to guide treatment decisions
5	The choice of the (composite) measure of disease activity and the target value should be influenced by comorbidities, patient factors. and drug-related risks
6	Measures of disease activity must be obtained and documented regularly, as frequently as monthly for patients with high/moderate disease activity or less frequently (such as every six months) for patients in sustained low disease activity or remission
7	Structural changes, functional impairment and comorbidity should be considered when making clinical decisions, in addition to assessing composite measures of disease activity
8	Until the desired treatment target is reached, drug therapy should be adjusted at least every three months
9	The desired treatment target should be maintained throughout the remaining course of the disease
10	The rheumatologist should involve the patient in setting the treatment target and the strategy to reach this target

Reproduced from Smolen JS, Breedveld FC, Burmester GR, et al. Treating rheumatoid arthritis to target: 2014 update of the recommendations of an international task force. *Annals of the Rheumatic Diseases* 2016;75:3–15.

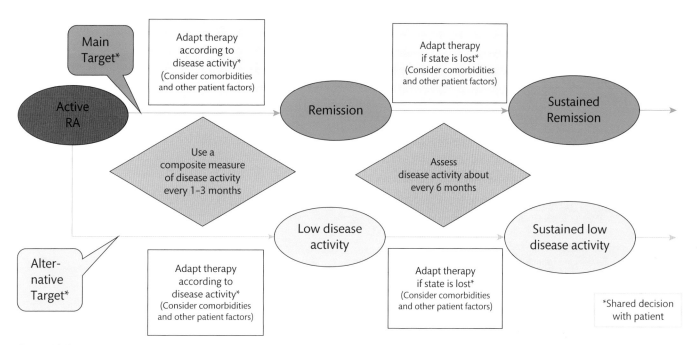

Figure 41.1 Treat-to-target algorithm for rheumatoid arthritis, as endorsed by the European League Against Rheumatism (EULAR). The recommended main treatment target is disease remission, though an alternative treatment target of low disease activity may be appropriate for some patients.

Reproduced from Smolen JS, Breedveld FC, Burmester GR, et al. Treating rheumatoid arthritis to target: 2014 update of the recommendations of an international task force. *Annals of the Rheumatic Diseases* 2016;75:3–15.

section the challenges that arise are first summarized in general terms, before a more detailed discussion covering the cardinal established measures and targets, along with patient-reported outcome measures and the currently recommended remission criteria.

General considerations and pitfalls

Current recommendations advocate a state of **clinical remission**—defined by a composite measure of disease activity that incorporates tender and swollen joint counts—as the preferred target (**Table 41.1**). However, although an increasingly achievable aspiration, remission is not necessarily a suitable target for all patients—particularly those with more long-standing disease in whom its dogged pursuit may achieve little besides accumulated drug reactions; here, the goal of low disease activity (LDA) may be more appropriate.[10] In addition, both LDA and remission have proved surprisingly difficult to define—a situation that is not helped by the diversity of composite measures available to do so (**Table 41.2**).

For example, dichotomous tools like the American College of Rheumatology (ACR)[24] or European League Against Rheumatism (EULAR) response criteria[25] have been developed alongside continuous scores such as the DAS,[2] DAS28,[26] simplified disease activity index (SDAI),[27] and clinical disease activity index (CDAI)[28] (**Table 41.2**).

Importantly, the performance of such scoring systems for defining treatment targets is impacted by variation in the relative weighting between objective measures (e.g. C-reactive protein (CRP), ESR, swollen joint count) *versus* parameters which are arguably more subjective in nature (tender joint count and patient VAS). This issue has been thrown into sharp relief with the increased use of therapies that target biological pathways directly affecting laboratory acute phase markers, as is the case for IL-6 signal blockers and Jak

inhibitors. Here, 'remission' is more easily achieved using a measure in which CRP or ESR is heavily weighted (such as the DAS28) than one that excludes acute phase parameters altogether (such as the CDAI). The apparent efficacy of an IL-6-blocking agent or Jak inhibitor may therefore be exaggerated if an inappropriate criterion is selected—a consequence that has important implications for the interpretation of clinical trials.[38,39]

The implementation of T2T recommendations also has a significant impact on patients' experience, aside from rheumatology service delivery. The composite measures described so far rely upon direct input from specialist healthcare professionals for their calculation, but monthly assessments in secondary care settings demanded for this purpose may not be acceptable to all patients. Interest has therefore grown in the compatibility of RA **patient-reported outcomes** (PROs) with the T2T strategy—including the collection of PRO data 'remotely' via secure web applications accessible by secondary care teams, for example. Such considerations further emphasize the central importance of sharing decisions with patients when selecting disease activity measures and treatment targets as part of a T2T strategy in RA management. Indeed, there may be specific instances in which a functional target, such as the ability to complete a particular physical task or leisure activity, is agreed as an acceptable goal, although this should not normally be prioritized without consideration of otherwise unsuppressed inflammatory disease and its potential destructive consequences.

Clinical measures

As the first widely used composite disease activity measure for RA, the DAS[2] continues to be used in clinical trials, retaining the advantage over other such measures of taking small joints of the lower limbs into account when assessing tenderness and swelling. The feet

Table 41.2 Summary of dichotomous and continuous disease activity evaluation measures, along with select patient-reported outcome measures

Composite measure	Components	Calculation	Cut points				Ref
			Remission	LDA	MDA	HDA	
Dichotomous tools (with joint counts)							
ACR 70 Response	Tender joint count (of 28), swollen joint count (of 28), patient global assessment VAS, physician global assessment VAS (both in cm/10), patient self-assessed disability, CRP (in mg/dL) or ESR (in mm/hr)	Response if TJC28 and SJC28 and one of remaining 3 criteria fall by ≥70% from baseline	–	–	–	–	24
EULAR 'Good' response	DAS or DAS28-ESR	Response if DAS (or DAS28-ESR) falls by ≥1.2 from baseline and reaches value of ≤2.4 (≤3.2 for DAS28-ESR)	–	–	–	–	25, 29
ACR-EULAR Boolean Remission	Tender joint count (of 28), swollen joint count (of 28), patient global assessment VAS, physician global assessment VAS (both in cm/10), CRP (in mg/dL)	Remission defined if all components ≤1	See *calculation*	–	–	–	30
Continuous scores (with joint counts)							
DAS	Ritchie articular index, swollen joint count (of 44), patient global health VAS (in mm/100), erythrocyte sedimentation rate (in mm/hr)	$0.53938 \times \sqrt{(RAI)} + 0.06465 \times \sqrt{(SJC44)} + 0.330 \times \log(ESR) + 0.00722 \times VAS_{patient}$	< 1.6	1.6 ≤ score ≤2.4	2.4 < score ≤3.7	> 3.7	2
DAS28-ESR	Tender joint count (of 28), swollen joint count (of 28), patient global health VAS (in mm/100), erythrocyte sedimentation rate (in mm/hr)	$0.56 \times \sqrt{(TJC28)} + 0.28 \times \sqrt{(SJC28)} + 0.70 \times \log_e(ESR) + 0.014 \times VAS_{patient}$	< 2.6	2.6 ≤ score ≤ 3.2	3.2 < score ≤5.1	>5.1	26
DAS28-CRP	Tender joint count (of 28), swollen joint count (of 28), patient global health VAS (in mm/100), C-reactive protein (in mg/dL)	$0.56 \times \sqrt{(TJC28)} + 0.28 \times \sqrt{(SJC28)} + 0.36 \times \log_e(CRP+1) + 0.014 \times VAS_{patient} + 0.96$	< 2.6 < 2.4*	2.6 ≤ score ≤ 3.2 2.4 < *score* ≤ 2.9*	3.2 < score ≤5.1 2.9 < *score* ≤ 4.6†	> 4.6	31-33
SDAI	Tender joint count (of 28), swollen joint count (of 28), patient global assessment VAS, physician global assessment VAS (both in cm/10), C-reactive protein (in mg/dL)	$TJC28 + SJC28 + VAS_{patient} + VAS_{physician} + CRP$	≤ 3.3	3.3 < score ≤ 11	11 < score ≤ 26	> 26	27
CDAI	Tender joint count (of 28), swollen joint count (of 28), patient global assessment VAS, physician global assessment VAS (both in cm/10),	$TJC28 + SJC28 + VAS_{patient} + VAS_{physician}$	≤ 2.8	2.8 < score ≤ 10	10 < score ≤ 22	> 22	28
Select patient-reported outcome scores							
RAPID3	HAQ-DI, patient global assessment, and patient pain assessment (both in cm/10)	$3.33 \times (HAQ-DI) + VAS_{patient} + Pain$	≤ 1	1 < score ≤ 2	2 < score ≤ 4	> 4	34,35
RADAI-5	Patient arthritis activity score over 6 months VAS, patient current disease activity VAS, patient pain VAS, patient general health VAS, patient hand stiffness VAS (all in cm/10)	(Sum of 5 components)/5	≤ 1.4	1.6 ≤ score ≤ 3.0	3.2 ≤ score ≤ 5.4	≥ 5.6	36, 37

are frequently involved in the disease and, when excluded from assessments otherwise determining remission, have been shown to harbour residual inflammatory activity in some patients with potentially destructive consequences.[40,41] Although undoubtedly important for such individuals, the additive value of including foot assessments in joint counts is not obvious when considering long-term radiographic and functional outcomes at a population level.[42] Moreover, the relative ease with which an abbreviated form of the DAS that ignores ankles and feet, now known as the DAS28-ESR,[26] may be determined, has cemented its popularity in clinical trials and daily practice since its development—including as the basis of EULAR treatment response criteria.[25] A modification of the DAS28 allows for use of CRP in place of ESR as an arguably more sensitive and specific marker of inflammation in RA (DAS28-CRP).[31] Although the cut points of these abbreviated forms are interchangeable by convention, close scrutiny demonstrates that a given DAS28-CRP score slightly understates the equivalent DAS28-ESR.[32] Despite widespread usage, definitions of remission based on DAS measurements (whether abbreviated or not) have been criticised as treatment targets in RA. This is primarily because residual disease activity can be clinically observed in a significant proportion of patients with scores below accepted remission cut points,[43] and those in sustained DAS remission continue to experience radiographic progression 20–40% of cases.[30,44]

The SDAI was originally developed as a sensitive, fully validated measure of RA disease activity for application in day-to-day clinical practice without the need for a calculator. It comprises a simple sum of five core variables: tender and swollen joint counts (of the same joints covered by the DAS28), CRP (measured in g/dl), and VAS-derived subjective measures of global disease activity on 10 cm scales obtained from both the patient and the physician. The measure receives a lesser acute phase marker contribution than do DAS measurements (5% *versus* approximately 15%), arguably making SDAI treatment targets more suited to the era of IL-6/Jak-targeting drugs.[28,32] Indeed, CRP was observed to add little independent information beyond the combination of clinical variables included in the SDAI, and the 4-variable CDAI is now also in common use and can be calculated without waiting for blood results.[28] Despite these apparent advantages progressive structural damage may still occur in the presence of SDAI and/or CDAI remission, albeit is less likely if sustained over time.[45]

Patient-reported outcome measures

PROs including pain, fatigue, work instability, and physical function reflect important effects of RA on the daily lives of patients living with the condition. Despite incorporation of PROs into most composite clinical scores (global health VAS in the DAS28, for example), those outcomes of most importance to patients may not be fully captured by standard RA disease activity metrics. This observation, coupled with the logistical challenge of regularly recording joint count components of such metrics, has led to an interest in using 'pure' PRO measures for defining treatment targets. For example, the Health Assessment Questionnaire Disability Index (HAQ-DI) is a long-established PRO measure capturing elements of impaired physical function highly relevant to RA[46] that has been combined with global health and pain VAS measurements to form the routine assessment of patient index data-3 (RAPID3) tool,[34] and cut points equivalent to those used as treatment targets in clinical scoring systems have

been proposed.[34] Similarly, a rheumatoid arthritis disease activity index combines patient-derived VAS measurements for current perceived disease activity, perceived disease activity over preceding six months, general health, pain and hand stiffness (RADAI-5); this may also be used to define states of LDA and/or remission[36,47] (see also Table 41.2). Tantalizing though they may be as potential cost-reducing means of 'remote' T2T implementation—circumventing the need for frequent hospital visits on the part of patients using **eHealth** technologies, for example[48]—treatment targets based solely upon PRO measures are not yet wholly endorsed for clinical practice.[10] Particular concern relates to their apparent discordance from clinical scores at low levels of inflammatory disease activity, where they have a tendency to underestimate remission thereby risking unnecessary treatment escalation decisions if used in isolation.[10,49]

ACR/EULAR remission criteria

In 2011, the ACR and EULAR published joint criteria, aiming to establish consensus definitions of remission in RA that are 'stringent but achievable'. They incorporate a Boolean definition alongside an index definition drawn from the existing SDAI score (Table 41.2).[30] Swollen and tender joint counts are on average lower when remission is defined using ACR/EULAR criteria compared with the DAS28 score,[16,50] and the definition appears to be able to predict favourable radiological outcomes using data from prospective clinical trials.[51,52] Yet achieving ACR/EULAR remission does not preclude the possibility of structural progression, and new erosions develop in a small but significant proportion of patients who consistently fulfil the Boolean definition developing new erosions over time.[45] Any suggestion that the criteria are insufficiently stringent on this basis must be balanced against the counter-argument, that excessive stringency of the patient global assessment threshold in particular may lead to *under*-diagnosis of remission in practice.[53–55] Therefore, notwithstanding the undoubted value of consensus remission criteria and their application as clinical trial outcomes, debate over the optimal definition of this state for use as a treatment target in RA continues. It has recently acquired added dimensions with proposals to incorporate novel parameters based on imaging and/or biomarkers of pathobiological relevance. Such issues will be considered further in the section that follows.

Remission: New concepts and controversies

The profound impact of widespread T2T strategy adoption in RA over recent years is perceived keenly by many rheumatologists, even if it is difficult to quantify precisely. For a once inexorably progressive disease, the fact that remission is now the subject of lively discussion as a treatment target, shown to be attainable for over a third of patients,[56] should surely be cause for celebration. Observational data is particularly illustrative in this regard: the proportion of RA patients found to be in SDAI remission in a large, unselected Norwegian cohort increased from 6% to 32% between 2004 and 2015, the corresponding increase in respect of LDA being from 41% to 83% (**Figure 41.2**).[57,58] Even taking into account the burgeoning use of biologic therapies it is hard to conceive that T2T has not played its role in this success. However, reductions in PROs appear to have been less sustained. For example, despite comparable temporal reductions in inflammatory disease activity among RA patients in a recent UK survey, disability as measured using HAQ scores remained worryingly static.[59] The argument that residual disease among patients considered to be in remission by current definitions contributes to the accrual of 'silent' joint damage may be relevant here, and will be discussed. So too will related debates over the need to target ever 'deeper' remission to improve RA outcomes in the future, and proposed tools for supplementing clinical assessments to this end.

A role for imaging in defining remission?

The progression of joint damage despite fulfilment of clinical remission criteria in many patients suggests that synovitis, whether or not clinically overt, remains prevalent and drives ongoing tissue destruction in this group. Available musculoskeletal ultrasound (MSUS) data certainly appears to be consistent with this hypothesis. A meta-analysis of 19 studies including 1369 RA patients in clinical remission demonstrated that, irrespective of the stringency by which remission was defined, almost half had MSUS evidence of residual peripheral joint synovitis.[60] Employing magnetic resonance imaging (MRI) of the dominant hand in a similar setting, bone marrow oedema was present in a comparable proportion but overall rates of subclinical pathology appear even higher.[61] A further meta-analysis of 13 longitudinal studies of RA patients in clinical remission clearly linked the presence of power Doppler synovitis (PDS) on ultrasound with both future arthritis flare and the development of bone erosions in affected joints.[62] Although less well characterized, the finding of bone marrow oedema on MRI is probably equally predictive.[63] Finally, limited data from synovial biopsies of RA patients in whom contemporaneous MSUS findings were recorded identify increased leukocyte infiltration in PDS-positive joints, and has been invoked to suggest absence of PDS is better than fulfilment of clinical remission criteria alone at predicting the absence of histological synovitis.[64]

Given this growing evidence base, together with increasingly widespread access to MSUS in particular, it was entirely logical to propose inclusion of an imaging component into RA remission criteria. Technical and practical challenges to doing so in a feasible format for routine application are not insurmountable, if by no means trivial, and such an approach has indeed been advocated by experts.[65,66] Two recent prospective clinical trials have sought to define a formal role for MSUS as part of a T2T strategy targeting 'imaging remission' in the light of this. In the open-label Targeting Synovitis in Early Rheumatoid Arthritis (TaSER) study, newly diagnosed RA patients were randomized to a strategy targeting either DAS28-ESR<3.2 or a combined DAS28-ESR/US construct (intervention arm), with equivalent DMARD escalation schedules in both arms.[67] The Aiming for Remission in rheumatoid arthritis: a randomized controlled trial examining the benefit of ultrasound in a TIght Control regimen (ARCTIC) study had similar objectives, employing a more ambitious clinical remission target of DAS<1.6 in both arms[68]: no overt advantage to incorporation of PDS parameters in the remission definition was observed in either study, including in terms of radiographic progression over up to 2 years. The authors of both studies concluded that the additional cost and treatment burden of an imaging-targeted escalation protocol are not currently justified. Conceivably, larger trials and/ or longer periods of follow-up, perhaps employing more discriminatory MSUS screening algorithms still to be defined, may yet carve a niche for this modality as an adjunctive tool for targeting remission in clinical practice.[69] An alternative view is that the focus of investigation should now shift to their potentially valuable role in **preventing** treatment escalation rather than triggering it, for example among patients confirmed to **lack** synovitis despite elevated composite disease activity attributable solely to joint tenderness and global health perception.[66]

A role for biomarkers in defining remission?

Although disease remission remains a conceptually enticing treatment goal, its practical realization in RA continues to be hampered

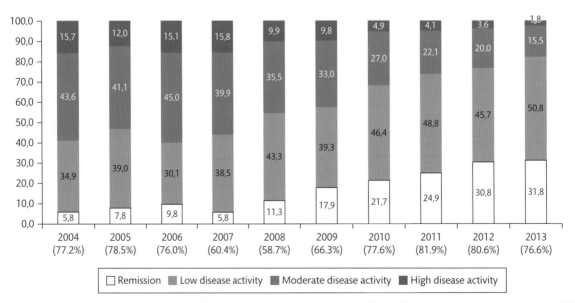

Figure 41.2 Percentage of patients with rheumatoid arthritis in remission, low, moderate, and high disease activity according to the simplified disease activity index (SDAI) in a Norwegian cohort over a ten-year period. The percentage of the cohort where SDAI measurements were available is indicated below the respective year.

Reproduced from Haugeberg G, Hansen IJ, Soldal DM, Sokka T. Ten years of change in clinical disease status and treatment in rheumatoid arthritis: results based on standardized monitoring of patients in an ordinary outpatient clinic in southern Norway. *Arthritis Research & Therapy*. 2015;17:219.

by imprecise definitions. As the molecular and cellular processes that underpin this heterogeneous disease are unravelled, might not biomarkers that reflect fundamental pathogenetic mechanisms provide an ultimate and wholly objective measure of disease activity for therapeutic targeting? This aspiration is not new but still proves elusive, exemplified by experience with the multibiomarker disease activity (MBDA) test (Vectra DA™). This yields a 0–100 score calculated based on read-outs of 12 simultaneously-measured serum analytes, themselves intended to reflect diverse components of RA pathophysiology.[70] Despite early promise, results of studies seeking to validate the measure as a viable treatment target have been at best conflicting and, ultimately, disappointing.[71] One difficulty with such tools is that the sensitivity of their readout to treatment is often intrinsically related to therapeutic choice—akin to the peculiar sensitivity of CRP to Jak inhibition discussed previously. Hence, since the MBDA panel includes IL-6, whose levels paradoxically **increase** with anti-IL-6 receptor monoclonal antibody treatment, its ability to reflect reduced disease activity in this therapeutic context is relatively blunt.[72] Disentangling biomarkers' true relationship with disease activity from their differential sensitivity to various drugs remains a stumbling block to their development as 'real-world' treatment targets. Here, it is also pertinent to recall RA as a disease of immune dysregulation first and foremost, in which persistent inflammation and tissue destruction, albeit driven by targetable cytokines, are probably consequences rather than underlying drivers. As in other autoimmune diseases where the ultimate therapeutic goal is restoration of immune tolerance, biomarkers of remission may ultimately look very similar—even identical—to biomarkers of tolerance.[73] The search for them is intense in the research arena, but has yet to deliver validated treatment targets of value to the clinic.

Remission depth: How deep should the target be?

As is evident from the foregoing discussion, RA remission may be conceptualized at a number of levels: it may be defined clinically (according to various thresholds discussed), linked to imaging findings, and/or assessed according to serological or tissue markers of relevant

pathobiological processes. It has even been suggested that remission in seropositive RA can never be reached until autoantibodies are no longer detectable in the circulation—a state of 'immunological remission' that is only very rarely described in the clinic (**Figure 41.3**).[74] In considering this it is critical to understand both the benefits and the costs of treating to targets that reflect ever-decreasing disease activity, or remission 'depth'. The comparative value of various LDA and remission measures as T2T goals is far from fully defined, yet the criterion selected will profoundly influence not only the intensity, but also any undesired effects, of the therapeutic intervention required to achieve it.[25] For now, we consider current T2T recommendations, advocating 'a composite measure of disease activity that incorporates tender and swollen joint counts' as a treatment target, to be an excellent guide for clinical practice whose implementation should harness evidence-based benefits for patients.[10] In the future, well-designed trials to appraise the value of each newly proposed target in RA should be pursued with the same rigour as those assessing the efficacy of novel therapies—assigning equal importance to the costs and the benefits of any change in strategy.

A final frontier?

How should RA be managed once remission has been achieved—and sustained over time? The question is far from hypothetical. Sustained drug-free remission (DFR) has become a reality for a substantial minority of patients, raising important risk-benefit questions in which the advantages of remission must be balanced against the side effects, risks, and costs of indefinite therapeutic intervention. Expert consensus on whether, when and how DMARDs should be discontinued in patients with stably controlled disease is only now beginning to emerge. Sustained DFR affords researchers a tantalizing opportunity to investigate mechanisms of 'immune resetting' by which some individuals revert from a state of immune dysregulation to one of tolerance, perhaps even offering a window on a cure for this disease.

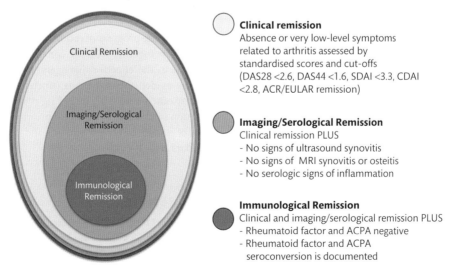

Figure 41.3 The 'shell model' of rheumatoid arthritis remission.

Reproduced from Schett G, Emery P, Tanaka Y, Burmester G, Pisetsky DS, Naredo E, et al. Tapering biologic and conventional DMARD therapy in rheumatoid arthritis: current evidence and future directions. *Annals of the Rheumatic Diseases*. 2016;75(8):1428–37 with permission from the BMJ Publishing Group.

Drug-free remission

Observational studies have reported DFR rates of between 9 and 16% in RA cohort populations overall, with higher rates reported among those more recently diagnosed.[75-77] Importantly, after DMARD cessation and over a minimum 1 year follow-up, these studies identified no appreciable progression in radiographic or disability scores (HAQ), the latter remaining commensurate with those seen in the general population.[77] The picture whereby increased sustained DFR rates have become achievable with passing decades is recapitulated in randomized controlled trials (RCTs), when studied as a primary end-point following csDMARD cessation among patients already in remission. In an early RCT the rate was only 20% following penicillamine discontinuation,[78] but the equivalent figure rises to 50–60% in more recent studies.[79,80] A similar DFR rate appears possible when stopping bDMARDs, providing a state of stable remission (as opposed to mere LDA) has been achieved prior to their cessation[81,82]; nonetheless, optimal tapering strategies in this setting in particular require refinement, and are the primary focus of active RCTs (for a comprehensive summary of DMARD cessation studies and their outcomes, see reference[74]). A key concern to be considered when contemplating treatment discontinuation is the likelihood of recapturing a state of remission following its reinstatement in the event of flare. A handful of studies have captured long-term outcomes of the 50% or so of patients who flare following DMARD withdrawal, indicating that the majority regain remission within 6 months of resuming their previous treatment without incurring significant radiographic progression.[83,84] Although formal recommendations on the subject of DMARD cessation for RA patients in clinical remission are limited and founded on a relatively immature evidence base, messages for clinical practice published by experts in the field in a recent review are reproduced in Box 41.1.

Predicting drug-free remission

Currently, the decision to discontinue treatment among RA patients in stable remission should be informed by careful discussion between the patient and rheumatologist, taking into account the pros and cons of each course of action.[15] The ability to accurately predict sustained DFR among such individuals would be a major advance.

The presence of anticitrullinated peptide autoantibodies (ACPA) and/or rheumatoid factor (RF) have both consistently been associated with lower rates of sustained DFR across multiple studies, with successful DMARD cessation perhaps more than five times as likely following treatment cessation in seronegative individuals.[76,79,80,85,86] Other clinical predictors of a favourable outcome probably include shorter disease duration, a more stringent definition of remission and male sex, but consistency across studies is lacking in these areas. Current data also suggests that the presence of ultrasound-detected PDS is likely to carry a greater risk of flare,[87] with only limited data indicating that MRI may be less helpful in this setting,[88] but more comprehensive evaluations of imaging for this purpose are awaited. Finally, early indications are that certain circulating inflammatory mediators contributing to the MBDA test mentioned previously, including CRP, are predictive of flare if present at the time of DMARD discontinuation.[89] The study of biomarkers is in its infancy in this context, but timely: as well as aiding clinical decision-making, readily measurable immune parameters that presage DFR *versus* flare may themselves offer insight into regulatory pathways of relevance to RA pathogenesis more generally, and they are the subject of active investigation.

> **Box 41.1** Key messages for clinical practice when considering disease-modifying antirheumatic drug withdrawal in rheumatoid arthritis remission
>
> **Eligible patients**
> Disease-modifying antirheumatic drug (DMARD) tapering should be considered if patients (a) fulfil standardized clinical criteria for remission state (disease activity score (DAS)28 <2.6; DAS44 <1.6; simplified disease activity index (SDAI) <3.3; Clinical Disease Activity Index <2.8; American Colleague of Rheumatology (ACR)/European League Against Rheumatism (EULAR) remission), (b) show sustained remission for at least 6 months documented by appropriate disease activity instruments at three sequential visits, (c) use stable DMARD treatment with respect to type and dose of DMARDs over the last 6 months and (d) do not use glucocorticoids to maintain their remission state.
>
> **Risk and predictors for relapse**
> Some rheumatoid arthritis patients can successfully taper or even stop DMARD treatment. Anticitrullinated autoantibody negativity and presence of 'deep' remission such as absence of ultrasound synovitis and/or normal serum markers of inflammation are associated with higher chances to achieve drug-free remission.
>
> **Mode of DMARD tapering/withdrawal**
> Both direct DMARD withdrawal and dose tapering protocols were studied. Patients need to be informed about the mode and how to taper their DMARD. For practical reasons, gradual withdrawal with an initial dose tapering phase may be preferable over immediate withdrawal. This concept applies to both biological and synthetic DMARDs.
>
> **Monitoring and relapse management**
> Particularly when starting DMARD tapering and/or withdrawal regular monitoring needs to be scheduled in order to early detect relapses. Patients need to be instructed about the risks of relapse as well as the way to manage them. Reintroduction of the former DMARD regimen has shown to recapture remission in virtually all patients relapsing.
>
> Reproduced from Schett G, Emery P, Tanaka Y, Burmester G, Pisetsky DS, Naredo E, et al. Tapering biologic and conventional DMARD therapy in rheumatoid arthritis: current evidence and future directions. *Annals of the Rheumatic Diseases*. 2016;75(8):1428–37 with permission from the BMJ Publishing Group

Summary

Building on the progress of recent decades, a consideration of treatment targets together with the concept of disease remission is fundamental to the effective management of RA in the modern era. Building evidence-based management strategies for patients that optimize outcomes for all, including effective cure rates through the induction of DFR, must now be a priority. The potential rewards in terms of quality of life for patients and cost savings for healthcare providers are self-evident.

REFERENCES

1. Ritchie DM, Boyle JA, McInnes JM, et al. Clinical studies with an articular index for the assessment of joint tenderness in patients with rheumatoid arthritis. *Q J Med* 1968;37(147):393–406.
2. van der Heijde DM, van 't Hof MA, van Riel PL, et al. Judging disease activity in clinical practice in rheumatoid arthritis: first

step in the development of a disease activity score. *Ann Rheum Dis* 1990;*49*(11):916–20.

3. van der Heide A, Jacobs JW, Bijlsma JW, et al. The effectiveness of early treatment with 'second-line' antirheumatic drugs. A randomized, controlled trial. *Ann Int Med* 1996;*124*(8):699–707.

4. Boers M, Verhoeven AC, Markusse HM, et al. Randomised comparison of combined step-down prednisolone, methotrexate and sulphasalazine with sulphasalazine alone in early rheumatoid arthritis. *Lancet* 1997;*350*(9074):309–18.

5. Lard LR, Visser H, Speyer I, et al. Early versus delayed treatment in patients with recent-onset rheumatoid arthritis: comparison of two cohorts who received different treatment strategies. *Am J Med* 2001;*111*(6):446–51.

6. Diabetes Control and Complications Trial Research Group, Nathan DM, Genuth S, et al. The effect of intensive treatment of diabetes on the development and progression of long-term complications in insulin-dependent diabetes mellitus. *N Engl J Med* 1993;*329*(14):977–86.

7. Grigor C, Capell H, Stirling A, et al. Effect of a treatment strategy of tight control for rheumatoid arthritis (the TICORA study): a single-blind randomised controlled trial. *Lancet* 2004;*364*(9430):263–9.

8. Schoels M, Knevel R, Aletaha D, et al. Evidence for treating rheumatoid arthritis to target: results of a systematic literature search. *Ann Rheum Dis* 2010;*69*(4):638–43.

9. Stoffer MA, Schoels MM, Smolen JS, et al. Evidence for treating rheumatoid arthritis to target: results of a systematic literature search update. *Ann Rheum Dis* 2016;*75*(1):16–22.

10. Smolen JS, Breedveld FC, Burmester GR, et al. Treating rheumatoid arthritis to target: 2014 update of the recommendations of an international task force. *Ann Rheum Dis* 2016;*75*(1):3–15.

11. Fransen J, Moens HB, Speyer I, van Riel PL. Effectiveness of systematic monitoring of rheumatoid arthritis disease activity in daily practice: a multicentre, cluster randomised controlled trial. *Ann Rheum Dis* 2005;*64*(9):1294–8.

12. Pope JE, Haraoui B, Rampakakis E, Psaradellis E, Thorne C, Sampalis JS. Treating to a target in established active rheumatoid arthritis patients receiving a tumor necrosis factor inhibitor: results from a real-world cluster-randomized adalimumab trial. *Arthritis Care Res (Hoboken)* 2013;*65*(9):1401–9.

13. Graudal N, Hubeck-Graudal T, Faurschou M, Baslund B, Jürgens G. Combination therapy with and without tumor necrosis factor inhibitors in rheumatoid arthritis: a meta-analysis of randomized trials. *Arthritis Care Res (Hoboken)* 2015;*67*(11):1487–95.

14. Kuijper TM, Luime JJ, de Jong PH, et al. Tapering conventional synthetic DMARDs in patients with early arthritis in sustained remission: 2-year follow-up of the tREACH trial. *Ann Rheum Dis* 2016;*75*(12):2119–23.

15. Smolen JS, Landewe R, Bijlsma J, et al. EULAR recommendations for the management of rheumatoid arthritis with synthetic and biological disease-modifying antirheumatic drugs: 2016 update. *Ann Rheum Dis* 2017;*76*(6):960–77.

16. Kuriya B, Sun Y, Boire G, et al. Remission in early rheumatoid arthritis—a comparison of new ACR/EULAR remission criteria to established criteria. *J Rheumatol* 2012;*39*(6):1155–8.

17. Wailoo A, Hock ES, Stevenson M, et al. The clinical effectiveness and cost-effectiveness of treat-to-target strategies in rheumatoid arthritis: a systematic review and cost-effectiveness analysis. *Health Technol Assess* 2017;*21*(71):1–258.

18. Singh JA, Saag KG, Bridges SL, Jr., et al. 2015 American College of rheumatology guideline for the treatment of rheumatoid arthritis. *Arthritis Rheumatol (Hoboken)* 2016;*68*(1):1–26.

19. National Institute for Health and Care Excellence (NICE). Rheumatoid Arthritis in Adults: Management. *NICE Guideline [NG100]*. London, UK: National Institute for Health and Care Excellence, 2009. Available at: https://www.nice.org.uk/guidance/ng100

20. Akdemir G, Heimans L, Bergstra SA, et al. Clinical and radiological outcomes of 5-year drug-free remission-steered treatment in patients with early arthritis: IMPROVED study. *Ann Rheum Dis* 2018;*77*(1):111–18.

21. Verstappen SM, Jacobs JW, van der Veen MJ, et al. Intensive treatment with methotrexate in early rheumatoid arthritis: aiming for remission. Computer Assisted Management in Early Rheumatoid Arthritis (CAMERA, an open-label strategy trial). *Ann Rheum Dis* 2007;*66*(11):1443–9.

22. Harrold LR, Reed GW, John A, et al. Cluster-randomized trial of a behavioral intervention to incorporate a treat-to-target approach to care of us patients with rheumatoid arthritis. *Arthritis Care Res (Hoboken)* 2018;*70*(3):379–87.

23. Solomon DH, Losina E, Lu B, et al. Implementation of treat-to-target in rheumatoid arthritis through a learning collaborative: results of a randomized controlled trial. *Arthritis Rheumatol* 2017;*69*(7):1374–80.

24. Felson DT, Anderson JJ, Boers M, et al. American College of Rheumatology. Preliminary definition of improvement in rheumatoid arthritis. *Arthritis Rheum* 1995;*38*(6):727–35.

25. van Gestel AM, Prevoo ML, van 't Hof MA, et al. Development and validation of the European League Against Rheumatism response criteria for rheumatoid arthritis. Comparison with the preliminary American College of Rheumatology and the World Health Organization/International League Against Rheumatism Criteria. *Arthritis Rheum* 1996;*39*(1):34–40.

26. Prevoo ML, van 't Hof MA, Kuper HH, van Leeuwen MA, van de Putte LB, van Riel PL. Modified disease activity scores that include twenty-eight-joint counts. Development and validation in a prospective longitudinal study of patients with rheumatoid arthritis. *Arthritis Rheum* 1995;*38*(1):44–8.

27. Smolen JS, Breedveld FC, Schiff MH, et al. A simplified disease activity index for rheumatoid arthritis for use in clinical practice. *Rheumatology (Oxf)* 2003;*42*(2):244–57.

28. Aletaha D, Nell VP, Stamm T, et al. Acute phase reactants add little to composite disease activity indices for rheumatoid arthritis: validation of a clinical activity score. *Arthritis Res Ther* 2005;*7*(4):R796–806.

29. van Gestel AM, Haagsma CJ, van Riel PL. Validation of rheumatoid arthritis improvement criteria that include simplified joint counts. *Arthritis Rheum* 1998;*41*(10):1845–50.

30. Felson DT, Smolen JS, Wells G, et al. American College of Rheumatology/European League Against Rheumatism provisional definition of remission in rheumatoid arthritis for clinical trials. *Arthritis Rheum* 2011;*63*(3):573–86.

31. Fransen J, Welsing PMJ, De Keijzer RMH, van Riel PLCM. Development and validation of the DAS28 using CRP. *Ann Rheum Dis* 2003;*62*(Suppl. 1):10.

32. Fleischmann R, van der Heijde D, Koenig AS, et al. How much does Disease Activity Score in 28 joints ESR and CRP calculations underestimate disease activity compared with the Simplified Disease Activity Index? *Ann Rheum Dis* 2015;*74*(6):1132–7.

33. Fleischmann RM, van der Heijde D, Gardiner PV, Szumski A, Marshall L, Bananis E. DAS28-CRP and DAS28-ESR cut-offs for high disease activity in rheumatoid arthritis are not interchangeable. *RMD Open* 2017;*3*(1):e000382.

34. Pincus T, Swearingen CJ, Bergman M, Yazici Y. RAPID3 (Routine Assessment of Patient Index Data 3), a rheumatoid arthritis index without formal joint counts for routine care: proposed severity categories compared to disease activity score and clinical disease activity index categories. *J Rheumatol* 2008;*35*(11):2136–47.

35. Pincus T, Bergman MJ, Yazici Y, Hines P, Raghupathi K, Maclean R. An index of only patient-reported outcome measures, routine assessment of patient index data 3 (RAPID3), in two abatacept clinical trials: similar results to disease activity score (DAS28) and other RAPID indices that include physician-reported measures. *Rheumatology (Oxf)* 2008;*47*(3):345–9.

36. Rintelen B, Haindl PM, Sautner J, Leeb BA, Deutsch C, Leeb BF. The rheumatoid arthritis disease activity index-5 in daily use. Proposal for disease activity categories. *J Rheumatol* 2009;*36*(5):918–24.

37. Leeb BF, Haindl PM, Maktari A, Nothnagl T, Rintelen B. Patient-centered rheumatoid arthritis disease activity assessment by a modified RADAI. *J Rheumatol* 2008;*35*(7):1294–9.

38. Kawashiri SY, Kawakami A, Iwamoto N, et al. Disease activity score 28 may overestimate the remission induction of rheumatoid arthritis patients treated with tocilizumab: comparison with the remission by the clinical disease activity index. *Modern Rheumatology* 2011;*21*(4):365–9.

39. Schoels M, Alasti F, Smolen JS, Aletaha D. Evaluation of newly proposed remission cut-points for disease activity score in 28 joints (DAS28) in rheumatoid arthritis patients upon IL-6 pathway inhibition. *Arthritis Res Ther* 2017;*19*(1):155.

40. Wechalekar MD, Lester S, Hill CL, et al. Active foot synovitis in patients with rheumatoid arthritis: unstable remission status, radiographic progression, and worse functional outcomes in patients with foot synovitis in apparent remission. *Arthritis Care Res (Hoboken)* 2016;*68*(11):1616–23.

41. Bakker MF, Jacobs JW, Kruize AA, et al. Misclassification of disease activity when assessing individual patients with early rheumatoid arthritis using disease activity indices that do not include joints of feet. *Ann Rheum Dis* 2012;*71*(6):830–5.

42. van Tuyl LH, Britsemmer K, Wells GA, et al. Remission in early rheumatoid arthritis defined by 28 joint counts: limited consequences of residual disease activity in the forefeet on outcome. *Ann Rheum Dis* 2012;*71*(1):33–7.

43. van der Heijde D, Klareskog L, Boers M, et al. Comparison of different definitions to classify remission and sustained remission: 1 year TEMPO results. *Ann Rheum Dis* 2005;*64*(11):1582–7.

44. Cohen G, Gossec L, Dougados M, et al. Radiological damage in patients with rheumatoid arthritis on sustained remission. *Ann Rheum Dis* 2007;*66*(3):358–63.

45. Lillegraven S, Prince FH, Shadick NA, et al. Remission and radiographic outcome in rheumatoid arthritis: application of the 2011 ACR/EULAR remission criteria in an observational cohort. *Ann Rheum Dis* 2012;*71*(5):681–6.

46. Bruce B, Fries JF. The Stanford Health Assessment Questionnaire: dimensions and practical applications. *Health Qual Life Outcomes* 2003;*1*:20.

47. Rintelen B, Sautner J, Haindl P, Mai H, Brezinschek HP, Leeb BF. Remission in rheumatoid artshritis: a comparison of the 2 newly proposed ACR/EULAR remission criteria with the rheumatoid arthritis disease activity index-5, a patient self-report disease activity index. *J Rheumatol* 2013;*40*(4):394–400.

48. Pincus T. Electronic eRAPID3 (Routine Assessment of Patient Index Data): opportunities and complexities. *Clin Exp Rheumatol* 2016;*34*(5 Suppl 101):S49–s53.

49. Curtis JR, Churchill M, Kivitz A, et al. A randomized trial comparing disease activity measures for the assessment and prediction of response in rheumatoid arthritis patients initiating certolizumab pegol. *Arthritis Rheumatol (Hoboken)* 2015;*67*(12):3104–12.

50. Thiele K, Huscher D, Bischoff S, et al. Performance of the 2011 ACR/EULAR preliminary remission criteria compared with DAS28 remission in unselected patients with rheumatoid arthritis. *Ann Rheum Dis* 2013;*72*(7):1194–9.

51. Klarenbeek NB, Koevoets R, van der Heijde DM, et al. Association with joint damage and physical functioning of nine composite indices and the 2011 ACR/EULAR remission criteria in rheumatoid arthritis. *Ann Rheum Dis* 2011;*70*(10):1815–21.

52. Sakellariou G, Scire CA, Verstappen SM, Montecucco C, Caporali R. In patients with early rheumatoid arthritis, the new ACR/EULAR definition of remission identifies patients with persistent absence of functional disability and suppression of ultra-sonographic synovitis. *Ann Rheum Dis* 2013;*72*(2):245–9.

53. Vermeer M, Kuper HH, van der Bijl AE, et al. The provisional ACR/EULAR definition of remission in RA: a comment on the patient global assessment criterion. *Rheumatology (Oxf)* 2012;*51*(6):1076–80.

54. Baker KF, Pratt AG, Thompson B, Isaacs JD. Let's not fool ourselves. In RA, the ACR/EULAR remission criteria are not perfect! *Ann Rheum Dis* 2017;*76*(6):e12.

55. Masri KR, Shaver TS, Shahouri SH, et al. Validity and reliability problems with patient global as a component of the ACR/EULAR remission criteria as used in clinical practice. *J Rheumatol* 2012;*39*(6):1139–45.

56. Ma MH, Scott IC, Kingsley GH, Scott DL. Remission in early rheumatoid arthritis. *J Rheumatol* 2010;*37*(7):1444–53.

57. Aga AB, Lie E, Uhlig T, et al. Time trends in disease activity, response and remission rates in rheumatoid arthritis during the past decade: results from the NOR-DMARD study 2000–2010. *Ann Rheum Dis* 2015;*74*(2):381–8.

58. Haugeberg G, Hansen IJ, Soldal DM, Sokka T. Ten years of change in clinical disease status and treatment in rheumatoid arthritis: results based on standardized monitoring of patients in an ordinary outpatient clinic in southern Norway. *Arthritis Res Ther* 2015;*17*:219.

59. Mian AN, Ibrahim F, Scott IC, et al. Changing clinical patterns in rheumatoid arthritis management over two decades: sequential observational studies. *BMC Musculoskelet Disord* 2016;*17*:44.

60. Nguyen H, Ruyssen-Witrand A, Gandjbakhch F, Constantin A, Foltz V, Cantagrel A. Prevalence of ultrasound-detected residual synovitis and risk of relapse and structural progression in rheumatoid arthritis patients in clinical remission: a systematic review and meta-analysis. *Rheumatology (Oxf)* 2014;*53*(11):2110–18.

61. Lisbona MP, Pamies A, Ares J, et al. Association of bone edema with the progression of bone erosions quantified by hand magnetic resonance imaging in patients with rheumatoid arthritis in remission. *J Rheumatol* 2014;*41*(8):1623–9.

62. Han J, Geng Y, Deng X, Zhang Z. Subclinical synovitis assessed by ultrasound predicts flare and progressive bone erosion in rheumatoid arthritis patients with clinical remission: a systematic review and metaanalysis. *J Rheumatol* 2016;*43*(11):2010–18.

63. Gandjbakhch F, Foltz V, Mallet A, Bourgeois P, Fautrel B. Bone marrow oedema predicts structural progression in a 1-year follow-up of 85 patients with RA in remission or with low disease activity with low-field MRI. *Ann Rheum Dis* 2011;*70*(12):2159–62.

64. Ramirez J, Celis R, Usategui A, et al. Immunopathologic characterization of ultrasound-defined synovitis in rheumatoid arthritis patients in clinical remission. *Arthritis Res Ther* 2015;*18*:74.

65. Wakefield RJ, D'Agostino MA, Naredo E, et al. After treat-to-target: can a targeted ultrasound initiative improve RA outcomes? *Ann Rheum Dis* 2012;*71*(6):799–803.

66. D'Agostino MA, Terslev L, Wakefield R, et al. Novel algorithms for the pragmatic use of ultrasound in the management of patients with rheumatoid arthritis: from diagnosis to remission. *Ann Rheum Dis* 2016;*75*(11):1902–8.

67. Dale J, Stirling A, Zhang R, et al. Targeting ultrasound remission in early rheumatoid arthritis: the results of the TaSER study, a randomised clinical trial. *Ann Rheum Dis* 2016;*75*(6):1043–50.

68. Haavardsholm EA, Aga AB, Olsen IC, et al. Ultrasound in management of rheumatoid arthritis: ARCTIC randomised controlled strategy trial. *BMJ* 2016;*354*:i4205.

69. D'Agostino MA, Boers M, Wakefield RJ, Emery P, Conaghan PG. Is it time to revisit the role of ultrasound in rheumatoid arthritis management? *Ann Rheum Dis* 2017;*76*(1):7–8.

70. Centola M, Cavet G, Shen Y, et al. Development of a multi-biomarker disease activity test for rheumatoid arthritis. *PLoS One* 2013;*8*(4):e60635.

71. Fleischmann R, Connolly SE, Maldonado MA, Schiff M. Brief report: estimating disease activity using multi-biomarker disease activity scores in rheumatoid arthritis patients treated with abatacept or adalimumab. *Arthritis Rheumatol* 2016;*68*(9):2083–9.

72. Reiss WG, Devenport JN, Low JM, Wu G, Sasso EH. Interpreting the multi-biomarker disease activity score in the context of tocilizumab treatment for patients with rheumatoid arthritis. *Rheumatol Int* 2016;*36*(2):295–300.

73. Baker KF, Isaacs JD. Prospects for therapeutic tolerance in humans. *Curr Opin Rheumatol* 2014;*26*(2):219–27.

74. Schett G, Emery P, Tanaka Y, et al. Tapering biologic and conventional DMARD therapy in rheumatoid arthritis: current evidence and future directions. *Ann Rheum Dis* 2016;*75*(8):1428–37.

75. Tiippana-Kinnunen T, Paimela L, Kautiainen H, Laasonen L, Leirisalo-Repo M. Can disease-modifying anti-rheumatic drugs be discontinued in long-standing rheumatoid arthritis? A 15-year follow-up. *Scand J Rheumatol* 2010;*39*(1):12–18.

76. van der Woude D, Young A, Jayakumar K, et al. Prevalence of and predictive factors for sustained disease-modifying antirheumatic drug-free remission in rheumatoid arthritis: results from two large early arthritis cohorts. *Arthritis Rheum* 2009;*60*(8):2262–71.

77. Ajeganova S, van Steenbergen HW, van Nies JA, Burgers LE, Huizinga TW, van der Helm-van Mil AH. Disease-modifying antirheumatic drug-free sustained remission in rheumatoid arthritis: an increasingly achievable outcome with subsidence of disease symptoms. *Ann Rheum Dis* 2016;*75*(5):867–73.

78. Ahern MJ, Hall ND, Case K, Maddison PJ. D-penicillamine withdrawal in rheumatoid arthritis. *Ann Rheum Dis* 1984;*43*(2):213–17.

79. ten Wolde S, Breedveld FC, Hermans J, et al. Randomised placebo-controlled study of stopping second-line drugs in rheumatoid arthritis. *Lancet* 1996;*347*(8998):347–52.

80. Haschka J, Englbrecht M, Hueber AJ, et al. Relapse rates in patients with rheumatoid arthritis in stable remission tapering or stopping antirheumatic therapy: interim results from the prospective randomised controlled RETRO study. *Ann Rheum Dis* 2016;*75*(1):45–51.

81. Tanaka Y, Hirata S, Kubo S, et al. Discontinuation of adalimumab after achieving remission in patients with established rheumatoid arthritis: 1-year outcome of the HONOR study. *Ann Rheum Dis* 2015;*74*(2):389–95.

82. Emery P, Hammoudeh M, FitzGerald O, et al. Sustained remission with etanercept tapering in early rheumatoid arthritis. *N Engl J Med* 2014;*371*(19):1781–92.

83. Kuijper TM, Lamers-Karnebeek FB, Jacobs JW, Hazes JM, Luime JJ. Flare rate in patients with rheumatoid arthritis in low disease activity or remission when tapering or stopping synthetic or biologic DMARD: a systematic review. *J Rheumatol* 2015;*42*(11):2012–22.

84. Verhoef LM, Tweehuysen L, Hulscher ME, Fautrel B, den Broeder AA. bDMARD dose reduction in rheumatoid arthritis: a narrative review with systematic literature search. *Rheumatol Ther* 2017;*4*(1):1–24.

85. El Miedany Y, El Gaafary M, Youssef S, et al. Optimizing therapy in inflammatory arthritis: prediction of relapse after tapering or stopping treatment for rheumatoid arthritis patients achieving clinical and radiological remission. *Clin Rheumatol* 2016;*35*(12):2915–23.

86. Klarenbeek NB, van der Kooij SM, Guler-Yuksel M, et al. Discontinuing treatment in patients with rheumatoid arthritis in sustained clinical remission: exploratory analyses from the BeSt study. *Ann Rheum Dis* 2011;*70*(2):315–19.

87. Naredo E, Valor L, De la Torre I, et al. Predictive value of Doppler ultrasound-detected synovitis in relation to failed tapering of biologic therapy in patients with rheumatoid arthritis. *Rheumatology (Oxf)* 2015;*54*(8):1408–14.

88. Oliveira I, Mensing W, Figueiredo C, et al. FRI0082 subclinical MRI inflammation does not predict relapse risk in rheumatoid arthritis patients tapering DMARDS. *Ann Rheum Dis* 2016;*75*(Suppl 2):456.

89. Rech J, Hueber AJ, Finzel S, et al. Prediction of disease relapses by multibiomarker disease activity and autoantibody status in patients with rheumatoid arthritis on tapering DMARD treatment. *Ann Rheum Dis* 2016;*75*(9):1637–44.

42

Clinical outcomes

David L. Scott

Introduction

Scope of clinical outcomes

Each disease has its own natural history. These histories reflect what would happen without medical interventions. Clinical outcomes assess differences between the overall benefits of medical treatments and the natural histories of untreated disease. Although effective treatment generally improves outcomes, some patients have poor outcomes due to adverse events. Clinical outcomes must therefore focus on groups of patients, with successful management giving substantially more positive than negative outcomes.[1-5]

In short-term diseases of sudden onset, it is simple to assess relationships between clinical interventions and disease outcomes. However, in long-term diseases such as rheumatoid arthritis (RA), outcomes reflect a large range of influences in addition to the disease itself and its treatment. These multiple confounding factors create challenges for judging the overall impact of treatment on outcomes.

Types of clinical outcomes

Clinical outcomes can be classified in several ways, including the nature of the outcome, whether it is defined in distinct categories or as a continuous variable and when it occurs.

The types of clinical outcomes measured fall into several broad areas:

- Disease measures: reflecting the presence and severity of the underlying disease, such as the presence and severity of joint inflammation in arthritis.
- End-organ damage: indicating the severity of the unwanted consequences of disease, such as the extent and severity of joint damage in arthritis.
- Quality of life measures: these more general assessments made by patients indicate the impact of their disease on their lives in general. Some are disease specific; for example, the Health Assessment Questionnaire (HAQ) assesses disability in arthritis. Others are generic and are applicable in all diseases; examples include the Short Form 36 (SF-36) and EuroQol.

Some crucial outcomes are of limited relevance in rheumatic diseases. The best example is death. Mortality rates associated with different medical interventions, though useful guides to the value of treatments, are only relevant in diseases with high mortality rates. In most rheumatic diseases, death is uncommon. Another example, the ability to work, is an increasingly important assessment of the overall impact of disease, but is not relevant in diseases affecting elderly patients who will usually have retired.

The scales on which clinical outcomes are assessed is a second issue. Some outcomes are categorical, which range from binary outcomes, like alive or dead, to longer scales dividing patients into three, four, or five categories. Some outcomes have longer numeric scales; examples include joint counts, radiographic scores, and quality of life measures like HAQ scores. Their apparent simplicity hides complex analytical issues. For instance, in measures like the HAQ, increments in scores along the scale from 0 to 3, although numerically similar, may not equate to identical changes in the disability.

The final domain is time. Outcomes can be short term—weeks and months—or long term, extending over years and decades. Short-term outcomes, though readily related to treatment, are often less relevant to patients. Clinical trials focus on short-term outcomes whereas observational studies explore longer-term outcomes.

This chapter focuses on disability and quality of life measures rather than disease activity and imaging outcomes. However, it is impossible to make sense of disability and quality of life without giving some consideration to the other outcome assessments, so they are mentioned briefly within the overview of outcomes.

International collaboration on outcomes

Since 1992 there have been regular meetings of the Outcome Measures in Rheumatoid Arthritis Clinical Trials (OMERACT) group. Although it initially started looking at outcomes for clinical trials in RA, it has been gradually transformed into a group evaluating outcome measures in rheumatology in general. Its work is widely disseminated.[6] As well as expanding beyond trials in RA, OMERACT has also involved patient partners, who have crucial roles in identifying key outcomes.[7]

OMERACT applies a filter to assess potential outcome measures. The original filter focussed on three key areas determine the relevant of the outcome measures used.[8] These comprised:

Box 42.1 American College of Rheumatology core data set for clinical trials

1 Tender joint count
2 Swollen joint count
3 Patient's assessment of pain
4 Patient's global assessment of disease activity
5 Physician's global assessment of disease activity
6 Patient's assessment of physical function
7 Acute-phase reactant value
8 Radiography or other imaging technique (for trials of one year or longer)

Reprinted from Felson DT et al. (1993) 'The American College of Rheumatology preliminary core set of disease activity measures for rheumatoid arthritis clinical trials. The Committee on Outcome Measures in Rheumatoid Arthritis Clinical Trials'. *Arthritis Rheum* 36: 729–40 with permission from Wiley and Sons.

- Truth: is the measure truthful, does it measure what is intended? Is the result unbiased and relevant? This area involves issues of face, content, construct, and criterion validity.
- Discrimination: does the measure discriminate between situations of interest? The situations can be states at one time (for classification or prognosis) or states at different times (to measure change). This area involves issues of reliability and sensitivity to change.
- Feasibility: can the measure be applied easily, given constraints of time, money, and interpretability? This area involves an essential element in the selection of measures, one that may be decisive in determining a measure's success.

This initial filter has been amended considerably over the years, and there is now a second agreed filter,[9] which is preferentially used by OMERACT. The second filter spans structure and process, and includes a methodological approach for introducing new outcome measures.

The first OMERACT meeting in 1992 resulted in agreement to introduce an internationally accepted core data set for clinical trials in RA, and this was widely adopted in future years.[10,11] These clinical outcomes are shown in **Box 42.1**. By 2017 most trials reported these outcomes. Kirkham et al.[12] evaluated 273 randomized trials of drug interventions for the treatment of RA registered in ClinicalTrials.gov between 2002 and 2016. Full publications were identified for completed studies from information in the trial registry or from an internet search. The full RA core outcome set was reported in 81% (116/143) of trials identified on the registry as completed (or terminated) for which results were found in either the published literature or the registry. They concluded that the uptake of the RA core outcome set in clinical trials has continued to increase over time, though not all trials report them.

Range of clinical outcomes in rheumatoid arthritis

Overview

The RA outcome matrix spans five domains (Table 42.1). Outcomes include symptoms and assessments of disease activity,[13] damage, and quality of life, the overall result—remission—and end results like joint replacement and death. There is no need to record all outcomes. A few measures can capture the impact of treatment. Joint counts and acute-phase measures like the erythrocyte sedimentation rate (ESR) are most useful in short-term studies whereas joint replacement and death are more relevant in long-term studies.

Symptoms and disease activity

Disease activity is in essence the severity of symptoms of RA. Although much has been written on how to assess disease activity, starting off with the development of integrated clinical assessments like the disease activity score (DAS),[14] the exact nature of disease activity is implied rather than clearly defined. However, patients with high activity disease have many swollen and tender joints, while patients with low disease activity have few. Historically, many individual measures were assessed, but it became self-evident about 30 years ago that the different measures needed to be combined in a single index.[15]

Using the internationally agreed core data set (Box 42.1), two approaches have been taken to define changes in disease activity and assess disease activity levels. The first of these is the development of response criteria. The American College of Rheumatology (ACR) criteria define response in these domains varying from 20% to 70% (ACR20, ACR50, and ACR70 responses). ACR20 responses require 20% improvement in tender and swollen joint counts and 20% improvement in three of the five remaining core set measures (patient and physician global assessments, pain, disability, and an acute-phase reactant).[16] The ACR50 and ACR70 thresholds are substantially higher and potentially have less value in determining clinical effectiveness in trials.[17] There have been concerns about the overall value of dichotomizing patients into responders and nonresponders on the basis of ACR20 and similar assessments.[18] These response criteria were designed for clinical trials and are not readily transferable to routine clinical practice settings.

The second way of combining the core data set assessments is in an integrated score. The most widely used of these is the DAS, and particularly its variant the DAS for 28 joints—the DAS28—which initially used the ESR as its acute-phase reactant.[13] There are a multiplicity of variants of the DAS, including using C-reactive protein instead of the ESR.[19] Using DAS28 with the ESR it has been possible to divide patients into different disease activity levels (from active to

Table 42.1 Outcome matrix for rheumatoid arthritis

Symptoms	Damage	Quality of life	Overall	End result
Joint counts	New erosions	HAQ	Remission	Joint replacement
ESR	Sharp scores	AIMS2	Work disability	Death
C-reactive protein	Larsen scores	SF-36		
DAS28 scores		EuroQol		
		NHP		

AIMS2, Arthritis Impact Measurement Scale 2; ESR, erythrocyte sedimentation rate; HAQ, Health Assessment Questionnaire; NHP, Nottingham Health Profile; SF-36, Short Form 36.

remission) and to provide response criteria that are broadly equivalent to ACR responders. These are summarized in Table 42.2.

DAS28 scores require relatively complex arithmetical calculations and there are simpler ways to combine the core data set measures.[20,21] Aletaha and his colleagues[22] have developed the Clinical Disease Activity Index (CDAI) and the Simplified Disease Activity Index (SDAI). The CDAI does not require any blood tests. The SDAI requires measurement of the C-reactive protein. Both provide combined assessments which can readily be used in clinical practice and trials and do not require any complex calculations. These different measures all have their pros and cons. However, for all of them the benefits of regular clinical measurement outweigh any of their limitations. It is therefore preferable for clinicians to use one of them routinely, and for pragmatic reasons it seems sensible to keep using one measure. In terms of the extent of their use, DAS28 currently dominates the field.

Finally, patient self-assessment can be used to replace the traditional measures such as DAS28 in which joint counts are assessed by clinicians. One of the best known of these measures is the RAPID3 (Routine Assessment of Patient Index Data 3),[23] which gives similar results to DAS28 and CDAI.

Joint damage

Assessing damage to the joints is an important clinical outcome assessment in RA, though it is often undertaken separately from measures of disease activity and disability and quality of life. It is the key measure of end-organ damage in RA, and is related to the need for joint replacement surgery in established disease. There are three different ways to assess joint damage. The conventional approach is to use radiological assessments. However, magnetic resonance imaging (MRI) and ultrasound all have additional roles.

Plain radiology uses standard imaging methods such as Sharp scores, and their various modifications, and Larsen scores.[24] In clinical trials the van der Heijde modified Sharp method has become the dominant scoring method. Systematic reviews show effective treatment substantially reduces the progression of erosive damage; there is no evidence one form of intensive treatment is superior to another.[25,26] In individual patients the value of measuring progressive joint damage is less certain. However, X-ray changes remain important for decisions about diagnosis and joint replacement surgery.

There is evidence that the progression of radiographic joint damage has decreased over recent decades. A cohort study of radiographic disease progression in patients with disease onset in the 1970s to 1990s evaluated changes in 418 patients.[27] Those treated in earlier decades used fewer disease-modifying antirheumatic drugs (DMARDs), had longer disease durations and higher joint counts at their first visit. The rates of radiographic progression differed between decades with a significant trend towards less radiographic progression in more recent times. These findings suggested reduced erosive damage is more effective antirheumatic treatment and not the result of a secular trend. These temporal declines in X-ray damage have been confirmed in other cohort studies.[28]

A systematic review of 44 trials of tumour necrosis factor inhibitors in RA with study entry dates from 1993 to 2008 showed significant decreases over time in baseline swollen joint counts, C-reactive protein levels, and Sharp or van der Heijde modified Sharp radiological scores.[29] This study shows that erosive damage is a declining problem over time. However, the balance of expert opinion stills favours using X-ray scores as a clinical outcome is trials and observational studies.[30] This view is supported by evidence that minimal treatment of RA fails to control the progression of joint damage.[31]

Ultrasound and MRI are increasingly used to diagnose and assess RA and their value is accepted by international experts.[32] One problem with these highly sensitive methods is that they often show changes in symptom-free persons who do not have RA. A systematic review of 31 studies of MRI findings in 516 symptom-free people found MRI features of RA, particularly erosions, occur frequently in people without symptoms of RA.[33] The introduction of these new methods will have several challenges of this sort to overcome. Ultrasound is also particularly useful in assessing active synovitis as well as erosive damage, and this is likely to be its main role in future years.[34] Nevertheless, a systematic review of ultrasound in assessing erosive damage in RA provided strongly positive findings.[35] Defining the present and future roles of these imaging assessments lie beyond the goals of this chapter.

Disability and quality of life

Patients assess their disability, function, and quality of life. Consequently these measures are termed 'patient-related outcome measures' (PROMs).[36] In many health systems, such as the United Kingdom National Health Service (NHS), PROMs have assumed central positions. One reason is that they are easily measured. In addition, treatment should result in improvements noticed by patients.

The main limitation of PROMs is that they are highly subjective. If patients believe they are disabled or have major health problems, their scores will reflect these health beliefs. In addition, generic outcome measures were not designed for patients with arthritis and therefore are relatively insensitive in detecting improvements in health status. The various measures may not give identical findings. Patients may record poor outcomes in some scores but not in

Table 42.2 Patient-related outcome measures for function and quality of life

Measure	Health Assessment Questionnaire	Short Form 36	EuroQol
Abbreviation	HAQ	SF-36	EQ-5D
Use	Disease specific	Generic	Generic
Components	Function	Function Pain General health, Vitality Social role Mental health	Mobility Self-care Usual activities Pain Mental health

others. Finally, the various PROMs have scales of differing lengths with views on how to describe normal. Some consider normal function should be scored as zero, with limitations of quality of life-giving higher scores. The HAQ and the Nottingham Health Profile (NHP) are examples of such positive scoring. Others consider normal function should be classified as scoring 100% or 1 (on a 0–1 scale), with limitations of quality of life-giving lower scores. The Short Form 36 (SF-36) and EuroQol are examples of such negative scoring.

Patient-related outcome measures

There are three dominant measures. These are the HAQ, the medical outcomes survey Short Form 36 (SF-36), and the EuroQol (EQ5D). They are summarized in Table 45.3. These measures have been used in observational studies, clinical trials, and to a growing extent in routine clinical practice settings. There are also many other measures, which provide useful information but are less commonly used. The main outcomes differ in how they are scaled. Conventionally disability scores start with normal function being zero and worst function being the highest score. Conversely, quality of life scores usually start with normal scores being high (1 on a zero to one scale and 100 on a zero to 100 hundred scale). As quality of life decreases, the results fall. This divergence in direction between the scores can create complexities when explaining results using different scoring methods.

Health Assessment Questionnaire (HAQ)

HAQ scores, also termed the HAQ Disability Index (HAQ-DI), assesses function by asking questions across eight categories—dressing, rising, eating, walking, hygiene, reach, grip, and usual activities.[37] Patients respond on four-point scales, ranging from 0 (no disability) to 3 (completely disabled). These are added to give the HAQ score on a 0–3 scale. The smallest increment is 0.125. It is a disease-specific measure, designed for patients with arthritis, and is used mainly in RA. The HAQ has been widely translated into many different languages. There are floor and ceiling effects in that HAQ scores of zero can still mean some disability is present and HAQ scores of 3 cover quite a range of possible disability levels.

Studies of using HAQ have highlighted two general principles which are relevant across all outcome measures. The first of these is the nature of the scale. There is substantial evidence it is an 'ordinal' rather than an 'interval' scale.[38] This means that changes at different points in the scale are not all identical. This means that incremental units of the raw score at the margins of the scale reflect an increasing level of disability compared to similar units towards the centre of the scale. The measurement properties of HAQ may be less robust than those of other outcome assessments because of these variations.[39]

The second general principle is the minimal clinically important difference. Conventionally this is considered to be 0.22 for the HAQ.[40] However, there is evidence it may be somewhat smaller in routine clinical practice settings.[41] An additional complexity is that the ordinal nature of HAQ scores calls into question some of the assumptions underlying the use of minimally important clinical differences with the HAQ.[42] Despite these reservations and doubts, it is clinically helpful to have a general agreement on the size of change likely to be clinically relevant for patients.

Short Form 36

The SF-36 gives eight scaled scores based on patients' responses to 36 questions. Each domain is transformed into 0–100 scales. The eight domains are physical function, physical role, bodily pain, general health, vitality, social role, emotional role, and mental health.[43] The first four can be combined into a physical component summary score and the latter four into a mental component summary score. There are also shorter similar scores, such as the SF-12, which are brief but less sensitive to changing health. The SF-36 is a generic measure, designed to capture health status in many different conditions. Like the HAQ, the SF-36 has been widely translated. There are many data sets available for SF-36 scores in healthy control groups. The SF-36 scores are scaled from 0 to 100; 0 is the worst possible score while 100 is completely normal.

EuroQol

The EuroQol or EQ-5D consists of the EQ-5D descriptive system and the EQ visual analogue scale. The EQ-5D descriptive system has five dimensions: mobility, self-care, usual activities, pain/discomfort, and anxiety/depression.[44] Each dimension has three levels: no problems, some problems, extreme problems. EQ-5D can be presented for each dimension. Recently an extended 5-point scoring scale has been introduced. Usually the scores are combined in an index which ranges from 1 (completely healthy) to 0 (no health at all, which can be viewed as being equivalent to death); for technical reasons, some patients have scores below 0. The EQ visual analogue score assesses patients' current health as a 100 mm visual analogue score. The EuroQol is another generic measure which has been widely translated. Scores for normal healthy controls are widely available.

Others

There are many other disease-specific and generic PROMs. Examples of long-established but infrequently used measures include the Arthritis Impact Measurement Scale (AIMs-2),[45] the Nottingham Health Profile (NHP),[46] and the Rheumatoid Arthritis Quality of Life (RAQoL) questionnaire.[47] All have strong points and are useful and valid. However, for a variety of reasons, they are less widely used.

It is possible that some new PROMs may gain greater traction. One potential candidate to be more widely adopted is Patient-Reported Outcome Measurement Information System (PROMIS) physical function item bank, which has excellent measurement properties in RA.[48] It is a content-driven 20-item short form tool that can be used to assess patients' physical function. Another candidate is the Rheumatoid Arthritis Impact of Disease (RAID) score, which is a European League Against Rheumatism (EULAR) initiative.[49] It covers a range of outcomes with seven domains spanning pain, functional disability, fatigue, emotional well-being, and sleep, coping, and physical well-being. It has performed well when evaluated in a range of patients seen in a variety of clinical settings.[50] One final PROM has been promoted by Arthritis Research UK—the Arthritis Research UK Musculo-Skeletal Health Questionnaire (MSK-HQ).[51] It covers a similar range of domains including pain severity, physical function, work interference, social interference, sleep, fatigue, emotional health, physical activity, independence, understanding, confidence to self-manage, and overall impact. It is intended to be used across a broad range of musculoskeletal disorders and not be restricted to RA or inflammatory arthritis. The existence of so many different patient-reported outcome measures (PROMs) suggests that none are ideal. Whether one or other of these new measures becomes a dominant measure is difficult to predict. Although it may be preferable to have international agreement to use a single measure, it is likely to be challenging obtaining such agreement.

Outcomes in context

Interrelationships between outcomes

Different clinical outcomes are closely interrelated. Patients with arthritis who have good clinical outcomes usually have reduced joint counts, less joint damage, and better quality of life. The converse is equally true. As a consequence, there is no need to measure all outcomes; a few carefully chosen outcomes can capture the overall response to treatment. Reducing the number of outcomes measured has some limitations. Several other factors are involved in determining individual outcomes. For example, in patients with RA the presence of rheumatoid factor increases the likelihood of erosive joint damage irrespective of the response to treatment. Similarly, the presence of comorbidities worsens patients' quality of life irrespective of their responses to treatment.

One crucial issue is whether some outcomes provide more useful information than others. Outcomes which capture issues of direct importance to patients are preferable to overtly medical outcomes. For instance, most experts believe it is more important to assess quality of life than laboratory measures like the ESR or erosive damage on radiographs. However, these patient-related outcomes have drawbacks: they can be highly subjective, they may show marked variations between patients, and their accuracy and reproducibility may be limited.

An associated issue is the generalizability of outcome measurements. Generic measures like the SF-36 and EuroQol can be applied across a wide range of diseases, including arthritis, connective tissue diseases, and non-rheumatological disorders. They provide comparable measures of the benefits of medical treatment in many patients. Such broad comparability is offset by reductions in sensitivity to changes in arthritis and a lack of specificity in detecting treatment effects.

Despite the close interrelationship between outcomes, caution is needed when using one outcome to assess possible changes in another. For example, using HAQ scores to assess potential changes in EuroQol raises several methodological complexities.[52] It is possible to take this approach provided other variables, such as pain are factored into the transformation.[53,54] The rationale for wanting to make such changes is to compare studies when undertaking health economic analyses and other assessments involving health utilities.

Confounding factors

Clinical outcomes attempt to capture the impact of treating rheumatic diseases. However, many other factors, often not directly related to the disease itself, are of equal importance. These confounding factors can make it challenging to compare outcomes between centres, because they may have very different confounding factors, which may not be unravelled by attempts to correct for them. Key confounding factors are:

• **Demography**: age, gender, and ethnicity are all relevant. Outcomes are worse in elderly patients, in women and patients from ethnic minorities.[55–57] HAQ also worsens with disease duration, though the interrelationships are complex.[58]
• **Deprivation**: poverty and deprivation worsen disease outcomes and to an extent these factors may explain relationships between ethnicity and poor outcome.[59–61]
• **Comorbidities**: patients with multiple comorbid conditions usually have worse quality of life and their outcomes are poorer for all diseases. The impact of depression is particularly important and has been studied in most detail for HAQ scores.[62–64]

These multiple confounding factors mean that comparing outcomes across units without adjustment will often show substantial differences. As it will be difficult to make appropriate adjustments, comparisons across centres may be flawed. Rather than treatment being similar at all units it ought to show considerable centre-by-centre variation.

Outcomes for health economics

PROMs inform health economic assessments. They are useful in the first steps of such analyses, which involve identifying the impact of an intervention on patients' quality of life.[65,66] Utility scores (on scales of 0–1, like EuroQol) when combined with information about time, can generate quality-adjusted life years (QALY). These are based on the number of years of life added by treatment based on the concept of perfect health being assigned the value of 1.0 down to a value of 0.0 for death.[67] Multiplying the average utility score by the time spent in this health state generates QALYs. Health economic analyses then compare the difference in QALYs attributable to treatment. The EuroQol can be used to directly measure QALYs, the SF-36 and SF-12 scores can be used to generate utility data, and HAQ scores can be used in modelling studies to provide data on QALYs. The potential role of these PROMs in judging the cost-effectiveness of treatments is an important part of their role in assessing health.

Integrated outcomes

Ideally outcomes should be captured using a single score or profile. This would have the benefits of simplicity and speed and would also allow comparisons to be made across units and countries. However, simple assessments may be inadequate and superficial and there is a complex balance between straightforward, easy approaches and oversimplifying complex problems.

Electronic capture, 'big data'

There is a growing belief that capturing PROMs such as HAQ electronically will add substantially to our understanding of RA and improve clinical management decisions. One example of this approach is the Measurement of Efficacy of Treatment in the Era of Outcome in Rheumatology (METEOR) database, which has collected information on data from 46 005 visits in 12 487 patients with RA.[68] It found it was possible to collect, store, and retrieve simple clinical data. Analysing the information collected in this way helped assess the quality of care given to patients with RA in a multinational setting within routine clinical practice.

Using PROMS to guide treatment decisions

There is also evidence that HAQ and other PROMs can be used to drive treatment decisions. Hendrikx and colleagues[69] found that a PROM-based algorithm was able to help specialists screen patients' disease activity before they attended routine outpatient visits. Using such an off-site monitoring system based on PROMs has the potential to rationalize the number and the timing of face-to-face consultations between patients and rheumatologists. It could also enable patients to manage their disease in a more proactive manner and increase their ability to make shared decisions with their specialists.

Limitations of patient self-assessment

The focus on self-assessment and PROMs has been accompanied by increasing understanding of the limitations of this approach. Studies of patient global assessments have highlighted the challenges involved. Firstly, there are wide variations in what patients are asked and this can lead to variability in findings.[70] Secondly, there are disparities between patients' perceptions and assessors' views.[71] Thirdly, patient recorded measures fluctuate substantially over time.[72] Finally, while patient global assessments are related to generic measures like SF-36, objective measures such as joint counts are less closely linked.[73] These limitations mean that self-assessments alone should not be the only outcome measures used. They also mean that caution is required when interpreting change in patient self-assessments.

Studies using the Health Assessment Questionnaire

Early rheumatoid arthritis

HAQ scores are often relatively high at disease onset and improve over the next 6–12 months due to the impact of treatment. Thereafter, they gradually increase over time. This has been termed the 'J-shaped' curve. There is some evidence that the nature of RA is changing over time, though this is controversial. Some groups have found that the pattern of change is similar, but more recent patients have lower mean HAQ scores, which may reflect changes in the disease itself, better treatment, and differences in referral patterns.[74] Other groups have found that the pattern of change and the degree of disability have remained similar over time, though disease activity levels have fallen due to improved treatment.[75] An example of these changes is shown in **Figure 42.1**.

Established rheumatoid arthritis

After the initial treatment has been completed, mean HAQ scores in established RA gradually increase over time.[58,76] The rate of increase varies between studies: it reflects the severity of disease, the extent of erosive damage, the effectiveness of treatment, and the presence of comorbidities. Historically the annual rate of increase in HAQ scores is in the region of 0.03 per year. This equates to an average 1% increase.[77] However, recent analyses suggest the rate of progression may be substantially less than 1% annually.[78] One reason for this uncertainty is that average increases in HAQ simplify a complex pattern of change. There is evidence from long-term observational studies that there are as many as four distinct HAQ trajectory subgroups, which vary from virtually no progression to fast rates of progression over time.[79] These patterns of progression are shown in **Figure 42.2**. Mean changes in HAQ scores do not show individual variation over short time periods, which can be marked. Mean changes hide the marked fluctuation in HAQ scores over months in individual patients.[80]

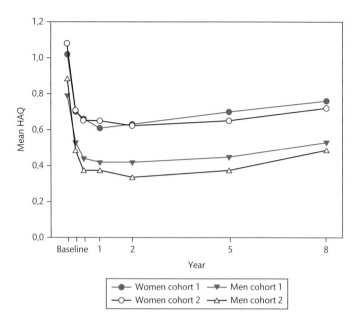

Figure 42.1 Functional disability during 8 years of follow-up. Cohort 1 is patients included between 1992 and 1999. Cohort 2 is patients included between 2000 and 2006. Data are reported separately for women and men. From the BARFOT study.

Reprinted from Andersson MLE et al (2017). Patients with Early Rheumatoid Arthritis in the 2000s Have Equal Disability and Pain Despite Less Disease Activity Compared with the 1990s: Data from the BARFOT Study over 8 Years. *J Rheumatol*; 44: 723–31with permission from the *Journal of Rheumatology*.

Clinical trials

HAQ scores fall with effective treatment, particularly with disease-modifying antirheumatic drugs and biologics. The changes are maximal by 6 months and thereafter stabilize. Systematic reviews show broadly similar falls with both simple treatment with disease-modifying drug monotherapy and intensive treatments with combinations of these drugs and biologics in more severe disease.[81]

However, the benefits of biologic treatments on HAQ may not be that dramatic. A systematic review of 28 trials of biologics by Barra et al.[82] evaluated treatments with five tumour necrosis factor inhibitors and three other types of biologic (abatacept, rituximab, and tocilizumab). The mean difference in HAQ scores after treatment was −0.22 (95% confidence intervals −0.24, −0.20) in patients who had failed disease-modifying drugs. In early RA the difference was −0.19 (95% confidence intervals −0.26, −0.13). As these differences were at the same level or below the minimally clinically important difference for HAQ, there was some uncertainty about the clinical significance of these differences. Another Cochrane systematic review provided broadly similar findings; in some analyses the impact of biologics is not necessarily clinically significant.[83]

Trials with the new Janus kinase inhibitors tofacitinib and baricitinib have also evaluated their impact on HAQ scores. Analyses of individual trials with these drugs show that in the initial months of treatment there are significant and clinically relevant improvements in HAQ scores with active treatment compared to placebo controls over 3 months.[84,85] There is insufficient research to know whether these new drugs are similar in their effectiveness than biologics or potentially give greater improvements. The differences could be due to the patients studied or the drugs themselves.

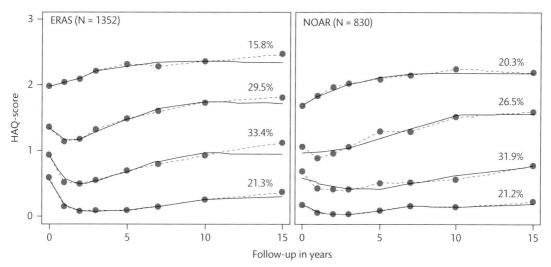

Figure 42.2 Long-term observational studies show four distinct HAQ trajectory subgroups varying from virtually no progression to fast rates of progression over time. ERAS—Early Rheumatoid Arthritis Study, NOAR—Norfolk Arthritis Register.
Reprinted from Norton S, et al (2014) 'Health Assessment Questionnaire disability progression in early rheumatoid arthritis: systematic review and analysis of two inception cohorts'. *Semin Arthritis Rheum* 44: 131–44 with permission from Elsevier.

Changes in HAQ scores are closely related to improvements in disease activity assessments. Data from three RA trials using conventional disease-modifying drugs (methotrexate, leflunomide, and sulfasalazine) found changes in mean HAQ scores occurred rapidly, and were noted after 1 month of treatment.[86] Further evaluation of this trial data showed changes in HAQ were highly suggestive that patients were receiving active treatment compared to placebo therapy.[87]

An analysis of over 7000 patients from 84 centres across 30 countries[88] found the proportion of variances attributable to recruiting centre was lower for patient-reported outcomes such as HAQ compared with objective measures such as joint counts and the ESR. This may explain the superior performance of measures like HAQ in assessing treatment response as these is far lower intercentre variability using this measure. Despite these apparent benefits of HAQ scores as a primary clinical assessment, it is unlikely to replace conventional disease activity measures.

Fibromyalgic rheumatoid arthritis

Some patients with RA have high levels of pain and fatigue and features of fibromyalgia. These patients form a distinct subset and their clinical features indicate an excess of tender joints compared to the number of swollen joints present. About 10–15% of patients have fibromyalgic rheumatoid and these patients have substantially higher HAQ scores compared to their disease activity levels.[89] These patients have increased pain sensitivity which may explain some of their clinical features.[90] Despite these differences patients with fibromyalgic disease have similar responses to treatment to other patients with RA.[91]

Treating to target

There is a strong international consensus that treating patients so that they achieve the therapeutic target of remission or low disease activity significantly improves their clinical outcomes. This approach is considered to benefit both early and established disease.[92] There is evidence from both a systematic review of clinical trials

and from observational studies that this approach reduces HAQ and improves other health status measures.[93,94] Whether low disease activity or remission are the optimal target, particularly in established RA has yet to be fully resolved.

Studies with the Short Form 36 health survey

The SF-36 shows a complex profile of outcomes in RA. Functional domains show marked changes, with very low scores. Mental health domains show less severe changes, though these are reduced compared to healthy individuals.[95] There is some evidence that mental health domains show similar changes to those seen in major treated psychological diseases like depression. These changes are shown in **Figure 42.3**.

A systematic review of observational studies of SF-36 scores in RA analysed findings in 31 studies.[96] In total 31 studies were studied; they included 22 335 patients. Pooled mean scores for the SF-36 physical component summary was 34 (95% confidence intervals 22, 46) and mental component summary was 46 (95% confidence intervals 30, 61). Increased age was associated with reduced physical function and physical component summary scores but improved mental health and mental component summary scores. Longer disease duration was associated with improved mental component summary scores. These results show patients with RA have substantially reduced health-related quality of life assessed by on the SF36.

Many trials have included the SF-36. A systematic review by Frendl and Ware[97] identified 151 trials in which primary clinical and SF-36 outcomes were concordant. Among clinically efficacious trials, 58% reported mean SF-36 improvements above the minimal clinically important difference threshold. However, SF-36 changes were often modest. This review showed that the SF-36 responds to treatment impact, distinguishing drug therapies that, on average, produce meaningful functional health benefits.

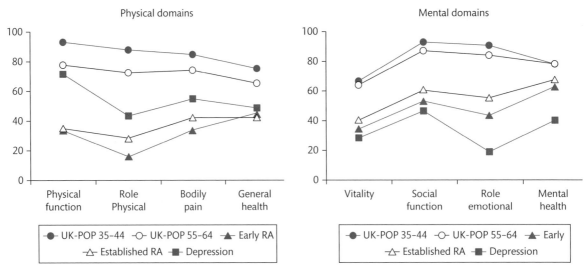

Figure 42.3 SF-36 scores from physical and mental domains in 913 patients with rheumatoid arthritis, healthy people, and patients with depression. Reprinted from Lempp H, et al (2011) 'Comparative quality of life in patients with depression and rheumatoid arthritis'. *Int Rev Psychiatry* 23: 118–24 with permission from Taylor and Francis.

Studies with the EuroQol

There have been relatively fewer studies using the EuroQol. There are also complexities due to recent changes in scoring. The traditional EuroQol had three scoring levels, but this is being changed to five scoring levels; the impact of these changes are uncertain but they may affect the use of the EuroQol in health economic studies.[98] Although some trials assess EuroQol most of the information about its role in assessment comes from observational studies. One unusual feature of the EuroQol is that it has a biphasic distribution, which is because some patients consider their disease causes major health problems for them.[99]

Recent observational studies show EuroQol scores improve considerably when patients are treated with biologics. The improvements occur in the early months of treatment and thereafter they plateau.[100] There is also evidence from using the EuroQol in a clinical registry that patients who take disease-modifying drugs inconsistently have worse clinical outcomes than consistent users.[101] Finally, in some clinical trials the EuroQol has been used to show intensive treatment with disease-modifying drug combination gives more overall benefit than methotrexate monotherapy[102] and with Janus kinase inhibitors and tumour necrosis factor inhibitors compared to placebo.[103]

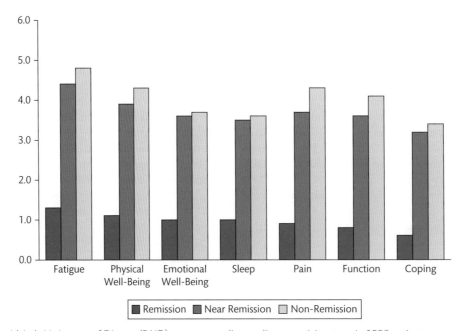

Figure 42.4 Rheumatoid Arthritis Impact of Disease (RAID) scores according to disease activity states in 1558 patients. Source: data from Ferreira RJO, et al (2017) 'Drivers of patient global assessment in patients with rheumatoid arthritis who are close to remission: an analysis of 1588 patients'. *Rheumatology* 56: 1573–8.

Other measures

New outcome measures such as the RAID and PROMIS assessments are just being introduced into clinical practice settings. The early studies using them have given positive results[50,104,105] and it is likely they will gradually become more widely used. They are simple to use but whether they will replace current assessments is uncertain. An example for RAID scores in one clinical study is shown in Figure 42.4.

Conclusions

Measuring disease outcomes is an essential for good medical care, which can only improve when clinicians know the results of their treatments and incorporate patients' views. Rheumatologists need to appreciate who they are seeing as patients and what happens as a consequence of their treatments. These sentiments are widely held but rarely followed. However, change seems inevitable with the widespread use of electronic records and the linking of records within and between institutions.

It is tempting to use outcome assessments to compare individual clinicians or units. However, this approach may be inappropriate and misleading. The diversity of patients and resources means heterogeneity is inevitable between and even within units. Rather than comparing absolute outcomes, we should focus on changes in outcomes. Despite the heterogeneity between units, clinicians should all be showing improved outcomes over time. The real cause of concern is not variations in absolute outcomes but differences in the direction of change. Poor performance is not having bad outcomes, so much as having worsening outcomes over time.

While clinical assessments, such as joint counts, reflect mainly what is happening to patients with RA, assessments of disability and health-related quality of life reflect a broader range of problems. They are influenced by disease activity and severity and also by comorbidities, age, and patients' views on the nature of their illness. When patients have many active joints, their arthritis is likely to be poorly controlled. However, when they have poor health-related quality of life many factors could be involved apart from their arthritis.

REFERENCES

1. Scott DL, Smith C, Kingsley G. What are the consequences of early rheumatoid arthritis for the individual? *Best Pract Res Clin Rheumatol* 2005;*19*:117–36.
2. Fransen J, van Riel, PL. Outcome measures in inflammatory rheumatic diseases. *Arthritis Res Ther* 2009;*11*:244.
3. Wells GA. Patient-driven outcomes in rheumatoid arthritis. *J Rheumatol Suppl* 2009;*8* 2:33–8.
4. Taylor RS, Elston J. The use of surrogate outcomes in model-based cost-effectiveness analyses: a survey of UK Health Technology Assessment reports. *Health Technol Assess* 2009;*13*:1–50.
5. Kingsley G, Scott IC, Scott DL. Quality of life and the outcome of established rheumatoid arthritis. *Best Pract Res Clin Rheumatol* 2011;*25*:585–606.
6. Outcome Measures in Rheumatology (OMERAT). Available at: https://www.omeract.org
7. Hsiao B, Fraenkel L. Incorporating the patient's perspective in outcomes research. *Curr Opin Rheumatol* 2017;*29*:144–9.
8. Boers M, Brooks P, Strand CV, Tugwell P. The OMERACT filter for Outcome Measures in Rheumatology. *J Rheumatol* 1998;*25*:198–9.
9. Boers M, Kirwan JR, Wells G, et al. Developing core outcome measurement sets for clinical trials: OMERACT filter 2.0. *J Clin Epidemiol* 2014;*67*:745–53.
10. Boers M, Tugwell P, Felson DT, et al. World Health Organization and International League of Associations for Rheumatology core endpoints for symptom modifying antirheumatic drugs in rheumatoid arthritis clinical trials. *J Rheumatol Suppl* 1994;*41*:86–9.
11. Felson DT, Anderson JJ, Boers M, et al. The American College of Rheumatology preliminary core set of disease activity measures for rheumatoid arthritis clinical trials. The Committee on Outcome Measures in Rheumatoid Arthritis Clinical Trials. *Arthritis Rheum* 1993;*36*:729–40.
12. Kirkham JJ, Clarke M, Williamson PR. A methodological approach for assessing the uptake of core outcome sets using ClinicalTrials.gov: findings from a review of randomised controlled trials of rheumatoid arthritis. *BMJ* 2017;*357*:j2262.
13. van Riel, PL, Fransen J. DAS28: a useful instrument to monitor infliximab treatment in patients with rheumatoid arthritis. *Arthritis Res Ther* 2005;*7*:189–90.
14. van der Heijde DM, van 't Hof MA, van Riel PL, et al. Judging disease activity in clinical practice in rheumatoid arthritis: first step in the development of a disease activity score. *Ann Rheum Dis* 1990;*49*:916–20.
15. Scott DL, Dacre JE, Greenwood A, Treasure L, Huskisson EC. Can we develop simple response criteria for slow acting antirheumatic drugs? *Ann Rheum Dis* 1990;*49*:196–8.
16. Felson DT, Anderson JJ, Boers M, et al. American College of Rheumatology. Preliminary definition of improvement in rheumatoid arthritis. *Arthritis Rheum* 1995;*38*:727–35.
17. Felson DT, Anderson JJ, Lange ML, Wells G, LaValley MP. Should improvement in rheumatoid arthritis clinical trials be defined as fifty percent or seventy percent improvement in core set measures, rather than twenty percent? *Arthritis Rheum* 1998;*41*:1564–70.
18. Felson DT, LaValley MP. The ACR20 and defining a threshold for response in rheumatic diseases: too much of a good thing. *Arthritis Res Ther* 2014;*16*:101.
19. Disease Activity Score (DAS). Available at: http://www.das-score.nl/das28/en/introduction-menu.html
20. van Gestel AM, Prevoo ML, van 't Hof MA, van Rijswijk MH, van de Putte LB, van Riel PL. Development and validation of the European League Against Rheumatism response criteria for rheumatoid arthritis. Comparison with the preliminary American College of Rheumatology and the World Health Organization/International League Against Rheumatism Criteria. *Arthritis Rheum* 1996;*39*:34–40.
21. van Riel PL, Renskers L. The Disease Activity Score (DAS) and the Disease Activity Score using 28 joint counts (DAS28) in the management of rheumatoid arthritis. *Clin Exp Rheumatol* 2016;*34* (5 Suppl 101):S40–4.
22. Aletaha D, Bécède M, Smolen JS. Information technology concerning SDAI and CDAI. *Clin Exp Rheumatol* 2016;*34*(5 Suppl 101):S45–8.
23. Pincus T, Furer V, Keystone E, Yazici Y, Bergman MJ, Luijtens K. RAPID3 (Routine Assessment of Patient Index Data 3) severity categories and response criteria: similar results to DAS28 (Disease Activity Score) and CDAI (Clinical Disease Activity Index) in the RAPID 1 (Rheumatoid Arthritis Prevention of

Structural Damage) clinical trial of certolizumab pegol. *Arthritis Care Res* 2011;*63*:1142–9.

24. van der Heijde DM. Plain X-rays in rheumatoid arthritis: overview of scoring methods, their reliability and applicability. *Baillieres Clin Rheumatol* 1996;*10*:435–53.

25. Graudal N, Jürgens G. Similar effects of disease-modifying antirheumatic drugs, glucocorticoids, and biologic agents on radiographic progression in rheumatoid arthritis: meta-analysis of 70 randomized placebo-controlled or drug-controlled studies, including 112 comparisons. *Arthritis Rheum* 2010;*62*:2852–63.

26. Graudal N, Hubeck-Graudal T, Tarp S, Christensen R, Jürgens G. Effect of combination therapy on joint destruction in rheumatoid arthritis: a network meta-analysis of randomized controlled trials. *PLoS One* 2014;*9*:e106408.

27. Finckh A, Choi HK, Wolfe F. Progression of radiographic joint damage in different eras: trends towards milder disease in rheumatoid arthritis are attributable to improved treatment. *Ann Rheum Dis* 2006;*65*:1192–7.

28. Carpenter L, Norton S, Nikiphorou E, et al. Reductions in radiographic progression in early rheumatoid arthritis over twenty-five years: changing contribution from rheumatoid factor in two multicenter UK inception cohorts. *Arthritis Care Res (Hoboken)* 2017;*69*(12):1809–17.

29. Rahman MU, Buchanan J, Doyle MK, et al. Changes in patient characteristics in anti-tumour necrosis factor clinical trials for rheumatoid arthritis: results of an analysis of the literature over the past 16 years. *Ann Rheum Dis* 2011;*70*:1631–40.

30. van der Heijde D, Landewé R. Should radiographic progression still be used as outcome in RA? *Clin Immunol* 2018;*186*:79–81.

31. Jansen JP, Vieira MC, Bradley JD, Cappelleri JC, Zwillich SH, Wallenstein GV. Meta-analysis of long-term joint structural deterioration in minimally treated patients with rheumatoid arthritis. *BMC Musculoskelet Disord* 2016;*17*:348.

32. Colebatch AN, Edwards CJ, Østergaard M, et al. EULAR recommendations for the use of imaging of the joints in the clinical management of rheumatoid arthritis. *Ann Rheum Dis* 2013;*72*:804–14.

33. Mangnus L, Schoones JW, van der Helm-van Mil AH. What is the prevalence of MRI-detected inflammation and erosions in small joints in the general population? A collation and analysis of published data. *RMD Open* 2015;*1*:e000005.

34. Takase-Minegishi K, Horita N, Kobayashi K, et al. Diagnostic test accuracy of ultrasound for synovitis in rheumatoid arthritis: systematic review and meta-analysis. *Rheumatology (Oxf)* 2018;*57*(1):49–58.

35. Szkudlarek M, Terslev L, Wakefield RJ, et al. Summary findings of a systematic literature review of the ultrasound assessment of bone erosions in rheumatoid arthritis. *J Rheumatol* 2016;*43*:12–21.

36. Marshall S, Haywood K, Fitzpatrick R. Impact of patient-reported outcome measures on routine practice: a structured review. *J Eval Clin Pract* 2006;*12*:559–68.

37. Fries JF, Spitz PW, Young DY. The dimensions of health outcomes: the health assessment questionnaire, disability and pain scales. *J Rheumatol* 1982;*9*:789–93.

38. Tennant A, Hillman M, Fear J, Pickering A, Chamberlain MA. Are we making the most of the Stanford Health Assessment Questionnaire? *Br J Rheumatol* 1996;*35*:574–8.

39. Taylor WJ, McPherson KM. Using Rasch analysis to compare the psychometric properties of the Short Form 36 physical function score and the Health Assessment Questionnaire disability index

40. Wells GA, Tugwell P, Kraag GR, Baker PR, Groh J, Redelmeier DA. Minimum important difference between patients with rheumatoid arthritis: the patient's perspective. *J Rheumatol* 1993;*20*:557–60.

41. Pope JE, Khanna D, Norrie D, Ouimet JM. The minimally important difference for the health assessment questionnaire in rheumatoid arthritis clinical practice is smaller than in randomized controlled trials. *J Rheumatol* 2009;*36*:254–9.

42. Doganay Erdogan B, Leung YY, Pohl C, Tennant A, Conaghan PG. Minimal clinically important difference as applied in rheumatology: an OMERACT rasch working group systematic review and critique. *J Rheumatol* 2016;*43*:194–202.

43. Ware JE, Sherbourne CD. The MOS 36-Item Short-Form Health Survey (SF-36). I. Conceptual framework and item selection. *Med Care* 1992;*30*:473–83.

44. Rabin R, de Charro, F. EQ-5D: a measure of health status from the EuroQol group. *Ann Med* 2001;*33*:337–43.

45. Meenan RF, Mason JH, Anderson JJ, Guccione AA, Kazis LE. AIMS2. The content and properties of a revised and expanded Arthritis Impact Measurement Scales Health Status Questionnaire. *Arthritis Rheum* 1992;*35*:1–10.

46. Hunt SM, McEwen J, McKenna SP. Measuring health status: a new tool for clinicians and epidemiologists. *J Roy Coll Gen Pract* 1985;*35*:185–8.

47. de Jong, Z, van der Heijde, D, McKenna SP, Whalley D. The reliability and construct validity of the RAQoL: a rheumatoid arthritis-specific quality of life instrument. *Br J Rheumatol* 1997;*36*:878–83.

48. Oude Voshaar MA, Ten Klooster PM, Glas CA, et al. Validity and measurement precision of the PROMIS physical function item bank and a content validity-driven 20-item short form in rheumatoid arthritis compared with traditional measures. *Rheumatology* 2015;*54*:2221–9.

49. Gossec L, Dougados M, Rincheval N, et al. Elaboration of the preliminary rheumatoid arthritis impact of disease (RAID) score: a EULAR initiative. *Ann Rheum Dis* 2009;*68*:1680–5.

50. Salaffi F, Di Carlo M, Vojinovic J, et al. Validity of the rheumatoid arthritis impact of disease (RAID) score and definition of cut-off points for disease activity states in a population-based European cohort of patients with rheumatoid arthritis. *Joint Bone Spine* 2018;*85*(3):317–22.

51. Hill JC, Kang S, Benedetto E, et al. Development and initial cohort validation of the Arthritis Research UK Musculoskeletal Health Questionnaire (MSK-HQ) for use across musculoskeletal care pathways. *BMJ Open* 2016;*6*:e012331.

52. Scott DL, Khoshaba B, Choy EH, Kingsley GH. Limited correlation between the Health Assessment Questionnaire (HAQ) and EuroQol in rheumatoid arthritis: questionable validity of deriving quality adjusted life years from HAQ. *Ann Rheum Dis* 2007;*66*:1534–7.

53. Hernández-Alava M, Wailoo A, Wolfe F, Michaud K. The relationship between EQ-5D, HAQ and pain in patients with rheumatoid arthritis. *Rheumatology (Oxf)* 2013;*52*:944–50.

54. Kim HL, Kim D, Jang EJ, et al. Mapping health assessment questionnaire disability index (HAQ-DI) score, pain visual analog scale (VAS), and disease activity score in 28 joints (DAS28) onto the EuroQol-5D (EQ-5D) utility score with the KORean Observational study Network for Arthritis (KORONA) registry data. *Rheumatol Int* 2016;*36*:505–13.

in patients with psoriatic arthritis and rheumatoid arthritis. *Arthritis Rheum* 2007;*57*:723–9.

55. Camacho EM, Verstappen SM, Lunt M, Bunn DK, Symmons DP. Influence of age and sex on functional outcome over time in a cohort of patients with recent-onset inflammatory polyarthritis: results from the Norfolk Arthritis Register. *Arthritis Care Res* 2011;63:1745–52.

56. Camacho EM, Verstappen SM, Symmons DP. Association between socioeconomic status, learned helplessness, and disease outcome in patients with inflammatory polyarthritis. *Arthritis Care Res* 2012;64:1225–32.

57. Bruce B, Fries JF, Murtagh KN. Health status disparities in ethnic minority patients with rheumatoid arthritis: a cross-sectional study. *J Rheumatol* 2007;34:1475–9.

58. Wolfe F. A reappraisal of HAQ disability in rheumatoid arthritis. *Arthritis Rheum* 2000;43:2751–61.

59. Katz PP, Barton J, Trupin L, Schmajuk G, Yazdany J, Ruiz PJ, Yelin E. Poverty, depression, or lost in translation? ethnic and language variation in patient-reported outcomes in rheumatoid arthritis. *Arthritis Care Res* 2016;68:621–8.

60. Baldassari AR, Cleveland RJ, Luong MN, et al. Socioeconomic factors and self-reported health outcomes in African Americans with rheumatoid arthritis from the Southeastern United States: the contribution of childhood socioeconomic status. *BMC Musculoskelet Disord* 2016;17:10.

61. Hifinger M, Norton S, Ramiro S, Putrik P, Sokka-Isler T, Boonen A. Equivalence in the Health Assessment Questionnaire (HAQ) across socio-demographic determinants: analyses within QUEST-RA. *Semin Arthritis Rheum* 2018;47(4):492–500.

62. Krishnan E, Häkkinen A, Sokka T, Hannonen P. Impact of age and comorbidities on the criteria for remission and response in rheumatoid arthritis. *Ann Rheum Dis* 2005;64:1350–2.

63. Scott DL, Wolfe F, Huizinga TW. Rheumatoid arthritis. *Lancet* 2010;376:1094–108.

64. Euesden J, Matcham F, Hotopf M, et al. The relationship between mental health, disease severity, and genetic risk for depression in early rheumatoid arthritis. *Psychosom Med* 2017;79:638–45.

65. Kobelt G. Thoughts on health economics in rheumatoid arthritis. *Ann Rheum Dis* 2007;66 (Suppl 3):35–9.

66. Schoels M, Wong J, Scott DL, et al. Economic aspects of treatment options in rheumatoid arthritis: a systematic literature review informing the EULAR recommendations for the management of rheumatoid arthritis. *Ann Rheum Dis* 2010;69:995–1003.

67. La Puma, J, Lawlor EF. Quality-adjusted life-years. Ethical implications for physicians and policymakers. *J Am Med Ass* 1990;263:2917–21.

68. Navarro-Compán V, Smolen JS, Huizinga TW, et al. Quality indicators in rheumatoid arthritis: results from the METEOR database. *Rheumatology (Oxf)* 2015;54:1630–9.

69. Hendrikx J, Fransen J, van Riel PL. Monitoring rheumatoid arthritis using an algorithm based on patient-reported outcome measures: a first step towards personalised healthcare. *RMD Open* 2015;1:e000114.

70. Nikiphorou E, Radner H, Chatzidionysiou K, et al. Patient global assessment in measuring disease activity in rheumatoid arthritis: a review of the literature. *Arthritis Res Ther* 2016;18:251.

71. Desthieux C, Hermet A, Granger B, Fautrel B, Gossec L. Patient-physician discordance in global assessment in rheumatoid arthritis: a systematic literature review with meta-analysis. *Arthritis Care Res* 2016;68:1767–73.

72. Studenic P, Stamm T, Smolen JS, Aletaha D. Reliability of patient-reported outcomes in rheumatoid arthritis patients: an observational prospective study. *Rheumatology* 2016;55:41–8.

73. Scott IC, Ibrahim F, Lewis CM, Scott DL, Strand V. Impact of intensive treatment and remission on health-related quality of life in early and established rheumatoid arthritis. *RMD Open* 2016;2:e000270.

74. Welsing PM, Fransen J, van Riel, PL. Is the disease course of rheumatoid arthritis becoming milder? Time trends since 1985 in an inception cohort of early rheumatoid arthritis. *Arthritis Rheum* 2005;52:2616–24.

75. Andersson MLE, Forslind K, Hafström I; BARFOT Study Group. Patients with early rheumatoid arthritis in the 2000s have equal disability and pain despite less disease activity compared with the 1990s: data from the BARFOT Study over 8 Years. *J Rheumatol* 2017;44:723–31.

76. Drossaers-Bakker, KW, de Buck M, van Zeben D, Zwinderman AH, Breedveld FC, Hazes JM. Long-term course and outcome of functional capacity in rheumatoid arthritis: the effect of disease activity and radiologic damage over time. *Arthritis Rheum* 1999;42:1854–60.

77. Scott DL, Garrood T. Quality of life measures: use and abuse. *Baillieres Best Pract Res Clin Rheumatol* 2000;14:663–87.

78. Stevenson MD, Wailoo AJ, Tosh JC, et al. The cost-effectiveness of sequences of biological disease-modifying antirheumatic drug treatment in England for patients with rheumatoid arthritis who can tolerate methotrexate. *J Rheumatol* 2017;44:973–80.

79. Norton S, Fu B, Scott DL, et al. Health Assessment Questionnaire disability progression in early rheumatoid arthritis: systematic review and analysis of two inception cohorts. *Semin Arthritis Rheum* 2014;44:131–44.

80. Greenwood MC, Doyle DV, Ensor M. Does the Stanford Health Assessment Questionnaire have potential as a monitoring tool for subjects with rheumatoid arthritis? *Ann Rheum Dis* 2001;60:344–8.

81. Ma MH, Kingsley GH, Scott DL. A systematic comparison of combination DMARD therapy and tumour necrosis inhibitor therapy with methotrexate in patients with early rheumatoid arthritis. *Rheumatology* 2010;49:91–8.

82. Barra L, Ha A, Sun L, Fonseca C, Pope J. Efficacy of biologic agents in improving the Health Assessment Questionnaire (HAQ) score in established and early rheumatoid arthritis: a meta-analysis with indirect comparisons. *Clin Exp Rheumatol* 2014;32:333–41.

83. Singh JA, Hossain A, Mudano AS, et al. Biologics or tofacitinib for people with rheumatoid arthritis naive to methotrexate: a systematic review and network meta-analysis. *Cochrane Database Syst Rev* 2017;5:CD012657.

84. Keystone EC, Taylor PC, Tanaka Y, et al. Patient-reported outcomes from a phase 3 study of baricitinib versus placebo or adalimumab in rheumatoid arthritis: secondary analyses from the RA-BEAM study. *Ann Rheum Dis* 2017;76:1853–61.

85. Strand V, Kremer JM, Gruben D, Krishnaswami S, Zwillich SH, Wallenstein GV. Tofacitinib in combination with conventional disease-modifying antirheumatic drugs in patients with active rheumatoid arthritis: patient-reported outcomes from a phase iii randomized controlled trial. *Arthritis Care Res* 2017;69:592–8.

86. Scott DL, Strand V. The effects of disease-modifying antirheumatic drugs on the Health Assessment Questionnaire score. Lessons from the leflunomide clinical trials database. *Rheumatology* 2002;41:899–909.

87. Strand V, Cohen S, Crawford B, Smolen JS, Scott DL; Leflunomide Investigators Groups. Patient-reported outcomes better discriminate active treatment from placebo in randomized

controlled trials in rheumatoid arthritis. *Rheumatology* 2004;*43*:640–7.

88. Khan NA, Spencer HJ, Nikiphorou E, et al. Intercentre variance in patient reported outcomes is lower than objective rheumatoid arthritis activity measures: a cross-sectional study. *Rheumatology* 2017;*56*:1395–400.

89. Pollard LC, Kingsley GH, Choy EH, Scott DL. Fibromyalgic rheumatoid arthritis and disease assessment. *Rheumatology* 2010;*49*:924–8.

90. Joharatnam N, McWilliams DF, Wilson D, Wheeler M, Pande I, Walsh DA. A cross-sectional study of pain sensitivity, disease-activity assessment, mental health, and fibromyalgia status in rheumatoid arthritis. *Arthritis Res Ther* 2015;*17*:11.

91. Durán J, Combe B, Niu J, Rincheval N, Gaujoux-Viala C, Felson DT. The effect on treatment response of fibromyalgic symptoms in early rheumatoid arthritis patients: results from the ESPOIR cohort. *Rheumatology* 2015;*54*:2166–70.

92. Smolen JS, Breedveld FC, Burmester GR, et al. Treating rheumatoid arthritis to target: 2014 update of the recommendations of an international task force. *Ann Rheum Dis* 2016;*75*:3–15

93. Stoffer MA, Schoels MM, Smolen JS, et al. Evidence for treating rheumatoid arthritis to target: results of a systematic literature search update. *Ann Rheum Dis* 2016;*75*:16–22.

94. de Andrade NPB, da Silva Chakr RM, Xavier RM, et al. Long-term outcomes of treat-to-target strategy in established rheumatoid arthritis: a daily practice prospective cohort study. *Rheumatol Int* 2017;*37*:993–7.

95. Lempp H, Ibrahim F, Shaw T, et al. Comparative quality of life in patients with depression and rheumatoid arthritis. *Int Rev Psychiatry* 2011;*23*:118–24.

96. Matcham F, Scott IC, Rayner L, et al. The impact of rheumatoid arthritis on quality-of-life assessed using the SF-36: a systematic review and meta-analysis. *Semin Arthritis Rheum* 2014;*44*:123–30.

97. Frendl DM, Ware JE Jr. Patient-reported functional health and well-being outcomes with drug therapy: a systematic review

of randomized trials using the SF-36 health survey. *Med Care* 2014;*52*:439–45.

98. Hernández-Alava M, Pudney S. Econometric modelling of multiple self-reports of health states: the switch from EQ-5D-3L to EQ-5D-5L in evaluating drug therapies for rheumatoid arthritis. *J Heanalth Econ* 2017;*55*:139–52.

99. Wolfe F, Hawley DJ. Measurement of the quality of life in rheumatic disorders using the EuroQol. *Br J Rheumatol* 1997;*36*:786–93.

100. Gülfe A, Wallman JK, Kristensen LE. EuroQol-5 dimensions utility gain according to British and Swedish preference sets in rheumatoid arthritis treated with abatacept, rituximab, tocilizumab, or tumour necrosis factor inhibitors: a prospective cohort study from southern Sweden. *Arthritis Res Ther* 2016;*18*:51.

101. Mjaavatten MD, Radner H, Yoshida K, et al. Do rheumatologists know best? An outcomes study of inconsistent users of disease-modifying anti-rheumatic drugs. *Semin Arthritis Rheum* 2015;*44*:399–404.

102. de Jong PH, Hazes JM, Buisman LR, et al. Best cost-effectiveness and worker productivity with initial triple DMARD therapy compared with methotrexate monotherapy in early rheumatoid arthritis: cost-utility analysis of the tREACH trial. *Rheumatology* 2016;*55*:2138–47.

103. Keystone EC, Taylor PC, Tanaka Y, et al. Patient-reported outcomes from a phase 3 study of baricitinib versus placebo or adalimumab in rheumatoid arthritis: secondary analyses from the RA-BEAM study. *Ann Rheum Dis* 2017;*76*:1853–61.

104. Ferreira RJO, Dougados M, Kirwan JR, et al. Drivers of patient global assessment in patients with rheumatoid arthritis who are close to remission: an analysis of 1588 patients. *Rheumatology* 2017;*56*:1573–8.

105. Bingham CO 3rd, Bartlett SJ, Merkel PA, et al. Using patient-reported outcomes and PROMIS in research and clinical applications: experiences from the PCORI pilot projects. *Qual Life Res* 2016;*25*:2109–16.

43

Clinical recommendations

Anna-Birgitte Aga, Espen A. Haavardsholm, Till Uhlig, and Tore K. Kvien

Management of early arthritis

The first EULAR recommendation for the management of early arthritis was published in 2007,[1-6] followed by a 2016 update.[7] The first version dealt with therapeutic aspects more strongly than the update, mainly since EULAR had not published treatment recommendations at that time.

The updated recommendations comprise three overarching principles and 12 recommendations for managing early arthritis (see Box 43.1). The selected statements involve the recognition of arthritis, referral, diagnosis, prognostication, treatment (information, education, pharmacological, and non-pharmacological interventions), monitoring, and strategy. Eighteen items were identified as relevant for future research. These recommendations provide both rheumatologists, general practitioners, health professionals, patients, and other stakeholders with an updated EULAR consensus on the entire management of early arthritis. The recommendations may be considered particularly important for rheumatoid arthritis (RA) since early diagnosis and treatment are important elements in a successful treatment strategy.

Management of rheumatoid arthritis

Treat-to-target

Reaching the therapeutic target of remission or low disease activity has improved outcomes in patients with RA. The main pillars of the treat-to-target recommendations are the definition of treatment target, namely clinical remission or at least low disease activity, the assessment of disease activity using composite measures that include joint counts, and adjusting therapy accordingly if the treatment target is not achieved within a particular timeframe. Abrogation of inflammation is the most important way to achieve these goals. The treatment of RA must be based on a shared decision between patient and rheumatologist, and the primary goal of treating patients with RA is to maximize long-term health-related quality of life through control of symptoms, prevention of structural damage, normalization of function, and participation in social and work-related activities.[8]

The treat-to-target recommendations are generic as they do not advocate any particular type of intervention, but just the principle that should be adhered to. The treat-to-target recommendations are based on systematic literature reviews[9,10] and an international expert opinion; they were first developed in 2010,[11] and updated in 2014.[8] See Table 43.1 for the updated 2014 treat-to-target recommendations, including comparison with the 2010 version.

Clinical remission is defined as the absence of signs and symptoms of significant inflammatory activity. Composite measures, in particular Clinical Disease Activity Index (CDAI), Disease Activity Score (DAS), DAS28, or Simplified Disease Activity Index (SDAI), should be generally used to assess disease activity, and the preferred target should be ACR/EULAR Boolean remission, alternatively DAS or DAS28 remission (see Chapter 16).

While remission should be a clear target, low disease activity may be an acceptable alternative therapeutic goal, particularly in long-standing disease.

The choice of the composite measure of disease activity and the target value should be influenced by comorbidities, patient factors, and drug-related risks. The therapeutic goal has to be individualized in patients with comorbidities, such as severe cardiovascular disease, uncontrolled diabetes, recurrent infections, or impairment of renal or hepatic function. Likewise, the treatment target and choice of composite measure of disease activity may be adjusted according to patient factors such as perception of pain, anxiety, and depression.[12,13]

EULAR recommendations

In recent years several efficacious agents treating RA have become available. Among the conventional synthetic (cs) disease-modifying antirheumatic drugs (DMARDs) rheumatologists adopted methotrexate in optimal doses as the anchor drug. In addition, a number of biological (b) DMARDs have been approved, and recently followed by targeted synthetic (ts) DMARD, with more drugs in development (see Section 7, Drug treatment).

New classification criteria of RA (see Chapter 2, Diagnosis) allow for identification of patients in their earlier disease course, and DMARD treatment should be started as soon as the diagnosis of RA is verified. The treatment should be aimed at reaching a target of sustained clinical remission (see Chapter 16, Disease activity assessment) or low disease activity in every patient within a particular time frame. The first step in the treatment strategy is methotrexate with rapid escalation to 25 mg/week plus short-term glucocorticoid aiming at >50% improvement within 3 months and target attainment within 6 months. Monitoring

Overarching principles

Management of early arthritis should aim at the best care and
must be based on a shared decision between the patient and the
rheumatologist

Rheumatologists are the specialists who should primarily care for patients with early arthritis

A definitive diagnosis in a patient with early arthritis should only
be made after a careful history taking and clinical examination, which
should also guide laboratory testing and additional procedures

Recommendations

Patients presenting arthritis (any joint swelling, associated with pain or
stiffness) should be referred to, and seen by, a rheumatologist, within
6 weeks after the onset of symptoms

Clinical examination is the method of choice for detecting arthritis,
which may be confirmed by ultrasonography

If a definite diagnosis cannot be reached and the patient has early undifferentiated arthritis, risk factors for persistent and/or erosive disease,
including number of swollen joints, acute phase reactants, rheumatoid
factor, ACPA, and imaging findings, should be considered in management decisions

Patients at risk of persistent arthritis should be started on DMARDs as
early as possible (ideally within 3 months), even if they do not fulfil classification criteria for an inflammatory rheumatologic disease

Among the DMARDs, methotrexate is considered to be the anchor
drug and, unless contraindicated, should be part of the first treatment
strategy in patients at risk of persistent disease

NSAIDs are effective symptomatic therapies but should be used at the
minimum effective dose for the shortest time possible, after evaluation of
gastrointestinal, renal, and cardiovascular risks

Systemic glucocorticoids reduce pain, swelling, and structural progression, but in view of their cumulative side effects, they should be used at
the lowest dose necessary as temporary (<6 months) adjunctive treatment. Intra-articular glucocorticoid injections should be considered for
the relief of local symptoms of inflammation

The main goal of DMARD treatment is to achieve clinical remission, and regular monitoring of disease activity, adverse events, and
comorbidities should guide decisions on choice and changes in treatment strategies to reach this target

Monitoring of disease activity should include tender and swollen
joint counts, patient and physician global assessments, erythrocyte
sedimentation rate (ESR), and C-reactive protein (CRP), usually by applying a composite measure. Arthritis activity should be assessed at
1-month to 3-month intervals until the treatment target has been
reached. Radiographic and patient-reported outcome measures, such
as functional assessments, can be used to complement disease activity
monitoring

Non-pharmacological interventions, such as dynamic exercises and
occupational therapy, should be considered as adjuncts to drug treatment in patients with early arthritis

In patients with early arthritis smoking cessation, dental care,
weight control, assessment of vaccination status, and management of
comorbidities should be part of overall patient care

Patient information concerning the disease, its outcome (including
comorbidities) and its treatment is important. Education programmes
aimed at coping with pain, disability, maintenance of ability to work and
social participation may be used as adjunct interventions

ACPA, anticitrullinated peptide antibodies; CRP, C reactive protein;
DMARD, disease-modifying antirheumatic drug; ESR, erythrocyte sedimentation rate; EULAR, European League Against Rheumatism; NSAIDs,
non-steroidal anti-inflammatory drugs.

should be frequent in active disease (every 1–3 months), and therapy
should be adjusted if improvement or target is not achieved. Without
unfavourable prognostic markers, switching to, or adding, another
csDMARD (plus short-term glucocorticoid) is suggested. In the presence of unfavourable prognostic markers (autoantibodies, high disease
activity, early erosions, failure of two csDMARDs) any bDMARD or
Janus kinase (JAK)-inhibitor should be added to the csDMARD. If this
fails, any other bDMARD or tsDMARD is recommended. See **Figure
43.1** for the updated EULAR treatment algorithm for RA, and see
Table 43.2 for the four overarching principles and 12 recommendations
for management of RA with DMARDs.[14]

EULAR developed the first set of recommendations for the management of RA with DMARDs in 2010,[15] and they were updated in
2013[16], 2016, and will be updated in 2020.[14] These recommendations
are based on systematic literature reviews,[17–19] international expert
opinions, and adherence to EULAR standard operating procedures
for the development of recommendations and to the Appraisal of
Guidelines for Research and Evaluation (AGREE II).

ACR guidelines

In 2015 the American College of Rheumatology (ACR) published a
new evidence-based, pharmacologic treatment guideline for RA.[20]
The guideline was based on systematic reviews to synthesize the evidence for the benefits and harms of various treatment options, using
the Grading of Recommendations Assessment, Development and
Evaluation (GRADE) methodology to rate the quality of evidence. The
strength of recommendations was graded as either strong (clinicians
are certain that the benefits of an intervention far outweigh the harms)
or conditional (uncertainty over the balance of benefits and harms).

The 2015 ACR guideline covers the use of traditional DMARDs,
biologic agents, tofacitinib, and glucocorticoids in early (<6 months)
and established (≥6 months) RA. In addition, the guideline covers the
application of a treat-to-target approach, tapering and discontinuing
medications, and the use of biologic agents and DMARDs in patients
with comorbidities such as hepatitis, congestive heart failure, malignancy, and serious infections. The guideline also addresses vaccines,
screening for tuberculosis, and laboratory monitoring for traditional
DMARDs. Topics related to diagnosis, monitoring of disease activity,
surgical interventions, or physical therapy interventions are not
covered by the guideline. In total, the 2015 ACR guideline includes 74
recommendations of which 23% are strong and 77% are conditional.

The ACR guideline addresses adult RA patients, defined as adults
≥18 years, meeting the ACR RA classification criteria (1987 or 2010
revised criteria).[21,22] The recommendations for treatment of early
RA applies to RA patients with duration of disease/symptoms of
<6 months, where 'duration' denotes the length of time the patient
has had symptoms/disease, not the length of time since RA diagnosis. The recommendations for treatment of established RA applies
to RA patients with duration of disease/symptoms of ≥6 months **or**
meeting 1987 ACR RA classification criteria.[20]

Six key principles and provisos were established as part of the
guideline development process:

1. Focus on common clinical scenarios, not exceptional cases.
2. Cost is a consideration in these recommendations; however, explicit cost-effectiveness analyses were not conducted.

Table 43.1 The updated recommendations (2014), including a comparison with the 2010 version

Overarching principles*		
2014		**2010**†
A.	The treatment of rheumatoid arthritis must be based on a shared decision between patient and rheumatologist	A. The treatment of rheumatoid arthritis must be based on a shared decision between patient and rheumatologist
B.	The primary goal of treating patients with rheumatoid arthritis is to maximize long-term health-related quality of life through control of symptoms, prevention of structural damage, normalization of function, and participation in social and work-related activities	B. The primary goal of treating the patient with rheumatoid arthritis is to maximize long-term health-related quality of life through control of symptoms, prevention of structural damage, normalization of function, and social participation
C.	Abrogation of inflammation is the most important way to achieve these goals	C. Abrogation of inflammation is the most important way to achieve these goals
D.	Treatment to target by measuring disease activity and adjusting therapy accordingly optimizes outcomes in rheumatoid arthritis	D. Treatment to target by measuring disease activity and adjusting therapy accordingly optimizes outcomes in rheumatoid arthritis
Final set of ten recommendations on treating rheumatoid arthritis to target based on both evidence and expert opinion*		
2014		**2010**
1	The primary target for treatment of rheumatoid arthritis should be a state of clinical remission	1 The primary target for treatment of rheumatoid arthritis should be a state of clinical remission
2	Clinical remission is defined as the absence of signs and symptoms of significant inflammatory disease activity	2 Clinical remission is defined as the absence of signs and symptoms of significant inflammatory disease activity
3	While remission should be a clear target, low disease activity may be an acceptable alternative therapeutic goal, particularly in long-standing disease	3 While remission should be a clear target, based on available evidence low disease activity may be an acceptable alternative therapeutic goal, particularly in established long-standing disease
4	The use of validated composite measures of disease activity, which include joint assessments, is needed in routine clinical practice to guide treatment decisions	6 The use of validated composite measures of disease activity, which include joint assessments, is needed in routine clinical practice to guide treatment decisions
5	The choice of the (composite) measure of disease activity and the target value should be influenced by comorbidities, patient factors, and drug-related risks	9 The choice of the (composite) measure of disease activity and the level of the target value may be influenced by consideration of comorbidities, patient factors, and drug-related risks
6	Measures of disease activity must be obtained and documented regularly, as frequently as monthly for patients with high/moderate disease activity or less frequently (such as every six months) for patients in sustained low disease activity or remission	5 Measures of disease activity must be obtained and documented regularly, as frequently as monthly for patients with high/moderate disease activity or less frequently (such as every 3–6 months) for patients in sustained low disease activity or remission
7	Structural changes, functional impairment and comorbidity should be considered when making clinical decisions, in addition to assessing composite measures of disease activity	7 Structural changes and functional impairment should be considered when making clinical decisions, in addition to assessing composite measures of disease activity
8	Until the desired treatment target is reached, drug therapy should be adjusted at least every three months*	4 Until the desired treatment target is reached, drug therapy should be adjusted at least every three months
9	The desired treatment target should be maintained throughout the remaining course of the disease	8 The desired treatment target should be maintained throughout the remaining course of the disease
10	The rheumatologist should involve the patient in setting the treatment target and the strategy to reach this target	10 The patient has to be appropriately informed about the treatment target and the strategy planned to reach this target under the supervision of the rheumatologist

*As worded, these recommendations constitute solely a brief summary of the discussions on individual aspects of the task force's activity. The task force specifies that these recommendations must not be interpreted without taking the respective text accompanying each item into account.

†The numbers at the left of the 2010 recommendations refer to the original numbering at that time.

Reprinted from Smolen J S et al (2016) 'Treating rheumatoid arthritis to target: 2014 update of the recommendations of an international task force'. *Ann Rheum Dis* 75(1):3–15 with permission from the BMJ Publishing Group Ltd.

3. Disease activity measurement using an ACR-recommended measure should be performed in a majority of encounters for RA patients.

4. Functional status assessment using a standardized, validated measure should be performed routinely for RA patients, at least once per year, but more frequently if disease is active.

5. If a patient has low RA disease activity or is in clinical remission, switching from one therapy to another should be considered only at the discretion of the treating physician in consultation with the patient. Arbitrary switching between RA therapies based only on a payer/insurance company policy is not recommended.

6. A treatment recommendation favouring one medication over another means that the preferred medication would be the recommended first option. However, favouring one medication over the other does not imply that the non-favoured medication is contraindicated for use in that situation; it may still be a potential option under certain conditions.

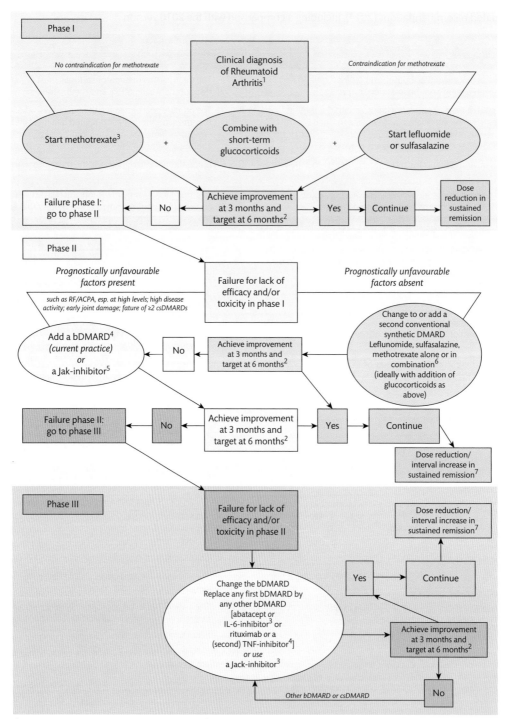

Figure 43.1 Algorithm based on the 2016 European League Against Rheumatism (EULAR) recommendations on rheumatoid arthritis (RA) management. ACPA, anticitrullinated protein antibody; ACR, American College of Rheumatology; bDMARD, biological DMARD; bsDMARD, biosimilar DMARDs; csDMARDs, conventional synthetic DMARDs; DMARDs, disease-modifying antirheumatic drugs; EMA, European Medicines Agency; FDA, Food and Drug Administration; IL, interleukin; MTX, methotrexate; RF, rheumatoid factor; TNF, tumour necrosis factor; tsDMARDs, targeted synthetic DMARDs.

Reprinted from Smolen JS et al (2017) 'EULAR recommendations for the management of rheumatoid arthritis with synthetic and biological disease-modifying antirheumatic drugs: 2016 update'. *Ann Rheum Dis* 76(6):960–77 with permission from the BMJ Publishing Group Ltd.

Table 43.2 The 2016 EULAR updated recommendations

Overarching principles

A	Treatment of RA patients should aim at the best care and must be based on a shared decision between the patient and the rheumatologist.
B	Treatment decisions are based on disease activity and other patient factors, such as progression of structural damage, comorbidities, and safety issues.
C	Rheumatologists are the specialists who should primarily care for RA patients.
D	RA incurs high individual, medical, and societal costs, all of which should be considered in its management by the treating rheumatologist.

Recommendations

1	Therapy with DMARDs should be started as soon as the diagnosis of RA is made.
2	Treatment should be aimed at reaching a target of sustained remission or low disease activity in every patient.
3	Monitoring should be frequent in active disease (every 1–3 months); if there is no improvement by at most 3 months after the start of treatment or the target has not been reached by 6 months, therapy should be adjusted.
4	MTX should be part of the first treatment strategy.
5	In patients with a contraindication to MTX (or early intolerance), leflunomide or sulfasalazine should be considered as part of the (first) treatment strategy.
6	Short-term glucocorticoids should be considered when initiating or changing csDMARDs, in different dose regimens and routes of administration, but should be tapered as rapidly as clinically feasible.
7	If the treatment target is not achieved with the first csDMARD strategy, in the absence of poor prognostic factors, other csDMARDs should be considered.
8	If the treatment target is not achieved with the first csDMARD strategy, when poor prognostic factors are present, addition of a bDMARD[1,2] or a tsDMARD[3] should be considered; current practice would be to start a bDMARD.
9	bDMARDs[1,2] and tsDMARDs[3] should be combined with a csDMARD; in patients who cannot use csDMARDs as comedication, IL-6 pathway inhibitors, and tsDMARDs may have some advantages compared to other bDMARDs.
10	If a bDMARD or tsDMARD has failed, treatment with another bDMARD or a tsDMARD should be considered; if one TNF inhibitor therapy has failed, patients may receive another TNF inhibitor or an agent with another mode of action.
11	If a patient is in persistent remission after having tapered glucocorticoids, one can consider tapering bDMARDs, especially if this treatment is combined with a csDMARD.
12	If a patient is in persistent remission, tapering the csDMARD could be considered.

DMARDs, disease-modifying antirheumatic drugs; boDMARDs, biological originator DMARDs; bsDMARD, biosimilar DMARDs; csDMARDs, conventional synthetic DMARDs; tsDMARDs, targeted synthetic DMARDs

1TNF-inhibitors: adalimumab, certolizumab pegol, etanercept, golimumab, infliximab boDMARDs or the respective EMA/FDA approved biosimilars; 2abatacept, rituximab (as first bDMARD under special circumstances), or tocilizumab or respective FDA/EMA approved biosimilars, as well as other IL-6 pathway inhibitors, sarilumab and/or sirukumab, once approved. 3 Jak-inhibitors (where approved)

Reprinted from Smolen J S et al (2017) 'EULAR recommendations for the management of rheumatoid arthritis with synthetic and biological disease-modifying antirheumatic drugs: 2016 update' *Ann Rheum Dis* 76(6):960–77 with permission from the BMJ Publishing Group Ltd.

Recommendations for the treatment of patients with early RA

The recommendations for treatment of early RA (disease duration less than 6 months) patients are provided in **Figure 43.2**.

Recommendations for the treatment of patients with established RA

Recommendations for treatment of established RA patients (disease duration ≥6 months), including tapering therapy, are provided in **Figure 43.3**. A treatment recommendation favouring one DMARD over another means that the preferred drug would be the recommended first option and the non-preferred drug may be the second option. There are several recommendations related to tapering therapy, in which 'Tapering' is defined as scaling back therapy, one medication at a time (reducing dose or dosing frequency). It is emphasized that patients' values and preferences should drive decisions related to tapering. A comprehensive plan to monitor disease activity and address possible flares should be implemented, and prior to tapering, RA patients should be informed of the risk of flare.

Recommendations in RA patients with high-risk comorbidities

Recommendations are provided in **Figure 43.4**, covering several high-risk conditions (congestive heart failure, hepatitis B and C, malignancies, lymphoproliferative disorders, and previous serious infections).

Recommendations for the use of vaccines in RA patients on DMARD and/or biologic therapy

Recommendations for use of vaccines in RA patients on DMARD and/or biologic therapy are provided in **Figure 43.5**.

Differences and similarities EULAR recommendations and ACR guidelines

Compared to earlier version of the ACR guidelines and EULAR recommendations for the management of adult RA, the 2015 ACR update, and the 2016 EULAR update have come much closer together.[14,20] Both apply prognostic factors for stratification, and adhere to the principles of the treat-to-target strategy,[8] aiming for ACR/EULAR remission.[23] Compared to the ACR, the EULAR recommendations are somewhat clearer regarding glucocorticoid use,

Recommendations for patients with symptomatic <u>Early RA</u>	Level of Evidence (evidence reviewed)
1. **Regardless of disease activity level, use a treat-to-target strategy rather than a non-targeted approach (PICO A.1).**	**Low (17)**
2. **If the disease activity is low, in patients who have never taken a DMARD:** • **use DMARD monotherapy (MTX preferred) over double therapy (PICO A.2).** • **use DMARD monotherapy (MTX preferred) over triple therapy (PICO A.3).**	**Low (18-21)** **Low (22-25)**
3. *If the disease activity is moderate or high, in patients who have never taken a DMARD:* • *use DMARD monotherapy over double therapy (PICO A.4).* • *use DMARD monotherapy over triple therapy (PICO A.5).*	*Moderate (18,20,21)* *High (22-25)*
4. **If disease activity remains moderate or high despite DMARD monotherapy (with or without glucocorticoids), use combination DMARDs <u>or</u> a TNFi <u>or</u> a non-TNF biologic (all choices with or without MTX, in no particular order of preference), rather than continuing DMARD monotherapy alone (PICO A.7).**	**Low (26-28)**
5. *If disease activity remains moderate or high despite DMARDs:* • *use a TNFi monotherapy over tofacitinib monotherapy (PICO A.8).* • *use a TNFi + MTX over tofacitinib + MTX (PICO A.9).*	*Low (29)* *Low (30)*
6. *If disease activity remains moderate or high despite DMARD (PICO A.6) or biologic therapies (PICO A.12), add low-dose glucocorticoids.*	*Moderate (31-37)* *Low (31-37)*
7. *If disease flares, add short-term glucocorticoids at the lowest possible dose and for the shortest possible duration (PICO A.10, A.11).*	*Very low (38-43)*

Figure 43.2 Summary of 2015 American College of Rheumatology recommendations for the treatment of early rheumatoid arthritis (RA). Green and bolded = strong recommendation. A strong recommendation means that the panel was confident that the desirable effects of following the recommendation outweigh the undesirable effects (or vice versa), so the course of action would apply to most patients, and only a small proportion would not want to follow the recommendation. Yellow and italicized = conditional recommendation: The desirable effects of following the recommendation probably outweigh the undesirable effects, so the course of action would apply to the majority of the patients, but some may not want to follow the recommendation. Because of this, conditional recommendations are preference sensitive and always warrant a shared decision-making approach. A treatment recommendation favouring one medication over another means that the preferred medication would be the recommended first option and the non-preferred medication may be the second option. Favouring one medication over the other does not imply that the non-favoured medication is contraindicated for use; it is still an option. Therapies are listed alphabetically; azathioprine, gold, and cyclosporine were considered but not included. Disease-modifying antirheumatic drugs (DMARDs) include hydroxychloroquine, leflunomide, methotrexate (MTX), and sulfasalazine. PICO = population, intervention, comparator, and outcomes; TNFi = tumour necrosis factor inhibitor.
Reprinted from Singh J et al (2016) '2015 American College of Rheumatology Guideline for the Treatment of Rheumatoid Arthritis'. *Arthritis & Rheumatology* 68(1):1–26 with permission from John Wiley and Sons.

especially in early RA concerning bridging therapy. Also the EULAR recommendations state that bDMARDs should be used in combination with csDMARDs (methotrexate) rather than as monotherapy. Also notably, the EULAR recommendations do not distinguish RA patients by disease duration (early versus established), but by three treatment phases (csDMARD-naïve, csDMARD-experienced, bDMARD-experienced). The ACR guidelines are more specific regarding treatment of RA with comorbidities, and addresses in more detail screening procedures, laboratory monitoring, and vaccination before and during DMARD treatment.

Other aspects

Biosimilars

Consensus recommendations for the use of biosimilars have been published by an expert group of specialists in rheumatology, dermatology and gastroenterology, and pharmacologists, patients, and a regulator from ten countries.[24] Five overarching principles and eight consensus recommendations were generated, encompassing considerations regarding clinical trials, immunogenicity, extrapolation of indications, switching between bio-originators and biosimilars and among biosimilars, and cost, see Table 43.3. The level of evidence and grade of recommendation for each varied according to available published evidence.

It is highlighted that the availability of biosimilars must significantly lower the cost of treating an individual patient and increase access to optimal therapy for all patients with rheumatic diseases. However, the discounts differ across different countries which also seem to be associated with the motivation to prescribe a biosimilar and especially to switch from the reference to the biosimilar product.

This consensus statement aimed to raise awareness about biosimilars and to discuss the key issues that healthcare providers must consider when using biosimilars to treat their patients. The assembled group of experts and patients achieved a high level of agreement about the evaluation of biosimilars and their use to treat rheumatological diseases.

Cardiovascular risk management

Cardiovascular disease risk is increased in patients with RA and this elevated risk is on the same level as in patients with diabetes mellitus.[25] This comorbidity problem motivated EULAR to publish recommendations for cardiovascular disease risk management in

Recommendations for patients with <u>Established RA</u>[1]	Level of Evidence (evidence reviewed)
1. **Regardless of disease activity level, use a treat-to-target strategy rather than a non-targeted approach (PICO B.1).**	**Moderate (44-46)**
2. **If the disease activity is low, in patients who have never taken a DMARD, use DMARD monotherapy (MTX preferred) over a TNFi (PICO B.2).**	**Low (47,48)**
3. *If the disease activity is moderate or high in patients who have never taken a DMARD:* • *use DMARD monotherapy (MTX preferred) over tofacitinib (PICO B.3).* • *use DMARD monotherapy (MTX preferred) over combination DMARD therapy (PICO B.4).*	*High (49)* *Moderate (18,20-25)*
4. **If disease activity remains moderate or high despite DMARD monotherapy, use combination traditional DMARDs _or_ add a TNFi _or_ a non-TNF biologic _or_ tofacitinib (all choices with or without MTX, in no particular order of preference), rather than continuing DMARD monotherapy alone (PICO B.5).**	**Moderate to Very low (23,26,29,30,47,48,50-59)**
5. **If disease activity remains moderate or high despite TNFi therapy in patients who are currently not on DMARDs, add one or two DMARDs to TNFi therapy rather than continuing TNFi therapy alone (PICO B.6).**	**High (60-65)**
6. *If disease activity remains moderate or high despite use of a single TNFi:* • *use a non-TNF biologic, with or without MTX, over another TNFi with or without MTX (PICO B.12 and B.14).* • *use a non-TNF biologic, with or without MTX, over tofacitinib with or without MTX (PICO B.13 and B.15).*	*Low to Very low (66-72)* *Very low[4]*
7. *If disease activity remains moderate or high despite use of a single non-TNF biologic, use another non-TNF biologic, with or without MTX, over tofacitinib, with or without MTX (PICO B.16 and B.17).*	*Very low[4]*
8. *If disease activity remains moderate or high despite use of multiple (2+) sequential TNFi therapies, first use a non-TNF biologic, with or without MTX, over another TNFi or tofacitinib (with or without MTX) (PICO B.8, B.9, B.10 B.11).*	*Very low (73-75)*
9. *If the disease activity still remains moderate or high despite the use of multiple TNFi therapies, use tofacitinib, with or without MTX, over another TNFi, with or without MTX, if use of a non-TNF biologic is not an option (PICO B.23 and B.24).*	*Low (29,30)*
10. *If disease activity remains moderate or high despite use of at least one TNFi and at least one non-TNF-biologic:* • *first use another non-TNF biologic, with or without MTX, over tofacitinib (PICO B.21 and B.22).* • *If disease activity remains moderate or high, use tofacitinib, with or without MTX, over another TNFi (PICO B.19 and B.20).*	*Very low (29,30)* *Very low (29)*
11. *If disease activity remains moderate or high despite use of DMARD, TNFi, or non-TNF biologic therapy, add short-term, low dose glucocorticoid therapy (PICO B.26 and B.27).*	*High to Moderate (33,41,76,77)*
12. *If disease flares in patients on DMARD, TNFi, or non-TNF biologic therapy, add short-term glucocorticoids at the lowest possible dose and the shortest possible duration (PICO B.28 and B.29).*	*Very low (40-43)*
13. *If the patient is in remission:* • *taper DMARD therapy (PICO B.31)[2].* • *taper TNFi, non-TNF biologic, or tofacitinib (PICO B.33, B.35, B.37) (please also see #15).*	*Low[3] (78)* *Moderate to Very low[3] (79,80)*
14. **If disease activity is low:** • **continue DMARD therapy (PICO B.30).** • **continue TNFi, non-TNF biologic or tofacitinib rather than discontinuing respective medication (PICO B.32, B.34 and B.36).**	**Moderate (78)** **High to Very low (79,80)**
15. *If the patient's disease is in remission, <u>do not</u> discontinue all RA therapies (PICO B.38).*	*Very low[4]*

Figure 43.3 Summary of 2015 American College of Rheumatology (ACR) recommendations for the treatment of established rheumatoid arthritis (RA). Green and bolded = strong recommendation. A strong recommendation means that the panel was confident that the desirable effects of following the recommendation outweigh the undesirable effects (or vice versa), so the course of action would apply to most patients, and only a small proportion would not want to follow the recommendation. Yellow and italicized = conditional recommendation: The desirable effects of following the recommendation probably outweigh the undesirable effects, so the course of action would apply to the majority of the patients, but some may not want to follow the recommendation. Because of this, conditional recommendations are preference sensitive and always warrant a shared decision-making approach. A treatment recommendation favouring one medication over another means that the preferred medication would be the recommended first option and the non-preferred medication may be the second option. Favouring one medication over the other does not imply that the non-favoured medication is contraindicated for use; it is still an option. Therapies are listed alphabetically; azathioprine, gold, and cyclosporine were considered but not included. Disease-modifying antirheumatic drugs (DMARDs) include hydroxychloroquine, leflunomide, methotrexate (MTX), and sulfasalazine. 1 = definition of established RA is based on the 1987 ACR RA classification criteria, since the 2010 ACR/European League Against Rheumatism RA classification allows classification of a much earlier disease state. 2 = tapering means scaling back therapy (reducing dose or dosing frequency), not discontinuing it. Tapering should be considered an option and not be mandated. If done, tapering must be conducted slowly and carefully, watching for increased disease activity and flares. Even for patients whose RA is in remission, there is some risk of flare when tapering. 3 = evidence is rated low quality or moderate to very low quality because some evidence reviewed for this recommendation was indirect and included studies with discontinuation rather than tapering of therapy or since studies involved patients achieving low disease activity rather than remission. 4 = no studies were available, leading to very low-quality evidence, and the recommendation was based on clinical experience. PICO = population, intervention, comparator, and outcomes; TNFi = tumour necrosis factor inhibitor.

Reprinted from Singh J et al (2016) '2015 American College of Rheumatology Guideline for the Treatment of Rheumatoid Arthritis'. *Arthritis & Rheumatology* 68(1):1–26 with permission from John Wiley and Sons.

High-risk condition	Recommendation	Level of Evidence (evidence reviewed)
Congestive heart failure[1]		
CHF	*Use combination DMARDs or non-TNF biologic or tofacitinib over TNFi (PICO C.1, C.2 and C.3).*	*Moderate to Very low (83,84)*
CHF worsening on current TNFi therapy	*Use combination DMARDs or non-TNF biologic or tofacitinib over another TNFi (PICO C.4, C.5 and C.6).*	*Very low[7]*
Hepatitis B[2]		
Active Hepatitis B infection and receiving/received effective antiviral treatment	**Same recommendations as in patients without this condition (PICO D.1).**	**Very low (85-92)**
Hepatitis C[2]		
Hepatitis C infection and receiving/received effective antiviral treatment	*Same recommendations as in patients without this condition (PICO E.1).*	*Very low (92-103)*
Hepatitis C infection and not receiving or requiring effective antiviral treatment	*Use DMARDs over TNFi (PICO E.2)[3].*	*Very low (92-103)*
Past history of treated or untreated malignancy[4]		
Previously treated or untreated skin cancer (non-melanoma or melanoma)	*Use DMARDs over biologics in melanoma (PICO F.1).* *Use DMARDs over tofacitinib in melanoma (PICO F.2).* *Use DMARDs over biologics in non-melanoma (PICO F.3).* *Use DMARDs over tofacitinib in non-melanoma (PICO F.4).*	*Very low (104-106)*
Previously treated lymphoproliferative disorder	**Use rituximab over TNFi (PICO G.1).**	**Very low (105,107)**
Previously treated lymphoproliferative disorder	*Use combination DMARD or abatacept or tocilizumab over TNFi (PICO G.2, G.3 and G.4).*	*Very low (105,107)*
Previously treated solid organ malignancy	*Same recommendations as in patients without this condition (PICO H.1).*	*Very low (105,108)*
Previous Serious Infection(s)[5]		
Previous Serious infection(s)	*Use combination DMARD over TNFi (PICO I.1)[5].* *Use abatacept over TNFi (PICO I.2)[6].*	*Very low (109-116)*

Figure 43.4 Summary of 2015 American College of Rheumatology recommendations for high-risk patients with established rheumatoid arthritis with moderate or high disease activity and congestive heart failure (CHF), hepatitis B or C, past history of malignancy, or serious infection(s). Green and bolded = strong recommendation. A strong recommendation means that the panel was confident that the desirable effects of following the recommendation outweigh the undesirable effects (or vice versa), so the course of action would apply to most patients, and only a small proportion would not want to follow the recommendation. Yellow and italicized = conditional recommendation. The desirable effects of following the recommendation probably outweigh the undesirable effects, so the course of action would apply to the majority of the patients, but some may not want to follow the recommendation. Because of this, conditional recommendations are preference sensitive and always warrant a shared decision-making approach. A treatment recommendation favouring one medication over another means that the preferred medication would be the recommended first option and the non-preferred medication may be the second option. Favouring one medication over the other does not imply that the non-favoured medication is contraindicated for use; it is still an option. 1 = conditional recommendations supported by evidence level ranging from moderate level to no evidence, supported by clinical experience and the Food and Drug Administration safety warning with tumour necrosis factor inhibitors (TNFi). 2 = strong recommendations for hepatitis B were largely based upon the recent American Association for the Study of Liver Diseases practice guidelines 85, 86, and clinical experience; conditional recommendations for hepatitis C were largely supported by very low-level evidence based upon case series and clinical experience. 3 = consider using DMARDs other than methotrexate or leflunomide, such as sulfasalazine or hydroxychloroquine. 4 = conditional recommendations supported by level of evidence ranging from very low to no evidence, are largely based upon expert opinion and clinical experience. 5 = conditional recommendation was supported by very low-level evidence. 6 = there was no consensus for making recommendations regarding the use of rituximab over TNFi or the use of tocilizumab over TNFi in this setting, due to indirect evidence (e.g. no comparison to TNFi or including patients with tuberculosis) and differences of opinion. In one study, compared to patients who restarted their previous TNFi following hospitalized infections, patients who switched to abatacept exhibited lower risk of subsequent hospitalized infections among the therapies examined. 7 = no studies were available, leading to very low-quality evidence, and the recommendation was based on clinical experience. DMARDs = disease-modifying antirheumatic drugs; PICO = population, intervention, comparator, and outcomes.

	Killed vaccines			Recombinant vaccine	Live attenuated vaccine
	Pneumococcal[1]	Influenza (intramuscular)	Hepatitis B[2]	Human Papilloma	Herpes Zoster[3]
Before initiating therapy					
DMARD monotherapy	✓	✓	✓	✓	✓
Combination DMARDs	✓	✓	✓	✓	✓
TNFi biologics	✓	✓	✓	✓	✓ (PICO J.1)[5]
Non-TNF biologics	✓	✓	✓	✓	✓ (PICO J.1)[5]
While already taking therapy					
DMARD monotherapy	✓	✓	✓	✓	✓
Combination DMARDs	✓	✓	✓	✓	✓
TNFi biologics	✓	✓	✓ (PICO J.4, J.5)[6]	✓	Not recommended (PICO J.2, J.3)[7]
Non-TNF biologics[4]	✓	✓	✓ (PICO J.4, J.5)[6]	✓	Not recommended (PICO J.2, J.3)[7]

Figure 43.5 2015 American College of Rheumatology (ACR) recommendations update regarding the use of vaccines in patients with rheumatoid arthritis (RA) starting or currently receiving disease-modifying antirheumatic drugs (DMARDs) or biologics. ✓ = recommend vaccination when indicated (based on age and risk). Red indicates vaccinations not recommended. The panel endorsed all 2012 RA treatment recommendations for vaccination with one exception (see footnote 6), and re-voted only for certain immunization recommendations in patients receiving biologics. All recommendations were conditional, except that the panel strongly recommended (in green) using appropriately indicated killed/inactivated vaccines in patients with early or established RA who are currently receiving biologics. Evidence level was very low for recommendations based on population, intervention, comparator, and outcomes (PICOs) J.1, J.2, J.3, J.4, and J.5. Evidence level for the remaining recommendations that were endorsed from the 2012 ACR RA treatment guideline was similar (on a different scale). 1 = the Centers for Disease Control and Prevention (CDC) also recommends a one-time pneumococcal revaccination after 5 years for persons with chronic conditions such as RA. The CDC recommends pneumococcal conjugate vaccine (PCV13 or Prevnar 13) for all children younger than 5 years of age, all adults ≥65 years, and persons 6–64 years of age with certain medical conditions. Pneumovax is a 23-valent pneumococcal polysaccharide vaccine (PPSV23) that is currently recommended for use in all adults ≥65 years old and for persons who are ≥2 years old and at high risk for pneumococcal disease (e.g. those with sickle cell disease, HIV infection, or other immunocompromising conditions). PPSV23 is also recommended for use in adults 19–64 years of age who smoke cigarettes or who have asthma (http://www.cdc.gov/vaccines/vpd-vac/pneumo/default.htm?s_cid=cs_797). 2 = if hepatitis B risk factors are present (e.g. intravenous drug abuse, multiple sex partners in the previous 6 months, healthcare personnel). 3 = the panel conditionally recommended that in RA patients ages ≥50 years, the herpes zoster vaccine should be given before the patient receives biologic therapy or tofacitinib for their RA. 4 = response to certain killed vaccines may be reduced after rituximab therapy. 5 = the panel conditionally recommended giving the herpes zoster vaccine before the patient receives biologic therapy or tofacitinib for their RA in both early or established RA patients ages ≥50 years (PICO J.1). The panel also voted that after giving the herpes zoster vaccine, there should be a 2-week waiting period before starting biologics. 6 = the panel strongly recommended that in patients with early or established RA who are currently receiving biologics, appropriately indicated killed/inactivated vaccines should be used (PICOs J.4 and J.5). 7 = the panel conditionally recommended that in early or established RA patients who are currently receiving biologics, live attenuated vaccines such as the herpes zoster (shingles) vaccine should not be used (PICOs J.2 and J.3). TNFi = tumour necrosis factor inhibitor.

Reprinted from Singh J et al (2016) '2015 American College of Rheumatology Guideline for the Treatment of Rheumatoid Arthritis'. *Arthritis & Rheumatology* 68(1):1–26 with permission from John Wiley and Sons.

patients with RA and other forms of inflammatory joint diseases in 2009.[26] A 2015–2016 update was published in 2017.[27] Much more evidence was available during these years. Based on the systematic literature review ten recommendations were defined, see Table 43.4.

Importantly, the rheumatologist is responsible for cardiovascular disease risk management in patients with RA (principle B). However, the organization will vary from hospital to hospital and country to country. A preventive cardiorheuma clinic may be an optimal, but resource demanding system.[28]

Pregnancy and lactation

Females during pregnancy experience an increased risk for adverse outcomes in mother and fetus. Drug treatment during pregnancy may be necessary to control maternal disease, and the risk of leaving a mother with active disease untreated during the whole pregnancy must be weighed against any potential harm through drug exposure of the fetus.

Adjustment of therapy in a patient planning a pregnancy aims to use medications that support disease control in the mother and are considered safe for the fetus. However, only a limited number of antirheumatic/immunosuppressive drugs fulfil these requirements. A EULAR task force updated available data from the literature and from several databases to reach expert consensus on their compatibility during pregnancy and lactation, resulting in EULAR points to consider for use of antirheumatic drugs during pregnancy and lactation (see Table 43.5).[29]

The observed association between non-steroidal anti-inflammatory drugs (NSAIDs) and miscarriage is controversial because confounding factors often have not been addressed in the studies. The majority of data relate to first trimester exposure. Exposures in the second and third trimesters have been reported for medications either regarded as compatible with pregnancy (examples glucocorticoids, azathioprine, antimalarials) or when serious maternal disease requires therapy during pregnancy (e.g. cyclophosphamide).

Table 43.3 Overarching principles (A–E) and consensus recommendations (1–8) for biosimilars

		Agreement* (%)	Level of evidence[†]	Grade of recommendations[‡]
Overarching principles				
A	Treatment of rheumatic diseases is based on a shared decision-making process between patients and their rheumatologists.	100	5	D
B	The contextual aspects of the healthcare system should be taken into consideration when treatment decisions are made.	100	5	D
C	A biosimilar, as approved by authorities in a highly regulated area, is neither better nor worse in efficacy and not inferior in safety to its bio-originator.	88	5	D
D	Patients and healthcare providers should be informed about the nature of biosimilars, their approval process, and their safety and efficacy.	96	5	D
E	Harmonized methods should be established to obtain reliable pharmacovigilance data, including traceability, about both biosimilars and bio-originators.	100	5	D
Consensus recommendations				
1	The availability of biosimilars must significantly lower the cost of treating an individual patient and increase access to optimal therapy for all patients with rheumatic diseases.	100	5	D
2	Approved biosimilars can be used to treat appropriate patients in the same way as their bio-originators.	100	1b	A
3	As no clinically significant differences in immunogenicity between biosimilars and bio-originators have been detected, antidrug antibodies to biosimilars need not be measured in clinical practice.	100	2b	B
4	Relevant preclinical and phase I data on a biosimilar should be available when phase III data are published.	100	5	D
5	Since the biosimilar is equivalent to the bio-originator in its physicochemical, functional, and pharmacokinetic properties, confirmation of efficacy and safety in a single indication is sufficient for extrapolation to other diseases for which the bio-originator has been approved.	100	5	D
6	Currently available evidence indicates that a single switch from a bio-originator to one of its biosimilars is safe and effective; there is no scientific rationale to expect that switching among biosimilars of the same bio-originator would result in a different clinical outcome but patient perspectives must be considered.	96	1b	A
7	Multiple switching between biosimilars and their bio-originators or other biosimilars should be assessed in registries.	100	5	D
8	No switch to or among biosimilars should be initiated without the prior awareness of the patient and the treating healthcare provider.	91	5	D

* Agreement indicates percentage of experts who approved the recommendation during the final voting round of the consensus meeting.

[†] 1a: systematic review of randomized clinical trials (RCTs); 1b: individual RCT; 2a: systematic review of cohort studies; 2b: individual cohort study (including low-quality RCT, e.g. <80% follow-up); 3a: individual case-control study; 4: case series (and poor quality cohort and case-control studies); 5: expert opinion without explicit clinical appraisal or based on physiology, bench-research, or 'first principles'

[‡] A: based on consistent level 1 evidence; B: based on consistent level 2 or 3 evidence or extrapolations from level 1 evidence; C: based on level 4 evidence or extrapolations from level 2 or 3 evidence; D: based on level 5 evidence or on troublingly inconsistent or inconclusive studies of any level

Reprinted from Kay J et al (2018) 'Consensus-based recommendations for the use of biosimilars to treat rheumatological diseases' *Ann Rheum Dis* 77(2):165–74 with the permission of the BMJ Publishing Group Ltd.

Available data from the literature and from registries show that a large proportion of medications can be taken by pregnant and lactating women with rheumatic disease without causing measurable harm to the fetus and child. Especially new evidence from the last decade strengthens the evidence for glucocorticoids, sulfasalazine, antimalarials, azathioprine, colchicine, ciclosporin, tacrolimus, and intravenous immunoglobulin (IVIGs) as being compatible with pregnancy and lactation. A practical consequence of the update is support for the use of tumour necrosis factor (TNF) inhibitor in the first half of pregnancy.

The difference in placental transfer related to molecule structure and half-life needs to be taken into account when selecting a TNF inhibitor for women of fertile age, and infliximab and adalimumab may preferentially be stopped at 20 weeks, and etanercept at week 30–32 of pregnancy. The CRIB and CRADLE studies have demonstrated that certolizumab pegol does not pass into placenta during pregnancy and that transfer to breast milk is also minimal.[30,31] Sound evidence for fetal/child safety is still lacking for golimumab, abatacept, tocilizumab, rituximab, belimumab, and anakinra.

Statements on lactation were restricted to compatibility, and included no detailed advice on timing, short-term discontinuation of breastfeeding, or discarding milk on days of drug administration.

The points to consider presented provide confidence that, in spite of limitations, effective drug treatment of active rheumatic disease is possible with reasonable safety for the fetus/child during pregnancy and lactation.

Table 43.4 Overarching principles and recommendations for cardiovascular disease risk in patients with RA

		Level of evidence	Strength of recommendation	Level of agreement (SD)
Overarching principles				
A	Clinicians should be aware of the higher risk for CVD in patients with RA compared with the general population. This may also apply to AS and PsA			
B	The rheumatologist is responsible for CVD risk management in patients with RA and other IJD			
C	The use of NSAIDs and corticosteroids should be in accordance with treatment-specific recommendations from EULAR and ASAS			
Recommendations				
1	Disease activity should be controlled optimally in order to lower CVD risk in all patients with RA, AS, or PsA	2b–3	B	9.1 (1.3)
2	CVD risk assessment is recommended for all patients with RA, AS, or PsA at least once every 5 years and should be reconsidered following major changes in antirheumatic therapy	3–4	C	8.8 (1.1)
3	CVD risk estimation for patients with RA, AS, or PsA should be performed according to national guidelines and the SCORE CVD risk prediction model should be used if no national guideline is available	3–4	C–D	8.7 (2.1)
4	TC and HDLc should be used in CVD risk assessment in RA, AS, and PsA and lipids should ideally be measured when disease activity is stable or in remission. Non-fasting lipids measurements are also perfectly acceptable	3	C	8.8 (1.2)
5	CVD risk prediction models should be adapted for patients with RA by a 1.5 multiplication factor, if this is not already included in the model	3–4	C	7.5 (2.2)
6	Screening for asymptomatic atherosclerotic plaques by use of carotid ultrasound may be considered as part of the CVD risk evaluation in patients with RA	3–4	C–D	5.7 (3.9)
7	Lifestyle recommendations should emphasize the benefits of a healthy diet, regular exercise, and smoking cessation for all patients	3	C	9.8 (0.3)
8	CVD risk management should be carried out according to national guidelines in RA, AS, or PsA, antihypertensives, and statins may be used as in the general population	3–4	C–D	9.2 (1.3)
9	Prescription of NSAIDs in RA and PsA should be with caution, especially for patients with documented CVD or in the presence of CVD risk factors	2a–3	C	8.9 (2.1)
10	Corticosteroids: for prolonged treatment, the glucocorticoid dosage should be kept to a minimum and a glucocorticoid taper should be attempted in case of remission or low disease activity; the reasons to continue glucocorticoid therapy should be regularly checked	3–4	C	9.5 (0.7)

AS, ankylosing spondylitis; ASAS, Assessment of Spondyloarthritis International Society; CVD, cardiovascular disease; EULAR, European League against Rheumatism; HDLc, high-density lipoprotein cholesterol; IJD, inflammatory joint disorder; NSAID, non-steroidal anti-inflammatory drug; PsA, psoriatic arthritis; RA, rheumatoid arthritis; SCORE, Systematic Coronary Risk Evaluation; TC, total cholesterol.
Reprinted from Agca R et al (2017) 'EULAR recommendations for cardiovascular disease risk management in patients with rheumatoid arthritis and other forms of inflammatory joint disorders: 2015/2016 update' *Ann Rheum Dis* 76(1):17–28 with permission from the BMJ Publishing Group Ltd.

Glucocorticoid-induced osteoporosis

Glucocorticoids (GCs) play an important role in the treatment of many inflammatory conditions, but can cause toxicity, including bone loss and fractures. The highest rate of bone loss occurs within the first 3–6 months of GC treatment. Often GC use is described for two categories: low (prednisone ≤7.5 mg/day) or high (>7.5 mg/day).

Updated ACR recommendations for the prevention and treatment of osteoporosis and fractures in patients receiving glucocorticoid treatment were published in 2017[32] and included therapies for the treatment of osteoporosis (OP) approved by the US Food and Drug Administration before 2015.

Panels agreed that the scope for recommendations should be the assessment, prevention, and treatment of OP and fractures in children and adults taking glucocorticoids (prednisone at ≥2.5 mg/day for >3 months), including patients with organ transplants, women of childbearing potential, and people receiving very high-dose GCs.

The recommendations were designed to optimize identification of patients at risk of GC-induced fractures so that they can

be appropriately treated, at the same time that risks and burden of testing and treatment were limited (see **Figure 43.6**).

The recommendations for glucocorticoid-induced osteoporosis (GIOP) cover:

- Reassessment of fracture risk
- Recommendations for initial treatment for prevention of GIOP in adults (women not of childbearing potential and men) beginning
- Long-term GC treatment
- Initial pharmacologic treatment for adults
- Recommendations for initial treatment for prevention of GIOP in special populations of patients beginning long-term GC treatment
- Recommendations for follow-up treatment for prevention of GIOP

Oral bisphosphonates were the preferred first-line therapy in the majority of clinical situations given their antifracture benefit, safety, and low cost, unless there are contraindications or concerns about patient adherence to treatment. Due to limitations in studies, most

Table 43.5 The EULAR points to consider for use of antirheumatic drugs before pregnancy and during pregnancy and lactation

		Grade of recommendation†
Overarching principles		
A	Family planning should be addressed in each patient of reproductive age and adjustment of therapy considered before a planned pregnancy.	
B	Treatment of patients with rheumatic disease before/during pregnancy and lactation should aim to prevent or suppress disease activity in the mother and expose the fetus/child to no harm.	
C	The risk of drug therapy for the child should be weighed against the risk that untreated maternal disease represents for the patient and the fetus or child.	
D	The decision on drug therapy during pregnancy and lactation should be based on agreement between the internist/ rheumatologist, gynaecologist/obstetrician, and the patient, and including other healthcare providers when appropriate.	
Points to consider for use of antirheumatic drugs in pregnancy*		
1	csDMARDs‡ proven compatible with pregnancy are hydroxychloroquine, chloroquine, sulfasalazine, azathioprine, ciclosporin, tacrolimus, and colchicine. They should be continued in pregnancy for maintenance of remission or treatment of a disease flare.	B
2	csDMARDs‡ methotrexate, mycophenolate mofetil, and cyclophosphamide are teratogenic and should be withdrawn before pregnancy.	B
3	Non-selective COX inhibitors (non-steroidal anti-inflammatory drugs, NSAIDs) and prednisone should be considered for use in pregnancy if needed to control active disease symptoms. NSAIDs should be restricted to the first and second trimesters.	B
4	In severe, refractory maternal disease during pregnancy methylprednisolone pulses, intravenous immunoglobulin, or even second or third trimester use of cyclophosphamide should be considered.	D
5	csDMARDs‡, tsDMARDs§ and anti-inflammatory drugs with insufficient documentation concerning use in pregnancy should be avoided until further evidence is available. This applies to leflunomide, mepacrine, tofacitinib, and selective COX II inhibitors.	B–D
6	Among bDMARDs¶ continuation of tumour necrosis factor (TNF) inhibitors during the first part of pregnancy should be considered. Etanercept and certolizumab may be considered for use throughout pregnancy due to low rate of transplacental passage.	B
7	bDMARDs¶ rituximab, anakinra, tocilizumab, abatacept, belimumab and ustekinumab have limited documentation on safe use in pregnancy and should be replaced before conception by other medication. They should be used during pregnancy only when no other pregnancy-compatible drug can effectively control maternal disease.	D
Points to consider for use of antirheumatic drugs during lactation*		
1	csDMARDs‡ and anti-inflammatory drugs compatible with breastfeeding should be considered for continuation during lactation provided the child does not have conditions that contraindicate it. This applies to hydoxychloroquine, chloroquine, sulfasalazine, azathioprine, ciclosporin, tacrolimus, colchicine, prednisone, immunoglobulin, non-selective COX inhibitors, and celecoxib.	D
2	csDMARDs‡, tsDMARDs§ and anti-inflammatory drugs with no or limited data on breastfeeding should be avoided in lactating women. This applies to methotrexate, mycophenolate mofetil, cyclophosphamide, leflunomide, tofacitinib, and cyclooxygenase II inhibitors other than celecoxib.	D
3	Low transfer to breast milk has been shown for infliximab, adalimumab, etanercept, and certolizumab. Continuation of TNF inhibitors should be considered compatible with breastfeeding.	D
4	bDMARDs¶ with no data on breastfeeding such as rituximab, anakinra, belimumab, ustekinumab, tocilizumab, and abatacept should be avoided during lactation if other therapy is available to control the disease. Based on pharmacological properties of bDMARDs¶, lactation should not be discouraged when using these agents, if no other options are available.	D

†**A** Category I evidence from meta-analysis of randomized controlled trials (1A) or from at least one randomized controlled trial (1B)
B Category II evidence from at least one controlled study without randomization (2A) or from at least one type of quasi-experimental study (2B), or extrapolated recommendations from category I evidence.
C Category III evidence from descriptive studies, such as comparative studies, correlation studies or case-control studies (3), or extrapolated recommendation from category I or II evidence.
D Category IV evidence from expert committee reports or opinions and/or clinical experience of respected authorities (4), or extrapolated recommendation from category II or III evidence.10
‡Conventional synthetic DMARDs.
§Targeted synthetic DMARDs.
¶Biologic DMARDs.
Reprinted from Götestam S C et al (2016) 'The EULAR points to consider for use of antirheumatic drugs before pregnancy, and during pregnancy and lactation' *Ann Rheum Dis* 75(5):795–810 with permission from the BMJ Publishing Group Ltd.

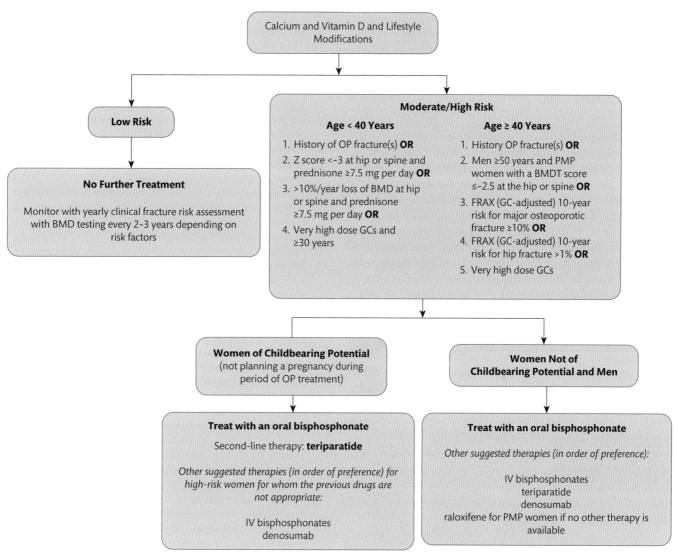

Figure 43.6 Initial pharmacologic treatment for adults. Recommended doses of calcium and vitamin D are 1000–1200 mg/day and 600–800 IU/day (serum level ≥20 ng/ml), respectively. Lifestyle modifications include a balanced diet, maintaining weight in the recommended range, smoking cessation, regular weight-bearing and resistance training exercise, and limiting alcohol intake to 1–2 alcoholic beverages/day. Very high-dose glucocorticoid (GC) treatment was defined as treatment with prednisone ≥30 mg/day and a cumulative dose of >5 gm in the past year. The risk of major osteoporotic (OP) fracture calculated with the FRAX tool (https://www.shef.ac.uk/FRAX/tool.jsp) should be increased by 1.15, and the risk of hip fracture by 1.2, if the prednisone dose is >7.5 mg/day (e.g. if the calculated hip fracture risk is 2.0%, increase to 2.4%). It is recognized that in some cases, bone mineral density (BMD) testing may not be available. PMP = postmenopausal; IV = intravenous.

Reprinted from Buckley L et al (2017) '2017 American College of Rheumatology Guideline for the Prevention and Treatment of Glucocorticoid-Induced Osteoporosis'. *Arthritis & Rheumatology* 69(8):1521–37 with permission from Wiley and Sons.

of the recommendations in these are conditional or recommend good clinical practice, and further studies are needed to examine differences in fracture risk in people with different OP risk factors.

Perioperative management

A collaboration between the ACR and the American Association of Hip and Knee Surgeons developed an evidence-based guideline for the perioperative management of antirheumatic drug therapy for adults with RA and other inflammatory rheumatic diseases undergoing elective total hip arthroplasty (THA) or total knee arthroplasty (TKA).[33] The following recommendation concern RA with respect to perioperative management of antirheumatic drug therapy in patients undergoing THA or TKA:

1. Continue the current dose of methotrexate, leflunomide, hydroxychloroquine, and/or sulfasalazine (non-biologic DMARDs) for patients undergoing elective THA or TKA.
2. Withhold all current biologic agents prior to surgery in patients undergoing elective THA or TKA, and plan the surgery at the end of the dosing cycle for that specific medication.
3. Withhold tofacitinib for at least 7 days prior to surgery in patients undergoing THA or TKA.
4. Restart biologic therapy in patients for whom biologic therapy was withheld prior to undergoing THA and TKA once the wound shows evidence of healing (typically ~14 days), all sutures/staples are out, there is no significant swelling, erythema,

or drainage, and there is no clinical evidence of non–surgical site infections, rather than shorter or longer periods of withholding.

5. Continue the current daily dose of glucocorticoids in patients who are receiving glucocorticoids for their rheumatic condition and undergoing THA or TKA, rather than administering perioperative supraphysiologic glucocorticoid doses (so-called stress dosing).

With respect to the important question of determining the withholding interval of biological agents before surgery, meta-analysis had shown that serum half-life may not correspond to the duration of the immunosuppressant effect. Therefore, the dosing cycle was chosen as more relevant in determining the withholding interval.

All recommendations in this guideline are conditional due to the mainly low quality of the evidence. A conditional recommendation means for the clinician that the desirable effects of a recommendation probably outweigh the undesirable effects, and would thus apply to the majority of the patients. Therefore, the panel cautioned against extrapolation to other orthopaedic procedures until further data are available.

Conclusion

The amount of evidence for effective and safe management of patients with RA is increasing. At the same time, new therapies are emerging. We are also facing an increasing focus on using stringent criteria in a treat-to-target approach. All these factors will indicate a further increase in available evidence supporting therapeutic decisions, which again will necessitate regular updates of evidence-based recommendations.

REFERENCES

1. Klareskog L, Catrina AI, Paget S. Rheumatoid arthritis. *Lancet* 2009;373(9664):659–72.
2. Smolen JS, Aletaha D, McInnes IB. Rheumatoid arthritis. *Lancet* 2016;388(10055):2023–38.
3. Aga AB, Lie E, Uhlig T, et al. Time trends in disease activity, response and remission rates in rheumatoid arthritis during the past decade: results from the NOR-DMARD study 2000–2010. *Ann Rheum Dis* 2015;74(2):381–8.
4. Grigor C, Capell H, Stirling A, et al. Effect of a treatment strategy of tight control for rheumatoid arthritis (the TICORA study): a single-blind randomised controlled trial. *Lancet* 2004;364(9430):263–9.
5. Verstappen SM, Jacobs JW, Van D, et al. Intensive treatment with methotrexate in early rheumatoid arthritis: aiming for remission. Computer Assisted Management in Early Rheumatoid Arthritis (CAMERA, an open-label strategy trial). *Ann Rheum Dis* 2007;66(11):1443–9.
6. Combe B, Landewe R, Lukas C, et al. EULAR recommendations for the management of early arthritis: report of a task force of the European Standing Committee for International Clinical Studies Including Therapeutics (ESCISIT). *Ann Rheum Dis* 2007;66(1):34–45.
7. Combe B, Landewe R, Daien CI, et al. 2016 update of the EULAR recommendations for the management of early arthritis. *Ann Rheum Dis* 2017;76(6):948–59.
8. Smolen JS, Breedveld FC, Burmester GR, et al. Treating rheumatoid arthritis to target: 2014 update of the recommendations of an international task force. *Ann Rheum Dis* 2016;75(1):3–15.
9. Schoels M, Knevel R, Aletaha D, et al. Evidence for treating rheumatoid arthritis to target: results of a systematic literature search. *Ann Rheum Dis* 2010;69(4):638–43.
10. Stoffer MA, Schoels MM, Smolen JS, et al. Evidence for treating rheumatoid arthritis to target: results of a systematic literature search update. *Ann Rheum Dis* 2016;75(1):16–22.
11. Smolen JS, Aletaha D, Bijlsma JW, et al. Treating rheumatoid arthritis to target: recommendations of an international task force. *Ann Rheum Dis* 2010;69(4):631–7.
12. Hammer HB, Uhlig T, Kvien TK, Lampa J. Pain catastrophizing is strongly associated with subjective outcomes, but not with inflammatory assessments in rheumatoid arthritis patients. *Arthritis Care Res (Hoboken)* 2018;70(5):703–12.
13. Michelsen B, Kristianslund EK, Sexton J, et al. Do depression and anxiety reduce the likelihood of remission in rheumatoid arthritis and psoriatic arthritis? Data from the prospective multicentre NOR-DMARD study. *Ann Rheum Dis* 2017;76(11):1906–10.
14. Smolen JS, Landewe R, Bijlsma J, et al. EULAR recommendations for the management of rheumatoid arthritis with synthetic and biological disease-modifying antirheumatic drugs: 2016 update. *Ann Rheum Dis* 2017;76(6):960–77.
15. Smolen JS, Landewe R, Breedveld FC, et al. EULAR recommendations for the management of rheumatoid arthritis with synthetic and biological disease-modifying antirheumatic drugs. *Ann Rheum Dis* 2010;69(6):964–75.
16. Smolen JS, Landewe R, Breedveld F, et al. EULAR recommendations for the management of rheumatoid arthritis with synthetic and biological disease-modifying antirheumatic drugs: 2013 update. *Ann Rheum Dis* 2014;73(3):492–509.
17. Nam JL, Takase-Minegishi K, Ramiro S, et al. Efficacy of biological disease-modifying antirheumatic drugs: a systematic literature review informing the 2016 update of the EULAR recommendations for the management of rheumatoid arthritis. *Ann Rheum Dis* 2017;76(6):1113–36.
18. Ramiro S, Sepriano A, Chatzidionysiou K, et al. Safety of synthetic and biological DMARDs: a systematic literature review informing the 2016 update of the EULAR recommendations for management of rheumatoid arthritis. *Ann Rheum Dis* 2017;76(6):1101–36.
19. Chatzidionysiou K, Emamikia S, Nam J, et al. Efficacy of glucocorticoids, conventional and targeted synthetic disease-modifying antirheumatic drugs: a systematic literature review informing the 2016 update of the EULAR recommendations for the management of rheumatoid arthritis. *Ann Rheum Dis* 2017;76(6):1102–7.
20. Singh JA, Saag KG, Bridges SL, Jr., et al. 2015 American College of Rheumatology Guideline for the Treatment of Rheumatoid Arthritis. *Arthritis Rheumatol* 2016;68(1):1–26.
21. Arnett FC, Edworthy SM, Bloch DA, et al. The American Rheumatism Association 1987 revised criteria for the classification of rheumatoid arthritis. *Arthritis Rheum* 1988;31(3):315–24.
22. Aletaha D, Neogi T, Silman AJ, et al. 2010 rheumatoid arthritis classification criteria: an American College of Rheumatology/European League Against Rheumatism collaborative initiative. *Ann Rheum Dis* 2010;69(9):1580–8.
23. Felson DT, Smolen JS, Wells G, et al. American College of Rheumatology/European League against Rheumatism

provisional definition of remission in rheumatoid arthritis for clinical trials. *Ann Rheum Dis* 2011;*70*(3):404–13.

24. Kay J, Schoels MM, Dorner T, et al. Consensus-based recommendations for the use of biosimilars to treat rheumatological diseases. *Ann Rheum Dis* 2018;*77*(2):165–74.

25. Lindhardsen J, Ahlehoff O, Gislason GH, et al. The risk of myocardial infarction in rheumatoid arthritis and diabetes mellitus: a Danish nationwide cohort study. *Ann Rheum Dis* 2011;*70*(6):929–34.

26. Peters MJ, Symmons DP, McCarey D, et al. EULAR evidence-based recommendations for cardiovascular risk management in patients with rheumatoid arthritis and other forms of inflammatory arthritis. *Ann Rheum Dis* 2010;*69*(2):325–31.

27. Agca R, Heslinga SC, Rollefstad S, et al. EULAR recommendations for cardiovascular disease risk management in patients with rheumatoid arthritis and other forms of inflammatory joint disorders: 2015/2016 update. *Ann Rheum Dis* 2017;*76*(1):17–28.

28. Rollefstad S, Kvien TK, Holme I, Eirheim AS, Pedersen TR, Semb AG. Treatment to lipid targets in patients with inflammatory joint diseases in a preventive cardio-rheuma clinic. *Ann Rheum Dis* 2013;*72*(12):1968–74.

29. Götestam Skorpen C, Hoeltzenbein M, Tincani A, et al. The EULAR points to consider for use of antirheumatic drugs before pregnancy, and during pregnancy and lactation. *Ann Rheum Dis* 2016;*75*(5):795–810.

30. Mariette X, Forger F, Abraham B, et al. Lack of placental transfer of certolizumab pegol during pregnancy: results from CRIB, a prospective, postmarketing, pharmacokinetic study. *Ann Rheum Dis* 2018;*77*(2):228–33.

31. Clowse ME, Forger F, Hwang C, et al. Minimal to no transfer of certolizumab pegol into breast milk: results from CRADLE, a prospective, postmarketing, multicentre, pharmacokinetic study. *Ann Rheum Dis* 2017;*76*(11):1890–6.

32. Buckley L, Guyatt G, Fink HA, et al. 2017 American College of Rheumatology guideline for the prevention and treatment of glucocorticoid-induced osteoporosis. *Arthritis Rheumatol* 2017;*69*(8):1521–37.

33. Goodman SM, Springer B, Guyatt G, et al. 2017 American College of Rheumatology/American Association of Hip and Knee Surgeons guideline for the perioperative management of antirheumatic medication in patients with rheumatic diseases undergoing elective total hip or total knee arthroplasty. *J Arthroplasty* 2017;*32*(9):2628–38.

44

European biologics registers

Angela Zink and Anja Strangfeld

Background

During the past 15 years, the insights gained from the European biologics registers have increasingly been incorporated into daily clinical decision making. When the first two TNF inhibitors were licensed in the beginning of this century, randomized clinical trials (RCTs) had convincingly shown their clinical efficacy and short-term safety. However, there was a lack of information on their long-term safety and effectiveness, in particular when used in daily practice with unselected patients. Therefore, individual researchers as well as scientific societies for rheumatology felt the need to join forces and raise robust evidence on the long-term effects of these new substances when used in daily practice. Since then, biologics registers increasingly fill the knowledge gap between the questions raised by an RCT: 'Can it work?', and the clinical question in daily practice: 'Does it work in my patients?'

Of course, the evidence raised by registers is different from that gained by RCTs. Large randomized, double-blind studies and meta-analyses of these RCTs are considered to produce the highest level of evidence due to the abundant comparability of cases and controls. However, even large RCTs and meta-analyses leave important clinical questions open. These may refer to risk increases in rare adverse events with an incidence below 1:1000 or events with a long latency (e.g. solid cancer and lymphomas). They may also refer to specific risks of patient groups seen in daily care resulting from comorbidity, comedication, age, or gender. It was shown in the past that patients enrolled in the large clinical trials that led to the approval of biologic agents represented only between 23 and 33% of those patients seen in daily practice.[1] RCTs use sophisticated inclusion and exclusion criteria concerning the level of disease activity, disability, age, comorbidity, and comedication, selecting out a majority of real-life patients. These selections result in highly homogenous study populations, enabling comparisons of study arms with small sample sizes. RCTs have a high internal validity due to randomization and blinding but they have a poor external validity due to their limited generalizability. Compared to that, epidemiologic cohort studies such as the biologics registers have a limited internal validity due to confounding by indication but a clearly higher external validity due to inclusion of unselected patients. Both study designs therefore have their place in the assessment of drugs, and they complement each other.

This has also been acknowledged by the European Medicines Agency (EMA) which has made the support of independent biologics registers mandatory in the framework of post-approval risk management plans of companies with new substances for the treatment of rheumatoid arthritis already from 2007 onwards.

When analysing and interpreting long-term real-life data, we face several challenges: the first and most important challenge results from the fact that physicians make treatment decisions depending on the clinical need and state of a patient. Therefore, groups of patients treated either with biologic agents or conventional synthetic (cs)disease-modifying antirheumatic drug (DMARD) therapy cannot be expected to be straightforward comparable. However, due to the large sample sizes in observational studies, subgroups of patients with similar background risk can be found that enable comparisons (e.g. by methods like propensity score matching, exact matching, or inverse probability weighting). In any case, it is far more challenging to extract valid information on the comparative effectiveness of different treatments from an observational study than from an RCT where we can ignore heterogeneity.

Closely connected to the challenge mentioned earlier is the problem that we need to consider all possible factors that may differently influence the outcome in treatment arms. This makes it necessary to collect data not only on different aspects of the disease and possible risk factors, such as disease activity, disability, quality of life, health behaviour, but also the full spectrum of chronic comorbidity, important comedication, and social factors such as education or income.

The third challenge is that we have to collect all this information in a longitudinal manner. Therefore, physicians and patients must be willing to adhere to standard documentation, either specifically for the register or by participating in standardized clinical record systems. One of the most important quality indicators of longitudinal studies in daily life is completeness of data and of follow-up. The credibility of results from real-life data strongly depends on the question for which percentage of patients' valid information is available. It is always preferable to have real data than to impute missing values.

There are several models for biologics registers in rheumatology in Europe (see also Table 44.1):

Table 44.1 Examples of biologics registers in Europe

Name	Start	Country	Design	Comparator
ARTIS (antirheumatic therapies in Sweden)[5,85]	1999	Sweden	Routine web-based data collection, integrated into clinical practice, no fixed time points of follow-up	Linkage to external population-based registers
BSRBR (British Society for Rheumatology Biologics register)[6,11,86]	2001	United Kingdom	National cohort study; initially mandatory with drug prescription, fixed time points of data collection	Comparison group of patients treated with csDMARDs, linkage with mortality and cancer registers
RABBIT (Rheumatoid Arthritis Observation of Biologic therapies)[1,7,10]	2001	Germany	National cohort study, fixed time points of data collection	Internal comparison group of patients at onset of csDMARD therapy after failure of at least one other
DANBIO (Danish National Registry for Biologic Therapies)[4,8]	2000	Denmark	Web-based clinical register in all rheumatologic hospitals in Denmark	Linkage to external population-based registers
SCQM-RA (Swiss Clinical Management Programme for Rheumatoid Arthritis)[15,87]	1997	Switzerland	Collection of treatment data within a system of quality management	No defined comparator group, internal comparisons
AIR (autoimmunity and rituximab), ORA (Orencia in RA), REGATE (Registry RoActemra)[88–90]	2005, 2008, and 2011	France	Individual registers for rituximab, abatacept, tocilizumab	No defined comparator cohorts
NOR-DMARD (Norwegian DMARD registry)[91]	2000	Norway	DMARD prescriptions to patients with inflammatory arthropathies	No defined comparator group, internal comparisons
ATTRA (Czech national registry of patients treated with anti-TNF drugs)[92]	2002	Czech Republic	Prospective multicenter cohort of patients with inflammatory rheumatic diseases	No defined comparator group, internal comparisons
reuma.pt (The Rheumatic Diseases Portuguese Register)[93]	2008	Portugal	National web-based platform, data collection during routine clinical care, all inflammatory rheumatic diseases	No defined comparator group, internal comparisons
BIOBADASER (Spanish register on adverse events of biological therapies in rheumatic diseases)[42,59]	2000	Spain	Multicenter platform to collect adverse events in patients starting biologic therapies	EMECAR cohort of non-biological treated patients as external comparator group

1. The Scandinavian model with routine registration of patients seen in daily care, such as the Swedish ARTIS register and the Danish DANBIO register. Their big advantage is the enrolment of patients as part of clinical routine and the possibility to link the data to national registries for cancer, drug prescription, hospitalization, or death. Therefore, the registers have a high completeness in capturing events covered by any of the national registers. Their disadvantage is that they have to rely on the data that are collected during routine visits. The frequency of these visits can vary greatly depending on patient characteristics, clinical status, and disease activity.

2. The model of specifically designed cohort studies observing all licensed drugs for rheumatoid arthritis (RA) treatment with regular, fixed time points of follow-up, careful monitoring for missing data and intensive queries back to the rheumatologist. Examples for this model are the British Society for Rheumatology Biologics Register (BSRBR) or the German Biologics register for rheumatoid arthritis (RABBIT). Similar concepts are followed by the Spanish BIOBADASER register or the Portuguese Reuma register.

3. The model of the French registers that are dedicated to particular drugs, such as Orencia in RA (ORA), autoimmunity and rituximab (AIR), and REGATE or to specific events like lymphomas or opportunistic infections, such as the RATIO register.

Each type of register has its specific advantages and limitations. Population-based registers such as the Scandinavian ones allow calculation of incidence rates compared to the general population or to patients with the same disease without the exposure of interest. This enables to detect a possible problem and to estimate the size of the problem. In contrast, specifically conducted cohort studies are better suited to look into details of risk factors and risk constellations because they collect exposures and outcomes usually in a more comprehensive and complete manner. Their strength is therefore that they are able to explain which subgroups of patients may be at increased risk or how benefits and risks resulting from the same disease may balance out.

Compared to other systems of real-world pharmacovigilance such as spontaneous reporting systems or long-term extensions of trials, the registers have invaluable advantages. Spontaneous reporting systems are unable to estimate the true incidence of adverse events since they cannot refer to a known denominator. Long-term extension studies of randomized controlled trial (RCTs), on the other hand, have the problem of limited external validity, according to their origin in highly selected trial populations.

Most of the biologics registers in rheumatology are a mixture of exposure and disease registers. They observe patients exposed to an entire class of drugs (not only one substance) and should have comparator groups exposed to conventional therapies in order to put the results into perspective. Usually these registers include patients at onset of exposure to any of the drugs under observation. On the other hand, they are disease registers since they follow the patients during the course of their disease, usually for at least 5, often even 10 years, irrespective of exposure to certain treatments at follow-up.

The registers have given insights into a large number of questions related to the effectiveness and safety of biologic agents. Recently, this also includes biosimilars and Janus kinase (JAK) inhibitors. In the following, we will highlight some of the most significant findings.

Real-world effectiveness

Registers allow comparison of patient groups treated with a variety of different treatments. However, it has always to be taken into account that there is channelling of patients to specific treatments which may influence treatment outcome. For instance, TNF inhibitors were licensed first, and until today they are usually applied as first (and often second) biologic agent whereas drugs with other modes of action often are applied in patients with one or more prior treatment failures. Patients with treatment failures tend to have more severe disease or more complications from comorbidity and poorer functional capacity.[2] Therefore, direct comparison of treatments without taking the line of treatment (first prescribed biologic DMARD, or second or third) into account may bias results.

In addition, the case mix of patients treated with biologic agents and thus the case mix of patients observed in the registers changed over time due to the availability of a variety of substances and the increased experience with these treatments.[3] For instance, the DANBIO register showed a shift in patient case mix of bDMARD users over time towards less severe cases and better clinical response.[4]

There are several outcomes measuring aspects of effectiveness, such as achievement of European League Against Rheumatism (EULAR) response, low disease activity, or remission on the one hand or drug survival, a combined surrogate marker for effectiveness and safety, on the other hand. Further, outcomes with economic implications such as work disability can be observed. In all comparisons of treatments, the problem of confounding by indication has to be kept in mind.

Drug survival and switching of therapies

In the Swedish register ARTIS, half of all patients starting infliximab, adalimumab, or etanercept during the period 2005–2012 discontinued treatment for various reasons.[5] Already within 2 months, one-third switched to a second TNFi. Around 35% of all patients on the second TNFi treatment achieved low disease activity or remission at 6 months.

The British, German, Swedish, and Danish registers found higher drug survival rates in RA for etanercept and adalimumab than for infliximab.[5–9]

Several analyses have shown that combination therapy with methotrexate leads to higher treatment continuation on most of the biologic agents.[6,7,10–13] However, biologic monotherapy may be mandatory due to prior intolerance to methotrexate. Higher drug survival rates for etanercept or infliximab in combination with methotrexate than for each substance alone were found in the British and German registers.[6,10] Survival rates for the combination of TNFi with leflunomide were comparable to methotrexate.[10] In DANBIO, all monotherapy courses with the exception of infliximab showed acceptable remission and drug adherence rates, with somewhat lower response rates than known from combination therapy.[14] Tocilizumab which has a different mode of action seems to have similar clinical effectiveness in mono- as in combination therapy.[15]

In one study rituximab showed equal clinical effectiveness in monotherapy and in combination with either methotrexate or leflunomide in patients who remained on therapy. However, there was a lower continuation rate on monotherapy, indicating that this (off-label) treatment option is not sufficient for all patients.[12] The CERRERA collaboration found a slightly higher effectiveness of rituximab in combination with leflunomide than with methotrexate.[16] There are only few hints on a differential effectiveness of therapies in individual patients. Two substances, abatacept and rituximab, seem to have better effectiveness in patients positive for rheumatoid factor and/or ACPA.[17–19]

Today, with the increasing availability of biosimilars and requested quota for their prescription by the health authorities or insurances in some countries, and limited healthcare resources in other countries, switching therapies has become more frequent also for non-medical reasons. So far, only one register reported on the clinical outcomes after mandated non-medical switch for all patients being treated with the originator infliximab to the biosimilar CT-P13.[20] In 802 patients with inflammatory diseases (403 RA, 120 psoriatic arthritis, and 279 axial spondyloarthritis) no negative effect of switching on disease activity after 6 months as well as on treatment discontinuation rates was found.

Other outcomes

An important question when prescribing novel drugs is whether these treatments can lead to a reduction in societal cost due to work disability and early retirement. Since today in most countries biologic agents are given relatively late in the course of disease when decisions about leaving the labour force are already made, it is difficult to show cost reductions from novel treatments. The ARTIS register recently has published data on patients starting TNFi, with either full or no work ability before start of treatment.[21] During 3 years of treatment, 35% of patients with no work ability at baseline and a disease duration of less than 5 years regained work ability compared to only 14% of those with longer disease duration. It can be expected that with more patients treated earlier in the course of the disease work disability can be prevented in a significant proportion of patients.

Safety of biologic agents

The driving force behind the initiation of all biologics registers was the initial uncertainty about the long-term safety and the potentially increased risk of rare but serious adverse events. These risks might be restricted to subgroups of patients with specific comorbidities or comedications, or they might only show up after several years of treatment. In any case, these potential risks could not be precluded after the initial clinical trials. Specific concerns were raised whether the immunosuppressive agents would increase the risk for serious infections, lymphoproliferative disorders, solid tumours, or autoimmune diseases. Today, we have a plethora of data concerning these risks and can provide robust answers on many of these questions.

Serious bacterial infections

One of the first questions that were addressed by several biologics registers was the potentially increased risk of serious bacterial infection by TNFi. The overall risk in patients treated with TNFi was 1.3

to 2.1 times higher than on conventional csDMARD therapy.[22–24] The risk of serious infection was highest in the first 3–6 months after start of treatment and declined thereafter.[25–27] However, it could be shown that this declining overall risk was attributable partly to a loss of patients at higher risk of infection from the observation and partly to an improved clinical status of the patients and tapering of glucocorticoids over time.[28] Taking drop-out processes as well as changing risk profiles of individual patients into account, the RABBIT Risk Score for serious infection was developed[28] and evaluated.[29] The RABBIT Risk Score is accessible in German and English at the website https://www.biologika-register.de.

The most recent report on the risk of serious infections stems from the BSRBR. Patients who switched to either another TNFi or to RTX after failure of a first TNFi were followed for one year. The overall standardized incidence (SI) risk was 5.9 per 100 patients-years on TNFi and 6.6 on RTX, resulting in an adjusted hazard ratio of 1.0.[30]

Data from the RABBIT register showed that patients who were exposed to biologic agents at the time of a serious bacterial infection had a significantly lower risk of subsequent sepsis and of death from the sepsis.[31] In agreement with experimental studies,[32] this can be explained by the beneficial role of immunosuppression in the prevention of uncontrolled host response. This complex analysis confirmed an observation that had been made years earlier by the British Register BSRBR[33] but could not be explained at that time.

Cardiovascular morbidity

Patients with RA are at increased risk of cardiovascular morbidity and mortality.[34] The risk increase is attributed to the role of chronic inflammation in the development of atherosclerosis. Several registers investigated whether this increased risk can be reverted by successful treatment with biologics agents. The BSRBR-RA first showed that patients who responded to TNFi treatment within 6 months had a significantly lower rate of myocardial infarction (MI) compared to those who did not.[35] The Swedish register ARTIS investigated 47 cases of acute coronary syndrome in 6592 patient-years. They found that among patients initiating TNFi those with EULAR good response had half the risk of acute coronary syndrome compared to those with only moderate response or non-responders. Non-responders had double the risk of the general population whereas in good responders there was no difference in risk compared to the general population.[36] A recent analysis from the BSRBR-RA of 252 verified first MIs found a decreased risk of MI in patients receiving TNFi compared to those receiving csDMARDs. The authors concluded that this might be attributed to a direct action of TNFi on the atherosclerotic process or to better overall disease control.[37]

In the German register RABBIT, 112 cases of MI occurred during follow-up among 11 285 patients.[38] In a nested case-control study a strong association was found between inflammation (levels of C-reactive protein at baseline and at follow-up) and the risk of MI. Further, insufficient treatment of comorbidities associated with increased cardiovascular risk (e.g. hypertension) was significantly more often found in cases with MI than in controls. This underlines the need for tight control of disease activity but also strict management of cardiovascular risk factors.

Patients with RA are also at increased risk of stroke.[39] In patients recruited to the BSRBR between 2001 and 2009, 127 incident ischaemic strokes were found. There was no association between exposure to TNFi and the risk of ischaemic stroke.[40] This could be confirmed by results from the German register.[41] In this analysis incident adverse events (especially serious infections) and untreated cardiovascular comorbidity were additionally identified as major risk factors for stroke.

Mortality

Already in 2007, the Spanish register BIOBADASER reported a decrease in mortality from cardiovascular events in TNFi-treated patients compared to that of a clinical cohort of conventionally treated patients.[42] In 12 672 patients treated with biologics and 3522 patients on csDMARDs, the BSRBR-RA did not find any difference in mortality risk.[43] The RABBIT register found that high disease activity as well as higher dosages of glucocorticoids were strong and independent risk factors of mortality. The data also showed a significantly reduced mortality in patients treated with TNFi or other biologic agents compared to those treated with csDMARDs only, even after control for disease activity, concomitant treatment, comorbidity, and other risk factors.[44]

Patients with RA are at increased risk of interstitial lung disease (ILD), and this extraarticular feature is associated with increased mortality. Guidelines in the United Kingdom caution the use of TNFi in patients with ILD since they can lead to exacerbations of the lung disease. The BSRBR investigated the mortality risk in patients with RA-ILD who received either TNFi or RTX as their first biologic agent.[45] The mortality risk was halved in the RTX cohort, suggesting a protective effect of RTX. However, due to small numbers of cases, this difference was not statistically significant. It should be further investigated by replication studies whether RTX is the safer choice in these high-risk patients.

Solid malignancies and lymphomas

Incident malignancies

A particular strength of registers is their ability to assess rare but serious adverse events that require large samples sizes as well as events with a long latency between exposure and outcome. Both features apply to the risk of malignancy.

Patients with RA are at increased risk of lymphomas[46,47] and a number of solid malignancies, such as lung and skin cancer.[48,49] The risk of lymphomas is closely related to the cumulative disease activity over time.[50] Lymphomas and solid malignancies were among the major events of specific interest in the registers, and some of the registers were powered to detect at least a doubling in risk.

An early report from ARTIS with 26 incident lymphomas did not find an increased risk of lymphomas in TNFi exposed compared to unexposed RA patients.[51] However, compared to the population, the risk in RA patients was nearly threefold. Other registers confirmed that there seems to be no increased overall risk of lymphomas conveyed by TNFi treatment or other biologic agents.[52,53] The French RATIO register compared different TNF inhibitors and found a higher risk of lymphomas in patients treated with monoclonal antibodies than with the fusion protein.[54] Until recently it was not entirely clear whether there may be a switch in the subtype distribution of lymphomas in RA linked to specific antirheumatic treatments. The Study Group on Biologics Registers of the EULAR jointly analysed data from 11 European registers.[55] Among nearly 125 000 patients, 533 lymphomas were observed. The majority (84%) were B-cell non-Hodgkin lymphomas, and only 7% were T-cell non-Hodgkin lymphomas. This is in line with the previous observation of an increased risk of B-cell lymphomas in patients with RA and does not suggest a shift in subtypes by biologic therapies.

Solid malignancies were addressed by several biologics registers. By linking data from ARTIS, from the Swedish RA register, and the Swedish cancer register, no increase in the cancer risk was seen over the first six years of treatment in 6366 patients with RA who started therapy with TNFi between 1999 and 2006.[56] The Italian LOHREN register found a risk of solid cancer comparable to the general population in 1064 patients exposed to TNFi.[57]

There was also no difference in the incidence of cancer in the RABBIT register between patients being exposed or not to TNFi.[58] In the Spanish BIOBADASER register, the age- and sex-adjusted incidence rate for cancer was even lower in patients exposed to biologics than in an unexposed population cohort. [59]

A 30% increased risk of solid malignancies was found in the BSRBR control group of patients never exposed to TNFi compared to the general population.[48] DANBIO reported the same risk increase over the population, irrespective of whether the patients had been exposed or unexposed to biologic agents.[53] If patients treated with TNFi or csDMARDs were compared, the BSRBR-RA did not find any difference in the risk of solid malignancy and also no risk difference among the TNF inhibitors etanercept, adalimumab, and infliximab.[60]

ARTIS found a slight increase in the incidence of basal cell cancer and squamous cell cancer in biologics-naïve RA patients compared to the population and an additional 30% increase for those treated with TNFi.[61] However, it could not be ruled out that this increase originates from patient characteristics of those treated with TNFi and not from the treatment.

All data indicate a generally increased risk of skin cancer in patients with RA. The BSRBR found a doubled risk for all kinds of skin cancer in patients with RA, independent of exposure to biologic agents or csDMARDs.[62] This finding was confirmed by DANBIO.[53] After a signal from Sweden of a 50% increased risk for malignant melanoma in patients exposed to TNFi,[63] the Study Group on Biologics Registers of EULAR performed a joint data analysis with seven European registers. Incidence rates of malignant melanoma were compared to the respective population rates of each country. The Swedish signal was not confirmed in the other countries, only Denmark had insignificantly increased rates.[64] The still conflicting results may be attributable to different skin types and different behaviour concerning sun exposure in the European countries.

A recent study from the Swedish population registers investigated the risk of malignant neoplasms in 15 129 patients starting treatment with TNFi and 7405 patient starting biologic agents with other modes of action compared to those on csDMARDs.[65] Initiators of a first or second TNFi, other bDMARDs or csDMARDs did not differ in their overall risk for solid malignancies. However, an increased risk of squamous cell skin cancer was found in patients treated with abatacept. Since this finding is based upon 17 cases only, it needs re-evaluation in other registers.

Recurrent malignancies

In 2010, the BSRBR[66] as well as RABBIT[58] reported on the recurrence risk in patients with prior tumours. In both registers, the percentages of patients with prior malignancies were twice as high in the control groups as in the TNFi exposed groups, indicating channelling of risk

patients to conventional therapies. Both registers did not find significant differences in recurrence rates between TNFi exposed and unexposed patients. However, the BSRBR found an insignificantly decreased and RABBIT observed an insignificantly increased risk in patients exposed to TNFi, attributable to different treatment styles in British and German rheumatologists. German rheumatologists prescribed TNFi in a majority of cases (77%) within the first ten years after cancer diagnosis, while in the United Kingdom only 42% of patients were treated within this time window.

Today, a majority of patients with RA and a history of cancer are prescribed rituximab (RTX), since this substance is used in the treatment of lymphomas and not considered to be tumour promoting. Data from the British Register BSRBR indicate that RA patients in the United Kingdom with prior malignancy selected to receive either TNFi or RTX do not have a higher risk of recurrent or new incident malignancies compared to patients receiving csDMARD treatment.[67]

In a case-control study with female patients with prior breast cancer in ARTIS, the same numbers of recurrences were found in patients exposed or unexposed to TNFi.[68] When data from ARTIS, the Swedish clinical RA registers and national registers on cancer, hospitalization, and outpatient care were linked, patients treated with TNFi had similar stages at cancer diagnosis and similar post-cancer survival rates to biologics-naïve patients.[69] DANBIO reported no evidence of an increased risk of malignant progression of precancerous lesions of the uterine cervix following biological treatment.[70]

Various safety issues

Tuberculosis and opportunistic infections

Already in the first years after their initiation, several registers found that TNFi, mainly the monoclonal antibodies, increase the risk for reactivation of latent tuberculosis.[71–73] It was shown that the risk can be significantly reduced by systematic screening.[74] Data suggest that there is an increased risk of viral infection, in particular herpes zoster, in patients treated with monoclonal antibodies.[75,76] In the BSRBR, an increased risk of septic arthritis was found in patients treated with TNFi.[25]

A higher occurrence rate of uncommon opportunistic infections such as listeriosis, atypical mycobacteriosis, non-typhoid salmonellosis, pneumocystis or histoplasmosis was found in the French RATIO register in patients treated with the monoclonal antibodies compared to the fusion protein. Further risk factors were oral steroid use >10 mg or intravenous boluses during the past year.[73,76] The BSRBR-RA showed a doubling in risk for pneumocystis jirovecii pneumonia of 2.0 per 10 000 patient-years of exposure in the TNFi cohort compared to 1.1 in patients exposed to csDMARDs.[77]

Lower gastrointestinal perforations

Recent data from the RABBIT register support the observation from randomized trials of an increased risk of lower intestinal perforations in patients treated with tocilizumab.[78] The crude incidence rate was 2.7/1000 patient-years on tocilizumab and 0.2–0.6/1000 PY in all other biologic or conventional DMARD treatments. Interestingly, one-third of the patients on tocilizumab presented without any of the typical symptoms of lower intestinal perforation. This may result in delayed treatment and explain the higher mortality of these patients (5/11 compared to 4/24 in other DMARD treatments). The British register compared the risk of gastrointestinal perforation between patients on TNFi and csDMARDs. In agreement with the German findings there was no increased risk conveyed by TNF inhibition.[79]

Lupus-like events

The BSRBR investigated the risk of incident lupus-like events and vasculitis-like events in patients exposed to TNFi compared to the csDMARD comparator group.[80] In 12 937 patients exposed to adalimumab, etanercept, infliximab or certolizumab and 3673 biologics-naïve patients the overall incidence rates for lupus-like events were 10 and 2 in 10 000 patient-years of exposure to TNFi and csDMARDs, respectively. The incidence rates for vasculitis-like events were 15 and 7 per 10 000 patient-years. Even though the crude rates were higher in patients exposed to TNFi, after adjustment for differences in baseline characteristics, there was no significant risk difference between TNFi and csDMARDs for these very rare events.

Pregnancy outcomes

Women of childbearing age are advised to use effective contraception during biological therapy. Nevertheless, incidental exposure to TNFi during pregnancy was observed in the registers. In an early report from the BSRBR[81] on 32 patients directly exposed to TNFi during or immediately prior to pregnancy, 23 women were exposed at the time of conception, 9 had discontinued TNFi on average 5 months earlier. Three-quarters of pregnancies (76%) ended with the birth of healthy babies, in 24% of pregnancies a first-trimester miscarriage occurred. Of the 23 patients who had been treated with TNFi at the time of conception, nine had additionally received methotrexate and two leflunomide. No malformations were observed.

In a more comprehensive analysis of the BSRBR,[82] 130 pregnancies were reported in patients ever exposed TNFi and 10 pregnancies in patients who had never received these substances. Based on exposure, the pregnancies were stratified in four groups according to the exposure status at the time of conception: (I) on TNFi and a concomitant therapy with methotrexate (MTX) and/or leflunomide; (II) monotherapy with TNFi; (III) previous TNFi discontinued; (IV) never exposed to bDMARDs. Higher abortion rates were found in groups I (23%) and II (24%) compared to group III (17%) and group IV (10%). However, biologics-naïve patients (group IV) had significantly lower disease activity, as measured by DAS28, than patients in the groups treated with TNFi. A total of 41% of patients who discontinued TNFi prior to conception (group III) had been treated with steroids at the time of conception. In comparison, this was only the case in 29% of group I patients. However, it was not possible to determine whether the increased rate of spontaneous abortions in patients treated with TNFi was caused by therapy or higher disease activity.

Further pregnancy data from biologics registers exist only in abstract form, for example from the German RABBIT register. 106 pregnancies were reported, of which 57 patients were exposed to biologics at the time of conception (46 × TNF inhibitors, 5 × tocilizumab, 3 × rituximab, 3 × abatacept), 38 patients had received the biologic at least 4 weeks prior to conception and 11 patients were biologic-naïve. This analysis did not confirm the widespread assumption of an improvement in disease activity in RA patients during pregnancy. On the contrary, only 43% of women who were in remission prior to conception were able to maintain them during pregnancy. Of those who were not in remission at the time

of conception, only 7% achieved such a state. All patients who were exposed to biologics at the time of conception were discontinued when pregnancy became known. However, a quarter of the patients started a TNFi again in the second or third trimester due to high disease activity. The rate of spontaneous abortions in patients exposed to TNFi at conception was 19% compared to 13% who had stopped at least 4 weeks prior to conception. No spontaneous abortions were reported in the biologic-naïve group.[83]

The current biologics registers in RA are only partially suited to answer the clinically important questions in relation with pregnancy. Only few patients are enrolled at childbearing age and the follow-up time points are not completely suitable to capture pregnancy courses. Observation during pregnancy and the first years of the child requires a specific approach as it is followed by the recently established European pregnancy registers. For instance, the German Rhekiss register has enrolled more than 800 pregnant patients with inflammatory rheumatic diseases since 2015, among them >250 patients with RA. We can expect that in the near future the pregnancy registers will significantly increase our knowledge on the safety of various biologic agents in this groups of highly vulnerable patients.

Summary and conclusions

With the European biologics registers, a novel generation of pharmaco-epidemiologic cohort studies has been successfully established. Different in methodology, they all have contributed to our understanding of the long-term risks and benefits of novel treatments. By including all patients treated in real practise without exclusion criteria, they have tremendously contributed to our knowledge what can be expected when patients are treated with these substances that would never have been included in a randomized clinical trial due to age, comorbidity, pregnancy, or severe functional disability.

All registers have shown an increased risk of serious infection on biologic agents which materializes most strongly in the first months after treatment onset and then decreases due to selective drop-out of high-risk patients as well as improvement in clinical status. They have also shown that risks arising from specific treatment have to be balanced out against risk from other treatments, comorbidity, or uncontrolled disease activity. The data concerning the overall risk of cancer are reassuring. However, independent of exposure, the generally increased risk of lymphoma and skin cancer in patients with RA has to be kept in mind. Further observation will also show whether with more patients treated successfully with TNFi the overall risk of lymphomas will decrease due to a lower percentage of patients with long-standing high disease activity. Further observation should also consider potentially increased risks in subgroups of patients such as older patients or those undergoing specific additional treatments.

The registers have shown beneficial effects of treatment with biologic agents such as the TNF inhibitors and also substances with other modes of action. Successful treatment with biologics decreases the risk for MI, other cardiovascular events, and overall mortality. Exposure to biologic agents at the time of a serious infection seems to decrease the risk of subsequent sepsis. In the light of this finding, further studies are needed to investigate whether it is always the best decision to stop biologics before planned surgeries.

Fortunately, initial concerns about an increase in the development of other autoimmune or demyelinating diseases have not materialized so far. However, given the insignificantly increased risk of lupus-like and vasculitis-like events in the BSRBR reported recently, more observation over longer periods of time is necessary. It might still be that 20 or more years of continuous immunosuppression by cytokine blockade or depletion of cells may have adverse effects not seen so far. This makes long-term observation of these patients so important, in particular if the treatment has already started at young age.

The registers also contribute to the further development of research methodology. Differences in results between registers have driven analyses leading to more complex explanations of time-dependent risks. It is of utmost clinical value that we have different registers in Europe that produce their results independent of each other but collaborate closely. In most cases parallel analyses of country-specific data are superior to pooling of raw data since the differences in healthcare systems and access to treatment produce additional heterogeneity and potential confounding.

Increasingly, new registries are set up in many countries for various indications. In order to get the best scientific value from these complex cohort studies, it is vital to ensure a high quality by exchange of methodologies. Under the umbrella of the EULAR the Subcommittee on Biologics Registries, which builds upon the work of a previous task force,[84] holds open meetings every 2 years. The aim is to coordinate the efforts throughout Europe and to make best use of the existing data sources.

In order to assess possible increases even in very small risks, international collaboration will continue to be required. The methodological challenge in performing joint analyses of data from different countries goes beyond the problem of confounding by indication. In addition, we have to take into account the heterogeneity resulting from differences in healthcare provision and access to treatment or from the ethnic and genetic background.

To conclude, with the data from the biologics registers and their increasing clinical use, rheumatologists prescribing the new biologic agents now have better information on the balance of benefits and risks, including aspects of costs to society. When new treatments arise, either entirely new substances or biosimilars, it is necessary to both evaluate them in the same manner as those currently on the market and compare the effectiveness and safety of the different agents. With longer exposure to multiple biologic treatments and more frequent switches, however, it will be increasingly difficult to establish unequivocally the influence of individual substances. Sophisticated methodology will be required to deal with the challenges of these data.

REFERENCES

1. Zink A, Strangfeld A, Schneider M, et al. Effectiveness of tumor necrosis factor inhibitors in rheumatoid arthritis in an observational cohort study: comparison of patients according to their eligibility for major randomized clinical trials. *Arthritis Rheum* 2006;54(11):3399–407.
2. Codullo V, Iannone F, Sinigaglia L, et al. Comparison of efficacy of first- versus second-line adalimumab in patients with rheumatoid arthritis: experience of the Italian biologics registries. *Clin Exp Rheumatol* 2017;35(4):660–5.
3. Zufferey P, Dudler J, Scherer A, Finckh A. Disease activity in rheumatoid arthritis patients at initiation of biologic agents and 1 year of treatment: results from the Swiss SCQM registry. *Joint Bone Spine* 2013;80(2):160–4.
4. Hetland ML, Lindegaard HM, Hansen A, et al. Do changes in prescription practice in patients with rheumatoid arthritis treated with biological agents affect treatment response and adherence to therapy? Results from the nationwide Danish DANBIO Registry. *Ann Rheum Dis* 2008;67(7):1023–6.
5. Chatzidionysiou K, Askling J, Eriksson J, Kristensen LE, van Vollenhoven R, ARTIS group. Effectiveness of TNF inhibitor switch in RA: results from the national Swedish register. *Ann Rheum Dis* 2015;74(5):890–6.
6. Hyrich KL, Symmons DP, Watson KD, Silman AJ, British Society for Rheumatology Biologics R. Comparison of the response to infliximab or etanercept monotherapy with the response to cotherapy with methotrexate or another disease-modifying antirheumatic drug in patients with rheumatoid arthritis: results from the British Society for Rheumatology Biologics Register. *Arthritis Rheum* 2006;54(6):1786–94.
7. Strangfeld A, Hierse F, Kekow J, et al. Comparative effectiveness of tumour necrosis factor alpha inhibitors in combination with either methotrexate or leflunomide. *Ann Rheum Dis* 2009;68(12):1856–62.
8. Hetland ML, Christensen IJ, Tarp U, et al. Direct comparison of treatment responses, remission rates, and drug adherence in patients with rheumatoid arthritis treated with adalimumab, etanercept, or infliximab: results from eight years of surveillance of clinical practice in the nationwide Danish DANBIO registry. *Arthritis Rheum* 2010;62(1):22–32.
9. Neovius M, Arkema EV, Olsson H, et al. Drug survival on TNF inhibitors in patients with rheumatoid arthritis comparison of adalimumab, etanercept and infliximab. *Ann Rheum Dis* 2015;74(2):354–60.
10. Zink A, Listing J, Kary S, et al. Treatment continuation in patients receiving biological agents or conventional DMARD therapy. *Ann Rheum Dis* 2005;64(9):1274–9.
11. Hyrich KL, Lunt M, Watson KD, Symmons DP, Silman AJ, British Society for Rheumatology Biologics R. Outcomes after switching from one anti-tumor necrosis factor alpha agent to a second anti-tumor necrosis factor alpha agent in patients with rheumatoid arthritis: results from a large UK national cohort study. *Arthritis Rheum* 2007;56(1):13–20.
12. Richter A, Strangfeld A, Herzer P, et al. Sustainability of rituximab therapy in different treatment strategies: results of a 3-year follow-up of a German biologics register. *Arthritis Care Res (Hoboken)* 2014;66(11):1627–33.
13. Manders SH, Kievit W, Jansen TL, et al. Effectiveness of tumor necrosis factor inhibitors in combination with various csDMARD in the treatment of rheumatoid arthritis: data from the DREAM Registry. *J Rheumatol* 2016;43(10):1787–94.
14. Jorgensen TS, Kristensen LE, Christensen R, et al. Effectiveness and drug adherence of biologic monotherapy in routine care of patients with rheumatoid arthritis: a cohort study of patients registered in the Danish biologics registry. *Rheumatology (Oxf)* 2015;54(12):2156–65.
15. Gabay C, Riek M, Hetland ML, et al. Effectiveness of tocilizumab with and without synthetic disease-modifying antirheumatic

drugs in rheumatoid arthritis: results from a European collaborative study. *Ann Rheum Dis* 2016;75(7):1336–42.

16. Chatzidionysiou K, Lie E, Nasonov E, et al. Effectiveness of disease-modifying antirheumatic drug co-therapy with methotrexate and leflunomide in rituximab-treated rheumatoid arthritis patients: results of a 1-year follow-up study from the CERERRA collaboration. *Ann Rheum Dis* 2012;71(3):374–7.

17. Gottenberg JE, Courvoisier DS, Hernandez MV, et al. Brief report: association of rheumatoid factor and anti-citrullinated protein antibody positivity with better effectiveness of abatacept: results from the pan-European registry analysis. *Arthritis Rheumatol* 2016;68(6):1346–52.

18. De Keyser F, Hoffman I, Durez P, Kaiser MJ, Westhovens R. Long-term follow-up of rituximab therapy in patients with rheumatoid arthritis: results from the Belgian MabThera in Rheumatoid Arthritis registry. *J Rheumatol* 2014;41(9): 1761–5.

19. Oldroyd AGS, Symmons DPM, Sergeant JC, et al. Long-term persistence with rituximab in patients with rheumatoid arthritis. *Rheumatology (Oxf)* 2018;57(6):1089–96.

20. Glintborg B, Sorensen IJ, Loft AG, et al. A nationwide nonmedical switch from originator infliximab to biosimilar CT-P13 in 802 patients with inflammatory arthritis: 1-year clinical outcomes from the DANBIO registry. *Ann Rheum Dis* 2017;76(8):1426–31.

21. Olofsson T, Petersson IF, Eriksson JK, et al. Predictors of work disability after start of anti-TNF therapy in a national cohort of Swedish patients with rheumatoid arthritis: does early anti-TNF therapy bring patients back to work? *Ann Rheum Dis* 2017;76(7):1245–52.

22. Listing J, Strangfeld A, Kary S, et al. Infections in patients with rheumatoid arthritis treated with biologic agents. *Arthritis Rheum* 2005;52(11):3403–12.

23. Dixon WG, Watson K, Lunt M, et al. Rates of serious infection, including site-specific and bacterial intracellular infection, in rheumatoid arthritis patients receiving anti-tumor necrosis factor therapy: results from the British Society for Rheumatology Biologics Register. *Arthritis Rheum* 2006;54(8):2368–76.

24. Askling J, Fored CM, Brandt L, et al. Time-dependent increase in risk of hospitalisation with infection among Swedish RA patients treated with TNF antagonists. *Ann Rheum Dis* 2007;66(10):1339–44.

25. Galloway JB, Hyrich KL, Mercer LK, et al. Risk of septic arthritis in patients with rheumatoid arthritis and the effect of anti-TNF therapy: results from the British Society for Rheumatology Biologics Register. *Ann Rheum Dis* 2011;70(10):1810–14.

26. Dixon WG, Symmons DP, Lunt M, et al. Serious infection following anti-tumor necrosis factor alpha therapy in patients with rheumatoid arthritis: lessons from interpreting data from observational studies. *Arthritis Rheum* 2007;56(9):2896–904.

27. Galloway JB, Hyrich KL, Mercer LK, et al. Anti-TNF therapy is associated with an increased risk of serious infections in patients with rheumatoid arthritis especially in the first 6 months of treatment: updated results from the British Society for Rheumatology Biologics Register with special emphasis on risks in the elderly. *Rheumatology (Oxf)* 2011;50(1):124–31.

28. Strangfeld A, Eveslage M, Schneider M, et al. Treatment benefit or survival of the fittest: what drives the time-dependent decrease in serious infection rates under TNF inhibition and what does this imply for the individual patient? *Ann Rheum Dis* 2011;70(11):1914–20.

29. Zink A, Manger B, Kaufmann J, et al. Evaluation of the RABBIT Risk Score for serious infections. *Ann Rheum Dis* 2014;73(9):1673–6.

30. Silva-Fernandez L, De Cock D, Lunt M, et al. Serious infection risk after 1 year between patients with rheumatoid arthritis treated with rituximab or with a second TNFi after initial TNFi failure: results from The British Society for Rheumatology Biologics Register for Rheumatoid Arthritis. *Rheumatology (Oxf)* 2018;57(9):1533–40.

31. Richter A, Listing J, Schneider M, et al. Impact of treatment with biologic DMARDs on the risk of sepsis or mortality after serious infection in patients with rheumatoid arthritis. *Ann Rheum Dis* 2016;75(9):1667–73.

32. Tracey KJ, Fong Y, Hesse DG, et al. Anti-cachectin/TNF monoclonal antibodies prevent septic shock during lethal bacteraemia. *Nature* 1987;330(6149):662–4.

33. Galloway JB, Hyrich KL, Mercer LK, et al. Anti-TNF therapy is associated with an increased risk of serious infections in patients with rheumatoid arthritis especially in the first 6 months of treatment: updated results from the British Society for Rheumatology Biologics Register with special emphasis on risks in the elderly. *Rheumatology (Oxf)* 2011;50(1):124–31.

34. Avina-Zubieta JA, Thomas J, Sadatsafavi M, Lehman AJ, Lacaille D. Risk of incident cardiovascular events in patients with rheumatoid arthritis: a meta-analysis of observational studies. *Ann Rheum Dis* 2012;71(9):1524–9.

35. Dixon WG, Watson KD, Lunt M, et al. Reduction in the incidence of myocardial infarction in patients with rheumatoid arthritis who respond to anti-tumor necrosis factor alpha therapy: results from the British Society for Rheumatology Biologics Register. *Arthritis Rheum* 2007;56(9):2905–12.

36. Ljung L, Rantapaa-Dahlqvist S, Jacobsson LT, Askling J. Response to biological treatment and subsequent risk of coronary events in rheumatoid arthritis. *Ann Rheum Dis* 2016;75(12):2087–94.

37. Low AS, Symmons DP, Lunt M, et al. Relationship between exposure to tumour necrosis factor inhibitor therapy and incidence and severity of myocardial infarction in patients with rheumatoid arthritis. *Ann Rheum Dis* 2017;76(4):654–60.

38. Meissner Y, Zink A, Kekow J, et al. Impact of disease activity and treatment of comorbidities on the risk of myocardial infarction in rheumatoid arthritis. *Arthritis Res Ther* 2016;18(1):183.

39. Wiseman SJ, Ralston SH, Wardlaw JM. Cerebrovascular disease in rheumatic diseases: a systematic review and meta-analysis. *Stroke* 2016;47(4):943–50.

40. Low AS, Lunt M, Mercer LK, et al. Association between ischemic stroke and tumor necrosis factor inhibitor therapy in patients with rheumatoid arthritis. *Arthritis Rheumatol* 2016;68(6):1337–45.

41. Meissner Y, Richter A, Manger B, et al. Serious adverse events and the risk of stroke in patients with rheumatoid arthritis: results from the German RABBIT cohort. *Ann Rheum Dis* 2017;76(9):1583–90.

42. Carmona L, Descalzo MA, Perez-Pampin E, et al. All-cause and cause-specific mortality in rheumatoid arthritis are not greater than expected when treated with tumour necrosis factor antagonists. *Ann Rheum Dis* 2007;66(7):880–5.

43. Lunt M, Watson KD, Dixon WG, et al. No evidence of association between anti-tumor necrosis factor treatment and mortality in patients with rheumatoid arthritis: results from the British Society for Rheumatology Biologics Register. *Arthritis Rheum* 2010;62(11):3145–53.

44. Listing J, Kekow J, Manger B, et al. Mortality in rheumatoid arthritis: the impact of disease activity, treatment with glucocorticoids, TNFalpha inhibitors and rituximab. *Ann Rheum Dis* 2015;*74*(2):415–21.

45. Druce KL, Iqbal K, Watson KD, Symmons DPM, Hyrich KL, Kelly C. Mortality in patients with interstitial lung disease treated with rituximab or TNFi as a first biologic. *RMD Open* 2017;*3*(1):e000473.

46. Smedby KE, Askling J, Mariette X, Baecklund E. Autoimmune and inflammatory disorders and risk of malignant lymphomas—an update. *J Intern Med* 2008;*264*(6):514–27.

47. Ekstrom K, Hjalgrim H, Brandt L, et al. Risk of malignant lymphomas in patients with rheumatoid arthritis and in their first-degree relatives. *Arthritis Rheum* 2003;*48*(4):963–70.

48. Mercer LK, Davies R, Galloway JB, et al. Risk of cancer in patients receiving non-biologic disease-modifying therapy for rheumatoid arthritis compared with the UK general population. *Rheumatology (Oxf)* 2013;*52*(1):91–8.

49. Buchbinder R, Barber M, Heuzenroeder L, et al. Incidence of melanoma and other malignancies among rheumatoid arthritis patients treated with methotrexate. *Arthritis Rheum* 2008;*59*(6):794–9.

50. Baecklund E, Iliadou A, Askling J, et al. Association of chronic inflammation, not its treatment, with increased lymphoma risk in rheumatoid arthritis. *Arthritis Rheum* 2006;*54*(3):692–701.

51. Askling J, Baecklund E, Granath F, et al. Anti-tumour necrosis factor therapy in rheumatoid arthritis and risk of malignant lymphomas: relative risks and time trends in the Swedish Biologics Register. *Ann Rheum Dis* 2009;*68*(5):648–53.

52. Wolfe F, Michaud K. Biologic treatment of rheumatoid arthritis and the risk of malignancy—Analyses from a large US observational study. *Arthritis Rheum* 2007;*56*(9):2886–95.

53. Dreyer L, Mellemkjaer L, Andersen AR, et al. Incidences of overall and site specific cancers in TNFalpha inhibitor treated patients with rheumatoid arthritis and other arthritides—a follow-up study from the DANBIO Registry. *Ann Rheum Dis* 2013;*72*(1):79–82.

54. Mariette X, Tubach F, Bagheri H, et al. Lymphoma in patients treated with anti-TNF: results of the 3-year prospective French RATIO registry. *Ann Rheum Dis* 2010;*69*(2):400–8.

55. Mercer LK, Regierer AC, Mariette X, et al. Spectrum of lymphomas across different drug treatment groups in rheumatoid arthritis: a European registries collaborative project. *Ann Rheum Dis* 2017;*76*(12):2025–30.

56. Askling J, van Vollenhoven RF, Granath F, et al. Cancer risk in patients with rheumatoid arthritis treated with anti-tumor necrosis factor alpha therapies: does the risk change with the time since start of treatment? *Arthritis Rheum* 2009;*60*(11):3180–9.

57. Pallavicini FB, Caporali R, Sarzi-Puttini P, et al. Tumour necrosis factor antagonist therapy and cancer development: analysis of the LORHEN registry. *Autoimmun Rev* 2010;*9*(3):175–80.

58. Strangfeld A, Hierse F, Rau R, et al. Risk of incident or recurrent malignancies among patients with rheumatoid arthritis exposed to biologic therapy in the German biologics register RABBIT. *Arthritis Res Ther* 2010;*12*(1):R5.

59. Carmona L, Abasolo L, Descalzo MA, et al. Cancer in patients with rheumatic diseases exposed to TNF antagonists. *Semin Arthritis Rheum* 2011;*41*(1):71–80.

60. Mercer LK, Lunt M, Low AL, et al. Risk of solid cancer in patients exposed to anti-tumour necrosis factor therapy: results from the British Society for Rheumatology Biologics Register for Rheumatoid Arthritis. *Ann Rheum Dis* 2015;*74*(6):1087–93.

61. Raaschou P, Simard JF, Asker Hagelberg C, Askling J, ARTIS Study Group. Rheumatoid arthritis, anti-tumour necrosis factor treatment, and risk of squamous cell and basal cell skin cancer: cohort study based on nationwide prospectively recorded data from Sweden. *BMJ* 2016;*352*:i262.

62. Mercer LK, Green AC, Galloway JB, et al. The influence of anti-TNF therapy upon incidence of keratinocyte skin cancer in patients with rheumatoid arthritis: longitudinal results from the British Society for Rheumatology Biologics Register. *Ann Rheum Dis* 2012;*71*(6):869–74.

63. Raaschou P, Simard JF, Holmqvist M, Askling J, ARTIS Study Group. Rheumatoid arthritis, anti-tumour necrosis factor therapy, and risk of malignant melanoma: nationwide population based prospective cohort study from Sweden. *BMJ* 2013;*346*:f1939.

64. Mercer LK, Askling J, Raaschou P, et al. Risk of invasive melanoma in patients with rheumatoid arthritis treated with biologics: results from a collaborative project of 11 European biologic registers. *Ann Rheum Dis* 2017;*76*(2):386–91.

65. Wadström H, Frisell T, Askling J. Malignant neoplasms in patients with rheumatoid arthritis treated with tumor necrosis factor inhibitors, tocilizumab, abatacept, or rituximab in clinical practice: a nationwide cohort study from Sweden. *JAMA Int Med* 2017;*177*(11):1605–12.

66. Dixon WG, Watson KD, Lunt M, et al. Influence of anti-tumor necrosis factor therapy on cancer incidence in patients with rheumatoid arthritis who have had a prior malignancy: results from the British Society for Rheumatology Biologics Register. *Arthritis Care Res (Hoboken)* 2010;*62*(6):755–63.

67. Silva-Fernandez L, Lunt M, Kearsley-Fleet L, et al. The incidence of cancer in patients with rheumatoid arthritis and a prior malignancy who receive TNF inhibitors or rituximab: results from the British Society for Rheumatology Biologics Register-Rheumatoid Arthritis. *Rheumatology (Oxf)* 2016;*55*(11):2033–9.

68. Raaschou P, Frisell T, Askling J, ARTIS Study Group. TNF inhibitor therapy and risk of breast cancer recurrence in patients with rheumatoid arthritis: a nationwide cohort study. *Ann Rheum Dis* 2015;*74*(12):2137–43.

69. Raaschou P, Simard JF, Neovius M, Askling J. Does cancer that occurs during or after anti-tumor necrosis factor therapy have a worse prognosis? A national assessment of overall and site-specific cancer survival in rheumatoid arthritis patients treated with biologic agents. *Arthritis Rheum* 2011;*63*(7):1812–22.

70. Cordtz R, Mellemkjaer L, Glintborg B, Hetland ML, Dreyer L. Malignant progression of precancerous lesions of the uterine cervix following biological DMARD therapy in patients with arthritis. *Ann Rheum Dis* 2015;*74*(7):1479–80.

71. Gomez-Reino JJ, Carmona L, Valverde VR, Mola EM, Montero MD. Treatment of rheumatoid arthritis with tumor necrosis factor inhibitors may predispose to significant increase in tuberculosis risk: a multicenter active-surveillance report. *Arthritis Rheum* 2003;*48*(8):2122–7.

72. Dixon WG, Hyrich KL, Watson KD, et al. Drug-specific risk of tuberculosis in patients with rheumatoid arthritis treated with anti-TNF therapy: results from the British Society for Rheumatology Biologics Register (BSRBR). *Ann Rheum Dis* 2010;*69*(3):522–8.

73. Tubach F, Salmon D, Ravaud P, et al. Risk of tuberculosis is higher with anti-tumor necrosis factor monoclonal antibody therapy than with soluble tumor necrosis factor receptor

therapy: the three-year prospective French Research Axed on Tolerance of Biotherapies registry. *Arthritis Rheum* 2009;60(7):1884–94.

74. Carmona L, Gomez-Reino JJ, Rodriguez-Valverde V, et al. Effectiveness of recommendations to prevent reactivation of latent tuberculosis infection in patients treated with tumor necrosis factor antagonists. *Arthritis Rheum* 2005;52(6):1766–72.

75. Strangfeld A, Listing J, Herzer P, et al. Risk of herpes zoster in patients with rheumatoid arthritis treated with anti-TNF-alpha agents. *JAMA* 2009;301(7):737–44.

76. Salmon-Ceron D, Tubach F, Lortholary O, et al. Drug-specific risk of non-tuberculosis opportunistic infections in patients receiving anti-TNF therapy reported to the 3-year prospective French RATIO registry. *Ann Rheum Dis* 2011;70(4):616–23.

77. Bruce ES, Kearsley-Fleet L, Watson KD, Symmons DP, Hyrich KL. Risk of Pneumocystis jirovecii pneumonia in patients with rheumatoid arthritis treated with inhibitors of tumour necrosis factor alpha: results from the British Society for Rheumatology Biologics Register for Rheumatoid Arthritis. *Rheumatology (Oxf)* 2016;55(7):1336–7.

78. Strangfeld A, Richter A, Siegmund B, et al. Risk for lower intestinal perforations in patients with rheumatoid arthritis treated with tocilizumab in comparison to treatment with other biologic or conventional synthetic DMARDs. *Ann Rheum Dis* 2017;76(3):504–10.

79. Zavada J, Lunt M, Davies R, et al. The risk of gastrointestinal perforations in patients with rheumatoid arthritis treated with anti-TNF therapy: results from the BSRBR-RA. *Ann Rheum Dis* 2014;73(1):252–5.

80. Jani M, Dixon WG, Kersley-Fleet L, et al. Drug-specific risk and characteristics of lupus and vasculitis-like events in patients with rheumatoid arthritis treated with TNFi: results from BSRBR-RA. *RMD Open* 2017;3(1):e000314.

81. Hyrich KL, Symmons DP, Watson KD, Silman AJ. Pregnancy outcome in women who were exposed to anti-tumor necrosis factor agents: results from a national population register. *Arthritis Rheum* 2006;54(8):2701–2.

82. Verstappen SM, King Y, Watson KD, Symmons DP, Hyrich KL. Anti-TNF therapies and pregnancy: outcome of 130 pregnancies in the British Society for Rheumatology Biologics Register. *Ann Rheum Dis* 2011;70(5):823–6.

83. Strangfeld A, Pattloch D, Spilka M, et al. *Pregnancies in Patients with Long-Standing Rheumatoid Arthritis and Biologic DMARD Treatment: Course of Disease During Pregnancy And Pregnancy Outcomes.* ACR, San Francisco, 7—11 November 2015. *Arthritis Rheumatol* 2015;67(Suppl. 10). Available at: https://acrabstracts.org/abstract/pregnancies-in-patients-with-long-standing-rheumatoid-arthritis-and-biologic-dmard-treatment-course-of-disease-during-pregnancy-and-pregnancy-outcomes/

84. Dixon WG, Carmona L, Finckh A, et al. EULAR points to consider when establishing, analysing and reporting safety data of biologics registers in rheumatology. *Ann Rheum Dis* 2010;69(9):1596–602.

85. Askling J, Fored CM, Geborek P, et al. Swedish registers to examine drug safety and clinical issues in RA. *Ann Rheum Dis* 2006;65(6):707–12.

86. Watson K, Symmons D, Griffiths I, Silman A. The British Society for Rheumatology biologics register. *Ann Rheum Dis* 2005;64 Suppl 4:iv42–3.

87. Uitz E, Fransen J, Langenegger T, Stucki G. Clinical quality management in rheumatoid arthritis: putting theory into practice. Swiss Clinical Quality Management in Rheumatoid Arthritis. *Rheumatology (Oxf)* 2000 May;39(5):542–9.

88. Couderc M, Gottenberg JE, Mariette X, et al. Efficacy and safety of rituximab in the treatment of refractory inflammatory myopathies in adults: results from the AIR registry. *Rheumatology (Oxf)* 2011;50(12):2283–9.

89. Lahaye C, Soubrier M, Mulliez A, et al. Effectiveness and safety of abatacept in elderly patients with rheumatoid arthritis enrolled in the French Society of Rheumatology's ORA registry. *Rheumatology (Oxf)* 2016;55(5):874–82.

90. Morel J, Constantin A, Baron G, et al. Risk factors of serious infections in patients with rheumatoid arthritis treated with tocilizumab in the French Registry REGATE. *Rheumatology (Oxf)* 2017;56(10):1746–54.

91. Olsen IC, Haavardsholm EA, Moholt E, Kvien TK, Lie E. NOR-DMARD data management: implementation of data capture from electronic health records. *Clin Exp Rheumatol* 2014;32(5 Suppl 85):S-158–162.

92. Horak P, Skacelova M, Hejduk K, Smrzova A, Pavelka K. Abatacept and its use in the treatment of rheumatoid arthritis (RA) in the Czech Republic-data from the ATTRA registry. *Clin Rheumatol* 2013;32(10):1451–8.

93. Santos MJ, Canhao H, Mourao AF, et al. Reuma.pt contribution to the knowledge of immune-mediated systemic rheumatic diseases. *Acta Rheumatol Port* 2017;42(3):232–9.

45

Voluntary patient registries

Jeff Greenberg and Sheetal Patel

Introduction

Voluntary patient registries for patients with rheumatoid arthritis (RA) have existed for many years, with many of these launched soon after the approval of the first biologic drugs. Over the years we have seen an increase in the number and size of voluntary registries.

With the number of approved drugs now available for the treatment of RA, there is an ever-increasing need for real world, objective data to shed light on the comparative effectiveness and comparative safety of newly approved drugs versus other standard of care older medications. This chapter will provide an overview of voluntary RA registries that currently recruit patients and actively publish research findings. This chapter will also highlight some of the key clinical insights derived from these voluntary registries.

Voluntary registries have their own strengths and limitations compared to population-based registries. Unlike pharmaceutical sponsored clinical trials, the majority of these voluntary registries do not exclude patients based on comorbidities. Additionally, clinical trials are not always feasible on a large scale and have limited duration. Observational registries do not typically have these limitations.

At this time numerous registries exist all over the United States, Latin America, Canada, Europe, and Asia which continue to provide invaluable epidemiologic data regarding utilization, safety, efficacy, and cost-effectiveness of the medications in common use. For this chapter, we will focus on some of the voluntary registries such as CORRONA, VARA, NDB, IORRA, BIOBADASAR, and RISE that have furthered this cause and have been the source for numerous peer-reviewed publications. In chronic disorders such as RA, these clinical registries have been very effective in demonstrating the long-term benefit and safety of these now routinely used medications.

The Consortium of Rheumatology Researchers of North America (CORRONA) RA Registry

This registry was founded by a group of academic US rheumatologists in 2001 and began collecting data in 2002. It has since evolved to become the largest prospective rheumatoid arthritis (RA) registry in the world. It has enrolled more than 42 000 patients across 40 states and this number is increasing every day. It is a large observational cohort with 130 000+ patient-years of detailed clinical observational data. It is the only US national registry that collects data from both the physician as well as the patient at the enrolment visit as well as subsequent follow-up encounters. Both the patient as well as rheumatologist complete questionnaires with emphasis on disease activity at the time of clinical encounter as well as pertinent information that has changed during the period of each subsequent visit. Data are collected approximately every 6 months. Collected data includes joint counts, visual analogue scales for patient and physicians, laboratory values such as acute phase reactants as well as diagnostic tests including rheumatoid factor and anticitrullinated protein antibody (ACPA) status. In addition, radiographic outcomes are recorded in categories ranging from normal, to joint space narrowing and erosions. Classical patient-reported outcomes (PROs) are also collected including the Health Assessment Questionnaire (HAQ). Patient habits including smoking, alcohol consumption, and demographics including employment, disability, insurance type and status, marital status, and time lost from work are routinely recorded. Reasons are reported by physician regarding start or switching of medications.[1]

Contributions to the literature from the CORRONA RA registry

The CORRONA RA registry data have been used for more than peer-reviewed 100 manuscripts over the past 15 years. Contributions to the literature have focused on a number of key thematic areas. The first major research area has been cardiovascular disease. Four papers have been published, advancing our knowledge relating to risk factors, risk prediction, and drug effects. The first paper by Solomon et al demonstrated that RA—related risk factors were independent predictors of incident CV events.[2]

A second study developed and internally validated a disease specific cardiovascular risk prediction score.[3] In addition, Greenberg et al published one of the first reports that anti-TNF biologics reduce the risk of cardiovascular events versus non-biologic disease-modifying antirheumatic drugs (DMARD).[4] Finally, a fourth paper demonstrated that patients with higher cumulative disease activity over time incurred a higher risk of CV events.[5]

In addition to studies of cardiovascular disease and other drug safety manuscripts, the registry has also been used for comparative effectiveness research. Among these publications, Harold et al. demonstrated that switching to rituximab versus a subsequent anti-TNF biologic was associated with improved clinical response outcomes.[6] This observation has been replicated in other registries, including by Finkh et al.[7] In contrast, Harold et al. also demonstrated that switching to abatacept versus a subsequent anti-TNF biologic was not associated with improved clinical outcomes.[8]

The Veteran's Affair's Rheumatoid Arthritis (VARA) registry

The veteran's registry, called VARA, offers an important source of information in the study of men suffering from RA. Conventionally most of the research regarding rheumatoid arthritis pathophysiology and outcomes has focused on women as RA is more common in women. However epidemiological data shows that men with RA tend to experience a more severe clinical course with more frequent extra-articular manifestations than women. In spite of this difference in prognosis, we have scarce information on predominantly male RA cohorts and the VARA registry addresses this gap.

Men account for almost 90% of the roughly 900 veterans with information in VARA. The VARA was established in 2002 with its first patient enrolled in early 2003 and now includes more than 2200 veterans. It is a prospective, observational, multicentre study that includes VA medical centres in 12 cities (Birmingham, Alabama; Brooklyn, New York; Dallas, Texas; Denver, Colorado; Jackson, Mississippi; Iowa City, Iowa; Little Rock, Arkansas; Omaha, Nebraska; Portland, Oregon; Philadelphia, Pennsylvania; Salt Lake City, Utah; and Washington, DC). Another unique advantage of this registry is the inclusion of US military veterans and active-duty personnel have traditionally been underrepresented in RA research partly due to the challenges involved in conducting investigations across federal facilities

In addition to support from VA research, VARA has been supported by the VA Office of Research Development, the National Institutes of Health, industry, and non-profit foundations. The database contains clinical and biological information about the patients who volunteer to submit data to VARA. All patients need to provide informed consent, be 18 years of age or older and should meet the American College of Rheumatology (ACR) classification criteria for RA. Serum, plasma, and DNA samples are collected at enrolment and banked in a central bio repository housed at the Nebraska Western-Iowa VA Health Care System in Omaha. The VARA Scientific and Ethics Advisory Committee (SEAC) provides ethical and scientific review as well as oversees bio specimen access. Upon receipt of specimens, standardized laboratory assays on serum, including C-reactive protein (CRP), rheumatoid factor (RF), and anticyclic citrullinated (anti-CCP) antibody are performed and these data are made available for all future investigations. Clinical data are entered by investigators during routine rheumatologic care. The VARA has served as a valuable resource for clinical and clinical-translational research, ranging from studies of disease outcomes and their determinants, genetic, and environmental risk factors, the validation of biomarkers, and healthcare resource utilization.

Contributions to the literature from VARA

Using these data, researchers have been able to examine specific medical and biological information about male RA patients to see what genetic and environmental factors may have played a role in the patients' disease and outcomes. There were several interesting outcomes noted. There was an observed twofold increase in mortality risk among men with RA compared with age-matched men without RA in the general US population (standardized mortality ratio [SMR] 2.1; 95% confidence interval, 1.8–2.5), a risk that seems to be higher than that observed in other RA cohorts that have focused on women. Of the variables associated with mortality in this group, several potentially modifiable factors were identified including high erythrocyte sedimentation rate (ESR); elevated Disease Activity Score (DAS)-28 (a composite measure of disease activity including assessments of 28 joints); prednisone use; and low body weight. In a multivariate analysis that included medication use and disease activity, factors associated with mortality included: Caucasian race, prednisone use, higher disease activity as measured on the Routine Assessment of Patient Index Data, increased ESR, greater RF concentration, and presence of subcutaneous nodules. In contrast, the use of methotrexate was associated with a 40% decreased mortality risk. This reduction was independent of confounders including disease activity, and was postulated to be likely from a decrease in cardiovascular deaths. Of note the finding of increased risk with prednisone use may be confounded by the fact that steroid use is associated with independent risks or could reflect more severe disease or treatment more focused on comfort than long-term safety.[9]

The National Data Bank (NDB) for Rheumatic Diseases

The NDB was founded as a non-profit research organization in 1998 by Dr Frederick Wolfe. It is a longitudinal observational patient-driven database and is the largest patient-reported research data bank for rheumatic disorders in the United States. The NDB obtains its information from patients with rheumatic diseases, and when required validates this information from hospital and physician sources and from national death records. Comprehensive self-reported questionnaires are sent out twice a year to patients with rheumatic diseases. These self-reported data have provided valuable insight into therapeutic response, long-term outcomes and the real-world burden of people who live with these chronic rheumatic conditions.

Since 1998 more than 100 000 patients with more than 100 various rheumatic diseases have consented to participate and more than 50 000 of whom have completed at least one 6-month questionnaire. Participating patients have been under the care of more than 1500 rheumatologists from the United States and Canada. The NDB obtains participants primarily by referral from US and Canadian rheumatologists where the treating rheumatologist provides the diagnosis. A minority of participants enrol from other sources, including self-referral, after obtaining information from physicians, societies, and websites. Funding for the NDB is derived from individual donations, public and private research grants, and from pharmaceutical; companies for conducting postmarketing drug safety registries. No reimbursement is provided for this involvement. The name 'data bank' highlights the multiple uses and wide scope than would be expected in a single registry study. In that essence, a database can be thought of a collection of registries. Databases are also very effective in assessing the risk of development of comorbid conditions, for example, cardiovascular and malignant disease. They also help determine the rates and predictors of direct and indirect costs, work disability, and mortality.[10]

Contributions to the literature from the NDB

Many important publications concerning RA, osteoarthritis, systemic lupus erythematosus, fibromyalgia, and pharmacoepidemiology have resulted from NDB research. A study by Kaleb et al. analysed the relationship between health status and all-cause mortality in 10 319 RA patients selected from the NDB, using the HAQ and the Medical Outcomes Study Short Form-36 questionnaire (SF-36). Results showed that the HAQ and the SF-36 PCS were both strongly associated with mortality risk in patients with RA.[11]

Wolfe et al published one of the first papers assessing increased risk of lymphoma after anti-TNFα treatment using data from the National Data Bank for Rheumatic Diseases. In this study 18 572 patients with RA were followed. Investigators concluded that even though the standardized incidence ratio for lymphoma was greatest for anti-TNF therapies, this may have been a result of channelling bias, whereby patients with the highest risk of lymphoma preferentially receive anti-TNF therapy.[12]

The Institute of Rheumatology Rheumatoid Arthritis cohort (IORRA)

The IORRA cohort is a large observational cohort established in 2000 at the Institute of Rheumatology at Tokyo Women's Medical University in Japan. The main goal of this study is to investigate the current status as well as changes in the treatment of RA in Japan. Tokyo Women's Medical University treats approximately 1% of all rheumatoid arthritis patients in Japan and the IORRA study is a clinical study of ambulatory RA patients treated there. Essentially, all RA patients were registered and clinical parameters were assessed with survey conducted every 6 months. Patients undergo an evaluation of swollen or painful joints by physicians twice a year (in spring and Autumn). Approximately 5000–5800 patients participate with more than 11 000 patients having been enrolled at least once. After blood tests, patients are given a survey form of about 30 pages that they can fill at home and mail back. Data are both patient-reported and physician-reported, and include disease activity, general health information, treatment data and new disease events, and selected laboratory data. Selected patient-reported health outcomes are validated using medical records.

Contributions to the literature from IORRA

Analysis of the IORRA cohort has yielded at least 36 papers in English.

Interestingly a large observational study of mortality and cause of death in 7926 Japanese patients with RA ((81.9% females; mean age 56.3 ± 13.1 years; mean disease duration 8.5 ± 8.3 years) who enrolled in IORRA from October 2000 to April 2007 showed that mortality of Japanese RA patients is comparable to that in previous reports from western countries, even though the causes of death were different. Another 14-year observational study analysed trends in the occurrence of malignancy in Japanese patients with RA based on data from the IORRA cohort. Among 11 106 Japanese patients with RA 507 malignancies (72 breast cancers, 68 malignant lymphomas, 65 stomach cancers, 60 lung cancers, 54 colorectal cancers) were confirmed. However, occurrence of overall and site-specific malignancies in Japanese patients with RA did not increase with the expanding use of methotrexate (MTX) and biological agents in the time frame observed.[13] An IORRA cohort study in 2010 analysed risk factors of lymphoproliferative disorders among patients with RA treated with methotrexate. It found that among RA patients concomitantly treated with MTX, high disease activity, but not methotrexate dose, were risk factors for the occurrence of lymphoproliferative disorder.[14]

BIOBADASER (Spanish Registry for Adverse Events of Biological Therapy in Rheumatic diseases)

This is a prospective registry of rheumatic patients treated with biological therapies that was created in February 2000 with 100 centres in Spain. It was established with the objective of identifying the relevant adverse events that could appear during the treatment of rheumatic diseases with biologic therapy, to identify the unexpected adverse events and to know the survival of the drug as an effective measure. It is essentially a registry involving patients that are being treated with biologics in the participating centres and collects information on the patients, the treatment as well as adverse events. A relevant adverse event is defined as any event related or not to the treatment that, independent of dose, produces death, puts the life of the patient in danger, merits hospitalization or prolongs it, or causes persistent or significant incapacity. Also included are the adverse events that the physician considered important. BIOBADASER 2.0 is a national drug safety registry of patients with rheumatic diseases starting treatment with any biologic and followed thereafter. BIOBADASER 2.0 is an adaptation of the former made in 2006, which includes all data, since February 2000, from 14 large public hospitals, as a way to reinforce quality and consistency and facilitate monitoring. Patients entering the registry are followed prospectively and evaluated at the time an adverse event or a change in the biologic therapy occurs; thus providing specific cohorts for specific analyses. The process of data entry is done directly on the internet by each participating centre every time there is a change in treatment of the registered patient or occurrence of an adverse events. Participation in BIOBADASER is completely voluntary and there is no payment involved. Data is monitored weekly and a more comprehensive review of the data is done randomly on 10% of the registered centres.

Contributions from BIOBADASER

The analysis of this registry was reassuring regarding increased rate of infections with biological therapies. A study by

Cobo-Ibáñez et al. analysed RA or other immune-mediated connective tissue diseases patients on anti-TNF or rituximab included in the Spanish registry BIOBADASER 2.0 (2000–2011). Incidence rate of serious infections was higher in non-RA immune-mediated connective tissue diseases (ICTD) than in RA, with an international ratio (IR) ratio of 3.15 (95% CI 1.86, 5.31) before adjustment and 1.96 (95% CI 1.06, 3.65) after adjustment for age, comorbidity, and corticosteroid use. Mortality due to infections was higher in ICTD although it did not reach statistical significance. Age, disease duration, comorbidities, corticosteroids, and ICTD different to RA were all independently associated with serious infections.[15]

Other studies have revealed that the rates of neoplasm or cardiac failure are not significantly increased with these therapies. Also, analysis did not provide sufficient data to implicate increased TNF antagonists use to incidence of demyelinating diseases in patients with rheumatic diseases. Differences between cases depending on the pharmacovigilance source could be explained by selective reporting bias outside registries.[16]

The Rheumatology Informatics System for Effectiveness (RISE) registry

The ACR launched the Rheumatology Informatics System for Effectiveness (RISE) in 2014. It is a US-based electronic health record (EHR)-enabled voluntary registry and is the first and largest national EHR-enabled rheumatology registry in the United States. Rheumatologists need to enter data only once and RISE will there on passively collect information from integrated EHR systems. It is officially recognized as a Qualified Clinical Data Registry by the Centers for Medicare & Medicaid Services. It allows for the collection of data on quality of care without individual patient informed consent. RISE currently includes data on numerous quality measures regarding RA, drug safety, allows osteoporosis prevention and treatment, low back pain, and preventive healthcare (e.g. smoking, blood pressure management). It relies upon whatever data is included in the medical record, and therefore may have missing data if different electronic medical records (EMRs) capture different data elements, or are not completed by the physician. It is aimed to help US rheumatologists effectively face some of the challenges of an evolving healthcare environment including adapting to new payment models, meeting changing certification requirements, and to fulfil national performance reporting requirements. The benchmarking tool users to compare the details of their patient population against established and validated rheumatology quality metrics. RISE also offers access to de-identified aggregate data from other participating sites so users can view the characteristics of their patient population and compare them with other participants' patient populations. RISE includes patients with all diagnoses seen by participating rheumatologists, and is free for all ACR and Alliance for Human Research Protection (AHRP) members. Additionally, it is compliant with the Health Insurance Portability and accountability Act. As of August 11, 2016, data has been collected from over 400 rheumatologists involving more than 650 000 patients and over 3 million encounters.

Contributions from RISE

Few studies have been published to date from RISE. Among the subset with RA, 34.4% of patients were taking a biologic or targeted synthetic DMARD at their last encounter, and 66.7% were receiving a non-biologic DMARD. Examples of quality measures include that 55.2% had a disease activity score recorded, 53.6% a functional status score, and 91.0% were taking a DMARD in the last year. RISE provides valuable infrastructure for improving the quality of care in rheumatology and is a unique data source to generate new knowledge. This can lead to more efficient care as well as more predictable payments in the future. It can also help decrease treatment gaps across the country. Data validation and mapping are ongoing.[17]

Conclusion

The establishment of voluntary registries for RA patients have provided valuable additional data on the postapproval comparative safety and comparative effectiveness of newly approved biologics.[18]

REFERENCES

1. Kremer J. The CORRONA database. *Clin Exp Rheumatol* 2005;23 Suppl 4:S172–177.
2. Solomon DH, Kremer J, Curtis JR, et al. Explaining the cardiovascular risk associated with rheumatoid arthritis: traditional risk factors versus markers of rheumatoid arthritis severity. *Ann Rheum Dis* 2010;69(11):1920–5.
3. Solomon DH, Greenberg J, Curtis JR, et al. Derivation and internal validation of an expanded cardiovascular risk prediction score for rheumatoid arthritis: a consortium of rheumatology researchers of North America Registry Study. *Arthritis Rheumatol* 2015;67(8):1995–2003.
4. Greenberg JD, Kremer JM, Curtis JR, et al. Tumour necrosis factor antagonist use and associated risk reduction of cardiovascular events among patients with rheumatoid arthritis. *Ann Rheum Dis* 2011;70(4):576–82.
5. Solomon DH, Reed GW, Kremer JM, et al. Disease activity in rheumatoid arthritis and the risk of cardiovascular events. *Arthritis Rheumatol* 2015;67(6):1449–55.
6. Harrold LR, Reed GW, Magner R, et al. Comparative effectiveness and safety of rituximab versus subsequent anti-tumor necrosis factor therapy in patients with rheumatoid arthritis with prior exposure to anti-tumor necrosis factor therapies in the United States CORRONA registry. *Arthritis Res Ther* 2015;17(1):256.
7. Finckh A, Ciurea A, Brulhart L, et al. B cell depletion may be more effective than switching to an alternative anti-tumor necrosis factor agent in rheumatoid arthritis patients with inadequate response to anti-tumor necrosis factor agents. *Arthritis Rheum* 2007;56(5):1417–23.
8. Harrold LR, Reed GW, Kremer JM, et al. The comparative effectiveness of abatacept versus anti-tumor necrosis factor switching for rheumatoid arthritis patients previously treated with an anti-tumor necrosis factor. *Ann Rheum Dis* 2015;74(2):430–6.
9. Mikuls TR, Reimod A, Kerr GS, Cannon GW. Insights and implications of the VA rheumatoid arthritis registry. *Fed Pract* 2015 May;32(5):24–9.

10. Wolfe F, Michaud K. The National Data Bank for rheumatic diseases: a multi-registry rheumatic disease data bank. *Rheumatology (Oxf)* 2011;*50*:16–24.

11. Michaud K, Vera-Llonch M, Oster GMortality risk by functional status and health-related quality of life in patients with rheumatoid arthritis. *J Rheumatol* 2012;*39*(1):54–9.

12. Wolfe F, Michaud K. Lymphoma in rheumatoid arthritis: the effect of methotrexate and anti-tumor necrosis factor therapy in 18,572 patients. *Arthritis Rheum* 2004;*50*:1740–51.

13. Nakajima A, Inoue E, Tanaka E, et al. Mortality and cause of death in Japanese patients with rheumatoid arthritis based on a large observational cohort, IORRA. *Scand J Rheumatol* 2010;*39*:360–7.

14. Shimizu Y, Nakajima A, Inoue E, et al. Characteristics and risk factors of lymphoproliferative disorders among patients with rheumatoid arthritis concurrently treated with methotrexate: a nested case-control study of the IORRA cohort. *Clin Rheumatol* 2017;*36*(6):1237–45.

15. Cobo-Ibáñez T, Descalzo MA, Loza-Santamaría E, et al. Serious infections in patients with rheumatoid arthritis and other immune-mediated connective tissue diseases exposed to anti-TNF or rituximab: data from the Spanish registry BIOBADASER 2.0. *Rheumatol Int* 2014;*34*:953–61.

16. Fernandez-Espartero MC, Perez-Zafrilla B, Naranjo A, Esteban C, Ortiz AM, Gomez-Reino JJ. Demyelinating disease in patients treated with TNF antagonists in rheumatology: data from BIOBADASER, a pharmacovigilance database, and a systematic review. *Semin Arthritis Rheum* 2011;*40*:330–37.

17. Yazdany J, Bansback N, Clowse M, et al. Rheumatology informatics system for effectiveness: a national informatics-enabled registry for quality improvement. *Arthritis Care Res (Hoboken)* 2016;*68*(12):1866–73.

18. Curtis JR, Jain A, Askling J, et al. A comparison of patient characteristics and outcomes in selected European and U.S. rheumatoid arthritis registries. *Semin Arthritis Rheum* 2010;*40*(1):2–14.e1.

Index

abatacept 47, 134, 436, 474, 477, 479
absenteeism 271, 273–7, 278
accelerometers 287
acetaminophen 334
acetylation 67
acid-dissociation
    radioimmunoassay 427
ACPA-negative arthralgia 114, 125,
    488, 490
ACPA-negative RA 45, 47, 49, 67,
    111, 116
ACPA-positive arthralgia 37, 125,
    126, 127, 488, 490
ACPA-positive RA 38, 45, 47, 49, 65,
    67, 87–8, 116, 124
ACR20/50/70 164, 498, 508
ACR/EULAR
    2010 classification criteria 18–19,
        24–5, 109–11
    remission criteria 497, 498, 499
activities of daily living 315
activity diaries 287, 313
activity logs 287
activity monitors 287
acute phase reactants 18, 162–3, 392
adalimumab 371, 372, 374–5, 431, 473
adaptive immunity 100–1
administration reactions 478–9
adrenal insufficiency 345–6
adverse effects/events 333, 344–9,
    359–60,
        361, 362, 377–82, 395, 404–6,
        436,
        449–50, 471–81, 537–40
aerobic capacity 285, 287
Aggregatibacter actinomy
    cetemcomitans 36, 38, 66
agranulocytosis 361
Aircast Pneumatic Walkers 303
air pollution 34
airway diseases, *see* pulmonary
    disease
airway exposures 34, 36, 37, 38, 122
alarmins 95
alcohol use 36
alopecia 476
American College of
    Rheumatology (ACR)
    ACR20/50/70 164, 498, 508
    ACR/EULAR 2010 classification
        criteria 18–19, 24–5, 109–11
    ACR/EULAR remission
        criteria 497, 498, 499
    classification criteria 18, 23–4, 109
    clinical guidelines 520–4
    improvement criteria 164

American Rheumatism
    Association (ARA)
    diagnostic criteria 7, 109
    functional class 1–4 224, 225
aminopterin 8
amyloidosis 117
anaemia 140
    aplastic 377
    of chronic disease 140, 392
    iron deficiency 140
analgesics 331–6
angiogenesis 169, 171–2, 372
animal models 465
ankle disease 298
ankle injections 304–6
antiacetylated protein
    antibodies 65, 67
anticarbamylated protein
    antibodies 65, 67
anti-CD20 molecules 407; *see also*
    rituximab
anticitrullinated protein antibodies
    (ACPA) 18, 37, 65, 66–8,
    87–8, 124
anticyclic citrullinated peptide
    (anti-CCP) antibodies 18, 468
antidepressants 335–6
antidouble stranded DNA
    antibodies 436
antidrug antibodies 381, 425
    detection 426
    tolerance 437
antigen presentation 73–4, 79
antigen recognition 74–5
antigen-specific
    immunotherapy 79–80
anti-idiotype antibodies 425
antimalarials 8
antineutrophil cytoplasmic
    antibodies 436
antinuclear antibodies 436
anti-TNF therapy, *see* tumour
    necrosis factor inhibitors
anxiety 142
aplastic anaemia 377
apps 323–4
APRIL 100–1, 407
ARA 1–4 224, 225
arthralgia
    ACPA-negative 114, 125,
        488, 490
    ACPA-positive 37, 125, 126, 127,
        488, 490
    clinically suspect 111–12,
        121, 124–5
    primary care 113

Arthritis Impact Measurement Scales
    (AIMS) 227
Arthritis Prevention in the Preclincal
    Phase of RA with Abatacept
    (APIPPRA) 491
Arthritis Self-Management
    Programme 323
arthroscopic biopsy 170
aspergillosis 378
aspirin 8
atacicept 407
atlantoaxial subluxation 117, 138
'at risk' of RA 121, 124–6, 172–3,
    488–9, 490
aurothioglucose 363
autoantibodies 65–9, 87–8, 124
autoimmune adverse events 436, 481
autonomic dysfunction 255
azathioprine 363

back-translation 465
bacterial infections 36, 38, 66,
    377–8, 537–8
BAFF 100–1, 407
Baker's cyst 117
balance 285
baricitinib 446, 449, 474–5
basal ganglia 254
B cells 100–1, 389–90, 399
B-cell therapies 399–408
Berg Balance Scale 287
big data 511
binding bodies 425
BIOBADASER 547–8
biologic disease-modifying
    antirheumatic drugs
    (bDMARDs) 355
    adverse events 473–5, 476, 477,
        478, 479, 480–1
    combination therapy 458
    cost-effectiveness 264–7
    European registers 535–41
    immunogenicity 425–37
    safety 537–40
    tapering 266
biomarkers 467–8, 500–1
biomimics 411
biosimilars 411–21
    clinical guidelines 524
    clinical trials 414, 416–19
    demonstration of
        biosimilarity 414
    economic factors 266, 419–20
    European Medicines Agency
        approach 411–13
    Health Canada approach 414

immunogenicity 419, 436–7
international consensus 421
naming and labelling 420
postmarketing surveillance 420
rituximab 407
switch studies 417–19
TNF inhibitors 420
US Food and Drug Administration
    approach 411, 413–14
body composition 287
bone adverse events 347, 480,
    529, 531
bone comorbidities 141–2, 152–3
bone erosion
    autoantibodies 68, 87–8
    cytokines 86–7, 102
    IL-6 391–2
    immune cells 85–6
    mechanisms 85–9
    MRI 211
    osteoblasts 89
    osteoclasts 85
    radiography 5–6, 117, 178–80
    synovial fibroblast role 56–7, 86
    ultrasound 196, 200
bone marrow oedema 210–11
bone resorption 85
boutonnière deformity 117
Bradford Hill criteria 472
brain, fatigue 254–5
breastfeeding 349, 359, 361, 527–8
bridging ELISA test 426
Bristol Rheumatoid Arthritis
    Fatigue Multi-Dimensional
    Questionnaire (BRAF
    MDQ) 252
bronchiectasis 135, 149–50, 406
bronchiolitis 135
buprenorphine 335

C5 49
calcium pyrophosphate disease-
    related arthritis 198
callus debridement 303
calreticulin 65
Canadian Occupational Performance
    Measure 312–13
cancer risk 135–6, 140, 141, 151–2,
    380–1, 406, 449, 475, 538–9
candidate genes 46–8
candidiasis 378
Caplan syndrome 135
capsaicin, topical 336
carbamylation 67
cardiovascular adverse events 347,
    380, 395, 406, 475–6, 538

cardiovascular disease 102–3, 137, 147–8, 392, 524, 527
cartilage destruction
  chondrocytes 90–1
  cytokines 102
  MRI 211
  radiography 117
  synovial fibroblasts 56–7, 89–90
case-control studies 34–7, 46
case definition 23–6
cataract 348
causality 472
CD4+ T cells 48, 76–8
CD8+ cytotoxic T cells 79
CD20 399
CD20 antagonists 407; see also rituximab
CD40 ligand 95
CD68 170
CDAI 165, 497, 498, 499, 509
ceiling effects 240
celecoxib 333–4
central fatigue 253
centrally acting analgesics 335–6
central nervous system 103–4, 138
central sensitization 285, 335
central tolerance 77
certolizumab pegol 371, 372, 375, 431, 434, 473
cervical spine 117, 138, 211
Charlson Comorbidity Index 145
chemokines 96–7
chlorambucil 363
chloroquine 8
chromosome 6q23 49
chrondrocytes 90–1
chronic obstructive pulmonary disease 150–1
ciclosporin 362–3
Cimzia, see certolizumab pegol
cis-signalling 389
citrullination 65, 79
classification criteria
  ACR 18, 23–4, 109
  ACR/EULAR 2010 criteria 18–19, 24–5, 109–11
  diagnosis versus 19–20, 109
clazakizumab 394
clearing bodies 425
ClinHAQ 227
Clinical Disease Activity Index (CDAI) 165, 497, 498, 499, 509
clinical features of RA 109–17
clinical guidelines 519–32
clinically suspect arthralgia 111–12, 121, 124–5
clinical management decisions 511
clinical outcomes 507–15
clinical remission 213, 497, 499–501, 519
  drug-free 501–2
  MRI 213, 500
  ultrasound 200, 202, 500
clinical significance 241
clinical treatment targets 496–9
clinical trials
  adverse event identification 472
  biosimilars 414, 416–19
coccidioidomycosis 378
codeine 335
COG6 48

cognitive-behavioural fatigue programme 255–6
cognitive comorbidities 103–4
cohort studies 34–7
cold environment 34
combination therapy 264, 349, 355, 356, 363–5, 457–60
comorbidity 145–53, 277, 289
complement 68
composite measures 163–6
compression neuropathies 138
Consortium of Rheumatology Researchers of North America (CORRONA) RA registry 545–6
conventional (synthetic) disease-modifying antirheumatic drugs 355–65
  adverse events 473, 476–7, 478, 479, 480–81
  combination therapy 264, 355, 356, 363–5, 457–60
  cost-effectiveness 264, 266–7, 357–8
  currently use drugs 355
  impacts 355–6
  monitoring 356
  starting 356
  stopping 356–7
  tapering 357
  triple therapy 363–4
core data set 508
core set variables 161
corneal melt 117, 141
coronary artery disease 137
CORRONA RA registry 545–6
corticosteroids, see glucocorticoids
cortisone 8
cost-effectiveness of treatment 262–7, 357–8, 406–7, 458–9
cost of illness studies 259–62
COX-2 inhibitors 333–4
CpG sites 50
C-reactive protein 18, 162–3, 392
cricoarytenoid arthritis 135
criterion contamination 240
critical quality attributes 414
cryptococcus 378
crystal-induced arthritis 14
CT-P13 420
cultural issues, self-reports 241
cutaneous adverse events 349, 380, 476–7
cutaneous manifestations of RA 141
cutaneous vasculitis 117
cyclophosphamide 363
cyst, Baker's 117
cytochrome P450 340
cytokines 78, 95–104
  bone erosion 86–7, 102
  cartilage destruction 102
  JAK-STAT pathway 443–4
  pre-RA 97–9
  synovitis 99
  systemic features of RA 102–4
  TNF inhibitors effects 99, 372
cytomegalovirus 36, 379
cytopenias 377

DANBIO registry 418, 437
danger associated molecular patterns 74

DAS 164–5, 497, 498, 499
DAS28 164–5, 497, 498, 499, 508–9
daylight sign 297
demyelinating disease 380
dendritic cells 73–4, 79
dens dislocation 117
depression 142, 153, 277, 392
diabetes
  glucocorticoid-induced 347–8
  RA risk 147–8
diagnosis of RA 13–22, 109
  ARA criteria 7, 109
  classification versus 19–20, 109
  critical features 17–18
  delayed 13
  differential diagnosis 16–17, 115–16
  initial evaluation 14–16
  MRI 211–12
  ultrasound 196–8, 201
diaries of activity 287, 313
diet 36, 122
differential diagnosis 16–17, 115–16
digital technology 317, 323–4, 499
direct calorimetry 286
disability
  benefits of therapeutic exercise 288–90
  clinical outcome 509–10
  work 271, 273–7
disease activity assessment 161–6, 497–9, 508–9
disease activity monitoring
  MRI 212
  ultrasound 198–9
disease-modifying antirheumatic drugs
  classification 355
  early use 8
disease-specific questionnaires 225, 227
distress 239, 243
DKK-1 89
DNA methylation 50–1, 57, 90
doubly labelled water 286
DRESS syndrome 361
drug development 463–8
drug-free remission 501–2
drug-induced conditions
  anaemia 140
  lung disease 136–7
  neutropenia 140
dry eyes and mouth 140–1
dynamic biomarkers 467
dyslipidaemia 148

early rheumatoid arthritis
  clinical guidelines 519, 523
  combination therapy 365
  recognition 116
  synovial biopsy 172
economic factors
  absenteeism 278
  biosimilars 266, 419–20
  clinical outcomes 511
  cost-effectiveness of treatment 262–7, 357–8, 406–7, 458–9
  cost of illness studies 259–62
  physical activity and exercise programmes 289–90

presenteeism 278
productivity 278–9
ectopic lymphoid-like structures 76–7
education
  educational level of patients 34, 241, 276
  ergonomics 314–15
  foot health 302
  self-management 317
Educational Needs Assessment Tool 313
effector T cells 77–8
eHealth 499
electrochemiluminescence-based assays 427
electronic self-report questionnaires 241–2
ELISA test 426
Enbrel, see etanercept
endocrine adverse events 480–1
energy conservation techniques 314
enthesitis 196, 211
environmental risk factors 33–7, 38–9, 121–2
epidemiology 7, 23–30
epigenetics 45, 50–1, 57
epigenome-wide association studies 50
episcleritis 117, 141
Epstein–Barr virus 36
EQ-5D 510, 514
ergonomic approaches 314–15
erythrocyte sedimentation rate 18, 162–3, 392
etanercept 371, 372, 374, 434, 473, 480
ethics, self-report questionnaires 242
etoricoxib 333
European League Against Rheumatism (EULAR)
  ACR/EULAR 2010 classification criteria 18–19, 24–5, 109–11
  clinical guidelines 519–20, 523–4
  EULAR-OMERACT composite power Doppler ultrasonography (PDUS) score 198–9
  EULAR-OMERACT RA MRI reference image atlas 212
  remission criteria 497, 498, 499
EuroQol 510, 514
Evaluation of Daily Activity Questionnaire 313
evolution of RA 123–4
exercise 256, 285–91, 306, 315
experiments of nature 465
Expert Patients Programme 323
expression quantitative trait locus 48
extra-articular disease 117, 133–42, 392
eye
  adverse events 348–9, 362, 479–80
  manifestations of RA 117, 140–1

family studies 34, 45
FasL 95
fatigue 114–15, 251–6, 289, 392
Fc receptors 68, 88, 372
Felty's syndrome 140
fentanyl 335
fertility 359, 361

fibroblast-like synoviocytes 55–60, 86, 89–90, 101, 171
fibromyalgia 239, 513
filgotinib 451
finger deformities 117
flares 200, 213, 276, 331, 357, 502
flexibility 285, 287
floor effects 240
follicular bronchiolitis 135
foot 117, 297–306
    injections 304–6
    orthoses 299, 302, 304
Foot Function Index 300
FOOTSTEP 302
footwear 303–4
Forestier, Jacques 8
Foxp3 78–9, 86
friction cost approach 278
frontostriatal pathways 254
functional assays 414
fungal infections 378–9

gait 298–9
Garrod, Alfred Baring 3
gastrointestinal adverse events 333, 347, 449–50, 478, 539–41
Genant–Sharp score 183, 185–7
gender differences
    risk of RA 34
    work outcomes 275–6
general practitioners 324
generic questionnaires 225
genetic factors
    gene–environment interactions 37, 38–9, 66
    risk of RA 33–4, 45–9, 65–6
    severity of RA 49–50
    treatment response 50, 173, 404
genome editing 48
genome-wide association studies 46–8
geographical risk factors 34
glaucoma 348–9
global assessments 162
Global Burden of Disease study 28
glucocorticoids 339–49
    adverse events 344–9, 472–3, 476, 477–8, 479, 450, 481, 529, 531
    combination therapy 349
    DMARD effect 342–3
    dosing strategies 343
    history of use 8–9
    indications 341–3
    local injections 304–6, 343–4
    monitoring 349
    oral 343
    pharmacology 339–41
    pregnancy and lactation 349
    prophylactic measures 349
    pulse therapy 343
    stress regimes 346–7
    tapering 346
gold injections 8, 363
golimumab 371, 372, 375–6, 434, 473
granulocyte-macrophage colony-stimulating factor 55, 56, 73, 77, 95, 100, 102
granulocytes 372

haematological abnormalities 140, 479
haemochromatosis 115

hair 349
hallux valgus 297, 299
hand
    deformities 117
    ergonomics 314
    exercises 315
    function 311–12, 313
    orthoses 315
    osteoarthritis 17, 115
Health Assessment Questionnaire (HAQ) 163, 227, 228–9, 510, 512–13
    ClinHAQ 227
    HAQII 227
    modified HAQ 227
    multidimensional HAQ 227, 230–2, 241
health economics, see economic factors
health-enhancing physical activity 286, 287–8, 289–91
health literacy 241
heart failure 137, 380
heart rate monitoring 286–7
hepatic adverse events 478
hepatitis B 115, 379, 404–5, 474
hepatitis C 115, 379, 404–5
herpes simplex virus 379
herpes zoster 405, 449
hidradenitis suppurativa 381
high-throughput screening 466
hip arthroplasty 531–2
histone modification 57
histoplasmosis 378
history of RA 3–9
HIV 379
HLA B 49
HLA DPB1 49
HLA DRB1 46–7, 48–9, 65
homeostasis 391
hormonal factors 34
Hospital Anxiety and Depression Scale 313
human capital approach 278
human immunodeficiency virus 379
human leucocyte antigens 38, 46–7, 48–9, 65
Humira, see adalimumab
hydroxychloroquine 355, 362, 473, 477, 479, 480
hypercholesterolaemia 450
hypercitrullination 36, 38, 66
hypersensitivity 478–8
hypertension 147
hypogammaglobulinaemia 405–6
hypothalamic–pituitary–adrenal axis 345–6
hypoxia 169, 172

ibuprofen 333–4
IgG 88
Ig-type receptors 95–6
IL-1 99
IL-1β 87, 104
IL-6 55, 56, 87, 95, 97, 99, 101, 102, 389–92
IL-6 inhibitors 392–5; see also tocilizumab
IL6R 47
IL-7 101
IL-15 101

IL-17A 101
IL-21 101
IL-23 98–9
immune response
    adaptive immunity 100–1
    IL-6 389–91
    innate immunity 74, 390–1
immunogenicity 406, 419, 425–37, 446
incidence of RA 23, 25–7
indirect calorimetry 286
infection
    feet 303
    increased risk in RA 136, 152, 344–5, 377–80, 404–5, 449, 472–5, 537–8, 539
    postoperative 379–80
    risk factor for RA 36, 38, 66
inflammation
    anticitrullinated protein antibodies 67
    cardiovascular disease 148
    fatigue 252–3
    fibroblast role 56, 57–8
    final common pathway 68–9
    foot pathology 302
    hypoxia 169
    IL-6 391–2
    JAK-STAT pathway 443
    memory response 58
    physical activity and exercise 289
    physical function scores 239
    shared factors with other inflammatory diseases 124
    subclinical 126
    synovial tissues 169, 170
    tendon 198
inflammatory bowel disease 381
infliximab 371, 372, 373, 427–31, 473
infusion reactions
    rituximab 404
    TNF inhibitors 377
injection therapy
    glucocorticoids 304–6, 343–4
    gold 8, 363
    injection site reactions 377
    ultrasound-guided 202–3, 304–6
innate immunity 74, 390–1
Institute of Rheumatology Rheumatoid Arthritis (IORRA) cohort 547
'intake' questionnaires 225
interferons 101
interleukin-6 55, 56, 87, 95, 97, 99, 101, 102, 389–92
interleukin-6 inhibitors 392–5; see also tocilizumab
interstitial lung disease 133–5, 149, 406
intervention studies 491
invadosomes 90
invariant natural killer T cells 79
iron deficiency anaemia 140

JAK inhibitors 446–52, 474–5, 477, 479
JAK-STAT pathway 443–5
joint aspiration, ultrasound-guided 202–3
joint assessment 161
joint count 161

joint damage
    clinical outcome 509
    IL-6 391–2
    physical function scores 239, 243
joint deformities 117, 297–8
joint distribution 113–14
joint injections, see injection therapy
joint pattern 17–18
joint protection 314
joint range-of-motion 285, 287
joint space 5–6, 180–1

knee arthroplasty 531–2
knee deformities 117

lactation 349, 359, 361, 527–8
lead generation 466
lead optimization 466–7
Leeds Foot Impact Scale 300
leflunomide 264, 355, 361–2, 473, 477, 479
Legionella pneumophila 378
leisure rehabilitation 316
leukocytes 56, 372, 391
leukotoxin A 66
lifestyle
    impact of RA 311
    risk factor for RA 33–7, 121–2
Lifestyle Management for Arthritis Programme 315, 317
lining layer 59–60
linkage disequilibrium 47–8
lipid paradox 102
lipid profile 450
Listeria monocytogenes 378
literacy 241
Löfgren's syndrome 17
lung disease 117, 124, 133–7, 149–51, 406, 477
lupus-like events 540
Lyme arthritis 17, 115
lymphocytes 171
lymphoma 140, 151, 381, 538–9

macrophage colony-stimulating factor 85, 100, 390
macrophages 100, 170
magnetic resonance imaging 207–13
    clinical outcome 509
    diagnosis of RA 211–12
    disease activity monitoring 212
    dynamic contrast-enhanced 208
    extremity MRI units 207
    fatigue 254–5
    gadolinium contrast 207–8
    outcome prediction 213
    pathology in RA 208–11
    remission 213, 500
    structural damage monitoring 212
    whole-body 208
malignancy risk 135–6, 140, 141, 151–2, 380–1, 406, 449, 475, 538–9
Manchester Foot Pain and Disability Questionnaire 300
matrix metalloproteinases 56, 57, 60, 90, 101, 102, 169, 372–3
Measurement of Efficacy of Treatment in the Era of Outcome in Rheumatology (METEOR) database 511
mechanistic biomarkers 467

memory response 58
mental health 142, 153, 277, 392
mepacrine 8
metabolic adverse events 347–8, 480–2
metabolic equivalent 286
metabolic syndrome 102–3
metabolism
  fatigue 254
  fibroblasts 58–9
  IL-6 391
  synovial 172
  T cells 77
metatarsophalangeal joints 297, 300
METEOR database 511
methotrexate 8, 355, 358–60
  adverse events 359–60, 473, 476, 477, 478, 480
  clinical use 359
  mechanism of action 358
  starting 356
  vaccinations 360
methylprednisolone 343
MHC class II genes 37, 38
mHealth 317
microbiome 36, 66, 124
micro-CT 200
microRNAs 51, 57
mobile health technology 317
modified HAQ 227
monoarthritis 114
monocytes 100, 170
morning stiffness 114, 125
mortality 30, 243, 538
MR spectroscopy 254
mucosal surfaces 124
multidimensional HAQ 227, 230–2, 241
Multimorbidity Index 145
multiplex biomarkers 468
multisensory monitors 287
muscle strength and endurance 285, 287
muscle weakness 138, 140
Musculo-Skeletal Health Questionnaire (MSK-HQ) 510
myeloid lineage 99–100
myocarditis 137
Myocrisin 363
myopathy
  glucocorticoid-induced 347
  manifestation of RA 138, 140

nail care 302
naproxen 333–4
National Data Bank 546–7
needle arthroscopic biopsy 170
nefopam 336
NETosis 68, 390–1
network science 468
neurological adverse events 477–8
neurological manifestations of RA 103–4, 138, 302
neuromuscular disorders 138, 140
neuromuscular function 285, 287
neutralizing bodies 425
neutropenia 140, 377, 405
neutrophil extracellular traps 68, 390–1
neutrophils 100
new-onset arthritis 14–16
NF-&B 58, 74, 391–2
nintedanib 149

NK cells 450
non-articular manifestations of RA 117, 133–42, 392
non-clinical safety evaluation 467
non-Hodgkin's lymphoma 140, 151
non-lymphocytic stromal memory 58
non-steroidal anti-inflammatory drugs 332–4
NOR-SWITCH 418, 437
nuclear factor of activated T-cell c1 86
nurses 324

obesity 36, 37, 122, 148
obinutuzumab 407
occupational therapy 311–17
ocular adverse events 348–9, 362, 479–80
ocular manifestations of RA 117, 140–1
ofatumumab 407
off-loading 303
oily fish 36
olokizumab 394
omega-3 fatty acids 36, 122
OMERACT, see Outcome Measures in Rheumatoid Arthritis Clinical Trials
online platforms 317, 323
onychocryptosis 302
ophthalmic adverse events 348–9, 362, 479–80
ophthalmic manifestations of RA 117, 140–1
opioids 334–5
opportunistic infections 136, 404, 449, 539
oral manifestations of RA 140–1
orthopaedic surgery 379–80, 531–32
orthoses
  foot 299, 302, 304
  hand and wrist 315
osteoarthritis 17, 115, 198
osteoblasts 89, 102
osteoclasts 68, 85, 102
osteonecrosis 347
osteopenia 141
osteophytes 196
osteoporosis 141, 152–3, 347, 392, 480, 529, 531
osteoprotegerin 86
Outcome Measures in Rheumatoid Arthritis Clinical Trials (OMERACT) 507–8
  EULAR-OMERACT composite power Doppler ultrasonography (PDUS) score 198–9
  EULAR-OMERACT RA MRI reference image atlas 212
  RA MRI scoring system (RAMRIS) 212
outcomes 213, 507–15
oxycodone 335

PAD enzymes 65, 66, 87
pain
  anticitrullinated protein antibodies 68
  benefits of therapeutic exercise 289
  drug management 331–6

IL-6 392
  increased sensitivity to 285, 335
  mechanisms in RA 331
paleopathology 4–5
palindromic rheumatism 17–18, 114, 116, 126
pancytopenia 377
pannus 55, 169, 391
paracetamol 334
paradoxical adverse events 381
parvovirus 16, 36, 115
pathogen associated molecular patterns 74
patient education, see education
Patient-Reported Outcome Measurement Information System (PROMIS) 232, 236–7, 241, 510, 515
patient-reported outcome measures 497, 498, 499, 509–10, 511–12
  fatigue 249
  foot-specific 300
pedometers 287
peer-led support 323
peficitinib 451
penicillamine 363
peptidyl-arginine deaminase (PAD) enzymes 65, 66, 87
performance-based measures 225
pericarditis 137
periodontitis 36, 38, 66, 123, 124
perioperative management 379–80, 530–32
peripheral arterial disease 302
peripheral fatigue 253
peripheral neuropathy 138, 302
peripheral sensitization 335
peripheral spondyloarthropathy 16–17
peripheral tolerance 77
peripheral ulcerative keratitis 117, 141
personalized medicine 464, 468
Personalized Risk Estimator of Rheumatoid Arthritis (PRE-RA) Family Study 487
pes planovalgus deformity 297
pharmacodynamics 467
pharmacogenetics 50
pharmacokinetics 467
phases of RA development 37
pH-shift-anti-idiotype ABT (PIA) method 427
physical activity 36, 256, 285–91
physical fitness measures 287
physical function 163, 221–43
physical inactivity 286, 287–8
piano key phenomenon 117
pirfenidone 149
plantar pressures 299–300
pleural lung disease (effusions) 135
Pneumocystis jirovecii (pneumocystis pneumonia) 136, 378–9, 474
pneumonitis 117
podiatrists 301–2
polymorphonuclear cells 99–100
polymyalgia rheumatica 17, 115
popliteal bursitis 117
Porphyromonas gingivalis 36, 38, 66
postmarketing surveillance 420, 472
prediction of disease progression/ outcome

models 123
MRI 213
ultrasound 196–8
predictive biomarkers 468
prednisolone 8–9, 339
prednisone 8–9, 339
  equivalents 340
  modified-release 349
pregnancy 349, 359, 361, 376, 527–8, 540
pre-rheumatoid arthritis 97–9, 121–8, 487–8
presenteeism 273–5, 277–8
prevalence of RA 23, 27–30
prevention of RA 39, 126–8, 487–91
primary care 113, 324
primary prevention 489
productivity 278–9
prognostic biomarkers 467–8
progressive multifocal leukoencephalopathy 405, 473
PROMIS 232, 236–7, 241, 510, 515
proof of concept 467
proof of mechanism 467
proprioception 285
proton pump inhibitors 333
psoriasis 381
psoriatic arthritis 16–17, 115, 198
psychiatric adverse events 349, 477–8
psychological assessment 313
psychological interventions 316–17
psychological manifestations of RA 142, 153, 277, 392
psychometrics 240
PTPN22 37, 46–7, 49, 65–6, 74
pulmonary arterial hypertension 135
pulmonary disease 117, 124, 133–7, 149–51, 406, 477
pulmonary hypertension 135
pure red cell aplasia 140
putamen 254

quality-adjusted life years 262–3, 511
quality of life 163, 509–10

RABBIT Risk Score 377, 472
RADAI 166, 498, 499
RADAR 165, 166
radiography 177–93
  bone erosions 5–6, 117, 178–80
  classification criteria 18–19
  clinical outcome 509
  detection of pathology in RA 178–81
  foot assessment 301
  joint space 5–6, 180–1
  scoring methods 181–7
radioimmunoassay 426–7
RAID score 510, 515
RANKL (receptor activator of nuclear factor-kappa B ligand) 56, 85–6, 95, 372–3
RAPID3 166, 222, 498, 499, 509
Rapid Assessment of Disease Activity in Rheumatology (RADAR) 165, 166
rate of perceived exertion 287
reactive oxygen species 77
Regional Examination of the Musculoskeletal System (REMS) 301

registries 472, 545–8
regulatory T cells 78–9
rehabilitation 316
remission, *see* clinical remission
remitting, seronegative, symmetric
      synovitis with pitting
      oedema 115
renal impairment 446
research questionnaires 225
respiratory symptoms 117, 124, 133–
      7, 149–51, 406, 477
retrocalcaneal bursitis 306
reverse signalling 371
Rheumatic Diseases Comorbidities
      Index 145
Rheumatoid Arthritis Disease
      Activity Index (RADAI) 166,
      498, 499
Rheumatoid Arthritis Impact of
      Disease (RAID) score 510, 515
Rheumatoid Arthritis Observation
      of Biologic Therapy (RABBIT)
      Risk Score 377, 472
Rheumatoid Arthritis Self-efficacy
      Scale 313
rheumatoid factor 6–7, 18, 65,
      66, 68, 87
rheumatoid nodules
      cardiac 137
      lung 135
      subcutaneous 6, 117, 141
Rheumatology Informatics System
      for Effectiveness (RISE)
      registry 548
risk factors for RA 33–9, 65–6, 121–3
risk stratification 488, 490
rituximab 399–408
      adverse events 404–6, 473–4,
            477, 479
      biosimilars 407
      clinical efficacy 400
      cost-effectiveness 406–7
      dose 403
      immunogenicity 406, 434
      immunoglobulin levels 406
      infusion reactions 404
      interstitial lung disease 134, 149
      non-response 403
      pretreatment screening 406
      radiographic outcomes 401
      repeat cycles 401–2
      response prediction 403
      retreatment strategies 402–3
      vaccinations 406
rofecoxib 333
Routine Assessment of Patient Index
      Data 3 (RAPID3) 166, 222, 498,
      499, 509
RS3PE 115

salicylate therapy 8
Salmonella infections 378
salt intake 36
sarcoid arthritis 17, 116
sarilumab 393–4
scleritis 117, 141
screening
      comorbidities 153
      pre-rituximab treatment 406
SDAI 165, 497, 498, 499, 509
secondary prevention 489
sedentary behaviour 286, 287–8

self-efficacy 313
self-management 321–5
      foot health 302
      occupational therapy 317
self-reports
      disease activity 165–6
      outcomes 512
      physical activity 287
      physical function 221–43
      see also patient-reported outcome
            measures
sensory/sensorimotor
      neuropathies 138, 302
septic arthritis 14
serious adverse event/reaction 471
serology 18
sex differences
      risk of RA 34
      work outcomes 275–6
sexual issues 315
SF-36 163, 232, 233–5, 510, 513
shared epitope 49, 65
Sharp score 182–3
Sheffield RA economic model 263
shoes 303–4
Short Form 36 163, 232, 233–5,
      510, 513
short text messages 287
shoulder deformities 117
sicca syndrome 140–1
silica dust 34, 36, 37, 38, 122
Simplified Disease Activity Index
      (SDAI) 165, 497, 498,
      499, 509
Simponi, *see* golimumab
single nucleotide polymorphisms 46,
      47–8, 65
sirukumab 396
Sjogren's syndrome 140–1
skin
      adverse events 349, 380, 476–7
      cancer 141, 381
      manifestations of RA 141
smartphone apps 323–4
smoking 34, 36, 37, 38, 50–1, 66,
      122, 148
social media 317
socioeconomic risk factors 34
sodium aurothiomalate 363
sodium chloride 36
Solganol 363
soluble gp130 395
solvent exposure 34
spinal involvement 117, 138, 211
spondyloarthropathy 16, 115, 198
spontaneous pharmacovigilance 472
squeeze test 114
Statins to Prevent RA (STAPRA) 491
statistical significance 241
STATs 442, 445
steroids, *see* glucocorticoids
stomatitis 476
Strategy to Prevent the Onset of
      Clinically Apparent Rheumatoid
      Arthritis (Stop-RA) 491
strenuous work 36
Streptococcus pneumoniae 377
stress, risk of RA 37
stromal cells 101
structural assays 414
sublining layer 59–60
subtalar joint injections 306

sulfasalazine (sulphasalazine) 8, 355,
      360–1, 473, 476–7, 478–9
sustaining bodies 425
swan neck deformity 117
switch studies 417–19
symmetric (poly)arthritis 114
synovial biopsy 169–73, 203
synovial effusion 195
synovial fibroblasts (FLS) 55–60, 86,
      89–90, 101, 171
synovial fluid analysis 14–15
synovial hyperplasia 55–6
synovial hypertrophy 195
synovial inflammation 169, 170
synovitis
      cytokines 99
      MRI 209–10
      ultrasound 200
systemic lupus
      erythematosus 17, 382

talonavicular joint injections 306
tapering
      biologics 266
      conventional (synthetic)
            DMARDs 357
      glucocorticoids 346
targeted synthetic disease-
      modifying antirheumatic drugs
      (tsDMARDs) 355, 458
target identification 463–4, 465–6
target validation 466
T-cell receptors 74–6, 79
T cells 74–9
      CD4+ 48, 76–8
      CD8+ cytotoxic 79
      IL-6 389
      innate (invariant natural killer) 79
      regulatory 78–9
      Th17 65, 69, 74, 79, 86, 101,
            171, 389
TCR excision circles 77
technology 317, 323–4, 499
telomeres 77
temperature-shift
      radioimmunoassay 427
tendons, ultrasound 198, 200
tenosynovial effusion 196
tenosynovial hypertrophy 196
tenosynovitis 198, 210
tertiary adrenal insufficiency 345–6
tertiary prevention 489
textile dust 34, 38, 122
text messages 287
T helper 17 (Th17) cells 65, 69, 74, 79,
      86, 101, 171, 389
therapeutic exercise 286, 288–91
thrombocytosis 392
thromboembolic events 135, 436,
      449, 479
thymus 77
tibialis posterior tendon pathology 298
tibialis posterior tendon sheath
      injections 306
tocilizumab 47, 392–3, 434, 436, 473,
      476, 477, 479
toe deformities 117, 297
toenails 302
tofacitinib 446–8, 474–5
tolerance 77, 437
tool compounds 465
topical capsaicin 336

topical NSAIDs 334
total hip/knee arthroplasty 531–32
toxicology 467
TRAF1 49
tramadol 335
translation, self-reports 241
translational research 464–5
trans-signalling 56, 389
TREAT EARLIER 491
treatment
      cost-effectiveness 262–7, 357–8,
            406–7, 458–9
      history of 7–9
      PROMIS-led decisions 511–12
      targets 495–9
treatment response
      epigenetics 51
      genetic factors 50, 173, 404
      ultrasound assessment 200, 201–2
treat-to-target 199–200, 495–6,
      513, 519
Tregs 78–9
triamcinolone 343
tricyclic antidepressants 335–6
tropism 59–60
tuberculosis 136, 377–8, 404, 449, 539
tumour necrosis factor (TNF) 95, 371
      bone erosion 87, 89, 102
      cardiovascular risk 102
      neuron function 104
      synovitis 99
tumour necrosis factor
      inhibitors 371–82
      adverse events 377–82, 473, 475,
            476, 477, 478, 479, 481
      antidrug antibodies 381
      biosimilars 420
      cellular effect 372–3
      guidelines for starting therapy 376
      immunogenicity 425, 427–34
      mechanism of action 99, 371–2
      'originators' 373–6
      perioperative 379–80
      pregnancy 376
twin studies 33–4, 45, 65

ulceration
      foot 302–3
      peripheral ulcerative
            keratitis 117, 141
ulcer 302–3
ultrasound 195–203
      bone erosion 196, 200
      clinical outcome 509
      diagnosis of RA 196–8, 201
      disease activity
            monitoring 198–9
      foot assessment 301
      joint aspiration and
            injections 202–3, 304–6
      low disease activity 202
      non-RA arthritides 198
      normality definition 200–1
      predictive role 196–8
      remission assessment 200, 202, 500
      structural damage
            assessment 200
      synovial biopsy 170, 203
      treatment response 200, 201–2
      treat-to-target 199–200
undifferentiated arthritis 14, 15–16,
      114, 121
upadacitinib 450–51

upper airway obstruction 135
usual interstitial pneumonia 149

vaccinations
    RA therapy 360, 406, 523
    risk factor for RA 36
valgus rearfoot deformity 298, 302
van der Heijde–Sharp score 183,
        185–7, 509
varicella zoster 379
varus rearfoot deformity 298, 299–300

vascular endothelial growth factor 372
vasculitis 117, 137–8, 302, 381–2
venous thromboembolism 135, 436,
        449, 479
Veteran's Affair's Rheumatoid
        Arthritis (VARA)
        registry 546
vimentin 67
viral infections
    mimics of RA 16, 115
    polyarthritis 16, 115

risk factor for RA 36
    TNF inhibitors 379
vitamin D 122
VO_{2max} 287, 289
vobarilizumab 394
voluntary patient registries 545–8

walking speed 298–9
whole synovial tissue explant
        model 171
work 271–9

Work Activities Limitations
        Scale 313
work disability 271, 273–7
Work Experience Survey Work–
        Rheumatic Conditions 313
work rehabilitation 316
wound care 302–3
wrist deformities 117
wrist orthoses 315

yellow card system 472